Current Review of Gastroenterology

1995

Published by Current Science Ltd,
34–42 Cleveland Street, London W1P 6LB, UK, and
Suite 700, 400 Market Street, Philadelphia, PA 19106, USA.

The reviews in this volume were originally published in *Current Opinion in Gastroenterology,* Volume 10, 1994.

ISBN 1-85922-787-2

Current Review of Gastroenterology

1995

Editor
Robert M. Donaldson, Jr. (USA)

Associate Editor
Tadataka Yamada (USA)

CS
CURRENT
SCIENCE

Contents

Nutrition

edited by Rosemarie L. Fisher

Liver

edited by Norman Gitlin and Johan Fevery

Inflammatory bowel disease

edited by Richard P. MacDermott

Esophagus

Edited by G.N.J. Tytgat

Pancreas

edited by Fred S. Gorelick

Biliary tract

edited by J. Thomas LaMont and Nezam H. Afdhal

Stomach and duodenum

edited by Mitchell L. Schubert

Immunology

edited by W. Allan Walker

Large intestine

Editorial overview

Victor W. Fazio, MD*, and Sidney F. Phillips, MD†

*Cleveland Clinic Foundation, Cleveland, Ohio, and
†Mayo Clinic and Medical School, Rochester, Minnesota, USA

Current Opinion in Gastroenterology 1994, **10**:1–3

Recent recognition that the colon can undergo subtle forms of inflammation (*eg*, collagenous colitis, microscopic colitis, and lymphocytic colitis) has increased greatly the relevance of ways in which inflammatory mediators and other bioactive compounds might influence absorption and secretion. Thus, it is not surprising that the capacity of a large bowel afflicted by pancolitis, with little or no normal mucosa, is greatly impaired. However, perhaps more subtle pathophysiologies need to be sought to explain the prominent diarrhea noted with these newer, milder forms of colitis. Timothy Gaginella in "Absorption and secretion in the colon" (pp 5–10), reviews recent literature on potential secretagogues and antisecretory peptides. Adding to the well-established, if circumstantial, association among prostaglandins, leukotrienes, and colonic inflammation are a number of comparative newcomers, such as platelet activating factor, pituitary adenylate cyclase activating peptide, endothelin 1, and guanelin, which may be an important activator of guanylate cyclase. The inhibitory peptides PYY and GLP-1, which are located in the distal small bowel and colon, certainly have been implicated in negative feedback control of the proximal gut; they may also have local effects as antisecretory peptides.

In his review of "Motility and functional diseases of the large intestine" Michael Kamm (pp 11–18) covers a wide spectrum of work, though an important general conclusion can be reached. These areas, which for so long have been the realm of art rather than clinical science, are advancing slowly but progressively, and on a broad front. Thus, intensive study of neuromuscular tissues from patients with motor failure ("intestinal pseudo-obstruction"), sometimes only as single case reports, continues to elucidate potential etiopathogeneses—enteric neuropathies, biochemical abnormalities of contractile proteins, even mitochondrial myopathies. The picture is still very fragmentary and tentative, but progress is apparent. Constipation continues to bother many patients and to frustrate physicians. Kamm touches upon many directions of current research—functions of the autonomic nervous system, manometry, measurements of transit, potential psychopathology and the role of surgical treatment in the most severe examples. Brief review of a very large literature on nitric oxide as an important mediator of relaxation (at the neural and perhaps muscular level) indicates a role for this system in relaxation of the internal anal sphincter.

In his review of the "Epidemiology and etiology of sporadic colorectal adenocarcinomas" (pp 19–26), William Karnes, Jr has focused on the role of diet and other components of the luminal milieu (*eg*, bile acids). He evaluates ways in which traditional epidemiologic techniques can be integrated (perhaps even reexamined) with exciting developments in the molecular genetics of colon neoplasia. Thus, a key question will be, how does the luminal milieu develop mutagenic potential and how does this facilitate the polyp-cancer sequence?

Following on the important theme of colorectal neoplasia Douglas McGill and Mark Larson (pp 27–33) review diagnostic and screening procedures. Screening and diagnosis are still firmly rooted in the traditional approaches; the double contrast barium enema, if performed carefully, is an excellent examination, albeit very small (and possibly trivial) lesions will be identified more often by endoscopy. Fecal markers and the biochemistry of biopsy samples, though of inherent appeal, do not appear to have the sensitivity and specificity

 ISBN 1-85922-606-X ISSN 0267–1379

to be of great value. The role of flow cytometry to quantify DNA aneuploidy offers an attractive addition to other screening techniques in high-risk individuals, though it may still be premature to recommend this widely. However, in the hands of experts, the results are impressive. Clearly, screening of high-risk groups will ultimately be influenced most by the further development of molecular strategies that will identify those individuals who require complete and frequent evaluation, separating them from those for whom screening programs can be less intense. Only then will society's resources be able to be apportioned more rationally and efficiently.

Thus, much of this past year's literature on colorectal endoscopy has focused on cost-effectiveness issues. For practical purposes, few will refute the superiority of large intestinal endoscopy as the procedure of choice in the diagnosis of cancerous and precancerous lesions. The challenge is the determination of what is reasonable value for a reasonable cost—or, to what extent can society afford expensive tests such as colonoscopy in specific situations, and in contemporary times. Current cancer screening strategies are far from ideal. Fecal occult blood testing—apparently inexpensive—is reported to miss as much as 70% of asymptomatic colorectal cancers, and more than 90% of colonic polyps. As mentioned, the benchmark for diagnosis, colonoscopy, has been and is expensive. The optimum frequency as well as extent of endoscopic screening remains both unclear and controversial.

David Ahlquist (pp 41–48) has provided an illuminating point-counterpoint review of this year's literature, underscoring the need for reexamination of screening guidelines. The concept of "routine" colonoscopy at 1 year following adenoma removal, as opposed to three yearly intervals, has been challenged. A compelling argument for the latter strategy has been made in one large multi-institutional study. Also, because curable anastomotic recurrence of colorectal cancer is very rare, colonoscopic surveillance strategies need to be directed at detection of metachronous lesions. This implies a less expensive program—with greater intervals between surveillance studies—using the guidelines provided. It is probable that clinical outcome as opposed to say "earlier" diagnosis will ultimately become *the* critical endpoint of future studies.

Endoluminal ultrasonography of the large bowel—especially for preoperative assessment or extent of mural invasion of rectal cancer—has proven to be a valuable tool in certain settings. However, while endoluminal ultrasonography has shown a sensitivity advantage over other methods in the diagnosis of local tumor recurrence, no survivorship advantage has yet been demonstrated. Should other studies support the value of endoluminal ultrasonography in distinguishing ulcerative colitis from Crohn's disease, then a further modality to characterize more accurately those difficult indeterminate cases would be a welcome addition for clinicians. This is especially so for the appropriate selection of patients undergoing restorative proctocolectomy—where in as many as 10% of cases, a diagnostic dilemma exists. Regarding intraoperative techniques, it seems paradoxic that *few* endoscopists use CO_2 insufflation (vs air) where advantages have been proven regarding patient comfort; yet monitored pulse oximetry—the benefit for which has not been shown in analyzing clinical outcome—has "become a standard practice." (Certain subgroups, *eg*, the elderly, may benefit.)

Turning to large bowel surgery and colorectal cancer, Jeffrey Milsom (pp 34–40) has focused on several controversial issues including perioperative blood transfusion and recurrence rates; surgical techniques such as nerve-sparing pelvic sidewall dissection in rectal cancer and the role of absorbable mesh to quarantine small intestine so that postoperative pelvic irradiation can be done safely. While this latter technique may pose some technical difficulties in some patients, one is in agreement with the reviewer that this is a valuable adjunct.

Both Jeffrey Milsom and our other surgical reviewer, Scott Strong (pp 49–55), examined this year's studies on inflammatory bowel disease. New data on outcome of strictureplasty for stenotic areas of small bowel Crohn's disease, and outcome of the ileorectal anastomosis for Crohn's disease generally support a role for these procedures. The long-term functional results of restorative proctocolectomy at the Mayo Clinic were reported. An excellent quality of life in 90% was noted. Still not resolved or settled are the issues relating to technique of restorative proctocolectomy such as double-stapled anastomosis and ileostomy avoidance.

As predicted in last year's review, laparoscopic bowel surgery is emerging as a major area of discussion if not enthusiasm for many surgeons. Thus far, one can state that laparoscopic bowel resection and anastomosis is possible; the "learning curve" for surgeons is considerable; cost-effectiveness of laparoscopic bowel surgery has still to be established; concerns about the appropriateness of laparoscopic bowel surgery for cancer surgery have been voiced on the basis of adequacy of resection and risk of implantation of malignant cells in the trochar sites. Ongoing studies are addressing this issue. One will again predict a wealth of literature on this revolutionary modality over the next several years.

Victor Fazio, MD, Department of Colorectal Surgery, Cleveland Clinic Foundation, One Clinic Center, 9500 Euclid Avenue, Cleveland, OH 44195, USA

Sidney F. Phillips, MD, Mayo Clinic, 200 First Street, Gastroenterology Unit Rochester, MN 55905, USA.

Absorption and secretion in the colon

Timothy S. Gaginella, PhD

Aphton Corporation, Woodland, California, USA

New studies continue to define how colonic absorption and secretion are regulated by intracellular pH, peptides, inflammatory mediators, laxatives, and antidiarrheal agents. Additional work has addressed the influence of aldosterone on electrogenic sodium absorption and has shown the importance of nutritional status in the action of vitamin A on thyroid hormone modulation of aldosterone action. There is further evidence implicating platelet-activating factor as a mediator of intestinal secretion in inflammatory bowel disease and in the mechanism of action of anthraquinone laxatives. The activity of peptide YY, pituitary adenylate cyclase–activating polypeptide, endothelin 1, and guanylin suggest that these peptides may have physiologic or pathophysiologic effects on colonic transport. Studies on methods to enhance the absorption of peptides through the colonic mucosa indicate that it may be possible to improve systemic bioavailability of peptides via this route of administration.

Current Opinion in Gastroenterology 1994, **10**:5–10

Physiologic mechanisms

The importance of intracellular pH as a regulator of Na^+/H^+ and Cl^-/HCO_3^- parallel transport across the colonic mucosa continue to be investigated. Using rat apical membrane vesicles, Rajendran and Binder [1] found that Cl^- uptake probably involves two separate (HCO_3^- and OH^-) exchangers. Based on kinetic considerations, they proposed that both mechanisms operate under physiologic conditions; one facilitates Cl^- transport in concert with Na^+/H^+ exchange (resulting in net electrochemically neutral NaCl absorption) and the other acts as an intracellular regulator of pH. In whole tissue, in which intracellular acidification was accomplished by decreasing extracellular pH while maintaining constant PCO_2, other investigators [2•] concluded that Na^+ absorption in the distal colon is not stimulated by intracellular acidification per se, but requires CO_2. Furthermore, they suggested that carbonic anhydrase stimulates ion transport independent of its catalytic action. Definitive studies on the role of intracellular pH in colonic NaCl transport in human physiology will require studies in humans or with human tissue.

Porcine distal colon has many functional and morphologic similarities to the human colon and yet has not been studied extensively relative to the coupling of anion-cation transport. Traynor and O'Grady [3] have concluded from Ussing chamber studies that in the porcine distal colon epithelium, Na^+ transport is mediated by two distinct amiloride-sensitivity pathways. Cl^- absorption has an absolute requirement for HCO_3^-, and the exchanger for these anions operates independently of Na^+ absorption.

Studies on the rabbit cecum have demonstrated an electrogenic Na^+ conductance pathway with characteristics different from those previously reported [4•], particularly in regard to lack of inhibition by amiloride [5]. Cl^- secretion by this tissue is believed to be driven by K^+/Cl^- symport [6].

Aldosterone administered *in vivo* induces electrogenic Na^+ absorption. This effect has now been demonstrated *in vitro* [7]. In a physiologic concentration range (0.1 to 10 nmol/L), aldosterone (by 8 hours) significantly enhanced amiloride-sensitive increases in short-circuit current in the rat distal colon. In another study, fasting rats for 72 hours or reducing their nutritional intake by one third for 9 days resulted in enhanced electrogenic Na^+ absorption in the distal colon [8]. This effect was linked to aldosterone, as adrenalectomy prevented the enhanced absorption. Advances in molecular biology have now allowed the cloning of the epithelial Na^+ channel from rat colon [9]. This should help us to better understand how aldosterone modulates receptors or channels for Na^+ transport, and how differ-

Abbreviations

IBD—inflammatory bowel disease; **PAF**—platelet-activating factor; **VIP**—vasoactive intestinal polypeptide.

ISBN 1-85922-606-X ISSN 0267–1379

ent segments of the gut (*eg*, cecum) might express different ion transporters.

Nutritional status can alter electrolyte transport. Vitamin A–deficient rats were found to have a reduced secretory response in the distal colon to the cholinergic agonist bethanechol [10]. Animals supplemented with vitamin A were protected from this effect. The vitamin deficiency had no effect on the secretory response to dibutyryl cyclic AMP, but the vitamin A–deficient animals were unresponsive to luminal amiloride. The mechanism for these effects was found to involve thyroid hormone modulation of aldosterone (Fig. 1).

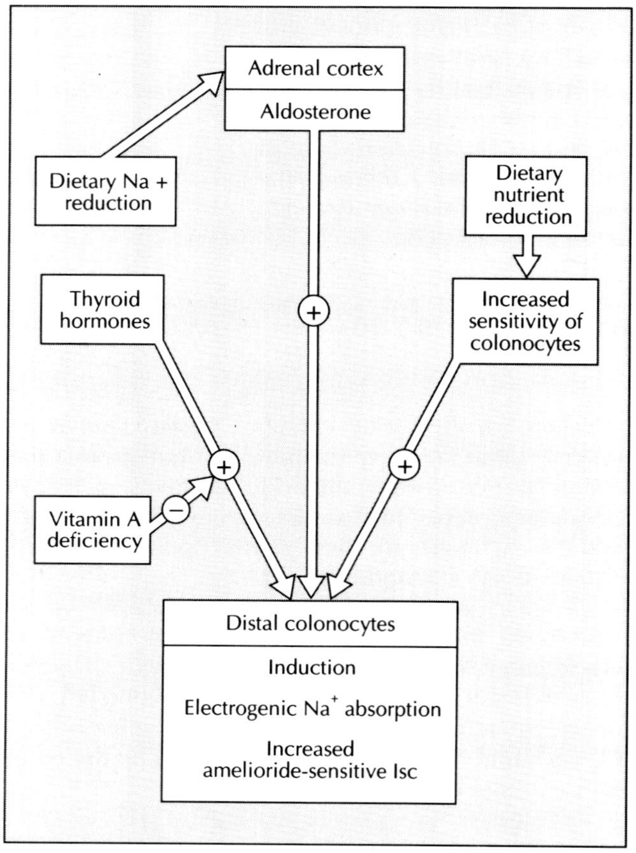

Fig. 1. Possible interrelation among diet, thyroid hormones, vitamin A, and aldosterone on induction of electrogenic Na^+ absorption in rat distal colon epithelial cells. Isc—short-circuit current (*From* Nzegwu and Levin [10]; with permission.)

Mechanisms responsible for potassium secretion by the colon continue to be pursued. Electron microprobe analysis of distal colonic mucosa (guinea pig) showed distribution of ion secretion along the crypts [11]. The secretion of K^+ was stimulated with prostaglandin E_2 and epinephrine. The pattern of cellular distribution of the electrolytes in the stimulated compared with unstimulated state indicated that most of the secretory cells were in the lower two thirds of the crypt and that most of the secretion was from vacuolated cells. The responding (nongoblet) cells were thought to express two different mechanisms for K^+ secretion, one responding to epinephrine and the other to prostaglandin E_2. It has been assumed that the major force driving the potassium secretion is Na^+/K^+ATPase [12]. Recently, a new ATPase, closely related to gastric H^+/K^+ATPase, has been isolated and characterized in the rat colon; this P-type ATPase is hypothesized to be responsible for K^+ absorption in the colon [13•].

The complicated interactions between cyclic AMP and Ca^{2+} as secretagogues in the rabbit distal colon were studied using a diverse group of agonists and antagonists [14•]. The experiments suggest a model for Cl^- secretion in which increased intracellular Ca^{2+} reduces cyclic AMP levels through effects on adenylate cyclase activity, without affecting phosphodiesterase or calmodulin-dependent mechanisms.

Pathophysiology

Inflammatory bowel disease (IBD) is often associated with secretory diarrhea. Previous studies have demonstrated impaired electrolyte absorption or secretion in patients in various stages of IBD. Jenkins and Milla [15] extended previous work by obtaining tissue from human infants and studying it *in vitro*. They compared tissue from infants with Hirschsprung's disease or anal atresia with or without diarrhea and inflammation of the colon. They found that the highly efficient NaCl absorption in noninflamed tissue was reversed to secretion in tissue that was inflamed. Although this study did not go into any depth regarding mechanism, it provides perhaps the first data from such a young group of patients.

Prostaglandins and leukotrienes are likely candidates as the mediators responsible for the secretory response of the mucosa in IBD. These eicosanoids are secretagogues in the small and large intestine [16]. Elevated concentrations of prostaglandins and leukotrienes occur in colonic specimens and stool of patients with ulcerative colitis [17]. Wardle *et al.* [18•] studied the effect of media obtained from cultured mucosal biopsy specimens from patients with ulcerative colitis on distal rat colonic mucosa *in vitro*. The media from the inflamed tissue had higher levels of prostaglandin E_2 and leukotriene D_4 than control media. It evoked an increase in short-circuit current that could be blocked by inhibition of cyclooxygenase and lipoxygenase, but only by about 57%. Additional manipulations resulted in the conclusion that other products of phospholipase A_2, such as serotonin, histamine, and platelet-activating factor (PAF) are also important in the secretory response.

The interactions among eicosanoids in IBD are complex. This is especially evident in two recent studies.

In control rabbit colon, prostaglandin E_2 evoked an increase in short-circuit current but was without effect in animals with experimental colitis [19]. There was no change in the responsiveness of the inflamed tissue to dibutyryl cyclic AMP. This indicates that prostaglandin E_2 responsiveness may have been lost due to a reduction in the affinity or the number of epithelial cell receptors or their ability to mediate an increase in cyclic AMP. In canine proximal colon, prostaglandin D_2 produced a complicated pattern of short-circuit responses [20]. Two different metabolites of prostaglandin D_2 were probably responsible for the variable effects, as one of the metabolites dose-dependently decreased, whereas the other dose-dependently increased short-circuit current. The differing responses may be due to different receptor subtypes. In human colitis (in which a plethora of prostanoids are present), the intensity of the secretory response of a given individual will depend on which metabolites are present or which receptors dominate.

Platelet-activating factor is increased in the colonic mucosa of patients with Crohn's disease [21]. This mediator stimulates anion secretion in the healthy rabbit distal colon but is ineffective in the cecum [22]. The epithelial cells themselves may be important contributors to the production of the PAF in ulcerative colitis [23•].

New animal models for IBD are under study. One of these involves the use of the antineoplastic antibiotic mitomycin C [24•]. After one intraperitoneal injection of mitomycin C, rats developed (at 7 days) diffuse colonic inflammation similar histologically to human ulcerative colitis. The small intestine was spared. The inflamed mucosa showed enhanced chemoluminescence, indicating the presence of high levels of oxygen-reactive metabolites; scavengers of these metabolites or inhibitors of their formation decreased the inflammation. This model shows promise because of its otherwise close similarity to human ulcerative colitis and the link to oxygen radicals, which probably occur in the mucosa of patients with ulcerative colitis [25]. Indeed, reactive oxygen metabolites are secretagogues, as supported by their direct effects on the epithelium and modulation of submucosal neural release of acetylcholine [26].

Peptide secretagogues

Vasoactive intestinal polypeptide (VIP) is a potent stimulator of intestinal secretion. Stimulation of adenylate cyclase is believed to be responsible for the secretory effect. A recently discovered 38-amino acid neuropeptide, pituitary adenylate cyclase–activating polypeptide, closely resembles VIP. The peptide is present in the submucosal plexus of the large intestine, and was found to stimulate chloride secretion in the guinea pig distal colon [27•]. Part of the effect is mediated by submucosal neurons and part through direct action on epithelial cells. Cross-desensitization with VIP showed that pituitary adenylate cyclase–activating polypeptide and VIP are probably recognized by the same epithelial cell receptor.

An alternative mechanism has been proposed for the secretory effect of another peptide, endothelin 1. This 21-amino-acid vasoconstrictor peptide evokes chloride secretion by the rat colon. The mechanism is partly due to activation of enteric nerves and may be mediated by cyclooxygenase products and calcium [28•,29]. The receptor subtype thought to be responsible for this effect is the ET_A receptor [28•]. Additional studies with newly developed antagonists should clarify whether the neural or non-neural actions of endothelin 1 are mediated by the same receptor type. It is also important to know whether its effects on colonic smooth muscle decreased contraction [29] are mediated by a different receptor than its action on electrolyte secretion.

There is a great deal of interest in a newly identified endogenous peptide of 15 amino acids that, like heat-stable *Escherichia coli* stable toxin, is a ligand for intestinal epithelial cell guanylate cyclase. The peptide, named *guanylin* (Fig. 2) [30••], stimulates chloride secretion across the rat colon in the same manner as heat-stable *E. coli*–stable toxin [31]. Additional work is ongoing to define the possible physiologic effects of guanylin as well as the factors that regulate its synthesis, release, and metabolism.

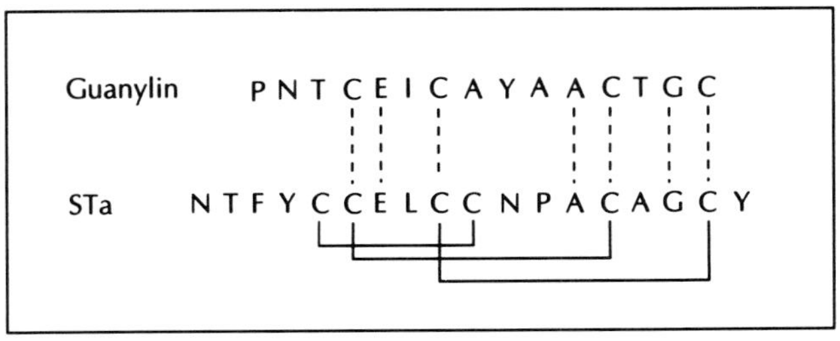

Fig. 2. Structures of guanylin and heat-stable *Escherichia coli* stable toxin (STa). *Dotted lines* indicate amino acid identity. *Solid lines* show alignment of disulfide bonds in STa. (*From* Currie *et al.* [30••]; with permission.)

Antisecretory peptides

The 36-amino-acid peptide, peptide YY, belongs to a family including pancreatic polypeptide and neuropeptide Y. Peptide YY was found to inhibit VIP-stimulated chloride secretion in the rabbit distal colon [32•]. The peptide also negated cyclic AMP increases produced by VIP or forskolin, as did neuropeptide Y and pancreatic polypeptide. It is conceivable that peptide YY acts physiologically to counterbalance the secretory action of VIP on the colon.

A synthetic analogue of somatostatin, octreotide, enhances the absorption of fluid and electrolytes by the intestine. It antagonizes secretion induced by several different secretagogues [33] and reduces the secretory diarrhea associated with AIDS and endocrinopathies [34]. Octreotide (50 μg twice daily subcutaneously) markedly improved diarrhea in a patient with insulin-dependent diabetes [35]. Paradoxically, octreotide had a marked stimulatory effect on prostanoid production and secretion in a patient with a fluid-secreting villous adenoma of the rectum [36].

Laxatives

The effects of senna-derived laxatives on rat colonic PAF content and the release of acid phosphatase into the lumen were studied and compared with the effects of castor oil [37]. Oral administration of senna or intraluminal perfusion with rhein or rhein-anthraquinone did not release PAF or acid phosphatase, but a single oral administration of castor oil did. The conclusion was that these anthraquinone laxatives are better tolerated by the colonic mucosa than is castor oil, in terms of mucosal injury. The results also suggest different mechanisms of action for the anthraquinones and ricinoleic acid (the active component of castor oil) in the rat colon.

Another study, conducted in rats with anthraquinone laxatives for 5 months, demonstrated a reduction in neuropeptide Y levels in mesenteric blood vessels. There were no changes in the levels of this peptide in the myenteric plexus [38]. The levels of other peptides (VIP, calcitonin gene–related peptide, and substance P) were unaffected in the mesenteric vessels and the myenteric plexus, and there was no histologic evidence for changes in tissue morphology or ultrastructure. Changes in enteric neurophysiology, which may have been affected by this treatment, were not studied. Nevertheless, this finding suggests that long-term administration of anthraquinone laxatives causes minimal or selective damage to the colonic mucosa.

Drug absorption

The colon is not ordinarily considered as an organ for absorbing drugs. Considerable research is underway, however, to find ways to enhance colonic drug absorption. Chemical modification of insulin with palmitic acid increased the lipophilicity of insulin and also reduced its degradation in the colon, resulting in an enhanced flux across closed loops of rat colon [39•]. In the absence of any enhancing agents, Beglinger *et al.* [40] were able to show that human calcitonin injected into the descending colon of normal subjects is absorbed rapidly, but only to the extent of a maximum of 2.7% of an intravenous dose. By comparison, the somatostatin analogue octreotide is absorbed by the colon only to the extent of about 1.28% in humans. The relevance of calcitonin absorption from the colon in therapeutics is somewhat obscure, but studies such as this and the one on insulin [39•] will help devise better systems for peptide delivery to the colon. Such modes of therapy may have relevance in therapeutics for IBD.

Comparison of the absorption rates for series of β-adrenergic blocking agents in the rat demonstrated rate constants of the same order in the small intestine and colon, indicating good transport of these drugs across the colonic membrane [41]. AZT (3′-azido-3′-dioxythymidine), currently being used in the treatment of AIDS, was studied to determine whether its absorption could be enhanced through the use of a mixed micelle formulation [42]. A micelle solution of palmitoyl-*DL*-carnitine chloride plus sodium glycocholate in isotonic phosphate buffer enhanced the absorption of AZT 5.4-fold; this mixture also enhanced the absorption of phenol red. The authors concluded that a paracellular pathway is therefore probably involved in the mechanism of the enhanced absorption of AZT.

References and recommended reading

Papers of particular interest, published within the annual period of review, have been highlighted as:

- • Of special interest
- •• Of outstanding interest

1. Rajendran VM, Binder HJ: **Cl-HCO3 and Cl-OH Exchanges Mediate Cl Uptake in Apical Membrane Vesicles of Rat Distal Colon.** *Am J Physiol* 1993, **264**:G874–G879.

2. • Dagher PC, Egnor RW, Charney AN: **Effect of Intracellular Acidification on Colonic NaCl Absorption.** *Am J Physiol* 1993, **264**:G569–G575.

Shows that a mechanism (possibly carbonic anhydrase or CO_2) independent of pH may contribute to sodium absorption in the rat distal colon.

3. Traynor TR, O'Grady SM: **Mechanisms of Na and Cl Absorption Across the Distal Colon Epithelium of the Pig.** *J Comp Physiol [B]* 1992, **162**:47–53.

4. • Sellin JH, Hall A, Cragoe EJ Jr, Dubinsky WP: **Characterization of an Apical Sodium Conductance in Rabbit Cecum.** *Am J Physiol* 1993, **264**:G13–G21.

Demonstrates that the cecum may absorb sodium by a similar yet distinctly different mechanism than the colon. The apical sodium channel could be regulated differently than the "classic" sodium channel.

5. Raijman I, Cragoe P, Sellin J: **Hormonal and Pharmacologic Regulation of Sodium Absorption in Rabbit Cecum In Vitro.** *Dig Dis Sci* 1992, **37**:1874–1881.

6. Ferreira KTG, Fernandes PL, Ferreira HG: **Ion Transport Across the Epithelium of the Rabbit Caecum.** *Biochim Biophys Acta* 1992, **1175**:27–36.

7. FROMM M, SCHULZKE JD, HEGEL U: **Control of Electrogenic Na^+ Absorption in Rat Late Distal Colon by Nanomolar Aldosterone Added In Vitro.** *Am J Physiol* 1993, **264**:E68–E73.

8. NZEGWU HC, LEVIN RJ: **Dietary Restriction Sensitizes the Rat Distal Colon to Aldosterone.** *J Physiol (Lond)* 1992, **447**:501–512.

9. CANESSA CM, HORISBERGER JD, ROSSIER BC: **Epithelial Sodium Channel Related to Proteins Involved in Neurodegeneration.** *Nature* 1993, **361**:467–470.

10. NZEGWU H, LEVIN RJ: **Vitamin A Deficiency and Small Intestinal Secretory Function in the Rat.** *Gut* 1991, **32**:1324–1328.

11. HALM DR, RICK R: **Secretion of K and Cl Across Colonic Epithelium: Cellular Localization Using Electron Microprobe Analysis.** *Am J Physiol* 1992, **262**:C1392–C1402.

12. FISHER KA, BINDER HJ, HAYSLETT JP: **Potassium Secretion by Colonic Mucosal Cells After Potassium Adaptation.** *Am J Physiol* 1976, **231**:987–994.

13. • CROWSON MS, SHULL GE: **Isolation and Characterization of a cDNA Encoding the Putative Distal Colon H+, K+-ATPase.** *J Biol Chem* 1992, **267**:13740–13748.

The application of this methodology could aid in the characterization of sodium channels in different segments of the gut, helping to determine if and how they differ.

14. • CALDERARO V, CHIOSI E, GRECO R, SPINA AM, GIOVANE A, QUAGLIUOLO L, SERVILLO L, BALESTRIERI C, ILLIANO G: **Role of Calcium in Chloride Secretion Mediated by cAMP Pathway Activation in Rabbit Distal Colon Mucosa.** *Am J Physiol* 1993, **264**:G252–G260.

Emphasizes the complexity of calcium and cyclic AMP interactions. Suggests that calcium is a major factor in the control of cyclic AMP-mediated colonic electrolyte secretion.

15. JENKINS HR, MILLA PJ: **The Effect of Colitis on Large-Intestinal Electrolyte Transport in Early Childhood.** *J Pediatr Gastroenterol Nutr* 1993, **16**:402–405.

16. GAGINELLA TS: **Eicosanoid-Mediated Intestinal Secretion.** In *Textbook of Secretory Diarrhea.* Edited by Lebenthal E, Duffey M. New York: Raven Press; 1990:15–30.

17. STENSON WF: **Role of Eicosanoids as Mediators of Inflammation in Inflammatory Bowel Disease.** *Scand J Gastroenterol* 1990, **25**:13–18.

18. • WARDLE TD, HALL L, TURNBERG LA: **Inter-Relationships Between Inflammatory Mediators Released From Colonic Mucosa in Ulcerative Colitis and Their Effects on Colonic Secretion.** *Gut* 1993, **34**:503–508.

Shows that although eicosanoids and other products of lipid metabolism contribute to colonic secretion in ulcerative colitis, other mediators such as serotonin, histamine, and bradykinin may also be involved.

19. GOLDHILL JM, BURAKOFF R, DONOVAN B, ROSE K, PERCY WH: **Defective Modulation of Colonic Secretomotor Neurons in a Rabbit Model of Colitis.** *Am J Physiol* 1993, **264**:G671–G677.

20. RANGACHARI PK, BETTI PA: **Biological Activity of Metabolites on PGD2 on Canine Proximal Colon.** *Am J Physiol* 1993, **264**:G886–G894.

21. SOBHANI I, HOCHLAF S, DENIZOT Y, VISSUZAINE C, RENE E, BENVENISTE J, LEWIN MMJ, MIGNON M: **Raised Concentrations of Platelet Activating Factor in Colonic Mucosa of Crohn's Disease Patients.** *Gut* 1992, **33**:1220–1225.

22. TRAVIS SPL, JEWELL DP: **Regional Differences in the Response to Platelet-Activating Factor in Rabbit Colon.** *Clin Sci* 1992, **82**:673–680.

23. • FERRARIS L, KARMELI F, ELIAKIM R, KLEIN J, FIOCCHI C, RACHMILEWITZ D: **Intestinal Epithelial Cells Contribute to the Enhanced Generation of Platelet Activating Factor in Ulcerative Colitis.** *Gut* 1993, **34**:665–668.

If it is confirmed that the epithelial cells furnish a major fraction of PAF released in IBD, this could be important to the more effective targeting of PAF antagonists or synthesis inhibitors in IBD therapy.

24. • KESHAVARZIAN A, DORIA MI, SEDGHI S, KANOFSKY JR, HECHT D, HOLMES EW, IBRAHIM C, LIST T, URBAN G, GAGINELLA T, FIELDS JZ: **Mitomycin C-Induced Colitis in Rats: a New Animal Model of Acute Colonic Inflammation Implicating Reactive Oxygen Species.** *J Lab Clin Med* 1992, **120**:778–791.

This new model of IBD shows that colonic inflammation, in association with diarrhea and oxygen radicals, closely resembles human ulcerative colitis. The method is simple and produces colitis in 7 days.

25. BABBS CF: **Oxygen Radicals in Ulcerative Colitis.** *Free Radic Biol Med* 1992, **13**:169–181.

26. GAGINELLA TS, GRISHAM MB, THOMAS DB, WALSH R, MOUMMI C: **Oxidant-Evoked Release of Acetylcholine From Enteric Neurons of the Rat Colon.** *J Pharmacol Exp Ther* 1992, **263**:1068–1073.

27. • KUWAHARA A, KUWAHARA Y, MOCHIZUKI T, YANAIHARA N: **Action of Pituitary Adenylate Cyclase-Activating Polypeptide on Ion Transport in Guinea Pig Distal Colon.** *Am J Physiol* 1993, **264**:G433–G441.

First demonstration that this peptide stimulates colonic secretion in a mammal.

28. • KIYOHARA T, OKUNO M, NAKANISHI T, SHINOMURA Y, MATSUZASA Y: **Effect of Endothelin 1 on Ion Transport in Isolated Rat Colon.** *Gastroenterology* 1993, **104**:1328–1336.

Extends the number of peptides known to stimulate colonic electrolyte secretion. Mechanism involves cyclooxygenase products and calcium (unlike VIP) and may be partially neural. Receptor subtype identified as ET_A.

29. MOUMMI C, XIE Y, KACHUR JR, GAGINELLA TS: **Endothelin-1 Stimulates Contraction and Ion Transport in the Rat Colon: Different Mechanisms of Action.** *J Pharmacol Exp Ther* 1992, **262**:409–414.

30. •• CURRIE MG, FOK KF, KATO J, MOORE RJ, HAMRA FK: **Guanylin: an Endogenous Activator of Intestinal Guanylate Cyclase.** *Proc Natl Acad Sci U S A* 1992, **89**:947–951.

Newly identified endogenous peptide agonist of guanylate cyclase. Mechanism on colonic secretion is apparently identical to *E. coli* stable toxin A.

31. KACHUR JF, WON-KIM S, MOUMMI C, FOK K, CURRIE MG: **Guanylin, a Newly Discovered Activator of Intestinal Guanylate Cyclase, Stimulates Ion Secretion Across Rat Colon [Abstract].** *Gastroenterology* 1992, **102**:A738.

32. • BALLANTYNE GH, GOLDENRING JR, FLEMING FX, RUSH S, FLINT JS, FIELDING LP, BINDER HJ, MODLIN IM: **Inhibition of VIP-Stimulated Ion Transport by a Novel Y-Receptor Phenotype in Rabbit Distal Colon.** *Am J Physiol* 1993, **264**:G848–G854.

Inhibition of VIP suggests a modulatory effect on physiologic regulation of fecal fluid. Defines required peptide fragment for activity.

33. FASSLER JE, O'DORISIO TM, MEKHJIAN HS, GAGINELLA TS: **Octreotide Inhibits Increases in Short-Circuit Current Induced in Rat Colon by VIP, Substance P, Serotonin and Aminophylline.** *Regul Pept* 1990, **29**:189–197.

34. GAGINELLA TS, O'DORISIO TM, FASSLER JE, MEKHJIAN HS: **Clinical Application of Somatostatin Analogues Part II.: Treatment of Endocrine and Nonendocrine Secretory Diarrheal States with Sandostatin.** *Metabolism* 1990, **39**:172–175.

35. Mourad FH, Gorard D, Thillainayagam AV, Colin-Jones D, Farthing MJG: **Effective Treatment of Diabetic Diarrhoea With Somatostatin Analogue, Octreotide.** *Gut* 1992, 33:1578–1580.

36. Smelt AHM, Meinders AE, Hoekman K, Noort WA, Keirse MJNC: **Secretory Diarrhea in Villous Adenoma of Rectum: Effect of Treatment with Somatostatin and Indomethacin.** *Prostaglandins* 1992, 43:567–572.

37. Mascolo N, Autore G, Izzo AA, Biondi A, Capasso F: **Effect of Senna and Its Active Compound Rhein and Rhein-Anthrone on PAF Formation by Rat Colon.** *J Pharm Pharmacol* 1992, 44:693–695.

38. Milner P, Belai A, Tomlinson A, Hoyle CHV, Sarner S, Burnstock G: **Effects of Long-Term Laxative Treatment on Neuropeptides in Rat Mesenteric Vessels and Caecum.** *J Pharm Pharmacol* 1992, 44:777–779.

39. • Hashizume M, Douen T, Murakami M, Yamamoto A, Takada K, Muranishi S: **Improvement of Large Intestinal Absorption of Insulin by Chemical Modification with Palmitic Acid in Rats.** *J Pharm Pharmacol* 1992, 44:555–559.
Data indicate that it may be possible to enhance peptide transport across the colonic mucosa by coupling to lipids.

40. Beglinger C, Born W, Muff R, Drewe J, Dreyfuss JL, Bock A, Mackay M, Fischer JA: **Intracolonic Bioavailability of Human Calcitonin in Man.** *Eur J Clin Pharmacol* 1992, 43:527–531.

41. Vila JI, Calpena AC, Obach R, Domenech J: **Gastric Intestinal and Colonic Absorption of a Series of β-Blockers in the Rat.** *Int J Clin Pharmacol Ther Toxicol* 1992, 30:280–286.

42. Park GB, Mitra AK: **Mechanism and Site Dependency of Intestinal Mucosal Transport and Metabolism of Thymidine Analogues.** *Pharm Res* 1992, 9:326–331.

Timothy S. Gaginella, PhD, Vice President, Aphton Corporation, PO Box 1049, Woodland, CA 95776, USA.

Motility and functional diseases of the large intestine

Michael A. Kamm, MD, MRCP, FRACP

St. Mark's Hospital, London, UK

Since the discovery in 1987 that it relaxes vascular smooth muscle, nitric oxide has emerged as an important inhibitory nonadrenergic noncholinergic neurotransmitter throughout the gastrointestinal tract. Immunohistochemical demonstration of its presence and its role in peristalsis, colonic relaxation, and sphincter function are discussed. Intestinal pseudoobstruction poses difficult diagnostic and management problems. However, new primary pathologies causing chronic disease are being identified and pharmacologic treatment of acute disease may be helpful. The repeatability and value of visceral evoked potentials in anorectal disease is discussed. Long-term data about the clinical spectrum of Hirschsprung's disease and immunohistochemical means of diagnosis are reviewed. An update is provided on the etiology and complications of severe constipation. Other areas reviewed include diarrhea and fat excretion, new motility pharmacotherapies, food and colonic motility, and optimum methods for measurement of colonic transit.

Current Opinion in Gastroenterology 1994, **10**:11–18

Nitric oxide

The discovery in 1987 by Palmer *et al.* [1] and Ignarro *et al.* [2], that NO (nitric oxide) derived from vascular endothelium caused vascular smooth muscle relaxation, unleashed enormous research activity. The importance of this neurotransmitter system in cell function and communication in many tissues soon became apparent. The substrate for NO synthesis is L-arginine and the enzyme responsible for its synthesis, NO synthase, depends on calcium, NADPH, and calmodulin for its activity. The demonstration in 1989 of NO synthase inhibition by L-NMMA (*N*-monomethyl-L-arginine) and L-NNA (*N*-nitro-L-arginine), structural analogues of L-arginine, allowed further detailed studies on the chemical pathways involved.

Later studies demonstrated that the NO system is responsible for a similar "dilator tone" in the gastrointestinal tract to that found in vascular endothelium, and that other constrictor and dilator influences act to produce further changes in tone and contractions (Fig. 1). NO, probably the major nonadrenergic noncholinergic inhibitory neurotransmitter, acts on intestinal muscle and influences intestinal blood flow and mucosal processes, including secretion.

To demonstrate that enteric neurons contain the necessary enzyme system, antibodies have been developed against NO synthase; alternatively, NO synthase has been shown to colocalize with NADPH diaphorase activity, a commonly used neural marker. Using both these techniques, Ward *et al.* [3••] have demonstrated the presence of this enzyme system in canine proximal colon. Positive labeling nerve trunks were identified throughout both the longitudinal and circular muscle coats, in addition to the submucosal pacemaker region.

Nitric oxide is also critically involved in sphincter function. Rattan *et al.* [4] studied relaxation of the internal anal sphincter in the opossum *in vivo*. Resting anal pressure, a reflection of smooth muscle internal sphincter tone, was monitored. The NO synthase inhibitor L-NNA caused a dose-dependent decrease in the amount of sphincter relaxation induced by intrarectal balloon distension, as well as in the relaxation induced by sacral nerve stimulation. Administration of the NO precursor L-arginine reversed this inhibition, restoring sphincter relaxation. Chakder and Rattan [5] further demonstrated that NO is directly released in response to stimulation of nonadrenergic noncholinergic inhibitory gut neurons. O'Kelly *et al.* [6•] have demonstrated *in vitro* that NO is involved in the neurogenic nonadrenergic noncholinergic relaxation of human internal anal sphincter.

Abbreviations

GABA—gamma aminobutyric acid; **VIP**—vasoactive intestinal polypeptide.

 ISBN 1-85922-606-X ISSN 0267–1379

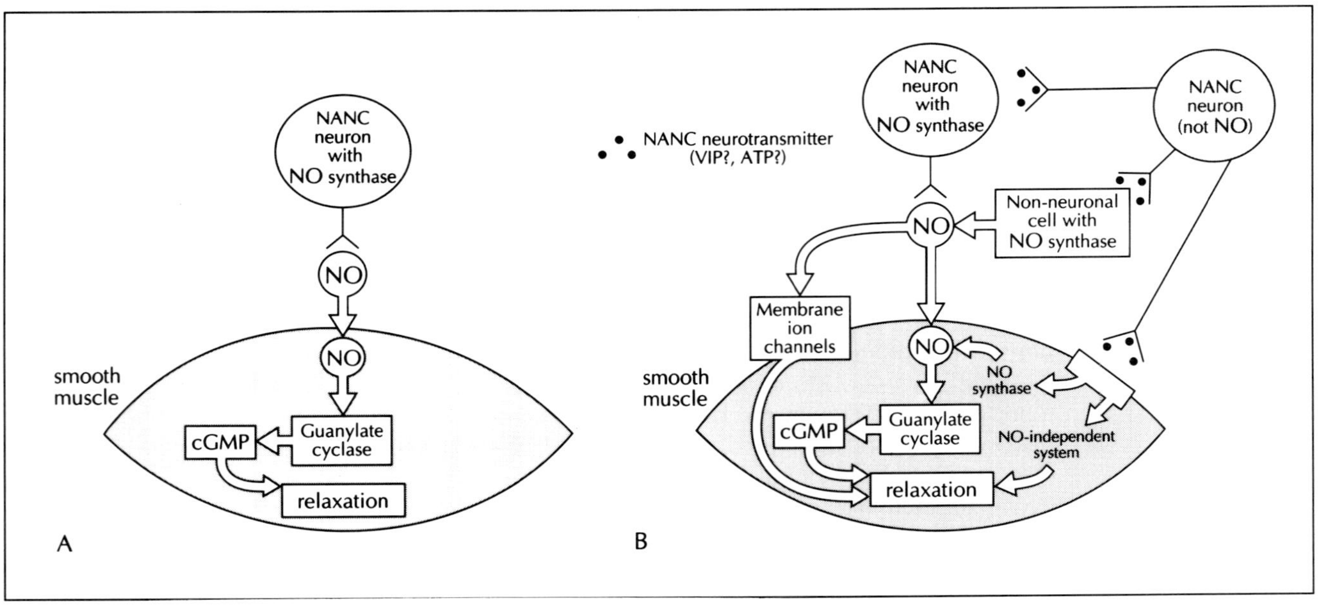

Fig. 1. Possible mechanisms by which nitric oxide (NO) can mediate NANC inhibition of smooth muscle. **A**, NO acts as a direct neurotransmitter. **B**, Other possible mechanisms for NANC inhibition, which may or may not involve NO. cGMP—cyclic GMP; NANC—nonaderenergic noncholernergic; VIP—vasoactive intestinal peptide. (*From* Stark and Szurszewski [12••]; with permission.)

Chakder and Rattan [7] also studied the second messengers that are involved in internal sphincter relaxation produced by NO, vasoactive intestinal polypeptide (VIP), and electric field stimulation. All three stimuli produced reduction in tone of sphincter muscle *in vitro*. The tissue levels of two second messengers, cyclic AMP and cyclic GMP, were increased by these stimuli, the extent of each rise being stimulus specific.

Grider [8] examined the mechanism underlying smooth muscle relaxation in rat colon. Both VIP and NO are important in reducing colonic smooth muscle tone, and in producing the descending relaxation phase of peristalsis. Field stimulation or radial stretch was accompanied by VIP release and NO production. NO production appeared to enhance VIP release. Relaxation appears to represent the combined effects of VIP and NO on muscle cells.

Grider and Makhlouf [9] also investigated the role of gamma aminobutyric acid (GABA) in the peristaltic reflex. GABA had no direct effect on isolated circular smooth muscle cells. Using a variety of agonists and antagonists on various preparations of rat colonic muscle the authors demonstrated that on release from myenteric neurons, GABA acts via GABAa receptors on cholinergic and VIP motor neurons responsible for the two components of the peristaltic reflex.

Boeckxstaens *et al.* [10•], by studying muscle strips *in vitro*, demonstrated that both NO and ATP appear to play a role in inhibitory nonadrenergic noncholinergic neurotransmission in the human colon.

Apart from a calcium-dependent enzyme, a second NO enzyme system has also been recognized in macrophage-polymorpholeukocytes and in the vascular endothelium. Lipopolysaccharides and cytokines activate this system, which is not calcium dependent. Middleton *et al.* [11••] obtained granulocytes and mononuclear cells from healthy subjects and demonstrated that they were able to relax distal colonic circular smooth muscle in a concentration-dependent manner, and showed that this was mediated by the release of NO. Inflammatory cells found in the mucosa during active inflammatory bowel disease may therefore play a role in these patients' altered bowel motility.

In what clinical circumstances might changes in NO activity be important? NO may be pathophysiologically involved whenever gastrointestinal tone is abnormally elevated, such as in achalasia, or excessively relaxed such as in gastroesophageal reflux or toxic megacolon. Even if the NO system is not of primary pathogenic importance, it offers an exciting possibility for pharmacologic manipulation of tone and motility. Stark and Szurszewski [12••] reviewed the role of NO in gastroenterologic and hepatic function (Fig. 2).

Chronic intestinal pseudoobstruction

In patients with chronic pseudoobstruction, silver staining to examine nerves and light and electron microscopic examination to examine muscle will often define an abnormality. However, these methods sometimes yield normal results in patients with characteristic clinical features of this syndrome.

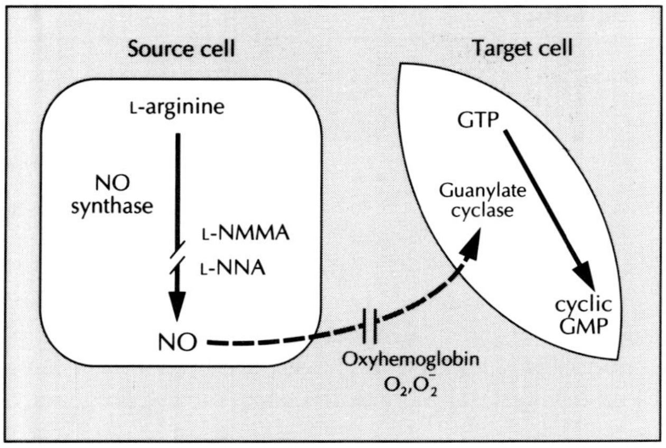

Fig. 2. Simplified representation of the synthesis and action of nitric oxide (NO). L-NMMA (*N*-monomethyl-L-arginine) and L-NNA (*N*-nitro-L-arginine) can inhibit NO synthase, whereas oxyhemoglobin, oxygen, or superoxide anion can inactivate NO. NO activates guanylate cyclase in the target cell. (*From* Stark and Szurszewski [12••]; with permission).

A variety of primary pathologies responsible for chronic intestinal pseudoobstruction continues to be unraveled using new methods. Smith *et al.* [13••] described a 48-year-old woman with constipation since childhood and episodes of nonmechanical obstruction. No abnormalities were detectable by light or electron microscopy, but immunostaining of enteric smooth muscle demonstrated an absence of smooth muscle α-actin confined to the circular muscle coat. Other contractile proteins were normal. This is the first description of a biochemical, as opposed to a structural, abnormality in chronic intestinal pseudoobstruction. A developmental block at one stage of embryogenesis could be responsible, as the two enteric muscle layers develop at different embryologic times.

Lowsky *et al.* [14] reported a 27-year-old man with visceral myopathy, ophthalmoplegia, and a peripheral limb myopathy. Molecular techniques demonstrated a striated muscle mitochondrial myopathy; although molecular techniques were not applied to the gut muscle, the combined lesions raised the possibility of a mitochondrial DNA mutation as the cause of the intestinal pathology.

Electron microscopic studies by Martin *et al.* [15] in a patient with visceral myopathy demonstrated that the intestinal fibrosis appears to derive from the transformation of smooth muscle fibers to myofibroblasts.

Krishnamurthy *et al.* [16] have studied the intestinal myenteric plexus from 26 children and infants, using cross sections stained with hematoxylin and eosin and frozen tangential sections processed using Smith's silver staining technique. Diverse abnormalities of the plexus were described, including an absence of the myenteric plexus (perhaps long-segment Hirschsprung's disease?), or a decrease in the myenteric argyrophilic neurons and axons.

It is often technically difficult to perform intestinal motility studies in patients with chronic pseudoobstruction; therefore, advances in noninvasive diagnosis must be welcomed. Surface electrogastrography was applied by Devane *et al.* [17••] in 11 children with chronic pseudoobstruction. Four had enteric neuropathy, three myopathy, and four indeterminate disease. Tachygastria (>5 cycles/min) was present in three patients with neuropathy. Irregular frequency was found in three patients with a neuropathy and two with undefined disease. One patient with a neuropathy and two with undefined pathology were normal. This study is particularly valuable because the diagnoses were primarily established with both histology and intestinal manometry.

The possible association between intestinal malrotation and pseudoobstruction was explored by Devane *et al.* [18•], who studied the small intestinal motor activity in eight children with persistent gut symptoms after surgical correction of malrotation. Seven children had a neuropathic motor pattern. The intrinsic nerve morphology was abnormal in three of four patients with full-thickness intestinal biopsies.

Colonic motility studies have rarely been performed in patients with pseudoobstruction. In a study of 30 children with pseudoobstruction documented with previous antroduodenal motility studies, those with constipation failed to generate a postprandial increase in colonic motility and most failed to demonstrate postprandial high-amplitude propagated contractions [19].

Acute colonic pseudoobstruction

Acute colonic pseudoobstruction (Ogilvie's syndrome) occurs most often in patients with other acute illnesses. Most patients can be treated conservatively. Jetmore *et al.* [20] retrospectively reported their experience of colonoscopic decompression in 48 patients. In sum, 84% were successfully treated by this method, 11% required an operation, and two patients died from "medical" causes. These studies should be interpreted cautiously; some studies have demonstrated a good outcome without any intervention, and the criteria for intervention (colonoscopic or surgical) usually vary in a retrospective series.

Hutchinson and Griffiths [21••] report the use of intravenous guanethidine (an adrenergic blocker) and neostigmine (a parasympathomimetic) in patients with acute colonic pseudoobstruction. Eight of the 11 patients, all with an acute illness predisposing them to this complication, responded within 10 minutes and did not experience a recurrence. Three patients without a predisposing factor did not respond. A cautious interpretation of these results has been voiced by Vantrappen [22].

Receptors

Ennes *et al.* [23••] have examined receptor-binding properties of freshly isolated and cultured rabbit colonic circular smooth muscle cells. Intracellular changes of cyclic AMP were observed in response to VIP and calcitonin gene–related peptide, and high levels of muscarinic receptors were demonstrated. However, major differences were observed between freshly isolated and cultured cells, suggesting that the former are damaged by the isolation procedure.

Presti and Gardner [24] have reviewed the current status of gastrointestinal peptide antagonists.

Measuring colonic motility

Twenty-four recordings of colonic motility have had a major impact on our knowledge of colonic motor function. A summary of the currently available data from these studies is presented by Bassotti *et al.* [25]. Jameson and Misiewicz [26], in a review of colonic motility testing, concluded that its role is limited in clinical practice but well established in research.

Epidemiology of functional symptoms

One quarter of the adult population have irritable bowel symptoms at any one time. But what is the natural history? A population study suggests that over a 1- to 2-year period, 10% lose their symptoms while a similar proportion gain new ones [27].

Diabetes and abnormal gut motility

Symptoms correlate poorly with demonstrable abnormalities of transit in patients with diabetes. Iber *et al.* [28] measured solid gastric emptying and small bowel and colonic transit in control subjects and asymptomatic and symptomatic patients with diabetes. Only colonic transit correlated with the symptom of severe constipation; other symptoms correlated poorly with objective findings.

Pregnancy

Although constipation is thought to be more common in pregnancy, there are few prospective studies about its true incidence or severity. A study of 1000 healthy women in an Israeli maternity ward showed that 55% noted no change in bowel frequency, 11% experienced a decrease, and 34% noted an increase in bowel frequency [29]. One third of those with decreased bowel frequency considered themselves constipated. Other studies have found a higher incidence of constipation. Baron *et al.* [30] have reviewed the literature relating to gastrointestinal motility disorders during pregnancy.

Bowel function in preterm infants

A study of 884 preterm infants has shown that delay in the passage of meconium occurs in about one third, and time to first bowel action is inversely related to gestational age [31•]. Infants demonstrated a minimum defecation rate of once per day, which increased in proportion to the amount of milk ingested.

Hirschsprung's disease

Rescorla *et al.* [32••] described the clinical history of 260 patients with Hirschsprung's disease treated in a pediatric center. One quarter of the patients were diagnosed after 1 year of age. In two thirds the aganglionic segment involved the rectum or rectosigmoid, whereas it involved the rectum in 15%, proximal colon in 9%, and the whole colon in 9%. The most common operation was the modified Duhamel procedure. In the 105 patients with long-term follow-up, two thirds had normal bowel function whereas most of the remainder had some constipation. Bowel function appeared to improve with time.

Total colonic (long segment) Hirschsprung's disease can be difficult to treat and has a high morbidity and mortality. Bickler *et al.* [33] reviewed their experience with 21 children (14 boys and seven girls) over a 31-year period. The transitional zone from ganglionic to aganglionic bowel was distal to midileum in 16, midileum in four, and midjejunum in one. Abdominal distension and constipation or delayed passage of meconium were the most common clinical findings. Two thirds were identified within the first 2 weeks of life, but one fifth were diagnosed after 20 weeks. Barium enema identified the transition zone in only one fifth of patients. Long-term follow-up of 10 years was available in six patients, five of whom had adequate bowel function.

Rectal biopsy is the main means of diagnosing Hirschsprung's disease. Full-thickness biopsies are often required in adults, although suction biopsies usually suffice in children. Diagnosis rests on demonstrating an absence of ganglion cells and an increase in cholinergic fibers in the lamina propria. Demonstration of the latter using the acetylcholinesterase technique requires fresh frozen tissue. Sams *et al.* [34••] have evaluated the efficacy of using the neuronal markers protein gene product 9.5, S100, and neuron-specific enolase in diagnosing Hirschsprung's disease. S100 was the most sensitive in demonstrating lamina propria fibers, but no one stain was reliable in this respect. Reproducibility was best using a combination of S100 and protein gene product 9.5, although further studies are required before these could be confidently used on their own to make a diagnosis.

Visceral evoked potentials

Measurement of evoked potential latency times has proved valuable in the diagnosis of neurologic disorders such as multiple sclerosis. With the increasing interest in the sensory and perceptive components of functional bowel disorders, many clinical investigators hoped that tests of sensory conduction from visceral structures might prove diagnostically useful. Cerebral recordings have been made after esophageal stimulation, but there is some controversy about their interpretation and reliability.

Speakman *et al.* [35•] studied 13 patients with either constipation or incontinence and 16 healthy control subjects. Somatosensory evoked potentials, from the tibial nerve or the dorsal genital nerve, were easily recorded and were reproducible. Rectal stimulation was performed using a bipolar ring electrode. Reproducible recordings were obtained from less than half the patients and similarly for control subjects. When latencies were obtained their range was too large to be of diagnostic value. There must be some doubt about the clinical value of such investigations.

Food and colonic motility

The ingestion of food increases colonic motility. Daly *et al.* [36] have shown that single-channel measured contractions are not substantially changed after food, but that contractions measured simultaneously along a length of bowel do increase substantially. Data from more than one channel may therefore be a more sensitive indicator of changes in motility than a single-channel motility index.

The colonic response to food relates not only to food ingestion, but also to cephalic stimulation: sight, smell, taste, and especially discussion about food. Rogers *et al.* [37] studied five healthy subjects with a range of stimuli, simultaneously measuring colonic motor activity.

Measurement of colonic transit

Are radiopaque markers inferior to radioisotope studies in assessing total and regional colonic transit? van der Sijp *et al.* [38•] compared the two methods simultaneously in healthy subjects and 12 patients with severe idiopathic constipation. Markers were surprisingly accurate at demonstrating sites of colonic delay, although radioisotopes incorporated into a meal allow the whole gut to be studied and multiple observations to be made without added radiation. The former appears increasingly important in view of the disturbance in upper gut motility in many patients with motility disorders apparently confined to the large bowel [39].

Diarrhea and fecal fat excretion

In an elegant study, Fine and Fordtran [40••] measured fecal fat excretion in normal subjects before and after diarrhea was experimentally induced. Fecal fat output went up from a mean of 3.4 g/d (normal upper limit, 6.4 g/d) to a mean of 7.7 g/d in those with severe diarrhea (fecal weight >800 g/d). This study sheds new light on the interpretation of elevated fecal fat excretion in patients with diarrhea.

New pharmacotherapies

Fedotozine, a peripherally acting opioid agonist, is attracting interest because of its effects on motility and potential for modifying functional pain. In a study on rats fedotozine reversed experimental ileus, an effect blocked by naloxone [41••]. This drug is worth watching.

The α-2 receptors mediate the inhibition of many gastrointestinal functions. Atipamezole, an α-2 antagonist, reversed laparotomy-induced ileus in experimental rats [42]. Pharmacologic manipulation of patients with ileus has been disappointing until now, but more selective drugs may be more successful.

Severe idiopathic constipation

Motility

Women with intractable constipation and documented slow intestinal transit have a decrease in the frequency of high-pressure peristaltic mass movements. Kamm *et al.* [43] colonoscopically inserted a multichannel manometric tube into the colon of five women with intractable constipation and induced motor activity using intraluminal bisacodyl. In all women this resulted in high-pressure peristaltic waves, which progressed around the colon and resulted in the effective evacuation of simultaneously instilled radioisotope. The ability to generate an appropriate pattern of motor activity therefore appears to be preserved in these women. van der Sijp *et al.* [39] documented disordered gastric and small bowel transit and the patterns of disordered colonic transit [38•] in severely constipated patients.

Autonomic function

Altomare *et al.* [44] injected acetylcholine into the dorsum of the foot, which was painted with a mixture of starch and iodine, to test autonomic integrity in a group of healthy subjects and severely constipated patients. The small black dots generated by sweating were photographed and counted. Patients demonstrated a significantly lower response, suggesting altered autonomic function.

Surgery and psychology

The variable results of surgery in these patients have been well documented in the literature over the past 5 years. Rex *et al.* [45•] present data from a slightly different angle: describing the selection of patients for surgery from their total group of severely constipated patients. Nineteen of 224 patients seen in a tertiary referral gastroenterologic practice underwent a subtotal colectomy, with 86% improved. Although this and other studies claim good results on the basis of predefined selection criteria, most of these criteria are subjective and unproved. The true value of such criteria could only be determined by randomized study. At a time when many patients are helped by biofeedback techniques [46] (not included in this series of 224 patients) such a study is unlikely to be performed. Despite stringent criteria for surgery, of the 16 patients with greater than 2 years' follow-up, two had experienced incontinence, one of whom required conversion to an ileostomy. Three patients had required further surgery for bowel obstruction.

In an editorial review of Rex *et al.*'s paper [45•], Devroede [47••] highlights the importance of psychologic assessment and long-term follow-up when treating patients with severe constipation and assessing the results of surgery.

The psychologic evaluation of patients with severely disordered transit by unstructured interview may be clinically useful, but for research purposes standardized questionnaires are valuable. But which questionnaire is best? Wald *et al.* [48] used the Hopkins Symptom Checklist and the Minnesota Multiphasic Personality Inventory to assess constipated patients. The two questionnaires provided similar information but the former was quicker to complete and score.

Complications of gallstones

Early this century the British surgeon Arbuthnot-Lane proposed that severe constipation was responsible for many of the afflictions that affect the human body; the cure was colectomy. Heaton *et al.* [49•] provide epidemiologic evidence that slow intestinal transit in women predisposes to gallstone formation. Cholecystosonography was performed in 1058 women in the population, and stones identified in 48 women. Fifteen of these women were normal body weight; their measured intestinal transit time was slower than age-matched control subjects. Gallstone formation may be favored by slow intestinal transit, leading to high biliary proportions of deoxycholate.

References and recommended reading

Papers of particular interest, published within the annual period of review, have been highlighted as:

- • Of special interest
- •• Of outstanding interest

1. PALMER RMJ, FERRIGE AG, MONCADA S: **Nitric Oxide Release Accounts for the Biological Activity of Endothelium-Derived Relaxing Factor.** *Nature* 1987, **327**:524–526.

2. IGNARRO LJ, BUGA GM, WOOD KS, BYRNS RE, CHAUDHURI G: **Endothelium-derived Relaxing Factor Produced and Released From Artery and Vein is Nitric Oxide.** *Proc Natl Acad Sci U S A* 1987, **84**:9265–9269.

3. •• WARD SM, XUE C, SHUTTLEWORTH W, BREDT DS, SNYDER SH, SANDERS KM: **NADPH Diaphorase and Nitric Oxide Synthase Colocalisation in Enteric Neurons of Canine Proximal Colon.** *Am J Physiol* 1992, **263**:G277–G284.

Demonstration of NO activity in canine colon, using NADPH diaphorase and antibodies directed against NO synthase.

4. RATTAN S, SARKAR A, CHAKDER S: **Nitric Oxide Pathway in Rectoanal Inhibitory Reflex of Opossum Internal Anal Sphincter.** *Gastroenterology* 1992, **103**:43–50.

5. CHAKDER S, RATTAN S: **Release of Nitric Oxide by Activation of Nonadrenergic Noncholinergic Neurons on Internal Anal Sphincter.** *Am J Physiol* 1993, **264**:G7–G12.

6. • O'KELLY T, BRADING A, MORTENSEN N: **Nerve Mediated Relaxation of the Human Internal Anal Sphincter: The Role of Nitric Oxide.** *Gut* 1993, **34**:689–693.

Evidence that NO is involved in neurally mediated internal anal sphincter relaxation in humans.

7. CHAKDER S, RATTAN S: **Involvement of cAMP and cGMP in Relaxation of Internal Anal Sphincter by Neural Stimulation, VIP, and NO.** *AM J Physiol* 1993, **264**:G702–G707.

8. GRIDER JR: **Interplay of VIP and Nitric Oxide in Regulation of the Descending Relaxation Phase of Peristalsis.** *Am J Physiol* 1993, **264**:G334–G340.

9. Grider JR, Makhlouf GM: **Enteric GABA: Mode of Action and Role in the Regulation of the Peristaltic Reflex.** *Am J Physiol* 1992, **262**:G690–G694.

10. • Boeckxstaens GE, Pelckmans PA, Herman AG, van Maercke YM: **Involvement of Nitric Oxide in the Inhibitory Innervation of the Human Isolated Colon.** *Gastroenterology* 1993, **104**:690–697.
In vitro studies of human colonic smooth muscle demonstrating involvement of NO in nonadrenergic noncholinergic neurotransmission.

11. •• Middleton SJ, Shorthouse M, Hunter JO: **Relaxation of Distal Colonic Circular Smooth Muscle by Nitric Oxide Derived From Human Leucocytes.** *Gut* 1993, **34**:814–817.
White cells release NO, which can then relax colonic muscle; this may be important in the relationship between inflammation and motility.

12. •• Stark ME, Szurszewski JH: **Role of Nitric Oxide in Gastrointestinal and Hepatic Function and Disease.** *Gastroenterology* 1992, **103**:1928–1949.
A comprehensive review about the role of NO in gastrointestinal function and disease.

13. •• Smith VV, Lake ED, Kamm MA, Nicholls RJ: **Intestinal Pseudo-Obstruction With Deficient Smooth Muscle Alpha-Actin.** *Histopathology* 1992, **21**:535–542.
The first description of a biochemical, as opposed to a structural, enteric abnormality in a patient with chronic intestinal pseudoobstruction.

14. Lowsky R, Davidson G, Wolman S, Jeejeebhoy KN, Hegele RA: **Familial Visceral Myopathy Associated With a Mitochondrial Myopathy.** *Gut* 1993, **34**:279–283.

15. Martin JE, Benson M, Swash M, Salih V, Gray A: **Myofibroblasts in Hollow Visceral Myopathy: The Origin of Gastrointestinal Fibrosis?** *Gut* 1993, **34**:999–1001.

16. Krishnamurthy S, Heng Y, Schuffler MD: **Chronic Intestinal Pseudo-Obstruction in Infants and Children Caused by Diverse Abnormalities of the Myenteric Plexus.** *Gastroenterology* 1993, **104**:1398–1408.

17. •• Devane SP, Ravelli AM, Bisset WM, Smith VV, Lake BD, Milla PJ: **Gastric Antral Dysrhythmias in Children With Chronic Idiopathic Intestinal Pseudoobstruction.** *Gut* 1992, **33**:1477–1481.
Noninvasive electrogastrography has been used to detect electrical rhythm disturbances in children with intestinal pseudoobstruction whose intestinal pathology and motility has been previously documented.

18. • Devane SP, Coorbes R, Smith VV, Bisset WM, Booth IW, Lake BD, Milla PJ: **Persistent Gastrointestinal Symptoms After Correction of Malrotation.** *Arch Dis Child* 1992, **67**:218–221.
Children with corrected malrotation continue to have symptoms, *eg*, abnormal intestinal motility and gut neuropathology, suggesting a link with pseudoobstruction.

19. Di Lorenzo C, Flores AF, Reddy SN, Snape WJ, Bazzocchi G, Hyman PE: **Colonic Manometry in Children With Chronic Intestinal Pseudo-Obstruction.** *Gut* 1993, **34**:803–807.

20. Jetmore AB, Timmcke AE, Gathright JB, Hicks TC, Ray JE, Baker JW: **Ogilvie's Syndrome: Colonoscopic Decompression and Analysis of Predisposing Factors.** *Dis Colon Rectum* 1992, **35**:1135–1142.

21. •• Hutchinson R, Griffiths C: **Acute Colonic Pseudo-Obstruction: A Pharmacological Approach.** *Ann Coll Surg Engl* 1992, **74**:364–367.
Intravenous autonomically active drugs may be an effective treatment for acute intestinal pseudoobstruction.

22. Vantrappen G: **Acute Colonic Pseudo-Obstruction [Commentary].** *Lancet* 1993, **341**:152–153.

23. •• Ennes HS, McRoberts JA, Hyman PE, Snape WJ: **Characterization of Colonic Circular Smooth Muscle Cells in Culture.** *Am J Physiol* 1992, **263**:G365–G370.
Freshly isolated and cultured smooth muscle cells exhibit different receptor characteristics.

24. Presti ME, Gardner JD: **Receptor Antagonists for Gastrointestinal Peptides.** *Am J Physiol* 1993, **264**:G399–G406.

25. Bassotti G, Crowell MD, Whitehead WE: **Contractile Activity of the Human Colon: Lessons From 24 Hour Studies.** *Gut* 1993, **34**:129–133.

26. Jameson JS, Misiewicz JJ: **Colonic Motility: Practice or Research.** *Gut* 1993, **34**:1009–1012.

27. Talley NJ, Weaver AL, Zinsmeister AR, Melton LJ: **Onset and Disappearance of Gastrointestinal Symptoms and Functional Gastrointestinal Disorders.** *Am J Epidemiol* 1992, **136**:165–177.

28. Iber FL, Parveen S, Vandrunen M, Sood KB, Reza F, Serlovsky R, Reddy S: **Relation of Symptoms to Impaired Stomach, Small Bowel, and Colonic Motility in Long-standing Diabetes.** *Dig Dis Sci* 1993, **38**:45–50.

29. Levy N, Lemberg E, Sharf M: **Bowel Habit in Pregnancy.** *Digestion* 1971, **4**:216–222.

30. Baron TH, Ramirez B, Richter JE: **Gastrointestinal Motility Disorders During Pregnancy.** *Ann Intern Med* 1993, **118**:366–375.

31. • Weaver LT, Lucas A: **Development of Bowel Habit in Preterm Infants.** *Arch Dis Child* 1993, **68**:317–320.
Time to first bowel action in preterm infants is inversely related to gestational age.

32. •• Rescorla FJ, Morrison AM, Engles D, West KW, Grosfeld JL: **Hirschsprung's Disease: Evaluation of Mortality and Long-Term Function in 260 Cases.** *Arch Surg* 1992, **127**:934–942.
Clinical description of a large series of children with Hirschsprung's disease: age at presentation, extent of disease, and follow-up after treatment.

33. Bickler SW, Harrison MW, Campbell TJ, Campbell JR: **Long-Segment Hirschsprung's Disease.** *Arch Surg* 1992, **127**:1047–1051.

34. •• Sams VR, Bobrow LG, Happerfield L, Keeling J: **Evaluation of PGP9.5 in the Diagnosis of Hirschsprung's Disease.** *J Pathol* 1992, **168**:55–58.
A critical assessment of the nerve stains S100 and protein gene product 9.5 in making a diagnosis of Hirschsprung's disease.

35. • Speakman CTM, Kamm MA, Swsah M: **Rectal Sensory Evoked Potentials: An Assessment of Their Clinical Value.** *Int J Colorectal Dis* 1993, **8**:23–28.
A study of the clinical value and reproducibility of visceral cerebral evoked potentials, suggesting that their role in clinical situations is limited.

36. Daly J, Bergin A, Sun WM, Read NW: **Effect of Food and Anti-Cholinergic Drugs on the Pattern of Rectosigmoid Contractions.** *Gut* 1993, **34**:799–802.

37. Rogers J, Raimundo AH, Misiewicz JJ: **Cephalic Phase of Colonic Pressure Response to Food.** *Gut* 1993, **34**:537–543.

38. • van der Sijp JRM, Kamm MA, Nightingale JMD, Britton KE, Granowska M, Akkermans LMA, Lennard-Jones JE: **Ra-**

dioisotope Determination of Regional Colonic Transit in Severe Constipation. *Gut* 1993, 34:402–408.
A comparison of radiopaque markers and radioisotopes in assessing regional colonic transit. The former is a reasonable screening test, the latter provides more detailed information and can be combined with upper gut studies.

39. van der Sijp, Kamm MA, Nightingale JMD, Walker E, Granowska M, Britton K, Akkermans LMA, Lennard-Jones JE: **Disturbed Gastric and Small Bowel Transit in Severe Idiopathic Constipation.** *Dig Dis Sci* 1993, 38:837–844.

40. Fine KD, Fordtran JS: **The Effect of Diarrhea on Fecal Fat**
•• **Excretion.** *Gastroenterology* 1992, 102:1936–1939.
The experimental production of diarrhea increases fecal fat excretion; clinical estimates may need to be modified in view of these findings.

41. Riviere PJM, Pascaud X, Chevalier E, Le Gallou B, Junien
•• JL: **Fedotozine Reverses Ileus Induced by Surgery or Peritonitis: Action at Peripheral K-Opioid Receptors.** *Gastroenterology* 1993, 104:724–731.
Opioid agonists may have a role in reversing postoperative ileus.

42. Tanila H, Kauppila T, Taira T: **Inhibition of Intestinal Motility and Reversal of Postlaparotomy Ileus by Selective Alpha2-Adrenergic Drugs in the Rat.** *Gastroenterology* 1993, 104:819–824.

43. Kamm MA, van der Sijp JRM, Lennard-Jones JE: **Observations on the Characteristics of Stimulated Defecation in Severe Idiopathic Constipation.** *Int J Colorectal Dis* 1992, 7:197–201.

44. Altomare D, Pilot MA, Scott M, Williams N, Rubino M, Ilincic L, Waldron D: **Detection of Subclinical Autonomic Neuropathy in Constipated Patients Using a Sweat Test.** *Gut* 1992, 33:1539–1543.

45. Rex DK, Lappas JC, Goulet RC, Madura JA: **Selection of**
• **Constipated Patients as Subtotal Colectomy Candidates.** *J Clin Gastroenterol* 1992, 15:212–217.
Description of a consecutive series of hospital patients with severe constipation.

46. Kamm MA: **Motility and Functional Diseases of the Large Intestine.** *Curr Opin Gastroenterol* 1993, 9:11–18.

47. Devroede G: **Constipation: A Sign of Disease to be Treated**
•• **Surgically, or a Symptom to be Deciphered as Nonverbal Communication? [Editorial].** *J Clin Gastroenterol* 1992, 15:189–191.
Editorial summarizing the importance of psychologic factors in the assessment of patients with severe constipation, and questions whether rigid treatment protocols that include surgery are appropriate for such functional disorders.

48. Wald A, Burgio K, Holeva K, Locher J: **Psychological Evaluation of Patients With Severe Idiopathic Constipation: Which Instrument to Use.** *Am J Gastroenterol* 1992, 87:977–980.

49. Heaton KW, Emmett PM, Symes CL, Braddon FEM: **An Ex-**
• **planation for Gallstones in Normal-Weight Women: Slow Intestinal Transit.** *Lancet* 1993, 341:8–10.
Gallstones are more common in normal weight women with slow intestinal transit than those women with normal transit.

Michael A. Kamm, MD, MRCP, FRACP, St. Mark's Hospital, City Road, London EC1V 2PS, UK.

Epidemiology and etiology of sporadic colorectal adenocarcinoma

William E. Karnes, Jr, MD

Mayo Clinic, Rochester, Minnesota, USA

Epidemiologic studies have shown that colorectal carcinoma is a disease of Western civilization, most likely related to diet. Diet probably plays a multifactorial role, containing both protective and promoting factors for colorectal carcinoma development. Sorting through the complexities of diet has been a major challenge to epidemiologists. Diets rich in fat and calories seem to contribute to colorectal carcinoma formation, whereas diets rich in plant fiber seem to be protective. Animal studies implicate bile acids, cholesterol, and fatty acids as promoters of colorectal carcinoma, whereas fiber and calcium antagonize cancer promoters. Based on the recent recognition that mutations of specific colon cancer–associated genes correlate with progression of normal mucosa through adenomatous polyps to frank carcinoma, we now approach the question of dietary influences from a new prospective. How do dietary factors affect the mutagenic potential colonic luminal contents? As the links between molecular biology and epidemiology begin to form, new preventative strategies will be developed and tested that may prove to dramatically reduce the incidence of colon carcinoma.

Current Opinion in Gastroenterology 1994, **10**:19–26

Adenocarcinoma of the colorectum is the second leading cause of death from cancer in the United States and generally affects both men and women equally, although some gender differences may exist between left- and right-sided cancers. In women, colon cancer is the third leading cause of cancer death behind lung and breast carcinoma; in men, colon carcinoma also ranks third behind lung and prostate carcinoma. Each year approximately 150,000 new cases of colon carcinoma are diagnosed and approximately 57,000 individuals die of the disease [1•]. Those who survive are diagnosed early and benefit from surgical resection. Those who are diagnosed too late for curative resection face little chance of meaningful response to available treatments and almost always die of their disease.

Clearly, novel approaches to the prevention, early detection, and treatment of colon carcinoma are needed. Accomplishing these goals will require a deeper understanding of the interrelationships between environmental factors and the genetics and biology of colorectal carcinoma. Epidemiologic studies have suggested that environmental factors influence risk of sporadic colorectal carcinoma. Identification of these factors should lead to effective preventative strategies. The dramatic flow of new information regarding cellular and genetic abnormalities associated with colorectal carcinoma development should lead to new screening tests of susceptibility, new markers of disease, and novel specific therapies. This article reviews current epidemiologic data as they relate to present theory regarding the etiology of sporadic (noninherited) colorectal carcinoma. The application of this information to screening and diagnostic strategies for colorectal carcinoma is covered in this issue by Douglas McGill and Mark Larson (pp 27–33).

Epidemiology

Sporadic colorectal carcinoma is a disease of Western society (Fig. 1) [2]. Although data are far from complete, the variable geographic incidence of colorectal carcinoma seems most impressive for the distal colon. In countries with a low incidence of colon carcinoma, right-side lesions predominate; in high-incidence countries, left-side carcinomas predominate [3]. Right- and left-side carcinomas also have different gender distributions, with women having more right-side colon car-

 ISBN 1-85922-606-X ISSN 0267–1379

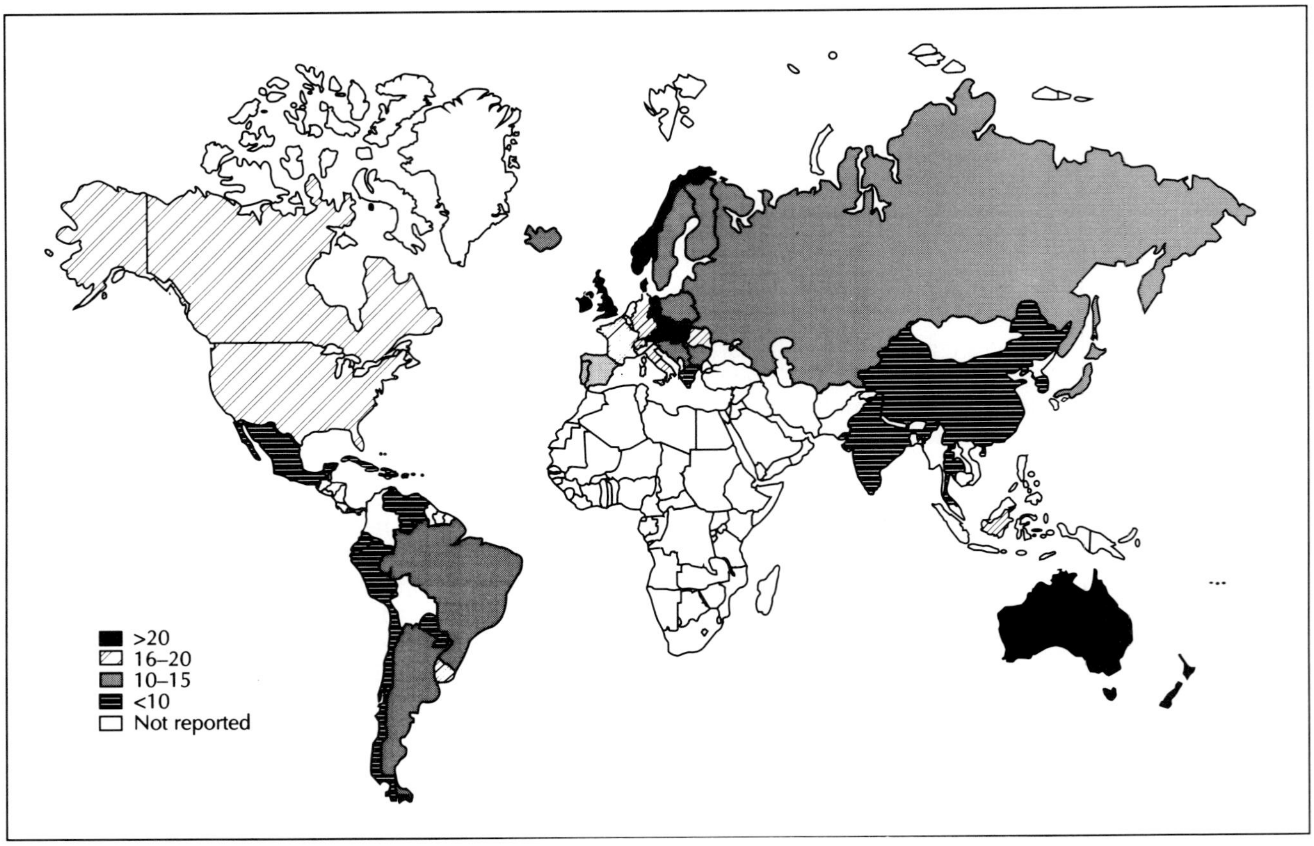

Fig. 1. Geographic representation of age-adjusted mortality rates from colorectal carcinoma per 100,000 population in 50 countries (*From* Boring *et al.* [1•]; with permission.)

cinomas than men [3]. Rectal carcinomas seem to follow a similar geographic pattern as left-side colon carcinomas. However, in contrast to left-side colon carcinomas, whose incidence had increased and then plateaued in the United States, rectal carcinomas have shown a declining incidence [4••,5]. Other evidence suggesting that proximal, distal, and rectal colon carcinomas may have different causes includes recent surveys of the prevalence of specific oncogenes and tumor suppressor gene abnormalities from adenomatous polyps and carcinomas from different regions of the colorectum [6]. Most analyses in epidemiologic studies have not properly considered these apparent differences between right- and left-side colorectal carcinomas.

Overall, the geographic pattern of risk for colorectal carcinoma is strikingly similar to that of breast carcinoma, suggesting common environmental risk factor(s) (Fig. 2*A*) [7]. In contrast to the positive correlation between the geographic incidences of breast and colorectal carcinoma, a significant negative correlation is seen between the geographic incidences of gastric and colorectal carcinoma (Fig. 2*B*). As has been described with gastric and breast carcinoma, immigrants from countries with a low incidence of colorectal carcinoma gradually acquire (over two to three decades) the risk of the country to which they move, and vice versa [8,9]. Apparently, some factor(s) in Western society reduce the incidence of gastric carcinoma while increasing the incidence of breast and colorectal carcinoma.

Geography alone does not appear to be an important independent risk factor for colorectal carcinoma. Even within a geographic region, subgroups tied together by strong ethnic, religious, or cultural traditions that maintain isolated and distinct lifestyles exhibit risks that often differ significantly from the surrounding population [10–12]. Colorectal carcinoma was a rare disease until the middle 19th century in Europe [13]. The adoption of modern Western lifestyles in the United States and Europe coincides with an increase in the incidence of left-side colon carcinoma. A similar trend is now being seen in countries like Japan that are in the midst of the same lifestyle changes [14].

The major challenge to epidemiologists has been to identify the independent component risk factors inherent in Western lifestyles. Correlative studies can be dismissed as providing such information. For example, one of the strongest correlations with risk of colorectal carcinoma is gross national product [15]. The most reliable studies are performed by prospectively segregating a given socioeconomic and regional population by the presence and absence of a hypothesized risk factor and prospectively testing for a difference in colorectal cancer incidence between the two groups (co-

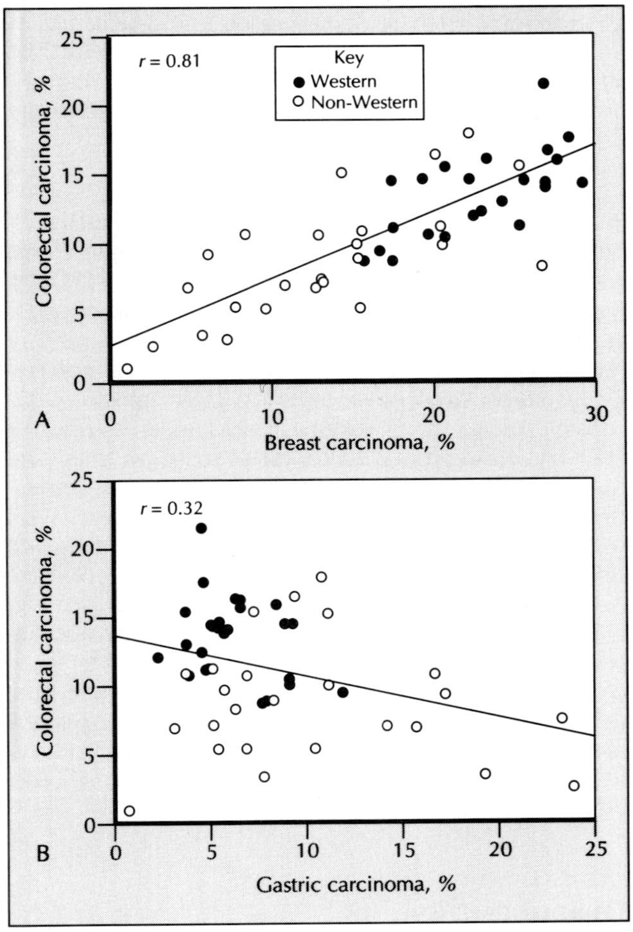

Fig. 2. **A**, Correlation between age-adjusted mortality rates per 100,000 population from 50 countries for colorectal and breast carcinoma ($r=0.81$, $P<0.0001$). **B**, Correlation between age-adjusted mortality rates per 100,000 population from 50 countries for colorectal and gastric carcinoma ($r=-0.32$, $P<0.01$). (*Data from* Boring *et al.* [1•].)

hort study). A more common and less expensive analytic approach is to retrospectively test for the presence of hypothesized risk factors in a group of individuals with colorectal carcinoma, using a control group without colorectal carcinoma from the same at-risk population (case-control study). Both approaches suffer from errors intrinsic to asking the right question. Case-control studies suffer from errors in selecting a proper control group and difficulties in obtaining accurate historic information.

What are the right questions? Compared with populations of low risk for colorectal carcinoma, Westerners have smaller, less-frequent bowel movements, are fatter and more sedentary, have fewer children, eat more fat, red meat, and refined carbohydrates, and eat less fiber-containing vegetables and fruits. Because these characteristics so tightly cosegregate between at-risk populations, it is not surprising that international correlative studies have shown each of these factors to be associated with increased risk of colorectal carcinoma. Furthermore, many of these characteristics go hand-in-hand (such as high fat and low fiber), making it nearly impossible to isolate independent effects. Even carefully performed, analytical, case-controlled and cohort studies have had a difficult time of separating independent effects.

Dietary risk factors

Burkitt [16] observed that residents of rural Bantu, Africa ingest a diet extremely high in fiber and low in fat, had enormous daily fecal mass, and had a small incidence of colon cancer. He hypothesized that foods deficient in fiber and high in refined carbohydrates and fat are responsible for colon cancer. Indeed, along with the increase in colorectal carcinoma incidence in the United States during the past 70 to 80 years has been an increase in fat and meat intake and reduction in complex carbohydrates [17]. The recent increase in the incidence of colorectal carcinoma in Japan (130% increase since 1985) has been accompanied by similar changes in diet, particularly fat, which has increased from 10% to 25% of energy over the same time period [18]. As a result of these observations, most investigators have focused their attention on the role of specific dietary elements and their downstream effect on stool mass and composition [19].

Dietary fat

A strong correlation exists between the geographic incidence of colorectal carcinoma and mean fat or cholesterol intake per capita (based on food disappearance data of the Food and Agriculture Organization) (Fig. 3) [20]. Most international and many national subgroup correlative studies agree with these observations. However, in case-controlled and cohort studies the relationship is not so clear. Seven of 11 case-control studies showed a significant positive correlation between fat or meat intake and colorectal carcinoma [21,22]. A notable positive case-control study of 80,000 women in the United States showed a significant correlation between colon cancer risk and high fat intake [23]. Two other recent case-control studies have shown significant associations between fat and meat intake and colorectal carcinoma [24••] or adenomatous polyps [25•,26••], and between colorectal carcinoma and egg (cholesterol) consumption [27••,28••]. However, none of seven cohort studies were able to show a positive correlation between meat or fat intake and colorectal cancer. In fact, two cohort studies found an inverse relationship [21,22]). Some have argued that different fats may pose variable risks with some forms even being protective [29,30••]. Unfortunately, most studies have made no attempt to dissect forms of fat in their analysis.

Several studies have shown a surprising inverse relationship between serum cholesterol and colorectal carcinoma, particularly in men [31]. A longitudinal analysis

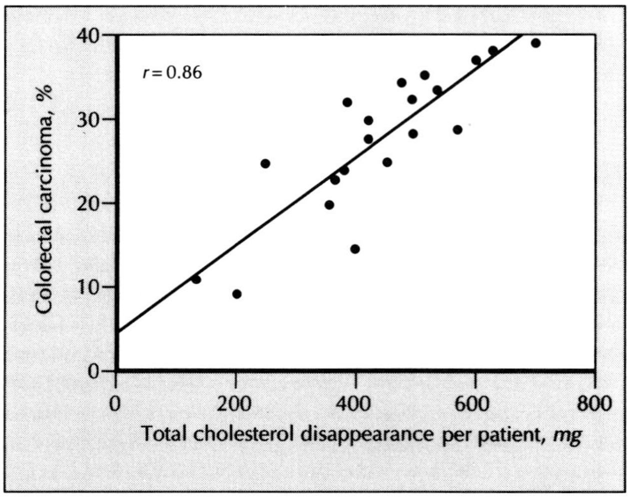

Fig. 3. Correlation between estimates of cholesterol consumption and colorectal carcinoma mortality rates per 100,000 population from 20 industrialized countries ($r=0.86$, $P<0.001$). Cholesterol data (daily cholesterol available for consumption per capita) are from the Food and Agriculture Organization; colorectal cancer mortality data are from the World Health Organization (averaged for years 1967, 1969, 1971, and 1973). (*Data from* Liu *et al.* [20].)

of Framingham Study subjects followed over 40 years showed that those who initially were in the first tertile of serum cholesterol and third tertile of body mass index had a fourfold increased risk of subsequent cancer of the colon but not rectum. This was not seen for women [32••]. A recent cross-sectional study showed a similar relationship between body mass index and risk of "high-risk" colorectal adenomas in men. However, in contrast to these earlier studies, men with adenomas tended to have higher serum cholesterol [33••]. The cholesterol issue is further complicated by a large cohort study from Finland with a 10-year follow-up [34], which showed that men initially in the highest four quintiles of serum cholesterol had an eight- to ninefold higher risk of subsequent development of colorectal carcinoma compared with those in the first quintile. The opposite was true for women. The disparate results of these studies may be explained by differential effects of different serum lipoprotein levels. Colorectal adenomas have been shown to be inversely related to high-density lipoprotein cholesterol and positively correlated to very low density lipoprotein and low-density lipoprotein cholesterol levels in a cross-sectional German study [35••].

Dietary fiber

Fiber is broadly defined as plant cellular material resistant to digestion by human beings. It includes, among others, the polysaccharides, *ie*, cellulose, hemicellulose, gums, and pectin; and the nonpolysaccharides, *ie*, lignin. Some are entirely digested by colonic bacteria (pectin) whereas others remain unaltered in the colon (lignin). Properties of fiber include absorption of water leading to increased stool bulk and reduced fecal transit time, absorption of cations, bile acids, and other organic compounds, and alterations in fecal pH, bacterial flora, short-chain fatty acids, and colonocyte proliferative indices [36]. Each type of fiber causes its own physiologic effects.

Investigations of the role of fiber in colorectal carcinoma risk have been plagued by its multiple forms and inability to precisely determine intake [37,38••]. For the most part, as with studies of fat intake, nonanalytical correlative studies have shown a significant relationship between increased fiber intake and reduced colon cancer risk [39]. Pre-1987 analytic case-control studies, with varying assessments of fiber or fiber-containing food intake, failed to show consistent results. In these studies, only vegetable intake seemed to have a reasonably consistent negative association with rate of colon carcinoma (six of nine). However, since 1987, with more standardized measures of fiber, nine of eleven case-control studies have shown significant negative associations between dietary fiber intake and rate of colorectal carcinoma [40••,41••]. Some of these latter studies also suggest that vegetable fiber may have protective effects superior to fruit or cereal fiber. Interestingly, two cohort studies showed protective effects of fruit intake but no specific effect of other dietary fiber [38••].

Dietary calcium

Calcium has been proposed to protect against colorectal carcinoma by binding known animal model promoters of colon carcinoma (bile acids and fatty acids) [42,43,44•]. Calcium is known to inhibit colon epithelial cell proliferation, reduce the cytotoxic potential of fecal water, and protect animals from developing colon tumors following exposure to carcinogens [45••]. A prospective 19-year longitudinal study of 1954 men in the United States found an inverse relationship between dietary calcium intake and colorectal carcinoma [46]. Additional case-controlled studies have shown similar results [24••,47]. In contrast, a prospective study of Japanese men in Hawaii [48] and a case-control study in Italy showed no significant association [49].

Other dietary factors

A number of other dietary factors have been examined including total energy intake, beer, vitamins, other micronutrients, food additives, and method of food preparation. Total caloric intake has been shown to be related to colorectal carcinoma risk [24••,41••]. Excessive beer drinking has been associated with a relative risk of 1.7 for rectal carcinoma in a cohort [50] and case-control study [51]. Neither study showed any relationship between beer drinking and colon carcinoma, al-

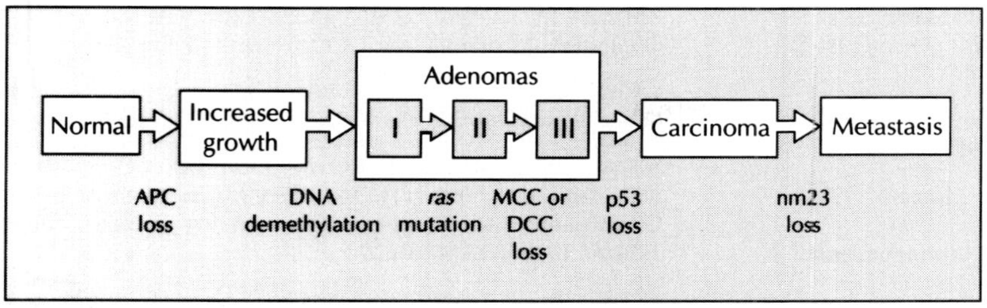

Fig. 4. Correlation between stages of stepwise progression of colorectal carcinoma and recognized mutational events affecting specific colon cancer–associated genes. Although a preferred sequence of mutational events is apparent, the accumulation of mutations is more important than the order in which they occur. APC—adenomatous polyposis coli tumor suppressor gene; DDC—deleted in colon cancer tumor suppressor gene; MCC—mutated in colon cancer tumor suppressor gene; nm23—nm23 metastasis suppressor gene; p53—p53 tumor suppressor gene; ras—Ki-*ras* oncogene. (*Adapted from* Vogelstein and Kinzler [56••]; with permission.)

though another study showed an increased risk of rectosigmoid adenomas with high beer consumption [52•]. Coffee has been studied in four cohort and four case-control studies. Only two showed relative risk above unity and four were below unity [53,54]. Historic parallels between the use of nitrate as a food preservative and the appearance of colorectal carcinoma have been observed [13]. Heavily browned fried meat was shown to be a more important determinant of risk than meat intake alone in a Swedish case-control study [55].

Etiologic considerations

According to present thinking, colorectal carcinoma results from mutational alteration of two or more genes important in the regulation of cell proliferation, differentiation, or programmed cell death (tumor suppressor genes and protooncogenes). Genetic abnormalities seem to follow a stepwise progression along the polyp-carcinoma sequence [56••] (Fig. 4). In inherited forms of colorectal carcinoma, the first mutation is already present through germ-line inheritance. In sporadic carcinoma, the mutations occur through environmental influences, related to carcinogens in the setting of mutational susceptibility (*ie*, during DNA synthesis and mitosis). Exogenous influences that combine to induce proliferation and damage DNA set the stage for the development of carcinoma.

What are the hypothesized mechanisms of action of dietary components on colorectal cancer risk? It can be assumed that risk components of diet facilitate mutational events whereas protective components inhibit or reverse these events [57••]. High dietary fats have been shown to increase intraluminal bile acids in animals. Certain fats and bile acids are cytotoxic, genotoxic, capable of stimulating colonocyte proliferation, can affect metabolism of carcinogens, and are known promoters of carcinogen-induced tumors in animals [58–60]. In humans, colorectal neoplasias are associated with increased fecal and serum concentrations of bile acids known to act as tumor promoters [61•]. Perhaps the observed inverse relationship between serum cholesterol and colon carcinoma is related to increased fecal bile acids. Heavily browned meats may increase the colonic load of carcinogenic heterocyclic amines [55]. Low fiber increases colonic transit time and prolongs exposure to intraluminal carcinogens whereas high fiber reduces transit time, dilutes carcinogens, binds bile acids, and alters the metabolism of bile acids known to promote carcinogen-induced colon cancer in animals [62•]. Calcium also binds and precipitates bile acids and luminal fats, and has been shown to reverse the cancer-promoting effects of bile acids. Finally, certain vegetables are rich in antioxidants and anticancer micronutrients that may directly counteract endogenous carcinogens.

Conclusions

In summary, there is no shortage of rationale to explain how suspected risk factors in the diet may influence the risk for colon cancer. However, we are still a long way from defining which of these, if any, are playing a critical role. The elements of Western diet that might be important in causing colon cancer may be the same elements that have reduced our risk of gastric carcinoma. Before any nutritional guidelines can be established, these possibilities must be adequately considered and tested in long-term, controlled, interventional studies.

Acknowledgments

The author wishes to thank Maureen Craft for her secretarial assistance and acknowledges funding support from the Mayo Foundation and grant number CA01674-02 from the National Cancer Institute. The contents of this manuscript are solely the responsibility of the author and do not necessarily represent the official views of the National Cancer Institute.

References and recommended reading

Papers of particular interest, published within the annual period of review, have been highlighted as:

- • Of special interest
- •• Of outstanding interest

1. Boring CC, Squires TS, Tong T: **Cancer Statistics, 1993.**
• *CA Cancer J Clin* 1993, 43:7–26.
A statistical tabulation of cancer incidence, mortality, and trends throughout the world.

2. Ziegler RG, Devesa SS, Fraumeni JF Jr: **Epidemiologic Patterns of Colorectal Cancer**. *Important Adv Oncol* 1986 :209–232.

3. Weisburger JH: **Causes, Relevant Mechanisms, and Prevention of Large Bowel Cancer**. *Semin Oncol* 1991, **18**:316–336.

4. Greenwald P: **Colon Cancer Overview**. *Cancer* 1992,
•• **70**:1206–1215.
A concise review covering epidemiology, prevention, screening, and treatment strategies for colorectal carcinoma.

5. Devesa SS, Chow WH: **Variation in Colorectal Cancer Incidence in the United States by Subsite of Origin**. *Cancer* 1993, **71**:3819–3826.

6. Delattre O, Olschwang S, Law DJ, Melot T, Remvikos Y, Salmon RJ, Sastre X, Validire P, Feinberg AP, Thomas G: **Multiple Genetic Alterations in Distal and Proximal Colorectal Cancer**. *Lancet* 1989, **ii**:353–356.

7. Howell MA: **The Association Between Colorectal Cancer and Breast Cancer**. *J Chronic Dis* 1976, **29**:243–261.

8. Henderson BE: **Summary Report of the Sixth Symposium on Cancer Registries and Epidemiology in the Pacific Basin**. *J Natl Cancer Inst* 1990, **82**:1186–1190.

9. McMichael AJ, McCall MG, Hartshorne JM, Woodings TL.: **Patterns of Gastrointestinal Cancer in European Migrants to Australia: The Role of Dietary Change**. *Int J Cancer* 1980, **25**:431–437.

10. Snowdon DA: **Animal Product Consumption and Mortality Because of All Causes Combined, Coronary Heart Disease, Stroke, Diabetes, and Cancer in Seventh-Day Adventists**. *Am J Clin Nutr* 1988, **48**:739–748.

11. Slattery ML, West DW, Robison LM, French TK, Ford MH, Schuman KL, Sorenson AW: **Tobacco, Alcohol, Coffee, and Caffeine as Risk Factors for Colon Cancer in a Low Risk Population**. *Epidemiology* 1990, **1**:141–145.

12. Thomas DB, Karagas MR: **Cancer in First and Second Generation Americans**. *Cancer Res* 1987, **47**:5771–5776.

13. Lauer K: **The History of Nitrite in Human Nutrition: A Contribution From German Cookery Books**. *J Clin Epidemiol* 1991, **44**:261–264.

14. Weisburger JH, Wynder EL: **Etiology of Colorectal Cancer With Emphasis on Mechanisms of Action and Prevention**. In *Important Advances in Oncology.* Edited by DeVita VTJ, Hellman S, Rosenberg SA. Philadelphia: JB Lippincott; 1987:197–220.

15. Armstrong B, Doll R: **Environmental Factors and Cancer Incidence and Mortality in Different Countries With Special Reference to Dietary Practices**. *Int J Cancer* 1977, **15**:617–631.

16. Burkitt DP: **Epidemiology of Cancer of the Colon and Rectum**. *Cancer* 1971, **28**:3–13.

17. **Diet, Nutrition and Cancer**. Washington: National Academy Press; 1982.

18. Willett W: **The Search for the Cause of Breast and Colon Cancer**. *Nature* 1989, **338**:389–394.

19. **Report of the Council on Scientific Affairs. Diet and Cancer:**
•• **Where Do Matters Stand?** *Arch Intern Med* 1993, **153**:50–56.
An up-to-date opinion of the role of diet in cancer risk. Specific forms of cancer are not discussed but the nature of the controversy as it relates to the complexity of dietary, biochemical, and molecular biological interactions is considered.

20. Liu K, Stamler J, Moss D, Garside D, Persky V, Soltero I: **Dietary Cholesterol, Fat, and Fiber, and Colon-Cancer Mortality: An Analysis of International Data**. *Lancet* 1979, **2**:782

21. Kolonel L: **Fat and Colon Cancer: How Firm Is the Epidemiologic Evidence?** *Am J Clin Nutr* 1987, **45**:336–341.

22. Vogel VG, McPherson RS: **Dietary Epidemiology of Colon Cancer**. *Hematol Oncol Clin North Am* 1989, **3**:35–63.

23. Willett WC, Stampfer MJ, Colditz GA, Rosner BA, Speizer FE: **Relation of Meat, Fat, and Fiber Intake to the Risk of Colon Cancer in a Prospective Study Among Women**. *N Engl J Med* 1990, **323**:1664–1672.

24. Peters RK, Pike MC, Garabrant D, Mack TM: **Diet and**
•• **Colon Cancer in Los Angeles County, California**. *Cancer Causes Control* 1992, **3**:457–473.
This is a report of a large case-control study of dietary factors on colon cancer risk involving 746 cancer patients and 746 controls. Control subjects were selected from the same neighborhood and matched for age, sex, race, and birth country. The study design analyzed multiple dietary components by a detailed questionnaire. The important findings were a positive risk assignment to total caloric intake and a negative risk assignment for calcium intake.

25. Kono S, Imanishi K, Shinchi K, Yanai F: **Relationship of**
• **Diet to Small and Large Adenomas of the Sigmoid Colon**. *Jpn J Cancer Res* 1993, **84**:13–19.
A case control study of dietary influences on sigmoid adenomatous polyps in Japanese men. Control subjects were selected from those with normal colonoscopy results. Dietary habits were ascertained by questionnaire prior to colonoscopy. Significant findings included a positive relationship with meat intake and a negative relationship with rice consumption.

26. Neugut AI, Garbowski GC, Lee WC, Murray T, Nieves JW,
•• Forde KA, Treat MR, Waye JD, Fenoglio-Preiser C: **Dietary Risk Factors for the Incidence and Recurrence of Colorectal Adenomatous Polyps**. *Ann Intern Med* 1993, **118**:91–95.
A case-control study of multiple dietary influences on the incidence and recurrence rates of adenomatous polyps. For both incident and recurrent polyps, consistent significant associations were only seen in women. Near significant positive odds ratios were seen for saturated fats and red meat to chicken ratios for incident polyps. A significant protective effect was seen with vitamin A for incident polyps. Dietary fiber was not protective for incident polyps but was significantly protective against recurrent polyps in women.

27. Steinmetz KA, Potter JD: **Food-Group Consumption and**
•• **Colon Cancer in the Adelaide Case-control Study. II. Meat, Poultry, Seafood, Dairy Foods and Eggs**. *Int J Cancer* 1993, **53**:720–727.
A case-control study of dietary factors and risk for colon carcinoma involving 220 patients with colon carcinoma and 438 age- and gender-matched control subjects identified randomly from the electoral roll. All completed detailed dietary questionnaires. The most impressive finding was a significant association between egg consumption and colon cancer in women, especially for proximal colon cancers.

28. Iscovich JM, Labbe KA, Castelleto R, Calzona A, Bernedo
•• A, Chopita NA, Jmelnitzsky AC, Kaldor J: **Colon Cancer in Argentina. I: Risk From Intake of Dietary Items**. *Int J Cancer* 1992, **51**:851–857.
This study analyzed meat, vegetable, and dairy product consumption. The significant findings were a positive association with egg consumption and a dose-related negative association with vegetable, fish, and poultry intake.

29. Kromhout D: **The Importance of N-6 and N-3 Fatty Acids in Carcinogenesis**. *Med Oncol Tumor Pharmacother* 1990, **7**:173–176.

30. Reddy BS: **Dietary Fat and Colon Cancer: Animal Model**
•• **Studies**. *Lipids* 1992, **27**:807–813.
A comprehensive review of the role of different forms of fat in carcinogen-induced colon cancer in animal models. Data are presented implicating high concentration of vegetable and animal fats as promoters of colon cancer, whereas coconut oil, fish oil, and trans-fatty acids do not promote colon carcinogenesis.

31. BROITMAN SA: **Dietary Cholesterol, Serum Cholesterol, and Colon Cancer: A Review.** *Adv Exp Med Biol* 1986, **206P137-52.**:137–152.

32. KREGER BE, ANDERSON KM, SCHATZKIN A, SPLANSKY GL: **Serum Cholesterol Level, Body Mass Index, and the Risk of Colon Cancer: The Framingham Study.** *Cancer* 1992, **70**:1038–1043.
•• This study examines the relationship between serum cholesterol and body mass index in members of the longitudinal Framingham Study. Serum cholesterol was inversely related to subsequent development of colorectal carcinoma in men. Body mass index was positively correlated. Together, these two factors produced a 4.5-fold increase in the risk of colorectal carcinoma.

33. BAYERDORFFER E, MANNES GA, OCHSENKUHN T, KOPCKE W, WIEBECKE B, PAUMGARTNER G: **Increased Risk of 'High Risk' Colorectal Adenomas in Overweight Men.**. Gastroenterology 1993, **104**:137–144.
•• A large cross-sectional study designed to determine the relationship between obesity and high- and low-risk adenomas (determined by size and histology). Men with high risk adenomas were significantly more obese and tended to have higher cholesterol levels.

34. KNEKT P, REUNANEN A, AROMAA A, HELIOVAARA M, HAKULINEN T, HAKAMA M: **Serum Cholesterol and Risk of Cancer in a Cohort of 39,000 Men and Women.** *J Clin Epidemiol* 1988, **41**:519–530.

35. BAYERDORFFER E, MANNES GA, WERNER OR, OCHSENKUHN T, SEEHOLZER G, KOPCKE W, WIEBECKE B, PAUMGARTNER G: **Decreased High-Density Lipoprotein Cholesterol and Increased Low-Density Cholesterol Levels in Patients with Colorectal Adenomas.** *Ann Intern Med* 1993, **118**:481–487.
•• This cross-sectional study involving 822 of 1124 consecutive patients undergoing colonoscopy examined the influence of cholesterol profiles on risk of adenomatous polyps. Patients with adenomas were found to have significantly lower high-density lipoprotein and higher low-density lipoprotein and very low density lipoprotein levels compared with those without adenomas.

36. KLURFELD DM: **Dietary Fiber-Mediated Mechanisms in Carcinogenesis.** *Cancer Res* 1992, **52(Suppl)**:2055s–2059s.

37. KLURFELD DM, KRITCHEVSKY D: **Dietary Fiber and Human Cancer: Critique of the Literature.** *Adv Exp Med Biol* 1986, **206**:119–135.

38. AUSMAN LM: **Fiber and Colon Cancer: Does the Current Evidence Justify a Preventive Policy?** *Nutr Rev* 1993, **51**:57–63.
•• An up-to-date review of epidemiological studies examining the role of dietary fiber in colorectal carcinoma and its impact on national policy. The various forms of fiber, their characteristics, and their content in different foods is summarized. The author concludes that the data to date are inconclusive and should not yet drive national policy.

39. TROCK BJ, LANZA E, GREENWALD P: **High Fiber Diet and Colon Cancer: A Critical Review.** *Prog Clin Biol Res* 1990, **346**:145–157.

40. BOLAND CR, KOLARS JC: **Fiber and Colon Cancer: The Weight of the Evidence [Editorial].** *Gastroenterology* 1992, **103**:1964–1967.
•• A particularly thoughtful and scholarly editorial that reviews the issue of fiber as a protective factor in colorectal carcinoma from the perspective of the cancer biology.

41. ISCOVICH JM, LABBE KA, CASTELLETO R, CALZONA A, BERNEDO A, CHOPITA NA, JMELNITZSKY AC, KALDOR J, HOWE GR: **Colon Cancer in Argentina. II: Risk From Fibre, Fat and Nutrients.** *Int J Cancer* 1992, **51**:858–861.
••

42. WELBERG JW, KLEIBEUKER JH, VAN DER MEER R, MULDER NH, DE VRIES EG: **Calcium and the Prevention of Colon Cancer.** *Scand J Gastroenterol Suppl* 1991, **188**:52–59.

43. WARGOVICH MJ, LYNCH PM, LEVIN B: **Modulating Effects of Calcium in Animal Models of Colon Carcinogenesis and Short-Term Studies in Subjects at Increased Risk for Colon Cancer.** *Am J Clin Nutr* 1991, **54**:202s–205s.

44. NEWMARK HL, LIPKIN M: **Calcium, Vitamin D, and Colon Cancer.** *Cancer Res* 1992, **52**:2067s–2070s.
• The proposed protective effects of calcium for colorectal carcinoma development are supported on several fronts including at the cellular level, carcinogen-induced colon cancers in animals, and human epidemiological studies. Proposed mechanisms of action are covered in detail.

45. LAPRE JA, DE VRIES HT, KOEMAN JH, VAN DER MEER R: **The Antiproliferative Effect of Dietary Calcium on Colonic Epithelium Is Mediated by Luminal Surfactants and Dependent on the Type of Dietary Fat.** *Cancer Res* 1993, **53**:784–789.
•• This paper describes experiments in animals designed to analyze dietary effects of high calcium and high fat on various fecal constituents (fatty acids and bile acids), epitheliolysis, colonocyte proliferation, and cytolytic activity of stool water. The key observation was that the antiproliferative effects of dietary calcium seemed to be mediated by its ability to precipitate intraluminal surfactants.

46. GARLAND C, BARRETT-CONNER E, ROSSOF AH, SHEKELLE RB, CRIGUI MH, PAUL O: **Dietary Vitamin D and Calcium and Risk of Colorectal Cancer: A 19-Year Prospective Study in Men.** *Lancet* 1985, **i**:307–309.

47. SORENSON AW, SLATTERY ML, FORD MH: **Calcium and Colon Cancer: A Review.** *Nutr Cancer* 1988, **11**:135–145.

48. HEILBRUN LK, HANKIN JH, NOMURA AMY, STEMMERMANN GN: **Colon Cancer and Dietary Fat, Phosphorus, and Calcium in Hawaiian-Japanese Men.** *Am J Clin Nutr* 1986, **43**:306–309.

49. NEGRI E, LA VECCHIA C, D'AVANZO B, FRANCESCHI S: **Calcium, Dairy Products, and Colorectal Cancer.** *Nutr Cancer* 1990, **13**:255–262.

50. CARSTENSEN JM, BYGREN LO, HATSCHEK T: **Cancer Incidence Among Swedish Brewery Workers.** *Int J Cancer* 1990, **45**:393–396.

51. RIBOLI E, CORNEE J, MACQUART MOULIN G, KAAKS R, CASAGRANDE C, GUYADER M: **Cancer and Polyps of the Colorectum and Lifetime Consumption of Beer and Other Alcoholic Beverages.** *Am J Epidemiol* 1991, **134**:157–166.

52. SANDLER RS, LYLES CM, MCAULIFFE C, WOOSLEY JT, KUPPER LL: **Cigarette Smoking, Alcohol, and the Risk of Colorectal Adenomas.** *Gastroenterology* 1993, **104**:1445–1451.
• A case-control study of 236 patients with colorectal adenomas. Beer drinking was shown to be a significant risk factor for adenomatous polyps, reaching fourfold between the highest and lowest quartiles.

53. LA VECCHIA C: **Epidemiological Evidence on Coffee and Digestive Tract Cancers: A Review.** *Dig Dis Sci* 1990, **8**:281–286.

54. ROSENBERG L: **Coffee and Tea Consumption in Relation to the Risk of Large Bowel Cancer: A Review of Epidemiologic Studies.** *Cancer Lett* 1990, **52**:163–171.

55. GERHARDSSON DE VERDIER M, HAGMAN U, PETERS RK, STEINECK G, OVERVIK E: **Meat, Cooking Methods and Colorectal Cancer: A Case-Referent Study in Stockholm.** *Int J Cancer* 1991, **49**:520–525.

56. VOGELSTEIN B, KINZLER KW: **the Multistep Nature of Cancer.** *Trends Genet* 1993, **9**:138–141.
•• This is the most recent of several nice reviews describing the mutational events that occur during the stepwise progression of colorectal carcinoma.

57. POTTER JD: **Reconciling the Epidemiology, Physiology, and Molecular Biology of Colon Cancer.** *JAMA* 1992, **268**:1573–1577.
•• A scholarly review of epidemiologic data as they relate to known biologic forces behind colon carcinogenesis.

58. KANDELL RL, BERNSTEIN C: **Bile Salt/Acid Induction of DNA Damage in Bacterial and Mammalian Cells: Implications for Colon Cancer.** *Nutr Cancer* 1991, **16**:227–238.

59. McMichael AJ, Potter JD: **Host Factors in Carcinogenesis: Certain Bile-Acid Metabolic Profiles That Selectively Increase the Risk of Proximal Colon Cancer.** *J Natl Cancer Inst* 1985, 75:185–191.

60. Tempero M: **Bile Acids, Ornithine Decarboxylase, and Cell Proliferation in Colon Cancer: A Review.** *Dig Dis Sci* 1986, 4:49–56.

61. Bayerdorffer E, Mannes GA, Richter WO, Ochsenkuhn T,
• Wiebecke B, Kopcke W, Paumgartner G: **Increased Serum Deoxycholic Acid Levels in Men with Colorectal Adenomas..** *Gastroenterology* 1993, **104**:145–151.

A small case-control study examining serum bile acids in men and women with and without colorectal adenomas. The level of deoxycholic acid was significantly higher in those with adenomas; this was most marked in men.

62. Korpela JT, Korpela R, Adlercreutz H: **Fecal Bile Acid**
• **Metabolic Pattern After Administration of Different Types of Bread.** *Gastroenterology* 1992, **103**:1246–1253.

The effects of different types of bread on fecal bile salt composition was studied in 12 Finnish women. Whole grain rye bread was shown to significantly reduce free lithocholic and deoxycholic acid in the stool by affecting the way they are conjugated. Both of these bile acids are known promoters of carcinogen-induced colon cancer in animals and some evidence suggests that their concentration in human stools may be markers of colon cancer risk.

William E. Karnes, Jr, MD, Center for Basic Research in Digestive Diseases, Mayo Clinic, 200 First Street, SW, Rochester, MN 55905, USA.

Diagnosis and screening of colorectal neoplasia

Mark V. Larson, MD, and Douglas B. McGill, MD

Mayo Clinic, Rochester, Minnesota, USA

Significant advances were made this past year in our understanding of the molecular genetics and pathogenesis of colorectal cancer. Direct applications of this information are being implemented into clinical practice. Divergent reports over the effectiveness of fecal occult blood testing have failed to clarify screening recommendations. As the emphasis on cost-effective screening for colorectal cancer increases, the future appears to lie in determining individual susceptibility with the use of genetic markers and the adjustment of screening recommendations accordingly.

Current Opinion in Gastroenterology 1994, **10**:27–33

The impact of colorectal cancer on the health care resources of the United States is staggering. About 5% of the American population will develop colon cancer that will prove fatal in about half of the cases. The molecular biology and genetics of colon cancer are being unraveled; scientists have determined the locations and sequences of genetic mutations that occur during the metamorphosis of cells from premalignancy to the cancerous stage. The populations at greatest risk of developing colon cancer are being identified and, in some situations, these can be disclosed by genetic tests that can be performed on the serum. Also, we more clearly understand the unique benefits and limitations of each screening and surveillance modality.

The vast majority of colorectal neoplasms are adenomas and carcinomas. The focus of this review will be on these lesions. It is important to keep in mind that other types of neoplasms can develop in the colon and can present with bleeding, abdominal pain, or a change in bowel habits in a fashion similar to adenocarcinomas, as recent reports on primary colonic lymphomas [1], histiocytomas [2], or even carcinoid tumors [3] indicate.

Diagnostic modalities

Patients in whom a colorectal neoplasm is suspected should have the entire colorectum examined either by colonoscopy or barium enema and proctosigmoidoscopy, in order to identify the primary site of disease and the presence of synchronous lesions. Whereas colonoscopy is considered more sensitive for the detection of smaller (<7 mm) neoplasia, a carefully performed barium enema is equally sensitive for detecting larger (>10 mm) polypoid lesions [4]. There is growing acceptance of double-contrast barium enemas over single-contrast barium enemas, as the former is more sensitive for detecting neoplasia and also adequately examines the rectum, which cannot be examined readily by the single-contrast technique [5]. Colonoscopic findings were compared with resected colon specimens and agreed with the pathologic findings 96% of the time for larger polyps (≥10 mm); when all polyps were included, colonoscopy detected only 89% [6]. This represents the true sensitivity of colonoscopy, and underscores the fact that colonoscopy is not the perfect "gold standard," as is often suggested when other imaging techniques are reviewed.

Abdominal imaging, including ultrasound, computed tomography, or magnetic resonance imaging, is useful in the demonstration of advanced disease such as hepatic metastases, is less useful for detecting extracolonic spread, and is not effective in primary detection. On the other hand, rectal ultrasonography has emerged as the most accurate method of staging rectal cancer, being superior to computed tomography and magnetic resonance imaging for the assessment of the extent of tumor invasion and lymph node involvement [7].

Hydrocolonic ultrasonography is a new technique that involves retrograde instillation of water into the colon before sonography [8]. In a prospective study, 300 consecutive patients with colorectal symptoms underwent hydrocolonic sonography followed by colonoscopy. A total of 28 of 29 (97%) colonoscopically verified carcinomas were detected by hydrocolonic sonography and specificity was 100%. In addition, 38 of 42 (91%) polyps greater than or equal to 7 mm in di-

Abbreviations

FAP—familial adenomatous polyposis; **FOBT**—fecal occult blood test; **HFAS**—hereditary flat adenoma syndrome; **HNPCC**—hereditary nonpolyposis colorectal cancer.

 ISBN 1-85922-606-X ISSN 0267–1379

ameter were detected by hydrocolonic sonography. The technique permits determination of the depth of tumor infiltration into the colonic wall, and in 82% of carcinomas, the T stage was correctly diagnosed. Whereas hydrocolonic ultrasonography will not supplant colonoscopy, its greatest application may be as a screening procedure, as it is well tolerated, noninvasive, and relatively inexpensive.

Immunoscintigraphy targets tumor sites with radiolabeled antibodies reactive with tumor-associated antigens. Multiple monoclonal antibodies have been used in cancer imaging, including those reactive with carcinoembryonic antigen and TAG-72, a glycoprotein expressed by most adenocarcinomas [9]. Recent reports confirm that immunoscintigraphy is more sensitive than computed tomography or magnetic resonance imaging for identification of extrahepatic sites of recurrent or metastatic colorectal cancer, whereas intrahepatic disease is better detected with computerized tomography [10,11]. Collier *et al.* [11] found that immunoscintigraphy detected only 41% of liver metastases (≥ 2 cm), whereas the sensitivity of computed tomography was 84% ($P < 0.001$). Unfortunately, it does not reliably identify early, primary cancers, and therefore, the principal role of immunoscintigraphy would be in postsurgical cancer surveillance.

Biologic markers or precursors of colorectal carcinoma

It is well accepted that carcinoembryonic antigen is not sensitive for use as a screening tool, but it has been widely, indeed routinely, used for detection of recurrence after colorectal cancer surgery. However, Moertel *et al.* [12••] report that even for this application, carcinoembryonic antigen monitoring is insensitive, lacks specificity, and has little impact on the cure rate with recurrent cancer. At this time, a more sensitive tumor marker is not imminent. CA-19-9, CA-50, and CA-195 were compared with carcinoembryonic antigen, and the diagnostic values of the new tumor markers were poorer than carcinoembryonic antigen for making a primary diagnosis of colorectal cancer [13].

Rectal mucosal ornithine decarboxylase activity has been reported to distinguish between patients with and patients without adenomatous polyps; however, the overlap in ornithine decarboxylase activity values is broad, suggesting limited usefulness [14]. In contrast, individuals with a family history of colorectal cancer demonstrated a significant difference in rectal mucosal proliferation assessed by the crypt cell production rate method when compared with a control population [15]. O'Brien *et al.* [16] reviewed a current list of putative biologic markers in colorectal mucosa of patients at risk, including abnormal cell proliferation (as determined by ornithine decarboxylase activity), alterations of mucin synthesis, and blood group and related carbohydrate antigen expression. The author concluded that the potential clinical applications for these and other biologic markers are still evolving.

Fecal markers have generally been reported to be unreliable for predicting the presence of large-bowel neoplasms [17]. Fecal occult blood has been reviewed previously in this journal, and its limitations will be discussed later in this review. Patients with colorectal cancers containing *ras* oncogene mutations frequently shed tumor material that contains *ras* oncogene mutations that can be detected in fecal material [18]. Calprotectin, a prominent neutrophil leukocyte protein that can be assessed in small spot samples of stools, was reported to be a highly sensitive marker of colorectal neoplasia [19]. A sum of 31 of 32 patients with colorectal cancer and 18 of 22 patients with colorectal neoplastic polyps had an elevated calprotectin level (sensitivity of 97% and 82%, respectively). Only one of 33 (3%) healthy controls had an elevated value, suggesting that calprotectin is also quite specific for colorectal neoplasia.

The issue of the association of hyperplastic rectosigmoid polyps with proximal colonic neoplasms is slowly being laid to rest; yet another report [20] failed to identify an increased prevalence of proximal neoplasms in patients with rectosigmoid hyperplastic polyps, while confirming the association between distal adenomatous polyps and proximal neoplasms. This further supports the recommendation that the finding of a distal adenoma but not a distal hyperplastic polyp warrants proceeding with full colonoscopy.

Inflammatory bowel disease

Chronic, extensive ulcerative colitis is well established as a predisposing condition for the development of colorectal adenocarcinoma. The risk of cancer may be equivalent in patients with Crohn's disease, given similar duration of disease and anatomic extent [21]. Although there are limitations in the use of epithelial dysplasia as a premalignant histologic marker, periodic surveillance colonoscopy with biopsies to detect dysplasia or early curable cancer is still widely recommended for managing patients with long-standing colitis [22]. The critical question of whether or not colonoscopic surveillance for dysplasia is a cost-effective practice for reducing cancer mortality in inflammatory bowel disease has remained controversial. However, Choi *et al.* [23•] provided convincing evidence that a surveillance program may reduce cancer mortality. In their study of 41 patients who developed carcinoma associated with ulcerative colitis, carcinoma was detected at a significantly earlier Duke's stage in the surveillance group. The 5-year survival rate was 77.2% in 19 patients who were under colonoscopic surveillance, and was 36.3% in 22 patients who were not ($P = 0.026$).

Aneuploidy is a quantitative alteration in the DNA content of cell nuclei that reflects genomic instability. Rubin *et al.* [24•] demonstrated that DNA aneuploidy is present in colonic mucosal biopsies in a minority of patients with chronic extensive ulcerative colitis, and that it was predictive of future development of dysplasia in patients without dysplasia initially. Thus, aneuploidy identifies a subset of ulcerative colitis patients who are more likely to develop dysplasia and perhaps more likely to require rigorous colonoscopic surveillance.

The p53 tumor suppressor gene is considered a pivotal influence on cell proliferation. The loss of a normal p53 allele in the presence of mutations within the remaining allele was previously demonstrated in sporadic colon carcinomas and has now been detected in patients with ulcerative colitis [25]. However, loss of a p53 allele appears to occur earlier in the histologic progression of neoplasia in ulcerative colitis than in sporadic colon cancer and was also found more often with more advanced degrees of dysplasia. Whereas the nondysplastic mucosa in sporadic colon cancer has not been shown to contain abnormalities at the p53 locus, nondysplastic mucosa in ulcerative colitis was found to be frequently aneuploid in DNA content and also contained clones of cells with p53 loss of heterozygosity [25]. The authors concluded from these observations that the pathogenesis of sporadic and ulcerative colitis–associated colorectal carcinomas differ in significant ways.

Inherited susceptibility

The genetic diagnosis of familial adenomatous polyposis (FAP) became possible with the localization of the FAP gene to chromosome 5, followed by isolation of the gene itself. Improved DNA markers linked to the FAP gene showed that a genetic diagnosis is now possible in 95% of individuals, with a predicted accuracy of greater than 98% [26,27]. These new markers now provide a level of efficacy appropriate for clinical testing.

Muto *et al.* [28] first described the flat adenoma, a minimally elevated colonic lesion with adenomatous tubules that spread laterally, resulting in flat rather than polypoid growth. Flat adenomas have a greater incidence of high-grade dysplasia than ordinary tubular adenomas of similar size, leading to speculation that it may be a higher risk precursor. Lynch *et al.* [29•] have described the clinical features of the hereditary flat adenoma syndrome (HFAS), which appears to be a hereditary colorectal cancer–prone disorder whose features are closer to FAP than to hereditary nonpolyposis colorectal cancer (HNPCC), although not typical of either. HFAS is similar to FAP in that both feature colonic adenomas have a high lifetime risk for colorectal cancer, and are linked to the same chromosome, 5q [30]. HFAS differs from FAP in that the colonic adenomas in HFAS are significantly fewer in number, are usually found in the right colon, and have distinctive endoscopic and histologic features as above. The colorectal cancers in this disorder have a later age of onset (average 55 years) than that associated with FAP and the HNPCC. Given its linkage to the FAP locus and the phenotypic parallels between HFAS and FAP, Spirio [30] concluded that HFAS is a variant of FAP.

One of the most exciting developments in human genetics in the past year provides further insight into the pathogenesis of familial colorectal cancer. In a cooperative effort, Aaltonen *et al.* [31••] examined numerous DNA markers in "familial" colon cancer such as the p53, K-*ras*, and FAP genes, and compared them with those of sporadic colon cancers. However, these studies were unrewarding. Unexpectedly, they identified "microsatellite DNA," which are short, repetitive DNA sequences that are interspersed throughout the genome, on chromosome 2 in the majority of patients with familial colon cancer. Whereas the few other genes linked to hereditary cancer susceptibility, including the FAP gene, are classic tumor suppressor genes, a totally different kind of abnormality was found in the region identified on chromosome 2. The microsatellite DNA at the chromosome 2 marker site varied from tumor to tumor, and there were similar changes in microsatellite DNA at several other chromosome sites in most of the familial cancers (11 of 14 cancers examined). Similar abnormalities were then identified in 13% (six of 46) of sporadic colon cancers. Other investigators almost simultaneously discovered a high degree of microsatellite DNA variation in a similar percentage (14%, 13 of 90) of sporadic colon cancers [32]. The authors concluded that there appears to have been an event in a single gene that causes mutations throughout the genome. They felt that they had identified a colon cancer "susceptibility gene" on chromosome 2, at least for familial cancer, and perhaps for some apparently sporadic colon cancers as well. This finding may help us not only in better understanding familial colorectal cancer, but in determining which families have a true familial predisposition and which families simply represent chance clustering. This has obvious implications for screening, especially if the gene itself can be isolated.

Screening

Colon cancer is not yet a preventable disease. However, colorectal cancers progress through a series of recognizable steps that eventuate in colorectal cancer. Therefore, secondary prevention, *ie*, early detection and removal of premalignant tumors at early stage cancers, is desirable and should reduce the mortality associated with colorectal cancer.

Increasingly accurate identification of selected populations at greatest risk for the development of colorectal cancer is now possible based on family history and phenotypic expression. It will soon be improved by the use of genetic markers now under development. Accordingly, appropriate screening strategies can now be developed for these subjects, including those with FAP, HNPCC, familial cancer syndromes, and inherited susceptibility to colorectal cancer.

Screening high-risk subjects

Colonoscopy is clearly the best available screening modality, as it can be at once both a diagnostic and therapeutic maneuver. How frequently and when to begin colonoscopic examinations in high-risk subjects is under debate; guidelines have not been validated in prospective, controlled trials. Nonetheless, the literature supports the following recommendations:

> 1) FAP—yearly examinations (flexible proctosigmoidoscopy versus colonoscopy) beginning at the onset of puberty in affected individuals based on positive genetic linkage analysis [33]. The emergence of adenomas can then be monitored and an appropriately timed colectomy planned. In those who test negatively, screening should still be done, but perhaps only every 3 years. Individuals suspected of having hereditary flat adenoma syndrome, a variant of FAP, should also undergo colonoscopic screening examinations, given the proximal colonic location and flat appearance of the adenomas that appear in this syndrome
>
> 2) HNPCC (including site-specific colorectal cancer and cancer family syndrome, *ie*, Lynch syndromes I and II, respectively)—colonoscopy every 1 to 2 years [34], beginning at 20 to 25 years of age. Screening examinations should be performed until age 70 to 75 years, although some advocate lifelong screening
>
> 3) Familial clustering—screening strategies for persons with familial risk should consider the number of affected first degree relatives and the age of tumor diagnosis in an index case. Until testing for the "susceptibility gene" can be applied clinically, interim guidelines recommend that if there are two affected first degree relatives, screening should be by colonoscopy, every 3 to 5 years beginning 5 to 10 years younger than the age of the earliest colon cancer in relatives [35].

The knowledge that nearly all colorectal cancers arise from preexisting adenomas, and from the high rate of synchronous and metachronous polyps, has led most physicians to practice colonoscopic surveillance after polypectomy. Ransohoff *et al.* [36] have questioned the cost effectiveness of colonoscopic surveillance at fixed and regular intervals, especially following the removal of small adenomas. Individuals found to have a tubular adenoma less than 1 cm, discovered during a screening examination, have a very low long-term risk for developing colorectal cancer, even in the absence of ongoing surveillance [37]. Winawer *et al.* [38•] randomly assigned patients to receive postpolypectomy follow-up colonoscopy at 1 and 3 years, or at 3 years only. The percentage of patients with adenomas with advanced pathologic features, *ie*, adenomas greater than 1.0 cm or containing high-grade dysplasia or invasive cancer, was the same (3.3%) in both groups. They concluded that repeat colonoscopy is not needed until 3 years after resection of a first adenomatous polyp, with earlier follow-up reserved for patients with numerous polyps or large, sessile adenomatous polyps.

Average-risk subjects

The appropriate screening schedule of subjects at average risk remains a hotly-debated topic, especially as the cost of medical care soars. The transfer of screening strategies appropriate for high-risk subjects to those at average risk would likely reduce the morbidity and mortality from colorectal cancer, but the cost would be considered prohibitive.

Fecal occult blood tests

Results concerning fecal occult blood tests (FOBT) continue to generate controversy. Sensitivity of four FOBTs (Hemoccult II [SmithKline Diagnostics, San Jose, CA], HemoccultSENSA [SmithKline Diagnostics, San Jose, CA], HemeSelect [SmithKline Diagnostics, San Jose, CA], and HemoQuant [Mayo Medical Laboratories, Rochester, MN, and SmithKline Beecham, Van Nuys, CA]) were compared in 107 patients with colorectal cancer, and in 81 patients with adenomas [39]. All tests were performed under optimal conditions with respect to diet and medications, sample collection, sample rehydration, and testing procedure. Sensitivity for detection of colorectal cancer varied from 71% to 97%, which was highest for HemeSelect, an immunochemical test specific for human hemoglobin. However, all patients had symptomatic colorectal cancers, and many had advanced tumors. Test sensitivity for all adenomas was 31% to 58% and now 42% to 76% for adenomas greater than or equal to 1 cm; again, the positivity rate was highest for HemeSelect. The authors acknowledge that positivity rates were higher than they would be in screening programs, but nonetheless the study provides comparative information regarding FOBTs.

Direct data on FOBT sensitivity for asymptomatic early-stage cancer or large premalignant adenomas, the intended targets of screening, have been sparse. Ahlquist *et al.* [40••] attempted to define the validity of FOBT in the screening setting by comparing yields by Hemoccult and HemoQuant against structural colorectal evaluations in subjects at risk for colorectal neoplasia.

Table 1. Fecal blood test sensitivities for colorectal cancer and polyps based on prospective comparison against structural colorectal studies in the surveillance setting*

	Cases, *n*	Sensitivity, %	
		Hemoccult†	HemoQuant‡§
Cancer¶	46	26	26
Intraluminal recurrence	29	21	24
New primary tumors	18	33	28
Duke's A or B	14	29	29
Polyps**			
≥2.0 cm	10	20	20
1.0–1.9 cm	46	11	8.7
0.5–0.9 cm	107	5.6	5.6
<0.5 cm	223	6.3	2.2
Adenomatous	255	8.6	5.9
Nonneoplastic	118	4.2	1.7

*From Ahlquist *et al.* [40••]; with permission.
†Hemoccult (SmithKline Diagnostics, San Jose, CA).
‡HemoQuant (Mayo Medical Laboratories, Rochester, MN, and SmithKline Beecham, Van Nuys, CA)
§HemoQuant was called positive if at least 2.1 mg of hemoglobin per gram of stool, which matched specificity of Hemoccult.
¶One patient had both new primary and intraluminal recurrences.
**Histologic examination was not available on all polyps.

In 1217 patients undergoing routine structural surveillance evaluations after resection of a colorectal tumor, the sensitivity for cancers was identical at 26% with both HemoQuant and Hemoccult (Table 1). The sensitivity for polyps 1.0 cm or larger was 11% by HemoQuant and was 13% by Hemoccult. Specificity for both Hemoccult and HemoQuant was 95%; however, the positive predictive value for colorectal cancer was only 5.9% for HemoQuant and 4.2% for Hemoccult. The authors believe that the low FOBT sensitivities in this study more accurately represent FOBT performance for the screen detection of colorectal neoplasia than do the much higher detection rates reported from selected groups of symptomatic referred patients.

Whether periodic FOBT reduces the mortality from colorectal cancer is being addressed in five trials with a combined enrollment of 309,000 subjects, some beginning as early as 1975; so far, one has demonstrated a reduction in mortality. Results from most of the studies are not yet reported; Mandel *et al.* [41••] conducted the Minnesota Colon Cancer Control Study, in which 46,551 participants were randomly assigned to be screened for FOB once a year, every 2 years, or not at all. Screening consisted of mailed-in guaiac-impregnated cards (Hemoccult) that were rehydrated with processing. This increases the sensitivity of the test. Participants who tested positively typically underwent a diagnostic evaluation that included colonoscopy. During the 13 years of follow-up, the cumulative incidence of colorectal cancer was virtually identical in the three groups, with 323 cases in both the annual and biennial screened groups, and 356 cases in the control group. However, at 13 years of follow-up, the cumulative annual mortality rate from colorectal cancer was specifically lower in the annually screened group (5.88 per 1000) than in the biennially screened group (8.33 per 1000) and in the control group (8.83 per 1000) (Fig. 1). Winawer [42], in an accompanying editorial, suggested that this is conclusive evidence that FOBT is an effective screening method and recommends its use on an annual basis in asymptomatic people over 50 years old who are at average risk for colorectal cancer.

The issue of rehydration of the hemoccult slides in Mandel *et al.*'s [41••] trial is important. Rehydration increased the sensitivity and resulted in positive tests in 10% of subjects tested and still more in those over 80 years old. Therefore, there were many colonoscopies performed. Specificity was low. The positive predictive value for colorectal cancer fell from 5.6% to 2.2%. The increased use of colonoscopy may have increased the likelihood that nonbleeding cancers in earlier stages were detected by chance in persons who tested positively for other reasons. This could in part explain the significant reduction in the group screened annually and the shift to detection at an earlier stage of cancer.

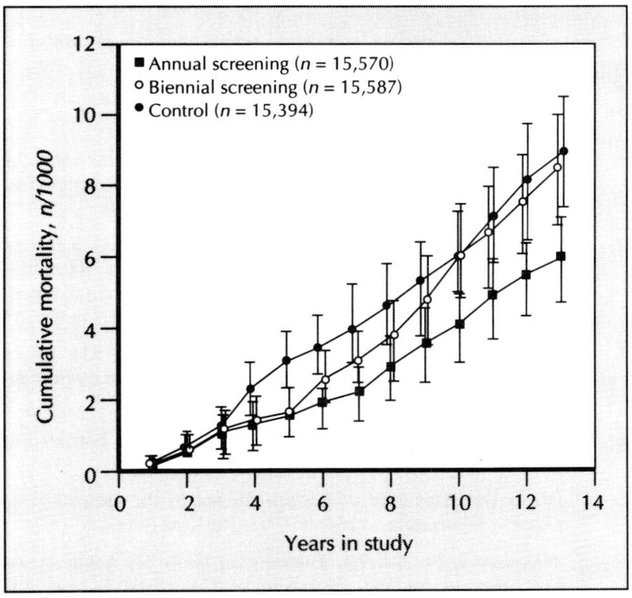

Fig. 1. Cumulative mortality from colorectal cancer, according to study group. *Bars* represent ±2 SE. (*From* Mandel *et al.* [41••]; with permission.)

These two important articles by Ahlquist *et al.* [40••] and Mandel *et al.* [41••], examining different aspects of the problem, draw divergent conclusions about the utility of FOBT for screening asymptomatic patients at average risk for colorectal cancer. By definition, screening tests applicable to the general population must be safe, inexpensive, and sensitive. Many argue that a test with so many false-positives is unacceptable for mass screening. The use of nonrehydrated specimens yields only approximately 2% positives in most studies with corresponding loss of sensitivity.

The only other screening tool test that might qualify for widespread application is flexible proctosigmoidoscopy. Selby *et al.* [43] demonstrated in a case control study that screening sigmoidoscopy can significantly reduce mortality from colorectal cancer arising within 20 cm of the anus. However, the majority of colorectal cancers lie above this region, limiting the usefulness of this procedure. To date, there have been no studies using either endoscopic or radiographic examinations of the more proximal colon that have demonstrated a similar reduction in colorectal cancer–associated mortality.

The most satisfactory and cost-effective approach to mass screening is not yet clear. Until it is, we must continue to apply screening strategies to high-risk groups, as well as emphasize case detection in concerned, asymptomatic individuals. In the latter group, complete structural examination of the colon, such as with a barium enema along with sigmoidoscopy conducted at 3- to 5-year intervals, seems appropriate.

References and recommended reading

Papers of particular interest, published within the annual period of review, have been highlighted as:

- • Of special interest
- •• Of outstanding interest

1. ZIGHELBOIM J, LARSON MV: **Primary Colonic Lymphoma: A Rare, Aggressive Tumor With Only a Marginal Response to Chemotherapy.** *Gastroenterology* 1993, **104**:A466.
2. SANTORO MJ, ABDULIAN JD, CHASE RL, GRIFFIN RA, SOLINGER MR, COLLEN MJ: **Malignant Fibrous Histiocytoma Metastatic to the Colon Presenting as a Lower Gastrointestinal Bleed.** *Am J Gastroenterol* 1992, **87**:1051–1053.
3. JETMORE AB, RAY JE, GATHRIGHT JB, MCMULLEN KM, HICKS TC, TIMMCKE AE: **Rectal Carcinoids—The Most Frequent Carcinoid Tumor.** *Dis Colon Rectum* 1992, **8**:717–725.
4. MCCARTY RL: **Colorectal Cancer: The Case for Barium Enema.** *Mayo Clinic Proc* 1992, **67**:253–257.
5. DODD GD: **The Role of Barium Enema in the Detection of Colonic Neoplasms.** *Cancer* 1992, **70**:1272–1275.
6. WARNEKE J, PETRELLI N, HERRERA L, NAVA H: **Accuracy of Colonoscopy for the Detection of Colorectal Polyps.** *Dis Colon Rectum* 1992, **35**:981–985.
7. HAWES RH: **New Staging Techniques: Endoscopic Ultrasound.** *Cancer* 1993, **71**:4207–4213.
8. LIMBERG B: **Diagnosis and Staging of Colonic Tumors by Conventional Abdominal Sonography as Compared With Hydrocolonic Sonography.** *N Engl J Med* 1992, **327**:65–69.
9. TEMPERO M: **Pitfalls in Antibody Imaging in Colorectal Cancer.** *Cancer* 1993, **71**:4248–4251.
10. GOLDENBERG DM, WLODKOWSKI TJ, SHARKEY RM, SILBERSTEIN EB, SERAFINI AN, GARTY II, VANHEERTUM RL, HIGGINBOTHAM-FORD EA, KOTLER JA, BALASUBRAMANIAN N, SWAYNE LC, HANSEN HJ, PINSKY CM: **Colorectal Cancer Imaging With Iodine-123-Labelled CEA Monoclonal Antibody Fragments.** *J Nucl Med* 1993, **34**:61–70.
11. COLLIER BD, ABDEL-NABI H, DOERR RJ, HARWOOD SJ, OLSEN J, KAPLAN EH, WINZELLBERG GG, GROSSMAN SJ, KRAG DN, MITCHELL EP: **Immunoscintigraphy Performed With IN-111-Labelled CYT-103 in the Management of Colorectal Cancer: Comparison With CT.** *Radiology* 1992, **185**:179–186.
12. •• MOERTEL CG, FLEMING TR, MCDONALD JS, HALLER DG, LAURIE JA, TANGEN C: **An Evaluation of the Carcinoembryonic Antigen (CEA) Test for Monitoring Patients With Resected Colon Cancer.** *JAMA* 1993, **270**:943–947.

A multicenter study that demonstrated that the carcinoembryonic antigen test is an insensitive and nonspecific marker of recurrent colorectal cancer. It ultimately had little impact on the low rate of recurrent cancer and proved to be a very expensive practice strategy, given the cost of the carcinoembryonic antigen test itself and the imaging studies ordered (computed tomography of the abdomen) if the carcinoembryonic antigen level was found to be elevated.

13. VAN DER SCHOUW YT, VERBEEK AL, WOBBES T, SEGERS MF, THOMAS CM: **Comparison of Four Serum Tumor Markers in the Diagnosis of Colorectal Carcinoma.** *Br J Cancer* 1992, **66**:148–154.
14. DESAI TK, PARIKH N, BRONSTEIN JC, LUK GD, BULL AW: **Failure of Rectal Ornithine Decarboxylase to Identify Adenomatous Polyp Status.** *Gastroenterology* 1992, **103**:1562–1567.
15. ROONEY PS, ROBINSON MHE, CLARKE PA, HARDCASTLE JD, ARMITAGE NC: **Individuals With a Strong Family History of Colorectal Cancer Demonstrate Abnormal Rectal Mucosal Proliferation.** *Br J Surg* 1993, **80**:249–251.
16. O'BRIEN MJ, O'KEANE JC, ZAUBER A, GOTTLIEB LS, WINAWER SJ: **Precursors of Colorectal Carcinoma.** *Cancer* 1992, **70**:1317–1327.
17. DUBROW R, YANNIELLI L: **Fecal Protein Markers of Colorectal Cancer.** *Am J Gastroenterol* 1992, **87**:854–858.
18. SIDRANSKY D, TOKINO T, HAMILTON SR, KINZLER KW, LEVIN B, FROST P, VOGELSTEIN B: **Identification Ras Oncogene Mutations in the Stool of Patients With Curable Colorectal Tumors.** *Science* 1992, **256**:102–105.
19. ROSETH AG, CHRISTINSSON J, AADLAND E, SCHJONSBY H, NYGAARD K, FAGERHOL MK: **Calprotectin: A Sensitive Marker of Gastrointestinal Neoplasia.** *Gastroenterology* 1993, **104**:A445.
20. BRADY PG, STRAKER RJ, MCCLAVE SA, NORD HJ, PINKAS M, ROBINSON BE: **Are Hyperplastic Rectosigmoid Polyps Associated With an Increase of Proximal Colonic Neoplasms?** *Gastrointest Endosc* 1993, **39**:481–485.
21. CHOI PM, ZELIG MP: **Similarity of Colorectal Cancer Complicating Crohn's Disease and Ulcerative Colitis.** *Gastroenterology* 1993, **104**:A682.
22. WOOLRICH AJ, DASILVA MD, KORELITZ BI: **Surveillance in the Routine Management of Ulcerative Colitis: The Predictive Value of Low-Grade Dysplasia.** *Gastroenterology* 1992, **103**:431–438.
23. • CHOI PM, NUGENT FW, SCHOETZ DJ, SILVERMAN ML, HAGGITT RC: **Colonoscopic Surveillance Reduces Mortality From Colorectal Cancer in Ulcerative Colitis.** *Gastroenterology* 1993, **105**:418–424.

An important study that sheds light on the issue regarding colonoscopic surveillance in ulcerative colitis. They have demonstrated the bottom line: there is a statistically significant improvement in survival in patients who undergo regular surveillance compared with those who do not.

24. • RUBIN CE, HAGGITT RC, BURMER GC, BRENTNALL TA, STEVENS AC, LEVINE DS, DEAN PJ, KIMMEY M, PERERA DR, RABINOVITCH PS: **DNA Aneuploidy in Colonic Biopsies Predicts the Future Development of Dysplasia in Ulcerative Colitis.** *Gastroenterology* 1992, **103**:1611–1620.

An important article that might have practice implications, in that it may help to identify a small subset of patients who require more frequent surveillance because they are more prone to the future development of dysplasia, and less frequent surveillance than those without aneuploidy. This practice could cost less and could prove more effective in finding curable lesions.

25. Burmer GC, Rabinovitch PS, Haggitt RC, Crispin DA, Brentnall TA, Kolli VR, Stevens AC, Rubin CE: **Neoplastic Progression in Ulcerative Colitis: Histology, DNA Content, and Loss of p53 Allele.** *Gastroenterology* 1992, **103**:1602–1610.

26. Burt RW, Ward K, Spirio L, Groden J, Joslyn G, Leppert M, DiSario J, White RL: **Accurate Identification of Familial Adenomatous Polyposis Coli Using Newly Developed Genetic Markers.** *Gastroenterology* 1992, **102**:347A.

27. Spirio L, Nelson L, Ward K, Burt RW, White R, Leppert M: **A CA Repeat Polymorphis Close to the Adenomatous Polyposis Coli (APC) Gene Offers Improved Diagnostic Testing for Familial APC.** *Am J Hum Genet* 1993, **52**:286–296.

28. Muto T, Kamiya J, Sawada T, Koaishi F, Sagihara K, Kubota Y: **Small "Flat Adenomas" of the Large Bowel With Special Reference to Its Clinical Pathologic Features.** *Dis Col Rectum* 1985, **28**:847–851.

29. • Lynch HT, Smyrk TC, Watson P, Lanspa SJ, Lynch PM, Jenkins JX, Rouse J, Cavalieri J, Howard L, Lynch B: **Hereditary Flat Adenoma Syndrome: A Variant of Familial Adenomatous Polyposis?** *Dis Colon Rectum* 1992, **35**:411–421.

An interesting description of the clinical and pathologic features of four kindreds with the hereditary flat adenoma syndrome, and a discussion of its similarities to familial adenomatous polyposis.

30. Spirio L, Otterud B, Stauffer D, Lynch H, Lynch P, Watson P: **Linkage of a Variant or Attenuated Form of Adenomatous Polyposis Coli to the Adenomatous Polyposis Coli (APC) Locus.** *Am J Hum Genet* 1992, **51**:92–100.

31. •• Aaltonen LA, Peltomaki P, Leach FS, Sistonen P, Pylkkanen L, Mecklin JP, Jarvinen H, Powell SM, Jen J, Hamilton SR, Petersen GM, Kinzler KW, Vogelstein B, de la Chapelle A: **Clues to the Pathogenesis of Familial Colorectal Cancer.** *Science* 1993, **260**:812–816.

A congestive effort by the molecular genetics laboratories of Vogelstein and de la Chapelle. They identified widespread alterations in short repeated DNA segments in chromosome 2 in familial cancers and also in a significant percentage of apparently sporadic cancers. They described this genetic abnormality as a "susceptibility gene." Its identification will help us to better understand familial colorectal cancer and may also have important implications in screening for colorectal cancer.

32. Thibodeau SN, Bren G, Schaid D: **Microsatellite Instability in Cancer of the Proximal Colon.** *Science* 1993, **260**:816–819.

33. Burt RW, Groden J: **The Genetic and Molecular Diagnosis of Adenomatous Polyposis Coli.** *Science* 1993, **104**:1211–1214.

34. Vasen HF, Mecklin JP, Watson P, Utsunomiya J, Bertarino L, Lynch P, Svensden B, Cristofaro G, Muller H, Khan PM, Lynch HT: **The International Collaborative Group on HNPCC Surveillance in Hereditary Colorectal Cancer and Nonpolyposis Colorectal Cancer and Internal Cooperative Study of 165 Families.** *Dis Colon Rectum* 1993, **36**:1–4.

35. Guillen JG, Forde KA, Treat MR, Neugent AI, O'Toole KM, Diamond BE: **Colonoscopic Screening for Neoplasms in Asymptomatic First-Degree Relatives of Colon Cancer Patients.** *Dis Col Rectum* 1992, **35**:523–529.

36. Ransohoff DF, Lang CA, Kho HS: **Colonoscopic Surveillance After Polypectomy: Considerations of Cost Effectiveness.** *Ann Intern Med* 1991, **114**:177–182.

37. Atkin WS, Morson BC, Cuzick J: **Long-Term Risk of Colorectal Cancer After Excision of Rectosigmoid Adenomas.** *N Engl J Med* 1992, **326**:658–662.

38. • Winawer SL, Zauber AG, O'Brien MJ, Ho MN, Gottlieb L, Sternberg SS, Wayne JD, Bond J, Schapiro M, Stewart ET, Panish J, Ackroyd F, Kurtz RC, Shike M: **The National Polyp Study Work Group: Randomized Comparison of Surveillance Intervals After Colonoscopic Removal of Newly Diagnosed Adenomatous Polyps.** *N Engl J Med* 1993, **328**:901–906.

A very important report from the National Polyp Study Work Group that offers follow-up recommendations based on prospectively collected data. Recommendations, if followed, should reduce the cost of postpolypectomy surveillance and screening.

39. St. John DJB, Young GP, Alexeyeff MA, Deacon MC, Cuthbertson AM, Macrae FA, Penfold JCB: **Evaluation of New Occult Blood Tests for Detection of Colorectal Neoplasia.** *Gastroenterology* 1993, **104**:1661–1668.

40. •• Ahlquist DA, Wieand HS, Moertel CG, McGill DB, Loprinzi CL, O'Connell MJ, Mailliard JA, Gerstner JB, Pandya K, Ellefson RD: **Accuracy of Fecal Occult Blood Screening for Colorectal Neoplasia.** *JAMA* 1993, **269**:1262–1267.

A prospective study evaluating the validity of Hemoccult and HemoQuant as markers for colorectal neoplasia in the screening setting. Low sensitivities and positive predictive values were reported for both tests for colorectal cancers and polyps. The authors felt that the low sensitivities more accurately represent FOBT performance for the screen detection of colorectal neoplasia than do the much higher detection rates reported from studies of symptomatic patients with more advanced neoplasms.

41. •• Mandel JS, Bond JH, Church TR, Snover DC, Bradley GM, Schuman LM, Ederer F: **Minnesota Colon Cancer Control Study: Reducing Mortality From Colorectal Cancer by Screening for Fecal Occult Blood.** *N Engl J Med* 1993, **328**:1365–1371.

A long-awaited report from the Minnesota Colon Cancer Control Study demonstrating that a reduction in mortality from colorectal cancer produced by testing for fecal occult blood.

42. Winawer SJ: **Colorectal Cancer Screening Comes of Age.** *N Engl J Med* 1993, **328**:1415–1417.

43. Selby JV, Friedman GD, Quesenberry CPJ, Weiss NS: **A Case-Control Study of Screening Sigmoidoscopy and Mortality From Colorectal Cancer.** *N Engl J Med* 1992, **326**:653–657.

Mark V. Larson, MD, Division of Gastroenterology, Department of Medicine, Mayo Clinic, 200 First Street SW, Rochester, MN 55905, USA.

Surgery of colorectal cancer and inflammatory bowel disease

Jeffrey W. Milsom, MD

The Cleveland Clinic Foundation, Cleveland, Ohio, USA

This review highlights the year's most important articles concerning surgical management of colorectal cancer and inflammatory bowel disease as well as examining the new and growing field of laparoscopic bowel surgery. As in the past, editorial comments pervade the text.

Current Opinion in Gastroenterology 1994, **10**:34–40

Perioperative care

Although there were very few articles appearing over the past year concerning perioperative care, one standout was the multicenter randomized trial led by Hoynck-Van-Papendrecht *et al.* [1•] that examined whether blood transfusions during surgery affected 5-year survival in colorectal cancer. In this study, the authors also evaluated whether the predeposition of two units of blood by patients about to undergo colorectal cancer surgery was feasible and could decrease use of homologous blood usage. A total of 310 patients were randomly assigned to either predeposit two units of blood or undergo the surgery with homologous blood available as necessary. Only 23% of the patients who predeposited blood, compared with 61% of the patients who did not, were exposed to homologous blood. Significant differences in the need for homologous blood were primarily noted in patients with left colon or rectal carcinomas undergoing surgery. The study solidly demonstrated that, in distal colonic or rectal lesions, deposition of two units of blood prior to surgery is feasible, and that it dramatically lowers the need for homologous blood transfusions. This simple concept should undoubtedly be used more widely in colorectal cancer surgery.

A second article, by Chung *et al.* [2•] of the Jewish General Hospital of Montreal, Canada, reviewed the need for perioperative blood transfusion and assessed outcome after resection for colorectal cancer. In reviewing over 20 papers evaluating more than 5000 patients, Chung *et al.* found cumulative odds ratios (95% confidence interval) of disease occurrence, death from cancer, and death from any cause of 1.80 (1.30 to 2.51), 1.76 (1.15 to 2.66), and 1.63 (1.12 to 2.38), respectively. They thus concluded that perioperative blood transfusion is associated with an increased risk of recurrence in colorectal carcinoma. I still believe the issue is multifaceted, but this article provides the reader with a comprehensive and up-to-date review of the topic. It is interesting that only last year, a similar article appearing in this review convincingly concluded that there was no evidence for causal association between transfusion and tumor growth [3].

Finally, Hammond *et al.* [4•], describe the process of preoperative endoscopic tattooing of the colon, which may be valuable in certain instances where a tumor is not palpable or visible at resectioned surgery. They note that indocyanine green, which remains visible in the colonic wall for up to 36 hours, is probably the most practical dye to use. Preoperative tattooing may prove especially useful in laparoscopic surgery, because it saves intraoperative time and avoids potential colonic distention, a difficult circumstance during laparoscopy.

Surgical challenges in colorectal cancer

Primary cancer surgery

MacFarlane *et al.* [5•] reviewed the local recurrence and survival data of 135 "high-risk" rectal cases (Dukes B and C) from the Basingstoke District Hospital in the United Kingdom. Despite the fact that combination therapy is becoming more and more popular in the management of advanced primary rectal cancer, they concluded that total mesorectal excision in rectal cancer leads to such a low local recurrence rate (5%) and overall recurrence rate (22%) at 5 years in Basingstoke patients that it is difficult to justify additional therapy beyond surgery. This radical surgical technique, long-supported by Heald and others, is probably very important in rectal cancer surgery. The study design espoused in this paper, however, directly comparing the Basingstoke data with that of the North Center Can-

Abbreviations

IPAA—ileal pouch–anal anastomosis; **RIGS**—radioimmunoguided surgery.

 ISBN 1-85922-606-X ISSN 0267–1379

cer treatment group data (which has much higher recurrence statistics), is flawed because a comparison of such disparate study groups cannot be used to justify the total mesorectal excision technique.

Two Scandinavian groups examined which type of therapy is best in the management of acute malignant large bowel obstruction [6•,7•]. Gandrup *et al.* [6•] studied 156 consecutive patients operated on for obstructing primary colorectal cancers. Their study population was elderly (median age 73 years), with 43 of the 95 patients undergoing primary resection and anastomosis, and 54 patients undergoing staged resection. There was an overall 30-day mortality of only 5%, with 61% of the patients having stage III or IV disease.

In a similar study by Sjödahl *et al.* [7•] from University Hospital in Linköping, Sweden, 115 patients with complete obstruction of the colon were studied retrospectively. This study population was also quite elderly (median age 73 years), with only 29 patients undergoing resection and primary anastomosis, and 40 patients undergoing primary resection. A staged resection was being undertaken in 48 patients, stomal formation in only 25 patients, and exploratory laparotomy in two. Postoperative mortality rate was 10% after primary resection and 15% after stage resections. The 5-year survival was 38% after primary and 29% after staged resections.

Both of these studies substantiate earlier reports that obstructing colorectal cancers occur in primarily elderly patients, but neither fully assesses whether primary resection, with or without anastomosis, is advisable or feasible. Most likely this complicated decision will continue to be made on a case-by-case basis by experienced surgeons.

In a turnabout from some of his previous surgical tactics, Enker [8•] of the Memorial Sloan-Kettering Cancer Center in New York City reported his results in the use of autonomic nerve-preserving, pelvic sidewall dissection in the operative treatment of rectal cancer. In this study of 42 men, he outlined his surgical technique in detail, finding 33 of 38 evaluable patients (86.7%) remaining potent, with 29 of 33 patients (87.9%) having normal ejaculation following surgery. Only one patient with an advanced cancer had local recurrence after a median follow-up of 20 months (range 4 to 85 months). The study design of this series, not being a prospective one, leaves something to be desired; nonetheless, the article is interesting for its detailed description of preserving the nerves around the rectum while performing a radical cancer operation (Fig. 1).

Because use of adjuvant pelvic radiation therapy continues to be popular, Thom *et al.* [9•] from the Robert Wood Johnson Medical School in New Brunswick, New Jersey reviewed the efficacy of placing a polyglycolic acid mesh to suspend the small bowel away from the pelvis in patients undergoing postoperative radiation therapy. This is done in an attempt to prevent radiation-associated small bowel injury. Thom *et al.* have reported on this technique in the past. In this study, they reviewed their perioperative experiences and the acute, toxic effects of postoperative radiation therapy in 53 patients undergoing rectal cancer surgery with sling placement. All patients had high-risk rectal cancers and were given a mean of 5100-cGy external beam radiotherapy after surgery. Significantly, at 1 to 6 years of follow-up (mean 2.1 years), there were no cases of radiation-associated small bowel injury. Only two of these high-risk patients developed pelvic recurrence, and no patients developed complications related to the polyglycolic acid mesh. The mesh was easily placed by securing it initially to the periosteum of the sacral promontory, then bringing it to the level of the umbilicus anteriorly by use of a running absorbable suture to ensure secure placement of the mesh circumferentially.

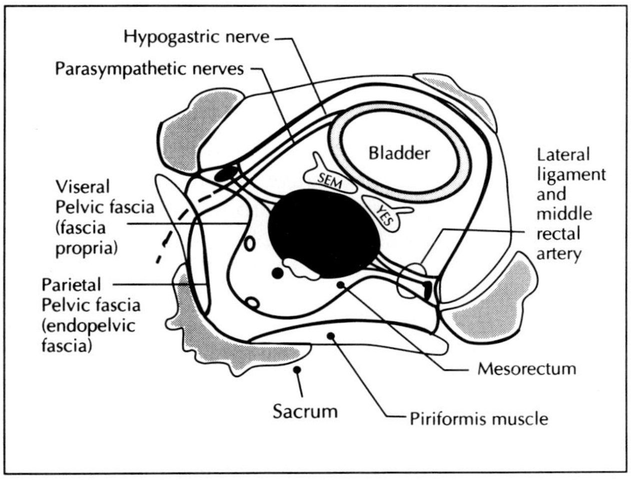

Fig. 1. Schematic cross sectional view of the pelvis, demonstrating the location of the parasympathetic and the sympathetic (hypogastric) nerves in relation to the rectum. (*From* Enker [8•]; with permission.)

Thom *et al.* [9•] believe that the intestinal sling procedure continues to be demonstrated as a safe apparatus to place at surgery, with a very low complication rate. I believe their conclusions are correct, and that this mesh should be considered for patients who will undergo postoperative radiation therapy for rectal cancer.

Although no major trials on rectal cancer were reported this year, Mendenhall *et al.* [10•] from the University of Florida Health Science Center in Gainesville, Florida have again retrospectively reported on a series of patients undergoing preoperative radiation therapy. In their study, they assessed 148 patients who underwent preoperative radiation therapy and surgery between 1975 and 1986. All patients had at least 5 years of follow-up. The radiotherapists used a variety of radiation therapy dosing regimens over this time period (from 3000 to 4500 cGy). They found a subset of 56 patients with locally advanced lesions (based on tethering or circumferential involvement of the rectal lumen), who were treated with preoperative radiation therapy and surgery, had significantly improved local recurrence–free survival (96% vs 67%), absolute survival (66% vs 40%), and cause-specific survival (77% vs 50%) compared with nonirradiated patients. All of these differences were statistically significant. They also noted no apparent increase in the incidence of postoperative complications in patients who were irradiated before surgery.

Although the report by Mendenhall *et al.* [10•] is a retrospective review, it does further substantiate the benefits of preoperative radiation therapy in patients with apparent advanced rectal cancers. It is hoped that through more reporting of multi-institutional studies, and by using preoperative endoluminal ultrasonography, more objective data regarding the use of preoperative radiation therapy will be forthcoming.

One of the year's more promising colorectal cancer studies was published by the Large Bowel Cancer Project in the United Kingdom, where Fielding *et al.* [11•] reported yet another study on the portal vein perfusion technique after curative resection for colorectal cancer. Encompassing the efforts of 11 hospitals in the United Kingdom between 1981 and 1984, 1075 patients were followed in the study, 613 of whom were not randomly assigned. All patients were followed for at least 5 years. After undergoing a curative colorectal cancer resection with insertion of a small catheter into a "conventional" radical of the portal vein, patients then received postoperative portal vein infusion of heparin (10,000 U/d) or heparin plus 5-fluorouracil (1000 mg/d). After 7 days of infusion, the treatment was stopped and patients were compared with a control group receiving no infusion. In patients who had stage II (Dukes' C or lymph node–positive) tumors, those who received the 5-fluorouracil plus heparin had a significant ($P < 0.03$) survival advantage of about 16% compared with surgery-only controls. This study, an important one, concludes that a much larger trial is necessary to elucidate the effects of this treatment on survival. It is hoped, as an editorial following this article suggests [12], that the AXIS trial of the UK Coordinating Committee on Cancer Research which is investigating the very same question, will be able to provide this in the next several years.

In the last article in the section, the use of radioimmunoguided surgery (RIGS) in primary colorectal cancer is evaluated. Arnold *et al.* [13•] from the Department of Surgery at Ohio State University explored whether the use of RIGS in combination with the antitumor-associated glycoprotein antibody, CC49, influenced therapeutic decisions in patients undergoing primary colorectal cancer surgery. In their study, 36 patients underwent preoperative injection of the CC49 glycoprotein antibody. Use of the hand-held gamma-detecting probe (Neoprobe 1000, Neoprobe Corp., Columbus, Ohio) was then evaluated after traditionally inspecting and palpating in the peritoneal cavity of patients undergoing colorectal cancer surgery. The gamma-detecting probe was used to discern "RIGS-positive" tissue. Overall, 30 patients (83%) had positive antibody localization at surgery with 24 (80%) patients having additional information procured from the use of the hand-held probe compared with gross findings at the time of surgery. Eleven (34%) patients had substantial changes in their surgical procedures as a result of the RIGS exploration.

The authors concluded that the RIGS system provided immediate staging information that impacted on therapeutic interventions, challenging the adequacy of traditional procedures alone for primary colorectal cancer surgery [13•]. This study, although intriguing, will not change the tactics of the vast majority of surgeons operating on colorectal cancer, because we really do not know the outcome of these RIGS patients compared with patients who are unable to undergo such surgery. Although this technique seems interesting, many more refinements in its use with follow-up data will be needed before it truly challenges the adequacy of traditional surgery.

Intraoperative evaluation of distant metastases in colorectal cancer

Two papers have appeared in the past year that discuss the use of intraoperative ultrasonography [14•,15•]. The first, from the University of Michigan [14•], discussed whether delayed computed tomography of the liver more accurately detects hepatic malignancy when compared with bolus contrast-enhanced dynamic computed tomography, also comparing this with intraoperative palpation and intraoperative ultrasonography of the liver in 51 patients requiring operation for intra-abdominal malignancy (92% with colorectal cancers). Whereas the sensitivities of delayed computed tomography and bolus contrast-enhanced dynamic computed tomography were 54% and 50%, respectively, the sensitivity of palpation alone for detection of metastases was 82%, equal to that of intraoperative ultrasonography. Both palpation and intraoperative ultrasonography were superior to any method of computed tomography, and the combination of the two was significantly more accurate in the detection of hepatic metastases than any single modality evaluated. This is not surprising, as the main failures of intraoperative ultrasonography are in the detection of surface lesions less than 1.0 cm in diameter. One weakness of the study may be that the intraoperative ultrasonography was performed using a 5.0-MHz probe, which is very poor at detecting lesions close to the probe. A higher frequency (7 to 7.5 MHz) probe would likely have improved the sensitivity of intraoperative ultrasound.

A similar study, performed by Boutkan *et al.* [15•] from the Free University Hospital in Amsterdam, compared intraoperative ultrasound with preoperative ultrasonography, computed tomography scan, and magnetic resonance imaging in patients with gastrointestinal malignancies and known hepatic metastases. Intraoperative ultrasonography supplied additional information in 38% of the 82 operations performed in this study, also allowing discrimination between solid versus cystic aspects of the tumors, and localizing the tumors in relation to vascular structures, especially important when resectional hepatic surgery was a consideration.

These and earlier studies have demonstrated the usefulness of intraoperative ultrasonography. Future studies will probably evaluate use of laparoscopic intraoperative ultrasonography in combination with laparoscopic intestinal surgery in order to thoroughly evaluate the liver.

Surgery of inflammatory bowel disease

Crohn's disease

The largest series of patients undergoing strictureplasties for the treatment of Crohn's disease was reported in the past year by the Department of Colorectal Surgery at the Cleveland Clinic Foundation. In this review, Fazio *et al.* [16••] examined 116 patients with obstructive Crohn's disease undergoing 452 primary strictureplasties (Heineke-Mikulicz, 405; Finney, 47). The median number of strictureplasties was three per patient with a range of one to 15. There were no mortalities, and septic complications occurred in only seven patients (6%). Reoperation for sepsis was only needed in two patients and relief of obstructive symptoms was achieved in all but two patients. After a median follow-up of 3 years, rates of restricture and new stricture/perforative disease were 2.5% and 24%, respectively. Over this time period, 17 patients (15%) required reoperation. This paper concludes that strictureplasty is a safe and credible surgical procedure for selected patients with small intestinal Crohn's disease. More long-term follow-up, however, will be critical to thoroughly evaluate its worth in this very difficult clinical situation.

The next study on Crohn's disease surgery, emanating from Johns Hopkins University, discusses patterns of ileal recurrence in Crohn's disease by randomly assigning 86 patients with ileal Crohn's undergoing their first ileocolic resection to receive either an end-to-end ($n=47$) or side-to-end ($n=39$) anastomosis [17•]. Cameron *et al.* reported no differences in documented ileal recurrences between the two groups. Interestingly, though, the recurrence spared the distal ileum in the patients who underwent a side-ileum-to-end-colon anastomosis, in other words sparing the blind pouch of the ileum. This study suggests that the fecal stream and reflux of colonic content may be important factors in determining the pattern of ileal recurrence after ileocolectomy for Crohn's disease.

Another interesting study looking at the excluded rectal segment after surgery for Crohn's colitis attempted to determine prognostic factors relating to the fate of the rectal segment. To do this, Guillem *et al.* [18•] of the Lahey Clinic in Burlington, Massachusetts studied 47 patients who underwent creation of an excluded rectal segment with colectomy and ileostomy for Crohn's disease. Disease developed in 33 patients (70%) in the excluded rectal segment by 5 years and over half of the patients in the study required completion proctectomy at a median of 2.4 years of follow-up. After a median follow-up of 6 years, only 14 patients were without clinical signs of disease in the rectum. This study found that neither initial involvement of the terminal ileum nor endoscopic inflammatory changes seen in the rectum predicted eventual disease of the excluded rectal segment. However, initial perianal disease, which complicated the Crohn's colitis, was strongly predictive of persistent excluded rectal segment disease and often led to proctectomy. This may be useful information in the care of such patients.

This study contrasts with another report looking at the low Hartmann's procedure for severe anorectal Crohn's disease from the Mt. Sinai Hospital of New York City. Sher *et al.* [19•] studied 25 patients with severe anorectal Crohn's disease and perineal fistulas whom they treated with a low Hartmann's procedure. In their study, 22 of 25 patients had a completely healed perineum at a mean follow-up period of 69 months. Their patient population, although unlikely to be significantly different from the Lahey Clinic study group in the previously discussed paper, certainly had almost completely different clinical outcomes. I can only say that, anecdotally, the experience at my institution has been that anorectal Crohn's disease tends to persistent even after diversion and thus I am reluctant to advocate use of the low Hartmann procedure in severe anorectal Crohn's disease.

A paper assessing the outcome of ileorectal anastomosis in Crohn's colitis, reported by Longo *et al.* [20•] from the Cleveland Clinic, assesses how well 132 patients who underwent this procedure fared after a follow-up period ranging from 6.2 months to 12.7 years (mean, 4.1 years). Preoperatively, 84 patients (63%) were found to have mild or moderate proctitis, with only 47 (37%) patients with complete rectal sparing. Nonetheless, most patients did extremely well, with only four anastomotic leaks and no operative deaths seen. A total of 118 patients eventually had functioning ileorectal anastomoses, with only 30 (23%) requiring proctectomy and 16 (13%) requiring proximal diversion during the study period. A small group of patients required re-resection and neoileorectal anastomosis. Overall, after a mean follow-up of 9.5 years, 72 patients (61%) retained their ileorectal anastomosis, with 44 patients being free of disease and 28 requiring steroids or antidiarrheal medicine. Although the study was retrospectively conducted, it solidly places ileorectal anastomosis into the armamentarium of the Crohn's disease surgeon, even if the rectum has mild-to-moderate proctitis. The main caveat offered by the study is that sphincter function should not be compromised in this group of patients if the ileorectal anastomosis option is used.

Ileal pouch surgery in mucosal ulcerative colitis

Schmitt *et al.* [20•], from the Department of Colorectal Surgery at the Cleveland Clinic Florida, evaluated 56 patients undergoing an ileoanal reservoir evaluated between 1988 and 1992. All patients underwent a double stapled ileal pouch–anal anastomosis (IPAA), with 0 to 2.5 cm of epithelium left above the dentate line. There was no evidence of dysplasia in any of the biopsied stapled lines just above the dentate line, and the distal resection line revealed active mucosal ulcerative colitis in only 19 patients. This paper cautions that, despite the fact that healing and function seem acceptable in the short term, the long-term effects of potentially retaining columnar epithelium just above the dentate line mandates periodic monitoring of this area.

The effect of anorectal eversion during restorative proctocolectomy on anal sphincter function in 26 patients was assessed by Lewis *et al.* [22•] from the Leeds Infirmary in Leeds, United Kingdom. In this study, the rectum was mobilized to the pelvic floor, transected at midrectal level, then everted, stapled closed, and anastomosed to the ileal pouch using a circular stapler. All patients had good functional results and anorectal manometric testing was not significantly changed before versus after surgery (except resting anal pressure). The article substantiates that eversion is a reasonable technique to use for IPAA.

Luukkohen and Jarvinen [23•] assessed treatment of the distal rectum by studying 40 consecutive patients randomly assigned to either hand-sutured or double-stapled ileoanal anastomosis. In this study, postoperative complications appeared to be the same, with one stapled anastomosis having to be converted to a hand-sutured one because of severe anastomotic stricture. Functional results were similar in both groups, as was the manometric mean resting anal pressure. Based on their results, the authors concluded that a double-stapled ileoanal anastomosis does not offer any functional or technical advantage over the hand-sutured technique. In my experience, however, the double-stapled technique is more quickly performed. The authors appear to dislike the stapling technique because it leaves traces of the disease behind and this is theoretically of concern. Again, long-term assessment of the double-stapled IPAA operation will be necessary, with periodic follow-up of the retained columnar epithelium.

The long-term functional results of the ileoanal reservoir were evaluated in three different papers from Japan and the United States this past year [24•–26•]. The study from Japan [24•] makes the following point: the assessment of quality of life in 80 patients undergoing the ileal J-pouch-anal anastomosis for colitis and polyposis was high, but appeared to have a close relationship to the personality factors of the patients. Thus, satisfaction with the surgery was not only associated with objective outcomes such as the number of bowel movements per day. This is not terribly surprising. The results of another Cleveland Clinic study, reported by Tjandra *et al.* [25•] demonstrated that, contrary to previous reports, familial polyposis patients and mucosal ulcerative colitis patients have very similar functional outcomes after IPAA surgery (median follow-up 32 months, range 6 months to 8.5 years). The major difference between 30 paired patients was that pouchitis was much more common in the colitis group than in the polyposis group (33% vs 10%).

Finally, in a study from the Mayo Clinic [26•], 971 patients with chronic ulcerative colitis undergoing IPAA were assessed for long-term functional results and quality of life. These patients were compared with a group of patients undergoing cholecystectomy during each of the same years as the study group up until 1990 (20 patients per year, totaling 160 patients). In spite of the alteration of their bowel habits, 90% of patients undergoing ileoanal anastomosis had a excellent overall quality of life and over 90% of patients had good performance scores in the areas examined. Results were similar to patients who had only undergone cholecystectomy. There was no evidence for a deterioration of this quality over time. This is the largest series with the longest follow-up to date on quality of life in IPAA patients. Table 1 highlights the major IPAA surgery papers.

Laparoscopic large intestine surgery

Reports on laparoscopic large bowel surgery have not proliferated rapidly over the past year, possibly because this surgery is much more difficult than laparoscopic cholecystectomy. The reports described below represent some of the largest and most interesting to date. Nonetheless, technical details as to how to perform efficient laparoscopic intestinal surgery remain largely unreported, and the possibilities of performing adequate cancer surgery are still unknown.

One of the largest laparoscopic intestinal surgical experiences to date has been reported by Franklin *et al.* [27•] of San Antonio, Texas. In a retrospective study of over 100 patients, they assert that all but a few pathologic situations in the intestine can be approached laparoscopically, and reported operating on all parts of the colon for a variety of indications. Of some concern is their policy for excising colorectal carcinomas. Although they state that carcinoma can be approached laparoscopically with the same precision and radicality as in open surgery, the paper lacks technical details of how this is accomplished. Nonetheless, they document considerable experience, with most patients being ready for discharge in less than 96 hours. I still think that this is a very prelimi-

Table 1. Reports on the ileal pouch–anal anastomosis operation

Study	Conclusions
Schmitt *et al.* [21•]	Double-stapling the reservoir is safe, but long-term effects or risks of retained columnar epithelium are unknown.
Lewis *et al.* [22•]	Eversion of the anorectum during restorative proctocolectomy does not impair sphincteric function.
Luukkonen *et al.* [23•]	A prospective randomized trial showed no difference in functional outcome between hand-sewn versus sutured ileal pouch anal anastomosis.
Fujita *et al.* [24•]	Quality of life and outcome after ileal J-pouch surgery correlates well with objective and subjective (personality) parameters.
Tjandra *et al.* [25•]	Familial polyposis and ulcerative colitis patients have very similar functional outcomes, except that pouchitis is more common in ulcerative colitis.
Kohler *et al.* [26•]	Quality of life and performance status remain very high in ileal pouch patients up to 9 years after surgery.

nary report, and will await reports of others with great interest.

A multi-institutional retrospective study evaluating laparoscopic colectomy was authored by Falk *et al.* [28•] of the United States. This study attempted to assess efficacy and safety of laparoscopy in colon and rectal surgery. In studying 66 patients, they found a conversion rate from laparoscopic colectomy to celiotomy of 41%, with a major morbidity of 24%. A comparison between patients undergoing laparoscopic procedures and patients undergoing conventional open surgical procedures was also performed. The authors concluded the following: 1) laparoscopic colon and rectal surgery can be accomplished with acceptable morbidity and mortality; 2) length of stay for laparoscopic colectomy appeared to be shorter than for conventional surgery; and 3) there was no proven total hospital cost benefit for this procedure. They also suggested that registries will be necessary to adequately assess long-term outcome. Unfortunately, in the preliminary stages of laparoscopic intestinal surgery, a study like this will do little to determine whether such surgery is advantageous; although this study is interesting it proves little except that laparoscopic techniques can be applied to the large intestine.

In their prospective evaluation of laparoscopic-assisted colectomy, Monson *et al.* [29•] of the United Kingdom take a cautious but optimistic approach to the use of laparoscopic techniques in 40 patients, 33 of whom had a "successfully completed" laparoscopic colectomy. A wide variety of diseases, including primary malignancy, were indications for surgery. These surgeons felt that early postoperative mobility and discharge from the hospital were notable features of laparoscopic patients. They concluded that laparoscopic colectomy was feasible in most patients (although most of their patients only underwent laparoscopic mobilization of the colon, with mesenteric division and anastomotic formation performed through a small laparotomy incision). Their conclusion that a substantial benefit accrues without compromising the surgical cure of the cancer is a premature one. This, as well as most benefits in laparoscopic intestinal surgery, awaits a prospective randomized study.

References and recommended reading

Papers of particular interest, published within the annual period of review, have been highlighted as:
- • Of special interest
- •• Of outstanding interest

1. • Hoynck-van-Papendrecht MA, Hop W, Langenhorst BL, Kothe FC, Marquet RL, Jeekel J: **Feasibility of a Predeposit Autologous Blood Donation Program in Colorectal Cancer Patients: Results From a Randomized Clinical Study.** *Vox Sang* 1992, **62**:102–107.

Predeposit of one or two units of autologous blood in colorectal cancer patients before surgery is largely possible.

2. • Chung M, Steinmetz OK, Gordon PH: **Perioperative Blood Transfusion and Outcomes After Resection for Colorectal Carcinoma [Review].** *Br J Surg* 1993, **80**:427–432.

A comprehensive review article that statistically demonstrates decreased survival after colorectal cancer surgery if transfusion is necessary.

3. Francis DMA: **Relationship between blood transfusion and tumour behaviour.** *Br J Surg* 1991, **78**:1420–1428.

4. • Hammond DC, Lane FR, MacKeigan JM, Passinault WJ: **Endoscopic Tattooing of the Colon - Clinical Experience.** *Am Surg* 1993, **59**:205–210.

An interesting article showing that tattooing of the colon with indocyanine green is safe and lasts 36 hours.

5. • MacFarlane JK, Ryall RDH, Heald RJ: **Mesorectal Excision for Rectal Cancer.** *Lancet* 1993, **341**:457–460.

The Basingstoke experience with "total mesorectal excision" in rectal cancer continues to be impressive with regard to local recurrence and survival.

6. • Gandrup P, Lung L, Balslev I: **Surgical Treatment of Acute Malignant Large Bowel Obstruction.** *Eur J Surg* 1992, **158**:427–430.

A retrospective review of surgical therapy in obstructing large bowel cancer. Little new information, but an interesting review.

7. • Sjodahl R, Franzen T, Nystrom PO: **Primary Versus Staged Resection for Acute Obstructing Colorectal Carcinoma.** *Br J Surg* 1992, **79**:685–688.

Another retrospective review of surgery in malignant large bowel cancer suggesting experience in this surgery is key.

8. • Enker WE: **Potency, Cure, and Local Control in the Operative Treatment of Rectal Cancer.** *Arch Surg* 1992, **172**:1396–1402.

An autonomic nerve-preserving operation is feasible in rectal cancer surgery.

9. • Thom A, Baumann J, Chandler JJ, Devereux DF: **Experience with High-Dose Radiation Therapy and the Intestinal Sling Procedure in Patients with Rectal Carcinoma.** *Cancer* 1992, **70**:581–584.

Polyglycolic acid mesh effectively holds the small intestine out of the pelvis, and may lessen the likelihood of small bowel radiation injury.

10. • Mendenhall WM, Bland KI, Copeland EM, Summers GE, Pfaff WW, Souba WW, Million RR: **Does Preoperative Ra-**

diation Therapy Enhance the Probability of Local Control and Survival in High-Risk Distal Rectal Cancer**. *Ann Surg* 1992, **215**:696–706.

Another study documenting possible efficacy of preoperative radiotherapy in advanced rectal cancers.

11. • FIELDING LP, HITTINGER R, GRACE RH, FRY JS: **Randomized Controlled Trial of Adjuvant Chemotherapy by Portal-Vein Perfusion after Curative Resection for Colorectal Adenocarcinoma**. *Lancet* 1992, **340**:502–506.

Postoperative portal vein 5-fluorouracil infusion after colorectal cancer surgery (with heparin) in Duke's C patients may enhance survival. A larger trial is needed.

12. GARTEN L, STENNING S, GRAY R: **Intraportal 5-Fluorouracil for Colorectal Cancer: the AXIS trial [Commentary]**. *Lancet* 340:985.

13. • ARNOLD MW, SCHNEEBAUM S, BERENS A, MOJZISIK C, HINKLE G, MARTIN EW JR: **Radioimmunoguided Surgery Challenges Traditional Decision Making in Patients with Primary Colorectal Cancer**. *Surgery* 1992, **112**:624–630.

A preliminary study suggesting radioimmunoguided surgery may provide additional information in many patients undergoing colorectal cancer surgery.

14. • KNOL JA, MARN CS, FRANCIS IR, RUBIN JM, BROMBERG J, CHANG AE: **Comparisons of Dynamic Infusion and Delayed Computed Tomography, Intraoperative Ultrasound, and Palpation in the Diagnosis of Liver Metastases**. *Am J Surg* 1993, **165**:81–88.

Intraoperative palpation and ultrasonography are more accurate than dye-enhanced computed tomography in detecting hepatic malignancies.

15. • BOUTKAN H, LUTH W, MEYER S, CUESTA M, VAN HEUZEN E, PREVOO W: **The Impact of Intraoperative Ultrasonography of the Liver on the Surgical Strategy of Patients with Gastrointestinal Malignancies and Hepatic Metastases**. *Eur J Surg Oncol* 1992, **18**:342–346.

Intraoperative ultrasonography of the liver is more accurate than preoperative ultrasonography, computed tomography scans, and magnetic resonance imaging in detecting liver metastases.

16. •• FAZIO VW, TJANDRA JJ, LAVERY IC, CHURCH JC, MILSOM JM, OAKLEY JR: **Long-Term Follow-up of Strictureplasty in Crohn's Disease**. *Dis Colon Rectum* 1993, **367**:355–361.

This is the largest series of single institution strictureplasties for Crohn's small bowel disease reported thus far. It documents safety and a 6% septic complication rate.

17. • CAMERON JL, HAMILTON SR, COLEMAN J, SITZMANN JV, BAYLESS TM: **Patterns of Ileal Recurrence in Crohn's Disease. A Prospective Randomized Study**. *Ann Surg* 1993, **215**:546–552.

The side-ileum-to-end-colic ileocolic anastomosis after resection of Crohn's ileal disease leads to, in instances of recurrence, sparing of the blind end of neoterminal ilium. Thus, does the fecal stream contribute to recurrence?

18. • GUILLEM JG, ROBERTS PL, MURRAY JJ, COLLER JA, VEIDENHEIMER MC, SCHOETZ DJ JR: **Factors Predictive of Persistent or Recurrent Crohn's Disease in Excluded Rectal Segments**. *Dis Colon Rectum* 1992, **35**:768–772.

The excluded rectal segment, after colectomy for Crohn's disease, often continues to cause significant symptoms, requiring removal in the majority of patients within 2.4 years.

19. • SHER ME, BAUER JJ, GORPHINE S, GELERNT I: **Low Hartmann's Procedure for Severe Anorectal Crohn's Disease**. *Dis Colon Rectum* 1992, **35**:975–980.

A low Hartmann procedure allowed complete perineal healing of anorectal Crohn's in 22 of 25 patients with mean follow-up of 69 months.

20. • LONGO WE, OAKLEY JR, LAVERY IC, CHURCH JM, FAZIO VW: **Outcome of Ileorectal Anastomosis for Crohn's Colitis**. *Dis Colon Rectum* 1992, **35**:1066–1071.

Ileorectal anastomosis after total abdominal colectomy for Crohn's disease led to retention of the anastomosis in 61% of 132 patients at a median of 9.5 years of follow-up, even in the face of some pouchitis.

21. • SCHMITT SL, WEXNER SD, LUCAS FV, JAMES K, NOGUERAS JJ, JAGELMAN DG: **Retained Mucosa after Double-Stapled Ileal Reservoir and Ileoanal Anastomosis**. *Dis Colon Rectum* 1992, **35**:1051–1056.

Retention of some columnar epithelium after ileal pouch surgery allows for acceptable postoperative function, but long-term follow-up is advised.

22. • LEWIS WG, HOLDSWORTH PJ, SAGAR PM, HOLMFIELD JHM, JOHNSTON D: **Effect of Anorectal Eversion During Restorative Proctocolectomy on Anal Sphincter Function**. *Br J Surg* 1993, **80**:121–123.

Anorectal eversion with stapling of the distal anorectal function and then circular-staple ileal pouch anastomosis allows for good functional results.

23. • LUUKKONEN P, JARVINEN H: **Stapled Hand-Sutured Ileoanal Anastomosis in Restorative Proctocolectomy. A Prospective, Randomized Study**. *Arch Surg* 1993, **128**:437–440.

Using a randomized study design, no differences in functional results were seen between hand-sewn versus stapled ileal pouch anastomoses.

24. • FUJITA S, KUSUNOKI M, SHOJI Y, OWADA T, UTSUNOMIYA J: **Quality of Life after Total Proctocolectomy and Ileal J-Pouch-Anal Anastomosis**. *Dis Colon Rectum* 1992, **35**:1030–1039.

Quality of life assessment after ileal pouch surgery is dependent on personality as well as physiologic factors.

25. • TJANDRA JJ, FAZIO VW, CHURCH JM, OAKLEY JR, MILSOM JW, LAVERY IC: **Similar Functional Results After Restorative Proctocolectomy in Patients with Familial Adenomatous Polyposis and Mucosal Ulcerative Colitis**. *Am J Surg* 1993, **165**:322–325.

Familial polyposis and ulcerative colitis patients have similar postoperative functional results after ileal pouch surgery, except that colitis patients more commonly have pouchitis (33% vs 10%).

26. • KOHLER LW, PEMBERTON JH, HODGE DO, ZINSMEISTER AR, KELLY KA: **Long-Term Functional Results and Quality of Life after Ileal Pouch-Anal Anastomosis and Cholecystectomy**. *World J Surg* 1992, **16**:1126–1132.

A total of 90% of 971 patients undergoing ileal pouch surgery rated their quality of life as excellent, with no deterioration over time.

27. • FRANKLIN ME, RAMOS R, ROSENTHAL D, SCHUESSLER W: **Laparoscopic Colonic Procedures**. *World J Surg* 1993, **17**:51–56.

Laparoscopic techniques are feasible to use in approaching many pathologic situations in all parts of the colon and rectum.

28. • FALK PM, BEART RW, WEXNER SD, THORSON AG, JAGELMAN DG, LAVERY IC, JOHANSEN OB, FITZGIBBONS RJ: **Laparoscopic Colectomy - A Critical Appraisal**. *Dis Colon Rectum* 1993, **36**:28–34.

This multi-institutional retrospective study demonstrated, in 66 patients, the feasibility of performing laparoscopic-assisted procedures on the large intestine with no demonstrable cost benefit and a possible shorter hospital stay.

29. • MONSON JR, DARZI A, CAREY PD, GUILLOU PJ: **Prospective Evaluation of Laparoscopic-Assisted Colectomy in an Unselected Group of Patients**. *Lancet* 1992, **340**:831–833.

This prospective evaluation of 40 patients undergoing laparoscopic or laparoscopic-assisted colectomy shows possible earlier discharge and postoperative mobility, but no comparison group was present.

Jeffrey W. Milsom, MD, Department of Colorectal Surgery/A111, Cleveland Clinic Foundation, 9500 Euclid Avenue, Cleveland, OH 44195, USA.

Colorectal endoscopy

David A. Ahlquist, MD

Mayo Clinic, Rochester, Minnesota, USA

Literature highlights from the past year pertaining to endoscopy of the colorectum are discussed. As most journal articles have dealt with applications in the screening, diagnosis, and management of colorectal neoplasia, the critique reflects this emphasis. Diagnostic and therapeutic advances, safety and monitoring information, and training issues in colonoscopy are also covered.

Current Opinion in Gastroenterology 1994, **10**:41–48

Rational use of instrumentation in the diagnosis and treatment of gastrointestinal disease depends not only on the clinical setting, but on demonstrated performance characteristics and cost of the technology employed. Increasingly, diagnostic algorithms must be supported by outcomes data to justify their application in patient care and to qualify for reimbursement. As such, it is imperative to evaluate both currently practiced and newer diagnostic approaches in terms of effectiveness, safety, quality control, and cost.

Colorectal cancer screening

Average-risk patients

Approximately 95% of all colorectal cancers occur in persons older than 50 years, and most patients found to have this common malignancy have no identifiable risk factors. Although early detection clearly translates into improved survival, current cancer screening strategies are far from ideal. Fecal blood testing, although noninvasive and seemingly inexpensive, lacks sensitivity and specificity. Based on prospective comparison against colonoscopy and other structural studies, fecal blood tests missed more than 70% of asymptomatic cancers and more than 90% of adenomas; the likelihood of finding a colorectal polyp was independent of fecal blood test results in a multicenter study [1]. Sigmoidoscopic [2•] and colonoscopic [3••] evaluations in asymptomatic persons 45 years old and over who were negative on fecal blood test screening, further reveal that colorectal neoplasms are commonly missed. In 621 such persons, Rex *et al.* [3••] observed adenomas in 27% and cancers in three instances on colonoscopy; importantly, more than 10% of persons older than 60 years had large adenomas (≥1 cm).

Although more expensive and invasive than fecal blood testing, colorectal endoscopy has clearly superior diagnostic accuracy and should be more effective as a primary screening approach. Indeed, in a case control study by Newcomb *et al.* [4••], the estimated risk of death from rectosigmoid cancer was significantly reduced among individuals having had at least one previous sigmoidoscopy screening compared with those who had never undergone one (odds ratio 0.21, 95% confidence interval 0.08 to 0.52). In contrast, neither fecal blood testing nor digital rectal examination was associated with a reduction in cancer mortality.

Controversy continues regarding the optimum frequency and extent of endoscopic colorectal screening. Aitkin *et al.* [5•] challenge current recommendations of sigmoidoscopic screening every 3 years and make a cogent argument for the cost-effectiveness of only one sigmoidoscopic screening at age 50 to 55 years based on a critique of the literature to date. Recent estimates that patients may harbor localized cancer for an average of 5 years before diagnosis, and much longer if the premalignant phase is included, lend further support for the adequacy of less frequent screening [6]. However, based on the case control study above [4••] and one reported earlier [7], the benefit of sigmoidoscopy is observed only for those distal cancers within its reach. Because half of all colorectal cancers occur proximal to the splenic flexure, a more logical structural screening approach would seem to require imaging the whole colorectum, such as by colon radiography or colonoscopy. Perhaps once-only or twice-only whole colorectal imaging will prove to be most cost effective. Current screening guidelines will require reexamination in view of our evolving understanding of practice outcomes.

High-risk patients

Predisposing conditions can be identified in about 20% of colorectal cancers. Persons with such conditions represent a group at high risk that qualifies for more in-

Abbreviation

HNPCC—hereditary nonpolyposis colorectal cancer.

tensive targeted screening with periodic structural colorectal evaluation.

Familial cancer

Few would disagree with the practice of regular early screening endoscopy for persons with familial adenomatous polyposis. Screening is more problematic with the other well-recognized autosomal dominant form, hereditary nonpolyposis colorectal cancer (HNPCC), which probably accounts for more than 5% of all colorectal cancer. Because there is no phenotype and the diagnosis must rely on a careful family history, identification of HNPCC probands represents a challenge. In a comprehensive review, Lynch *et al.* [8•] emphasize the early age onset, a proclivity for proximal colon lesions, and an excess of synchronous or metachronous cancers in HNPCC. Uncontrolled observations support the value of close colonoscopic surveillance in persons with HNPCC [9•]. X-Linked agammaglobulinemia appears to be another genetic condition predisposing to early-age colorectal cancer that would justify colonoscopic screening [10•]. Additional studies [11,12••] underscore the increased risk of colorectal neoplasia in those with a family history of sporadic colorectal cancer, especially if affected relatives are first degree. In the absence of rigorous outcomes data on screening relatives with sporadic cancer, structural colorectal evaluation every 3 to 5 years seems reasonable.

Colorectal polyps

Although both adenomatous and hyperplastic polyps represent focal lesions in a biochemically abnormal epithelium [13], the clinical relevance of these common polyps differs. Only adenomatous polyps undergo malignant transformation and have clear predictive value for synchronous or metachronous adenomas. In a prospective colonoscopic evaluation of asymptomatic patients following sigmoidoscopy, Brady *et al.* [14•] found proximal adenomas in significantly more patients with rectosigmoid adenomas (42%) than in those with rectosigmoid hyperplastic polyps (14%) or in controls (12%; $P = 0.006$). Some adenomas can be flat and difficult to identify endoscopically, as further characterized by Matsumoto *et al.* [15•], but it is unclear whether the natural history of flat adenomas differs from that of polypoid adenomas. In contrast to multiple juvenile polyposis, patients with solitary juvenile polyps do not appear to have an increased risk of developing colorectal cancer [16•].

In a multicenter, randomized comparison of surveillance intervals after colonoscopic removal of adenomas, Winawer *et al.* [17••] established that less frequent is not necessarily less effective. Although more adenomas were detected when surveillance colonoscopy was performed at both 1 and 3 years than at 3 years only, the percentage of patients found to have large or highly dysplastic adenomas did not differ between groups (Table 1). The authors advocate colonoscopy 3 years after polypectomy. Optimal surveillance intervals may be even longer, especially after removal of single small adenomas.

Previous colorectal cancer

In the perioperative period, preferably before surgery, full colonoscopy is indicated to screen for important synchronous neoplasms. In 65 patients undergoing colorectal cancer resection who did not have complete colon inspection, Brullet *et al.* [18•] performed successful intraoperative colonoscopy and found synchronous cancer in eight patients (12%) and polyps in 24 patients (36%). Despite the enormous resources invested and wide practice variations observed in postoperative follow-up, there is a striking paucity of data to direct management. Even with intensive postoperative colorectal endoscopic surveillance, curable anastomotic recurrences will be found in fewer than 1% of cases, as further corroborated by Safi *et al.* [19•]. Postoperative colonoscopic surveillance is justified more for detection of metachronous neoplasia than for meaningful salvage from recurrent disease. After one or two annual postoperative examinations, colorectal evaluations could reasonably be repeated at 3- to 5-year intervals.

Inflammatory bowel disease

In contrast to earlier reports from large referral centers, community-based estimates of colorectal cancer risk

Table 1. Comparison of findings on surveillance colonoscopy done either twice (1 and 3 years) or once (3 years only) following removal of an index adenoma*

	Patients, %			
	Colonoscopic surveillance twice ($n = 338$)	Colonoscopic surveillance once ($n = 428$)	Relative risk (95% CI)	*P* value
Any adenoma	42	32	1.3 (1.1–1.6)	0.006
Adenoma with advanced pathologic features†	3.3	3.3	1.0 (0.5–2.2)	0.99

*From Winawer *et al.* [17••]; with permission.
†Adenomas with high-grade dysplasia, invasive cancer, or size greater than 1.0 cm.
CI—confidence interval.

with ulcerative colitis have revealed small or absent increases, as in the recent Danish study by Langholz *et al.* [20••]. Among patients with ulcerative colitis, it would be most cost-effective to focus intensive surveillance on subgroups at greatest risk for cancer. Rubin *et al.* [21••] found that the presence of DNA aneuploidy on colonoscopic biopsies was highly predictive of subsequent dysplasia whereas its absence suggested a low likelihood of future dysplasia. It is not known what impact the identification of p53 point mutations in dysplastic biopsies will have on practice decisions [22••,23•]. Although Broome *et al.* [24•] have suggested that colorectal cancer risk is greater in those with primary sclerosing cholangitis, others [25] have been unable to confirm this association.

In a cohort study, Choi *et al.* [26••] found that colonoscopic surveillance in patients with ulcerative colitis was associated with a significantly reduced risk of fatal colorectal cancer. Of interest, dysplasia represented the sole endoscopic finding in only 32% of those found to have cancer during surveillance. Because of the predominance of rectosigmoid neoplasia with ulcerative colitis, Choi also suggests that more intensive distal sampling should be obtained in surveillance programs [27].

Other risk factors

Two well done studies support a mild excess risk for right-sided colorectal cancer following cholecystectomy, especially in women [28•,29••]. Accordingly, flexible sigmoidoscopy alone would be an inappropriate screening strategy in such persons. In a large Swedish study, Suadicani *et al.* [30••] observed a surprisingly high and strongly significant relative risk for colon cancer in persons regularly using antihypertensive or sedative medications even after adjusting for potential confounding factors [30••]. Because a large subset of our population is influenced by such drugs, these observations will need to be corroborated before guidelines are affected. Anal dysplasia is common in homosexual men [31•], but its natural history with respect to cancer progression is poorly understood and the role of anoscopic screening or therapy is unclear at present.

Diagnosis

Colonoscopy is indisputably the gold standard for the diagnosis of mucosal-based colorectal disease. Recently evaluated adjuncts promise to extend the diagnostic capacity of colorectal endoscopy. Schomacker *et al.* [32•,33•] have been able to distinguish adenomatous from hyperplastic polyps based on surface fluorescence differences, but the value of this technique in discriminating flat dysplasia and the extent to which electronic endoscopy can be programmed for such imaging remain to be established. Considering current limitations in locoregional tumor staging, Sudan *et al.* [34•] performed a study in dogs to explore the feasibility of colonoscopic indirect lymphoangiography by injecting contrast dye into the mucosa and observed encouraging early results. Colonoscopic injection of various dyes can safely mark lesions to create serosal-side tattoos that can then be used to target operative or laparoscopic resection [35].

Endoscopic and endoluminal ultrasound

Numerous studies over the past year confirm the accuracy of endoluminal ultrasound in assessing the depth of tumor invasion as well as its relative insensitivity in correctly classifying local lymph node involvement [36•–38•]. Endoluminal ultrasound can be used to safely direct needle biopsies into local lymph nodes and increase diagnostic accuracy [39•]. In women, transvaginal ultrasound may be more informative than the transrectal approach for highly stenosing cancers [40]. Although endoluminal ultrasound may be more sensitive than endoscopy alone in detecting local tumor recurrences [41•], improved survival without such diagnostic efforts has not been established. Endoscopic ultrasound may have a role in detecting invasive cancer within large villous adenomas, especially when nonsurgical therapy is contemplated [42•]. However, caution with such interpretation must be exercised following laser or electrocoagulative treatment, because such thermal injury can create transmural artifact that mimics invasive tumor [43]. Endoscopic ultrasound may enhance the discrimination between Crohn's disease and ulcerative colitis by demonstrating transmural involvement in the former [44•].

Therapy and technique

Polypectomy

Little new information has surfaced in the past year. Another small series supports the safety and efficacy of endoscopic resection of local sessile cancers and large polyps after local injections of hypertonic saline with epinephrine [45•]. Whereas the injected solution creates a cushion under such flat neoplasms to theoretically prevent mural thermal injury or bleeding, no prospective comparisons with other techniques have been reported. Laparoscopic removal has become an alternative to open resection for larger polyps not amenable to endoscopic therapy [46•,47].

Laser therapy

Additional uncontrolled series lend support to the safety and efficacy of endoscopic yttrium aluminum garnet laser for curative therapy of sessile villous adenoma [48•] or palliation of cancers [49]. In a retrospective comparison of endoscopic yttrium aluminum garnet laser with palliative surgery for advanced rectal cancer, Take *et al.* [50•] reported equal effectiveness and survival; they recommended laser palliation for incurable rectal cancer because morbidity and hospitalization were lower and rectal function was spared. Expanded series have been reported that further demonstrate the benefit and safety of endoscopic yttrium aluminum garnet [51•] or argon [52•] laser coagulation in the definitive management of transfusion-dependent bleeding from radiation proctopathy. In the absence of prospective comparisons, it is difficult to judge the cost-effectiveness of such laser therapy relative to established surgical approaches or to newly described approaches such as rectal formalin irrigation [53].

Miscellaneous techniques

Hiltunen *et al.* [54•] reported successful colonoscopic detorsion of sigmoid volvulus in 26 of 30 patients, but volvulus recurred in nearly one third of cases unless followed by corrective surgery. Fluoroscopy is used by some to facilitate the performance or teaching of colonoscopy, but equipment is expensive and accumulated radiation exposure can become a concern. An ingenuous nonradiologic technique involving an electromagnetic sensoring system has been developed by two groups [55•,56•] to allow real-time three-dimensional imaging of endoscopic position.

Colon preparation

Several approaches to colon purgation have proven to be comparably safe and effective, and selections are often based on physician or patient preference. Recent comparisons suggest that patients prefer flavored over plain oral lavage solutions [57•] and an oral sodium phosphate solution over the polyethylene glycol-electrolyte lavage [58•]. Supplementary enemas do not appear to improve the quality of colon preparation over oral lavage solutions alone and are usually unnecessary [59]. Patients in whom complete colonoscopy is not possible can undergo satisfactory air contrast barium enema the same day without additional preparation [60]. On a cautionary note, colorectal purgation can artifactually elevate serum carcinoembryonic antigen levels [61•].

Complications and monitoring

It is critical to balance the benefits of colonoscopic intervention against its complications. This is especially important, considering that the large majority of polyps removed will never progress to a malignant stage. In a large series of colonoscopies performed by expert colonoscopists in the ambulatory setting [62•], the overall complication rate was about 3%; however, the complication rate after polypectomy was 5%, with bleeding in 3% and perforation in 0.3%. Those perforations not associated with signs of peritonitis can often be managed conservatively with antibiotics and parenteral fluids, despite the presence of free air on abdominal radiography [63].

Although it is now well-established that postprocedural abdominal discomfort is lessened by use of carbon dioxide insufflation, few endoscopists or endoscopy manufacturers advocate this routinely. In a randomized comparison between carbon dioxide and air insufflation with respect to postcolonoscopy discomfort, Stevenson *et al.* [64••] noted a significant reduction in pain with carbon dioxide (two of 27) compared with air (17 of 29) ($P < 0.001$); objective measurements of gas distention were also significantly less in the carbon dioxide group [64••].

Whereas monitoring pulse oximetry has become a standard practice in many centers, its benefit has not been established with hard outcomes data. Iber *et al.* [65] observed that oxygen desaturation was significantly more likely in patients age 70 years or older, in persons with multi-systems illnesses, and in those undergoing endoscopic retrograde cholangiopancreatography; they suggest that pulse oximetry is especially indicated in such patient subgroups.

Training and certification

Both rigid and flexible sigmoidoscopy are widely performed by general physicians and surgeons. Because of the potentially enormous volume of sigmoidoscopies generated by population-based screening programs, many advocate an important role for nonphysician sigmoidoscopists. In a small randomized comparison, DiSario and Sanowski [66•] found no significant differences in the outcomes of insertion depth, time of procedure, or lesion recognition between patients sigmoidoscoped by medical residents and those done by nurses who had received the same hands-on training.

Controversy surrounds the issue of the increasing number of nongastroenterologists or nonformally trained physicians performing colonoscopy and other more complicated endoscopic procedures. Whereas some welcome this trend toward procedural decentralization as a potential benefit to patient access and physician compliance [67], others express alarm at the potential danger of compromised quality of care. Several retrospective reports of small colonoscopy series performed by practitioners who did not receive traditional mentored training in accredited programs suggest a high diagnostic yield and few complications [68–70]. These observations have led some to conclude that a postgraduate endoscopy fellowship is not necessary to achieve expertise in colonoscopy [68].

There are virtually no prospective data assessing technical and interpretive colonoscopy skill or patient outcomes with respect to the type of training or practice of the colonoscopist. Opinions have varied on the number of mentored procedures required to achieve clinical competency.

A prospective study by Cass *et al.* [71•] demonstrated that gastroenterology fellows achieved the cecum in only 84% of cases after having performed 100 mentored colonoscopies compared with a 94% success rate in cecal intubation among their mentors. In another report [72•], experienced colonoscopists were able to reach the cecum in more than 95% and with effort intubated the ileocecal valve in more than 70% of cases. Clearly, high level technical proficiency and, even more so, diagnostic acumen in colonoscopy increase with experience. Carefully designed studies are needed to help direct matters of quality control and credentialing in colonoscopy. For the most technically challenging diagnostic or therapeutic procedures, special advanced fellowships are now advocated by professional societies [73].

In an era of limited fiscal resources, the diagnostic and therapeutic armamentarium available to the colorectal endoscopist continues to expand. It is increasingly important to consider the appropriateness of instrumental interventions with respect to patient outcomes and cost in addition to the technique and quality of their application.

References and recommended reading

Papers of particular interest, published within the annual period of review, have been highlighted as:
- • Of special interest
- •• Of outstanding interest

1. AHLQUIST DA, WIEAND HS, MOERTEL CG, MCGILL DB, LOPRINZI CL, O'CONNELL MJ, MAILLIARD JA, GERSTNER JB, PANDYA K, ELLEFSON RD: **Accuracy of Fecal Occult Blood Screening for Colorectal Neoplasia: A Prospective Study Using Hemoccult and HemoQuant.** *JAMA* 1993, **269**:1262–1267.

2. • CAUFFMAN JG, HARA JH, RASGON IM, CLARK VA: **Flexible Sigmoidoscopy in Asymptomatic Patients With Negative Fecal Occult Blood Tests.** *J Fam Prac* 1992, 34:281–286.

Sigmoidoscopic findings in a group of 1000 asymptomatic persons 45 years or older with negative fecal occult blood test results.

3. •• REX DK, LEHMAN GA, ULBRIGHT TM, SMITH JJ, POUND DC, HAWES RH, HELPER DJ, WIERSEMA MJ, LANGEFELD CD, WEI LI MS: **Colonic Neoplasia in Asymptomatic Persons With Negative, Fecal Occult Blood Tests: Influence of Age, Gender, and Family History.** *Am J Gastroenterol* 1993, **88**:825–831.

Careful descriptive study of colonoscopic findings in 621 asymptomatic persons aged 50 to 75 years with negative fecal occult blood tests. Colorectal neoplasms were found in nearly 30%, including cancers in three persons.

4. •• NEWCOMB PA, NORFLEET RG, STORER BE, SURAWICZ TS, MARCUS PM: **Screening Sigmoidoscopy and Colorectal Cancer Mortality.** *J Natl Cancer Inst* 1992, **84**:1572–1575.

An excellent case-study demonstrating a significant benefit of periodic sigmoidoscopy, but not of fecal occult blood testing or digital examination, in reducing colorectal cancer mortality.

5. • ATKIN WS, CUZICK J, NORTHOVER JMA, WHYNES DK: **Prevention of Colorectal Cancer by One-Only Sigmoidoscopy.** *Lancet* 1993, **341**:736–740.

An editorial offering a cogent argument for the cost-effectiveness of once in a lifetime sigmoidoscopy screening at age 55 to 60 years.

6. KORETZ RL: **Malignant Polyps: Are They Sheep in Wolves' Clothing?** *Ann Intern Med* 1993, **118**:63–68.

7. SELBY JV, FRIEDMAN GD, QUESENBERRY CP JR, WEISS NS: **A Case-Control Study of Screening Sigmoidoscopy and Mortality From Colorectal Cancer.** *N Engl J Med* 1992, 326:653–657.

8. • LYNCH HT, SMYRK TC, WATSON P, LANSPA SJ, LYNCH JF, LYNCH PM, CAVALIERI J, BOLAND CR: **Genetics, Natural History, Tumor Spectrum, and Pathology of Hereditary Nonpolyposis Colorectal Cancer: An Updated Review.** *Gastroenterology* 1993, **104**:1535–1549.

A comprehensive update on the biology and chemical behavior of hereditary nonpolyposis colorectal cancer.

9. • VASEN JF, MECKLIN JP, WATSON P, UTSUNOMIYA J, BERTARIO L, LYNCH P, SVENDSEN LB, CRISTOFARO G, MULLER H, KHAN PM, LUNCH HT: **Surveillance in Hereditary Nonpolyposis Colorectal Cancer: An International Cooperative Study of 165 Families.** *Dis Colon Rectum* 1993, **36**:1–4.

A description of practice variations and diagnostic yields in surveillance programs for hereditary nonpolyposis colorectal cancer patients among nine major medical centers.

10. • VAN DER MEER JWM, WEENING RS, SCHELLEKENS PTA, VAN MUNSTER IP, NAGENGAST FM: **Colorectal Cancer in Patients With X-Linked Agammaglobulinaemia.** *Lancet* 1993, **341**:1439–1440.

Presentation of three unrelated cases of rapidly progressive colorectal cancer in three young adults with x-linked agammaglobulinaemia.

11. MEAGHER AP, STUART M: **Colonoscopy in Patients With a Family History of Colorectal Cancer.** *Dis Colon Rectum* 1992, **35**:315–321.

12. •• GUILLEM JG, FORDE KA, TREAT MR, NEUGUT AL, O'TOOLE KM, DIAMOND BE: **Colonoscopic Screening for Neoplasms in Asymptomatic First-Degree Relatives of Colon Cancer Patients. A Controlled, Prospective Study.** *Dis Colon Rectum* 1992, **35**:523–529.

A well done prospective comparison of colonoscopic findings in asymptomatic adults with and asymptomatic adults without a family history of colorectal cancer in first-degree relatives.

13. GISON PR, FOLINO M, ROSELLA O, FINCH CF, MOELLER I, ALEXEYEFF M, LINDLEY J, YOUNG GP: **Neoplasia and Hyperplasia of Large Bowel: Focal Lesions in an Abnormal Epithelium.** *Gastroenterology* 1992, **103**:1452–1459.

14. • BRADY PG, STRAKER RJ, MCCALVE SA, NORD HJ, PINKAS M, ROBINSON BE: **Are Hyperplastic Rectosigmoid Polyps Associated With an Increased Risk of Proximal Colonic Neoplasms?** *Gastrointest Endosc* 1993, **39**:481–485.

A prospective comparison of colonoscopic findings in asymptomatic persons aged 50 years or older whose screening sigmoidoscopy revealed diminutive hyperplastic polyps, diminutive adenomas, both, or neither.

15. • MATSUMOTO T, IIDA MITSUO, KUWANO Y, TADA S, YAO T, FUJISHIMA M: **Minute Non-Polypoid Adenoma of the Colon Detected by Colonoscopy: Correlation Between Endoscopic and Histologic Findings.** *Gastrointest Endosc* 1992, **38**:645–650.

A meticulous description of endoscopic and histologic findings in 34 nonpolypoid colorectal adenomas smaller than 5 mm.

16. • NUGENT KP, TALBOT IC, HODGSON SV, PHILLIPS RKS: **Solitary Juvenile Polyps: Not a Marker for Subsequent Malignancy.** *Gastroenterology* 1993, **105**:698–700.

The first long-term outcomes study of persons following removal of a solitary colorectal juvenile polyp. The risk of dying and of developing colorectal cancer was compared to that of an age- and sex-matched group from the general population.

17. •• WINAWER SJ, ZAUBER AG, O'BRIEN JM, HO MN, GOTTLIEB L, STERNBERG SS, WAYE JD, BOND J, SCHAPIRO M, STEWART ET, PANISH J, ACKROYD F, KURTZ RC, SHIKE M: **Randomized Comparison of Surveillance Intervals After Colonoscopic Removal of Newly Diagnosed Adenomatous Polyps.** *N Engl J Med* 1993, **328**:901–906.

A classically designed prospective study comparing the yield of metachronous adenomas in 1418 patients randomly assigned to surveillance colonscopy at either 1 and 3 years or 3 years only, following removal of an index adenoma.

18. BRULLET E, MONTANE JM, BOMBARDO J, BONFILL X, NOGUE
• M, BORDAS JM: **Intraoperative Colonoscopy in Patients With Colorectal Cancer**. *Br J Surg* 1992, 79:1376–1378.

A descriptive series of 67 consecutive patients with colorectal cancer undergoing intraoperative colonoscopy.

19. SAFI F, LINK KH, BEGER HG: **Is Follow-Up of Colorec-**
• **tal Cancer Patients Worthwhile?** *Dis Colon Rectum* 1993, 36:636–642.

An analysis of the salvage from intensive surveillance following colorectal cancer resection in 1045 consecutive patients.

20. LANGHOLZ E, MUNKHOLM P, DAVIDSEN M, BINDER V: **Colorec-**
•• **tal Cancer Risk and Mortality in Patients With Ulcerative Colitis**. *Gastroenterology* 1992, **103**:1444–1451.

A convincing cohort study of coloctomy rates, colorectal cancer risk in a general population based on the well-kept Danish statistics.

21. RUBIN CE, HAGGITT RC, BURMER GC, BRENTNALL TA, STEVENS
•• AC, LEVINE DS, DEAN PJ, KIMMEY M, PERERA DR, RABINOVITCH PS: **DNA Aneuploidy in Colonic Biopsies Predicts Future Development of Dysplasia in Ulcerative Colitis**. *Gastroenterology* 1992, **103**:1611–1620.

An excellent study describing DNA aneuploidy prevalence, its association with abnormal synchronous histology, and its predictive value for subsequent dysplasia in 81 patients with chronic ulcerative colitis undergoing regular surveillance colonoscopic biopsies.

22. BURMER GA, RABINOVITCH PS, HAGGIT RC, CRISPIN DA,
•• BRENTNALL TA, KOLLI VR, STEVENS AC, RUBIN CE: **Neoplastic Progression in Ulcerative Colitis: Histology, NDA Content, and Loss of a p53 Allele**. *Gastroenterology* 1992, **103**:1602–1610.

Careful molecular genetic analyses (single strand confirmation polymorphism analysis, DNA sequencing, and loss of heterozygosity studies) on colonoscopic biopsies showing dysplasia or cancer from 45 cancer patients with chronic ulcerative colities.

23. YIN J, HARPAZ N, TONY Y, HUANG Y, LAURIN J, GREENWALD
• BD, HONTANOSAS M, NEWKIRK C, MELTZER SJ: **p53 Point Mutations in Dysplastic and Cancerous Ulcerative Colitis Lesions**. *Gastroenterology* 1993, **104**:1633–1639.

A description of specific p53 point mutations in biopsies from a small number of ulcerative colitis patients with dysplasia and cancer.

24. BROOME U, LINDBERG G, LOFBERG R: **Primary Sclerosing**
• **Cholangitis in Ulcerative Colitis—A Risk Factor for the Development of Dysplasia and DNA Aneuploidy?** *Gastroenterology* 1992, **102**:1877–1880.

A comparison of colorectal cancer prevalence in a referred group of ulcerative colitis patients with and without primary scerlosing cholangitis.

25. CHOI PM, NUGENT FW, ROSSI RL: **Relationship Between Colorectal Neoplasia and Primary Sclerosing Cholangitis in Ulcerative Colitis**. *Gastroenterology* 1992, **103**:1707–1709.

26. CHOI PM, NUGENT FW, SCHOETZ DJ, SILVERMAN ML, HAGGIT
•• RC: **Colonoscopic Surveillance Reduces Mortality From Colorectal Cancer in Ulcerative Colitis**. *Gastroenterology* 1993, **105**:418–424.

An outcome analysis of 41 ulcerative colitis patients who developed colorectal cancer. Cancer stage and 5-year survival rates were compared between the 19 patients who had surveillance colonoscopies and the 22 patients who did not.

27. CHOI PM: **Predominance of Rectosigmoid Neoplasia in Ulcerative Colitis and Its Implication on Cancer Surveillance**. *Gastroenterology* 1993, **104**:666–667.

28. GIOVANNUCCI E, COLDITZ GA, STAMPFER MJ: **A Meta-Analysis**
• **of Cholecystectomy and Risk of Colorectal Cancer**. *Gastroenterology* 1993, **105**:130–141.

A meta-analysis of the nearly 60 studies addressing the relationship between cholecystectomy and colorectal cancer risk. Results were not adjusted for potentially confounding factors or for time since cholecystectomy.

29. EKBOM A, YUEN J, ADAMI HO, MCLAUGHLIN JK, CHOW WH,
•• PERSSON I, FRAUMENI JF: **Cholecystectomy and Colorectal Cancer**. *Gastroenterology* 1993, **105**:142–147.

A large population-based cohort study of 62,615 patients who underwent cholecystectomy and were followed long-term for the development of colorectal cancer. Proximal and distal colorectal cancers were evaluated separately.

30. SUADICANI P, HEIN HO, GYNTELBERG F: **Is the Use of Antihy-**
•• **pertensives and Sedatives a Major Risk Factor for Colorectal Cancer?** *Scnad J Gastroenterol* 1993, **28**:475–481.

An 18-year prospectively conducted cohort study of 5249 Danish men aged 40 to 59 years yielding the novel observation that the relative risk for colorectal cancer was significantly increased in the large subset of individuals chronically using sedative or anti hypertensitive medication. Results were adjusted for potentially confounding factors including smoke, alcohol, physical activity, and social class.

31. SURAWICZ CM, KIRBY P, CRITCHLOW C, SAYER J, DUNPHY
• C, KIVIAT N: **Anal Dysplasia in Homosexual Men: Role of Anoscopy and Biopsy**. *Gastroenterology* 1993, **105**:658–666.

A descriptive study of anoscopic findings in 90 selected gay men.

32. SCHOMACKER KT, FRISOLI JK, COMPTON CC, FLOTTE TJ,
• RICHTER JM, DEUTSCH TF, NISHIOKA NS: **Ultraviolet Laser-Induced Fluorescence of Colonic Polyps**. *Gastroenterology* 1992, **102**:1155–1156.

Using a probe fluorimeter, laser-induced native fluorescemce measurements were obtained of normal mucosa, hyperplastic polyps, and adenomas via colonoscopy.

33. SCHOMACKER KT, FRISOLI JK, COMPTON CC, FLOTTE TJ,
• RICHTER JM, NISHIOKA NS, DEUTSCH TF: **Ultraviolet Laser-Induced Fluorescence of Colonic Tissue: Basic Biology and Diagnostic Potential**. *Lasers Surg Med* 1992, **12**:63–78.

Laser-induced fluorescence of hyperplastic and neoplastic polyps were examined *in vivo* and *in vitro* with respect to tissue-specific fluorophores and to polyp morphology.

34. SUDAN DL, MELLINGER JD, MILLER SF, PETT JL: **Colono-**
• **scopic Indirect Lymphangiography**. *Gastrointest Endosc* 1993, **39**:179–181.

An ingenious approach to assesment of regional colonic lymph nodes. A new technique of colonoscopic mucosal injections of lymphangiographic dye is described in a dog model.

35. HAMMOND DC, LANE FR, MACKEIGAN JM, PASSINAULT WJ: **Endoscopic Tattooing of the Colon: Clinical Experience**. *Am Surg* 1993, **59**:205–210.

36. SOLOMON MJ, MCLEOD RS: **Endoluminal Transrectal Ultra-**
• **sonography: Accuracy, Reliability, and Validity**. *Dis Colon Rectum* 1993, **36**:200–205.

The accuracy of rectal cancer staging by endoluminal ultrasound is assessed based on a comprehensive review of reported studies.

37. HERZOG U, VON FLUE M, TONDELLI P, SCHUPPISSER JP: **How**
• **Accurate Is Endorectal Ultrasound in the Preoperative Staging of Rectal Cancer?** *Dis Colon Rectum* 1993, **36**:127–134.

A prospective descriptive study of the sensitivity, specificity, and predictive values of endoluminal ultrasound for staging rectal cancer.

38. SCIALPI M, ANDREATTA R, AGUGIARO S, ZOTTELE F, NICCOLINI
• M, PALMA FD: **Rectal Carcinoma: Preoperative Staging and Detection of Postoperative Local Recurrence With Transrectal and Transvaginal Ultrasound**. *Abdom Imaging* 1993, **18**:381–389.

Another prospective series of endoluminal ultrasound for staging rectal cancer. The additional diagnostic yield of the transvaginal approach is described.

39. MILSOM JW, LAVERY IC, STOLFI VM, CZYRKO C, CHURCH JM,
• OAKLEY JR, FAZIO VW: **The Expanding Utility of Endoluminal Ultrasonography in the Management of Rectal Cancer**. *Surgery* 1992, **112**:832–840.

A well-done prospective assessment of the accuracy of endorectal ultrasound for rectal cancer staging. results of ultrasound-guided lymph node biopsies are described.

40. SCIALPI M, ZOTTELE F, NICCOLINI M, DALLA PALMA F: **Transvaginal Echography in the Study of the Rectum. A New Method With Rectal Distension With Water.** *Radiologia Medica* 1993, **85**:203–208.

41. • ROMANO G, ESERCIZIO L, SANTANGELO M, VALLONE G, SANTANGELO ML: **Impact of Computed Tomography Vs. Intrarectal Ultrasound on the Diagnosis, Resectability, and Prognosis of Locally Recurrent Rectal Cancer.** *Dis Colon Rectum* 1993, 36:261–265.
The clinical utility of endoluminal ultrasound and computed tomography for the detection of locally recurrent rectal cancer are compared.

42. • HULSMANS FH, TIO TL, MATHUS-VLIEGEN EM, BOSMA A, TYTGAT GN: **Colorectal Villous Adenoma: Transrectal US in Screening for Invasive Malignancy.** *Radiology* 1992, **185**:193–196.
An assessment of the accuracy of transrectal ultrasound for the diagnosis of invasive cancer in large rectal villous adenomas in 81 patients.

43. HULSMANS FJ, MATHUS-VLIEGEN LM, BOSMAN S, BOSMA A, TYTGAT GN: **Colorectal Adenomas: Inflammatory Changes That Simulate Malignancy After Laser Coagulation—Evaluation With Transrectal US.** *Radiology* 1993, **187**:367–371.

44. • HILDEBRANDT U, KRAUS J, ECKER KW, SCHMID T, SCUDER G, FEIFEL G: **Endosonographic Differentiation of Mucosal and Transmural Non-Specific Inflammatory Bowel Disease.** *Endoscopy* 1992, 24:359–363.
An analysis of the accuracy of endoscopic ultrasound for distinguishing Crohn's disease (transmural inflammation) by comparison with histology on resected colorectal specimens.

45. • UCHIKAWA H, HIRAO M, YAMAGUTIO M: **Endoscopic Mucosal Resection Combined With Local Injection of Hypertonic Saline Epinephrine Solution for Early Colorectal Cancers and Other Tumors.** *Gastrointest Endosc* 1992, 39:606–607.
Another small series describing the safety and effectiveness of snare polypectomy following local injection of a hypertonic saline epinephrine solution into the polyp base.

46. • BECK DE, KARULF RE: **Laparoscopic-Assisted Full-Thickness Endoscopic Polypectomy.** *Dis Colon Rectum* 1993, 35:693–695.
A description of a laparoscopic approach to the removal of large colonic polyps in three patients.

47. FALK PM, BEART RW, WEXNER SD, THORSON AG, JAGELMAN DG, LAVERY IC, JOHANSEN OB, FITZGIBBONS RJ: **Laparoscopic Colectomy: A Critical Appraisal.** *Dis Colon Rectum* 1993, 36:28–34.

48. • AUBERT A, MEDURI B, FRITSCH J, AIME F, BAGLIN AC, BARBAGELATA B: **Colorectal Villous Tumors. Treatment by Electro-Resection and Laser Photocoagulation. 134 Cases.** *Presse Medical* 1992, **21**:2046–2049.
A description of a long-term outcome in a large series of patients with colorectal villous adenomas treated by the combination of electrosnare excision and laser coagulation.

49. ECKHAUSER ML, MANSOUR EG: **Endoscopic Laser Therapy for Obstructing and/or Bleeding Colorectal Carcinoma.** *Am Surg* 1992, **58**:358–363.

50. • TACKE W, PAECH S, KRUIS W, STUETZER H, MUELLER JM, ZIEGENHAGEN DJ, ZEHNTER E: **Comparison Between Endoscopic Laser and Different Surgical Treatments for Palliation of Advanced Rectal Cancer.** *Dis Colon Rectum* 1993, 36:377–381.
A nonrandomized retrospective comparison of palliative outcomes in patients with advanced rectal cancer who received either endoscopic laser or surgical therapy.

51. • VIGGIANO TR, ZIGHELBOIM J, AHLQUIST DA, GOSTOUT CJ, WANG KK, LARSON MV: **Endoscopic Nd:YAG Laser Coagulation of Bleeding From Radiation Proctopathy.** *Gastrointest Endosc* 1993, **39**:513–517.
A report of long-term outcomes in the largest single series of radiation proctopathy treated by a yttrium aluminum garnet laser. A total of 47 patients treated for medically refractory bleeding were followed for a mean of 13 months.

52. • TAYLOR JG, DISARIO JA, BUCHI KN: **Argon Laser Therapy for Hemorrhagic Radiation Proctitis: Long-Term Results.** *Gastrointest Endos* 1993, 39:641–644.
A description of outcomes in 14 patients with bleeding radiation proctopathy treated by argon laser.

53. SEOW-CHOEN F, HAK-SU G, EU KW, HO YH, TAY SK: **A Simple and Effective Treatment for Hemorrhagic Radiation Proctitis Using Formalin.** *Dis Colon Rectum* 1993, ??:135–138.

54. • HILTUNEN KM, SYRJA H, MATIKAINEN M: **Colonic Volvulus.** *Eur J Surg* 1992, **158**:607–611.
A retrospective population-based study of colonic volvulus with emphasis on radiographic diagnosis and endoscopic management.

55. • BLADEN JS, ANDERSON AP, BELL GD, RAMEH B, EVANS B, HEATLEY DJT: **Non-Radiological Technique for Three-Dimensional Imaging of Endoscopes.** *Lancet* 1993, **341**:719–722.
A clever new technique to display colonoscope position without radiography that employs an electromagnetic imaging system.

56. • WILLIAMS C, GUY C, GILLIES D, SAUNDERS B: **Electronic Three-Dimensional Imaging of Intestinal Endoscopy.** *Lancet* 1993, 341:724–725.
Another new technique for displaying colonoscope position.

57. • MATTER SE, RICE PS, CAMPBELL DR: **Colonic Lavage Solutions: Plain Versus Flavored.** *Am J Gastroenterol* 1993, **88**:49–52.
A randomized comparison of patient preference for flavored oral lavage solution.

58. • MARSHALL JB, PINEDA JJ, BARTHEL JS, KING PD: **Prospective, Randomized Trial Comparing Sodium Phosphate Solution With Polyethylene Glycol-Electrolyte Lavage for Colonoscopy Preparation.** *Gastrointest Endosc* 1993, **39**:631–634.
A randomized comparison of these two preparations in 153 patients. Outcomes of patients acceptance and quality of colonoscopic preparation were evaluated.

59. LEVER EL, WALTER MH, CONDON SC, BALASUBRAMANIAM K, CHEN YK, MITCHELL RD, HERBER R, COLLEN MJ: **Addition of Enemas to Oral Lavage Preparation for Colonoscopy Is Not Necessary.** *Gastrointest Endosc* 1992, **38**:369–372.

60. MARK DG, REX DK, LAPPAS JC: **Quality of Air Contrast Barium Enema Performed the Same Day As Incomplete Colonoscopy With Air Insufflation.** *Gastrointest Endosc* 1992, **38**:693–695.

61. • TURNER J, STURGEON CM: **Effect of Bowel Cleansing on Serum CEA Levels.** *J R Coll Surg Edinburg* 1993, **38**:89–91.
An interesting and novel observation of serum carcinoembryonic antigen elevations induced by colonoscopic preparations in patients with or without colorectal neoplasia.

62. • WAYE JD, LEWIS BS, YESSAYAN S: **Colonoscopy: A Prospective Report of Complications.** *Lancet* 1992, **15**:347–351.
A report of complications in a series of 2097 persons undergoing ambulatory colonoscopy by experienced colonoscopists.

63. DONCKIER V, ANDRE R: **Treatment of Colon Endoscopic Perforations.** *Acta Chirurgica Belgica* 1993, **93**:60–62.

64. •• STEVENSON GW, WILSON JA, WILKINSON J, NORMAN G, GOODACRE RL: **Pain Following Colonoscopy: Elimination With Carbon Dioxide.** *Gastrointest Endosc* 1992, **38**:564–567.
A carefully done and well-designed study prospectively comparing subjective responses (pain) and objective findings (radiographic gas distention) in patients undergoing colonoscopy that were randomly assigned to insufflation by air or by carbon dioxide.

65. IBER FL, SUTBERRY M, GUPTA R, KRUSS D: **Evaluation of Complications During and After Conscious Sedation for En-**

doscopy Using Pulse Oximetry. *Gastrointest Endosc* 1993, 39:620–625.

66. DISARIO JA, SANOWSKI RA: **Sigmoidoscopy Training for Nurses and Resident Physicians**. *Gastrointest Endosc* 1993, 39:29–32.
• A small, randomized comparison of patient outcomes with sigmoidscopy done by nurses or resident physicians who received comparable procedural training.

67. RODNEY NM: **Flexible Sigmoidoscopy and the Despecialization of Gastrointestinal Endoscopy. An Environmental Impact Report**. *Cancer* 1992, 70:1266–1271.

68. REED DN, COLLINS JD, WYATT WJ, HULL JE, PATTON ML, DAHM SO, DABIDEEN HH, HUDSON JC, ALLEN DB: **Can General Surgeons Perform Colonoscopy Safely?** *Am J Surg* 1992, **163**:257–259.

69. RODNEY WM, DABOV G, CRONIN C: **Evolving Colonoscopy Skills in a Rural Family Practice: The First 293 Cases**. *Fam Prac Res J* 1993, **13**:43–52.

70. GODREAU CJ: **Office-Based Colonoscopy in a Family Practice**. *Fam Prac Res J* 1992, **12**:313–320.

71. CASS CW, FREEMAN ML, PEINE CJ, ZERA RT, ONSTAD GR: **Objective Evaluation of Endoscopy Skills During Training**. *Ann Int Med* 1993, **118**:40–44.
• A nicely done prospective analysis of endoscopic technical skills relative to the extent of training.

72. MARSHALL JB, BARTHEL JS: **The Frequency of Total Colonoscopy and Terminal Ileal Intubation in the 1990's**. *Gastrointest Endosc* 1993, **39**:518–520.
• A description of the extent of colonoscopic intubation in a large consecutive series done by an expert colonoscopist at a single center.

73. SIVAK MV, VENNES JA, COTTON PB, GEENEN JE, BENJAMIN SB, LEHMAN GA: **Advanced Training Programs in Gastrointest Endoscopy**. *Gastrointest Endosc* 1993, **39**:462–464.

David A. Ahlquist, MD, Mayo Clinic, 200 First Street SW, 19th Floor, Rochester, MN 55905, USA.

Colorectal surgical conditions

Scott A. Strong, MD

The Cleveland Clinic Foundation, Cleveland, Ohio, USA

The past year's literature is replete with publications discussing a variety of colorectal topics. Many of the particularly useful articles concerning diverticulitis, the ileal pouch–anal anastomosis, laparoscopic colorectal surgery, rectal procidentia, stomas, surgical techniques, large bowel trauma, and assorted miscellaneous conditions are reviewed.

Current Opinion in Gastroenterology 1994, **10**:49–55

Diverticulitis

Diverticulitis is a well-recognized disease entity whose more virulent presentation in the younger population has been recently appreciated. Schauer *et al.* [1•] reported on 238 patients treated for diverticulitis, 61 were 40 years old or younger. The younger patients were primarily obese (82%) and more commonly required an urgent operation during their initial hospitalization for complications of diverticulitis. The most common surgical indication was perforation and recurrent disease for the younger and older age group, respectively. Moreover, the patients 40 years of age or younger had a sevenfold increase in the incidence of enteric fistulas compared with the older population. Conversely, Acosta *et al.* [2•] reviewed 86 patients admitted during a 6-year period for acute diverticulitis, 17 of whom were 40 years of age or younger. Whereas 41% of the younger patients and 54% of the older patients required urgent operation for their disease, the operative morbidity and mortality rates were equivalent.

To determine the better operative procedure for people with diffuse purulent or fecal peritonitis secondary to perforated left-sided colonic diverticulitis, Kronberg [3•] conducted a prospective, randomized trial. The patients were subjected to suture closure of the perforation with omental coverage and transverse colostomy ($n=31$) or resection and proximal end colostomy ($n=31$). Although no difference was found between the two groups in operative mortality associated with fecal peritonitis, the patients found to have purulent peritonitis demonstrated significantly better survival if suture closure and omental patching of the perforation with transverse colostomy was performed. The shorter length of stay noted in the resection group may, in part, reflect the higher mortality rate of this population.

Finally, as evidenced above, many patients undergoing emergent surgery for perforated diverticulitis warrant diversion with reconstitution of the alimentary tract at a later date. Pearce *et al.* [4•] reviewed the outcome of 80 patients undergoing reversal of their colostomy after a Hartmann's procedure. Multifactorial analysis indicated that the interval between the initial and secondary procedure was the most critical factor in predicting operative morbidity and length of hospitalization. Clinical evidence of anastomotic leak was found in six of 12 patients when the interval was less than 3 months, seven of 28 patients for an interval of 3 to 6 months, and zero of 40 patients when the interval was longer than 6 months. All deaths ($n=3$) and clinical septicemia ($n=4$) occurred in the earlier groups.

Ileal pouch–anal anastomosis

Total proctocolectomy and ileal pouch–anal anastomosis (IPAA) is considered by many to be the operation of choice for mucosal ulcerative colitis (MUC) warranting surgical intervention. However, in the severely toxic case, subtotal colectomy with ileostomy and preservation of the rectosigmoid stump remains the favored treatment. The stump can be matured as a mucous fistula, closed and left intraperitoneal, or closed and implanted

Abbreviations

BAR—biofragmentable anastomotic ring; **FAP**—familial adenomatous polyposis; **IPAA**—ileal pouch–anal anastomosis; **MUC**—mucosal ulcerative colitis.

 ISBN 1-85922-606-X ISSN 0267–1379

in the subcutaneous tissue. Ng *et al.* [5•] reported on 32 patients treated at two institutions where the stump was closed (23 stapled, four sutured, and five stapled and sutured) and implanted above the fascia level at the inferior aspect of the wound; a rectal drainage tube was placed transanally in 15 patients. Although seven patients experienced postoperative difficulties, only two required operative treatment (necrotizing fasciitis and intra-abdominal sepsis). At the time of restorative surgery, the rectosigmoid stump was readily identified in all cases. This technique offers an attractive alternative in the management of toxic colitis as long as surgical principles are recalled (*ie,* tension-free delivery of the rectosigmoid stump).

To see if this operation influenced the results of IPAA in patients with MUC, Penna *et al.* [6•] evaluated the effect of previous subtotal colectomy with ileostomy and sigmoidostomy on the outcome of IPAA. The group undergoing a three-stage IPAA ($n=55$) was compared with another population of colitics subjected to the conventional two-stage operation ($n=78$). The three-stage group underwent completion proctectomy, IPAA, and loop ileostomy within 6 months (median, 4 months) of their initial procedure. The incidence of pelvic abscess and postoperative occlusion was actually lower in the three-stage group, as was the average number of daily bowel movements (5.1 vs 5.9) 3 months postileostomy closure. After 1 year, the occurrence of daytime stools, nocturnal stools, incontinence, need for a pad, and use of antidiarrheals was equivalent between the two operative groups. Previous subtotal colectomy with ileostomy and sigmoidostomy did not adversely influence the outcome of subsequent IPAA in patients with MUC.

In familial adenomatous polyposis (FAP), the use of the IPAA, as opposed to ileoproctostomy, is more controversial because of concerns of compromised function. Accordingly, Penna *et al.* [7•] compared the functional results of FAP patients before and after conversion of an ileoproctostomy to an IPAA. For 21 patients with more than 12 months follow-up, the average number of daily stools was 3.8 before and 4.6 after conversion. Furthermore, daytime and nocturnal continence was unchanged. Overall, 90% of patients said that their lifestyle was the same or improved following the conversion. The authors suggest that an IPAA be recommended to polyposis patients at relatively increased risk for rectal carcinoma.

The question left unanswered by Penna *et al.* [7•] was how the results of IPAA in FAP compared with those in MUC; however, Tjandra *et al.* [8•] were able to retrospectively examine this issue. In FAP ($n=39$) and MUC ($n=39$) groups matched for demographics, pouch configuration, pouch construction, and duration of follow-up (median of 32 months), the duration of operation, length of hospital stay, and operative blood loss were similar. And, although the overall and pouch-related complication rates were higher in the MUC group, the functional results (*ie,* daytime stools, nighttime stools, time to defer defecation, nocturnal seepage, and use of antidiarrheals) were no different. Moreover, an analog scale estimating quality of life, health, and satisfaction with outcome was identical for the two disease groups, scoring 9 out of a possible 10 (10 representing the highest level).

While acceptance of the procedure grows, debate over techniques employed for the construction of a pelvic reservoir continues with a report from Luukkonen and Jarvinen [9••]. The authors prospectively randomly assigned 40 consecutive patients to a hand-sutured anastomosis with mucosectomy ($n=19$) or a double-stapled anastomosis without mucosectomy ($n=21$). Although the group numbers were small, there was no significant difference in the occurrence of anastomotic leakage, anastomotic stricture, or pouch-vaginal fistula. At both 3 and 6 months follow-up, stool frequency, nighttime evacuation, and mucous leakage were similar for the two operative groups. The relative decrease in maximal resting pressure was 30% and 27% for the hand-sewn and stapled group, respectively. In conclusion, the authors found no advantage associated with a double-stapled IPAA, rather, the need for annual surveillance is eliminated with mucosectomy and hand-sutured IPAA.

A temporary ileostomy is traditionally created in patients who undergo IPAA to lessen the risk of pelvic sepsis while the pouch and anastomosis heal. Grobler *et al.* [10•], however, performed a randomized study of 45 patients to examine the role of loop ileostomy in patients receiving a totally stapled IPAA. Entry criteria required the absence of anastomotic leak on intraoperative testing and technical satisfaction on the part of the surgeon, although this was not objectively defined. Of patients with an ileostomy ($n=23$) and those nondiverted ($n=22$), the incidence of anastomotic wound infection, pelvic sepsis, and pouchitis were similar. No mortalities occurred, but ileostomy complications affected 52% of patients. Although the relative risk of pelvic sepsis is low in IPAA without diversion, objective criteria (*eg,* steroid and immunosuppressant dosages, albumin levels) are not mentioned and the study numbers are too small to draw significant conclusions.

In a nonrandomized fashion, Sagar *et al.* [11•] similarly compared patients who underwent IPAA with ($n = 28$) and without ($n = 30$) the use of a temporary, diverting loop ileostomy. The decision for or against an ileostomy was made at the completion of the procedure based on urgency of the procedure, toxemia, anastomotic tension, pelvic hemostasis, and integrity of anastomoses. High dosages of preoperative steroids were not a contraindication to ileostomy omission. The two operative groups were similar in demographics, diagnoses, duration of disease, disease distribution, and steroid usage. The length of stay (excluding the hospitalization for ileostomy closure) and incidence of pelvic sepsis, anastomotic stricture, and bowel obstruction were no different between the groups. As in the study cited earlier, the small numbers make meaningful interpretation of the data difficult. However, it would appear from these two reports that fecal diversion may be safely omitted in select patients subjected to IPAA by surgeons experienced with this procedure.

The anastomotic stricturing and anovaginal fistula that sometimes complicate restorative proctocolectomy do not necessarily mandate a poor outcome or pouch loss; rather, Fazio and Tjandra [12•] described an operative technique useful in these cases. Following mechanical and antibiotic bowel preparation, a circumferential incision is made just distal to the anastomotic stricture or internal os of the fistula. The dissection then continues in the plane between the ileal pouch and underlying sphincter muscles. The fully mobilized pouch can be delivered beyond the anal verge and the diseased segment amputated. A hand-sutured neopouch–anal anastomosis is subsequently created. This technique was successfully used in three patients, although one person experienced minor nocturnal seepage.

Laparoscopy

As the experience with laparoscopy increases, its use in large bowel surgery will become more defined. A prospective evaluation of laparoscopic ($n = 29$) versus open appendectomy ($n = 36$) was conducted with randomization precluded by instrument availability [13••]. Of the patients studied, the two operative groups were demographically similar. Although two of the laparoscopic cases were converted to open cases because of technical difficulties, the average operative time did not differ between groups. However, the average length of stay, the wound infection rate, and the median number of analgesic injections were significantly less in the laparoscopic group. The results suggest that emergent laparoscopic appendectomy by experienced surgeons may be an improvement over open appendectomy.

Whereas prospective, randomized studies have been performed for laparoscopic cholecystectomy and appendectomy, no such studies exist for colectomies. However, a few retrospective, multicenter series have been published. Phillips *et al.* [14] presented their experience with 51 consecutive patients who underwent laparoscopic colectomies for carcinoma ($n = 24$), diverticulitis ($n = 13$), villous adenoma ($n = 6$), sessile polyp ($n = 3$), and other miscellaneous conditions ($n = 5$). Of these laparoscopic surgeries, 14% were converted to facilitated procedures and 8% were converted to open operations. The surgeries lasted an average of 2.3 hours (range 1.25 to 6.5 hours), with all but two patients passing flatus on the first postoperative day. No parenteral medications were prescribed after the second postoperative day as they were discontinued when the patient was able to tolerate oral medications. The length of hospitalization averaged 4.6 days (range 1 to 30 days) and the major morbidity and mortality rates were 8% and 2%, respectively.

Falk *et al.* [15], representing four institutions, described 66 laparoscopic or laparoscopic-assisted operations including sigmoid colectomy ($n = 19$), right hemicolectomy ($n = 15$), low anterior resection ($n = 6$), colectomy with IPAA ($n = 5$), and abdominoperineal resection ($n = 3$). The conversion, major morbidity, and mortality rate were 41%, 24%, and 0%, respectively. The average length of stay for laparoscopic right hemicolectomies and sigmoid colectomies was approximately 5 days. Obviously, laparoscopic colectomies can be performed by experienced surgeons but the overall benefit and appropriateness for tumor resection remains undocumented.

Rectal procidentia

The preferred operation for rectal procidentia and its accompanying dysfunctional complaints remains unclear, due in part to a poor understanding of the disease components. For example, persistent rectoanal inhibition has been suggested as a cause for associated fecal incontinence. To test this notion, Farouk *et al.* [16] compared 22 patients with rectal prolapse to 17 control patients. All subjects underwent anal manometry and ambulatory fine-wire electromyography of the internal sphincter, external sphincter, and puborectalis. In the prolapse group, the patients were studied before and 3 to 4 months after transabdominal resection and rectopexy with bilateral division of the lateral stalks. Although the internal anal sphincter electromyography frequency and canal resting pressures were improved postoperatively, the levels were still significantly lower than the control population. However, of the 16 patients with a preoperatively absent rectoanal inhibitory reflex, all subjects recovered the reflex postoperatively. Unfortunately, the authors omitted the information necessary to correlate the objective data with functional outcome in these patients with corrected rectal prolapse.

Transperineal correction of rectal prolapse is advocated by some, particularly in the elderly patient. Williams *et al.* [17•] performed perineal proctosigmoidectomy for complete rectal prolapse in 114 patients, the majority of whom were aged over 70 years. Whereas the median hospital stay was 4 days, only 12% of the patients suffered significant postoperative complications. Eleven patients (10%) developed recurrent full thickness rectal prolapse during the follow-up period that averaged 12 months. Of importance, fecal incontinence affected 67 patients preoperatively with 11 treated by concomitant levatorplasty; perineal proctosigmoidectomy and levatorplasty dramatically improved fecal incontinence (91%) compared with proctosigmoidectomy alone (46%).

In search of the better abdominal operation, Luukkonen *et al.* [18••] prospectively randomly assigned 30 patients undergoing transabdominal repair of rectal prolapse to either rectopexy and sigmoid resection ($n=15$) or polyglycolic acid mesh rectopexy alone ($n=15$). A single mortality occurred in the rectopexy with resection group whereas there was safe and effective control of the procidentia in both groups. After 6 months of follow-up, anal pressures were similarly elevated between the two operative groups and the rates of improved fecal continence were equivalent. However, five of the 15 patients treated by rectopexy alone experienced severe constipation postoperatively, a condition which did not occur in the rectopexy with resection group. Although the group numbers were small, the results suggest that rectopexy with sigmoid resection can safely correct rectal prolapse without risking the severe constipation associated with mesh rectopexy alone.

Stomas

Although the construction and use of colostomies has been detailed for decades, some traditional notions have been recently challenged. For instance, Majno *et al.* [19•] retrospectively reviewed 67 loop transverse colostomies (26 right upper quadrant and 41 right iliac fossa) created over a 4-year period. Although no patients with stomas sited in the iliac fossa complained of problems, many with right upper quadrant colostomies experienced difficulties visualizing the stoma and three of the 26 ostomates had problems with the appliance restricting their lifestyle. Despite past teachings, the right iliac fossa may be the preferred location for a loop transverse colostomy.

Furthermore, a laparotomy may not be necessary for colostomy creation. Trephine stoma formation, in which an end stoma is constructed without formal laparotomy, was successfully performed by Anderson *et al.* [20•] in 24 of 27 patients. Of this group, 22 colostomies and two ileostomies were created. To ease sigmoid colostomy construction, the bowel was delivered to the skin level at a previously marked site and the rectum was insufflated to identify the distal limb. Compared with patients undergoing laparotomy solely for stoma construction during the same 4-year period, the trephine stoma was associated with a shorter operative time and the patients required a smaller dosage of opiates postoperatively. At a median follow-up of 12 months, two patients suffered stomal prolapse; one of these also demonstrated a parastomal hernia.

Finally, in order to determine the optimal timing of sigmoid colostomy maturation, Roed-Petersen *et al.* [21••] randomly assigned 100 patients to immediate (created at laparotomy) or delayed maturation (opened on day 1 and matured on day 10). The mortality rate was equal (4%) between the two treatment groups with the length of stay and incidence of stoma gangrene, retraction, and separation similar. Although follow-up was too brief to adequately determine the occurrence of stenosis and parastomal herniation, the authors of this study now advocate immediate colostomy maturation.

Techniques

The usefulness of the biofragmentable anastomotic ring (BAR) anastomosis continues to be championed by some authors. A randomized, prospective study was designed by Gullichsen *et al.* [22••] to determine the efficacy of the BAR anastomosis ($n=79$) compared with a two-layer sutured anastomosis ($n=71$) in 150 consecutive patients undergoing surgery of the large intestine. Patients were excluded if the bowel diameter was too narrow to accommodate the smallest BAR device (28 mm). Whereas the duration of postoperative ileus and length of stay were similar between the two groups, the overall mortality rates were 1% and 6% for the BAR and sutured anastomoses, respectively. Clinically evident anastomotic leaks occurred in two patients with a BAR anastomosis and three patients with a sutured anastomosis; a single anastomotic stricture complicated each group. The BAR anastomosis appears to be a safe alternative in patients undergoing colonic surgery.

Despite the employment of sophisticated mechanical devices, anastomotic breakdown continues to complicate colorectal anastomoses. In order to obviate this problem, Yalin *et al.* [23•] prospectively evaluated end-to-end stapled colorectal anastomoses, correlating a positive air test and completeness of the doughnuts with clinical evidence of an anastomotic leak. In 21 consecutive patients, 11 high, six low, and four very low coloproctostomies were constructed. Only one patient demonstrated incomplete doughnuts, but with anastomotic disruption confirmed by air testing, another four patients demonstrated an air leak. Three of the air leaks were repaired by suture reinforcement and the remaining two disruptions (both in very low anastomoses) were treated by proximal diversion. The only clinical anastomotic leak developed in the patient who had a very low anterior resection, incomplete doughnuts, positive air leak, and proximal diversion. Although the study does not prove an untreated air leak will result in a clinically apparent anastomotic disruption, the association seems empirically valid.

Nonpalpable lesions of the colon can be difficult to locate intraoperatively making appropriate resection arduous and frustrating. Hammond *et al.* [24•] employed endoscopic tattooing in 12 patients for 15 lesions (one in the right colon, four in the transverse colon, three in the descending colon, and seven in the sigmoid colon). Approximately 1 to 2 mL of 1% indocyanine green was injected in two to three sites around each lesion. Tattooing was performed within 36 hours of the planned resection and was considered successful in all cases as a large serosal stain was readily visualized on the surface of the injected bowel. In one case, penetration of the needle through the bowel wall had occurred without an untoward reaction. In another instance, an inflammatory infiltrate was noted histologically at the injection site; the injections did not otherwise effect pathologic interpretation of the tattooed lesions. Of particular importance, unlike many other agents, indocyanine green is approved for this use by the US Food and Drug Administration.

Trauma

Falcone *et al.* [25••] studied colorectal trauma in a prospective, randomized, controlled manner to determine a preferred method of managing severe colon and intraperitoneal rectal injury. The study inclusion criteria consisted of injuries occupying more than 25% of the bowel circumference, hypotension on arrival or intraoperatively, blood loss exceeding 1500 mL, at least three associated organ injuries, fecal contamination, and the degree of injury mandated colon resection. Patients expiring within 24 hours of presentation, operated on elsewhere, and presenting more than 8 hours after injury were excluded. Patients were randomized intraoperatively to group 1—primary repair or anastomosis with intracolonic bypass using the Coloshield (Deknatel, Fall River, MA) ($n=11$) or group 2—colostomy ($n=11$). The two groups possessed similar demographics, mechanisms of injury, severities of injury, and operative morbidity rates. The colostomy group tended to have a longer length of stay and cost of hospitalization. Although the study numbers are small, primary repair or anastomosis with intracolonic bypass appears to be a safe alternative to colostomy in severe large bowel trauma.

Ivatury *et al.* [26•] also studied penetrating injuries of the colon in a prospective manner with definitive management emphasized. Injuries in the 252 patients were managed by repair ($n=159$), resection and anastomosis ($n=26$), or exteriorized repair ($n=34$). Colostomy ($n=33$) was reserved for left-sided injuries requiring resection or for delayed treatment. As expected, the injury severity indices were higher in the exteriorized repair group than the simple repair population. Of the 219 patients treated without a colostomy, 205 (94%) did well. In the repair and resection with anastomosis groups, only three patients developed an anastomotic leak; eight of the 34 exteriorized repairs experienced suture-line breakdown necessitating conversion to a colostomy. In conclusion, the majority of penetrating midgut colon injuries can be safely managed without diversion in hemodynamically stable patients.

Miscellaneous

Setya *et al.* [27•] reported one of the largest series of massive lower gastrointestinal hemorrhage managed by blind subtotal colectomy when localization of the bleeding source was unsuccessful despite multiple and varied diagnostic modalities. Although the bleeding was controlled in all 12 cases, four patients died and five of the eight survivors experienced complications; diverticulosis was suspected to be the leading cause of the hemorrhage. The results indicate that blind subtotal colectomy for massive lower gastrointestinal hemorrhage is an effective yet formidable procedure with serious morbidity and mortality.

Medich *et al.* [28•] detailed the role of laparotomy in the treatment of severe pseudomembranous colitis. Over a 27-month period, 12 patients required 14 laparotomies for *Clostridium difficile* colitis. Most patients demonstrated pyrexia, abdominal tenderness, leukocytosis, and ileus. However, only six patients (50%) suffered from diarrhea. Operative treatment of the patients included nontherapeutic laparotomy ($n = 7$), segmental resection ($n = 3$), and subtotal colectomy with ileostomy ($n = 4$). Although the APACHE II (Acute Physical and Chronic Health Evaluation) scores were not significantly different between the three groups, the treatment failure rates were 57%, 67%, and 0%, respectively. If operative therapy is indicated for severe pseudomembranous colitis unresponsive to medical therapy, subtotal colectomy with ileostomy should be considered.

Diversion colitis is a well-recognized entity that affects bypassed large intestine. However, the actual incidence of this entity and its adverse impact on colostomy closure was unclear until Orsay *et al.* [29••] studied these questions prospectively. After excluding those with Crohn's disease and ulcerative colitis, 34 asymptomatic patients underwent endoscopy with biopsy of their bypassed segment prior to colostomy closure. After an average of 26 weeks of diversion, 74% of patients demonstrated mild-to-severe colitis with biopsies displaying varying degrees of inflammation. The complication rate associated with colostomy closure was not significantly different between the diversion colitis patients and the normal population.

References and recommended reading

Papers of particular interest, published within the annual period of review, have been highlighted as:

- • Of special interest
- •• Of outstanding interest

1. • SCHAUER PR, RAMOS R, GHIATAS AA, SIRINEK KR: **Virulent Diverticular Disease in Young Obese Men.** *Am J Surg* 1992, **164**:443–448.

A review of 238 patients with diverticulitis revealed that those under the age of 40 years more commonly required an urgent operation during their initial hospitalization.

2. • ACOSTA JA, GRABENC ML, DOBERNECK RC, MCCARTHY JD, FRY DE: **Colonic Diverticular Disease in Patients 40 Years Old or Younger.** *Am Surg* 1992, **58**:605–607.

A report of 86 patients with diverticulitis showed age did not influence the need for urgent operation, operative morbidity, or operative mortality.

3. • KRONBERG O: **Treatment of Perforated Sigmoid Diverticulitis: A Prospective Randomized Trial.** *Br J Surg* 1993, **80**:505–507.

A prospective, randomized trial to elucidate the better treatment of perforated diverticulitis. If purulent peritonitis was present, patients subjected to suture closure of the perforation, omental coverage, and proximal diversion did better than those treated by resection and colostomy.

4. • PEARCE NW, SCOTT SD, KARRAN SJ: **Timing and Method of Reversal of Hartmann's Procedure.** *Br J Surg* 1992, **79**:839–841.

A retrospective report studied 80 patients undergoing reversal of their Hartmann's procedure. The best outcome occurred with waiting at least 6 months, as opposed to sooner, between the initial and secondary procedure.

5. • NG RLH, DAVIES AH, GRACE RH, MORTENSEN NJ: **Subcutaneous Rectal Stump Closure After Emergency Subtotal Colectomy.** *Br J Surg* 1992, **79**:701–703.

Subcutaneous implantation of the rectosigmoid stump after colectomy for toxic colitis possesses an acceptable rate of attributable complications.

6. • PENNA C, DAUDE F, PARC R, TIRET E, FRILEUX P, HANNOUN L, NORDLINGER B, LEVY E: **Previous Subtotal Colectomy With Ileostomy and Sigmoidostomy Improves the Morbidity and Early Functional Results After Ileal Pouch-Anal Anastomosis in Ulcerative Colitis.** *Dis Colon Rectum* 1993, **36**:343–348.

A total of 55 patients undergoing a three-stage ileal pouch–anal anastomosis for ulcerative colitis had similar functional results and lower morbidity than a demographically matched group who underwent a traditional two-stage procedure.

7. • PENNA CP, TIRET E, KARTHEUSER AH, FRILEUX P, HANNOUN L, NORDLINGER B, PARC R: **Comparison of Functional Results of Ileorectal and Ileo-Anal Anastomoses in Familial Adenomatous Polyposis. Conversions of Ileorectal Anastomoses Into Ileo-Anal Anastomoses.** *Gastroenterol Clin Biol* 1992, **16**:401–405.

Of 21 patients with familial adenomatous polyposis who had conversion of their ileoproctostomy to a pelvic reservoir, 90% experienced a comparable or improved lifestyle.

8. • TJANDRA JJ, FAZIO VW, CHURCH JM, OAKLEY JR, MILSOM JW, LAVERY IC: **Similar Functional Results After Restorative Proctocolectomy in Patients With Familial Adenomatous Polyposis and Mucosal Ulcerative Colitis.** *Am J Surg* 1993, **165**:322–325.

Patients who received a pelvic pouch for familial adenomatous polyposis were compared with a matched cohort of ulcerative colitics undergoing the same procedure; although the morbidity rate was higher in the later group, the functional outcome was similar.

9. •• LUUKKONEN P, JARVINEN H: **Stapled Vs Hand-Sutured Ileoanal Anastomosis in Restorative Proctocolectomy. A Prospective, Randomized Study.** *Arch Surg* 1993, **128**:437–440.

The double-stapled ileal pouch-anal anastomosis provides no advantages compared with a hand-sewn anastomosis.

10. • GROBLER SP, HOSIE KB, KEIGHLEY MRB: **Randomized Trial of Loop Ileostomy in Restorative Proctocolectomy.** *Br J Surg* 1992, **79**:903–906.

A prospective, randomized study suggests that a diverting loop ileostomy can be safely omitted in select patients requiring a restorative proctolectomy.

11. Sagar PM, Lewis W, Holdsworth PJ, Johnston D: **One-Stage Restorative Proctocolectomy Without Temporary Defunctioning Ileostomy.** *Dis Colon Rectum* 1992, 35:582–588.
• This prospective, nonrandomized study suggests that a diverting loop ileostomy can be safely omitted in select patients requiring a restorative proctolectomy.

12. Fazio VW, Tjandra JJ: **Pouch Advancement and Neoileoanal Anastomosis for Anastomotic Stricture and Anovaginal Fistula Complicating Restorative Proctocolectomy.** *Br J Surg* 1992, 79:694–696.
• The authors describe a technique of ileal pouch advancement whereby pelvic reservoirs complicated by anastomotic stricture or anovaginal fistula may be salvaged.

13. McAnena OJ, Austin O, O'Connell PR, Hederman WP, Gorey TF, Fitzpatrick J: **Laparoscopic Versus Open Appendectomy: A Prospective Evaluation.** *Br J Surg* 1992, 79:818–820.
•• A prospective, randomized study showing that laparoscopic appendectomy may be an improvement over the open procedure because of shorter hospital stays and less postoperative pain.

14. Phillips EH, Franklin M, Carroll BJ, Fallas MJ, Ramos R, Rosenthal D: **Laparoscopic Colectomy.** *Ann Surg* 1992, 216:703–708.

15. Falk PM, Beart RW Jr, Wexner SD, Thorson AG, Jagelman DG, Lavery IC, Johansen OB, RJ Jr: **Laparoscopic Colectomy: A Critical Appraisal.** *Dis Colon Rectum* 1993, 36:28–34.

16. Farouk R, Duthie GS, Bartolo DCC, MacGregor AB: **Restoration of Continence Following Rectopexy for Rectal Prolapse and Recovery of the Internal Anal Sphincter Electromyogram.** *Br J Surg* 1992, 79:439–440.

17. Williams JG, Rothenberger DA, Madoff RD, Goldberg SM: **Treatment of Rectal Prolapse in the Elderly by Perineal Proctosigmoidectomy.** *Dis Colon Rectum* 1992, 35:830–834.
• This paper reviews 114 patients treated by transperineal correction of rectal prolapse showing the procedure can be safely performed with acceptable recurrence rates.

18. Luukkonen P, Mikkonen U, Jarvinen H: **Abdominal Rectopexy With Sigmoidectomy Vs Rectopexy Alone for Rectal Prolapse.** *Int J Colorectal Dis* 1992, 4:219–222.
•• A prospective, randomized study suggesting that rectopexy with sigmoid resection can safely correct rectal prolapse without risking the severe constipation associated with polyglycolic acid mesh rectopexy alone.

19. Majno PE, Lees VC, Goodwin K, Everett WG: **Siting a Transverse Colostomy.** *Br J Surg* 1992, 79:576–577.
• Loop transverse colostomies may be more appropriately sited in the right iliac fossa than in the traditional right upper quadrant location.

20. Anderson ID, Hill J, Vohra R, Schofield PF, Kiff ES: **An Improved Means of Faecal Diversion: The Trephine Stoma.** *Br J Surg* 1992, 79:1080–1081.
• Trephine stoma formation may safely obviate the need for a laparotomy incision.

21. Roed-Petersen K, Andersen B, Baden H, Burcharth: **Morbidity After Immediate and Delayed Opening of Sigmoid End Colostomy: A Randomised Trial.** *Eur J Surg* 1992, 158:495–497.
•• This randomized, prospective study indicates that a sigmoid colostomy can be primarily matured without subjecting the patient to additional sequelae.

22. Gullichsen R, Havia T, Ovaska J, Rantala A: **Colonic Anastomosis Using the Biofragmentable Anastomotic Ring and Manual Suture: A Prospective Randomized Trial.** *Br J Surg* 1992, 79:578–580.
•• The biofragmentable anastomotic ring compared favorably with a two-layered sutured anastomosis in a prospective, randomized trial.

23. Yalin R, Aktan O, Yegen C, Dosluoglu H, Okboy N: **Importance of Testing Stapled Rectal Anastomoses With Air.** *Eur J Surg* 1993, 159:49–51.
• Testing of rectal anastomoses with air insufflation may identify otherwise unnoticed leaks that may be clinically significant.

24. Hammond DC, Lane FR, Mackeigan JM, Passinault WJ: **Endoscopic Tattooing of the Colon: Clinical Experience.** *Am Surg* 1993, 59:205–210.
• Endoscopic tattooing of colonic lesions with idocyanine green safely assists in identifying nonpalpable lesions.

25. Falcone RE, Wanamaker SR, Santanello SA, Carey LC: **Colorectal Trauma: Primary Repair or Anastomosis With Intracolonic Bypass Vs. Ostomy.** *Dis Colon Rectum* 1992, 35:957–963.
•• In a randomized fashion, the authors showed that primay repair or anastomosis with intracolonic bypass appears to be a safe alternative to colostomy in severe large bowel trauma.

26. Ivatury RR, Gaudino J, Nallathambi MN, Simon RJ, Kazigo ZJ, Stahl WM: **Definitive Treatment of Colon Injuries: A Prospective Study.** *Am Surg* 1993, 59:43–49.
• The majority of penetrating right and transverse colon injuries can be safely managed without diversion in hemodynamically stable patients.

27. Setya V, Singer JA, Minken SL: **Subtotal Colectomy As a Last Resort for Unrelenting, Unlocalized, Lower Gastrointestinal Hemorrhage.** *Am Surg* 1992, 58:295–299.
• Blind subtotal colectomy for massive lower gastrointestinal hemorrhage is an effective yet formidable procedure with serious morbidity and mortality.

28. Medich DS, Lee KK, Simmons RL, Grubbs PE, Yang HC, Showalter DP: **Laparotomy for Fulminant Pseudomembranous Colitis.** *Arch Surg* 1992, 127:847–853.
• If operative therapy is indicated for severe pseudomembranous colitis unresponsive to medical therapy, subtotal colectomy with ileostomy should be considered.

29. Orsay CP, Kim DO, Pearl RK, Abcarian H: **Diversion Colitis in Patients Scheduled for Colostomy Closure.** *Dis Colon Rectum* 1993, 36:366–367.
•• Diversion colitis, a common sequela of fecal diversion, has no untoward effects when bowel continuity is restored.

Scott A. Strong, MD, Department of Colorectal Surgery, The Cleveland Clinic Foundation, 9500 Euclid Avenue, Cleveland, OH 44195-5044, USA.

Gastrointestinal infections

Editorial overview

Sherwood L. Gorbach, MD

Tufts University School of Medicine, Boston, Massachusetts, USA

Current Opinion in Gastroenterology 1994, **10**:57–58

The field of gastrointestinal infections has seen significant progress during the past year. Not only have there been good clinical and therapeutic studies, but what is particularly encouraging is the application of molecular biology to our basic understanding of these illnesses. Laboratory science has elucidated the pathogenesis of several types of intestinal infections. In addition, the techniques of polymerase chain reaction (PCR) and genetic probes have provided new diagnostic tests for the infectious agents.

Christine Wanke (pp 59–65) has reviewed infections involving the small intestine, including infections in HIV-positive persons and in travelers. The immunocompromised status of HIV-infected patients makes them susceptible to intestinal pathogens of all types. Bacteremia caused by *Salmonella*, *Campylobacter* and *Shigella* has been observed in AIDS patients. Many of these individuals go on to develop chronic, persistent infections with recurrent waves of bacteremia. New protozoan pathogens have been described in AIDS patients, including two genera of *Microsporidia.* A coccidian organism recently named *Cyclospora* has recently been described. Infections in travelers continue to be investigated, and new pathogens have been identified. US troops in Operation Desert Storm had a 57% incidence of diarrheal disease after 2 months in Saudi Arabia. Water- and food-borne outbreaks of diarrhea have been associated with *Salmonella* and *Escherichia coli* O157:87. A massive epidemic of cryptosporidiosis was reported in Milwaukee, Wisconsin, involving 200,000 individuals.

Colonic infections, reviewed by Jeffrey Griffiths (pp 66–73), involve several types of organisms, such as *Shigella*, *Clostridium difficile*, *Campylobacter*, *Entamoeba histolytica*, and *E. coli* O157:87. The pathogenesis of shigellosis has been elegantly described by using molecular techniques. *E. coli* O157:87 has emerged as a major pathogen in the United States. The illness is hemorrhagic colitis, often associated with hemolytic-uremic syndrome. Resistance of *Salmonella* and *Campylobacter* to antibiotics, including the new fluoroquinolones, is increasingly reported.

Viruses are arguably the most common causes of gastrointestinal infection. Robert Shaw (pp 74–79) summarizes developments in this important field. Norwalk-like viruses have recently been designated members of the *Calciviridae.* Important advances in the cloning and characterization of these agents, as well as astroviruses, will facilitate our understanding of the epidemiology and pathogenesis of infections by these agents. *Rotavirus* is the most common viral pathogen in young children. A new classification has been described using antibodies directed VP7 and VP4 proteins. Whereas important leads on the development of a *Rotavirus* vaccine have been described, field trials of candidate vaccines have thus far been disappointing.

Important developments were seen in the study of parasitic infections, reviewed by Ana Maria Cevallos and Michael Farthing (pp 80–87). New immunodiagnostic tests for identifying *E. histolytica* have been developed and appear to be rather promising. *Cryptosporidium* is known to cause acute and chronic diarrhea in children that is invariably self-limited, but it can cause a debilitating diarrheal illness in AIDS patients. Other pathogens infecting AIDS patients include *Cyclospora* and *Microsporidia.* An important development in treatment of *Trichuris trichiura* was reported. It seems that successful treatment of this infection can restore the cognitive deficit present in children with trichuriasis.

Children are more susceptible to gastrointestinal infections than adults. As reviewed by Michael Gracey (pp 88–97), several classes of *E. coli* can cause intestinal infection. Despite the expanding number of microorganisms that cause intestinal infection, many such infections in children go undiagnosed. Fecal samples from these so-called pathogen-free episodes cause cytotoxicity when exposed to tissue cultures, suggesting the presence of a microbial toxin. The usual toxins such as those produced by *C. difficile*, *Shigella*, and *E. coli*, have been excluded, but the putative pathogen has not been identified. Risk factors for gastrointestinal infections in children have been described. Many relate to environmental contamination and poor hygiene practices in the home.

Abbreviation

PCR—polymerase chain reaction.

 ISBN 1-85922-606-X ISSN 0267–1379

Helicobacter pylori causes ulceration of the stomach and duodenum. Dino Vaira *et al.* (pp 98–104) review the current status of this organism. An exciting development is the identification of a cytotoxin. In addition, production of ammonium appears to be important in pathogenesis. Several diagnostic tests have been developed in order to reduce the need for upper intestinal endoscopy. Although the preferred antibiotic regimen is bismuth, metronidazole, and tetracycline for 2 weeks, several new regimens involving omeprazole with antibiotics are being studied. Some development in vaccine production has been reported, but considerable work is still needed.

Susan Cookson and Robert Edelman (pp 105–111) have reviewed treatments for gastrointestinal infection. For traveler's diarrhea, fluoroquinolones are preferred in most locations, although many strains of *E. coli* in Mexico remain sensitive to the older antibiotics. Loperamide, when used with antibiotics, shortens the course of shigellosis. Treatment of cytomegalovirus colitis in AIDS patients has proven difficult with ganciclovir because the clinical improvement was rather minimal. In patients infected with *Cryptosporidium*, a trial of paromomycin seems justified.

Diagnostic tests have seen major advances, as reported by Grace Thorne (pp 112–118). PCR and molecular genetic techniques have produced more sensitive and specific tests for various pathogens. Pathogenic *E. histolytica* can be separated from nonpathogenic strains. New techniques for isolating *Salmonella* and *Shigella*, using immunomagnetic beads followed by PCR, have been described. PCR has also been used to diagnose Norwalk virus. Improved methods for diagnosis of *C. difficile* and *Cryptosporidium* are being evaluated.

Gastrointestinal infections remain among the most common illnesses affecting human beings. Children suffer the most frequent and most severe intestinal infections, but intestinal pathogens can cause illness in people of all ages. Immunocompromised patients, such as those with HIV infection, are particularly prone to such pathogens. The advances in these various areas have been reviewed by a distinguished panel of experts, and they present an encouraging story of advancement in our understanding and treatment of these disorders.

Sherwood L. Gorbach, MD, Professor of Community Health and Medicine, Tufts University School of Medicine, 136 Harrison Avenue, Arnold Room 205, Boston, MA 02111, USA.

Small intestinal infections

Christine A. Wanke, MD

New England Deaconess Hospital and Harvard Medical School, Boston, Massachusetts, USA

Diarrheal disease has long been recognized as a cause of morbidity and mortality in children in the developing world. Small bowel infections play a major role in this diarrheal disease. With the advent of the AIDS epidemic, diarrheal disease is gaining importance as a syndrome that may severely compromise the quality of life of these patients. In addition, in the past year several dramatic outbreaks of diarrheal disease related to contaminated food or water have occurred. This review examines recent papers that discuss infectious causes of diarrheal disease in AIDS patients, travelers, and individuals who may have been exposed to contaminated food or water, and touches on treatment modalities.

Current Opinion in Gastroenterology 1994, **10**:59–65

Diarrhea in HIV-positive patients

Acute and chronic diarrhea in HIV-positive patients have remained issues of concern and controversy [1••,2•]. Whereas the exact incidence and prevalence of diarrheal disease in HIV-positive patients in the United States is not clear, the diarrhea-wasting syndrome has been the AIDS-defining illness in at least 17% of newly reported cases. The true prevalence of diarrheal disease is probably much higher; although it may not approach the 80% to 90% incidence seen in AIDS patients in Africa, it may well compromise the quality of life of more than half of the AIDS patients in the United States [3••,4•].

Acute diarrheal disease (defined for HIV patients as a diarrheal illness lasting <1 month) has received less attention in this population than chronic diarrheal illness accompanied by wasting, but it is worthy of attention. There is a tendency for an increased rate of complications with enteric bacterial illnesses in AIDS patients [5•]. Salmonellosis has been particularly problematic in the HIV population, with bacteremia occurring in nearly 50% of AIDS patients in one study. Salmonellosis has also been complicated by a high relapse rate, especially in bacteremic patients. The dramatically increased incidence of *Salmonella* infections in HIV-positive patients noted previously appears to have decreased recently, perhaps because of the common usage of zidovudine and trimethoprim sulfamethoxazole in this population, both of which provide some protection against *Salmonella* bacteria.

Bacteremias and increased relapse rate are increased in patients with lower CD4 counts. Enteric infections with *Campylobacter* and *Shigella* have also been more complicated in patients with advanced HIV. In one study of human immunodeficiency positive-patients, 8% of the patients infected with *Campylobacter* and 50% of the patients infected with *Shigella* had bacteremia with the same enteric organism [5•]. Patients with AIDS and either *Campylobacter*- or *Shigella*-based enteritis were more likely to have relapsing illness than those patients who were HIV positive but without a diagnosis of AIDS. The optimal drug of choice and duration of treatment for these enteric bacterial illnesses have not yet been defined. Although the quinolone antibiotics are often empirically chosen for therapy, several reports of resistance and clinical relapse of *Campylobacter* enteritis in patients with HIV while on therapy with these agents have appeared.

Enteric illness caused by *Clostridium difficile* in the HIV-positive population is also of interest and some controversy [1••,6]. There has been speculation that patients with HIV might be more susceptible to *C. difficile*–caused diarrhea, with fewer days of antibiotics required to precipitate diarrheal illness by this organism in this population. It has also been postulated that disease caused by *C. difficile* in this population might be more refractory to therapy, with a slower cessation of diarrhea once treatment with either metronidazole or oral vancomycin has begun; however, there are few data to support this. There is one study that suggests that patients with HIV have the same nosocomial risk

© 1994 Current Science ISBN 1-85922-606-X ISSN 0267–1379

of acquiring *C. difficile* as HIV. HIV-positive patients, however, acquire strains of *C. difficile* in hospital that are distinct from the strains usually seen in nosocomial situations. The clinical significance of this is not clear [6].

The role that viral pathogens may play in causing either acute or chronic diarrheal disease in patients with HIV is also not clear. There may be geographic variation in the occurrence of various viral pathogens. The epidemiologic data from different geographic locales are divergent. Studies done to date in the United States have not documented a significant role for *Rotavirus* or the Norwalk-like agents in diarrheal disease in patients with HIV, as these pathogens occur with equal frequency in the nondiarrheal population as in the symptomatic population [1••]. In Australia and Europe, however, *Rotavirus* does seem to be associated more often with acute diarrheal disease in HIV-positive populations, as it is identified with less frequency in the nondiarrheal HIV-positive controls [7].

More attention has been directed toward chronic, wasting diarrhea in HIV-positive patients. The etiology, best method of evaluation, and the possibility of identifying a treatable cause for this syndrome remain controversial [1••,2•,3••,4•]. It is possible that a subgroup, perhaps 20% to 40%, of HIV-positive patients with diarrhea and malnutrition do not have a readily identifiable extrinsic pathogen, but rather an AIDS enteropathy [1••,3••]. The possible etiologies of this syndrome include HIV infection of the enterocytes, dysregulation of the enteric autonomic nerves, small bowel overgrowth, dysregulation of lymphokines within the intestinal lymphatic tissue, or intestinal immune dysfunction. Attempts to correlate detection of HIV within the enterocytes by *in situ* hybridization or p24 antigen detection have met with mixed success, as have attempts to correlate histopathologic changes with the presence of infection or parasites, or with the presence of HIV in the enterocyte [3••]. It is possible that additional unrecognized enteric pathogens will be identified that will explain some of the diarrheal illnesses in these otherwise pathogen-negative patients.

The recent identification of a second microsporidial species as a cause of a significant number of chronic wasting diarrheal illnesses in the HIV-positive population is an exciting development [8•,9••]. The incidence and prevalence of microsporidial diarrhea is not clear, but as the facility of microscopists and clinical laboratories in identifying the organism increases, the number of recognized cases is rising sharply and additional epidemiologic information should become available rapidly. Whereas electron microscopic examination of small bowel tissue, duodenal fluid, or stool is required for speciation of the organisms, organisms can be readily identified by light microscopy in small bowel tissue or identified in stool by the modified trichrome stain by an experienced observer. Speciation of microsporidia into one of the two genera that commonly infect the bowel, *Enterocytozoon bineusi* or *Septada intestinalis,* also requires an experienced microscopist [10•].

The epidemiologic factors that place an individual at risk for acquiring microsporidia are not known. Although it is clear that the disease caused by *Microsporidium* becomes obvious when HIV is advanced, whether the organism is carried asymptomatically by individuals with competent immune systems is not known. The clinical course of microsporidial diarrhea is a chronic, intermittent one, accompanied by bloating and weight loss. Functionally, individuals with microsporidia often malabsorb fat, carbohydrates, and vitamin B_{12} [9••]. Microsporidia have been documented as a cause of acalculous cholecystitis, and disease caused by *S. intestinalis* appears to be disseminated with organisms frequently seen in the urine and demonstrated in renal epithelium and pulmonary tissue at autopsy [8•,11•,12]. Attempts to treat microsporidia with either metronidazole or albendazole have had mixed results. Patients infected with *S. intestinalis* appear to respond readily to therapy with albendazole, clearing the organism from their stool; the response of patients infected with *E. bineusi* has been much more difficult to judge. Treatment with metronidazole has transiently improved symptoms in some patients, but these reports did not provide speciation of organisms, so whether there is also a differential response of the two species to metronidazole is not clear. Patients treated with metronidazole do not clear the organisms from their stool. Therapy with antimotility, anti-secretory agents has also been intermittently successful, with some patients reporting improvement in symptoms with oral agents such as loperamide or Imodium (Janssen Pharmaceutica, Beerse, Belgium) or with somatostatin analogue.

A coccidian cyanobacterium-like organism recently named *Cyclospora cayetanensis* has been identified in stools of both HIV-positive patients with chronic diarrhea and in travelers [13••,14•,15]. This organism was originally thought to be a blue-green algae, but subsequent investigations revealed that these organisms can excyst and release sporozoites [13••]. *Cyclospora* bacteria are identified in stool by the modified acid-fast stain, and may be described as looking like a large *Cryptosporidium*. They have been noted to be associated with mild inflammation when biopsies have been done [14•]. Patients complain of abdominal cramping, bloating and weight loss; diarrhea has been self-limited in immune-competent patients but has been protracted in HIV-positive patients [16•]. Many of the HIV patients with *Cyclospora*-based diarrhea have also reported travel: *Cyclospora* has infected individuals from

Chicago, and travelers to or natives of Nepal, Peru, Puerto Rico, and Mexico.

Cryptosporidium parvum has long been recognized as a pathogen in HIV-positive patients with diarrhea. It causes a profuse watery diarrhea with cramps and weight loss and has been very resistant to therapy. The mechanism by which *Cryptosporidium* causes diarrhea is still not clear. This year, published reports suggested that there is not a clear association between the number of cryptosporidial oocysts in the stool or those seen on duodenal biopsy and the severity of diarrhea [17•]. Additionally, a study reviewing the natural history of cryptosporidial diarrhea demonstrated that the duration of symptoms in the HIV-positive population is correlated inversely with the total lymphocyte count, as has been previously suggested [18]. Patients in these studies were frequently coinfected with additional pathogens.

Cytomegalovirus remains a significant pathogen in patients with HIV and those severely immunocompromised and has multiple presentations within the gastrointestinal tract. Infiltrative intestinal disease such as that caused by *Mycobacterium avium* intracellulare complex also causes chronic diarrheal and wasting syndromes in HIV patients. As the definitive diagnosis of these two syndromes must be made by biopsy and histopathologic examination of the small bowel, many cases are treated presumptively if evidence of the organisms is found elsewhere. The true incidence of these syndromes is therefore not clear.

The most appropriate or most cost-effective evaluation for HIV patients with diarrhea is not clear [4•]. However, it appears that management, if not cure, of diarrheal disease is often possible if a pathogen is known. Nutritional evaluation and adjustment of diet may also be important in improving the quality of life of these patients (Table 1).

Table 1. Suggested evaluation of HIV-positive patients with diarrhea.

History
Travel
Exposures: pets, diet*
Drugs, including antibiotics†
Number of stools, presence of blood, mucus
Physical examination
Temperature
Postural signs
Weight
Abdominal exam
Laboratory
Diarrhea
≤7 d
Stool culture—*Campylobacter, Salmonella, Shigella*
Stool exam—Leukocyte, *Giarda, Clostridium difficile* toxin
>7 d
CD4 count>200 stool culture, stool exam
CD4 count<200 stool culture, stool exam plus stool exam for *Cryptosporidium, Microsporidium*
>28 d
With weight loss, cramping: stool culture, stool exam for *Cryptosporidium, Microsporidium* plus consider upper endoscopy and biopsy
Functional evaluation: iron, zinc, vitamin B_{12}, fecal fat, D-xylose
Nutritional counseling
No weight loss, with blood, tenesmus: stool culture, stool exam plus consider colonoscopy and biopsy, consider blood cultures for *Mycobacterium avium* complex cytomegalovirus

*Raw shellfish: consider viral agents, noncholera vibrios; unpasteurized dairy products: consider *Salmonella, Campylobacter, Cryptosporidium*; herbal medicines: consider *Salmonella*; undercooked pork: consider *Yersinia*.

†If patient is taking antibiotics, consider *C. difficile* as well as medication side effect, *ie*, zidovudine, didanosine.

Traveler's diarrhea

Availability of food and water uncontaminated by bacterial, viral, or parasitic organisms capable of causing diarrheal disease is of great importance to travelers to the developing world. However, sporadic problems with contamination of foodstuffs or community water supplies within the developed world also occur. It is possible to educate a traveler about eating habits that place him at a greater risk of acquiring diarrheal pathogens; however, the extent of contaminated food and water supplies makes it unlikely that an individual can completely protect himself against all possible contamination, either in the developing world or the developed world [19••] (Table 2).

For travelers, the greatest risk of acquiring enteric pathogens is from contaminated drinking water or from fresh fruits and vegetables. The majority of traveler's diarrhea is caused by bacterial pathogens; the enterotoxigenic *Escherichia coli, Salmonella, Shigella, Campylobacter*, noncholera vibrios, *Aeromona*, and *Pleisiomona*. Other groups of *E. coli* such as the enteropathogenic *E. coli* and the recently described enteroaggregative *E. coli* have also been associated with diarrheal disease in travelers [20]. With the continuation of the cholera pandemic throughout the western hemisphere, cholera has become more of a concern for travelers, and 102 cases of cholera were identified in 12 of the United States in 1992 [21]. Cholera remains a very uncommon cause of diarrhea in travelers and is associated with less than 1% of all cases of traveler's diarrhea. A new outbreak of severe cholera-like diarrheal illness has been reported from southern India and Bangladesh and is associated with a new organism, *Vibrio cholera* non 01, strain 139. Viral agents such as *Rotavirus* and the Norwalk-like agents play a fairly prominent role as pathogens in traveler's diarrhea as well, although they are more common in some geographic areas such as Africa, and display marked seasonal variation. Parasitic agents such as *Giardia, Cryptosporidium*, and *Cy-*

clospora are also reported as etiologic agents of traveler's diarrhea; these organisms also display a marked geographic variation.

Table 2. Dietary recommendations for travelers.

Drink	Avoid
Boiled water	Fresh fruit juices
Bottled carbonated water	Ice
Bottled carbonated soda	Milk products, if not pasteurized
Beer	
Hot tea or coffee	
Eat	**Avoid**
Freshly cooked, hot foods	Steam table foods
Peeled fruits	Prepared stored foods
Cooked vegatables	Salads
	Rare meats
	Raw shellfish

Diarrheal disease in travelers has received increased attention since the incidence rates of diarrheal disease in the US troops in Operation Desert Storm were published. These data revealed that 57% of troops suffered from diarrheal symptoms after 2 months in Saudi Arabia and that 20% of the troops were temporarily unable to perform their usual duties because of diarrheal symptoms. Similar studies have shown that diarrheal disease is common in US military personnel participating in exercises in South America and West Africa [22•].

Water- and food-borne outbreaks of diarrhea

There have been numerous attempts to track the source of food-borne outbreaks of diarrheal pathogens in the developed world. The nontyphoidal *Salmonella* remain a common cause of contaminated food and dairy products. It was previously thought that transmission of *Salmonella* occurred primarily by nonpasteurized dairy products or cracked shell eggs, but it has recently become clear that there are many sources of transmission including intact shell eggs and pasteurized dairy products such as mozzarella cheese [23•–25•]. Other sources of *Salmonella* recently reported have included infected pork, poultry, and raw milk cheeses [26–28]. Multiple serotypes have been involved in outbreaks including *Salmonella typhimurium, Salmonella dublin, Salmonella enteriditis* group D, *Salmonella infantis, Salmonella javiana,* and *Salmonella oranienburg* in Great Britain, the Netherlands, and the United States.

Another recent, well-documented and publicized outbreak of contaminated food in the United States was the association of hamburger meat and *Escherichia coli* O157:H7 [29]. This organism is classified as an enterohemorrhagic *E. coli* and has been associated with a spectrum of illness ranging from mild diarrhea to severe dysentery with hemolytic-uremic syndrome. *Campylobacter* has also been a common cause of food-associated diarrheal disease, and has been particularly linked to the consumption of contaminated dairy products or poultry [30].

Table 3. Medical conditions that warrant prophylaxis of traveler's diarrhea.

Use of H_2 blockers, reduced gastric acid
Presence of inflammatory bowel disease
Immunocompromised patient
Organ transplant recipient
HIV-positive patient
Presence of severe cardiovascular or vascular disease
Prosthetic valve recipient
Long-term antibiotic use

The community water supply in Milwaukee, Wisconsin became contaminated with *Cryptosporidium* early in 1993 and as many as 200,000 individuals developed diarrheal illness consistent with cryptosporidiosis [31•]. Nearly half of the HIV-infected patients in Milwaukee that were surveyed reported symptoms consistent with cryptosporidiosis. Outbreaks of this type, whether caused by cryptosporidium or by other pathogens such as *Salmonella*, are of particular concern to members of the community that are debilitated by other serious medical illness, the elderly, and the immune compromised.

Treatment

There are no vaccines yet available to prevent all diarrheal disease [32]. Prophylaxis may be feasible for some travelers, but is not recommended except in extraordinary circumstances because of the potential side effects of antibiotics, cost, and the increasing resistance of enteric pathogens to available oral antibiotics (Table 3). The cornerstone of therapy for diarrheal disease remains adequate oral rehydration with electrolyte solutions, but new approaches to prevention and treatment are being investigated.

The quinolone antibiotics have become the drugs of choice for empiric therapy of diarrheal illness in adults when a bacterial pathogen is suspected. The antimicrobial spectrum of these drugs makes them useful in this setting, as they are bactericidal against *E. coli, Salmonella, Shigella,* and *Campylobacter,* as well as the less common bacterial pathogens such as *Yersinia, Vibrio cholera,* and the noncholera vibrios. These agents are not presently considered appropriate for children and should not be used in pregnant women. Additionally, the emergence of resistance of bacteria with clinical relapse of disease, particularly *Campylobacter,* during the course of therapy has complicated treatment with these agents [33•,34].

Alternate therapies with antisecretory agents such as loperamide have also proven to be successful. The combination of loperamide and quinolone antibiotics has been used more successfully in diarrheal disease than either agent alone. There is one report of the success of this combination in treating adult patients with dysenteric illness, for which the use of antimotility drugs has otherwise been avoided [35•]. A trial using zaldaride maleate, an intestinal calmodulin inhibitor, demonstrated that this agent was more successful than placebo in shortening the severity and duration of traveler's diarrhea [36•]. As mediators of intestinal secretion, calcium and calmodulin offer promising targets for inhibition and reduction of intestinal fluid losses without the use of opiates or drugs that directly affect intestinal motility.

A variety of binding agents are also of potential interest in preventing or treating diarrheal disease caused by various enteric pathogens. A case report noted that the use of oral immunoglobulin A was successful in treating a child with refractory and relapsing *C. difficile* diarrhea. The yolks of eggs from hens immunized with enterotoxigenic *E. coli* were successful in preventing enterotoxigenic *E. coli* infection in an animal model in which these immunoglobulin preparations were given orally [37•]. Additionally, whereas the immunoglobulin in breast milk has been previously shown to be protective against diarrheal pathogens, a report recently documented that the nonimmunoglobulin portion of human milk mucin was also successful in preventing rotaviral gastroenteritis in an animal model [38•]. The effects of these preparations are presumed to be associated with their ability to bind to pathogens or to small intestinal receptors. *Saccharomyces boulardii* has been investigated extensively as an alternate agent to treat or prevent *C. difficile* diarrhea; a yeast-secreted protease has been shown to reduce toxin A binding to enterocytes [39].

References and recommended reading

Papers of particular interest, published within the annual period of review, have been highlighted as:

- • Of special interest
- •• Of outstanding interest

1. •• BARTLETT JG, BELITSOS PC, SEARS CL: **AIDS Enteropathy.** *Clin Infect Dis* 1992, **15**:726–735.

A comprehensive review of the current state of knowledge about chronic diarrhea in advanced HIV. This review discusses the results of clinical studies of chronic diarrhea in patients with AIDS and summarizes the information to date about HIV enteropathy.

2. • BELITSOS PC, GREENSON JK, YARDLEY JH, SISLER JR, BARTLETT JG: **Association of Gastric Hypoacidity With Opportunistic Enteric Infections in Patients With AIDS.** *J Infect Dis* 1992, **166**:277–284.

A small, but controlled, study looking extensively for causes of infectious diarrhea in patients with HIV and correlating those infections to abnormal gastric pH and small bowel overgrowth.

3. •• KOTLER DP, REKA S, CHOW K, ORENSTEIN JM: **Effects of Enteric Parasitoses and HIV Infection Upon Small Intestinal Structure and Function in Patients With AIDS.** *J Clin Gastroenterol* 1993, **16**:10–15.

A comprehensive, pathologic retrospective study which reports the results of functional studies, as well as infectious pathogens in HIV-positive patients with and without diarrhea. This study included intestinal tissue examinations for HIV by *in situ* hybridization and enzyme-linked immunosorbent assay and found no correlation of HIV with intestinal injury or infection.

4. • RABENECK L: **Diagnostic Workup Strategies for Patients With HIV-Related Chronic Diarrhea.** *J Clin Gastroenterol* 1993, **16**:245–250.

A commentary summarizing problems with previous studies that have suggested evaluation strategies for patients with HIV and chronic diarrhea. This commentary stresses the fact that not enough information is currently available to develop an appropriate evaluation scheme while outlining avenues of research that should be undertaken.

5. • NELSON MR, SHANSON DC, HAWKINS DA, GAZZARD BG: **Salmonella, Campylobacter and Shigella in HIV-Seropositive Patients.** *AIDS* 1992, **6**:1495–1498.

This is one of the few studies in the literature about bacterial enteric pathogens in patients with HIV. This study is a retrospective review of the diagnosis, clinical course, complication rate, and treatment of patients with *Salmonella, Campylobacter,* and *Shigella.*

6. BARBUT F, DEPITRE C, DELMEE M, CORTHIER G, PETIT JC: **Comparison of Enterotoxin Production, Cytotoxin Production, Serogrouping, and Antimicrobial Susceptibilities of *Clostridium difficile* Strains Isolated From AIDS and Human Immunodeficiency Virus-Negative Patients.** *J Clin Microbiol* 1993, **31**:740–742.

7. ALBRECHT H, STELLBRINK HJ, FENSKE S, ERMER M, RAEDLER A, GRETEN H: **Rotavirus Antigen Detection in Patients With HIV Infection and Diarrhea.** *Scand J Gastroenterol* 1993, **28**:307–310.

8. • ORENSTEIN JM, DIETERICH DT, KOTLER DP: **Systemic Dissemination by a Newly Recognized Intestinal Microsporidia Species in AIDS.** *AIDS* 1992, **6**:1143–1150.

A pathologic description of the dissemination of what this paper calls the second microsporidial species, which is probably *Septada intestinalis.* The report describes the small bowel, gall bladder, and renal findings in these patients.

9. •• MOLINA JM, SARFATI C, BEAUVAIS B, LEMANN M, LESOURD A, FERCHAL F, CASIN I, LAGRANGE P, MODIGLIANI R, DEROUIN F, MODAI J: **Intestinal Microsporidiosis in Human Immunodeficiency Virus-Infected Patients With Chronic Unexplained Diarrhea: Prevalence and Clinical and Biologic Features.** *J Infect Dis* 1993, **167**:217–221.

The most comprehensive clinical report to date describing the differences between patients with HIV and chronic diarrhea infected with microsporidia and those with other pathogens. The patients with intestinal microsporidia had abnormal D-xylose absorption, lower Karnofsky scores, and lower CD4 counts than did patients with chronic diarrhea but without microsporidia.

10. • CALI A, KOTLER DP, ORENSTEIN JM: ***Septata intestinalis* n.g., n. sp., an Intestinal Microsporidian Associated With Chronic Diarrhea and Dissemination in AIDS Patients.** *J Eur Microbiol* 1993, **40**:101–112.

A parasitologic description of *Septada intestinalis,* the new microsporidial species which has the potential to disseminate but may also be more responsive to therapy.

11. • Pol S, Romana CA, Richard S, Amouval P, Desportes-Livage I, Carnot F, Pays JF, Berthelot P: **Microsporidia Infection in Patients With the Human Immunodeficiency Virus and Unexplained Cholangitis.** *N Engl J Med* 1993, **328**:95–99.
A clinical description of eight patients with HIV who were found to have colangitis and biliary microsporidiosis documented by electron microscopy.

12. Beaugerie L, Teilhac MF, Deluol AM, Fritsch J, Girard PM, Rozenbaum W, LeQuintree Y, Chatelet FP: **Cholangiopathy Associated With *Microsporidia* Infection of the Common Bile Duct Mucosa in a Patient With HIV Infection.** *Ann Intern Med* 1992, **117**:401–402.

13. •• Ortega YR, Sterling CR, Gilman RH, Cama VA, Diaz F: **Cyclospora Species: A New Protozoan Pathogen of Humans.** *N Engl J Med* 1993, **328**:1308–1312.
A description of the cyclospora organisms found to be associated with diarrheal disease in two cohorts of children followed prospectively in Peru.

14. • Bendall RP, Locas S, Moody A, Tovey G, Chiodini PL: **Diarrhoea Associated With Cyanobacterium-Like Bodies: A New Coccidian Enteritis of Man.** *Lancet* 1993, **341**:590–592.
This paper contains a description of the clinical disease caused by *Cyclospora cayetanensis* as well as the clinical course of diarrheal disease associated with the new organism. This study is from Nepal, where the majority of patients with *Cyclospora* have been identified to date.

15. Hoge CW, Shlim DR, Rajah R, Triplett J, Shear M, Rabold JG, Echeverria P: **Epidemiology of Diarrhoeal Illness Associated With Coccidian-Like Organism Among Travellers and Foreign Residents in Nepal.** *Lancet* 1993, **341**:1175–1179.

16. • Wurtz RM, Kocka FE, Peters CS, Weldon-Linne CM, Kuritza A, Yungbluth P: **Clinical Characteristics of Seven Cases of Diarrhea Associated With a Novel Acid-Fast Organism in the Stool.** *Clin Infect Dis* 1993, **16**:136–138.
A comparison of the clinical course of cyclospora diarrhea in HIV-positive and HIV-negative patients.

17. • Goodgame RW, Genta RM, White AC, Chappell CL: **Intensity of Infection in AIDS-Associated Cryptosporidiosis.** *J Clin Infect Dis* 1993, **167**:704–709.
A prospective examination of stools from patients with known cryptosporidium attempting to correlate severity of disease and number of stools with the immune status of the patient. This report documents no association with the number of organisms seen and severity of disease, but does report increased duration of disease with suppression of the total lymphocyte count.

18. McGowan I, Hawkins AS, Weller IVD: **The Natural History of Cryptosporidial Diarrhoea in HIV-Infected Patients.** *AIDS* 1993, 7:349–354.

19. •• DuPont HL, Ericsson CD: **Prevention and Treatment of Traveler's Diarrhea.** *N Engl J Med* 1993, **328**:1821–1828.
A comprehensive review of the prophylaxis and treatment of traveler's diarrhea. The authors have extensive experience with studies of traveler's diarrhea. Drug recommendations and dosage charts for both prophylactic and treatment regimens are given in the paper.

20. Cohen MB, Hawkins JA, Weckbach LS, Staneck JL, Levine MM, Heck JE: **Colonization by Enteroaggregative *Escherichia coli* in Travelers With and Without Diarrhea.** *J Clin Microbiol* 1993, **31**:351–353.

21. Centers for Disease Control: **Cholera—International Travel, 1992.** *MMWR* 1992, **268**:1648–1649.

22. • Bourgeois AL, Gardiner CH, Thornton SA, Batchelor RA, Burr DH, Escamilla J, Echeverria P, Blacklow NR, Hermann JE, Hyams KC: **Etiology of Acute Diarrhea Among United States Military Personnel Deployed to South America and West Africa.** *Am J Trop Med Hyg* 1993, **48**:243–248.
A prospective study of acute diarrhea in US military personnel. This report not only exhaustively examines stools for etiologic agents but looks at the resistance patterns of organisms from South America and West Africa. This report concludes that because of resistance patterns, quinolones may be the therapy of choice for traveler's diarrhea.

23. • Centers for Disease Control: **Outbreak of *Salmonella enteritidis* Infection Associated With Consumption for Raw Shell Eggs.** *JAMA* 1992, **267**:3263–3264.
A brief report of the association of *Salmonella* with raw, intact shell eggs which also summarizes some of the Centers for Disease Control surveillance data about *Salmonella enteritidis* infections.

24. • Hedberg CW, KorlathJA, D'Aoust JY, White KE, Schell WL, Miller MR, Cameron DN, MacDonald KL, Osterholm MT: **A Multistate Outbreak of *Salmonella javiana* and *Salmonella oranienburg* Infections Due to Consumption of Contaminated Cheese.** *JAMA* 1992, **268**:3203–3207.
A report tracing the source of a *Salmonella enteritidis* outbreak related to contaminated but pasteurized cheese. This paper discusses the possible routes of contamination during manufacture and cheese processing.

25. • Vugia DJ, Mishu B, Smith M, Tavris DR, Hickman-Brenner FW, Tauxe RV: ***Salmonella enteritidis* Outbreak in a Restaurant Chain: The Continuing Challenges of Prevention.** *Epidemiol Infect* 1993, **110**:49–61.
A case control study looking at association of intact egg shells with the acquisition of *Salmonella* infection.

26. van de Giessen AW, Dufrenne JB, Ritmeester WS, Berkers PATA, van Leeuwen WJ, Notermans SHW: **The Identification of *Salmonella enteritidis*-Infected Poultry Flocks Associated With an Outbreak of Human Salmonellosis.** *Epidemiol Infect* 1992, **109**:405–411.

27. Maguire H, Cowden J, Jacob M, Rowe B, Roberts D, Bruce J, Mitchell E: **An Outbreak of *Salmonella dublin* Infection in England and Wales Associated With a Soft Unpasteurized Cows' Milk Cheese.** *Epidemiol Infect* 1992, **109**:389–396.

28. Maguire HCF, Codd AA, Mackay VE, Rowe B, Mitchell E: **A Large Outbreak of Human Salmonellosis Traced to a Local Pig Farm.** *Epidemiol Infect* 1993, **109**:239–246.

29. Centers for Disease Control: **Preliminary Report: Foodborne Outbreak of *Escherichia coli* 157:H7 Infections From Hamburgers—Western United States, 1993.** *MMWR Morb Mortal Wkly Rep* 1993, **42**:85–86.

30. Wood RC, MacDonald KL, Osterholm MT: ***Campylobacter* Enteritis Outbreaks Associated With Drinking Raw Milk During Youth Activities: A 10 Year Review of Outbreaks in the United States.** *JAMA* 1992, **268**:3228–3230.

31. • McCarthy M: **USA: Cryptosporidiosis Outbreak.** *Lancet* 1993, **341**:1084.
An extremely brief report of the outbreak of *Cryptosporidium* in Milwaukee in April of 1993 documenting potential contamination of a community's water system.

32. Holmgren J, Svennerholm AM: **Bacterial Enteric Infection and Vaccine Development.** *Gastroenterol Clinics North Am* 1993, **21**:283–302.

33. • Wretlind B, Stromberg A, Ostlund L, Sjogren E, Kaijser B: **Rapid Emergence of Quinolone Resistance in *Campylobacter jejuni* in Patients Treated With Norfloxacin.** *Scand J Infect Dis* 1992, **24**:685–686.

A small clinical trial of patients with *Campylobacter jejuni* diarrheal disease treated with a quinolone. These patients had both relapsing disease and the emergence of resistant organisms in the stool while on therapy.

34. REINA J, BORRELL N, SERRA A: **Emergence of Resistance to Erythromycin and Fluoroquinolones in Thermotolerant *Campylobacter* Strains Isolated From Feces 1987-1991**. *Eur J Clin Microbiol* 1992, **11**:1163–1166.

35. • MURPHY GS, BODHILTA L, ECHEVERRIA P, TANSUPHASWADIKUL S, HOGE CW, IMLARP S, TAMURA K: **Ciprofloxacin and Loperamide in the Treatment of Bacillary Dysentery**. *Ann Intern Med* 1993, **118**:8582–8586.

A prospective, controlled trial of 88 adult patients in Thailand with dysentery treated with a quinolone and placebo or a quinolone and loperamide. Patients were infected with *Shigella*, invasive *E. coli*, and other invasive pathogens. Those patients receiving the loperamide in addition to the antibiotic had much more rapid resolution of diarrhea. This study stands alone against previous literature that suggested antimotility agents should not be used in invasive diarrheal disease.

36. • DUPONT HL, ERICSSON CD, MATHEWSON JJ, MARANI S, KNELLWOLF-COUSIN AL, MARTINEZ-SANDOVAL FG: **Zaldaride Maleate, an Intestinal Calmodulin Inhibitor, in the Therapy of Travelers' Diarrhea**. *Gastroenterology* 1993, **104**:709–715.

A controlled clinical trial of zaldaride maleate alone versus placebo for control of traveler's diarrhea in Mexico. This is the first report of a calmodulin inhibitor decreasing the severity and duration of traveler's diarrhea. This group of agents has exciting potential for opening new pathways of controlling intestinal secretion in patients who should not be given the more classic antidiarrheal agents.

37. • O'FARRELLY C, BRANTON D, WANKE CA: **Oral Ingestion of Egg Yolk Immunoglobulin From Hens Immunized With an Enterotoxigenic *Escherichia coli* Strain Prevents Diarrhea in Rabbits Challenged With the Same Strain**. *Infect Immun* 1992, **60**:2593–2597.

An animal study describing the use of a specific immunoglobulin prepared from egg yolks of immunized hens and the ability of this preparation to prevent enterotoxigenic diarrheal disease.

38. • YOLKEN RH, PETERSON JA, VONDERFECHT SL, FOUTS ET, MIDTHUN K, NEWBURG DS: **Human Milk Mucin Inhibits Rotavirus Replication and Prevents Experimental Gastroenteritis**. *J Clin Invest* 1992, **90**:1984–1991.

An animal study describing the identification of a non immunoglobulin human milk mucin glycoprotein associated with protection against rotaviral infection.

39. POTHOULAKIS C, KELLY CP, JOSHI MA, GAO N, O'KEANE CJ, CASTAGLIUOLO I, LAMONT JT: ***Saccharomyces boulardii* Inhibits *Clostridium difficile* Toxin A Binding and Enterotoxicity in Rat Ileum**. *Gastroenterology* 1993, **104**:1108–1115.

Christine A. Wanke, MD, Division of Infectious Diseases, New England Deaconess Hospital and Harvard Medical School, 185 Pilgrim Road, Boston, MA 02215, USA.

Colonic infections

Jeffrey K. Griffiths, MD, MPH&TM

St. Elizabeth's Medical Center, Boston, Massachusetts, USA

Epidemics of enterohemorrhagic *Escherichia coli* O157:H7 in the Pacific Northwest of the United States have highlighted the presence of colonic pathogens in the food chain. Risk factors for the disease and the properties of similar *E. coli* and *Shigella* are discussed, and advances in our understanding of *Clostridium difficile*–associated colitis and diarrhea, *Campylobacter*-induced dysentery, and illness due to *Entamoeba histolytica* are presented. New insights into how bacteria survive stomach acidity and how they may be affected by breast milk, as well as modes of intracellular spread may provide the basis for new therapeutic modalities. The direct colonic damage HIV, itself, causes is discussed.

Current Opinion in Gastroenterology 1994, **10**:66–73

Shigella and *Escherichia coli*

Breast feeding is important in protecting infants from shigellosis; both specific and nonspecific immune factors are thought to be important. Shiga and Shiga-like toxins (made by *Shigella* and enterohemorrhagic *Escherichia coli*, respectively) bind to a glycolipid (globotriaosylceramide, or Gb3) on the surface of colonocytes. Globotriaosylceramide has now been found in breast milk [1•]. Thus Shiga toxin or Shiga-like toxins made by infecting bacteria could be made unavailable via globotriaosylceramide binding, conferring some protection to an infant.

The uniquely low oral inoculum of *Shigella* (10 to 500 bacteria) required for disease has remained unexplained for years; most bacteria are killed by stomach acid. In a simple yet elegant paper, Gordon and Small [2••] have found that most *Shigella* species and *E. coli*, but not *Salmonella* species, survive at pH 2.5 for at least 2 hours if they are in stationary phase. Log phase growth bacteria are markedly more sensitive to acid. Thus a few acid-resistant, stationary-phase *Shigella* are probably more dangerous than millions of acid-sensitive, growth-phase organisms.

Shigella flexneri appears to travel from cell to cell by using two separate mechanisms. In the first, the bacterium shoots through the basolateral walls of one cell into an adjacent one; cometlike structures of polymerized actin form behind the pathogen as it moves. The energy for this movement may be provided by actin polymerization. The second form of travel is along the intracellular perijunctional actin ring, a sort of railroad track along the perimeter of the cell. Figure 1 is reproduced from the very fine paper by Vasselon *et al.* [3••] in Sansonetti's group in Paris, in which the latter form of movement is also documented to require de novo actin polymerization.

Inhibitors of microbial invasion and cellular travel may become powerful therapeutic tools. Intracellular signal transduction pathways, such as calcium modulation and the phosphorylation of regulatory proteins, are increasingly recognized as linked. For example, intracellular calcium is a crucial mediator of the dynamic reorganization of the cellular cytoskeleton (which may be how *Shigella* zooms into adjacent cells). Zaldaride maleate, a calmodulin inhibitor, has been shown to decrease the severity and duration of traveler's diarrhea [4•]. In addition, invasive *Salmonella* bacteria are known to stimulate protein phosphorylation within target host cells [5••]. Gut function may be disrupted by bacterial damage to intracellular regulation, alteration of the cytoskeleton, or gross disruption of cell integrity; agents that blunt this process may ameliorate the clinical sequelae of infection.

Although no earth-shaking advances in the treatment of dysentery occurred this past year, loperamide was shown to reduce the median duration of diarrhea from 42 to 19 hours, and the median number of subsequent stools from 6.5 to 2.0, in those treated with ciprofloxacin for dysentery primarily caused by ciprofloxacin-sensitive *Shigella* [6•]. Others have found loperamide useful in the treatment of traveler's diarrhea, which is usually watery and not dysenteric [7]. The danger, of course, is to give both drugs to someone infected with a quinolone-resistant organism; there is some evidence that opiates increase morbidity and mortality when used alone in dysentery [8,9]. As the number of clinically available quinolones increases, we can expect to see increasing numbers of studies documenting their efficacy in diarrheal diseases. One re-

  ISBN 1-85922-606-X ISSN 0267–1379

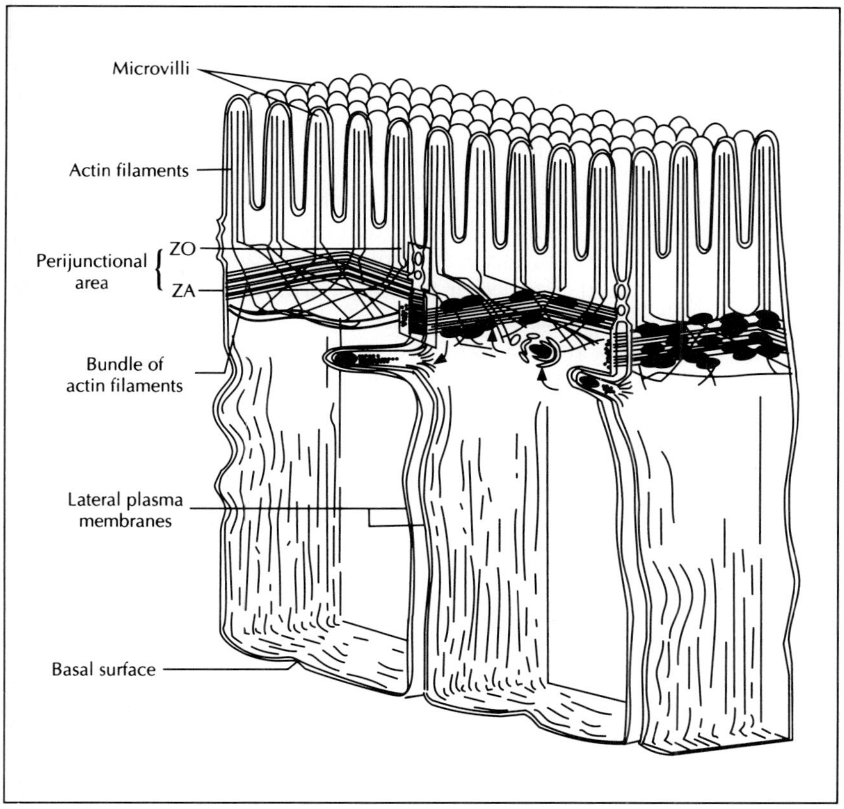

Fig. 1. Schema of colonization of an epithelial cell monolayer by *Shigella flexneri*. ZA—zonula adherens; ZO—zonula occludens. (*From* Vasselon *et al.* [3••]; with permission.)

cent study suggests that a single dose of the long-acting (half-life, 9 to 12 hours) fluoroquinolone fleroxacin may be equivalent to a 3-day course [10•] for infections caused by *Shigella*, *Vibrio cholera*, and *Vibrio parahaemolyticus*.

Several epidemics of *E. coli* O157:H7-induced disease occurred in the Northwest United States during 1993, associated with contaminated hamburgers that were not cooked thoroughly [11]. Hundreds became ill, and at least three people died of hemolytic-uremic syndrome and hemorrhagic colitis [12]. Many cases appeared to be due to secondary spread within households. In Ottawa [13•], children with hemolytic-uremic syndrome were retrospectively found to have had contact with another individual with diarrhea more often than controls; moreover, eating raw hamburger was marginally significant (P=0.05) as a risk factor.

Astoundingly, investigation of an epidemic in Minnesota found the secondary attack rate in children attending daycare centers to be 22% overall, and up to 63% in one facility. Temporary exclusion of children until two consecutive stool cultures were negative prevented transmission [14•]. Another study from Canada [15•] found a stronger association between consumption of pink ground beef in noncommercial settings, reporting the rate of ingestion (odds ratio) in those with *E. coli* O157:H7 disease to be 3.5 that of controls with no disease. Eating raw hamburgers and exposure to others with bloody diarrhea are the major risk factors identified for this disease in North America.

During an investigation of bloody diarrhea and hemolytic-uremic syndrome in Massachusetts, *E. coli* O157:H7 was found to have been transmitted by fresh-pressed apple cider [16•].Apples are not routinely washed, nor cider pasteurized, nor preservatives added in small cider mills. *E. coli* O157:H7 survive for 20 days in unpreserved refrigerated apple cider (in stationary phase, no doubt); the addition of 0.1% sodium benzoate reduces survival to less than 7 days. Though the US Food and Drug Administration does not consider foods with a pH less than 4.6 to be potentially hazardous, apple cider (pH 3.5 to 4.0) will support the survival of both *Salmonella* and *E. coli*.

Sorbital-fermenting *E. coli* O157:H bacteria were often found as the pathogen in a prospective, cooperative study of 147 children at 28 pediatric centers in Europe. This well-done study by Bitzan *et al.* [17••] documented at least 11 different serotypes causing hemolytic uremic syndrome. A common screening technique for enterohemorrhagic *E. coli* is sorbitol fermentation; the O157:H7 serotype is usually sorbitol negative. Thus the usual North American screening techniques may miss a non-O157:H7 serotype. Smith and Scotland [18•] have published a useful guideline to the isolation and identification of *E. coli* O157:H7 and non-O157 toxin-producing strains.

Shiga-like toxin production by *E. coli* is strongly linked to hemorrhagic colitis and hemolytic uremic syndrome. In a study of two cohorts of calves in Sri Lanka, 91 of 171 consecutive calf fecal specimens (from calves both ill and well) were positive for a variety of *E. coli* serotypes that were documented to synthesize Shiga-like toxin [19•]. The Western-diet food chain includes an important reservoir of these organisms, and all beef eaters are at risk if meat is not cooked until no longer pink. Other recent reports have shown toxin-producing *E. coli* can be found in pigs [20•].

Willshaw *et al.* [21•] in London investigated 48 strains of toxin-producing *E. coli*, and found toxin production to be the only common characteristic among all the strains. Only 13 showed localized adherence to HEp-2 cells and hybridized with the attaching and effacing gene probe; five were probe positive but did demonstrate localizing adherence; none hybridized with the enteropathogenic *E. coli* factor. Thus it may be most accurate to think of categories of pathogenic *E. coli* (*eg*, enteropathogenic *E. coli*, enterohemorrhagic *E. coli*, enterotoxigenic *E. coli*, enteroinvasive *E. coli*, and enteroaggregative *E. coli*) as idealized, Platonic paradigms: the bacteria care not a whit, and share characteristics back and forth. When a particular congruence of factors—contact with a reservoir (cattle), vector exposure (pink hamburger), age, inoculum dose, and the assembled genetic characteristics of the serotype come together, human disease occurs. Serotype O157:H7 is well represented in the food chain in North American and has the requisite repertory of factors to cause disease, thus, we see it commonly in North America. In other areas, other serotypes are represented, and hemorrhagic colitis and hemolytic uremic syndrome may therefore be produced by a wider spectrum of serotypes.

Along this line of discourse, two recent reports have documented possible molecular mimicry by *Citrobacter freundii*. This organism was found to produce Shiga-like toxin II-related toxins in two isolates from humans with diarrhea; once realized, the investigators in Germany further examined isolates obtained from beef samples, and found five of 81 also positive [22]. Thus, *Citrobacter*, as well as *E. coli* and *Shigella*, may make Shiga toxin or Shiga-like toxin; does this mean they could potentially cause hemorrhagic colitis and hemolytic uremic syndrome? In Australia, some *C. freundii* carries the *E. coli* O157 antigen, demonstrating the need to identify pathogens with biochemical as well as serologic tests [23•].

The actual pathophysiology of infection with enterohemorrhagic *E. coli* is not well understood. Two important bacterial factors are thought to be the Shiga-like toxins and adherence factors. Li *et al.* [24••] studied the effects of enterohemorrhagic *E. coli* infection in infant rabbits: in addition to mucosal disease (colonocyte necrosis and epithelial cell loss, neutrophil invasion, and goblet cell depletion), colonic Na^+ absorption was inhibited, and $C1^-$ secretion was stimulated, resulting in diarrhea. Interestingly, they found (using deletion mutant studies) that strains without Shiga-like toxins (verotoxins) or the 60-MD plasmid-encoded adhesion factor are still capable of producing mucosal disease, separate from the ion transport changes. Tzipori *et al.* [25,26] had similar results using gnotobiotic piglet model and O157:H7 and non-O157:H7 serotypes. This reinforces the message that we still do not have the full picture on how enterohemorrhagic *E. coli* bacteria cause disease.

The accurate diagnosis of an enteric pathogen is often impossible after treatment has begun, preventing the clinician from confirming a *Shigella* or *E. coli* infection. Even after treatment with ciprofloxacin, *Shigella*, or enteroinvasive *E. coli*, infections can be diagnosed by polymerase chain reaction amplification of either chromosomal or invasion plasmid DNA in fecal material, despite feces being culture-negative [27•]. Although this technique is still a research tool, polymerase chain reaction diagnostics may not be far off for colonic infections, and may allow accurate and specific diagnosis after treatment has been initiated.

Campylobacter, Yersinia, and *Salmonella* infections

Campylobacter jejuni and *Campylobacter coli* are among the most common bacterial causes of acute enteritis. These organisms are often transmitted to humans from animals. Dysenteric symptoms are frequent. In a clinical report from Norway of 135 patients with culture-confirmed infection, 30% had bloody diarrhea and a third had tenesmus [28••]. Convalescent carriage was common (mean, 38 days) after the onset of illness; antimicrobial treatment reduced the likelihood of carriage, but was so often administered late in the disease that no therapeutic effect was ascertainable. Diarrhea was common in the households of the patients (*eg*, possible secondary cases) and two cases of neonatal infection acquired from the mother at the time of delivery were noted.

Resistance to fluoroquinolones by *Campylobacter* organisms has been reported from Europe, perhaps because of increased veterinary use [29•]. For example, in Spain there has been a progressive increase in ciprofloxacin resistance of isolates from children [30•], although this age group is not commonly exposed to this drug. It is likely that these isolates acquired resistance to quinolones in companion or food animals, and were then transmitted to the children. Erythromycin remains a drug of choice, although the newer macrolides azithromycin and clarithromycin show excellent *in vitro* activity and have superior pharmacologic properties [31•].

Yersinia enterocolitica causes colitis and diarrhea, among other disorders. Reactive arthritis often occurs after infection. A large series of cases in Norway [32••] was recently reported; interestingly, bloody diarrhea occurred only in those less than 18 years old, but joint pain was much more common in adults. In 10% of patients, symptoms continued for over a year. Convalescent carriage of *Y. enterocolitica* 0:3 strains was common and prolonged. Invasive serobiogroups of this organism produce heat-stable enterotoxin (*Yersinia* heat-stable toxin), which may factor in the development of diarrhea. In a recent prospective study of yersiniosis in children in Chile, a noninvasive strain was isolated that produces a new enterotoxin, called YST-II; its prevalence is yet to be determined [33•].

The mechanism of post-yersiniosis arthritis is unclear. Probst *et al.* [34•] cloned T cells from reactive arthritis synovial fluid, and found a multiclonal, individually different response to bacterial antigens in the cells. Finding these cells in the fluid of an inflamed joint strongly argues for the presence of either bacterial antigens that have reached the joints in a still unclear way, or multiple cross-reactive epitopes in the joint tissues.

Because most sequelae of *Salmonella* infections involve the small bowel, I will only remind the reader of the ileitis and colitis that *Salmonella* cause, and note just two bits of news. First, porins (pore-forming proteins) produced by *Salmonella* species induce the release of cytokines (tumor necrosis factor, interleukin-1, interleukin-6, gamma interferon, and interleukin-4) by monocytes and lymphocytes [35•]. This effect is independent of lipopolysaccharide-dependent cytokine induction. Porins also activate complement, cause the release of histamine, and function as chemoattractants. Many gram-negative bacteria contain porins. As these proteins are part of endotoxin, their presence may also account for the failure of monoclonal antibodies to lipopolysaccharide to prevent the sepsis syndrome.

The spread of highly resistant *Salmonella typhi* continues unabated. A recent series from Karnataka India reports that 78% of *S. typhi*-infected patients had isolates resistant to ampicillin, chloramphenicol, or trimethoprim-sulfamethoxazole [36•]. Travelers returning from the Indian subcontinent should be presumed to have a resistant strain if typhoid is diagnosed [37•]. Fluoroquinolones are being championed as rational, albeit expensive, alternatives to traditional and inexpensive agents; a number of trials have shown very encouraging results indeed for the fluoroquinolones [38•]. In Calcutta, a comparative randomized trial of furazolidone and chloramphenicol in 133 children bacteriologically proven to have *S. typhi* infection demonstrated that furazolidone was an effective, inexpensive agent in this age group [39•]. Furazolidone use was not associated with any persistent typhoid carriage, and the time to an afebrile state was similar to that of chloramphenicol [39•].

Clostridium difficile–associated diarrhea and pseudomembranous colitis

An excellent succinct review of *Clostridium difficile*–associated diarrhea and pseudomembranous colitis was written by Fekety and Shah [40••], and complements John Bartlett's super missive on the 10 most commonly asked questions about this disease [41••]. Much of the damage associated with CD is mediated by the two protein exotoxins, toxins A and B. Toxin A is a potent cause of diarrhea, and toxin B is a virulent cytotoxin. Many studies have shown that a variety of nonpathogenic yeast confer a protective effect in this infection, including *Saccharomyces boulardii.* Pothoulakis, *et al.* [42••] at Boston University have shown that this yeast inhibits toxin A binding to, and enterotoxicity in, rat ileum, as measured by radiolabeled toxin binding, fluid secretion, and mannitol permeability. This provides some rationale for the protective effects seen in animal models and in humans. Toxin B is thought to cause the depolymerization of actin inside model cell lines, disorganizing the cytoskeleton. A new study has shown that toxin B profoundly impairs the phagocytic function of macrophages. Moreover, cytokine (tumor necrosis factor) production by macrophages is greatly amplified in the presence of toxin B [43•]. The authors speculate that the tumor necrosis factor production in affected gut could explain the "septic shock"-like effect seen in some elderly people afflicted with *C. difficile*-associated pseudomembranous colitis but having no gram-negative bacteremia. The idea is intriguing but speculative.

Accurate laboratory testing for *C. difficile* toxins, and their cytopathic effects may avert the need for diagnostic sigmoidoscopy. Readers may be interested in diagnostic methods involving more sensitive cell lines [44•] and the polymerase chain reaction technique [45•]. Inhibitory substances in stool may prove problematic for the latter technique, requiring additional (expensive) steps to remove inhibitory extraneous DNA materials [46•].

In a novel study [47•], the strains from 49 HIV-seronegative patients were compared with the strains from 50 AIDS patients; serogroup C was very common in the latter (66% vs 18%, $P<0.0001$). This serogroup is often quite resistant to antimicrobials, and the authors theorize it may have been selected for by the multiple course of antibiotics AIDS patients commonly receive. Will we see metronidazole-or vancomycin-resistant *C. difficile* colitis in the future?

Parasitic infections

Entamoeba histolytica remains a primary cause of dysentery. A concise case report from Australia [48•] describes a man in whom colectomy was required despite eradication of amoebae; the paper review the indications for colectomy in this rare circumstance. Another species of amoeba, *Entamoeba chattoni* (nomen nudum *E. polecki*), was found in two reports to cause sporadic infections in Venezuela [49•] and infections after close contact with monkeys [50•]. It may well be that all "amoebic dysentery" is not *E. histolytica* infection, as the two amoebae are very easily confused. The number of case reports is so small that no conclusions can be drawn about differences in presentation.

Colonic infections in AIDS patients

Gastrointestinal symptoms are common in HIV-seropositive individuals, and become more frequent with declining immune function and the passage of time. Indeed, some have speculated that the intestinal mucosa may be a preferred site of HIV proliferation and T-cell death.

Clayton *et al.* [51••] have conducted an excellent, careful study of rectal mucosal biopsy specimens from 75 HIV-seropositive patients and 16 HIV-seronegative control subjects. They report a previously undescribed, characteristic progression of histologic changes in the rectal (colonic) mucosa that appears to directly relate to HIV disease progression. Using immunohistopathologic methods, they found that four distinct stages were seen in HIV-seropositive patients: 1) an early, nearly normal phase in Walter Reed stage 1 to 2 subjects with low p24 antigen levels; 2) an inflammatory phase with lymphocytic infiltrates, plasma cells, eosinophils with degranulation, and abundant markers of HIV replication (*eg*, p24 antigen), seen in Walter Reed stage 3 to 4 individuals; 3) a transitional stage, where normal lymphocyte populations are seen, but with subtle inflammatory changes, usually in Walter Reed stage 5 and some stage 6 subjects; and 4) a lymphoid depletion stage, with decreased lymphocytes but often with endothelial cell activation and apoptosis, mostly found in Walter Reed stage 6 subjects. This stage correlates to severe loss of immune deficiency, and is seen in the majority of AIDS autopsies; it is the stage complicated by cytomegalovirus colitis or cryptosporidiosis. Moreover, the authors report that in subjects with the final stage of mucosal changes, the presence of altered bowel habits was common and tissue levels of tumor necrosis factor, interleukin 1, prostaglandin E_2, and leukotriene B_4 were altered. The general level of inflammation correlated with the presence and amount of HIV in rectal tissue determined histologically and by enzyme-linked immunosorbent assay, and was maximal before overt immunodeficiency became apparent.

This suggests that HIV infection, itself, in the absence of opportunistic infections, causes a characteristic mucosal process with inflammation, activation, and destruction of T lymphocytes, and the recruitment and infection of peripheral lymphocytes. Positivity of p24 antigen immunohistochemical stain was localized to eosinophils and eosinophil degranulation; eosinophil granules contain potent cytotoxins that are associated with gut epithelial damage. HIV infection alone may increase the general permeability of the gut [52]: increased exposure to bacterial toxins (*eg*, endotoxin) through the "leaky" gut may lead to HIV activation, presumably by inducing tumor necrosis factor secretion. In sum, a locally self-promoting inflammatory process may occur, and may serve as a reservoir of HIV production and lymphocyte infection.

Colonic epithelial cells do not express CD4 antigens, which are the HIV receptor on lymphocytic cells, yet are known to be directly susceptible to HIV infection. A neutral glycolipid related to galactosylceramide (GalCer) may be the receptor for HIV, and blocking antibody to this molecule prevent HIV infection of HT-29 cells, (a model cell line derived from a colonic tumor). Rates of infection are directly related to the levels of this glycolipid [53•]. The presence of an alternative receptor for HIV on colonic cells may provide a mechanism for anorectal transmission of the virus.

Cytomegalovirus infection in the population at large is ubiquitous, yet overt intestinal infection is rare; in contrast, cytomegalovirus is the most serious and most common specific colonic opportunistic infection seen in HIV-seropositive people residing in the developed world. In the developing world, pathogens such as *Microsporidium* and *Cryptosporidium* may be more prevalent, but adequate data is lacking. Establishing the diagnosis of cytomegalovirus infection is problematic, as no single technique (*eg*, culture, *in situ* hybridization with biotinylated probes, histology, and polymerase chain reaction) is faultless. Though some have championed the use of polymerase chain reaction [54•] as a best tool, most clinicians still feel that, "Clinical suspicion, earnest evaluation of histology, and the judicious use of staining techniques and viral cultures continue to be the mainstays of diagnosis" [55•].

As a coda to this review, we note the increasing recognition of cytomegalovirus appendicitis in AIDS patients, and point the reader towards a concise case report and review of the literature [56•]; duration of symptoms (16 hours to 3 weeks) is usually longer than in typical appendicitis, and edema of the appendix may be demonstrated via ultrasonography or computed tomography [56•].

References and recommended reading

Papers of particular interest, published within the annual period of review, have been highlighted as:

- • Of special interest
- •• Of outstanding interest

1. NEWBURG DS, ASHKENAZI S, CLEARY TG: **Breast Milk Contains**
• **the Shiga Toxin and Shiga-Like Toxin Receptor Glycolipid Gb3.** *J Infect Dis* 1992, 166:832–836.

Solid paper demonstrating the natural occurrence of what may be receptor blockade against the toxins of pathogens.

2. GORDON J, SMALL PLC: **Acid Resistance in Enteric Bacteria.**
•• *Infect Immun* 1993, 61:364–367.

A simple, elegant, and short paper. The authors demonstrate that metabolically inactive, near stationary phase bacteria survive acid conditions much better than do active, log phase bacteria, and may have provided a mechanism to explain how low inoculums of enteroinvasive *E. coli* and *Shigella* bypass the usual defensive mechanism.

3. •• VASSELON T, MOUNIER J, HELLIO R, SANSONETTI PJ: **Movement Along Actin Filaments of the Perijunctional Area and De Novo Polymerization of Cellular Actin are Required for *Shigella Flexneri* Colonization of Epithelial Caco-2 Cell Monolayers.** *Infect Immun* 1992, **60**:1031–1040.

Well done, and the discussion of bacterial movement inside mammalian cells (the gut) is quite good.

4. • DUPONT HL, ERICSSON CD, MATHEWSON JJ, MARANI S, KNELLWOLF-COUSIN AL, MARTINEZ-SANDOVAL FG: **Zaldaride Maleate, an Intestinal Calmodulin Inhibitor, in the Therapy of Travelers' Diarrhea.** *Gastroenterology* 1993, **104**:709–715.

A nice practical result that connects to a basic understanding of intracellular events in the infected gut.

5. •• GALAN JE, PACE J, HAYMAN MJ: **Involvement of the Epidermal Growth Factor Receptor in the Invasion of Cultured Mammalian Cells by *Salmonella typhimurium*.** *Nature* 1992, **357**:588–589.

A major advance in our understanding of how this bacterium interacts with the target host cell. It may have quite an influence on new therapeutic modalities.

6. • MURPHY GS, BODHIDATTA L, ECHEVERRIA P, TANSUPHASWADIKUL S, HOGE CW, IMLARP S, TAMURA K: **Ciprofloxacin and Loperamide in the Treatment of Bacillary Dysentery.** *Ann Intern Med* 1993, **118**:582–586.

A well-designed and controlled study showing clearcut benefit to individuals treated with both drugs compared with ciprofloxacin alone. No doubt this will provoke some discussion about the risks in areas with fluoroquinolone-resistant organisms.

7. VAN LOON FP, BENNISH ML, SPEELMAN P, BUTLER C: **Double Blind Trial of Loperamide for Treating Acute Watery Diarrhoea in Expatriates in Bangladesh.** *Gut* 1989, **30**:492–495.

8. FORMAL SB, ABRAMS GD, SCHNEIDER H, SPRINZ H: **Experimental *Shigella* Infections: VI. Role of the Small Intestine in an Experimental Infection in Guinea Pigs.** *J Bacteriol* 1963, **85**:119–125.

9. DUPONT HL, HORNICK RB: **Adverse Effect of Lomotil Therapy in Shigellosis.** *JAMA* 1973, **226**:1525–1528.

10. • BUTLER T, LOLEKHA S, RASIDI, KADIO A, DEL-ROSAL PL, ISKANDAR H, RUBINSTEIN E, PASTORE G: **Treatment of Acute Bacterial Diarrhea: a Multicenter International Trial Comparing Placebo With Fleroxacin Given as a Single Dose or Once Daily for 3 Days.** *Am J Med* 1993, **94**(Suppl 3A):187–194.

This paper suggests that a single dose of fleroxacin is functionally equivalent to longer dosing; experience has shown that when epidemic cholera strikes, a single dose of doxycycline or tetracycline may shorten infection, and so the result is not unexpected.

11. MACDONALD KL, OSTERHOLM MT: **Editorial. The Emergence of *Escherichia coli* O157:H7 Infection in the United States. The Changing Epidemiology of Foodborne Disease.** *JAMA* 1993, **269**:2264–2266.

12. ANONYMOUS: **Preliminary Report: Foodborne Outbreak of *Escherichia coli* O157:H7 Infections From Hamburgers - Western United States.** *MMWR Morb Mortal Wkly Rep* 1993, **42**:85–86.

13. • ROWE PC, ORRBINE E, LIOR H, WELLS GA, MCLAINE PN: **Diarrhoea in Close Contacts as a Risk Factor for Childhood Haemolytic Uraemic Syndrome.** *Epidemiol Infect* 1993, **110**:9–16.

One of three papers addressing an aspect of the recent epidemics of enterohemmorhagic *E. coli* O157:H7 in North American, and painting a wider canvas together than individually.

14. • BELONGIA EA, OSTERHOLD MT, SOLER JT, AMMEND DA, BRAUN JE, MACDONALD KL: **Transmission of *Escherichia coli* O157:H7 Infection in Minnesota Child Day-Care Facilities.** *JAMA* 1993, **269**:883–888.

One of three papers addressing an aspect of the recent epidemics of EHEC O157:H7 in North America, and painting a wider canvas together than individually.

15. • LE SAUX N, SPIKA JS, FRIESEN B, JOHNSON I, MELNYCHUCK D, ANDERSON C, DION R, RAHMAN M, TOSTOWARKY W: **Ground Beef Consumption in Noncommercial Settings is a Risk Factor for Sporadic *Escherichia Coli* O157:H7 Infection in Canada.** *J Infect Dis* 1993, **167**:500–502.

One of three papers addressing an aspect of the recent epidemics of EHEC O157:H7 in North American, and painting a wider canvas together than individually.

16. • BESSER RE, LETT SM, WEBER JT, DOYLE MP, BARRETT TJ, WELLS JG, GRIFFIN PM: **An Outbreak of Diarrhea and Hemolytic Uremic Syndrome From *Escherichia coli* O157:H7 in Fresh-Pressed Apple Cider.** *JAMA* 1993, **269**:2217–2220.

I was impressed not only by the investigative work, but also by the authors' investigation of cider as a potential haven for *E. coli* O157:H7. The latter made much more sense to me after having read Gordon and Small's paper (*Infect Immun* 1993, 61:364–367).

17. •• BITZAN M, LUDWIG K, KLEMT M, KONIG H, BUREN J, MULLER-WIEFEL DE: **The Role of *Escherichia coli* 0:157 Infections in the Classical (Enteropathic) Haemolytic Uraemic Syndrome: Results of a Central European, Multicentre Study.** *Epidemiol Infect* 1993, **110**:183–196.

Well-done, complete, and large study of hemolytic uremic syndrome in Europe, where both the pathogens and the epidemiology are a bit different from North America.

18. • SMITH HR, SCOTLAND SM: **ACP Broadsheet 135: Isolation and Identification Methods for *Escherichia coli* O157 and Other Vero Cytoxin-Producing Strains.** *Br Med J* 1993, **??**:10–17.

Not the lightest of reading, but both useful to the laboratory and useful to the reader trying to learn more about these colonic pathogens.

19. • TOKHI AM, PEIRIS JSM, SCOTLAND SM, WILLSHAW GA, SMITH HR, CHEASTY T: **A Longitudinal Study of Vero Cytotoxin Producing *Escherichia coli* in Cattle Calves in Sri Lanka.** *Epidemiol Infect* 1993, **110**:197–208.

A clever study that documents the intimate association between Shiga-like toxin (Verotoxin)-producing *E. coli* and domestic cattle.

20. • CAPRIOLI A, NIGRELLI A, GATTI R, ZAVANELLA M: **Isolation of Verotoxin-Producing *Escherichia coli* From Slaughtered Pigs.** *Eur J Clin Microbiol Infect Dis* 1993, **12**:227–228.

Further documents the presence of EHEC-associated organisms from another important food animal.

21. • WILLSHAW GA, SCOTLAND SM, SMITH HR, ROWE B: **Properties of Vero Cytotoxin-Producing *Escherichia coli* of Human Origin of O Serogroups other than O157.** *J Infect Dis* 1992, **166**:797–802.

Documents the large array of phenotypic and genotypic properties that Shiga-like toxin producing organisms can display. This should trouble anyone who believes that *E. coli* stay within the boundaries of the organizational boxes in which we place them!

22. SCHMIDT H, MONTAG M, BOCKEMUHL J, HEESEMANN J, KARCH H: **Shiga-Like Toxin II-Related Cytotoxins in *Citrobacter freundii* Strains From Humans and Beef Samples.** *Infect Immun* 1993, **61**:534–543.

23. • BETTELHEIM KA, EVANGELIDIS H, PEARCE JL, SOWERS E, STROCKBINE NA: **Isolation of a *Citrobacter freundii* Strain Which Carries the *Escherichia coli* O157 Antigen.** *J Clin Microbiol* 1993, **31**:760–761.

Only time will tell if the presence of Shiga-like toxin, and the presence of the O:157 serotype, in some *Citrobacter freundii* indicate potential new pathogenic possibilities.

24. •• LI Z, BELL C, BURET A, ROBINS-BROWNE R, STIEL D, O'LOUGHLIN E: **The Effect of Enterohemorrhagic *Escherichia coli* O157:H7 on Intestinal Structure and Solute Transport in Rabbits.** *Gastroenterology* 1993, **104**:467–474.

This group used deletion mutants to confirm the results of Tzipori *et al.* (see the two papers below), who used naturally occurring strains that lacked specific genetic material, that factors *other* than Shiga-like toxin and the attachment genes contribute to the intense inflammation seen in EHEC infections. We obviously have a lot to learn about these organisms.

25. Tzipori S, Wachsmuth KI, Smithers J, Jackson C: **Studies in Gnotobiotic Piglets on Non-O157:H7 *Escherichia coli* Serotypes Isolated From Patients With Hemorrhagic Colitis.** *Gastroenterology* 1988, 94:590–597.

26. Tzipori S, Karch H, Wachsmuth KI, Robins-Browne RM, O'Brien AD, Lior H, Cohen ML, Smithers J, Levine MM: **The Role of a 60-Megadalton Plasmid and Shiga Like Toxins in the Pathogenesis of Infection Caused by *Enterohemorrhagic Escherichia coli* O157:H7 in Gnotobiotic Piglets.** *Infect Immun* 1987, **55**:3117–3125.

27. • Sethabutr O, Venkatesan M, Murphy G, Eampokalap B, Hoge CW, Echeverria P: **Detection of *Shigellae* and *Enteroinvasive Escherichia coli* by Amplification of the Invasion Plasmid Antigen H DNA Sequence in Patients With Dysentery.** *J Infect Dis* 1993, **167**:458–461.

I love the idea of being able to make a posttreatment etiologic diagnosis, feeling quite frustrated when cultures are negative after treatment is begun. Polymerase chain reaction is uniquely suited to this purpose.

28. •• Kapperud G, Lassen J, Ostroff SM, Aasen S: **Clinical Features of Sporadic *Campylobacter* in Norway.** *Scand J Infect Dis* 1992, **24**:741–749.

For *Campylobacter* students, this paper extends our concepts about the range of disease, and manifestations in different age groups. Estimates of the costs to the Norwegian economy are also given, helping to place this infection in perspective.

29. • Endtz HP, Ruijs JR, van Klingeren B, Jansen WH, van der Reyden T, Mouton RP: **Quinolone Resistance in Campylobacter Isolated from Man and Poultry Following the Introduction of Fluoroquinolones in Veterinary Medicine.** *J Antimicrob Chemother* 1991, **27**:199–208.

Campylobacter organisms have been reported to develop resistance to fluoroquinolones during treatment, so the issue of resistance is not academic.

30. • Reina J, Borrell N, Serra A: **Emergence of Resistance to Erythromycin and Fluoroquinolones in Thermotolerant *Campylobacter* Strains Isolated From Feces 1987-1991.** *Eur J Clin Microbiol Infect Dis* 1992, **11**:1163–1166.

Campylobacter organisms have been reported to develop resistance to fluoroquinolones during treatment, so the issue of resistance is not academic.

31. • Endtz HP, Broeren M, Mouton RP: **In Vitro Susceptibility of Quinolone-Resistant *Campylobacter jejuni* to New Macrolide Antibiotics.** *Eur J Clin Microbiol Infect Dis* 1993, **12**:48–50.

Campylobacter organisms have been reported to develop resistance to fluoroquinolones during treatment, so the issue of resistance is not academic.

32. •• Ostroff SM, Kapperud G, Lassen J, Aasen S, Tauxe RV: **Clinical Features of Sporadic *Yersinia enterocolitica* Infections in Norway.** *J Infect Dis* 1992, **166**:812–817.

Of interest to readers will be the documentation of prolonged disease (greater than a year) in some, and the differences in age-specific symptomatology.

33. • Robins-Browne RM, Takeda T, Fasano A, Bordun AM, Dohi S, Kasuga H, Fong G, Prado V, Guerrant RL, Morris JG Jr: **Assessment of Enterotoxin Production by *Yersinia enterocolitica* and Identification of a Novel Heat-Stable Enterotoxin Produced by a Noninvasive *Y. enterocolitica* strain Isolated From Clinical Material.** *Infect Immun* 1993, **61**:764–767.

Careful work in describing and characterizing a new bacterial toxin from a noninvasive strain.

34. • Probst P, Hermann E, Meyer zum Buschenfelde K-H, Fleischer B: **Multiclonal Synovial T-Cell Response to *Yersinia enterocolitica* in Reactive Arthritis: The *Yersinia* 61-kDa Heat-Shock Protein is Not the Major Target Antigen.** *J Infect Dis* 1993, **167**:385–391.

The multiclonal nature of the T-cell response may indicate that reactive arthritis in yersiniosis is not all dependent on a single bacterial antigen or epitope.

35. • Galdiero F, Cipollaro de L'Ero G, Benedetto N, Galdiero M, Tufano MA: **Release of Cytokines Induced by *Salmonella typhimurium porins*.** *Infect Immun* 1993, **61**:155–161.

The latest in a progression of papers describing the pathologic sequelae of porins; this business about cytokine induction is intriguing, given current knowledge about how central cytokines are in the development of inflammation and sepsis.

36. • Rao PS, Rajashekar V, Varghese GK, Shaivananda PG: **Emergence of Multidrug-Resistant *Salmonella typhi* in Rural Southern India.** *Am J Trop Med Hyg* 1993, **48**:108–111.

A well-written and well-done study that documents the spread of multidrug resistant typhoid, and the clinical efficacy of both fluoroquinolones in adults and furazolidone in children.

37. • Threlfall EJ, Ward LR, Rowe B, Raghupathi S, Chandrasekaran V, Vandepitte J, Lemmens P: **Widespread Occurrence of Multiple Drug-Resistant *Salmonella typhi* in India.** *Eur J Clin Microbiol Infect Dis* 1992, **11**:990–993.

A well-written and well-done study that documents the spread of multidrug resistant typhoid, and the clinical efficacy of both fluoroquinolones in adults and furazolidone in children.

38. • Arnold K, Hong C-S, Nelwan R, Zavala-Trujillo I, Kadio A, Barros MA, de Garis S: **Randomized Comparative Study of Fleroxacin and Chloramphenicol in Typhoid Fever.** *Am J Med* 1993, **94(Suppl 3A)**:195–200.

A well-written and well-done study that documents the spread of multidrug resistant typhoid, and the clinical efficacy of both fluoroquinolones in adults and furazoldone in children.

39. • Dutta P, Rasaily R, Saha MR, Mitra U, Manna B, Chakraborty S, Mukherjee A: **Randomized Clinical Trial of Furazolidone for Typhoid Fever in Children.** *Scand J Gastroenterol* 1993, **28**:168–172.

A well-written and well-done study that documents the spread of multidrug resistant typhoid, and the clinical efficacy of both fluoroquinolones in adults and furazolidone in children.

40. •• Fekety R, Shah AB: **Diagnosis and Treatment of *Clostridium difficile colitis*.** *JAMA* 1993, **269**:71–75.

Clinical wisdom distilled for the pleasure of the reader to imbibe.

41. •• Bartlett JG: **The 10 Most Common Questions About *Clostridium difficile*-Associated Diarrhea/Colitis.** *Infect Dis Clin Pract* 1992, **1**:254–259.

Clinical wisdom distilled for the pleasure of the reader to imbibe.

42. •• Pothoulakis C, Kelly CP, Joshi MA, Gao N, O'Keane CJ, Castagliuolo I, Lamont JT: ***Saccharomyces boulardii* Inhibits *Clostridium difficile* Toxin A Binding and Enterotoxicity in Rat Ileum.** *Gastroenterology* 1993, **104**:1108–1115.

Nice science delineating the benefits of a yeast in *C. difficile*-associated disease by examining the mechanisms by which we believe toxin A does its damage.

43. • Siffert J-C, Baldacini O, Kuhry J-G, Wachsmann D, Benabdelmoumene S, Faradji A, Monteil H, Poindron P: **Effects of *Clostridium difficile* toxin B on Human Monocytes and Macrophages: Possible Relationship With Cytoskeletal Rearrangement.** *Infect Immun* 1993, **61**:1082–1090.

Whoa! Toxin B appears to both activate cytokine production (instigating inflammation) and render the phagocytic macrophage impotent at the same time via cytoskeletal derangements.

44. • Walpita P, Billman GF, Krous HF: **Mammalian Epithelial Cell Line Kit for Detection of *Clostridium difficile* Toxin.** *J Clin Microbiol* 1993, **31**:315–317.

Of interest to anyone trying to increase their diagnostic abilities for *C. difficile* toxins.

45. GUMERLOCK PH, TANG YJ, WEISS JB, SILVA J JR: **Specific Detection of Toxigenic Strains of *Clostridium difficile* in Stool Specimens.** *J Clin Microbiol* 1993, **31**:507–511.
•
Of interest to anyone trying to increase their diagnostic abilities for *C. difficile* toxins.

46. KATO N, OU C-Y, KATO H, BARTLEY SL, LUO CC, KILLGORE GE, UENO K: **Detection of Toxigenic *Clostridium difficile* in Stool Specimens by the Polymerase Chain Reaction.** *J Infect Dis.* 1993, **167**:455–458.
•
Of interest to anyone trying to increase their diagnostic abilities for *C. difficile* toxins.

47. BARBUT F, DEPITRE C, DELMÉE M, CORTHIER G, PETIT J-C: **Comparison of Enterotoxin Production, Cytotoxin Production, Serogrouping,and Antimicrobial Susceptibilities of *Clostridium difficile* Strains Isolated From AIDS and Human Immunodeficiency Virus-Negative Patients.** *J Clin Microbiol* 1993, **31**:740–742.
•
For the life of me I can't figure out why the authors did this study, but it is interesting. Why serogroup C was so much more common in AIDS patients is not clear - is it because of antibiotic pressure, as the authors suggest, or some ecologic alteration in the gut of HIV patients?

48. CAMPBELL SF, WYNNE JM, MCCORMACK JG: **Severe Amoebic Colitis Requiring Colonic Resection.** *Aust N Z J Surg* 1992, **62**:405–407.
•
Reminds us that medical treatment is not adequate in some patients with amebic colitis. Alerts us to the pathogenic potential of other *Entamoeba* species.

49. ***Entamoeba polecki*: Human Infections in Venezuela.** *Trans R Soc Trop Med Hyg* 1992, **86**:633–634.
•
Reminds us that medical treatment is not adequate in some patients with amebic colitis. Alerts us to the pathogenic potential of other *Entamoeba* species.

50. SARGEAUNT PG, PATRICK S, O'KEEFE D: **Human Infections of *Entamoeba chattoni* Masquerade as *Entamoeba histolytica*.** *Trans R Soc Trop Med Hyg* **86**:633–634.
•
Reminds us that medical treatment is not adequate in some patients with amebic colitis. Alerts us to the pathogenic potential of other *Entamoeba* species.

51. CLAYTON F, REKA S, CRONIN WJ, TORLAKOVIC E, SIGAL SH, KOTLER DP: **Rectal Mucosal Pathology Varies With Human Immunodeficiency Virus Antigen Content and Disease Stage.** *Gastroenterology* 1992, **103**:919–933.
••
This superb study ties together the pathologic, viral, and immunologic characteristics of gut tissue during the progression of disease in HIV-seropositive individuals, and does so in a way that may help explain the prevalence of "nonspecific" symptoms and the sequelae of increased mucosal permeability. Highly recommended.

52. KAPEMBWA MS, HEMING SC, SEWANKAMBO N, SERWADDA D, LUCAS S, MOODY A, GRIFFIN GE: **Altered Small Intestinal Permeability Associated With Diarrhea in Human-Immunodeficiency-Virus-Infected Caucasian and African Subjects.** *Clin Sci* 1991, **81**:327–334.

53. FANTINI J, COOK DG, NATHANSON N, SPITALNIK SL, GONZALEZ-SCARANO F: **Infection of Colonic Epithelial Cell Lines by Type 1 Human Immunodeficiency Virus is Associated With Cell Surface Expression of Galactosylceramide, a Potential Alternative gp120 Receptor.** *Proc Natl Acad Sci U S A* 1993, **90**:2700–2704.
•
There is a large body of research being conducted on the entry of HIV into cells other than lymphocytes, and this well-done study strongly suggests that the colonic mucosa can be directly invaded by HIV without the presence of glycoprotein 120.

54. GOODGAME RW, GENTA RM, ESTRADA R, DEMMLER G, BUFFONE G: **Frequency of Positive Tests for Cytomegalovirus in AIDS Patients: Endoscopic Lesions Compared With Normal Mucosa.** *Am J Gastroenterol* 1993, **88**:338–343.
•
Deals with active issues in the diagnosis of cytomegalovirus colitis, which is often problematic. Reports an unusual manifestation of cytomegalovirus colitis.

55. BONACINI M, LAINE L: **Editorial. Detection of Cytomegalovirus in the Gastrointestinal Tract: Seeking a Gold Standard.** *Am J Gastroenterol* 1993, **88**:332–333.
•
Deals with active issues in the diagnosis of cytomegalovirus colitis, which is often problematic. Reports an unusual manifestation of cytomegalovirus colitis.

56. NEUMAYER LA, MAKAR R, AMPEL NM, ZUKOSKI CF: **Cytomegalovirus Appendicitis in a Patient With Human Immunodeficiency Virus Infection. Case Report and Review of the Literature.** *Arch Surg* 1993, **128**:467–468.
•
Deals with active issues in the diagnosis of cytomegalovirus colitis, which is often problematic. Reports an unusual manifestation of cytomegalovirus colitis.

Jeffrey K. Griffiths, MD, Division of Infectious Diseases, St. Elizabeth's Medical Center, 736 Cambridge Street, Boston, MA 02135, USA.

Viral infections of the gastrointestinal tract

Robert D. Shaw, MD

Newport Veterans Administration Medical Center, Northport, New York, USA

Viral infections of the gastrointestinal tract are a major worldwide cause of morbidity and mortality, especially in underdeveloped settings. *Rotavirus* is the leading cause of severe gastroenteritis in children and has been the object of intensive vaccine development efforts for several years. Although much has been learned, a satisfactory vaccine strategy has yet to be reported and many investigators are now testing alternative strategies. Recent advances in the study of gastroenteritis viruses include the cloning and characterization of the genomes of Norwalk-like viruses (now designated members of the *Caliciviridae*) and astroviruses, which have spawned a variety of epidemiologic studies and portend many more.

Current Opinion in Gastroenterology 1994, **10**:74–79

Viral gastroenteritis

Astroviruses

Astroviruses are nonenveloped particles with a distinctive star-shaped surface structure that have been detected in the stools of humans and animals with gastroenteritis. Recently obtained information on the genomic and capsid structure of astroviruses has resulted in classification of these viruses in a distinct family, the *Astroviridae* [1•,2••]. As a result, it has been only in the past 1 to 2 years that suitable diagnostic assays have become available that have permitted astroviruses to be identified as a significant cause of diarrheal disease. The importance of this virus as a human pathogen is probably substantial because the frequency of the syndrome of viral gastroenteritis is so great; however, astroviruses are not as important as rotaviruses because they less frequently cause disease, especially with severe symptoms. Several recent epidemiologic studies are now providing data with which to place this issue into perspective. Children in Nigeria suffering from diarrhea were found to be infected with *Astrovirus* 1.5% when *Rotavirus* was found in 26% [3•]. (Both infections appear to be seasonal in temperate climates, although this may not be the case in tropical regions.) A 5-year prospective study of *Rotavirus*, enteric *Adenovirus*, and *Astrovirus* found that about 8% of viral enteritis was caused by *Astrovirus* [4•]. Children in the rural highlands of Guatemala had *Astrovirus* associated with 7.3% of 361 diarrheal stools [5•]. Investigators in Baltimore found *Astrovirus* to be an infrequent cause of diarrhea requiring medical attention [6•].

An outbreak of gastroenteritis in Marin County, California in 1978 was caused by a viral agent that was isolated and later administered to volunteers. Immunoassays were recently prepared to detect antibodies to this agent, which has now been recognized as an astrovirus, but this virus could not be implicated as a cause in 32 other outbreaks of nonbacterial gastroenteritis that were screened with this assay. However, prevalence of antibody to this strain of *Astrovirus* was approximately 13% in children 6 months to 3 years old and increased to 41% in older children and young adults [7•].

Caliciviruses

The recent classification of Norwalk and Norwalk-like viruses as caliciviruses has greatly simplified the nomenclature of gastroenteritis viruses [8•]. There are ongoing efforts to use the newly acquired genetic information to investigate epidemiologic questions and develop diagnostic reagents and assays. Several recent reports have described the development of polymerase chain reaction–based assays for detection of Norwalk virus in stool samples [9•,10•].

Adenoviruses

Enteric adenoviruses, especially types 40 and 41, are recognized as major causes of gastroenteritis in children and occasional pathogens in immunocompromised adults. Polymerase chain reaction–based assays for all groups of adenoviruses and also for enteric adenoviruses have been developed, and have been shown to be highly sensitive and specific [11].

Ongoing epidemiologic studies continue to identify *Adenoviridae* as an important gastroenteritis pathogen, although significantly less important than *Rotavirus*. The relative contributions of adenoviruses to overall morbidity seems similar in temperate, developed countries or in less developed, tropical regions such as Nigeria. One aspect of *Adenoviridae* infection that distinguishes the syndrome from that caused by *Rotavirus* and *Astrovirus* is that it may occur throughout the year even in temperate climates where the other viral infections are more common in winter [3•,4•,12•]. As is often the case with gastroenteritis viruses, many of the infections are subclinical [13•].

Monoclonal antibodies have been characterized that will be useful in improving the typing of enteric adenoviruses [14•].

Rotavirus

Epidemiology

Rotavirus is the major cause of viral gastroenteritis in infants and young children, but can also cause disease in adults. This is especially true in special situations like close family contact or international travel. An example of the latter situation has been reported by Bourgeois *et al.* [15•], who report a surprising number of cases of *Rotavirus* (and less surprisingly) Norwalk gastroenteritis among military personnel traveling to South America. As expected, enterotoxigenic *Escherichia coli* were the most common pathogen identified in these patients with diarrhea.

The evolution of rotavirus classification has been underway for some time. Initially, *Rotavirus* serotypes were distinguished by antibodies directed at the VP7 protein. As understanding increased of the role of antibodies to VP4, a new classification scheme was proposed to account for this, and each *Rotavirus* strain was designated to have a G type (defined by VP7) and a P type (defined by antibodies to the protease-sensitive VP4) in a manner similar to the scheme used for influenza that identifies hemagglutinin and neuraminidase serologies. Approximately eight *Rotavirus* G types have been identified in humans, and six P types, although the numbers are frequently increased as most viruses are yet to have their P types identified [16•]. P typing has been somewhat difficult because of the predominant reactivity of hyperimmune serum to VP7, the cross-reactivity of many VP4-specific neutralizing monoclonal antibodies, and the low levels of discrimination of antisera to individual VP4 proteins expressed in recombinant molecular systems such as baculovirus. To facilitate this process, efforts to develop convenient monoclonal antibody-based P typing immunoassays are being reported [17••]. A more precise assessment of the serologic variety of circulating rotaviruses remains essential to the development of an effective vaccine strategy.

Signs and symptoms

The syndrome of viral gastroenteritis involves nausea and vomiting as well as diarrhea. In children infected with *Rotavirus*, investigators have identified a delay in gastric emptying that may explain prominent vomiting [18•]. However, as *Rotavirus* infects the small intestinal epithelium, it remains unclear by what mechanism gastric emptying is affected. De Boissieu *et al.* [19•] suggest that α-interferon stimulation during *Rotavirus* infection may be a mechanism that may cause symptoms.

The presence of fecal leukocytes or occult blood is often considered a marker for invasive bacterial enteritis. However, such findings are regularly found in *Rotavirus* infections. A recent observation of this phenomenon was reported by Huicho *et al.* [20•].

Pathophysiology

It is known that nonimmune defenses such as gastric acid are important in protecting against bacterial infection, but factors protecting against viral infection are less well characterized. Chen *et al.* [21•] have been studying the role of intestinal mucin in prevention of *Rotavirus* infection. Using a murine model of *Rotavirus* infection, they demonstrated that the inhibitory effect of intestinal mucin varied with location in the gastrointestinal tract. Inhibition was also affected by the structure of the viral hemagglutinin VP4. Inhibition of viral binding to enterocytes is probably responsible for the inhibitory effect.

A rise in endogenous α-interferon levels during *Rotavirus* infection has been documented by De Boissieu *et al.* [19•]. A role for cytokines in either the induction of symptoms or the limitation of infection is likely, but reports such as this are only the beginning of this story.

Vaccines

Recombinant adenoviruses have been studied as intestinal vaccine vectors for a variety of antigens, including hepatitis B [22]. Those investigating *Rotavirus* have reported the design of a recombinant *Adenovirus* vector that expresses a modified *Rotavirus* VP7, a major neutralization antigen that can induce protective immunity [23••].

Clinical strategies for the administration of an anticipated *Rotavirus* vaccine are under constant study. Crawley *et al.* [24•] have gathered data to support the proposition that vaccination will need to be performed well within the first 6 months of life, while Brussow *et al.* [25•] have determined that titers of anti-*Rotavirus* antibodies in breast milk from Mexican mothers were not sufficient to impair the immunity that is generated by live, attenuated viral vaccines.

Clinical markers of *Rotavirus* immunity have been difficult to obtain. Serum antibodies are not very good predictors of intestinal immune status. Therefore, it is of some interest that Matson *et al.* [26•] have found that fecal anti-*Rotavirus* immunoglobulin A correlated with resistance to infection among young children in daycare centers. Offit *et al.* [27•] identified children suffering a primary infection by the measurement of serum immunoglobulin A and *Rotavirus*-specific T-helper cells, a novel way to exclude the complicating factors of previous *Rotavirus* infection or maternal antibody contributions. They found that in eight children less than 2 years old, six developed immunoglobulin A responses directed to the VP4 protein and seven had convalescent helper T-cell activity. The principal determinants of the specificity of the neutralizing antibody response to *Rotavirus* have been the subjects of considerable conflicting data, and so it is not surprising that in the same time period that Richardson *et al.* [28•] measured serum responses to *Rotavirus* infection by different methods and determined that most of the children they studied had type-specific responses directed at VP7 (the other major neutralization protein). However, they also noted that all patients tested did have some antibodies to VP4.

Development of a useful *Rotavirus* vaccine has been imminent for quite some time now, but field trials of candidate vaccines have been disappointing. The principal difficulty has been the type-specific immunity induced by live attenuated vaccines, which affords inadequate disease prevention because of the several serotypes that tend to circulate simultaneously. Probably the only exception has been in Finland, where investigators have found candidate vaccines to be useful [29]. Interesting trials using live attenuated viruses remain ongoing, mostly using combinations of reassortant viruses designed to induce immunity to several serotypes, but little success has been reported this year.

Viral intestinal infections in the immunocompromised host

Adenoviruses seem to be important in immunocompromised patients. One recent report identified *Adenovirus* in large bowel mucosa of HIV-positive patients, although the contribution to disease was not very clear [30•]. An interesting study using a technique of *in situ* hybridization found that patients with pulmonary *Adenovirus* infection who also had *Adenovirus* cultured from the intestinal tract did not have evidence of invasive intestinal infection. Of course, these were not enteric *Adenovirus* types 40 and 41 [31•].

Rotaviruses have been variably found in the stools of immunocompromised individuals. A recent study has found a significant number of diarrheal illnesses in AIDS patients that seem to be associated with rotaviruses, but the infections were mild and self-limited [32•].

References and recommended reading

Papers of particular interest, published within the annual period of review, have been highlighted as:

• Of special interest

•• Of outstanding interest

1. • MATSUI SM, KIM JP, GREENBERG HB, YOUNG LM, SMITH LS, LEWIS TL, HERRMANN JE, BLACKLOW NR, DUPUIS K, *ET AL.*: **Cloning and Characterization of Human Astrovirus Immunoreactive Epitopes.** *J Virol* 1993, 67:1712–1715.

The authors reported the cloning of a protein-coding region of human astrovirus that appears to be common to most serotypes of human astrovirus. The authors can use this work as the basis of further progress, such as the development of convenient immunoassays for epidemiologic studies to more precisely evaluate the pathogenic role of astroviruses.

2. •• MONROE SS, JIANG B, STINE SE, KOOPMANS M, GLASS RI: **Subgenomic RNA Sequence of Human Astrovirus Supports Classification of Astroviridae as a New Family of RNA Viruses.** *J Virol* 1993, 67:3611–3614.

The molecular analysis of the *Astrovirus* genome has confirmed that the 2484-nucleotide RNA contains a single open reading frame, which encodes a protein with a predicted molecular mass of 88 kD. This protein is probably the capsid protein precursor present in infected cells. As it does not share amino acid similarities with capsid proteins of other viruses with similar genomic organizations, these viruses are now classified in an exclusive viral family, the *Astroviridae.*

3. • AVERY RM, SHELTON AP, BEARDS GM, OMOTADE OO, OYEJIDE OC, OLALEYE DO: **Viral Agents Associated With Infantile Gastroenteritis in Nigeria: Relative Prevalence of Adenovirus Serotypes 40 and 41, Astrovirus, and Rotavirus Serotypes 1 to 4.** *J Diarrhoeal Dis Res* 1992, 10:105–108.

Gastroenteritis pathogens seem to occur in similar frequencies in many parts of the world. Rotaviruses are almost always the most important cause of severe viral diarrhea regardless of the geographic area studied. In this study, which reported data from Nigeria and the United Kingdom, enteric adenoviruses and astroviruses were identified as significant pathogens, although far less often than rotaviruses.

4. • BATES PR, BAILEY AS, WOOD DJ, MORRIS DJ, COURIEL JM: **Comparative Epidemiology of Rotavirus, Subgenus F (Types 40 and 41) Adenovirus and Astrovirus Gastroenteritis in Children.** *J Med Virol* 1993, 39:224–228.

In a 5-year prospective study, episodes of *Rotavirus*, subgenus F *Adenovirus*, and *Astrovirus* gastroenteritis are reported, including 1426 total infections. The etiologic breakdown was 78.3% *Rotavirus*, 17.8% *Adenovirus*, and 7.9% *Astrovirus.* Adenoviruses were particularly common in victims less than 6 months old and showed no seasonal preference (rotaviruses and astroviruses are more common in winter).

5. • CRUZ JR, BARTLETT AV, HERRMANN JE, CACERES P, BLACKLOW NR, CANO F: **Astrovirus-Associated Diarrhea Among Guatemalan Ambulatory Rural Children.** *J Clin Microbiol* 1992, 30:1140–1144.

Astrovirus excretion was associated with 7.3% of diarrheal episodes in 321 Guatemalan children; 2.4% of stools from diarrhea-free periods also contained astroviruses; and, in symptomatic infections, up to two thirds of children also had other potential enteropathogens present. Diarrhea associated with astroviruses alone had a median duration of 5 days and was associated with vomiting in 8.6%, with fever in 17.1%, with dehydration in 5.7%, and with loss of appetite in 34.3% of the episodes. Diarrhea due to astroviruses was accompanied by weight loss. *Astrovirus*-caused diarrhea contributes to the high morbidity observed in young children living under poor conditions and has a deleterious effect on their nutritional status.

6. KOTLOFF KL, HERRMANN JE, BLACKLOW NR, HUDSON RW,
• WASSERMAN SS, MORRIS J JR., LEVINE MM: **The Frequency of Astrovirus as a Cause of Diarrhea in Baltimore Children.** *Pediatr Infect Dis J* 1992, **11**:587–589.

The authors use a monoclonal antibody-based immunoassay to detect *Astrovirus* in stool specimens from 424 children less than 2 years old at the University of Maryland Hospital. Some children were hospitalized with diarrhea, some were outpatients, and a small number of cases were nosocomial. A group of 309 controls were matched for age and date of illness. *Astrovirus* was identified in 2.8% of children with diarrhea and 1.6% of controls. In five of 12 cases of diarrhea associated with *Astrovirus*, another enteropathogen was found. The authors concluded that in the Baltimore area *Astrovirus* was an uncommon cause of diarrhea requiring medical attention.

7. MIDTHUN K, GREENBERG HB, KURTZ JB, GARY GW, LIN FY,
• KAPIKIAN AZ: **Characterization and Seroepidemiology of a Type 5 Astrovirus Associated With an Outbreak of Gastroenteritis in Marin County, California.** *J Clin Microbiol* 1993, **31**:955–962.

The Marin County agent, implicated in diarrheal outbreaks in 1978, has been further characterized as an *Astrovirus*. Also, the pathogenicity of the isolate was tested in a volunteer study (one of 19 developed illness, nine of 19 developed serologic responses). Astroviruses have been found in the feces of infants and young children with mild gastroenteritis, occurring in outbreaks in nurseries, daycare centers, and also in nursing homes. It is currently thought to be a common (2% to 8%) cause of epidemic gastroenteritis in children, but to generally cause mild disease, unlike *Rotavirus* and enteric *Adenovirus*. The present study screened stools in 32 outbreaks among older children and adults, but none of the gastroenteritis cases could be attributed to a type of *Astrovirus* that shares significant similarity to the Marin County agent.

8. LAMBDEN PR, CAUL EO, ASHLEY CR, CLARKE IN: **Sequence and**
• **Genome Organization of a Human Small Round-Structured (Norwalk-Like) Virus.** *Science* 1993, **259**:516–519.

The complete genomic nucleotide sequence of another Norwalk-like small, round-structured virus (the Southampton virus) has been determined. The 7696-nucleotide genome encodes three open reading frames that are structurally similar to caliciviruses, as was the Norwalk virus sequenced previously.

9. DELEON R, MATSUI SM, BARIC RS, HERMANN JE, BLACKLOW NR,
• GREENBERG HB, SOBSEY MD: **Detection of Norwalk Virus in Stool Specimens by Reverse Transcriptase-Polymerase Chain Reaction and Nonradioactive Oligoprobes.** *J Clin Microbiol* 1992, **30**:3151–3157.

A reverse transcriptase-polymerase chain reaction-oligoprobe, method was developed for the detection of the Norwalk virus. This assay appears to be very sensitive (100 times more sensitive than radioimmunoassay) and specific, and should provide an excellent means for research labs to improve epidemiologic studies of this noncultivatable virus. Further studies will be needed to determine optimal design of polymerase chain reaction primers to detect a wide range of Norwalk and Norwalk-like viruses.

10. JIANG X, WANG J, GRAHAM DY, ESTES MK: **Detection of Nor-**
• **walk Virus in Stool by Polymerase Chain Reaction.** *J Clin Microbiol* 1992, **30**:2529–2534.

The use of polymerase chain reaction to diagnose Norwalk virus in stools seems likely to be a good idea, especially for epidemiologic or environmental studies, because the virus is shed in small amounts from humans and may contaminate water at extremely low concentrations. In fact, the authors showed that polymerase chain reaction was very sensitive for antigen detection in the stools of volunteers challenged with Norwalk. It remains to be seen whether primers can be selected that will permit polymerase chain reaction detection of a wide range of related but varyingly dissimilar human caliciviruses that are serologically related to the prototype Norwalk virus.

11. ALLARD A, ALBINSSON B, WADELL G: **Detection of Adenoviruses in Stools From Healthy Persons and Patients With Diarrhea by Two-Step Polymerase Chain Reaction.** *J Med Virol* 1992, **37**:149–157.

12. VAN R, WUN CC, O'RYAN ML, MATSON DO, JACKSON L,
• PICKERING LK: **Outbreaks of Human Enteric Adenovirus Types 40 and 41 in Houston Day Care Centers.** *J Pediatr* 1992, **120**:516–521.

Daycare centers are well known as excellent locations for transmission of gastroenteritis viruses. This study defines the role of enteric adenoviruses in daycare center epidemics, identifying enteric adenoviruses in 10 outbreaks of 96 children tested. The infection is often asymptomatic and viral shedding occurred a mean of 2.6 days before symptoms and for 5.3 days after symptoms resolved.

13. NISHIO O, SAKAE K, ISHIHARA Y, ISOMURA S, INOUYE S:
• **Adenovirus Infection and Specific Secretory IgA Responses in the Intestine of Infants.** *Microbiol Immunol* 1992, **36**:623–631.

Infants were followed from birth to 7 years old, and frequent repeated infections with adenoviruses of different serotypes were identified. Fecal immunoglobulin A responses were commonly identified, demonstrating intestinal infection. Most infections were mild or asymptomatic.

14. DE JONG JC, BIJLSMA K, WERMENBOL AG, VERWEIJ-UIJTERWAAL
• MW, VAN DER AVOORT HGAM, WOOD DJ, BAILEY AS, OSTERHAUS ADME: **Detection, Typing, and Subtyping of Enteric Adenoviruses 40 and 41 From Fecal Samples and Observation of Changing Incidences of Infections With These Types and Subtypes.** *J Clin Microbiol* 1993, **31**:1562–1569.

The authors reported the selection and characterization of a group of monoclonal antibodies that have several advantages as serotyping and subtyping reagents. The ability to distinguish *Adenovirus* types and subtypes does not have clinical significance, but may have epidemiologic interest. Also, these antibodies can specifically identify a Canadian genotype that was not identified by a previous commercial assay. Preliminary epidemiology done on samples from the Netherlands indicated that 4% of children with diarrhea scored positively (vs 21% for *Rotavirus*). The illness is best characterized as endemic as the incidence is spread throughout the year.

15. BOURGEOIS AL, GARDINER CH, THORNTON SA, BATCHELOR
• RA, BURR DH, ESCAMILLA J, ECHEVERRIA P, BLACKLOW NR, HERRMANN JE, *ET AL.*: **Etiology of Acute Diarrhea Among United States Military Personnel Deployed to South America and West Africa.** *Am J Trop Med Hyg* 1993, **48**:243–248.

Many military personnel develop diarrhea while traveling. In this study of naval personnel serving in South America and West Africa, 289 cases of diarrhea were studied revealing specific pathogens in 51% (a typical number). Enterotoxigenic *E. coli* were most commonly found as the pathogen, which is the usual finding in adult populations. A surprising contribution from gastroenteritis viruses was also observed: 11% with *Rotavirus* and 10% with Norwalk. The bacteria had a high rate of resistance to trimethoprim or sulfamethoxazole, but not to quinalones (yet).

16. DUNN SJ, GREENBERG HB, WARD RL, NAKAGOMI O, BURNS
• JW, VO PT, PAX KA, DAS M, GOWDA K, *ET AL.*: **Serotypic and Genotypic Characterization of Human Serotype 10 Rotaviruses From Asymptomatic Neonates.** *J Clin Microbiol* 1993, **31**:165–169.

A report of the characterization of the 10th human rotavirus G serotype. This virus bears a strong genetic similarity to bovine rotaviruses and may be the result of interspecies transmission.

17. COULSON BS: **Typing of Human Rotavirus VP4 by an Enzyme**
•• **Immunoassay Using Monoclonal Antibodies.** *J Clin Microbiol* 1993, **31**:1–8.

The addition of P typing to the previously established G typing has theoretic advantages in determination of protective immunity, as the system accounts for antibodies directed against both outer capsid proteins that mediated disease protection (VP4 and VP7). Well characterized monoclonal antibodies have been available for several years that can be used in convenient immunoassays to G-type *Rotavirus* strains, but VP4-specific antibodies have not previously been characterized to provide the same service for P typing. This report begins this process, which will gradually evolve as better antibodies and more P types are identified.

18. BARDHAN PK, SALAM MA, MOLLA AM: **Gastric Emptying of**
• **Liquid in Children Suffering From Acute Rotaviral Gastroenteritis.** *Gut* 1992, **33**:26–29.

Delayed gastric emptying has been shown to be a feature of Norwalk virus infection in adults. This report has now documented that it is also part of the pathophysiology of *Rotavirus* gastroenteritis. In many cases, vomiting may be a more prominent symptom than diarrhea, especially early in the illness.

19. DE BOISSIEU D, LEBON P, BADOUAL J, BOMPARD Y, DUPONT C:
• **Rotavirus Induces Alpha-Interferon Release in Children With Gastroenteritis.** *J Pediatr Gastroenterol Nutr* 1993, **16**:29–32.

The intestinal cytokine response to infection is a factor that may have a role in the pathogenesis of *Rotavirus* symptoms. High interferon levels occurring within 2 days of the onset of illness are correlated to the number of vomiting episodes. Perhaps the observed reduction in gastric emptying (Bardham *et al. Gut* 1992, 33:26–29) may be mediated by alterations in cytokine levels such as the α-interferon peak reported in this paper.

20. HUICHO L, SANCHEZ D, CONTRERAS M, PAREDES M, MURGA H,
• CHINCHAY L, GUEVARA G: **Occult Blood and Fecal Leukocytes as Screening Tests in Childhood Infectious Diarrhea: An Old Problem Revisited.** *Pediatr Infect Dis* 1993, **12**:474–477.

The authors found fecal occult blood and fecal leukocytes to be insensitive markers of invasive bacterial enteritis, but also found both cell types frequently in the stools of patients with *Rotavirus*-caused diarrhea (16% and 39% for leukocytes and erthrocytes respectively).

21. CHEN CC, BAYLOR M, BASS DM: **Murine Intestinal Mucins In-**
• **hibit Rotavirus Infection.** *Gastroenterology* 1993, **105**:84–92.

Mucin, a population of polymeric glycoproteins, constitutes the primary component of the mucus layer that overlies the gastrointestinal tract. Murine intestinal mucins were purified by the authors and tested for viral inhibition in tissue culture assays. Colonic mucins were more potent inhibitors of *Rotavirus* replication in tissue culture systems than small intestinal mucins, and viral susceptibility to mucin inhibition correlated with the viral gene 4, which codes for the viral hemagglutinin. Mucins represent a barrier to certain *Rotavirus* infections.

22. TACKET CO, LOSONSKY G, LUBECK MD, DAVIS AR, MIZUTANI S, HORWITH G, HUNG P, EDELMAN R, LEVINE MM: **Initial Safety and Immunogenicity Studies of an Oral Recombinant Adenohepatitis B Vaccine.** *Vaccine* 1992, **10**:673–676.

23. BOTH GW, LOCKETT LJ, JANARDHANA V, EDWARDS SJ, BELLAMY
•• AR, GRAHAM FL, PREVAC L, ANDREW ME: **Protective Immunity to Rotavirus-Induced Diarrhoea is Passively Transferred to Newborn Mice From Naive Dams Vaccinated With a Single Dose of a Recombinant Adenovirus Expressing Rotavirus VP7sc.** *Virology* 1993, **193**:940–950.

VP7sc is a novel *Rotavirus* antigen engineered for presentation at the cell surface. VP7 is a major neutralization antigen, but artificial presentations of this antigen in several expression vectors have not resulted in antigenically intact neutralizing antigen. These authors report the use of a recombinant *Adenovirus* to express VP7 that is presented in the cell membrane. This system produced VP7 that appeared to be capable of inducing protective immunity in mice. Adenovirus vaccines now join a variety of other alternative vaccine approaches awaiting further testing to define the optimal strategy for vaccination against gastroenteritis viruses.

24. CRAWLEY JM, BISHOP RF, BARNES GL: **Rotavirus Gastroen-**
• **teritis in Infants Aged 0-6 Months in Melbourne, Australia: Implications for Vaccination.** *J Paediatr Child Health* 1993, 29:219–221.

Almost 600 gastroenteritis patients under the age of 6 months were hospitalized in Melbourne, Australia between April 1980 and April 1990. Rotaviruses of several (G) serotypes were found in specimens from 15.1% of the infants, adenoviruses in 12.4%, and other pathogens in 10.8%. This finding supports the imperative that *Rotavirus* vaccination will need to be given during the first 1 to 3 months of life in developed countries, as is recommended for developing countries.

25. BRUSSOW H, BENITEZ O, URIBE F, SIDOTI J, ROSA K, CRAVIOTO
• A: **Rotavirus-Inhibitory Activity in Serial Milk Samples From Mexican Women and Rotavirus Infections in Their Children During Their First Year of Life.** *J Clin Microbiol* 1993, 31:593–597.

The *Rotavirus* inhibitory titer was too low in the majority of Mexican breast milk samples to have a significant effect on *Rotavirus* infection (that is, it will not prevent or ameliorate symptoms) or vaccination (live attenuated vaccine strains will not be neutralized before the desired antigen presentation is made at the mucosal surface).

26. MATSON DO, O'RYAN ML, HERRERA I, PICKERING L, ESTES
• MK: **Fecal Antibody Responses to Symptomatic and Asymptomatic Rotavirus Infection.** *J Infect Dis* 1993, **167**:577–583.

Children who contracted *Rotavirus* infection at daycare centers were prospectively identified. Antirotavirus fecal immunoglobulin A was evaluated before and after infection to determine whether it might have a role in protection of children from natural *Rotavirus* infection. The first 50 cases excreting virus and a similar number of nonexcreting controls were evaluated. Antirotavirus fecal immunoglobulin A was detected in 90% of infected children (both symptomatic and asymptomatic). The authors reported that preexposure titers were higher in those not infected, and were therefore associated with disease protection. Most infected children had fourfold or greater rises in antirotavirus fecal immunoglobulin A titers after infection, regardless of presence or absence of symptoms.

27. OFFIT PA, HOFFENBERG EJ, SANTOS N, GOUVEA V: **Rotavirus-**
• **Specific Humoral and Cellular Immune Response After Primary, Symptomatic Infection.** *J Infect Dis* 1993, 167:1436–1440.

The humoral and cellular immune response after symptomatic primary *Rotavirus* infection was examined in eight children under 2 years old. *Rotavirus*-specific immunoglobulin A, *Rotavirus*-specific T-helper cells, and neutralizing antibody responses were evaluated at the time of illness, 2 to 8 weeks later, and 3 to 5 months later. In addition, *Rotavirus* strains associated with infection were tested by polymerase chain reaction analysis using oligos specific for gene 4 (P type) and 9 (G type). This approach avoids complications in interpretation that arise in the first few months of life from immunoglobulins of maternal origin. The absence of *Rotavirus*-specific immunoglobulin A or T-helper cell activity at the time of illness was consistent with a primary infection in seven of eight children. Two children were infected with serotype 1 (P1G1), three with serotype 3 (P1G3), and three with serotype 4 (P1G4). Neutralizing antibodies were directed against the gene 4 (P type) protein product (VP4). Because all infecting strains were P type 1, convalescent antisera did not distinguish between different *Rotavirus* G types. *Rotavirus*-specific immunoglobulin A responses were detected in six of eight children and *Rotavirus*-specific thorium cell responses were found in seven of eight children during convalescence. The authors have applied the binary classification system to the rotaviruses infecting theses patients, although the contribution of the P typing was not important in this case.

28. RICHARSON SC, GRIMWOOD K, BISHOP RF: **Analysis of Homotypic and Heterotypic Serum Immune Responses to Rotavirus Proteins Following Primary Rotavirus Infection by Using the Radioimmunoprecipitation Technique**. *J Clin Microbiol* 1993, **31**:377–385.
• Three sequential serum samples were collected from each of 20 children with natural *Rotavirus* infection. Radioimmunoprecipitation assay for immunoglobulin G to major structural proteins of the four major serotypes were performed. Homologous responses to VP7 were detected in 93% of those infected with type G1 and 50% of those with type G4. Heterologous VP7 responses were detected infrequently. All patients tested had VP4-specific antibodies.

29. VESIKARI T: **Clinical Trials of Live Oral Rotavirus Vaccines: The Finnish Experience**. *Vaccine* 1993, **11**:255–261.

30. MADDOX A, FRANCIS N, MOSS J, BLANSHARD C, GAZZARD B: **Adenovirus Infection of the Large Bowel in HIV Positive Patients**. *J Clin Pathol* 1992, **45**:684–688.
• Immunochemical staining and electron microscopy identified *Adenovirus* in the large intestine of 10 HIV-positive patients, including eight with AIDS, all of whom had diarrhea. Other pathogens were also present, and the inflammatory pattern was nonspecific (typically a mild to moderate chronic inflammatory infiltrate, with neutrophils only occasionally present). The contribution of *Adenovirus* to the disease condition was not clear.

31. STRICKLER JG, SINGLETON TP, COPENHAVER CM, ERICE A, SNOVER DC: **Adenovirus in the Gastrointestinal Tracts of Immunosuppressed Patients**. *Am J Clin Pathol* 1992, 97:555–558.
• Isolation of *Adenovirus* in the stool of immunosuppressed transplant recipients did not imply invasive intestinal disease. Rather, the virus derived from pulmonary infections and carried to the gut by swallowed secretions. Typing of *Adenovirus* may assist with this kind of discrimination as none of the viruses isolated from the stools in these patients were the enteric strains 40 and 41.

32. ALBRECHT H, STELLBRINK HJ, FENSKE S, ERMER M, RAEDLER A, GRETEN H: **Rotavirus Antigen Detection in Patients With HIV Infection and Diarrhea**. *Scand J Gastroenterol* 1993, **28**:307–310.
• *Rotavirus* was detected in the stools of 9 of 66 HIV-infected patients with diarrhea but in none of 35 without diarrhea. Symptoms were conducted by antidiarrheal medications and were self-limited. The role of *Rotavirus* as a pathogen in AIDS patients has been unclear, as some studies have not found the virus to be associated with disease but rather with immunosuppression. Although this study implies that the infection sometimes results in disease in adult HIV-infected individuals, the symptoms do not appear to be severe nor is the duration chronic.

Robert D. Shaw, MD, Assistant Professor of Medicine, Research Service, Building 61 (151), Department of VA Affairs Medical Center (632), Middleville Road, Northport, NY 11768, USA.

Parasitic infections of the gastrointestinal tract

Ana Maria Cevallos, MD, and Michael J.G. Farthing, MD, FRCP

St. Bartholomew's Hospital, London, UK

During the past year, there have been important advances in the field of parasitic diseases of the gut. An immunodiagnostic test that allows the rapid identification of pathogenic *Entamoeba histolytica* has been developed. Two new parasites that produce diarrhea have been characterized. *Cyclospora*, a cyanobacterium-like organism, is prevalent worldwide, affects immunocompetent individuals, and has been described as a cause of traveler's diarrhea. *Encephalitozoon* sp has been reported in patients with AIDS; however, unlike *Enterocytozoon bieneusi*, it has the potential for systemic dissemination. Treatment of *Trichuris trichiura* has been demonstrated to rapidly correct the cognitive deficit present in children with trichuriasis. Lastly, combined treatment of hydatid disease by percutaneous drainage plus albendazole has been shown to be an effective form of management.

Current Opinion in Gastroenterology 1994, **10**:80–87

Protozoa

Entamoeba histolytica

The diagnosis of amebiasis is routinely done by microscopic examination of feces. Examination of stools for ova and parasites is laborious and the results depend largely on the skill of the microscopist. Immunologic methods for diagnosis are being developed. The Enzymeba test [1•] is based on the detection of histolysain, the major cysteine proteinase of *Entamoeba histolytica*. The Enzymeba test showed 87.5% sensitivity and 100% specificity. However, cysteine proteinases are present in both pathogenic and nonpathogenic *E. histolytica*. It is unlikely that this assay will distinguish between them. This distinction is important as only infection with pathogenic *E. histolytica* requires treatment. An immunodiagnostic assay, which is based on monoclonal antibodies to the galactose-specific adhesin [2••], for detection of pathogenic *E. histolytica* has been reported. The assay is based on detection of epitopes of the adhesin present only in pathogenic strains of *E. histolytica*. Specificity and sensitivity of the assay for pathogenic *E. histolytica* were 97% and 100%, respectively. The assay clearly differentiated pathogenic from nonpathogenic *E. histolytica*.

Increased expression and excretion of cysteine-proteinases correlate with virulence of both axenic laboratory strains and clinical isolates of *E. histolytica*. It has recently been found that pathogenic *E. histolytica* has a unique proteinase gene, the ACP1 gene, not present in nonpathogenic *E. histolytica* [3••]. The presence of the ACP1 gene correlated with increased proteinase expression, activity and *in vitro* cytopathic effect. The presence of ACP1 in pathogenic *E. histolytica* is, therefore, a genetically predetermined virulence factor.

Entamoeba histolytica trophozoites are continuously exposed to the complement system during invasion of the colon and hematogenous spread to the liver. Although these pathogens activate the alternative pathway of complement, the trophozoites are resistant to killing by complement C5b-9 complexes deposited in the membrane surface. It has recently been shown that the galactose-specific adhesin of *E. histolytica* partly mediates complement resistance [4•]. *E. histolytica* resistance to lysis was blocked by antiadhesin monoclonal antibodies. Purified adhesin was shown to bind to C8 and C9 and inhibited lysis of C5b-9 sensitive amoeba at the step of C8 and C9 assembly. However, the adhesin is constitutively expressed and therefore the inhibition of the assembly of the complement membrane complex does not explain the differences in complement sensitivity between axenically cultured amoebae and amoebae grown in the presence of human sera or passaged through animals. In another study [5•], resistance of pathogenic *E. histolytica* to complement lysis was decreased by cytochalasin B, glutaraldehyde fixation, and trypsin. This suggests that an intact membrane mobility and a trypsin-

Abbreviation
VSP—variant surface protein.

 ISBN 1-85922-606-X ISSN 0267–1379

sensitive surface component are necessary to inhibit the activation of the alternative complement pathway. Nonpathogenic *E. histolytica* is always complement resistant. The mechanisms of resistance are different from those found in *E. histolytica* as cytochalasin B or trypsin did not affect resistance to complement.

Giardia lamblia

Giardia lamblia localize and multiply in the small intestine and may cause acute or chronic diarrhea with malabsorption. Abnormal pancreatic function has been documented in giardiasis. The effects of *Giardia* trophozoites on pancreatic trypsin, chymotrypsin, and amylase activity *in vitro* have been studied [6•]. *Giardia* trophozoites inhibited tryptic activity but had no effect on chymotrypsin or amylase activities. Inhibition of trypsin may enhance parasite survival in the small intestine by allowing trophozoites to escape destruction by luminal proteases and may also contribute to malabsorption.

The predominant protein on the trophozoite surface is one of a unique group of cysteine-rich proteins called variant surface proteins (VSPs). VSPs can vary spontaneously or in response to antibody or environmental pressures. Loss of a VSP leads to replacement with another cysteine-rich variant that is usually immunologically distinct. The biological relevance of these proteins is not known, although they are thought to contribute to the chronicity of giardiasis. Two groups have independently demonstrated that all known variants of these proteins bind zinc [7•,8•]. It has been speculated that metal binding by VSP may maintain the surface protein in a more compact conformation, shielding potential substrates from proteolysis and protecting the trophozoite from disruption by bile salts and lipases. VSPs may contribute to malabsorption by inhibition of metal-dependent intestinal enzymes.

The mechanisms involved in parasite clearance are poorly understood. The antibody response to *Giardia* antigens in children with persistent diarrhea and giardiasis has been studied [9•]. Anti-*Giardia* immunoglobulin M response was increased, but the levels of anti-*Giardia* immunoglobulin A and G antibodies were similar to controls. Unlike patients which clear infection, patients with chronic giardiasis had no immunoglobulin A response to a *Giardia* heat shock antigen. The association of high concentrations of *Giardia*-specific immunoglobulin M, low concentrations of *Giardia*-specific immunoglobulin G and A and inability to clear the infection suggest that the switch from an immunoglobulin M to an immunoglobulin G or A response is inefficient.

Cryptosporidium parvum

Cryptosporidium parvum is a common cause of diarrhea in both immunocompetent and immunodeficient individuals. During the past year, several articles regarding the natural history of infection have been published. Phillips *et al.* [10•] reviewed their experience with children with cryptosporidiosis. During a 6.5-year period, 123 children with cryptosporidiosis and no clinical evidence of immune deficiency were identified. Mixed infections with other pathogens were common (29% of the cases). There was an unexpectedly high incidence of chronic diarrhea; in 58% of the cases it lasted more than 2 weeks, in 39% more than 3 weeks, and in 8% more than 6 months. In all cases the diarrhea eventually resolved spontaneously. An increased risk of developing chronic diarrhea was found in children under 2 years old (63% vs 38%) and in those with mixed infections (77% vs 50%). In children with diarrhea due to *Cryptosporidium* only, chronic infection developed more frequently in children who acquired the infection abroad (82%) than those who acquired the infection in the United Kingdom (64%).

Two groups based in London reported their experience with *Cryptosporidium* in HIV-positive patients [11••,12••]. A retrospective study by Blanchard *et al.* [11••] involved 128 patients and described four clinical patterns of disease: asymptomatic (3.9%), transient (28.7%), chronic (59.7%) and fulminant (7.8%). McGowan *et al.'s* [12••] retrospective study of 38 patients with cryptosporidial diarrhea reported transient infection in 29% of the cases and presence of other enteric pathogens in 21% of their cases (three of 11 transient infections and five of 27 chronic infections). An interesting finding in both studies was that successful treatment of intercurrent enteric infection was associated with disappearance of the cryptosporidia and resolution of diarrhea. This finding suggests that although the presence of secondary pathogens appears not to be of prognostic value, the response to antimicrobial agents is predictive. In both studies chronic infection was associated with decreased survival and there was an inverse correlation between risk of developing chronic infection and number of CD4 cells. This correlation has also been found by another group [13•]. CD4 counts greater than 180 to 200 [11••,13•] reliably predict spontaneous resolution of diarrhea.

Sclerosing cholangitis that is AIDS related has been described in association with cryptosporidiosis. It is still not known if *Cryptosporidium* sp (and other infectious agents) are directly implicated in the pathogenesis of hepatobiliary disease in AIDS patients or if they are all independent aspects of an advanced stage of HIV infection [14••]. The prevalence of AIDS-related sclerosing cholangitis in patients with cryptosporidiosis has been reported to be 18% to 26% [11••,12••]. AIDS-related sclerosing cholangitis has been associated with both transient and chronic cryptosporidiosis [12••]. The prevalence of cryptosporidiosis in patients with AIDS-related sclerosing cholangitis has been reported at 65% [15••] and 74% [14••]. Coinfection with cytomegalovirus was common in both series.

The wide clinical spectrum of cryptosporidiosis depends substantially on the immunologic status of the host. However, parasite virulence factors may also play a role. In a recent study using a neonatal calf model of infection, significant differences in oocyst production and severity of disease were found between *C. parvum* isolates of human origin [16•].

No antimicrobial agent has proved to be consistently effective against *Cryptosporidium*. Two small, open nonrandomized trials using paromomycin in AIDS patients have been reported [17•,18•]. In one study [17•], five patients received paromomycin 1.5 to 2.0 g/d for either 10 days (one patient) or continuously (four patients). All patients improved although one patient later relapsed while receiving paromomycin. Three cleared *Cryptosporidium* from their stools. In the second trial, seven patients received paromomycin 2 g/d for an average of 12 days [18•]. All patients had a good symptomatic response and four cleared the infection. Recurrence developed in three patients. Paromomycin appears to be a promising agent for the treatment of cryptosporidiosis but prospective controlled trials are needed. Vapreotide, a somatostatin analogue, was not of benefit in the management of AIDS-related diarrhea in patients with cryptosporidiosis [19•].

Cyclospora

Diarrheal illness associated with this previously unrecognized organism was first described in travelers to Haiti and Mexico in 1986. Since then, cases have been reported worldwide in both immunocompetent and immunocompromised individuals. The organism was usually described as *Cryptosporidium muris*-like oocyst, a flagellate, an unsporulated coccidian, a cyanobacterium-like body, or a coccidian-like body. During the past year it has been proved that this organism is a new protozoon that belongs to the genus *Cyclospora*. Ortega *et al.* [20••] purified oocysts from feces of affected patients and induced their sporulation and excystation *in vitro* (Fig. 1). Each oocyst contains two sporocysts each of which encloses two sporozoites. Morphologic examination of both unsporulated and sporulated organisms by electron microscopy confirmed their identity. Prospective studies of the prevalence of *Cyclospora* have been reported from Peru [20]. In the first study (January 1988 to July 1989) involving 147 children (mean age 23 months), there was a prevalence of 18%. During this period, 32 episodes of infection were detected of which only nine (28%) were associated with diarrhea. In the second study (November 1989 to October 1991) involving 230 slightly younger children (mean age 15 months), the prevalence was 6% and 18 episodes of infection were detected of which only two (11%) were associated with diarrhea.

Bendall *et al.* [21•] report three cases of traveler's diarrhea due to *Cyclospora*. Histologic examination of jejunal biopsies demonstrated the presence of the parasite intracellularly but in an extranuclear location, unlike *Cyclospora carolytica*, the best documented mammalian cyclosporan, which is an intranuclear parasite.

Both studies emphasized that the unsporulated *Cyclospora* resembles *Cryptosporidium* oocysts and that to make a positive identification it is necessary to measure the oocysts that are 8 to 10 μm in diameter (*Cryptosporidium parvum* oocysts are 4 to 6 μm). When examined under ultraviolet epifluorescence, the *Cyclospora* organisms show strong green autofluorescence.

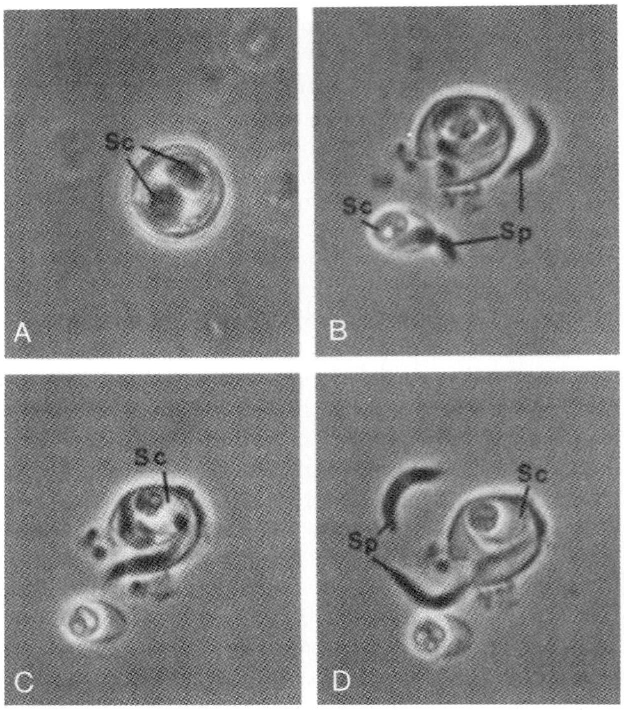

Fig. 1. Sporulation and excystation. **A**, Sporulated oocyst with two sporocysts (Sc). **B**, Excystation resulting in the liberation of two sporozoites (Sp) from the first sporocyst. **C**, One sporocyte liberated from the second sporocyst. **D**, Excystation completed, with the liberation of the second sporozoite from the second sporocyst. (*From* Ortega *et al.* [20•]; with permission.)

Microsporidia

Microsporidiosis is a well-recognized cause of chronic diarrhea in AIDS patients. In a study of 18 AIDS patients with unexplained chronic diarrhea and negative stool bacterial cultures and examination for ova and parasites, *Enterocytozoon bieneusi* was found in nine (50%) [22•]. In another study [23•] involving 180 consecutive HIV patients who underwent upper gastrointestinal endoscopy and multiple pinch biopsies, *E. bieneusi* was detected in 32 (31 of 109 patients with diarrhea and one of 71 patients without diarrhea). *E. bieneusi* has also been increasingly recognized in association with AIDS cholangiopathy. In a small series of eight cases of unexplained AIDS-related sclerosing cholangitis, examination of bile demonstrated the presence of spores of E. bieneusi in all [24••].

A new microsporidian has been recently identified in patients with AIDS [23•,25•]. Unlike *E. bieneusi*, this microsporidia appeared to develop within septated parasitophores vacuoles, and lack polar disks and clear clefts (Fig. 2) [25•]. It closely resembled, but was distinguishable from, members of the genus *Encephalitozoon* [23•,25•]. *Encephalitozoon*-like organisms were detected in four of 180 consecutive patients who underwent upper gastrointestinal endoscopy [23•]. Unlike *E. bieneusi*, infection with *Encephalitozoon*-like microsporidia is not confined to enterocytes. The organism has been found in gut lamina propria macrophages, portal vein, bronchial epithelium, and urine [26••].

There is no consistently effective treatment for microsporidial infection at any site. The results of a small therapeutic open trial of HIV-patients with diarrhea due to infection with *E. bieneusi* have been published [27•]. Six patients were treated with 400 mg twice daily for 4 weeks. Diarrhea resolved completely in all patients within 1 week of starting treatment and body weight stabilized or increased. Four patients relapsed at 19 to 31 days after stopping the treatment but responded to a second course of albendazole. Controlled trials are needed to evaluate the use of albendazole in the treatment of microsporidal diarrhea.

Helminths

Intestinal helminthiases are among the most prevalent human chronic infections. However, pathogenesis of intestinal helminth infection is poorly defined, particularly concerning diarrhea. In a recent article, Genta [28•] summarized all the current knowledge about the mechanisms by which some worms may cause diarrhea. The available evidence suggests that five helminthic parasites do cause diarrhea: *Trichinella spiralis* (early phases of infection), *Trichuris trichiura*, *Stronglyloides stercoralis*, *Capillaria philippinensis*, and *Schistosoma* (particularly *Schistosoma mansoni*). All these parasites have an invasive phase during which adult worms, their eggs, or their larvae establish intimate contact with the host's intestinal mucosa and elicit local inflammatory responses resulting in various structural and functional alterations of the gut. Although brief bouts of diarrhea have frequently been described in volunteers exposed to infective larvae of *Ancylostoma duodenale*, *Ancylostoma ceylonicum*, and *Necator americanus*, epidemiologic studies have failed to discover any relation between hookworm infection and diarrhea. Other helminths that may cause diarrhea include: *Hymenolepis nana*, *Diphyllobothrium latum*, and *Fasciolopsis buski*. There is no evidence to suggest that *Ascaris lumbricoides* or *Taenia* sp produce diarrhea.

Nematodes

The relationship between level of infection with *Trichuris trichiura* and antibody response at a population level has recently been studied [29•] in two communities, one of high endemicity and one of low endemicity. The age-related prevalence of infection peaked to 93% in the 6- to 8-year-olds in the high endemic area and to 54% in the 8- to 10-year-olds in the low endemic area. In both areas, prevalence levels remained high until adulthood followed by a decline after the age of 26. The age-related intensity of infection peaked at 6 to 8 years in the high endemic area (4000 eggs per gram of stool) and at 3 to 6 years of age (90 eggs per gram of stool) in the area of low endemicity. In both areas the levels of anti-*Trichuris* immunoglobulin G_1 and G_2 antibodies correlated with intensity of infection. Immunoglobulin G_4, E, and A an-

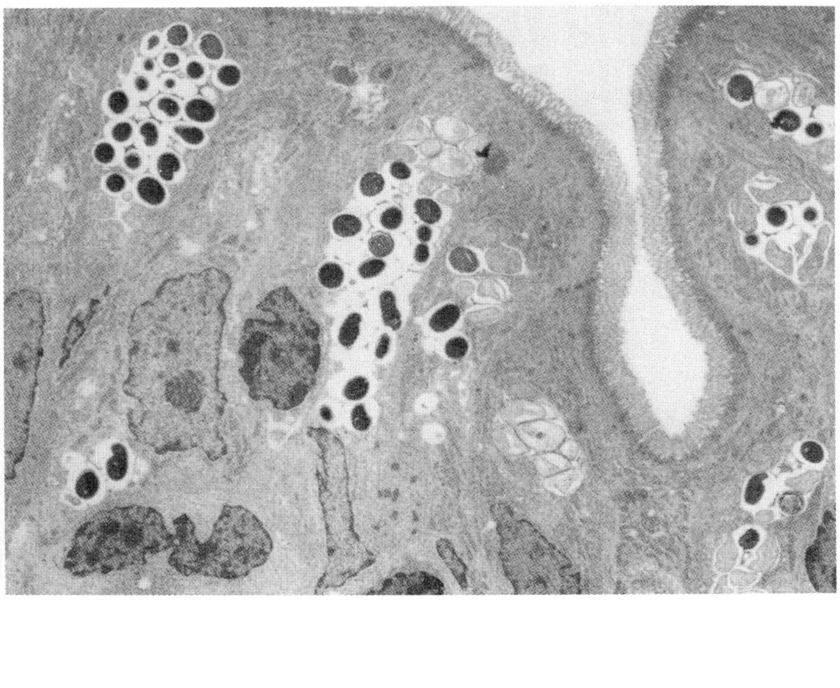

Fig. 2. Transmission electron micrograph. Septated vacuoles containing developing spores are especially concentrated in the apical cytoplasm of these duodenal enterocytes. Note the intraepithelial lymphocyte. (Magnification ×3330.)(*From* Orenstein *et al.* [25•]; with permission.)

tibodies persisted into early adulthood and the subsequent decline was gradual. However, in the low endemic area, lower levels of infection were reflected in lower parasite-specific antibody concentrations of all isotypes. The major difference was found in the immunoglobulin A response. In the low endemic area immunoglobulin A levels showed a slight increase with age. In contrast, the high endemic area demonstrated a vigorous immunoglobulin A response that persisted into early adulthood. These data suggest that production of immunoglobulin A requires a high exposure to be triggered and that it may be involved in determining protective immunity.

Until recently, the evidence that worms may affect cognitive performance is largely circumstantial. A double-blind placebo trial was conducted to determine the effect of moderate-to-high loads of *T. trichiura* infection on the cognitive functions of 159 school children (9 to 12 years old) in Jamaica [30••]. Infected children were randomly assigned to treatment (albendazole) or placebo groups. A third group of noninfected children was used as a control. A battery of eight cognitive function tests was administered before and after 9 weeks of treatment. In the initial test, noninfected children scored better than the infected groups. After treatment, the albendazole group had significant improvements in the test of auditory short-term memory and in the scanning and retrieval of long-term memory tests when compared with the placebo group. Unlike the placebo group, treated children were no longer significantly different from the noninfected control group.

The long-term solutions to malnutrition and geohelminth control lie in eradication of poverty and in community-based programs to improve health care living conditions. The enormous financial and logistic difficulties of implementing those improvements in most developing countries have made population-based chemotherapy the only way to reduce drastically the prevalence and intensity of geohelminth infection in the short-term future.

There is a large overlap in the geographic distributions of *A. lumbricoides*, *T. trichiura*, and hookworm and, therefore, multiple species infections may occur in the same region. A review of the published data that reported the simultaneous prevalence of two or more geohelminth infections has recently been summarized [31•]. There is a close correlation in the geographic distributions of *A. lumbricoides* and *T. trichiura*. The distribution of hookworm was largely independent of the other two parasites. The similar distributions and epidemiological characteristics of infection with *A. lumbricoides* and *T. trichiura* suggests that simultaneous control of these two parasites by the same strategy would not only be feasible but highly desirable. Multiple species control strategies that aim to control hookworm infection may require a more complicated protocol with more precise locality targeting.

When developing strategies for control of geohelminth infection, it is important to balance the growth and health benefits against the feasibility and economic costs of implementing them. A placebo-controlled trial comparing the growth in infected children after chemotherapy with placebo, one 600-mg dose of albendazole per school year, or two 600-mg doses of albendazole per school year has been published [32•]. At the end of the study, children receiving one dose of albendazole had a mean egg reduction rate of 84% for hookworm, 42% for *Trichuris* and 55% for *Ascaris*. Children receiving two doses had significantly bigger reductions in the rates of infection, 95% for hookworm, 32% for *Trichuris*, and 87% for *Ascaris*. There were no differences in the prevalence rates of infection in the placebo group. Regarding their nutritional status, the placebo group showed a significant decrease in percent weight-for-age and percent arm circumference-for-age, and no change in percent weight-for-height. In contrast, the two treated groups had a significant and identical improvement in all their anthropometric parameters. It is concluded that one or two doses of albendazole per year resulted in similar growth improvements, despite bigger reinfection rates in the one dose group.

Cestodes

Imaging procedures are widely used in the diagnosis of hydatid disease and its complications. Immunodiagnostic tests are useful in confirming the hydatid nature of the visualized cyst and in performing epidemiologic studies. Many antibody detection assays are available.

Table 1. Sensitivity, specificity, and predictive values of eight serologic tests for detection of antibodies in hydatid disease*

Parameter	IgG ELISA	IHA	Latex agglutination	IEP	IgA ELISA	RAST	IgE ELISA	Total IgE
Sensitivity, %	91	87	83	73	50	78	38	56
Specificity, %	99	98	94	97	85	93	97	71
+ Predictive value, %	99	98	95	98	82	97	94	79
– Predictive value, %	89	85	81	68	56	55	58	46

*From Force *et al.* [33]; with permission.
ELISA—enzyme-linked immunosorbent assay; IEP—immunoelectrophoresis; Ig—immunoglobulin; IHA—indirect hemagglutination; RAST—radioallergosorbent test; +, positive; –, negative.

The specificity and sensitivity of these tests vary according to the characteristics and location of hydatid cysts in the patient. The cross-reactivity of these tests with cisticercosis, schistosomiasis, filariasis, and other helminth infections are well documented.

In a study involving 131 patients with echinococcosis [33•], eight serological tests were evaluated regarding their sensitivity, specificity, and role in the follow-up of these patients after treatment (medical or surgical). Immunoglobulin G enzyme-linked immunosorbent assay and indirect hemagglutination were the most sensitive tests (Table 1) for the preoperative diagnosis of hydatid disease (91% and 87% sensitivity, respectively). When the data were analyzed according to site of involvement the sensitivity of all tests were low for lung lesions (18% to 62%). After treatment there was a decrease in the immunologic response in patients with clinical cure but this was also true in some patients who remained infected. Less than 57% of patients with a favorable outcome became antibody negative. A new immunodiagnostic test using a synthetic recombinant protein has been published [34•]. It had a sensitivity of 85% and specificity of 86% for immunoglobulin G-A-M responses. The specificity for immunoglobulin E response was 100%; however, only 60% of human hydatid sera were positive for immunoglobulin E.

The value of an assay for diagnosis of human hydatidosis based on the detection of free and immune-complex hydatid-specific antigens has been published [35•]. Two antigens of a molecular weight of 8 and 116 kD were evaluated. The sensitivity, specificity, and diagnostic efficiency for detection of either antigen in acid-treated serum samples was 100%. This assay may be of value in the follow-up of patients with hydatidosis after treatment.

The results of a prospective, randomized trial comparing percutaneous drainage (10 patients), albendazole (11 patients), and percutaneous drainage plus albendazole (12 cases) has been published [36••]. All the 22 cysts treated with percutaneous drainage and only two of 12 (18.2%) cysts treated with albendazole alone reduced in size. Maximum size reduction was observed in cysts treated with a combination of drainage and albendazole. Complications observed with drainage were cyst infection in two patients, fever in three, cyst biliary rupture in one, and urticaria in two. All complications were managed successfully without any mortality. The patient with biliary rupture required drainage through an endoscopic retrograde cholangiopancreatographic procedure.

Trematodes

The detection of *Schistosoma* egg excretion is too laborious for evaluation of mass chemotherapy campaigns. Unfortunately, the available immunodiagnostic tests do not separate active from past infection. The magnetic bead antigen capture enzyme-linked immunosorbent assay is a simple and quantitative screening test for detection of active infection. It specifically measures the amount of schistosomal circulating anodic antigen. Its use in the evaluation of response to treatment in 55 patients has been assessed [37•]. The amounts of circulating anodic antigen detected by the assay were positively correlated with the numbers of eggs per gram of feces. A significant reduction in circulating anodic antigen was measured after chemotherapy. The sensitivity was 88% to 89% in clinically significant cases excreting more than 100 eggs per gram. In light infections, the sensitivity was lower. The value of this test in the design of control programs in endemic areas for *Schistosoma mansoni* should be confirmed.

References and recommended reading

Papers of particular interest, published within the annual period of review, have been highlighted as:
- • Of special interest
- •• Of outstanding interest

1. • LUACES AL, PICO T, BARRETT AJ: **The Enzymeba Test: Detection of Intestinal *Entamoeba histolytica* Infection by Immuno-Enzymatic Detection of Histolysain.** *Parasitology* 1992, **105**:203–205.

Description of a diagnostic test based on the immunoadsorption of *E. histolytica* cysteine proteinase from fecal samples, and subsequent visual detection of the enzyme by a color reaction. The test has a sensitivity of 87.5% and specificity of 100%. The test does not differentiate pathogenic *E. histolytica* from nonpathogenic *E. histolytica.*

2. •• HAQUE R, KRESS K, WOOD S, JACKSON TFHG, LYERLY D, WILKINS T, PETRI WA, JR: **Diagnosis of Pathogenic *Entamoeba histolytica* Infection Using a Stool ELISA Based on Monoclonal Antibodies to the Galactose-Specific Adhesin.** *J Infect Dis* 1993, **167**:247–249.

Monoclonal antibodies directed against pathogen-specific epitopes of the galactose adhesin of *E. histolytica* were used in an enzyme-linked immunosorbent assay to detect antigen from pathogenic *E. histolytica.* Specificity and sensitivity of the assay were 97% and 100%, respectively. This test effectively distinguishes pathogenic from nonpathogenic *E. histolytica.*

3. •• REED S, BOUVIER J, POLLAK AS, ENGEL JC, BROWN M, HIRATA K, QUE X, EAKIN A, HAGBLOM P, GILLIN F, MCKERROW JH: **Cloning of a Virulence Factor of *Entamoeba histolytica.* Pathogenic Strains Possess a Unique Cysteine Proteinase Gene.** *J Clin Invest* 1993, **91**:1532–1540.

Cloning of three cysteine proteinase genes: ACP1, ACP2, and ACP3. ACP2 and ACP3 are present in both pathogenic and non-pathogenic *E. histolytica.* ACP1 is present only in pathogenic *E. histolytica.*

4. • BRAGA LL, NINOMIYA H, MCCOY JJ, EACKER S, WIEDMER T, PHAM C, WOOD S, SIMS PJ, PETRI WA JR: **Inhibition of the Complement Membrane Attack Complex by the Galactose-Specific Adhesion of *Entamoeba histolytica.*** *J Clin Invest* 1992, **90**:1131–1137.

Identification of the galactose-specific adhesin of *E. histolytica* as mediator of complement resistance in pathogenic *E. histolytica.* The adhesin shared sequence similarities and antigenic cross-reactivity with CD59, a membrane inhibitor of C5b-9 in human blood cells.

5. • HAMELMANN C, URBAN B, FOERSTER B, HORSTMANN RD: **Complement Resistance of Pathogenic *Entamoeba histolytica* Mediated by Trypsin-Sensitive Surface Component(s).** *Infect Immun* 1993, **61**:1636–1640.

The mechanisms of complement resistance of pathogenic and nonpathogenic are different. Pathogenic *E. histolytica* requires intact membrane motility and a trypsin-sensitive surface component to inhibit the activation of the alternative pathway of the complement.

6. • SEOW F, KATELARIS P, NGU M: **The Effect of *Giardia lamblia* Trophozoites on Trypsin, Chymotrypsin and Amylase *in vitro*.** *Parasitology* 1993, **106**:233–238.
Giardia lamblia trophozoites inhibit trypsin activity *in vitro*. They do not have any effect on chymotrypsin or amylase activities. Inhibition of trypsin may enhance parasite survival in the small intestine and may also contribute to malabsorption.

7. • NASH TE, MOWATT MR: **Variant-Specific Surface Proteins of *Giardia lamblia* Are Zinc-Binding Proteins.** *Proc Natl Acad Sci U S A* 1993, **90**:5489–5493.
Four of the reported five variant surface proteins contain a putative metal-binding domain that resembles other metal binding motifs. Three different native variant surface proteins bound Zn^{2+}. Co^{2+}, Cu^{2+}, and Cd^{2+} inhibited zinc binding.

8. • ZHANG Y-Y, ALEY SB, STANLEY SL, GILLIN FD: **Cysteine-Dependent Zinc Binding by Membrane Proteins of *Giardia lamblia*.** *Infect Immun* 1993, **61**:520–524.
Variant surface proteins bind zinc. Binding was inhibited by competition with other divalent ions.

9. • CHAR S, CEVALLOS AM, YAMSON P, SULLIVAN PB, NEALE G, FARTHING MJG: **Impaired IgA Response to *Giardia* Heat Shock Antigen in Children With Persistent Diarrhoea and Giardiasis.** *Gut* 1993, **34**:38–40.
Children with chronic giardiasis do not have an adequate immunoglobulin A response. Unlike children with acute giardiasis, they do not have an antibody immunoglobulin A response to a *Giardia* heat shock antigen.

10. • PHILLIPS AD, THOMAS AG, WALKER-SMITH JA: ***Cryptosporidium*, Chronic Diarrhoea and the Proximal Small Intestinal Mucosa.** *Gut* 1992, **33**:1057–1061.
Fifty percent of immunocompetent children with cryptosporidiosis had chronic diarrhea. All patients eventually recovered spontaneously.

11. •• BLANSHARD C, JACKSON AM, SHANSON DC, FRANCIS N, GAZZARD B: **Cryptosporidiosis in HIV-Seropositive Patients.** *Q J Med* 1992, **85**:813–823.
Cryptosporidiosis occurs in 5% of all patients with HIV and in 21% of those with AIDS. The median survival for patients with fulminant, chronic, and transient infection was 5, 20, and 36 weeks, respectively.

12. •• MCGOWAN I, HAWKINS AS, WELLER IV: **The Natural History of Cryptosporidial Diarrhoea in HIV-Infected Patients.** *AIDS* 1993, **7**:349–354.
Infection with *C. parvum* in HIV-infected patients is transient in 29% of the cases. The median survival for patients with transient infection was 66 weeks, and for chronic infection 11.5 weeks.

13. • FLANIGAN T, WHALEN C, TURNER J, SOAVE R, TOERNER J, HAVLIR D, KOTLER D: ***Cryptosporidium* Infection and CD4 Counts.** *Arch Intern Med* 1992, **116**:840–842.
In a series of 47 patients with HIV infection and cryptosporidiosis, a CD4 count greater than 180 cells/mm^3 was associated with spontaneous clearance of infection.

14. •• BENHAMOU Y, CAUMES E, GEROSA Y, CADRANEL JF, DOHIN E, KATLAMA C, AMOUYAL P, CANARD JM, AZAR N, HOANG C, LE CHARPENTIER Y, GENTILINI M, OPOLON P, VALLA D: **AIDS-Related Cholangiopathy. Critical Analysis of a Prospective Series of 26 Patients.** *Dig Dis Sci* 1993, **38**:1113–1118.
In this study two types of biliary tract involvement were detected: stenosis of terminal portion of the common bile duct (27% of the cases) and distal stenosis combined with diffuse irregularity of the extrahepatic biliary ducts (73% of the cases). Concomitant infection by cytomegalovirus or *Cryptosporidium* sp. was more frequent when intrahepatic duct irregularities were present (94%) than absent (14%).

15. •• FORBES A, BLANSHARD C, GAZZARD B: **Natural History of AIDS Related Sclerosing Cholangitis: A Study of 20 Cases.** *Gut* 1993, **34**:116–121.
The natural history of 20 consecutive patients with AIDS-related sclerosing cholangitis is reviewed. Of these patients, 13 had cryptosporidiosis, six had active cytomegalovirus and five had no gastrointestinal pathogen. Controls, matched for age, CD4 counts and opportunistic infections had identical outcome (mean survival 7.5 months). Increasing age, however, appeared protective in AIDS-related sclerosing cholangitis.

16. • POZIO E, GOMEZ MORALES MA, BARBIERI FM, LA ROSA G: ***Cryptosporidium*: Different Behaviour in Calves of Isolates of Human Origin.** *Trans R Soc Trop Med Hyg* 1992, **86**:636–638.
Three human isolates of *Cryptosporidium* differ in the severity of disease produced in neonatal calves.

17. • ARMITAGE K, FLANIGAN T, CAREY J, FRANK I, MACGREGOR RR, ROSS P, GOODGAME R, TURNER J: **Treatment of Cryptosporidiosis With Paromomycin. A Report of Five Cases.** *Arch Intern Med* 1992, **152**:2497–2499.
The treatment of 5 patients with cryptosporidiosis and AIDS has been reported. All patients had resolution of symptoms and normalization of bowel movements, although one patient later relapsed while receiving paromomycin.

18. • FICHTENBAUM CJ, RITCHIE DJ, POWDERLY WG: **Use of Paromomycin for Treatment of Cryptosporidiosis in Patients With AIDS.** *Clin Infect Dis* 1993, **16**:298–300.
Review of seven patients with cryptosporidiosis and AIDS treated with paromomycin. All patients had an initial symptomatic response. Eradication of the parasite was achieved in three patients.

19. • GIRARD PM, GOLDSCHMIDT E, VITTECOQ D, MASSIP P, GASTIABURU J, MEYOHAS MC, COULAUD JP, SCHALLY AV: **Vapreotide, a Somatostatin Analogue, in Cryptosporidiosis and Other AIDS-Related Diarrhoeal Diseases.** *AIDS* 1992, **6**:715–718.
Report of an open, non-comparative pilot trial on the efficacy and tolerance of vapreotide in the treatment of refractory AIDS-related diarrhea. Four of 34 patients demonstrated a complete response, 12 had a partial response, and 14 patients did not respond. Patients with conditions other than cryptosporidiosis had a significantly higher probability of response.

20. •• ORTEGA YR, STERLING CR, GILMAN RH, CAMA VA, DIAZ F: **Cyclospora Species—a New Protozoan Pathogen of Humans.** *N Engl J Med* 1993, **328**:1308–1312.
The "cyanobacterium-like" organisms isolated from feces in patients with diarrhea in Peru have been characterized. Sporulation of cysts and detailed morphologic examination of the parasites have revealed that this organism belongs to the genus *Cyclospora*.

21. • BENDALL RP, LUCAS S, MOODY A, TOVEY G, CHIODINI PL: **Diarrhoea Associated With Cyanobacterium-Like Bodies: A New coccidian Enteritis of Man.** *Lancet* 1993, **341**:590–592.
Description of three patients with traveler's diarrhea associated with cyanobacterioum-like bodies. Electromicroscopy of biopsy specimens revealed intraepithelial coccidia with morphologic characteristics suggestive of *Cyclospora*.

22. • MOLINA JM, SARFATI C, BEAUVAIS B, LEMANN M, LESOURD A, FERCHAL F, CASIN I, LAGRANGE P, MODIGLIANI R, DEROUIN F, *ET AL.*: **Intestinal Microsporidiosis in Human Immunodeficiency Virus-Infected Patients With Chronic Unexplained Diarrhea: Prevalence and Clinical and Biologic Features.** *J Infect Dis* 1993, **167**:217–221.
In a series of 18 patients with HIV infection and chronic unexplained diarrhea, nine (50%) had infection with *Enterocytozoon bieneusi*, other pathogens were found in four (22%), and in 6 (33%) patients diarrhea remained unexplained.

23. • FIELD AS, HING MC, MILLIKEN ST, MARRIOTT DJ: **Microsporidia in the Small Intestine of HIV-Infected Patients. A New Diagnostic Technique and a New Species.** *Med J Aust* 1993, **158**:390–394.
Microsporidiosis was demonstrated in 33% of patients with chronic diarrhea. In four cases (2%) an *Encephalitozoon*-like organism was identified. Staining of mucosal biopsies with Warthin-Starry stain was as effective as examination by electron microscopy.

24. •• POL S, ROMANA CA, RICHARD S, AMOUYAL P, DESPORTES-LIVAGE I, CARNOT F, PAYS JF, BERTHELOT P: **Microsporidia In-**

fection in Patients With the Human Immunodeficiency Virus and Unexplained Cholangitis. *N Engl J Med* 1993, **328**:95–99.
Microsporidiosis was found in eight cases of unexplained AIDS-related cholangitis.

25. • ORENSTEIN JM, TENNER M, CALI A, KOTLER DP: **A Microsporidian Previously Undescribed in Humans, Infecting Enterocytes and Macrophages, and Associated With Diarrhea in an Acquired Immunodeficiency Syndrome Patient.** *Hum Pathol* 1992, **23**:722–728.
Description of a case of chronic diarrhea due to a previously undescribed microsporidian, *Encephalitozoon* sp, in a patient with AIDS.

26. •• ORENSTEIN JM, DIETERICH DT, KOTLER DP: **Systemic Dissemination by a Newly Recognized Intestinal Microsporidia Species in AIDS.** *AIDS* 1992, **6**:1143–1150.
Two out of five patients with small intestinal infection due to *Encephalitozoon* had the organism demonstrable in urine. At the autopsy of one of these patients, parasites were also observed in the gall-bladder, in nonparenchymal liver cells and in bronchial epithelium.

27. • BLASNSHARD C, ELLIS DS, TOVEY DG, DOWELL S, GAZZARD BG: **Treatment of Intestinal Microsporidiosis With Albendazole in Patients With AIDS.** *AIDS* 1992, **6**:311–313.
In an open study, six patients with intestinal microsporidiosis were treated with albendazole. Diarrhea resolved completely in all patients. Four patients relapsed but responded to a second course of albendazole.

28. • GENTA RM: **Diarrhea in Helminthic Infections.** *Clin Infect Dis* 1993, **16(Suppl 2)**:S122–S129.
Review article on diarrhea in helminthic infections.

29. • NEEDHAM CS, BUNDY DA, LILLYWHITE JE, DIDIER JM, SIMMONS I, BIANCO AE: **The Relationship Between *Trichuris trichiura* Transmission Intensity and the Age-Profiles of Parasite-Specific Antibody Isotypes in Two Endemic Communities.** *Parasitology* 1992, **105**:273–283.
Study of the immune response to *T. trichiura* in two communities with high and low levels of transmission. Specific anti-*Trichuris* immunoglobulin G_1 and G_2 levels correlated to current intensity of infection (which peaked in small children). immunoglobulin G_4, E, and A levels persisted into early adulthood. In the low transmission area, lower infection levels were reflected in lower parasite-specific antibody levels. There was no significant increase in immunoglobulin A levels in the low transmission area.

30. •• NOKES C, GRANTHAM-MCGREGOR SM, SAWYER AW, COOPER ES, ROBINSON BA, BUNDY DA: **Moderate to Heavy Infections of *Trichuris trichiura* Affect Cognitive Function in Jamaican School Children.** *Parasitology* 1992, **104**:539–547.
A double-blind placebo trial to determine the effect of *Trichuris* infection on the cognitive function of school children. Children with trichuriasis performed less well in several cognitive tests compared with noninfected controls. After successful treatment, performance improved and was no longer different from noninfected controls.

31. • BOOTH M, BUNDY DA: **Comparative Prevalences of *Ascaris lumbricoides*, *Trichuris trichiura* and Hookworm Infections and the Prospects for Combined Control.** *Parasitology* 1992, **105**:151–157.
The study of the comparative distribution of *A. lumbricoides*, *T. trichiura*, and hookworm showed that *A. lumbricoides* and *T. trichiura* have closely related distributions, whereas hookworm infection is largely independent of the other two. Multiple species control strategies for *A. lumbricoides* and *T. trichiura* is not only possible but desirable.

32. • STEPHENSON LS, LATHAM MC, ADAMS EJ, KINOTI SN, PERTET A: **Weight Gain of Kenyan School Children Infected With Hookworm, *Trichuris trichiura* and *Ascaris lumbricoides* Is Improved Following Once- or Twice-Yearly Treatment With Albendazole.** *J Nutr* 1993, **123**:656–665.
One or two doses of albendazole per year were equally effective in improving growth in children infected with *T. trichiura*, *A. lumbricoides*, or both, despite the greater rate of reinfection in children who received only one dose.

33. • FORCE L, TORRES JM, CARRILLO A, BUSCA J: **Evaluation of Eight Serological Tests in the Diagnosis of Human Echinococcosis and Follow-up.** *Clin Infect Dis* 1992, **15**:473–480.
In a comparative study of eight serological tests in the diagnosis of hydatid disease, immunoglobulin G enzyme-linked immunosorbent assay was the most sensitive (91%) and specific (99%). The sensitivity for pulmonary disease was low for all tests. A combination of immunoglobulin G enzyme-linked immunosorbent assay, indirect hemagglutination and immunoglobulin A enzyme-linked immunosorbent assay was necessary to achieve a sensitivity of 81% in pulmonary echinococcosis.

34. • CHAMEKH M, GRAS-MASSE H, BOSSUS M, FACON B, DISSOUS C, TARTAR A, CAPRON A: **Diagnostic Value of a Synthetic Peptide Derived From *Echinococcus granulosus* Recombinant Protein.** *J Clin Invest* 1992, **89**:458–464.
The diagnostic value of an *Echinococcus*-derived synthetic peptide was tested with sera from patients with different parasites for their antibody reactivity with this peptide in enzyme-linked immunosorbent assay. A high-binding sensitivity and specificity of immunoglobulin G-A-M antibodies were obtained with patients infected with *E. granulosus.*

35. • KANWAR JR, VINAYAK VK: **The Significance of Free and Immune-Complexed Hydatid-Specific Antigens(s) as an Immunodiagnostic Tool for Human Hydatidosis.** *J Med Microbiol* 1992, **37**:396–403.
An enzyme-linked immunosorbent assay system was developed to detect hydatid-specific antigens in serum. This test may be used for diagnostic purposes and monitoring the response to treatment.

36. •• KHUROO MS, DAR MY, YATOO GN, ZARGAR SA, JAVAID G, KHAN BA, BODA MI: **Percutaneous Drainage Versus Albendazole Therapy in Hepatic Hydatidosis: A Prospective, Randomized Study.** *Gastroenterology* 1993, **104**:1452–1459.
A randomized trial of the treatment of hepatic hydatidosis demonstrated that percutaneous drainage plus albendazole is an effective form of treatment.

37. • GUNDERSEN SG, HAAGENSEN I, JONASSEN TO, FIGENSCHAU KJ, DE JONGE N, DEEDLER AM: **Quantitative Detection of Schistosomal Circulating Anodic Antigen by a Magnetic Bead Antigen Capture Enzyme-Lined Immunosorbent Assay (MBAC-EIA) Before and After Mass Chemotherapy.** *Trans R Soc Trop Med Hyg* 1992, **86**:175–178.
The magnetic bead antigen capture enzyme-linked immunosorbent assay has been applied to detect schistosomal circulating anodic antigen in pre- and posttreatment sera from 55 individuals. The assay had a specificity of 100% and a sensitivity of 88% to 89% in cases excreting more than 100 eggs per gram of feces. The test is rapid and simple to perform and could be used in the evaluation of mass chemotherapy campaigns.

Ana Maria Cevallos, MD, and Michael J.G. Farthing, MD, FRCP, Department of Gastroenterology, St. Bartholomew's Hospital, West Smithfield, London EC1A 7BE, United Kingdom.

Gastrointestinal infections in children

Michael Gracey, MD, PhD, FRACP

Health Department of Western Australia, Perth, Australia

Gastrointestinal infections are common and important in infants and young children, particularly where poor hygiene and living conditions allow the spread of infectious agents. With increasing information about microorganisms that cause these infections and improved methods to detect them, many episodes that were once undiagnosed can now be attributed to previously unrecognized viruses, bacteria, and other pathogens. These advances facilitate better management and will permit more effective control and preventive strategies. This review highlights some recent reports about enterovirulent classes of *Escherichia coli*, including *E. coli* O157:H7, which causes the hemolytic-uremic syndrome and hemorrhagic colitis; *Campylobacter* species and a new *Campylobacter*-like organism (*Arcobacter butzleri*); *Helicobacter pylori*; *Aeromonas* species; and rotavirus. Important new information about intestinal parasites, including *Giardia* and *Cryptosporidium*, has emerged that should prove of practical use in diagnosis and management in places where these parasites are prevalent in children, particularly in parts of the world where HIV infection has become established. A newly described organism, so far called coccidian-like or cyanobacterium-like body, has been found in patients with prolonged diarrhea (including travelers and expatriate residents) in several countries; the name *Cyclospora cayetanensis* has been proposed for this organism. This year's review concludes with a short commentary on some recent reports about risk factors that predispose children to gastrointestinal infections, *eg*, nutritional status, domestic hygiene, maternal hygiene behavior, and young children gathered in communal facilities like day care centers. Immune function status is also important, and deficiencies of single nutrients such as vitamin A, pyridoxine, folic acid, iron, and zinc may also play a role.

Current Opinion in Gastroenterology 1994, **10**:88–97

Etiology and pathogenesis

Escherichia coli strains that cause diarrhea in humans can be grouped according to the pathogenic mechanisms involved, such as enterotoxigenic, enteroinvasive, enterohemorrhagic, enteroaggregative, and enteropathogenic *E. coli* (EPEC). Epidemiologic and laboratory evidence of the diarrheagenic potential of *E. coli* strains that are adherent to tissue culture cells *in vitro* (enteroadherent *E. coli* [EAEC]) is appearing but is not universally accepted as proof of their role in human diarrheal disease. Excellent reviews about this subject have been published lately [1•,2••] including one about EPEC [3••], which may cause enterocyte skeletal damage by bacterial adherence through signal induction pathways that stimulate protein kinase activity [4].

Escherichia coli of nonenteropathogenic serogroups that adhere to HEp-2 or HeLa tissue cells in culture are referred to as EAEC or enteroadherent aggregative *E. coli*, and are becoming recognized as important causes of diarrhea among travelers and in infants and children. Strains of EAEC can be classified according to their *in vitro* adherence patterns, *ie*, whether they are diffusely adherent or locally adherent. EAEC were isolated from the feces of 19.7% of 218 hospitalized Indian infants

Abbreviations

CLB—coccidian-like or cyanobacterium-like body; **EAEC**—enteroadherent *Escherichia coli*; **ELISA**—enzyme-linked immunosorbent assay; **EPEC**—enteropathogenic *Escherichia coli*; **PCR**—polymerase chain reaction; **VTEC**—verotoxigenic *Escherichia coli*.

 ISBN 1-85922-606-X ISSN 0267–1379

under 6 months of age with acute diarrhea in Calcutta [5•]; none of the strains demonstrated conventional virulence factors including toxin production (heat-labile enterotoxin, heat-stable enterotoxin, verocytotoxin or Shiga-like toxin) or invasiveness. More than one third (37%) of the 43 EAEC isolates were EPEC with known O:K serogroups. Of the remainder, 41% had diffuse adherence; 37% showed localized adherence, and 22% showed both types of adherence, indicating the importance of heat-labile enterotoxin EAEC in these patients. Diffusely adherent EAEC and enteroaggregative *E. coli* were not significantly associated with diarrhea in 138 Aboriginal children less than 5 years of age in remote, tropical, northwest Australia [6••], but EAEC were significantly associated with diarrhea, mainly in children below 18 months of age [7•]. Sixteen children (23.5%) with diarrhea but only six (8.6%) without diarrhea showed a unique pattern of detachment of the HEp-2 cell monolayer from the glass coverslip when examined in the adhesion assay ($P \leq 0.05$). This feature, called cell detachment by the authors, may be a new virulence characteristic; these newly recognized cell-detaching *E. coli* may be another enterovirulent class of *E. coli*.

Escherichia coli O157:H7 has become recognized as an important human diarrhea pathogen over the past decade, and excellent reviews and commentaries about this subject have been published recently [8,9,10,11•]. Most patients have bloody diarrhea and abdominal cramps; in young patients there is a higher incidence of complications including the hemolytic-uremic syndrome, hemorrhagic colitis, and thrombotic thrombocytopenic purpura. This is not a common gastrointestinal infection and many clinical laboratories do not identify *E. coli* O157:H7 in fecal cultures because a selective culture medium is needed. However, this is a potentially very serious infection that warrants prompt detection because it should respond to antimicrobial therapy if detected sufficiently early. Outbreaks have been linked to contaminated ground (minced) meat, raw milk, and person-to-person spread. A recent case-control study involving 243 patients (12 were under 5 years of age, 23 were 5 to 17 years of age) in a small city in rural Missouri traced the infection to transmission by water for the first time; several of the affected persons were visitors to the city where the outbreak occurred [12•]. The number of new cases declined rapidly after residents were ordered to boil water and after the water supply was chlorinated (Fig. 1). This infection, which can cause bloody or nonbloody diarrhea, is probably often undiagnosed because routine microbiological methods fail to identify the organism. Verocytotoxigenic *E. coli* (VTEC) may also be a significant cause of sporadic or endemic diarrhea in children in the tropics [7•]. Person-to-person transmission of VTEC occurs in a substantial proportion of episodes of childhood hemolytic-uremic syndrome [13•].

A range of methods has been used to identify the Shiga-like toxin–producing or enterohemorrhagic strains of *E. coli* that are involved; these include cytotoxin detection and neutralization with specific antisera, hybridization of DNA probes, and various forms of immunodetection including enzyme-liked immunosorbent assay (ELISA). It has recently been shown that polymerase chain reaction (PCR) can be used to diagnose enterohemorrhagic *E. coli* infections from stool samples without prior culture of the specimens [14•].

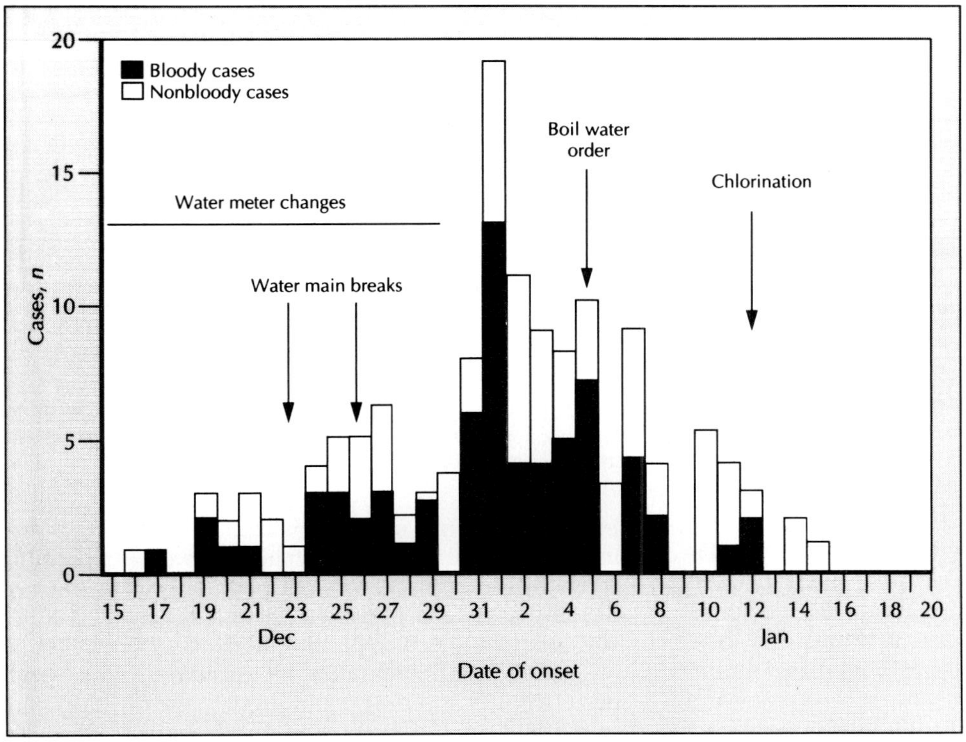

Fig. 1. Episodes of diarrheal illness among city residents by date of onset and character of stool in Cabool, Missouri, from 15 December 1989 to 20 January 1990. (*From* Swerdlow *et al.* [12•]; with permission.)

Campylobacteriosis

Campylobacter jejuni has become recognized as a major cause of enteritis in recent years. Consumption of contaminated water, unpasteurized milk, and inadequately cooked poultry and other meats has been implicated in its transmission. Campylobacteriosis is a particularly important cause of diarrhea in children; high carrier rates are associated with levels of community hygiene, and the infection is often believed to be caused by exposure to animals. A study of more than 200 human episodes compared with 526 controls in King County, Washington state, showed that exposure to animals with diarrhea was associated with a fourfold increase in the risk of *C. jejuni/coli* enteritis (odds ratio 4.3, 95% confidence interval 1.9 to 9.7) and that 6.3% of episodes were attributable to such exposure [15•]. A 10-year retrospective review of information from 51 state and territorial health departments in the United States involving preschool through college subjects identified 12 outbreaks of *Campylobacter* enteritis in 11 states; 458 episodes associated with these outbreaks occurred among 45% of the 1013 persons from the study who drank raw milk [16••]. Fourteen outbreaks (70%) occurred among children between kindergarten and third grade.

Therefore, drinking raw milk on school field trips or other youth activities remains an important risk factor for campylobacteriosis in the United States and requires appropriate public health measures and educational programs. The public health implications of *E. coli* O157:H7 disease in the United States, particularly in relation to food-borne infections, was the subject of a recent editorial [11•].

Campylobacter-like organisms have been implicated as a cause of recurrent abdominal cramps in Italian children [17•]. Recognized enteric pathogens were isolated from fecal specimens from none of the affected 10 patients, all of whom had the *Campylobacter*-like organisms detected and who, on epidemiologic grounds, probably acquired their infections by person-to-person transmission. By using sodium dodecyl sulfate–polyacrylamide gel electrophoresis of whole-cell proteins and cellular fatty acid analysis, this *Campylobacter*-like organism was identified as *A. butzleri.*

Helicobacter pylori

Helicobacter pylori infection is now generally accepted as an important cause of gastritis and peptic ulcer disease. There is increasing evidence that many persons acquire this infection during childhood [18•,19]; acquisition probably lasts for decades [20•] and may continue in adults with an age-related increase in frequency continuing up to 70 years [21]. The modes of transmission and acquisition of this infection are not fully established; fecal-oral transfer, person-to-person spread, and contamination of endoscopes have been proposed. An association between the prevalence of the infection and the metropolitan water supply has been reported from Peru [22•]. It seems that acquisition is earlier and more frequent in developing countries, and infections from these areas are more likely to be resistant to metronidazole (>90%) than in industrialized regions like Europe and Australia (<20%) [23•]. Although there are differences in prevalence of *H. pylori* infection in ecological and climatic zones, such as coastal areas, mountains, and jungles in Peru, these are probably much less important than differences in sanitation [23•]. *H. pylori* infection seems to be prevalent in China; a cross-sectional study from a large city (Guangzhou) and three rural areas in southern China (Guangdong) demonstrated an overall prevalence of 44.2% with a significantly higher rate in the urban population [24••]. That study clearly shows that early childhood is the critical period for acquisition of the infection (Fig. 2); by 5 years of age 23% of all children in the study were infected and the rate of seroprevalence continued to increase by about 1% annually. Density of living conditions was shown to be a prime determinant in the acquisition of *H. pylori.* The common practice of sending Chinese city children to kindergarten at 3 years of age, and the Chinese custom of eating from communal bowls and using chopsticks might also be important.

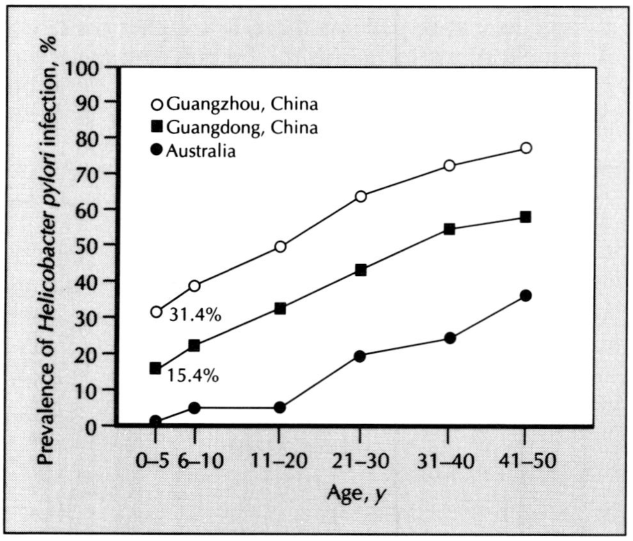

Fig. 2. Prevalence of *Helicobacter pylori* infection by age in the Provinces of Guangzhou and Guangdong in China compared with that found in Australia. (*From* Mitchell *et al.* [24••]; with permission.)

In clinical settings in industrialized countries, *H. pylori* infection in children has been investigated as a possible cause of recurrent abdominal pain. However, the evidence that *H. pylori*–related gastritis is involved is not yet convincing [25•,26•], although *H. pylori* infection or gastritis have often been demonstrated in such children [25•,27•] and thus might predate the development of chronic gastritis and peptic ulcer disease. In adults, treatment with bismuth compounds and antibiotics has proven effective in eradication of *H. pylori* infection, but because of concerns about possibly toxicity, bismuth preparations are not licensed for use in children in some countries. Combined therapy with amoxicillin and tinidazole was effective in a study of Italian children, with only a small proportion relapsing after 18 months [28•]. Microbiological culture can be considered as the gold standard to diagnose *H. pylori* infection in children, but noninvasive tests such as serology or ^{13}C-urea breath test are very acceptable alternatives, with 95% sensitivity and 92% specificity [29•]. Cytology and the rapid urease test on gastric biopsy specimens have been used effectively for prompt diagnosis [30•], and PCR has been developed for the specific detection of *H. pylori* and should be useful in helping to elucidate the role of this organism in gastroduodenal disease [31•].

Aeromonas spp

There is increasing evidence to implicate species of *Aeromonas* in human diarrheal disease, particularly in children. A recent study in England, involving more than 1000 fecal specimens from children with gastrointestinal symptoms over a 12-month period, confirmed that *Aeromonas* spp (especially *Aeromonas caviae*) can cause gastroenteritis in children (usually causing mild diarrhea for 2 to 3 days), and occurs most often in the warmer months of the year [32•]. A study of clinical and environmental isolates of *Aeromonas* spp in India showed that most isolates were enterotoxin-positive when tested for fluid accumulation in rabbit ileal loops [33•]. Most clinical and environmental isolates of *A. caviae* were enterotoxigenic but isolates of *Aeromonas hydrophila* and *Aeromonas sobria* caused more marked fluid accumulation. The environmental strains of *A. hydrophila* and *A. sobria* caused greater fluid accumulation than the clinical isolates. Strains of *Aeromonas* spp that produced little or no fluid accumulation initially became toxin producers after one to three passages through rabbit ileal loops, which suggests that all strains of these species of *Aeromonas* may be potentially enterotoxigenic, regardless of their source.

Fecal cytotoxicity

Despite advances in knowledge about how microorganisms cause diarrhea in humans and improved laboratory methods to detect them, a significant proportion of stool samples submitted for investigation from episodes of community-acquired diarrhea do not yield identifiable pathogens. Cytotoxicity in tissue culture can be associated with several enteric pathogens, which might be useful when further investigation is necessary to determine the cause of diarrhea in children. Cytotoxicity of fecal extracts was demonstrated in 47 of 88 children (54%) referred for microbiological investigation of stools in the hospital. Cytotoxic *Clostridium difficile* and VTEC were the pathogens identified most commonly, but cytotoxicity was also found in association with *C. jejuni, Salmonella* spp, *Shigella sonnei, Giardia lamblia,* rotavirus, and adenovirus [34]. In five of 13 patients with diarrhea and cytotoxic *C. difficile,* other pathogens were also present, supporting the view that *C. difficile* organisms are more readily recovered when the intestinal flora have been altered by colonization with other microorganisms. There was no correlation between previous treatment with antibiotics and isolation of *C. difficile.* Cytotoxicity neutralized by antitoxin, usually to *Clostridium sordellii,* is used to detect cytotoxic *C. difficile.* Cytotoxicity not neutralized in this way could be used as an indication for further investigation of stools for the presence of other pathogens such as VTEC or viruses. Another study of fecal cytotoxicity, from northern England, used fecal samples from community-acquired diarrheal episodes in subjects over 10 years of age from whom parasites, *Salmonella, Shigella, Campylobacter,* or *C. difficile* were not found. The ability of fecal cultures to produce cytotoxin was investigation by use of an *in vitro* toxin enhancement procedure [35•]. Twenty-eight percent of samples were cytotoxin-positive; nine were neutralized by antiverocytotoxin 1, 29 by anti-VT2, and eight by neither. In patients in whom neutralization by either verocytotoxins 1 or 2 or the combined antisera was negative, neutralization by *C. sordellii* antiserum was also tested. This report suggests that *E. coli* undetected by routine diagnostic methods may be significant causes of diarrhea in the community, and jointly these two reports show a need for further research into how enteric microorganisms cause childhood diarrhea and how they can be detected and identified in clinical and epidemiological settings.

Rotavirus

Rotavirus is an important cause of childhood gastrointestinal infection requiring hospitalization; infection is confined to the gut but there are serum as well as intestinal antibody responses that have incompletely defined roles in protection against symptomatic disease. Copro-immunoglobulin A conversion was investigated prospectively in 35 children who were recruited at the time of severe rotavirus illness [36•]. A total of 94% of the children experienced reinfection and 38% developed sustained elevations in specific copro-immunoglobulin A, which was a feature of children with higher mean annual rates of rotavirus infection and a lower ratio of symptomatic to total number of rotavirus infections, suggesting that production of a specific copro-immunoglobulin A plateau correlated with protection against an excess of infection and symptomatic disease. There have been many attempts to immunize infants and children, actively or passively, against rotavirus infections. A recent study evaluated orally administered live rhesus monkey rotavirus vaccine (RRV, VP7 serotype 3) and human-rhesus reassortant rotavirus vaccine (Dx RRV, VP7 serotype 7) in a placebo-controlled field trial of 223 US infants (predominantly suburban middle class) 2 to 4 months of age [37•]. A single dose (10^4 plaque-forming units) of either vaccine provided significant protection from rotavirus illness; serum antibody responses occurred in 78% and 71% of RRV and DxRRV vaccines, respectively, with efficacy rates of 66% ($P = 0.01$) and 77% ($P = 0.002$) against rotavirus-associated illness in the first season after vaccination.

The possible protective effects of anti-rotavirus and anti–*E. coli* milk antibodies against acute diarrheal diseases in children living in lower socioeconomic conditions in Santiago, Chile, were investigated prospectively over a 6-month period [38••]. The cohorts of 124 and 108 subjects were given either a commercial milk formula or the same formula containing 1% (weight for weight) bovine milk immunoglobulin concentrate from cows hyperimmunized with human rotaviruses and the major EPEC serogroups. No protective effect on diarrheal diseases was demonstrated. The authors believe that although increasing the immunoglobulin concentration in the milk formula is theoretically possible, the high cost and high numbers of hyperimmunized milking cows required will preclude the large-scale use of this approach and that promotion of breast-feeding is still a preferred strategy to reduce the burden of diarrheal diseases in infants in developing countries.

Parasites

Intestinal infection with the flagellated protozoan *G. lamblia* (or *Giardia duodenalis, Giardia intestinalis*) is prevalent in infants and young children in many parts of the world, particularly where conditions of personal and community hygiene are poor. Giardiasis is very prevalent in young Australian Aboriginal children in remote areas. A recently published, longitudinal 3-year study presents strong circumstantial evidence to implicate dogs in the cycle of transmission [39•]; this is supported by molecular characterization using PCR to epidemiologically map the DNA profiles of isolates of *Giardia* from humans and from dogs in northwest Australia [40•]. Many reported outbreaks of giardiasis have been traced to water-borne or person-to-person transmission. Several outbreaks have been found to be food-borne, and a recent report may be the first to trace an outbreak to a commercial food outlet [41•]. This outbreak involved 27 (75%) of 36 persons in a group who met in a restaurant in Washington state; circumstantial evidence suggests that ice contaminated by a food handler may have been the vehicle for transmission of the infection. Parasitic infestations, *eg, G. duodenalis* or *Strongyloides stercoralis*, are highly prevalent in children in tropical, developing countries and may contribute to persistent diarrhea and its associated malnutrition, in some instances through excessive protein losses from the gastrointestinal tract [42•].

In parts of the world where the HIV pandemic has become established, such as sub-Saharan Africa where as many as 1 million children have been infected [43], intestinal parasites may be an important cause of chronic diarrhea, further compromising their nutritional status. A prospective, cross-sectional study of 15-month to 5-year-old children with chronic diarrhea hospitalized in Dar es Salaam (Tanzania) showed that about 40% of these subjects were HIV-seropositive, many with diarrhea lasting less than 1 month [44•]. Overall, these children were severely malnourished and the association between chronic diarrhea and undernutrition may have diminished the difference between HIV-negative and HIV-positive groups, both of which had intestinal parasites in about 50% of subjects. Recognized diarrheagenic pathogens were found in nearly 40% of subjects with chronic diarrhea (including *Giardia, Cryptosporidium, Strongyloides, Trichuris trichiura*) but the only parasite found significantly more often in HIV-positive subjects with chronic diarrhea was *Blastocystis hominis*. Importantly, up to 40% of the subjects studied had diarrhea-causing parasites that could be diagnosed and treated in most developing countries and simple screening for fecal leukocytes should help in identification of such patients. Even without fecal concentration procedures, careful repeated stool microscopy could help improve the treatment of a significant proportion of patients like these.

A capture ELISA method was used to detect *G. lamblia* antigens in formalin-treated fecal samples stored for 18 months from Chilean schoolchildren [45•] and in the longitudinal follow-up of a cohort of 68 children below 6 years of age in a mountain village in the United Arab Emirates [46•]. The proportions of fecal samples positive for *Giardia* in the latter study were as follows: by routine microscopy, 8.8%; by formol-ether concentration, 14.7%; and by capture ELISA, 19.3%. The authors propose the method for use in clinical diagnosis as well as in epidemiologic investigations.

Cryptosporidium is another intestinal parasite that has come into prominence lately, owing to its association with chronic life-threatening illness in immunocompromised hosts and its ability to cause acute gastroenteritis and diarrheal outbreaks in children, *eg*, in day care centers. Cryptosporidiosis can affect children without clinical evidence of immune deficiency. A review of 123 such children investigated in a hospital in London, England, over a 6.5 year period showed that 50% of children excreting only *Cryptosporidium* had chronic diarrhea [47•]. All nine children who had intestinal biopsies done had a mild-to-moderate enteropathy and in seven of those nine patients, *Cryptosporidium* was identified adhering to the intestinal mucosa, on the villous, not crypt, epithelium. *Cryptosporidium* should be sought routinely in the investigation of children with chronic diarrhea and who fail to thrive. *Cryptosporidium* infection has become recognized only in the past few years as a potential cause of community-acquired diarrhea in the People's Republic of China, particularly in refractory or prolonged episodes. A survey of more than 5000 infants and children under 15 years of age in Jiangsu province found that 1.8% of subjects has oocysts detected in their stools; the highest isolation rate (3%) occurred between 1 and 5 years of age [48•]; intermittent or persistent diarrhea was the commonest symptom.

The newly described organism so far called coccidian-like or cyanobacterium-like body (CLB), was found in patients with prolonged diarrhea from several countries. A case-control study of travelers and expatriate residents at two outpatient clinics in Kathmandu, Nepal, investigated causes of diarrhea in 964 subjects with gastrointestinal symptoms and 96 symptom-free control subjects [49••]. CLB was identified in 11% of those with symptoms compared with only one (1%) of the control subjects ($P=0.0003$). The diarrheal illness associated with CLB lasted a median of 7 weeks compared with only 9 days for individuals with other causes of diarrhea ($P<0.0001$). Patients with CLB infections were, on average, four times more likely than control subjects to report consumption of untreated water; furthermore, organisms of the same appearance were identified in a water sample that was implicated, epidemiologically, with CLB infection. Another report about CLB concerns three patients with fecal cysts of CLB who had developed diarrhea after visiting North Africa or the Indian subcontinent [50••]. Upper intestinal aspirates from two of these three patients also yielded CLB, suggesting that they had enteritis; two patients had light microscopic evidence of jejunitis with increased numbers of inepithelial lymphocytes and villous blunting. Electron microscopy of the same biopsy specimens demonstrated that intraepithelial CLB appears to be a new water-borne enteric pathogen for humans. The name *Cyclospora cayetanensis* has been proposed for these organisms.

Risk factors

With improved outcomes from episodes of acute childhood diarrhea in developing countries, largely through more effective and widespread use of oral rehydration therapy, increased attention is being given to those acute episodes that become persistent (*ie*, last beyond 14 days). This is now a major cause of diarrheal deaths in such places. A recent study in impoverished populations in northeast Brazil reported that half of the diarrhea mortality was due to persistent diarrhea [51••]. As well, 11% of 14 or more diarrheal illnesses per child year in an urban slum setting last more than 14 days, a cut-off definition that clearly identified the children at high risk of heavy diarrhea morbidity. Such heavily affected children had impaired catch-up growth. Furthermore, malnutrition significantly predisposed children to increased incidence and duration of diarrhea and to a greater incidence of persistent diarrhea. In contrast to the usual predominance of enterotoxigenic *E. coli* and rotavirus as causal agents in diarrheal episodes in such settings, this study found that *Cryptosporidium* (in 13%) and EAEC (36% with aggregative, 29% with diffuse, 13% with localized adherence to HEp-2 cells) were the main pathogens isolated from fecal or upper intestinal samples.

In a rural indigenous population in Guatemala, six behaviors were found to have significant association with persistent diarrhea: presence of toys on the ground; presence of babies' bottles on the ground; mothers' hands being dirty; presence of a fecally soiled diaper on the ground in the household compound; presence of feces in the yard; and the wearing of fecally soiled diapers [52•]. In urban Brazilian infants the following were significant risk factors for diarrhea; hospitalization in the previous month, exposure to a day care center, prior diarrhea in another household member, and low family income [53•]. Breast-feeding in infants less than 6 months old and boiling household drinking water were protective.

The close association of malnutrition and diarrheal disease in children in developing countries has long been widely accepted. However, the degree of interaction and interdependence between these two factors is not universally agreed. Diarrheal disease contributes, not surprisingly, to malnutrition but the impact of malnutrition on diarrheal episodes seems to be variable. in general, malnutrition causes diarrhea of longer duration, and some studies have shown a higher diarrhea incidence [51••]. A community-based, longitudinal study in Matlab, a rural lowland area in Bangladesh, examined these interrelationships in a cohort of 705 children followed for 1 year [54•]. The diarrhea incidence rate was 4.6 episodes per year. About three quarters of the children were below 2 SD (Z scores) under weight and height for age and about one third were below -2 Z score weight for height. About 20% of the children were anergic and these children had a 50% increased incidence of diarrhea. There was only a modest association between undernutrition and the incidence of diarrhea; the history of diarrhea in a child in the previous 3 months was a strong predictor for diarrhea in the next 3-month interval. Statistical evaluation of their findings showed that malnutrition and impaired cell-mediated immunity were independent risk factors for the occurrence of diarrhea. Cell-mediated immune deficiency might result from protein-energy malnutrition or from deficiencies of single nutrients such as vitamin A, pyridoxine, folic acid, iron or zinc.

Increased risk of diarrheal episodes and other infectious episodes has previously been documented in children attending day care centers. A more recent study in the United States showed that the risk of clinic visits for diarrhea is roughly doubled in children receiving day care and was similar for those attending day care centers (odds ratio, 2.4), daycare homes (odds ratio, 2.0), or when cared for by a relative (odds ratio, 2.0). These increased risks of day care were highest in the first month of enrollment [55•].

References and recommended reading

Papers of particular interest, published within the annual period of review, have been highlighted as:

- • Of special interest
- •• Of outstanding interest

1. HART CA, BATT RM, SAUNDERS JR: **Diarrhoea Caused by *Escherichia coli*.** *Ann Trop Paediatr* 1993, **13**:121–131.
•
A review on the role of *E. coli* in diarrheal disease.

2. ECHEVERRIA P, SAVARINO SJ, YAMAMOTO T: ***Escherichia coli* Diarrhoea.** *Baillieres Clin Gastroenterol* 1993, 7:243–262.
••
A comprehensive and authoritative review about *E. coli* diarrhea in a monograph about infectious diarrhea.

3. DONNENBERG MS, KAPER JB: **Enteropathogenic *Escherichia coli*.** *Infect Immun* 1992, **60**:3953–3967.
••
An authoritative "minireview" about EPEC which includes a diagrammatic three-step scheme that summarizes the mechanisms involved.

4. MANJARREZ-HERNANDEZ HA, BALDWIN TJ, AITKEN A, KNUTTON S, WILLIAMS PH: **Intestinal Epithelial Cell Protein Phosphorylation in Enteropathogenic *Escherichia coli* Diarrhoea.** *Lancet* 1992, **339**:521–523.

5. GHOSH AR, NAIR GB, NAIK TN, PAUL M, PAL SC, SEN D: **Entero-Adherent *Escherichia coli* is an Important Diarrheagenic Agent in Infants Below 6 Months in Calcutta, India.** *J Med Microbiol* 1992, 36:264–268.
•
Escherichia coli adherent to HEp-2 and HeLa cells were isolated from the feces of 19.7% of hospitalized Indian infants under 6 months of age with acute diarrhea. More than one third of the isolates were of known enteropathogenic O;K serogroups (EPEC). This study showed that locally adherent EAEC was an important etiologic agent of acute diarrhea in these infants.

6. GUNZBURG ST, CHANG BJ, ELLIOTT SJ, BURKE V, GRACEY M: **Diffuse and Enteroaggregative Patterns of Adherence of Enteric *Escherichia coli* Isolated From Aboriginal Children From the Kimberley Region of Western Australia.** *J Infect Dis* 1993, **167**:755–758.
••
Reports community surveys of patterns of *in vitro* adherence of fecal *E. coli* in Aboriginal children up to 5 years of age in different seasons in parts of tropical northwest Australia. EAEC were significantly associated with diarrhea, mainly in children below 18 months of age. More than 20% of children with diarrhea, but less than 9% without diarrhea, showed a previously unreported pattern of detachment of the HEp-2 cell monolayer from the glass coverslip when examined in the adhesion assay. This feature has been called cell detachment, and it is suggested that cell-detaching *E. coli* are a new enterovirulent class of *E. coli*.

7. GUZBURG ST, CHANG BJ, BURKE V, GRACEY M: **Virulence Factors of Enteric *Escherichia coli* in Young Aboriginal Children in North-West Australia.** *Epidemiol Infect* 1992, 109:283–289.
•
Describes the patterns of virulence factors found in enteric *E. coli* isolated from young aboriginal communities in remote communities in far northwest Australia. Enterotoxigenic *E. coli* were the most frequently identified enteric pathogens, with an incidence similar to those from other tropical regions. Heat-stable toxin-producing strains were associated with diarrhea throughout the year, but heat-labile toxin-producing strains were more prevalent in the summer monsoon. VTEC and EAEC were significant causes of diarrhea.

8. MILFORD DV, TAYLOR CM, GUTTRIDGE B, HALL SM, ROWE B, KLEANTHOUS H: **Haemolytic Uraemic Syndromes in the British Isles 1985-8: Association With Verocytotoxin Producing Escherichia coli. Part 1: Clinical and Epidemiological Aspects.** *Arch Dis Child* 1990, **65**:716–721.

9. KLEANTHOUS H, SMITH HR, SCOTLAND SM, GROSS RJ, ROWE B, TAYLOR CM, MILFORD DV: **Haemolytic Uraemic Syndromes in the British isles, 1985-8: Association With Verocytotoxin Producing Escherichia coli. Part 2: Microbiological Aspects.** *Arch Dis Child* 1990, **65**:722–727.

10. GRIFFIN PM, TAUXE RV: **The Epidemiology of Infections Caused by *Escherichia coli* O157:H7; Other Enterohemorrhagic *E. coli*, and the Hemolytic Uremic Syndrome.** *Epidemiol Rev* 1991, **13**:60–98.

11. MACDONALD KL, OSTERHOLM MT: **The Emergence of *Escherichia coli* O157:H7 Infection in the United States. The Changing Epidemiology of Foodborne Disease [Editorial].** *JAMA* 1993, **269**:2264–2265.
•
An editorial on the emergence of *E. coli* O157:H7 infection in the United States, prompted by an outbreak involving 23 patients in Massachusetts, including four with the diagnosis of hemolytic-uremic syndrome, a well-recognized complication of this infection. This infection is easily overlooked but is emerging as a potentially important public health problem; *E. coli* O157:H7 is now a significant foodborne pathogen, which illustrates the changing epidemiology of foodborne disease in the United States and highlights many of the ensuing public health issues and the difficulties associated with prompt detection, control, and clinical management.

12. SWERDLOW DL, WOODRUFF BA, BRADY RC, GRIFFIN PM, TIPPENS S, DONNELL HD, GELDREICH E, PAYNE PJ, MEYER A, WELLS JG, GREENE KD, BRIGHT M, BEAN NH, BLAKE PA: **A Waterborne Outbreak in Missouri of *Escherichia coli* O157:H7 Associated With Bloody Diarrhea and Death.** *Ann Intern Med* 1992, **117**:812–819.
•
Reports an investigation that was done to describe and determine the source of a large outbreak of *E. coli* O157:H7 infections in Missouri that occurred in a rural township with an unchlorinated water supply. This was a very large outbreak, involving 243 patients, 32 of whom were hospitalized and four of whom died. The outbreak was believed to be transmitted by water and the number of new cases declined rapidly after the residents were ordered to boil water and after the water supply was chlorinated. This is a potentially very serious infection, which is probably underdiagnosed because routine methods will not detect the causative organism.

13. ROWE PC, ORRBINE E, LIOR H, WELLS GA, MCLAINE PN, CP-KDRC CO-INVESTIGATORS: **Diarrhoea in Close Contacts as a Risk Factor for Childhood Haemolytic Uraemic Syndrome.** *Epidemiol Infect* 1993, **110**:9–16.
•
A case-control study of 34 children hospitalized with hemolytic-uremic syndrome, 88% of whom were shown to have been exposed to VTEC. Evidence supports person-to-person transmission of these *E. coli* in a substantial proportion of such patients.

14. BRIAN MJ, FROSOLONO M, MURRAY BE, MIRANDA A, LOPEZ EL, GOMEZ HF, CLEARY TG: **Polymerase Chain Reaction for Diagnosis of Enterohemorrhagic *Escherichia coli* Infection and Hemolytic-Uremic Syndrome.** *J Clin Microbiol* 1992, 30:1801–1806.
•
Demonstrates that PCR can be used to diagnose enterohemorrhagic *Escherichia coli* infection without prior culture of fecal specimens. This should facilitate clinical diagnosis of this infection and could be particularly useful in the investigation of outbreaks of hemolytic-uremic syndrome.

15. SAEED AM, HARRIS NV, DIGIACOMO RF: **The Role of Exposure to Animals in the Etiology of *Campylobacter jejuni/coli* Enteritis.** *Am J Epidemiol* 1993, 137:108–114.
•
This case-control study in Washington state shows that exposure to animals with diarrhea was associated with a fourfold increase in the risk of *Campylobacter jejuni/coli* enteritis.

16. WOOD RC, MACDONALD KL, OSTERHOLM MT: ***Campylobacter* Enteritis Outbreaks Associated with Drinking Raw Milk: A 10-Year Review of Outbreaks in the United States.** *JAMA* 1992, **268**:3228–3230.
••
A 10-year retrospective survey in the United States and Puerto Rico to determine the incidence or recognized outbreaks of *Campylobacter* enteritis associated with drinking raw milk during youth activities such as school field trips. The investigation identified 20 outbreaks in 11 states, at least one each year, with 458 outbreak-associated episodes documented. *Campylobacter jejuni* is one of the commonest identified causes of acute infectious diarrhea in developed countries. There is a need for greater awareness of the potential risks associated with drinking raw milk, and more effective educational programs are needed to reduce these risks.

17. • Vandamme P, Pugina P, Benzi G, Van Elterijck R, Vlaes L, Kersters K, Butzler J-P, Lior H, Lauwers S: **Outbreak of Recurrent Abdominal Cramps Associated With *Arcobacter butzleri* in an Italian School**. *J Clin Microbiol* 1992, **30**:2335–2337.

An investigation of an outbreak of recurrent abdominal cramps in an Italian nursery and primary school. None of the affected children had diarrhea. Microbiologic and epidemiologic findings suggest that a *Campylobacter*-like organism, identified as *A. butzleri*, was the responsible etiologic agent.

18. • Mendall MA, Goggin PM, Molineaux N, Levy J, Toosy T, Strachan D, Northfield TC: **Childhood Living Conditions and *Helicobacter pylori* Positivity in Adult Life**. *Lancet* 1992, **339**:896–897.

A study that relates prevalence of IgG antibodies against *H. pylori* (determined by ELISA) to living conditions of these adult English subjects (mean age, 46 years) when they were 8 years of age. Absence of a fixed hot-water supply and domestic crowding in childhood were powerful independent risk factors for current *H. pylori* infection, implicating these factors and household contact in childhood in the pathogenesis of the disease.

19. Odera G, Vaira D, Holton J: **Age-Related Increase of *Helicobacter pylori* Frequency in Symptom-Free and Dyspeptic Children**. *Lancet* 1992, **340**:671–672.

20. • Parsonnet J, Blaser MJ, Perez-Perez GI, Hargett-Bean N, Tauxe RV: **Symptoms and Risk-Factors of *Helicobacter pylori* Infection in a Cohort of Epidemiologist**. *Gastroenterology* 1992, **102**:41–46.

A study of symptoms and risk factors associated with *H. pylori* infection in a group of 341 epidemiologists. The investigation used serum samples collected between 1969 and 1987 and one recent sample collected from each subject in 1988 and evaluated their *H. pylori* IgG levels by ELISA.

21. Karnes WE, Samloff IM, Siurala M, Kekki M, Sipponen P, Kim SWR, Walsh JH: **Positive Antibody and Negative Tissue Staining for *Helicobacter pylori* in Subjects With Atrophic Body Gastritis**. *Gastroenterology* 1991, **101**:167–174.

22. • Klein PD, Gastrointestinal Physiology Working Group, Graham DY, Gaillour A, Opekun AR, O'Brian Smith E: **Water Sources as Risk Factor for *Helicobacter pylori* Infection in Peruvian Children**. *Lancet* 1991, **337**:1503–1506.

An investigation of the prevalence of *H. pylori* infection in 407 children aged 2 months to 12 years in Lima, Peru, using ^{13}C-urea breath test. *H. pylori* was acquired early and the number of infected individuals increased rapidly with age; overall prevalence was 48% and was highly correlated with socioeconomic status. The municipal water supply was implicated in transmission.

23. • The Gastrointestinal Physiology Working Group of the Cayetano Heredia and the Johns Hopkins University: **Ecology of *Helicobacter pylori* in Peru: Infection Rates in Coastal, High Altitude, and Jungle Communities**. *Gut* 1992, **33**:604–605.

Reports rates of infection with *H. pylori* in endoscopic clinic patients investigated in three widely different geographic regions of Peru: the coast, the Andean Sierra, and the Amazon jungle.

24. •• Mitchell HM, Li YY, Hu PJ Liu Q, Chen M, Du GG, Wang ZJ, Lee A, Hazell SL: **Epidemiology of *Helicobacter pylori* in Southern China: Identification of Early Childhood as the Critical Period for Acquisition**. *J Infect Dis* 1992, **166**:149–153.

A large cross-sectional study to investigate the prevalence and possible modes of transmission of *H. pylori* in southern China. The investigation provides interesting information about the increasing seroprevalence of *H. pylori* after 5 years of age in urban and rural populations in that region in comparison with parallel data from Australia and against other published data. There is strong evidence from this study that density of living conditions is an important determinant of the acquisition of *H. pylori*.

25. • Maaroos H-I, Räga T, Sipponen P, Siurala M: ***Helicobacter pylori* and Gastritis in Children With Abdominal Complaints**. *Scand J Gastroenterol* 1991, **26**(suppl 186):95–99.

Reports the result of gastroscopy with biopsies in 178 Estonian children with upper abdominal pain. Gastritis and *H. pylori* infection prevalences showed a trend to increase with age, and although *H. pylori*-related gastritis may often cause abdominal pain in children, convincing proof of the association is lacking.

26. • Fiedorek SC, Castell HB, Pumphrey CL, Evans DJ Jr, Evans DG, Klein PD, Graham DY: **The Role of *Helicobacter pylori* in Recurrent, Functional Abdominal Pain in Children**. *Am J Gastroenterol* 1992, **87**:347–349.

An investigation of possible *H. pylori* infection as a cause of presumed functional recurrent abdominal pain in childhood. Results do not support the association as being common.

27. • Prieto G, Polanco I, Larrauri J, Rota L, Lama R, Carrasco S: ***Helicobacter pylori* Infection in Children: Clinical, Endoscopic, and Histologic Correlations**. *J Pediatr Gastroenterol Nutr* 1992, **14**:420–425.

Reports findings on 270 consecutive patients up to 20 years of age who had endoscopies performed for investigation of abdominal pain. Found correlation between *H. pylori* colonization and gastric histologic findings, which supports a possible role for *H. pylori* infection in gastroduodenal disease from childhood.

28. • Odera G, Vaira D, Ainley C: **Eighteen Month Follow Up of *Helicobacter pylori* Positive Children Treated With Amoxycillin and Tinidazole**. *Gut* 1992, **33**:1328–1330.

Reports that after eradication of *H. pylori* by use of combined amoxicillin and tinidazole treatment, only a small portion (about 10%) of children relapse during the following 18 months.

29. • Vandenplas Y, Blecker U, Devreker T, Keppens E, Nijs J, Cadranel S, Pipeleers-Marichal M, Goosseus A, Lawwers S: **Contribution of the ^{13}C-Urea Breath Test to the Detection of *Helicobacter pylori* Gastritis in Children**. *Pediatrics* 1992, **90**:608–611.

This study shows that noninvasive tests such as serology or ^{13}C-urea breath test can be used to diagnose *H. pylori* infection in children; each test had greater than 90% sensitivity and specificity.

30. • Debongnie JC, Delmee M, Mainguet P, Hoat CBJ, Legros G: **Cytology: A Simple, Rapid, Sensitive Method in the Diagnosis of *Helicobacter pylori***. *Am J Gastroenterol* 1992, **87**:20–23.

Describes how cytology and the rapid urease test on gastric biopsy specimens can be used to diagnose *H. pylori* infection within an hour. Touch cytology (imprints from biopsy specimens) was found to be simple, quick, sensitive, and reproducible, and did not adversely affect the biopsy specimens for later microbiologic culture or histologic examination.

31. • Clayton CL, Kleanthous H, Coates PJ, Morgan DD, Tabaqchali S: **Sensitive Detection of *Helicobacter pylori* by Using Polymerase Chain Reaction**. *J Clin Microbiol* 1992, **30**:192–200.

Reports PCR for the specific detection of *H. pylori*. In the reported studies of 50 strains of *H. pylori*, the method was 100% specific and capable of detecting as few as 10 *H. pylori* cells.

32. • Wilcox MH, Cook AM, Eley A, Spencer RC: ***Aeromonas* spp as a Potential Cause of Diarrhoea in Children**. *J Clin Pathol* 1992, **45**:959–963.

A report from England confirming that *Aeromonas* species, particularly *A. caviae*, may cause gastroenteritis in children, mostly during the warmer months of the year.

33. • Singh DV, Sanyal SC: **Enterotoxicity of Clinical and Environmental Isolates of *Aeromonas* spp**. *J Med Microbiol* 1992, **36**:269–272.

A study of enterotoxicity of clinical and environmental isolates of *Aeromonas* species in Varanasi, India. Adds evidence that these microorganisms are significant diarrheal pathogens for humans and suggests that all strains of the species *A. hydrophila* and *A. sobria* may be capable of producing enterotoxins.

34. Kennedy E, Burke V, Pearman J, Robinson J, Gracey M: **Cytotoxic Effects of Children's Faeces: Relation to Diarrhoea Due to *Clostridium difficile* and Other Enteric Pathogens**. *Ann Trop Paediatr* 1991, **11**:107–112.

35. • BURKE D, AL JUMAILI BJ, ALMARDINI H, RECORD CO: **Culture Negative Cytotoxin Positive Stools in Community Acquired Diarrhoea.** *Gut* 1993, 34:192–193.

A significant proportion of episodes of community-acquired diarrhea go undiagnosed. This study (see also Kennedy *et al.*, *Ann Trop Paediatr* 1991, 11:107–112) shows that many of these undetected infections (in this case 28%) may be associated with bacterial cytotoxins that are detectable in fecal samples.

36. • COULSON BS, GRIMWOOD K, HUDSON IL, BARNES GL, BISHOP RF: **Role of Coproantibody in Clinical Protection of Children During Reinfection With Rotavirus.** *J Clin Microbiol* 1992, 30:1678–1684.

Reports that copro-IgA conversion is a more sensitive marker of rotavirus reinfection and that frequent rotavirus infection in children seems to stimulate the production of a specific copro-IgA plateau, which correlates with protection against an excess of infection and symptomatic disease.

37. • MADORE HP CHRISTY C, PICHICHERO M, LONG C, PINCUS P, VOSEFOKY D, KAPIKIAN AZ, DOLIN R, THE ELMWOOD PANORAMA AND WESTFALL PEDIATRIC GROUPS: **Field Trial of Rhesus Rotavirus or Human-Rhesus Rotavirus Reassortant Vaccine of VP7 Serotype 3 or 1 Specificity in Infants.** *J Infect Dis* 1992, 166:235–243.

Findings of a field trial of rhesus rotavirus reassortant vaccine of VP7 serotype 3 or 1 specificity in infants. A single dose of these vaccines provided significant protection in 2- to 4-month-old infants against rotavirus-associated illness in the first season after vaccination, with rates of efficacy of 66% and 77%, respectively.

38. •• BRUNSER O, ESPINOZA J, FIGUEROA G, ARAYA M, SPENCER E, HILPERT H, LINK-AMSTER H, BRÜSSOW H: **Field Trial of an Infant Formula Containing Anti-Rotavirus and Anti-*Escherichia coli* Milk Antibodies From Hyperimmunized Cows.** *J Pediatr Gastroenterol Nutr* 1992, 15:63–72.

This study reports the results of a field trial of the use of an infant formula containing anti-rotavirus and anti–*E. coli* antibodies that were produced in hyperimmunized cows in comparison with the use of the same formula without the bovine milk immunoglobulin concentrate. The trial was conducted in Chilean children living in low socioeconomic circumstances in urban Santiago. No beneficial effect of the antibody-supplemented formula was demonstrated.

39. • MELONI BP, THOMPSON RCA, HOPKINS RM, REYNOLDSON JA, GRACEY M: **The Prevalence of Giardia and Other Intestinal Parasites in Children, Dogs and Cats From Aboriginal Communities in the Kimberley.** *Med J Aust* 1993, 158:157–159.

Giardia duodenalis (or *G. lamblia*) was found in 32% of Aboriginal children and in 12.5% of adults; other frequent intestinal parasites included *Hymenolepis nana* and *Entamoeba coli* in this 4-year parasitological survey of fecal samples from humans and from dogs and cats in remote communities in northwest Australia where childhood diarrhea is endemic. The dogs and cats in these communities were also frequently infected. The high prevalence of hookworm and *Giardia* infections in dogs and hookworm and *Toxoplasma* infection in cats is of potentia zoonotic significance for humans who live in such circumstances.

40. • THOMPSON RCA, REYNOLDSON JA, LYMBERY AJ: ***Giardia*: From Molecules to Disease and Beyond.** *Parasitology Today* 1993, 9:313–315.

Report from an international conference held in Fremantle, Australia, in December 1992 on *Giardia* and giardiasis.

41. • QUICK R, PAUGH K, ADDISS D, KOBAYASHI J, BARON R: **Restaurant-Associated Outbreak of Giardiasis.** *J Infect Dis* 1992, 166:673–676.

Describes an outbreak of giardiasis that occurred in three quarters of participants at a meeting in a restaurant in Washington state. Circumstantial evidence suggests that ice contaminated by a food handler may have been the vehicle for the outbreak.

42. • SULLIVAN PB, LUNN PG, NORTHROP-CLEWES CA, FATHING MJG: **Parasitic Infection of the Gut and Protein-Losing Enteropathy.** *J Pediatr Gastroenterol Nutr* 1992, 15:404–407.

An investigation of intestinal protein losses in children with and without parasitic infestation of the gut. Seventeen percent of children with persistent diarrhea had protein-losing enteropathy. This was particularly important in children infected with *S. stercoralis* but was infrequent in children with giardiasis.

43. GOLDFARB J: **AIDS in Africa: Impact on Children.** *Pediatr AIDS HIV Infect* 1991, 2:180–184.

44. • CEGIELSKI JP, MSENGI AE, DUKES CS, MBISE R, REDDING-LALLINGER R, MINJAS JN, WILSON ML, SHAO J, DURACK DT: **Intestinal Parasites and HIV Infection in Tanzanian Children With Chronic Diarrhea.** *AIDS* 1993, 7:213–221.

A prospective, cross-sectional study to determine whether particular intestinal parasites are associated with HIV infection in Tanzanian children with chronic diarrhea. Forty percent of subjects with chronic diarrhea were HIV-seropositive and diarrheagenic parasites were found in up to 40% of children with chronic diarrhea. *B. hominis* was detected only in HIV-infected patients. The prevalence of severity of malnutrition in non-HIV–infected children in the study population and its effects on immune function made difficult the distinction between HIV-infected and non-HIV–infected children.

45. • GOLDIN AJ, APT W, AGUILERA X, ZULANTAY I, WARHURST DC, MILES MA: **A Capture ELISA Detects *Giardia Lamblia* Antigens in Formalin-Treated Faecal Samples.** *Trans R Soc Trop Med Hyg* 1992, 86:164–165.

Describes results of a capture ELISA method to detect *G. lamblia* antigens in formalin-treated fecal samples from Chilean schoolchildren.

46. • ELKADI IA, SMITH DH, HOMMEL M: **Early Diagnosis of Giardiasis by Faecal Antigens Detection Using Capture ELISA in a Cohort of Children in the United Arab Emirates.** *Trans R Soc Trop Med Hyg* 1992, 86:520–521.

Reports the use of capture ELISA to diagnose giardiasis by detection of fecal antigens in a group of children in the United Arab Emirates; results suggest that the method has applicability for clinical diagnosis and epidemiologic surveys.

47. • PHILLIPS AD, THOMAS AG, WALKER-SMITH JA: ***Cryptosporidium*, Chronic Diarrhoea and the Proximal Small Intestinal Mucosa.** *Gut* 1992, 33:1057–1061.

A hospital-based review over more than 6 years into possible associations among cryptosporidiosis, chronic diarrhea in children, and upper intestinal histology. Findings showed a mild-to-moderate enteropathy with *Cryptosporidium* adherent to the villous epithelium in children who did not have immune deficiency and suggest that *Cryptosporidium* should be sought in children who fail to thrive, particularly those with a history of diarrhea.

48. • CHEN Y-G, YAO F-B, LI H-S, SHI W-S, DAI M-X, LU M: ***Cryptosporidium* Infection and Diarrhea in Rural and Urban Areas of Jiangsu, People's Republic of China.** *J Clin Microbiol* 1992, 30:492–494.

A cross-sectional screening survey of Chinese infants and children under 15 years of age for fecal *Cryptosporidium* oocysts conducted in more than 5000 subjects in a suburb of Xuzhou City and six rural areas of Jiangsu. The highest isolation rate (3%) occurred between 1 and 5 years of age; intermittent or persistent diarrhea was the commonest syndrome.

49. •• HOGE CW, SHLIM DR, RAJAH R, TRIPLETT J, SHEAR M, RABOLD JG, ECHEVERRIA P: **Epidemiology of Diarrhoeal Illness Associated With Coccidian-Like Organism Among Travellers and Foreign Residents in Nepal.** *Lancet* 1993, 341:1175–1179.

A report about CLBs in more than 100 patients with gastrointestinal symptoms (11% of those investigated) compared with only 1% in symptom-free control subjects investigated in Kathmandu, Nepal. This organism appears to cause prolonged diarrhea (median duration, 7 weeks) and consumption of untreated water has been implicated in its transmission.

50. •• BENDALL RP, LUCAS S, MOODY A, TOVEY G, CHIODINI PL: **Diarrhoea Associated With Cyanobacterium-Like Bodies: A New Coccidian Enteritis of Man.** *Lancet* 1993, 341:590–592.

Report about three patients who developed diarrhea while traveling in North Africa on the Indian subcontinent in whom stool samples detected CLB cysts. The findings suggest that these coccidia cause enteritis, which can cause gastrointestinal symptoms including diarrhea.

51. LIMA AM, FANG G, SCHORLING JB DE ALBUQUERQUE, MCAULIFFE JF, MOTA S, LEITE R, GUERRANT RL: **Persistent Diarrhoea in Northeast Brazil: Etiologies and Interactions With Malnutrition.** *Acta Paediatr* 1992, Suppl **381**:39–44.
•• An investigation into factors associated with persistent diarrhea in young children attending an outpatient clinic in Brazil's northeast region. Seventy percent of all deaths in those under 5 years of age were due to diarrhea and half of the diarrhea deaths were due to illness that lasted longer than 2 weeks. Diarrheal illnesses restricted catch-up growth in malnourished children and malnutrition significantly predisposed children to a greater incidence and duration of diarrhea as well as a greater incidence of persistent diarrhea. The predominant potential pathogens found in fecal specimens or intestinal contents were *Cryptosporidium* and EAEC.

52. BARTLETT AV, HURTUDO E, SCHROEDER DG, MENDEZ H: **Association of Indicators of Hygiene Behaviour With Persistent Diarrhea of Young Children.** *Acta Paediatr* 1992, Suppl **381**:66–71.
• A study of the association between water and hygiene-related behaviors and persistent diarrhea among children under 3 years of age in an indigenous rural Guatemalan community.

53. BLAKE PA, RAMOS S, MACDONALD KL, RASSI V, TANDELLI GOMES TA, IVEY C, BEAN NH, TRABULSI LR: **Pathogen-Specific Risk Factors and Protective Factors for Acute Diarrheal Disease in Urban Brazilian Infants.** *J Infect Dis* 1993, **167**:627–632.
• Reports on risk factors and protective factors associated with episodes of acute diarrhea in 500 urban infants in Brazil. Assesses factors associated with specific pathogens including enterovirulent *E. coli*, *Salmonella*, *Shigela*, and rotavirus.

54. BAQUI AH, BLACK RE, SACK RB, CHOWDHURY HR, YUNUS M, SIDDIQUE AK: **Malnutrition, Cell-Mediated Immune Deficiency, and Diarrhea: A Community-Based Longitudinal Study in Rural Bangladeshi Children.** *Am J Epidemiol* 1993, **137**:355–365.
• A community-based, longitudinal 12-month study in Bangladesh of 705 children to examine the associations between malnutrition, cell-mediated immune deficiency, and the incidence of diarrhea in children under 5 years of age. Malnutrition and cell-mediated immune deficiency were important independent risk factors, but other possible factors, particularly the role of inapparent micronutrient deficiencies, require closer investigation.

55. REVES RR, MORROW AL, BARTLETT AV, CARUSO CJ, PLUMB RL, LU BT, PICKERING LK: **Child Day Care Increases the Risk of Clinic Visits for Acute Diarrhea and Diarrhea Due to Rotavirus.** *Am J Epidemiol* 1993, **137**:97–107.
• A case-control study of risk factors for acute diarrhea in children under 3 years of age receiving day care in Houston, Texas.

Michael Gracey, MD, PhD, FRACP, Aboriginal Health Unit, Health Department of Western Australia, Second Floor, C Block, 189 Royal Street, East Perth WA, 6004 Australia.

Peptic ulcer disease and *Helicobacter pylori* infection

Dino Vaira, MD*, John Holton, MRCPath†, Mario Miglioli, MD*, Marcello Menegatti, MD*, Paolo Mulè, MD*, and Luigi Barbara, MD*

*University of Bologna, Bologna, Italy, and
†University College London Medical School, London, UK

The most significant epidemiologic findings over this review period have been the isolation of *Helicobacter pylori* from feces and the results of the Eurogast Study firmly linking colonization by *H. pylori* to the development of gastric carcinoma. With respect to the mechanisms of pathogenesis, the purification of the cytotoxin and an investigation of its mode of action are also important. Similarly, the demonstration of the effect of *H. pylori* on somatostatin and gastrin-releasing peptide levels open further avenues of research. Numerous serologic tests are currently available, and an increasing use in screening procedures to reduce endoscopy workloads can be anticipated. The current regimen giving the highest eradication rate is bismuth, metronidazole, and tetracycline for 2 weeks, although the use of omeprazole with antibiotics is becoming more prevalent. Finally, the development of a vaccine is likely to be a major research area for the future.

Current Opinion in Gastroenterology 1994, **10**:98–104

Infection with *Helicobacter pylori*, a gram-negative, microaerophilic bacterium that is found attached to the surface of gastric epithelial cells, is the most common infection worldwide. It is the cause of gastritis and ulceration and is a risk factor for the development of gastric cancer. The organism is found mainly in humans but its mode of transmission is poorly understood. The ways in which *H. pylori* induces inflammation and ulceration are not clear, although host and microbial factors are both important. Infection with the organism can be diagnosed using tests requiring endoscopy, or by serology and urea-breath tests. The present treatment is unsatisfactory because multiple drugs must be given for prolonged periods to ensure eradication of the organism. These drug combinations have a high rate of side effects, although successful eradication does lead to a much reduced ulcer relapse rate.

Epidemiology

Human infection with *H. pylori* can originate from another person, animals, or the environment. Abattoir workers are known to have a higher seroprevalence for *H. pylori* infection [1]. Despite this prevalence, food source animals are unlikely to be the source of *H. pylori* infection in humans. In a seroepidemiologic comparison of Asian meat eaters with Asian vegans, no difference could be detected in the seropositivity rate between the two groups [2]. This finding confirms previous seroepidemiologic studies of the prevalence of *H. pylori* infection in vegetarians. Person to person transmission of *H. pylori* is suggested by the clustering of infection found in families, institutions, and occupational groups having close person to person contact. Recently, a naturally acquired acute infection in an infant was reported, with serologic evidence presented that is consistent with sequential acquisition of *H. pylori* within the family group [3•]. Further evidence of intrafamilial transmission of *H. pylori* has been presented by Nwokolo *et al.* [4•], who detected a clonal variant of a strain of the organism in three family members from each of three generations. Person to person transmission is further supported by the demonstration that endoscopy staff have a higher seroprevalence of *H. pylori* than do matched control subjects, but interestingly, dentists, who also have a similar type of contact with patients, are not more prone to having *H. pylori* colonization [5]. Density of living conditions is a significant risk factor, with young age being a critical period for acquisition of the organism [6].

The route of transmission between individuals is not known. Evidence in favor of transmission by oral secre-

Abbreviations
ELISA—enzyme-linked immunosorbent assay; **NSAID**—nonsteroidal anti-inflammatory drug.

 ISBN 1-85922-606-X ISSN 0267–1379

tion is supported by the detection of *H. pylori* in dental plaque. Experimental evidence in support of the oral route of transmission was given by Lee *et al.* [7], who showed that *H. pylori* was transmitted from infected to noninfected Beagle puppies, but that *Helicobacter felis* was not transmitted between mice kept in the same cage. The latter do not have orooral contact like dogs nor do they vomit. Against the suggestion that oral secretions are an important route of transmission is the infrequency of detection of the organism in oral secretions and the lack of an excess prevalence of infection in dentists. The most significant finding to date in elucidating the epidemiology of *H. pylori* is its detection in feces [8••], which clearly strengthens the arguments for a fecooral route of transmission.

Under environmental stress, *H. pylori* converts to a coccoid form that can remain viable for up to 30 days when kept in river water [9•]. This finding clearly supports the epidemiologic evidence provided by Klein *et al.* [10] that municipal water supplies may be a vehicle for the transmission of *H. pylori.*

Clinical associations

When *H. pylori* is present in the stomach and duodenum it is almost always associated with either an acute or chronic inflammatory response. *H. pylori* can also be found associated with columnar epithelium in Barrett's esophagus, but in this location its presence is only nonspecifically linked to inflammation [11]. The inflammatory response caused by *H. pylori* does not necessarily lead to the presence of upper gastrointestinal symptoms in the patient. Conversely, in patients with upper gastrointestinal symptoms not due to ulceration (*ie,* nonulcer dyspepsia) it is controversial as to whether the presence of *H. pylori* is related to the symptoms or whether the symptoms improve with eradication of the organism. One study was able to demonstrate an improvement of the symptoms with eradication of *H. pylori* [12•], although another study was not able to demonstrate any correlation between eradication of the organism and improvement of symptoms in the short term [13•]. However, 1 year after initial treatment, patients who remained free of *H. pylori* did have fewer symptoms than patients in whom eradication had not been successful [13•].

Although there is some doubt about the causal link between *H. pylori* infection and nonulcer dyspepsia, there is little doubt about its causal link to peptic ulceration. A considerable body of evidence accumulated over several years has demonstrated this clinical association, which was recently summarized [14••]. However, two recent studies have raised queries about the link between *H. pylori* and the initiation of gastritis and relapse of duodenal ulceration [15•,16•]. In the first study [15•], involving 30 asymptomatic individuals, the authors demonstrated the presence of gastritis in the absence of *H. pylori* and suggested that the organism may colonize inflamed mucosa, exacerbating the inflammation but not initiating it. The study used only histologic stains to detect *H. pylori*; the stains may have missed small numbers of the organism. In the second study [16•], a longitudinal investigation of 74 patients with duodenal ulceration, the authors could find no statistical correlation between the presence of *H. pylori* and healing or relapse of ulceration. Both these studies raise doubts about a cause-effect relationship of *H. pylori* and inflammation.

The most important recent development is an increasing awareness of the causal link between chronic *H. pylori* infection and the progression to gastric carcinoma. Several seroepidemiologic studies have provided suggestive evidence for this link. A recent report from the Eurogast Study group [17••], which analyzed data from 13 countries, has demonstrated that statistically, a sixfold greater risk of gastric cancer would occur in a population with a 100% infection rate than in a population completely free of *H. pylori.* The evidence for *H. pylori* as a risk factor for the development of gastric cancer has recently been summarized in two excellent reviews [18•,19•]. The progression from chronic gastritis caused by *H. pylori* to gastric atrophy and intestinal metaplasia are seen as the link between the organism and the development of carcinoma.

Pathogenesis

On the one hand, all strains of *H. pylori* may have equal potential to cause ulceration, and the outcome may depend on such factors as the local density of infection or host factors. On the other hand, there may be specific ulcerogenic strains. The process whereby gastritis and ulceration are induced are still, in the main, to be elucidated, but the outcome of any infection is likely to depend on a balance between bacterial virulence factors and host factors. The first step in establishing an infection is adhesion of the organism to the substrate. The receptor for *H. pylori* is phosphatidylethanolamine, which is found preferentially in the antrum of the stomach [20•]. At the point of attachment, the gastric cells produce an adhesion pedestal with apparent fusion of the two cell surfaces. Although *H. pylori* is often regarded as only having a superficial location in the stomach, it was recently demonstrated *in vitro* that it can be internalized by epithelial cells by a process of receptor-mediated endocytosis [21•]. The authors suggest that if this process occurs *in vivo* it may be important in explaining the development of a sustained immune response and perhaps tissue damage.

The topographic distribution of the organism may also be important in determining disease progression. In a study by Leung *et al.* [22••], who used morphometric techniques to determine the density of colonization by *H. pylori* in both gastritis and ulceration, the results showed that high bacterial density and a high degree of concomitant epithelial degeneration correlated with gastric ulceration. This dependence of tissue damage on bacterial density may be related to high local concentrations of toxic factors.

The presence of *H. pylori* on the epithelial cells leads to changes of surface hydrophobicity of the gastric mucosa [23•]. These changes may be induced by the action of phospholipase A2, produced by the organism, although in a recent study no significant difference in phospholipase A2 activity was found between *H. pylori*–positive patients and *H. pylori*–negative patients [24]. However, a deleterious effect on mucus secretion caused by *H. pylori* has been demonstrated [25•]. *In vitro*, the secretory response of mucus cells was strongly inhibited, although glycoprotein synthesis was unaffected.

Further evidence of the importance of ammonia as a toxin has been presented [26•]. Using a cell monolayer, the authors compared the vacuolation of cells induced by a wild-type urease–positive organism with that by a urease-negative mutant, showing that the ammonia produced by the wildtype strains was essential for inducing disruption of intracellular junctions and vacuolation. In addition to having a direct toxic effect, ammonia has also been shown to enhance neutrophil-dependent gastric mucosal injury through the formation of monochloramine [27].

The production of a cytotoxin has been linked to the development of duodenal ulceration [28]. The cytotoxin induces vacuolation in the cells and these vacuoles are autophagosomal in nature [29•]. The process of vacuolation is enhanced by weak bases such as ammonia and nicotine [30•], and recently the toxin has been purified and shown to be a protein of molecular mass of approximately 80 kD [31••].

In addition to direct toxic effects on cells, *H. pylori* may bring about ulceration by disturbing the normal physiologic balance of acid and pepsin secretion. Infection is known to increase both gastrin and pepsinogen concentrations in the blood, and further evidence of this was recently presented [32]. Both hypergastrinemia and hyperpepsinogenemia can be reversed by eradicating *H. pylori* [33,34].

Recent work suggests possible mechanisms whereby *H. pylori* can bring about these alterations to gastrin and pepsin concentrations. Elevation in gastrin levels is principally due to an elevation in the G17 fraction [35•] that is produced by the antrum. This elevation is not caused by luminal changes in pH, nor by a decreased sensitivity of parietal cells to gastrin [36•]. Control of gastrin release by gastrin-releasing peptide and somatostatin is affected by *H. pylori* [37••,38••] and can be reversed by eradicating the organism. There is a decrease in the somatostatin messenger RNA in D cells, but there is no alteration in D or G cell numbers [39•] (although in children elevated G cell numbers have been recorded [40•]).

Diagnosis

Numerous commercial assays are available for the diagnosis of *H. pylori* infection, and comparison of them has been the subject of many recent publications. Pyloriset-immunoglobulin G (Orion Pharmaceutica, Espoo, Finland) was found to have a sensitivity of 92% and specificity of 84%, and it is considered a reliable test for the diagnosis of *H. pylori* infection [41]. Goossens *et al.* [42•] evaluated a commercially available complement fixation test against culture and histology, demonstrating differences in sensitivity and specificity depending on patient age and ethnic background. The study also showed a significant decrease in antibody levels 3 to 6 months after *H. pylori* had been eradicated from the patient.

Taha *et al.* [43•] evaluated Pyloriset, Helico-G (Porton, Cambridge, UK), Malakit (Biolab, Wavre, Belgium), and GAP-immunoglobulin G (BioRad, Milan, Italy) in patients who have either been receiving or not been receiving nonsteroidal anti-inflammatory drugs (NSAIDs). The authors found the specificity of all of these tests to be low in comparison with that of invasive tests and they found the specificity reduced even further in patients taking NSAIDs.

Talley *et al.* [44] evaluated Pyloristat (BioWhittaker, Walkersville, MD), Helico-G, and Premier (Meridian Diagnostics), concluding that all three tests were reliable diagnostic methods. However, Hoek *et al.* [45] compared three serologic assays (Pyloriset, GAP-immunoglobulin G, and Helico-G) and concluded that none of the tests had a significantly high sensitivity or specificity and that better commercial assays should be developed.

In one study, an enzyme-linked immunosorbent assay (ELISA) test using an unfractionated sonicate of *H. pylori* was compared with Western blotting and an ELISA using pure 120-kD protein as an antigen [46•]. It was concluded that the 120-kD protein can be used as an antigen, giving an acceptable sensitivity and specificity for diagnostic purposes. In addition to being used in diagnosis, serology can also be used to evaluate treatment [47] and as a screening procedure prior to endoscopy, either to admit or exclude patients for endoscopy [48,49•].

Treatment and prevention

Helicobacter pylori is very sensitive *in vitro* to many antibiotics and antiulcer agents, but due to the slow growth of the organism the results of *in vitro* sensitivity testing by disc diffusion may be unreliable. An alternative test is the E-test, which was found to be reproducible and closely correlated to the minimum inhibitory concentration [50•]. The E-test is not affected by inoculum size or incubation times and is a suitable alternative to disc testing for routine purposes. A multicenter survey of metronidazole resistance of *H. pylori* using both minimum inhibitory concentration determination and the E-test, demonstrated a 27% resistance overall, but resistance prevalence varied from 7% (in Madrid) to 47% (in Athens) [51•]. Resistant strains were more commonly found in women, a finding that may have related to a greater use of metronidazole to treat gynecologic conditions. Numerous combinations of antibiotics have been tried in eradication protocols for *H. pylori.* A meta-analysis of 27 studies has recently been reported and has shown eradication rates (averaged) of 18.6% (monotherapy), 48.2% (dual therapy), and 82.3% (triple therapy). Triple therapy with bismuth, metronidazole, and tetracycline gave the highest eradication rates (94.1%), compared with 73.1% for bismuth, metronidazole, and amoxicillin [52••].

Recently, 2-week courses of triple therapy have been investigated. In one study [53•] of 101 patients with *H. pylori*–positive peptic ulcers a triple regimen of bismuth, amoxicillin, and metronidazole showed an eradication rate of 84%. The eradication rate was dependent on the pretreatment metronidazole sensitivity of the isolate, and was 89% with metronidazole-sensitive strains and 61% with metronidazole-resistant strains. A similar result was found with the triple regimen of bismuth, tetracycline, and metronidazole given for 2 weeks to 40 patients [54]. The eradication rates were 90% for metronidazole-sensitive organisms but only 31% for metronidazole-resistant organisms. With even shorter courses of antibiotics (given for less than 8 days) an eradication rate of 58% was achieved if the organism was metronidazole sensitive and 0% if metronidazole resistant [55•]. Triple drug regimens (bismuth, amoxicillin, and metronidazole) given for 2 weeks gave the highest eradication rates.

With the current therapy combinations, 2 weeks seems to be the minimum length of treatment required to achieve acceptable eradication rates. The dependence of successful eradication on sensitivity of the isolate to metronidazole is also clearly demonstrated in these studies. The side effects of triple therapy can be reduced by giving more frequent, but lower doses of bismuth, metronidazole, and tetracycline. Doses were given five times a day for 2 weeks without compromising the eradication rate, which in this study was 96%, compared with 92% for the standard four times a day dosage [56•].

Omeprazole does not eradicate *H. pylori* if given as monotherapy but, if combined with antibiotics, can achieve good eradication rates. A regimen of omeprazole for 4 weeks with bismuth, tetracycline, and metronidazole for 1 week achieved a 95% eradication rate, but the rate was only 4% if given alone [57]. Omeprazole combined with erythromycin and bismuth and given for 1 week only showed a 15% eradication rate, compared with about 50% if given for 2 weeks combined with amoxicillin [58•]. The optimal treatment for *H. pylori*–associated disease is still being sought, and therapeutic trials with different agents are being evaluated. Recently, guidelines for conducting therapeutic trials of *H. pylori* anti-infective regimens have been published [59•].

Because of the link between long-term colonization with *H. pylori* and the ultimate development of gastric cancer, the possibility of developing a vaccine against *H. pylori* is being explored actively. Preliminary animal experiments give clear support for the feasibility of vaccine development, although the involvement of immunopathologic mechanisms of tissue damage caused by *H. pylori* raises a note of caution. This important and developing area of investigation was recently reviewed [60•].

References and recommended reading

Papers of particular interest, published within the annual period of review, have been highlighted as:
- • Of special interest
- •• Of outstanding interest

1. VAIRA D, D'ANASTASIO C, HOLTON J, DOWSETT JF, LONDEI M, BERTONI F, BELTRANDI E, GRAUENFELS P, SALMON PR, GANDOLFI L: **Campylobacter pylori in Abattoir Workers: Is It a Zoonosis?** *Lancet* 1988, ii:725–726.

2. WEBBERLEY MJ, WEBBERLEY JM, NEWELL DG, LOWE P, MELIKIAN V: **Sero-Epidemiology of Helicobacter pylori Infection in Vegans and Meat-Eaters.** *Epidemiol Infect* 1992, 108:457–462.

3. • MITCHELL JD, MITCHELL HM, TOBIAS V: **Acute Helicobacter Pylori Infection in an Infant, Associated With Gastric Ulceration and Serological Evidence of Intra-familial Transmission.** *Am J Gastroenterol* 1992, 87:382–386.

Evidence of person to person transmission of *H. pylori* is discussed.

4. • NWOKOLO CU, BICKLEY J, ATTARD AR, OWEN RJ, COSTAS M, FRASER IA: **Evidence of Clonal Variants of Helicobacter pylori in Three Generations of a Duodenal Ulcer Family.** *Gut* 1992, 33:1323–1327.

A restriction enzyme analysis of *H. pylori* DNA isolated from several members of the same family, the results of which are consistent with person to person transmission of *H. pylori* is discussed.

5. MALATY HM, EVANS DJ, ABRAMOVITCH K, EVANS DG, GRAHAM DY: **Helicobacter pylori Infection in Dental Workers: A Seroepidemiological Study.** *Am J Gastroenterol* 1992, 87:1728–1731.

6. MITCHELL HM, LI YY, HU PJ, LIU Q, CHEN M, DU GG, WANG ZJ, LEE A, HAZELL SL: **Epidemiology of Helicobacter pylori in Southern China: Identification of Early Childhood as the Critical Period for Acquisition.** *J Infect Dis* 1992, 166:149–153.

7. LEE A, FOX JG, OTTO G, HEGEDUS-DICK E, KRAKOWKA S: **Transmission of Helicobacter Spp.: A Challenge to the Dogma of Faecal-Oral Spread.** *Epidemiol Infect* 1991, 107:99–109.

8. •• THOMAS JE, GIBSON GR, DARBOE MK, DALE A, WEAVER LT: **Isolation of Helicobacter pylori From Human Feaces.** *Lancet* 1992, 2:1194–1195.

An important study recording the isolation of *H. pylori* from the feces of nine of 23 Gambian children and establishing the fecal-oral route of transmission as probable.

9. • SAHAMAT M, MAI U, PASZKO-KOLVA C, KESSEL M, COLWELL RR: **Use of Autoradiography to Assess Viability of Helicobacter pylori in Water.** *Appl Environ Microbiol* 1993, 59:1231–1235.

The authors labelled *H. pylori* in its noncultivatable form with ^{3}H-thymidine and showed that viability is preserved for up to 30 days. This is an important study because it gives experimental support to a possible environmental reservoir for *H. pylori.*

10. KLEIN PD, GRAHAM DY, GAILLOUR A, OPEKUN AR, O'BRIAN-SMITH E: **Water Source as a Risk Factor for *Helicobacter pylori* Infection in Peruvian Children.** *Lancet* 1991, 1:1503–1506.

11. LOEFFELD RJLF, TEN TIJE BJ, ARENDS JW: **Prevalence and Significance of *Helicobacter pylori* in Patients With Barrett's Oesophagus.** *Am J Gastroenterol* 1992, **87**:1598–1600.

12. • VAIRA D, HOLTON J, AINLEY C, FALZON M, OSBORN J, D'ANNA I, ROMANOS A, CHANDRAKUMARAN K, MCNEIL I: **Double Blind Trial of Colloidal Bismuth Subcitrate Versus Placebo in *H. pylori* Positive Patients With Nonulcer Dyspepsia.** *Ital J Gastroenterol* 1992, **24**:400–404.

A study that demonstrates the symptomatic improvement that follows eradication of *H. pylori* in patients suffering from nonulcer dyspepsia.

13. • LAINE L: **Helicobacter pylori and Nonulcer Dyspepsia.** *Gastroenterology* 1992, **103**:340–341.

A summary of the work relating to a possible link between *H. pylori* and nonulcer dyspepsia, with a reply by the author indicating a possible long-term benefit of eradication to symptom improvement.

14. •• MEGRAUD F, LAMOULLATTE H: **Helicobacter pylori and Duodenal Ulcer: Evidence Suggesting Causation.** *Dig Dis Sci* 1992, 37:769–772.

An excellent summary of the lines of evidence supporting the causal link between colonization by *H. pylori* and the development of ulceration based on modification of Koch's postulates.

15. • FALLINGBORG J, POULSEN LO, GROVE A, STUBBE-TEGLBJAERG P: **Frequency of Helicobacter pylori and Gastritis in Healthy Subjects Without Gastrointestinal Symptoms.** *Scand J Gastroenterol* 1992, 27:388–390.

A provocative study that suggests that *H. pylori* may not be the cause of gastric inflammation, as suggested by many other studies, including self-inoculation studies, but may perpetuate an already existing inflammation.

16. • RYE-CLAUSEN M, FRANZMANN MB, HOLST C, SORENSEN TIA, CHRISTOFFERSEN P, MATZEN P, KRAG E: **Longitudinal Study of Influence of *Helicobacter pylori* on Current Risk of Duodenal Ulcer Relapse.** *Scand J Gastroenterol* 1992, **27**:421–426.

A longitudinal study involving 74 patients with duodenal ulcers over a 2-year period in which a correlation was not found between the relapse of ulceration and the incidence of colonization by *H. pylori.*

17. •• EUROGAST STUDY GROUP: **An International Association Between *Helicobacter pylori* Infection and Gastric Cancer.** *Lancet* 1993, **341**:1359–1362.

A very important study that supports the clinical association between colonization by *H. pylori* and the risk of developing gastric cancer.

18. • SIPPONEN P: ***Helicobacter pylori* Infection: A Common Worldwide Environmental Risk Factor for Gastric Cancer?** *Endoscopy* 1992, **24**:424–427.

An excellent and concise overview of the study that demonstrates a link between colonization by *H. pylori* and the development of gastric cancer.

19. • FORMAN R: ***Helicobacter pylori* Infection and Gastric Carcinogenesis.** *Eur J Gastroenterol Hepatol* 1992, **4**(Suppl 2):S31–S35.

An excellent review of the evidence demonstrating that *H. pylori* colonization is a risk factor for gastric cancer.

20. • LINGWOOD CA, HUESCA M, KUKSIS A: **The Glycerolipid Receptor for *Helicobacter pylori* (and Exoenzyme S) Is Phosphatidylethanolamine.** *Infect Immun* 1992, **60**:2470–2474.

A review demonstrating the chemical identity of the receptor for *H. pylori* and showing that it is most abundant in the antral cells of the stomach.

21. • EVANS DG, EVANS DJ, GRAHAM DY: **Adherence and Internalization of *Helicobacter pylori* by HEp-2 Cells.** *Gastroenterology* 1992, **102**:1557–1567.

This paper shows that *H. pylori* can be taken up by cell monolayers suggesting that *in vivo* this may be important in the development of a sustained immune response.

22. •• LEUNG KM, HUI PK, CHAN WY, THOMAS TMM: ***Helicobacter pylori*-Related Gastritis and Gastric Ulcer: A Continuum of Progressive Epithelial Degeneration.** *Am J Clin Pathol* 1992, 98:569–574.

A very detailed study of 145 gastric biopsy specimens demonstrating a spectrum of cell damage that is dependent on density of infection, leading finally to ulceration.

23. • GOGGIN PM, MARRERO JM, SPYCAL RT, JACKSON PA, CORBISHELY CM, NORTHFIELD TM: **Surface Hydrophobicity of Gastric Mucosa in *Helicobacter pylori* Infection: Effect of Clearance and Eradication.** *Gastroenterology* 1992, 103:1486–1490.

A study showing that the surface hydrophobicity of gastric mucosa was reduced by *H. pylori* and returned to normal after eradication of the organism.

24. BERSTAD K, BERSTAD A, JR, SJODHAL R, WEBERG R, BERSTAD A: **Eosinophilic Cationic Protein and Phospholipase A2 Activity in Human Gastric Juice. With Emphasis on *Helicobacter pylori* status and effects of antacids.** *Scand J Gastroenterol* 1992, 27:1011–1017.

25. • MICOTS I, AUGERON C, LABOISSE CL, MUZEAU F, MEGRAUD F: **Mucin Exocytosis: A Major Target for *Helicobacter pylori*.** *J Clin Pathol* 1993, **46**:241–245.

This review shows that mucin biosynthesis is unaffected by *H. pylori*, but that secretion of mucus is inhibited. *In vivo* this inhibition would compromise the defense of the gastric mucosa.

26. • MEGRAUD F, NEMAN-SIMHA V, BRUGMANN D: **Further Evidence of the Toxic Effects of Ammonia Production by *Helicobacter pylori* Urease on Human Epithelial Cells.** *Infect Immun* 1992, **60**:1858–1863.

This study adds support to the role of locally produced ammonia as a toxic factor in *Helicobacter* species infections.

27. SUZUKI M, MIURA S, SUEMATSU M, FUKUMURA D, KUROSE I, SUZUKI H, KAI S, KUDOH Y, OHASHI M, TSUCHIYA M: ***Helicobacter pylori*-Associated Production Enhances Neutrophil Dependent Gastric Mucosal Cell Injury.** *Am J Physiol* 1992, 263:G719—G725.

28. FIGURA N, GUGLIELMETTI P, ROSSOLINI A, BARBERI A, CUSI G, MUSUMANNO RA, RUSSI M, QUARANTA S: **Cytotoxin Production by *Campylobacter pylori* Strains Isolated From Patients With Peptic Ulcers and From Patients With Chronic Gastritis Only.** *J Clin Microbiol* 1989, **27**:225–226.

29. • CATRENICH CE, CHESTNUT MH: **Character and Origin of Vacuoles Induced in Mammalian Cells by the Cytotoxin of *Helicobacter pylori*.** *J Med Microbiol* 1992, 37:389–395.

An ultrastructural and dynamic study of vacuoles produced by the cytotoxin of *H. pylori* suggest that they are autophagosomes.

30. • COVER TL, VAUGHN SG, CAO P, BLASER MJ: **Potentiation of *Helicobacter pylori* Vacuolating Toxin Activity by Nicotine and Other Weak Bases.** *J Infect Dis* 1992, **166**:1073–1078.

This study demonstrates that the process of vacuole production induced by the cytotoxin is enhanced by weak bases such as nicotine (from cigarette smoking) and ammonia (produced by urease).

31. •• COVER TL, BLASE MJ: **Purification and Characterization of the Vacuolating Toxin From *Helicobacter pylori*.** *J Biol Chem* 1993, 267:10570–10575.

This paper reviews biochemical purification and analysis of the cytotoxin of *H. pylori.*

32. MOSS S, MEYER-WYSS B, RENNER EL, MERKI HS, GAMBONI G, BEGLINGER C: **Influence of *Helicobacter pylori*, Sex and Age on Serum Gastrin and Pepsinogen Concentration in Subjects Without Symptoms and Patients With Duodenal Ulcers.** *Gut* 1993, 34:752–756.

33. Moss S, Calam J: **Acid Secretion and Sensitivity to Gastrin in Patients With Duodenal Ulcer: Effect of Eradication of *Helicobacter pylori*.** *Gut* 1993, **34**:888–892.

34. Fraser AG, Prewett EJ, Pounder RE, Samloff IM: **Twenty Four Hour Hyperpepsinogenaemia in *Helicobacter pylori* Positive Subjects is Abolished by Eradication of Infection.** *Aliment Pharmacol Ther* 1992, **6**:389–394.

35. • Mulholland G, Ardill JES, Fillmore D, Chittajallu RS, Fullarton GM, McColl KEL: ***Helicobacter pylori* Related Hypergastrinaemia is the Result of a Selective Increase in Gastrin 17.** *Gut* 1993, **34**:757–761.
Demonstration that the elevation of gastrin produced by *H. pylori* is in the gastrin 17 fraction and not the gastrin 34 fraction, which explains why the hypergastrinemia is principally post prandial.

36. • Chittajallu RS, Howie CA, McColl KEL: **Effect of *Helicobacter pylori* on Parietal Cell Sensitivity to Pentagastrin in Duodenal Ulcer Subjects.** *Scand J Gastroenterol* 1992, **27**:857–862.
This study shows that the hypergastrinemia caused by *H. pylori* is not a compensatory response to altered parietal cell function but may be due to the direct effects of inflammation.

37. •• Beardshall K, Moss S, Gill J, Levi S, Ghosh P, Playford RJ, Calam J: **Suppression of *Helicobacter pylori* Reduces Gastrin Releasing Peptide Stimulated Gastrin Release in Duodenal Ulcer Patients.** *Gut* 1992, **33**:601–603.
First demonstration that suppression of *H. pylori* reduces the gastrin 17 secretion induced by gastrin-releasing peptide, a nonluminal neuropeptide stimulant.

38. •• Moss SF, Legon S, Bishop AE, Polak JM, Calam J: **Effect of *Helicobacter pylori* on Gastric Somatostatin in Duodenal Ulcer Disease.** *Lancet* 1992, **340**:930–932.
This paper shows that the level of messenger RNA coding for somatostatin is decreased in D cells caused by *H. pylori* and provides a mechanism to explain the hypergastrinemia associated with infection.

39. • Graham DY, Lew GM, Lechago J: **Antral G-Cell and D-Cell Numbers in *Helicobacter pylori* Infection: Effect of *H. pylori* Eradication.** *Gastroenterology* 1993, **104**:1655–1660.
H. pylori–stimulated elevation of gastrin is not associated with alteration in either the number of G or D cells.

40. • Oderda G, Fiocca R, Villani L, Altare F, Morra I, Ansaldi N: **Gastrin Cell Hyperplasia in Childhood *Helicobacter pylori* Gastritis.** *Eur J Gastroenterol Hepatol* 1993, **5**:13–16.
The authors show that the number of gastrin-releasing cells is elevated in gastritis caused by *H. pylori* and that this elevation can be reversed by eradication of the organism. They support a local effect of *H. pylori* on the G cells.

41. Granberg C, Mansikka A, Lehtonen OP, Killari H, Gronfors R, Nurmi H, Raiha I, Stahlberg MR, Leino R: **Diagnosis of *Helicobacter pylori* Infection by Using Pyloriset EIA-G and EIA-A for Detection of Serum Immunoglobulin G (IgG) and IgA Antibodies.** *J Clin Microbiol* 1993, **31**:1450–1453.

42. • Goossens H, Glupczynski Y, Burette A, Van den Borre C, DePrez C, Bodenmann J, Keller A, Butzler JP: **Evaluation of a Commercially Available Complement Fixation Test for Diagnosis of *Helicobacter pylori* Infection and for Follow Up After Antimicrobial Therapy.** *J Clin Microbiol* 1992, **30**:3230–3233.
This paper demonstrates that the sensitivity and specificity of a serodiagnostic test depend on the age and ethnic background of the population tested, and that serum antibodies fall with time after successful eradication of the infecting organism.

43. • Taha AS, Reid J, Boothmann P, Gemmel CG, Lee FD, Sturrock RD, Russell RI: **Serological Diagnosis of *Helicobacter pylori*: Evaluation of Four Tests in the Presence and Absence of Non-Steroidal Anti-Inflammatory Drugs.** *Gut* 1993, **34**:461–465.
The authors found a poor specificity for the serodiagnostic tests used, which was further reduced in patients taking NSAIDs.

44. Talley NJ, Kost L, Haddad A, Zinmeister AR: **Comparison of Commercial Serological Tests for Detection of *Helicobacter pylori* Antibodies.** *J Clin Microbiol* 1992, **30**:3146–3150.

45. Hoek FJ, Noach LA, Rauws EAJ, Tytgat GNJ: **Evaluation of the Performance of Commercial Test Kits for the Detection of *Helicobacter pylori* Antibodies in Serum.** *J Clin Microbiol* 1992, **30**:1525–1528.

46. • Gerstenecker B, Eschweiler H, Vogele H, Koch HK, Hellerich U, Kist M: **Serodiagnosis of *Helicobacter pylori* Infection With an Enzyme Immunoassay Using the Chromatographically Purified 120kDa Protein.** *Eur J Clin Microbiol Infect Dis* 1992, **11**:595–601.
An ELISA test using a purified antigen of *H. pylori* was shown to be sensitive and specific as a diagnostic test.

47. Glupczynski Y, Burette A, Goossens H, DePrez C, Butzler JP: **Effect of Antimicrobial Therapy on the Specific Serological Response to *Helicobacter pylori* Infection.** *Eur J Clin Microbiol Infect Dis* 1992, **11**:583–588.

48. Sobala GM, Crabtree JE, Penrith JA, Rathbone BJ, Shallcross TM, Wyatt JI, Dixon MF, Heatley RV, Axon ATR: **Screening Dyspepsia by Serology to *Helicobacter pylori*.** *Lancet* 1991, **338**:94–96.

49. • Mendall MA, Goggin PM, Marrero IM, Molineaux N, Levy J, Badve S, Corbishley C, Finlayson C, Maxwell D, Northfield TC: **Role of *Helicobacter pylori* Serology in Screening Prior to Endoscopy.** *Eur J Gastroenterol Hepatol* 1992, **4**:713–717.
This study suggests that the use of serology as a screening procedure prior to endoscopy would reduce the endoscopy workload by 41%.

50. • Cederbrant G, Kahlmeter G, Ljungh A: **The E-Test for Antimicrobial Susceptibility of *Helicobacter pylori*.** *J Antimicrob Chemother* 1993, **31**:65–71.
A comparison of minimum inhibitary concentration determination and the E-test for determining *H. pylori* sensitivity to antibiotics shows that the E-test is a reliable *in vitro* method.

51. • Glupczynski Y: **Result of a Multicentre European Survey in 1991 of Metronidazole Resistance in *Helicobacter pylori*.** *Eur J Clin Microbiol Infect Dis* 1992, **11**:777–781.
A collaborative study from 11 centers in Europe measuring the local prevalence of *H. pylori* resistance to metronidazole and showing a wide variation in the rates. The study also showed that metronidazole-resistant *H. pylori* was more common in females.

52. •• Chiba N, Rao BV, Rademaker JW, Hunt RH: **Meta-Analysis of the Efficacy of Antibiotic Therapy in Eradicating *Helicobacter pylori*.** *Am J Gastroenterol* 1992, **87**:1716–1727.
This statistical analysis of the results of 27 treatment studies shows that triple therapy with bismuth, metronidazole, and tetracycline gives the highest eradication rates.

53. • Seppala K, Farkkila M, Nuutinen H, Hakala K, Vaananen H, Rautelin H, Kosunen TU: **Triple Therapy of *Helicobacter pylori* Infection in Peptic Ulcer: A 12 Month Follow Up Study of 93 Patients.** *Scand J Gastroenterol* 1992, **27**:973–976.
A study showing that 2-week treatment with bismuth, amoxicillin, and metronidazole achieved an eradication rate of 84% and that the success was dependent on the pretreatment sensitivity of *H. pylori* to metronidazole.

54. Bell GD, Powell K, Burridge SM, Pallecaros A, Jones PH, Gant PW, Harrison G, Trowell JE: **Experience With Triple Anti-*Helicobacter Pylori* Eradication Therapy: Side Effects and the Importance of Testing Pre-Treatment Isolates for Metronidazole Resistance.** *Aliment Pharmacol Ther* 1992, **8**:427–435.

55. • Burette A, Glupczynski Y, DePrez C: **Evaluation of Various Multi-Drug Eradication Regimens for *Helicobacter Pylori*.** *Eur J Gastroenterol Hepatol* 1992, **4**:817–823.

A comparison of various short-course eradication regimens showing that 2-week treatment gave the highest eradication rate.

56. • BORODY TJ: **Possibilities for *Helicobacter Pylori* Suppression/Eradication.** *Eur J Gastroenterol Hepatol* 1992, **4**(Suppl 2):S37–S40.

Reduced side effects of bismuth-containing triple therapy is achieved without reduction in eradication rates by more frequent and lower doses of the drugs.

57. HOSKINGS SW, LING TKW, YUNG MY, CHENG A, CHUNG SCS, LEUNG JWC, LI AKC: **Randomised Controlled Trial of Short Term Treatment to Eradicate *Helicobacter pylori* in Patients With Duodenal Ulcer.** *BMJ* 1992, **305**:502–504.

58. • BELL CD, POWELL KL, BURRIDGE SM, SPENCER C, BOLTONS G, PURSENS K, BROOKS S, PROSSER S, HARRISON G, GANT PW, JONES PH, TROWELL JE: **Omeprazole Plus Antibiotic Combinations for the Eradication of Metronidazole Resistant *Helicobacter pylori*.** *Aliment Pharmacol Ther* 1992, **6**:751–758.

A combination of omeprazole and amoxicillin is an effective treatment for *H. pylori* infection whether the organisms were metronidazole resistant or not, but omeprazole alone gave poor eradication rates.

59. • MURRAY DM, DUPONT HL, COOPERSTOCK M, CORRADO ML, FEKETY R: **Evaluation of New Anti-Infective Drugs for the Treatment of Gastritis and Peptic Ulcer Disease Associated With Infections by *Helicobacter pylori*.** *Clin Infect Dis* 1992, **15**(Supp 1):S268–S273.

Protocol for therapeutic trials of anti–*H. pylori* agents is discussed.

60. • GOODWIN CS: **The Possibility of a Vaccine Against *Helicobacter pylori*.** *Eur J Gastroenterol Hepatol* 1993, **5**:9–12.

A review of the work on vaccine development against *H. pylori*.

Dino Vaira, MD, 1st Medical Clinic, S. Orsola Hospital, Nuove Patologie, Via Massarenti 9, 40138 Bologna, Italy.

Treatment of gastrointestinal infections

Susan L. Cookson, MD, and Robert Edelman, MD

University of Maryland, Baltimore, Maryland, USA

Several new or reconfirmed strategies for the treatment of selected gastrointestinal infections have emerged from investigations published during 1992 and 1993. For traveler's diarrhea, fluoroquinolones are now preferred, except in Mexico where trimethoprim-sulfamethoxazole remains the antibiotic of choice. The efficacy of early treatment of *Escherichia coli* O157:H7-associated hemorrhagic enteritis remains unproven. One dose of ciprofloxacin is sufficient to treat shigellosis caused by strains other than *Shigella dysenteriae* type 1. Loperamide in combination with antibiotics shortens the clinical course of shigellosis. Treatment of *Salmonella*-associated gastroenteritis with antibiotics prolongs carriage and is thus not recommended. *Clostridium difficile* asymptomatic carriage should not be treated with antibiotics. The treatment of cytomegalovirus colitis in HIV patients remains unclear; ganciclovir shows improvement only in histopathology in a controlled trial. A trial of paromomycin may be considered for HIV-positive patients with refractory cryptosporidiosis.

Current Opinion in Gastroenterology 1994, **10**:105–111

Diarrheagenic *Escherichia coli*

Diarrheagenic *Escherichia coli* comprises six different categories of strains based on distinct virulence properties, interactions with intestinal mucosa, growth characteristics, and clinical syndromes. These categories are enteroinvasive, enterohemorrhagic, enterotoxigenic, enteropathogenic, enteroaggregative, and diffusely adherent. Three of the categories, enterotoxigenic *E. coli* (ETEC), enterohemorrhagic *E. coli*, and enteroaggregative *E. coli*, have been the subject of clinical investigations this year.

Enterotoxigenic *Escherichia coli*

Enterotoxigenic *E. coli* is a pathogen commonly encountered by travelers and by infants and children in developing countries.

Antibiotic resistance patterns

Enterotoxigenic *E. coli* resistance patterns are multiple and vary by locale. For example, more ETEC strains from South America and West Africa were resistant to trimethoprim-sulfamethoxazole than strains from Mexico [1,2••,3•]. Of 142 US military personnel with diarrhea in South America and West Africa, 20% had ETEC; 39% of isolates were resistant to trimethoprim-sulfamethoxazole [3•]. By contrast, less than 10% of Mexican ETEC isolates were resistant to trimethoprim-sulfamethoxazole, but substantially more strains were resistant to tetracyclines and ampicillin [1,2••]. None of the Mexican, South American, or African strains were resistant to norfloxacin. Continuous monitoring of *in vitro* antibiotic susceptibility facilitates selection of optimal drug therapy in countries where unrestricted use of antibiotics is associated with development of microbial resistance.

Treatment studies

In a well-designed study, 66 travelers were randomly assigned to receive either 3 or 5 days of ofloxacin or a placebo [4••]. Mean duration of diarrhea was shortest in the 3-day treatment group (26 hours) compared with the placebo group (66 hours; $P<0.05$), although ETEC was not more rapidly eradicated from the stool in the treatment group. In another study, 90% of patients had trimethoprim-sulfamethoxazole–resistant strains of ETEC, but only 20% failed treatment with trimethoprim-sulfamethoxazole [3•]. *In vitro* resistance to trimethoprim-sulfamethoxazole affected the clinical outcome minimally.

An intestinal calmodulin inhibitor, zaldaride maleate, has antisecretory properties but no antiperistaltic activity. Zaldaride maleate was used to treat ETEC-associated diarrhea [5•]. The three different dose regimens of zaldaride maleate produced no statistically significant difference in duration of diarrhea, although the highest

Abbreviation

ETEC—enterotoxigenic *Escherichia coli.*

 ISBN 1-85922-606-X ISSN 0267–1379

zaldaride maleate dose tended to shorten the duration of diarrhea compared with placebo. This drug warrants further study.

In conclusion, trimethoprim-sulfamethoxazole remains the antibiotic of choice for ETEC in Mexico. Quinolones are preferred elsewhere, and 3 days of treatment with quinolones are effective.

Enterohemorrhagic *Escherichia coli*

Escherichia coli O157:H7 causes a hemorrhagic colitis and is implicated in hemolytic-uremic syndrome in children. Whether antibiotics benefit the children with enteritis or precipitate the development of hemolytic-uremic syndrome remains unanswered. Recently, 47 patients with *E. coli* O157:H7-associated enteritis were randomly assigned to receive either trimethoprim-sulfamethoxazole starting on day 7 of diarrhea or no treatment [6•]. No significant difference in the duration of enteritic symptoms or development of hemolytic-uremic syndrome (8% in treated group and 16% in control group) was observed. Future studies must determine if instituting therapy earlier would be beneficial.

Enteroaggregative *Escherichia coli*

Enteroaggregative *E. coli* manifests an aggregative adherence pattern to cultures of HEp-2 cells and is associated with pediatric diarrhea in certain developing countries. Clinical isolates of enteroaggregative *E. coli* from Latin America and Thailand were tested for their resistance patterns [7•]. In 63 clinical isolates, high levels of resistance to penicillins, tetracycline, aminoglycosides, chloramphenicol, and trimethoprim-sulfamethoxazole were noted. The isolates were susceptible to all newer quinolones tested. These resistance patterns resemble those of ETEC.

Shigella

Shigella infection kills many children in developing countries and is one of the few causes of traveler's diarrhea that requires antimicrobial therapy. Enteroinvasive *E. coli* is very similar to *Shigella* and is often included in studies of *Shigella* species.

Antibiotic resistance patterns

In the past, ampicillin or trimethoprim-sulfamethoxazole were the treatments of choice, but now antibiotic choice is locale- and strain-dependent. Ampicillin or trimethoprim-sulfamethoxazole in developed countries, and quinolones in developing countries are now preferred for suspected shigellosis [8•].

In some developing countries, *Shigella* species retain a high sensitivity to trimethoprim-sulfamethoxazole. For example, from 1987 to 1989, only 8% of Mexican strains were resistant to trimethoprim-sulfamethoxazole compared with 23% of strains resistant to ampicillin [2••]. However, trimethoprim-sulfamethoxazole–resistant strains occurred more frequently in other countries, totaling 30% in Guatemala and Argentina [9•] and 80% in India [10•] and Thailand [11••]. In the Thai and Indian studies, all strains were susceptible to ciprofloxacin and nalidixic acid [11••,12].

Loperamide plus antibiotics

Loperamide use in dysentery is generally contraindicated, but its combination with antibiotics may be safe. Two important studies examine this question. In the first study, US students in Mexico with diarrhea were treated with three different dose regimens of trimethoprim-sulfamethoxazole plus loperamide as follows: 1) trimethoprim-sulfamethoxazole (320 mg/1600 mg) one dose, 2) trimethoprim-sulfamethoxazole (160 mg/800 mg) twice daily doses for 3 days, or 3) a trimethoprim-sulfamethoxazole (320 mg/1600 mg) first dose followed by twice daily doses (160 mg/800 mg) for 3 days [13•]. All subjects received loperamide after each loose stool; trimethoprim-sulfamethoxazole alone and loperamide alone were not assessed. All groups responded favorably to therapy, but group 3 responded most rapidly ($P<0.01$). In the second study, Thai adults presenting with *Shigella* or enteroinvasive *E. coli*–associated diarrhea for 2 days and less than 11 stools per day were treated for 3 days with ciprofloxacin plus loperamide [11••]. Addition of loperamide significantly decreased the duration of diarrhea to 19 hours compared with 42 hours in the placebo group (Table 1).

Antibiotics alone

Prado *et al.* [9•] examined the new, oral cephalosporin, ceftibuten, in a random, nonblind protocol in Latin America. In children with *Shigella* or enteroinvasive *E. coli*-associated dysentery, 13 received ceftibuten, and nine received trimethoprim-sulfamethoxazole. No difference in duration of diarrhea or fever was seen. In another study, norfloxacin and nalidixic acid were compared in 122 Indian adults with *Shigella*-associated diarrhea [10•]. No significant difference was found between the two treatment groups even though 13.3% of strains were resistant to nalidixic acid. Bennish *et al.* [8•] recommend initial empiric treatment with the established quinolone, nalidixic acid, and replacement of nalidixic acid with pivmecillinam if clinical failure occurs at 48 hours. Pivmecillinam is not available in the United States. As with ETEC, US travelers in Mexico with *Shigella*-associated diarrhea were treated with 3 or 5 days of ofloxacin or placebo [4••]. Three days of ofloxacin gave the most rapid post-treatment eradication (24 hours) compared with placebo (98 hours; $P<0.05$). Three rather than 5 days of ofloxacin is acceptable treatment, which suggests that even shorter therapy with fluoroquinolones may be efficacious.

Table 1. Recovery from dysentery by ciprofloxacin plus loperamide versus ciprofloxacin plus placebo*

	Shigella or enteroinvasive *Escherichia coli* groups		
Variable	Ciprofloxacin plus loperamide ($n=21$)	Ciprofloxacin plus placebo ($n=26$)	*P* value
Duration of diarrhea, *h* †‡	19 (6, 42)	42 (21, 46)	0.028§
Diarrheal stools after treatment, *n* ‡	2 (1, 5)	6.5 (2, 9)	0.016§
Time to resolution of diarrhea, % ¶			
12 h	38	12	0.043**
24 h	67	35	0.058††
36 h	71	46	0.148
48 h	90	77	0.269

*From Murphy *et al.* [11••]; with permission.
†Measured hours from time of enrollment to occurrence of last unformed stool.
‡Data are median (25th, 75th percentile).
§Mann-Whitney-Wilcoxon test.
¶Yates corrected chi-square or Fisher exact test, two-tailed, as appropriate.
**Difference = 26% (95% confidence interval, 2% to 50%).
††Difference = 32% (95% confidence interval, 5% to 59%).

The powerful fluoroquinolone, ciprofloxacin, has been shown to be efficacious after a single dose. Twenty-seven Indian adults presenting with diarrhea for less than 3 days with more than 10 stools per day were treated with one 1-g dose of ciprofloxacin [12]. Diarrhea was arrested by 24 hours after treatment. In Bangladesh, one dose (1 g), two doses (1 g, twice daily), and 10 doses (500 mg, twice daily) of ciprofloxacin were administered to adults suffering with shigellosis for less than 4 days [14••]. With most *Shigella* species, the 1-day courses of ciprofloxacin were as clinically (Fig. 1) and microbiologically effective as the 5-day course. However, in patients with *Shigella dysenteriae* type 1 there were six of 25 treatment failures with 1-day courses compared with zero of 15 failures after 5 days of treatment ($P=0.05$). Unfortunately, a single dose of ciprofloxacin is still prohibitively expensive for most people in developing countries.

In conclusion, one dose of ciprofloxacin in adults is probably adequate for all *Shigella* strains except *S. dysenteriae* type 1. Loperamide in adults is safe when combined with antibiotics and shortens the clinical course of shigellosis. Nalidixic acid is inexpensive, effective against shigellosis and in most countries has been approved for use in children. At our hospital, 500 mg of ciprofloxacin is 11 times more expensive than 500 mg of nalidixic acid; therefore nalidixic acid should be considered as alternative therapy for shigellosis in children or adults.

Salmonella

Gastroenteritis

The debate on whether to treat *Salmonella*-associated gastroenteritis with antibiotics continues. Quinolones may be associated with relapse and prolonged *Salmonella* carriage [15••]. For example, prolonged carriage was seen in a *Salmonella enteritidis* outbreak occurring after a British medical meeting [16]. In this case, 92% of those exposed to contaminated potato salad developed severe or mild symptoms and were treated with 5 days of ciprofloxacin. It took 6 to 10 weeks for the majority of patients to become culture negative and six patients needed 14 weeks to eradicate the organism! Similarly, in a Swedish, double-blind, randomized study of *Salmonella*-associated diarrhea, norfloxacin (400 mg twice daily for 5 days) was more effective in causing clinical cure or improvement (58% vs 35%, $P=0.03$), but *Salmonella* excretion was prolonged (50 days) compared with placebo (23 days) [17••].

Typhoid fever

Increasingly, antibiotic resistant organisms are being isolated in typhoid outbreaks. An Indian outbreak of multidrug-resistant *Salmonella typhi* occurred in 1990 [18•]. Forty-nine percent of isolates (18 of 37) had multidrug-resistant patterns compared with 10% (three of 30) of strains with such patterns isolated in 1988 and 1989. In 1990, resistance to ampicillin, streptomycin, tetracycline, and chloramphenicol occurred in 81% of strains and resistance to cotrimoxazole occurred in 40% of strains. Disturbingly, high-grade resistance is developing to relatively inexpensive antibiotics commonly used to treat enteric fever, such as chloramphenicol, ampicillin, and cotrimoxazole [18•]. Fortunately, no Indian strains were resistant to gentamicin, cefotaxime, and quinolones. Although quinolones are the treatment of choice of multiresistant *S. typhi*, high costs seriously limit their use in developing countries. Furazolidone, a synthetic antimicrobial nitrofuran, may offer an alternative [19••]. Of 133 *S. typhi* Indian isolates, all were susceptible to furazolidone and the cure rate was 86.2%. Furazolidone is a reasonable alternative to quinolones for multidrug-resistant *S. typhi*, given its low cost, safety in all age groups, few side effects, minimal resistance worldwide, and possible low risk of inducing *Clostridium difficile* colitis.

In summary, we do not recommend antibiotics for immunocompetent patients who have *Salmonella*-associated gastroenteritis. With treatment, the carrier state is prolonged. *Salmonella typhi* is becoming more resistant to many commonly used antibiotics. Quinolones are the drugs of choice for enteric fever in adults, but they are not recommended for children and are too expensive for routine use in developing countries. Furazolidone is a satisfactory alternative because of its efficacy, low cost, and safety in children.

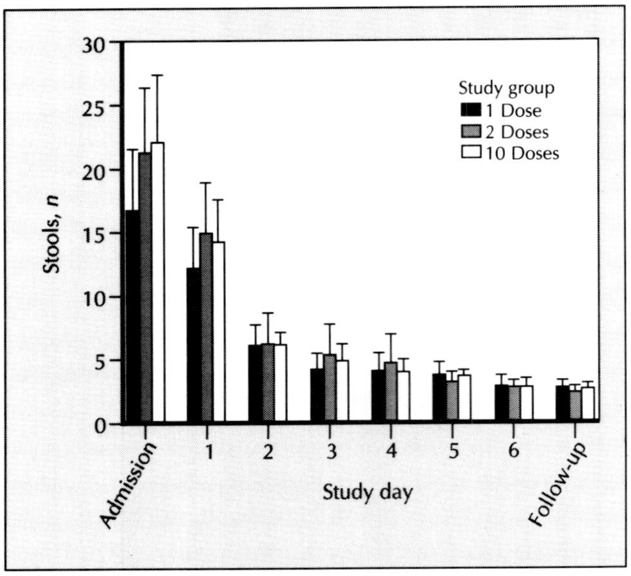

Fig. 1. Mean stool frequency by treatment group and study day. The error bars indicate the upper 95% confidence interval of the mean. No statistically significant differences between study groups in the mean number of stools were found for any of the study days. The mean number of stools before admission and on follow-up were determined by history. The preadmission period is the period from the midnight before admission until admission to the study. For follow-up, the time period was the 24 hours before the visit to the treatment center. For study days 1 to 6, there were 40 persons in the single-dose group, 43 in the two-dose group, and 35 in the 10-dose group. At follow-up, there were 34 persons in the single-dose group, 41 in the two-dose group, and 34 in the 10-dose group. Four patients in the one-dose group and two patients in each of the two- and 10-dose groups received open-label, 5-day therapy with ciprofloxacin starting on study day 4 or later. (*From* Bennish *et al.* [14••]; with permission.)

Campylobacter

If treatment is needed, erythromycin remains the antibiotic of choice for *Campylobacter*-associated diarrhea, especially with the worldwide increase of quinolone-resistant *Campylobacter* strains. For example, of 1240 strains of *Campylobacter* isolated in Great Britain, all strains were sensitive to ciprofloxacin in 1990, but by 1991, 3% (11 of 359) were resistant [20]. On the Mediterranean Balearic Islands, *Campylobacter* isolates identified before 1987 were not resistant to quinolones, but by 1991 30% were resistant [21]. Only 3% of these same isolates were resistant to erythromycin. The Swedish Study Group [17••] compared 5-day norfloxacin therapy to a placebo in patients infected with *Campylobacter* species. No difference occurred in the clinical cure rate. However, the rapid development of quinolone resistance in this cohort was dramatically shown by the fact that six of nine *Campylobacter* strains obtained after treatment had minimal inhibitory concentrations of at least 32, a fourfold increase compared with pretreatment levels. Another probable cause of antibiotic resistance is the use of fluoroquinolones in the poultry industry [20,21].

In summary, *Campylobacter* are developing greater resistance to quinolones; this fact together with the frequent therapeutic failure of quinolones leaves erythromycin as the treatment choice if any antibiotic is needed.

Antibiotic-associated diarrhea

Clostridium difficile colitis or pseudomembranous colitis occurs in 10% to 15% of hospitalized patients who develop diarrhea as a result of antimicrobial therapy [22••]. Antibiotic therapy of pseudomembranous colitis is required in some clinical settings.

Ciprofloxacin, which does not kill anaerobic intestinal bacteria and in one case report was associated with a cure, is unlikely to cause *C. difficile*–associated diarrhea [23]. In one study, the minimal inhibitory concentrations of ciprofloxacin for 205 *C. difficile* isolates ranged from 8 to 32 mg/L [24]. This is quite high, but because the concentration of ciprofloxacin in stool is much greater than in blood, ciprofloxacin may be adequate to eliminate intestinal organisms. In contrast to clindamycin, ciprofloxacin appears not to facilitate growth of *C. difficile* in fecal emulsions [24].

In a nonblinded, randomized study of 46 patients with *C. difficile*-associated diarrhea, teicoplanin was as efficacious as vancomycin in eliminating the diarrhea [25•]. The rates of microbiologic and clinical relapse and carriage were also similar [25•]. Twice-daily administration of teicoplanin seems as effective as four-times-daily vancomycin administration for *C. difficile*-associated diarrhea. However, the two treatment groups were not comparable clinically, which may have biased the results in favor of teicoplanin. Teicoplanin, which is available only for compassionate use, warrants future study as a treatment for *C. difficile*-associated diarrhea.

Vancomycin does not eradicate *C. difficile* carriage [26••]. At 2 months, 67% (four of six) of patients treated with vancomycin had positive cultures compared with only 11% (one of nine) in the placebo group. Because fecal excretion of *C. difficile* is transient in most asymptomatic individuals, we do not recommend treating such carriers. *Clostridium difficile*–associated diarrhea found in AIDS patients should be treated conventionally [27•].

Diarrheal diseases related to HIV

Acute and chronic diarrhea is common in patients with HIV. Although the virus itself is implicated, many common and novel infectious pathogens also have been identified as possible causes of the diarrhea. Enteric viruses may be more common than either enteric bacteria or parasites, which may explain why empiric treatment is often ineffective. In one cohort study, 35%, 11%, and 3% of patients, respectively, had viruses, bacteria, and parasites associated with their acute diarrhea [28••]. Because of the diversity of pathogens, a randomized, single-blind study of empiric combination chemotherapy was performed in 28 AIDS patients presenting with chronic diarrhea in Zambia [29•]. Placebo was dipyridamole, and combination chemotherapy for enteric bacteria and parasites consisted of 2 g of tinidazole for 2 days, 1 g of thiabendazole for 3 days, and 960 mg of cotrimoxazole twice daily for 7 days. No differences in clinical outcome were found between placebo and combination chemotherapy groups. This again reaffirms that empiric treatment of diarrhea in AIDS patients is not often efficacious.

Cytomegalovirus-associated colitis

In the only double-blind, placebo-controlled study of ganciclovir for the treatment of cytomegalovirus colitis reported to date, 62.5% of the ganciclovir group (n=32) had histopathologic improvement of colonic tissue compared with 36.7% of placebo group (n=30, P=0.042) after 14 days of treatment [30••]. However, diarrhea, abdominal pain, fever, and fatigue did not significantly improve. Ganciclovir is much less expensive than foscarnet and it remains the treatment of choice for gastrointestinal cytomegalovirus disease based on previous, uncontrolled studies [31,32]. In a retrospective, uncontrolled study, 28 patients with cytomegalovirus colitis treated with foscarnet were identified [33]. A total of 57% (16 of 28) had complete response to foscarnet within 2 to 3 weeks, and the remainder relapsed, failed therapy, or died. The most troublesome adverse effect was penile ulceration (6%, four of 66) with renal impairment being largely avoidable with hydration. Failure of ganciclovir after two induction attempts to cure cytomegalovirus colitis may prompt the use of foscarnet. There was 80% clinical response and 60% histopathologic response in patients treated with foscarnet after ganciclovir failure, but the sample size was small and the study was not blinded for clinical response [34•]. Randomized, controlled trials directly comparing foscarnet, ganciclovir, and placebo for therapy of cytomegalovirus colitis are needed. However, a companion placebo arm with long-term follow-up may be unethical.

Cryptosporidiosis

Cryptosporidium parvum causes a self-limiting diarrhea in immunocompetent individuals, but in AIDS patients it can cause a persistent enteritis complicated by malabsorption. Paromomycin is an oral, poorly absorbed aminoglycoside. In two recent papers, medical records were reviewed retrospectively for paromomycin use in the treatment of cryptosporidiosis [35,36•]. In the first study, all seven patients treated initially improved, but five had a recurrence [35]. In the second study, the diarrhea of all five patients significantly abated after a variety of treatment regimens, but one patient relapsed [36•].

In conclusion, 12 patients in these two studies initially responded to paromomycin, but recurrences and relapses were common. Given lack of other treatment for the intractable diarrhea of *Cryptosporidium*, an empiric trial of paromomycin can be considered by the physician and patient.

Continuing reports on hormonal therapy in AIDS patients with chronic diarrhea are being published. In an open, noncomparative pilot trial, patients received subcutaneous vapreotide, a synthetic somatostatin analogue [37•]. Patients with less than 10 stools per day and no *Cryptosporidium* isolated were more likely to respond initially. Two thirds of the patients on continuous therapy relapsed within 3 weeks to 5 months. In total, 13% of patients had complete remission, but duration of follow-up was not given. These results suggest vapreotide may initially benefit AIDS patients with noncryptosporidial diarrhea.

References and recommended reading

Papers of particular interest, published within the annual period of review, have been highlighted as:
- • Of special interest
- •• Of outstanding interest

1. Wistrom J, Gentry LO, Palmgren AC, Price M, Nord CE, Ljundh A, Norrby SR: **Ecological Effects of Short-Term Ciprofloxacin Treatment of Travellers' Diarrhea**. *J Antimicrob Chemother* 1992, **30**:693–706.

2. •• Bandres JC, Mathewson JJ, Ericsson CD, Dupont HL: **Trimethoprim/Sulfamethoxazole Remains Active Against Enterotoxigenic *Escherichia coli* and *Shigella* Species in Guadalajara, Mexico**. *Am J Med Sci* 1992, **303**:289–291.

This study of *E. coli* and *Shigella* isolates from 1980, 1987, 1988, and 1989 in US travelers reveals minimal change in resistance patterns over this time.

3. • Thorton SA, Wignall SF, Kilpatrick ME, Bourgeois AL, Gardiner C, Batchelor RA, Burr DH, Oprandy JJ, Garst P, Hyams KC: **Norfloxacin Compared to Trimethoprim/Sulfamethoxazole for the Treatment of Travelers' Diarrhea Among U.S. Military Personnel Deployed to South American and West Africa**. *Mil Med* 1992, **157**:55–58.

In a double-blind study of 142 patients, the authors demonstrate that both norfloxacin and trimethoprim-sulfamethoxazole were clinically effective in the treatment of travelers' diarrhea; however, there was a 20% failure rate in the trimethoprim-sulfamethoxazole group due to resistant strains of ETEC.

4. •• Dupont HL, Ericsson CD, Mathewson JJ, Dupont MW: **Five Versus Three Days of Ofloxacin Therapy for Traveler's Diarrhea: A Placebo-Controlled Study**. *Antimicrob Agents Chemother* 1992, **36**:87–91.

In a well-designed study, the authors show that 3 days rather than 5 days of ofloxacin was the preferred duration of treatment for travelers' diarrhea. Organisms isolated included *E. coli* and *Shigella*.

5. • Dupont HL, Ericsson CD, Mathewson JJ, Marani S, Knellwolf-Cousin AL, Martinez-Sandoval FG: **Zaldaride Maleate, an Intestinal Calmodulin Inhibitor, in the Therapy of Travelers' Diarrhea**. *Gastroenterology* 1993, **104**:709–715.

Zaldaride maleate was examined for the treatment of travelers' diarrhea. Of the three doses tested, only the highest dose, 20 mg, reduced the duration of diarrhea compared to placebo, though not significantly. The implication of this work is that intracellular calcium may be a mediator of diarrhea.

6. PROULX F, TURGEON JP, DELAGE G, LAFLEUR L, CHICOINE
• L: **Randomized, Controlled Trial of Antibiotic Therapy for *Escherichia coli* O157:H7 Enteritis.** *J Pediatr* 1992, **121**:299–303.

This study attempts to examine the effect of antibiotics on progression of hemolytic-uremic syndrome; however, therapy was begun after 7 days of enteritis and no significant effect was noted on the duration of gastroenteritis or development of hemolytic-uremic syndrome.

7. YAMAMOTO T, ECHEVERRIA P, YOKOTA T: **Drug Resistance**
• **and Adherence to Human Intestines of Enteroaggregative *Escherichia coli*.** *J Infect Dis* 1992, **165**:744–749.

This investigation of one of the newest categories of diarrheagenic *E. coli*, reveals highly antibiotic resistant strains. Enteroaggregative *E. coli* will continue to receive attention as a cause of diarrhea, especially in developing countries.

8. BENNISH ML, SALAM MA: **Rethinking Options for the**
• **Treatment of Shigellosis.** *J Antimicrob Chemother* 1992, **30**:234–247.

The authors provide a good review of treatment options in developing countries.

9. PRADO D, LOPEZ E, LIU H, DEVOTO S, WOLOJ M, CONTRINI
• M, MURRAY BE, GOMEZ H, CLEARY TG: **Ceftibuten and Trimethoprim-Sulfamethoxazole for Treatment of *Shigella* and Enteroinvasive *Escherichia coli* Disease.** *Pediatr Infect Dis J* 1992, **11**:644–647.

This study compares the effectiveness of a new, oral cephalosporin compared with trimethoprim-sulfamethoxazole. Trimethoprim-sulfamethoxazole was effective except in cases associated with resistant organisms, which occurred frequently.

10. BHATTACHARYA MK, NAIR GB, SEN D, PAUL M, DEBNATH A,
• NAG A, DUTTA D, DUTTA P, PAL SC, BHATTACHARYA SK: **Efficacy of Norfloxacin for Shigellosis: A Double-Blind Randomized Clinical Trial.** *J Diarrhoeal Dis Res* 1992, **10**:146–150.

This is another study examining the treatment of shigellosis with newer fluoroquinolones. Norfloxacin did no better clinically than the older quinolone, nalidixic acid, even though 13% of strains were resistant to nalidixic acid.

11. MURPHY GS, BODHIDATTA L, ECHEVERRIA P, TANSUPHASWAD-
•• IKUL S, HOGE CW, IMLARP S, TAMURA K: **Ciprofloxacin and Loperamide in the Treatment of Bacillary Dysentery.** *Ann Intern Med* 1993, **118**:582–586.

A well-designed, interesting study shows that loperamide was not deleterious and actually helpful in treating dysentery if administered with ciprofloxacin. Loperamide is contraindicated as monotherapy for dysentery.

12. BHATTACHARYA SK, BHATTACHARYA MK, DUTTA D, DUTTA P, PAUL M, SEN D, SARKAR S, SAHA A, PAL SC: **Single-Dose Ciprofloxacin for Shigellosis in Adults.** *J Infect* 1992, **25**:117–119.

13. ERICSSON CD, NICHOLLS-VASQUEZ I, DUPONT HL, MATHEWSON
• JJ: **Optimal Dosing of Trimethoprim-Sulfamethoxazole When Used With Loperamide to Treat Traveler's Diarrhea.** *Antimicrob Agents Chemother* 1992, **36**:2821–2824.

Another study examines the addition of loperamide to antibiotics, but unfortunately loperamide alone or trimethoprim-sulfamethoxazole alone were not examined. In this double-blind investigation, the optimal dose of trimethoprim-sulfamethoxazole was a single large dose followed by 3 days of a more standard dose of trimethoprim-sulfamethoxazole, accompanied by loperamide from the onset.

14. BENNISH ML, SALAM MA, KHAN WA, KHAN AM: **Treat-**
•• **ment of Shigellosis: III. Comparison of One- and Two-Dose Ciprofloxacin With Standard 5-Day Therapy.** *Ann Intern Med* 1992, **117**:727–734.

This well-designed study demonstrates that single-dose ciprofloxacin is effective treatment of non-*dysenteriae Shigella*. As expected, single-dose therapy is inferior to 10-day treatment for *S. dysenteriae* type 1.

15. WILCOX MH, SPENCER RC: **Quinolones and Salmonella Gas-**
•• **troenteritis.** *J Antimicrob Chemother* 1992, **30**:221–228.

A thoughtful review that discusses the problems of treating salmonella gastroenteritis with quinolones.

16. LEIGH DA: **The Treatment of a Large Outbreak of Acute Bacterial Gastroenteritis With Ciprofloxacin.** *J Antimicrob Chemother* 1992, **30**:733–735.

17. WISTROM J, JERTBORN M, EKWALL E, NORLIN K, SODERQUIST
•• B, STROMBERG A, LUNDHOLM R, HOGEVIK H, LAGERGREN L, ENGLUND G, NORRBY R, AND THE SWEDISH STUDY GROUP: **Empiric Treatment of Acute Diarrheal Disease With Norfloxacin.** *Ann Intern Med* 1992, **117**:202–208.

This study suggests the major limitations of treating acute diarrhea with quinolones are to prolong fecal shedding of salmonella and to induce resistance in campylobacter.

18. RAO RS, AMARNATH SK, SUJATHA S: **An Outbreak of Ty-**
• **phoid Due to Multidrug Resistant *Salmonella typhi* in Pondicherry.** *Trans R Soc Trop Med Hyg* 1992, **86**:204–205.

This study reveals a worrisome increase of resistance from 1988 to 1990.

19. DUTTA P, RASAILY R, SAHA MR, MITRA U, MANNA B,
•• CHAKRABORTY S, MUKHERJEE A: **Randomized Clinical Trial of Furazolidone for Typhoid Fever in Children.** *Scand J Gastroenterol* 1993, **28**:168–172.

A randomized, double-blind study showing that furazolidone was a satisfactory alternative to chloramphenicol in the treatment of typhoid fever caused by chloramphenicol-resistant strains.

20. BOWLER I, DAY D: **Emerging Quinolone Resistance in Campylobacters.** *Lancet* 1992, **340**:245.

21. REINA J: **Resistance to Fluoroquinolones in *Salmonella* non-*typhi* and *Campylobacter* spp.** *Lancet* 1992, **340**:1035–1036.

22. FEKETY R, SHAH AB: **Diagnosis and Treatment of *Clostridium***
•• ***difficile* Colitis.** *JAMA* 1993, **269**:71–75.

An excellent review that covers pathogenesis, diagnosis and treatment of *C. difficile*-associated diarrhea.

23. DANIELS J, PRISTAS A: **Successful Treatment of *Clostridium difficile* Colitis With Ciprofloxacin.** *J Clin Gastroenterol* 1992, **15**:176–177.

24. GOLLEDGE CL, CARSON CF, O'NEILL GL, BOWMAN RA, RILEY TV: **Ciprofloxacin and *Clostridium difficile*-Associated Diarrhea.** *J Antimicrob Chemother* 1992, **30**:141–147.

25. DELALLA F, NICOLIN R, RINALDI E, SCARPELLINI P, RIGOLI R,
• MANFRIN V, TRAMARIN A: **Prospective Study of Oral Teicoplanin Versus Oral Vancomycin for Therapy of Pseudomembranous Colitis and *Clostridium difficile*-Associated Diarrhea.** *Antimicrob Agents Chemother* 1992, **36**:2192–2196.

Teicoplanin and vancomycin were compared in 51 patients; clinical cures and failures, relapses, and carriage states were comparable.

26. JOHNSON S, HOMANN SR, BETTIN KM, QUICK JN, CLABOTS
•• CR, PETERSON LR, GERDING DN: **Treatment of Asymptomatic *Clostridium difficile* Carriers (Fecal Excretors) With Vancomycin or Metronidazole.** *Ann Intern Med* 1992, **117**:297–302.

A randomized, placebo-controlled nonblinded trial suggests that a higher rate of carriage occurs after treatment of asymptomatic fecal excretors. The authors recommend not treating such individuals. Metronidazole could not be evaluated because antibiotics were used after the metronidazole.

27. COZART JC, KALANGI SS, CLENCH MH, TAYLOR DR, BORUCKI
• MJ, POLLARD RB, SOLOWAY RD: ***Clostridium difficile* Diarrhea in Patients With AIDS Versus Non-AIDS Controls.** *J Clin Gastroenterol* 1993, **16**:192–194.

A hospital chart review found that *C. difficile*-associated diarrhea resolved with vancomycin or metronidazole treatment equally well in AIDS patients as in control non-AIDS patients. There was no follow-up search for relapses.

28. GROHMANN GS, GLASS RI, PEREIRA HG, MONROE SS,
•• HIGHTOWER AW, WEBER R, BRYAN RT, FOR THE ENTERIC

Opportunistic Infections Working Group: **Enteric Viruses and Diarrhea in HIV-Infected Patients**. *N Engl J Med* 1993, **329**:14–20.

An interesting study that identified a high rate of viral-associated acute and chronic diarrhea in HIV-infected patients. The enteric viruses are novel and include astrovirus and picobirnavirus.

29. Kelly P, Buve AP: **Chemotherapy of African AIDS Diarrhea: • A Preliminary Study**. *AIDS* 1993, 7:91–93.

Though the numbers of patients are small, this investigation suggests that empiric treatment of chronic diarrhea in AIDS patients is ineffective and that a high level of spontaneous remissions may occur.

30. Dieterich DT, Kotler DP, Busch DF, Crumpacker C, Du •• Mond C, Dearmand B, Buhles W: **Ganciclovir Treatment of Cytomegalovirus Colitis in AIDS: A Randomized, Double-Blind, Placebo-Controlled Multicenter Study**. *J Infect Dis* 1993, **167**:278–282.

First controlled study; histopathologic improvement was seen but the diarrhea did not improve after 14 days of treatment. Other symptoms, such as fever and weight loss, tended to improve. The authors speculate that ganciclovir may be effective if used for more than 14 days.

31. Chachoua A, Dieterich DT, Krasinski K: **Ganciclovir in the Treatment of Cytomegalovirus Gastrointestinal Disease With the Acquired Immunodeficiency Syndrome**. *Ann Intern Med* 1987, **107**:133–137.

32. Dieterech DT, Chachoua A, LaFleur F, Worrel C: **Ganciclovir Treatment of Gastrointestinal Infections Caused by Cytomegalovirus in Patients With AIDS**. *Rev Infect Dis* 1988, **10**(Suppl):S532–537.

33. Blanshard C: **Treatment of HIV-Related Cytomegalovirus Disease of the Gastrointestinal Tract With Foscarnet**. *J Acquir Immune Defic Syndr* 1992, **5**(**Suppl 1**):S25–S28.

34. Dieterich DT, Poles MA, Dicker M, Tepper R, Lew E: • **Foscarnet Treatment of Cytomegalovirus Gastrointestinal Infections in Acquired Immunodeficiency Syndrome Patients Who Have Failed Ganciclovir Induction**. *Am J Gastroenterol* 1993, **88**:542–548.

Foscarnet therapy of refractory cytomegalovirus disease induced remission when ganciclovir failed in at least 60% of this small cohort.

35. Fichtenbaum CJ, Ritchie DJ, Powderly WG: **Use of Paromomycin for Treatment of Cryptosporidiosis in Patients With Aids**. *Clin Infect Dis* 1993, **16**:2989–3000.

36. Armitage K, Flanigan T, Carey J, Frank I, MacGregor RR, • Ross P, Goodgame R, Turner J: **Treatment of Cryptosporidiosis With Paromomycin. A Report of Five Cases**. *Arch Intern Dis* 1992, **152**:2497–2499.

This series of cases suggests some benefit of paromomycin with follow-up periods of 3 to 6 months. Doses of drug varied from patient to patient.

37. Girard PM, Goldschmidt E, Vittecoq D, Massip P, • Gastiaburu J, Meyohas MC, Coulaud JP, Schally AV: **Vapreotide, a Somatostatin Analogue, in Cryptosporidiosis and Other AIDS-Related Diarrheal Diseases**. *AIDS* 1992, 6:715–718.

Another pilot study of a somatostatin analogue used in the treatment of chronic diarrhea in AIDS patients.

Susan L. Cookson, MD, and Robert Edelman, MD, University of Maryland, Division of Infectious Diseases and Geographic Medicine and Center for Vaccine Development, MSTF Building, Room 934, 10 South Pine Street, Baltimore, MD 21201, USA.

Diagnostic tests in gastrointestinal infections

Grace M. Thorne, PhD

Children's Hospital, Boston, Massachusetts, USA

Advances in the basic science technologies (monoclonal antibodies, polymerase chain reaction, and molecular genetic techniques) have lead to more sensitive and specific detection systems for gastrointestinal pathogens. In the past year, two different monoclonal-based, enzyme-linked immunosorbent assays have been described that specifically detect pathogenic *Entamoeba histolytica* in stool. A number of different pretreatment methods have been employed to improve polymerase chain reaction detection of pathogens in stool. Two studies have used immunomagnetic beads (*ie*, monoclonal antibody–coated) to selectively isolate salmonellae and shigellae followed by detection using polymerase chain reaction-based tests. Spin column chromatography isolation of Norwalk virus allowed for rapid detection of this virus by reverse transcriptase-polymerase chain reaction. A Quiagen procedure improved detection of the toxin A gene target for direct detection of *Clostridium difficile* by polymerase chain reaction methods. Results of recent evaluations of new commercially available products for detection of *Cryptosporidium* spp are evaluated. This report emphasizes tests with improved sensitivity, specificity, and utility in the clinical microbiology laboratory.

Current Opinion in Gastroenterology 1994, **10**:112–118

Escherichia coli O157:H7

The hamburger-borne outbreaks in January 1993 that occurred in Washington, Idaho, Nevada, and California have focused attention on the devastating public health impact of *Escherichia coli* O157:H7 in North America. In these outbreaks, over 500 culture-confirmed cases were identified. Forty-one persons developed hemolytic uremic syndrome and four children died [1]. Quick detection of this infection was hampered by the fact that most laboratories that culture stool do not test for *E. coli* O157:H7. Consequently, it is important that physicians request that stool samples from patients who suddenly have blood in their stool be cultured on MacConkey sorbitol agar.

Currently, commercial tests capable of detecting the Shiga-like cytotoxins (verotoxins) made by these pathogens are not available. Toxin detection methods employing probes or polymerase chain reaction (PCR) techniques are not routinely used in clinical laboratories. Various enzyme-linked immunosorbent assays (ELISAs) have been previously described, although none have been applied directly to stool samples. Recently Hull *et al.* [2•] described a direct screening immunoblot assay for Shiga-like cytotoxins producing organisms and tested it in a small study of stool samples in Thailand. The assay requires overnight growth of organisms in stool on nitrocellulose filters incubated on special mitomycin-containing agar. Specificity of the assay was found to be improved by using a monoclonal antibody that cross-reacts with the B subunits of both Shiga-like cytotoxins SLT-I and SLT-II. The test was able to identify the pathogen when present at ratios of 1:1000 to 1:5000 in the normal stool flora. Because this assay requires overnight growth on media containing a highly toxic (*ie*, carcinogenic and teratogenic) compound and a lengthy (4 hours and 15 minutes) enzyme immunoassay protocol, the method still lacks the rapidity, simplicity, and the ease of handling needed for a routine diagnostic laboratory. Direct detection in stool is a step in the right direction because other non-O157 serotypes of *E. coli* as well as *Citrobacter freundii* [3•] are known to produce these toxins. Further studies with new detection systems are needed to determine the role of these newly described Shiga-like cytotoxin producers in diarrhea and food-borne infections.

Entamoeba histolytica

Detection of pathogenic *Entamoeba histolytica* currently requires use of DNA probes or zymodeme analysis techniques that are not suitable for routine di-

Abbreviations

CFU—colony-forming units; **ELISA**—enzyme-linked immunosorbent assay; **PCR**—polymerase chain reaction.

 ISBN 1-85922-606-X ISSN 0267–1379

agnostic laboratories. A monoclonal antibody capable of distinguishing between invasive and noninvasive clinical isolates of *E. histolytica* has been developed by Gonzalez-Ruiz *et al.* [4••]. Using the monoclonal antibody in a immunofluorescence assay, the authors found 100% correlation between the new test and zymodeme characterization when 88 *E. histolytica* isolates were tested. The study collection comprised six reference strains and 82 clinical isolates from Bangladesh, Colombia, and Mexico. The clinical isolates were also characterized by zymodeme analysis and represented three different zymodeme types, two invasive and one noninvasive, from a total of six parent zymodemes. Preliminary characterization of the epitope detected by this pathogen-specific monoclonal antibody identified a previously undescribed 81- to 84-kD internal protein.

A second pathogen-specific ELISA has been develop based on monoclonal antibodies to the galactose-specific adhesin of *E. histolytica* [5••]. Preliminary studies of 74 patients in Bangladesh resulted in ELISA sensitivity and specificity of 100% and 97%, respectively. Although a more extensive series of isolates need to be tested with both monoclonal assays, the results are encouraging that a direct fecal test specific for invasive organisms employing either fluorescence microscopy or ELISA may be available in the near future.

Cryptosporidium spp

The latest outbreak of water-borne cryptosporidiosis in Milwaukee has focused more interest on this small coccidian parasite and points out the need for a rapid simple tests to detect the presence of *Cryptosporidium* in stools and environmental samples.

There have been new reports of various techniques for concentration and detection. Ungureanu and Dontu [6•] report a new staining technique using the fluorescent dye, mepacrine (quinacrine). This dye is much cheaper and less toxic than auramin-O, which has possible carcinogenic ability. The authors report that once fecal smears are stained they can be viewed under low magnification and the *Cryptosporidium* will fluoresce, whereas yeasts do not fluoresce after mepacrine staining. As with auramin-O, all suspect specimens should be subsequently stained by the modified Ziehl-Neelsen technique for confirmation.

Weber *et al.* [7•] at the Centers for Disease Control have developed an improved stool concentration procedure that includes formalin-ethyl acetate sedimentation followed by layering over hypertonic sodium chloride solution. The new procedure was compared with the standard formalin-ethyl acetate and although both procedures had similar sensitivities for diarrheal (*ie*, watery) stool specimens, the new method gave enhance detection of *Cryptosporidium* oocysts in formed stool samples with sensitivity of 70% to 90% vs 0% with the standard method. These studies were performed with human stool samples seeded with known numbers of oocysts and the limit of detection was 5000 oocysts per gram of stool. Further evaluation of this protocol for its ability to concentrate other enteric protozoa and helminth eggs is needed.

Evaluation of new commercially produced immunofluorescent assay and ELISA tests for detection of *Cryptosporidium* spp were published (Table 1). Garcia *et al.* [8•] found good correlation of immunofluorescent assay detection of both *Giardia* and *Cryptosporidium* with a dual reagent. Specimens were also examined by routine ova and parasite examination with *Giardia* detected by trichrome stain and modified acid-fast method used for detection of *Cryptosporidium*. There were also eight specimens found negative by routine stains and positive by immunofluorescent assay, which on reexamination were determined true positives. The authors felt that the immunofluorescent assay technique was at least 10-fold more sensitive than routine stain, and time for examination of slides was decreased from 20 minutes to 30 seconds using the immunofluorescent assay.

Rosenblatt and Sloan [9•] evaluated a commercial ELISA test (LMD Laboratories, Carlsbad, CA) in a study of 296 specimens submitted to the Mayo Clinic parasitology laboratory for routine examination. The majority (82%) of specimens were preserved in 10% formalin,

Table 1. *Cryptosporidium* detection by immunofluorescent assay and enzyme-linked immunosorbent assay methods

	Specimens, *n*	Sensitivity, %	Specificity, %	Study
IFA test				
Merifluor *Cryptosporidium/Giardia* (Meridian Diagnostics, Cincinnati, OH)	230	100	100	Garcia *et al.* [8•]
ELISA tests				
ELISA *Cryptosporidium* (LMD Laboratories, Carlsbad, CA)	296	93	99	Rosenblatt and Sloan [9•]
ELISA IDEIA *Cryptosporidium* (Dako, Santa Barbara, CA)	435	100	100	Siddons *et al.* [10•]

ELISA—enzyme-linked immunosorbent assay; IFA—immunofluorescent assay.

17% were stored frozen at -65°C, and 1% (4 specimens) were tested while fresh. ELISA results were compared with those obtained from indirect immunofluorescent antibody detection, Merifluor *Cryptosporidium/Giardia* (Meridian Diagnostics, Cincinnati, OH). The ELISA sensitivity was 93%, specificity was 99%, positive predictive value was 99%, and negative predictive value was 96%. It is important to know that the ELISA was compared with immunofluorescent assay testing performed on specimen sediments, whereas the ELISA was performed on diluted stool (*ie*, unconcentrated). In this study, storage conditions did not appear to affect the test results. There was no cross-reactivity with other parasites (*ie*, *Giardia lamblia* was present in 54 samples and 16 other pathogens were present in 37 other samples).

Siddons *et al.* [10•] have reported the sensitivity of another commercially available ELISA based on a monoclonal antibody to a genus-specific antigen. In this study, the ELISA was compared with routine ova and parasite microscopic exam and a British immunofluorescent assay test. Although it is difficult to estimate the limit of detection of these assays, the ELISA tests seem comparable to immunofluorescent assay, which are felt to detect approximately 5 x 10^3 oocysts per gram of stool.

Improved ELISA technology to aid in coprodiagnosis of cryptosporidiosis is still needed in order to detect low level shedding, which can occur particularly in asymptomatic individuals (AIDS patients). Currently all enzyme immunoassay tests for cryptosporidia reported to date are genus specific. A highly sensitive species-specific test is needed for environmental testing of water sources and for specific confirmation of *Cryptosporidium parvum* in feces.

Helicobacter pylori

Studies over the past decade have resulted in the emergence of *H. pylori* as a significant gastroduodenal pathogen. Further, this organism now appears linked to the development of gastric carcinoma [11]. Consequently, detection of infection with this organism is of increased importance. Diagnosis of peptic ulcer disease or gastritis is best accomplished by endoscopy that allows for histologic analysis of the gastric mucosa and detection of the organism directly by staining or following culture of biopsy tissue. The latter requires rapid transport in medium to prevent loss of viability, and isolation of the organism takes from 5 to 7 days following incubation at 37°C in a microaerophilic environment. PCR technology has shown promise in rapid sensitive detection of this pathogen. Sensitive and specific PCR-based tests have been described previously. Because no biochemical typing schemes have been devised, strain differentiation requires restriction endonuclease analysis of chromosomal DNA. Recently, a simpler method was reported by Foxall *et al.* [12••]. They have amplified a portion of the urease gene that could be further analyzed by restriction enzyme digestion. Using these techniques, 22 clinical isolates were found to group in 10 different patterns, allowing the relationship of the organisms to be determined. These techniques provide sensitive tools with which to detect this pathogen and study the epidemiology of infection.

Clostridium difficile

Most toxigenic strains of *Clostridium difficile* produce two toxins: an enterotoxin (toxin A) and a potent cytotoxin (toxin B). The role of toxigenic strains of *C. difficile* in antibiotic-associated diarrhea and colitis is now well established. Animal studies using purified preparations of the toxins have led many to the overall conclusion that the features of gastrointestinal disease can be reproduced by toxin A alone. However, others feel that toxin B is also important for disease production because vaccination of hamsters against both toxins is needed for complete protection.

Clostridium difficile strains have been classified into 21 serogroups by using typing methods based on polyacrylamide gel electrophoresis and serogrouping. Certain groups are homogeneous with regard to toxin production, whereas others include both toxigenic and nontoxigenic strains. There appears to be a link between toxin A and B production and genetic linkage of the two toxin genes on the chromosome has been described. With the exception of strain 8864, all toxigenic isolates found to date produced either both toxins or neither toxin.

The toxin A-/toxin B+ strain, designated 8864, was recently the subject of two reports. The strain is of interest because it remains capable of producing hemorrhage and bloody fluid in ligated ileal rabbit loops, as well as producing hemorrhage and diarrhea in the hamster model of disease. Borriello *et al.* [13•] reported that the strain was most likely deleted for the toxin A gene because the strain was unreactive with both gene A–specific DNA probe and a set of six toxin A–specific primers in PCR studies. These authors felt that the toxin B produced by the prototype strains was not responsible for the disease in the animal models because it remained neutralizable by antibodies. However, a second PCR product was found when toxin B–specific primers were used.

Lyerly *et al.* [14•] published their studies of this same strain and found that it did contain a region of the toxin A gene (*ie*, the 5′ end, which is the front portion). They also found that toxin B of this strain is more toxic and possesses small amounts of enterotoxin activity. The latter was interpreted as a potential cause of disease-producing ability in hamsters.

Depitre *et al.* [15••] found the phenotype of A-, B+ was not unique to strain 8864 but also found in serogroup F strains that are isolated primarily from asymptomatic infants. These authors found no evidence of biologic toxin A using three different ELISA assays; however, PCR techniques detected fragments of toxin A. In studies aimed at the pathogenicity of these isolates, the authors also found that the toxin B of group F strains was more similar to *Clostridium sordellii* lethal toxin than to the toxin B produced by *C. difficile* VPI 10463 a prototype A+/B+ toxigenic strain. The authors also found a protective effect of colonization with a serogroup F strain in axenic mice subjected to challenge with a lethal strain.

These studies still leave unanswered questions as to the best test (*ie*, "gold standard") for detection of disease caused by toxigenic *C. difficile*. The cytotoxicity assay remains the most sensitive and specific assay. Clearly, the cytotoxicity assay for toxin B performed on infants, colonized with serogroup F strains, could be misleading. The various ELISA assays for toxin A are less sensitive than the cytotoxicity assays, yet they will provide rapid detection of the enterotoxin; truly pathogenic toxin A–negative strains appear to be limited in number. More studies are needed to more thoroughly characterize isolates linked with pseudomembranous colitis, and antibiotic-associated diarrhea, and determine their toxin-producing abilities both genetically and phenotypically.

Vibrio cholerae O139

Beginning in late 1992, an epidemic of cholera-like illness had been identified and found to extend along a 1000 mile stretch of the Bay of Bengal from Madras, India to Bangladesh [16–18]. The strains of atypical *Vibrio cholerae* could not be identified as any of the known types and a new serogroup O139 was created [19]. The emergence of *V. cholerae* O139 represents a change in the recognized causes of epidemic cholera. Until now, only toxigenic *V. cholerae* serogroup O1 were recognized as having epidemic potential. The appearance of this "new" infectious agent expands this definition and currently the World Health Organization asks that all nations report illnesses caused by toxigenic *V. cholerae* O139 as cholera.

A case of *V. cholerae* O139 has been documented in a traveler returning to the United States from a stay in India [20•]. Although further spread in the United States is unlikely, the potential for further spread of this organism into parts of Asia and other developing countries is probable. This new strain should be considered along with typical *V. cholerae* O1 as the potential cause of any cholera-like illness in travelers returning from the Indian subcontinent. The strain is cultured on the same media *ie*, thiosulfate citrate-bile salts-sucrose medium used for isolation of all *V. cholerae*. Isolates of non-O1 should be further characterized and a specific diagnostic antiserum for *V. cholerae* O139 is being prepared for use in the United States. [20•]

Polymerase chain reaction–mediated detection of enteric pathogens

A variety of procedures have been used to eliminate inhibition of PCR reaction by stool constituents and thereby allow for direct detection of infectious agents in feces (Table 2). Use of immunomagnetic particles coated with monoclonal antibodies has recently been reported by two groups to improve the isolation of organisms in stool and allow for elimination of fecal debris and inhibitors. Widjojoatmodjo *et al.* [21•] used pooled monoclonal antibody-coated bead suspensions reactive against Salmonella serogroups A to E in an immunomagnetic test protocol with PCR detection of a common gene sequence. The level of detection was approximately 50 colony-forming units (CFU) per PCR reaction. No data was given on the level of detection of the organism with the beads alone. The authors also found that bilirubin was inhibitory to PCR reactions at 10 μg/mL and bile salts at 50 μg/mL.

Table 2. Summary of recent polymerase chain reaction–based tests for enteric pathogens

Organism	PCR pretreatment method	PCR target	Detection level (per gram feces)	Study
Campylobacter jejuni, Campylobacter coli	—	Flagellin A	4 CFU	Oyofo *et al.* [26••]
Helicobacter pylori	—	Urease gene	—	Foxall *et al.* [12••]
Yersinia enterocolitica	—	Attachment invasion locus	—	Kwaga *et al.* [27•]
Clostridium difficile	Quiagen procedure	Toxin A	—	Boonduthun *et al.* [28•]
Vibrio cholerae	—	Chlolera toxin	—	Fields *et al.* [24•]
Shigella dysenteriae 1, Shigella flexneri	Immunomagnetic isolation	Invasion associated locus	10–15 CFU	Islam and Lindberg [22••]
Salmonella serogroups A to E	Immunomagnetic isolation	Origin of replication	10^5 CFU	Widjojoatmodjo *et al.* [21•]
Norwalk virus*	Spin column chromatography	Immunogenic protein	<100 virions	De Leon *et al.* [23••]

*Reverse transcriptase-PCR
CFU—colony-forming units; PCR—polymerase chain reaction.

Islam and Lindberg [22••] used beads coated with a single monoclonal antibody that is directed against the common epitope of the O polysaccharide of *Shigella dysenteriae* type 1 and *Shigella flexneri*. Organisms bound to the bead were boiled in water, and the supernatant subjected to amplification using a primer pair specific for a gene coded on the invasion-associated locus found in the large virulence plasmid of all four Shigella species–as well as enteroinvasive strains of *E. coli*. The target amplicon was detected by an enzymed-labeled probe. The assay was very sensitive and could be performed in 7 hours.

DeLeon *et al.* [23••] have developed a highly sensitive and specific method for detection of Norwalk viruses using a reverse transcriptase PCR oligoprobe method. Their approach consisted of partial purification of virus from fecal material by exclusion chromatography on Sephadex G-200 spin-columns (Pharmacia, Piscataway, NJ) followed by reverse transcriptase-PCR amplification and confirmation of the Norwalk virus specific product by hybridization with digoxigenin (non-radioactive) oligoprobes. The authors compared reverse transcriptase-PCR amplification of two different viral genome regions, an RNA polymerase (260 bp fragment), and putative immunogenic protein (224 bp product). Testing was performed on well-characterized stool specimens and various tissue- and cell-culture propagated viruses. Tests using the immunogenic protein primers detected 95% (19 of 20) Norwalk positive samples versus only 75% detection (15 of 20) using the polymerase primers. The spin column appeared to adequately remove fecal PCR inhibitors and was more rapid, practical, and efficient than methods described previously, *ie*, phenol choloroform extraction followed by ethanol precipitation and cellulose fiber (CF-11) chromatography.

Polymerase chain reaction has also been successfully used to determine the toxin status of *V. cholerae* strains and, according to Fields *et al.* [24•], the PCR test is more rapid and less cumbersome than other established diagnostic methods for detection of cholera toxin. Olsvik *et al.* [25•] have also used automated sequencing linked to the PCR reaction to determine the DNA sequences of the cholera toxin B subunit in a worldwide strain collection. The sequencing data identified three types of cholera toxin B subunits. Such technology can provide useful epidemiologic information and it will be interesting to apply this technology to the *V. cholerae* O139 toxin producers.

References and recommended reading

Papers of particular interest, published within the annual period of review, have been highlighted as:
- • Of special interest
- •• Of outstanding interest

1. CDC: **Update: Multistate Outbreak of *Escherichia coli* O157:H7 Infection From Hamburgers–Western United States.** *MMWR Morb Mortal Wkly Rep* 1993, **42**:258–263.

2. • HULL AE, ACHESON DWK, ECHEVERRIA P, DONOHUE-ROLFE A, KEUSCH GT: **Mitomycin Immunoblot Colony Assay for Detection of Shiga-like Toxin-producing *Esherichia coli* in Fecal Samples Comparison with DNA Probes.** *J Clin Microbiol* 1993, **31**:1167–1172.

A direct screening immunoblot method for detection of Shiga-like cytotoxin producing organisms is described. The test employs mitomycin, which induces replication of bacteriophage and increases toxin yield. The assay detected toxin producing *E. coli* in background of normal stool flora in ratios of 1:1000 to 1:5000. In a field trial of the method, the sensitivity was 88% and specificity 89% when compared with DNA probe testing.

3. • SCHMIDT H, MONTAG M, BOCKEMUHL J, HEESEMANN J, KARCH H: **Shiga-like Toxin II-related Cytotoxins in *Citrobacter freundii* Strains from Humans and Beef Samples.** *Infect Immun* 1993, **61**:534–543 .

This is the first demonstration of the intergeneric occurrence of SLT-II related toxins in *C. freundii*. The relationship of this new marker to enteropathogenicity of this organism will require future epidemiologic studies.

4. •• GONZALEZ-RUIZ A, HAQUE R, REHMAN T, AGUIRRE A, JARAMILLO C, CASTANON G, HALL A, GUHL F, RUIZ-PALACIOS G, WARHURST DC, MILES MA: **A Monoclonal Antibody for Distinction of Invasive and Noninvasive Clinical Isolates of *Entamoeba histolytica*.** *J Clin Microbiol* 1992, **30**:2807–2813.

The authors describe the production of a monoclonal antibody against a previously undescribed internal protein of *E. histolytica*. When used in an immunofluorescence assay, the monoclonal antibody was 100% sensitive and specific in its reactions with 88 isolates previously characterized as invasive or noninvasive by zymodeme analysis.

5. •• HAQUE R, KRESS K, WOOD S, JACKSON TFHG, LYERLY D, WILKINS T, PETRI WA JR: **Diagnosis of Pathogenic *Entamoeba histolytica* Infection Using a Stool ELISA Based on Monoclonal Antibodies to the Galactose-specific Adhesin.** *J Infect Dis* 1993, **167**:247–249.

The use of pathogen-specific monoclonal antibodies directed against pathogen-specific epitopes of the galactose adhesin in an ELISA format offers promise of a rapid and sensitive method for detection of pathogenic *E.histolytica* in feces.

6. • UNGUREANU EM, DONTU GE: **A New Staining Technique for the Identification of *Cryptosporidium* Oocysts in Faecal Smears.** *Trans Roy Soc Trop Med Hyg* 1992, **86**:638.

The authors describe a new staining method using a fluorescent dye, mepacrine (quinacrine), which is readily available, and cheaper and less toxic than auramine O.

7. • WEBER R, BRYAN RT, JURANEK DD: **Improved Stool Concentration Procedure for Detection of *Cryptosporidium* Oocysts in Fecal Specimens.** *J Clin Microbiol* 1992, **30**:2869–2873.

The authors developed a new stool concentration technique which includes formalin-ethyl acetate sedimentation followed by layering and flotation over hypertonic sodium chloride solution. In studies of spiked stool, the new method outperformed the standard formalin-ethyl acetate technique resulting in 100% detection of oocysts in stool spiked with 50,000 oocysts per gram of feces.

8. • GARCIA LS, SHUM AC, BRUCKNER DA: **Evaluation of a New Monoclonal Antibody Combination Reagent for Direct Fluorescence Detection of *Giardia* Cysts and *Cryptosporidium* Oocysts in Human Fecal Specimens.** *J Clin Microbiol* 1992, **30**:3255–3257.

The authors document the excellent sensitivity and specificity offered by use of monoclonal antibody reagents over conventional staining methods for detection of *Giardia* and *Cryptosporidium*. The dual reagent was 100% sensitive and specific in this study of 230 human fecal specimens.

9. • ROSENBLATT JE, SLOAN LM: **Evaluation of an Enzyme-linked Immunosorbent Assay for Detection of *Cryptosporidium* spp. in Stool Specimens.** *J Clin Microbiol* 1993, **31**:1468–1471.

This is the first reported evaluation of the commercially available LMD brand ELISA (LMD Laboratories, Carlsbad CA). In 296 stool specimens, the ELISA sensitivity was 93% and the specificity was 99% when compared with test results using an immunofluorescence-assay method.

10. • SIDDONS CA, CHAPMAN PA, RUSH BA: **Evaluation of an Enzyme Immunoassay Kit for Detecting *Cryptosporidium* in Faeces and Environmental Samples.** *J Clin Pathol* 1992, **45**:479–482.

The authors evaluated a commercially available enzyme immunoassay based on a monoclonal antibody to a genus-specific *Cryptosporidium* antigen. The test was 100% sensitive and specific when compared with microscopy (testing was performed to arbitrate discrepant test samples). A few water samples were also tested and the enzyme immunoassay detected the organism when present at concentrations of 100 to 1000 oocysts/L.

11. **The Eurogast Study Group: An International Association Between *Helicobacter pylori* Infection and Gastric Cancer.** *Lancet* 1993, **341**:1359–1362.

12. •• FOXALL PA, HU L-T, MOBLEY HLT: **Use of Polymerase Chain Reaction-amplified *Helicobacter pylori* Urease Structural Genes for Differentiation of Isolates.** *J Clin Microbiol* 1992, **30**:729–741.

This paper describes a straight forward method for distinguishing different isolates of *H. pylori*. The procedure involves PCR amplification of a 2.4 kb PCR product which includes the urease structural genes. The product is then subjected to *HaeIII* restriction endonuclease digestion which produced 10 distinct patterns on agarose gels. Although only 22 isolates were studied, the method may serve as a sensitive epidemiologic tool for typing strains of *H. pylori*.

13. • BORRIELLO SP, WREN BW, HYDE S, SEDDON SV, SIBBONS P, KRISHNA MM, TABAQCHALI S, MANEK S, PRICE AB: **Molecular, Immunological, and Biological Characterization of Toxin A-negative, Toxin B-positive Strain of *Clostridium difficile*.** *Infect Immun* 1992, **60**:4192–4199.

The authors report on the characterization of a naturally occuring strain that is cytotoxic (toxin B+) but fails to produce toxin A. The authors demonstrate that the strain was capable of causing hemorrhage and bloody fluid accumulation in rabbit loops and hemorrhage and diarrhea in hamsters.

14. • LYERLY DM, BARROSO LA, WILKINS TD, DEPITRE C, CORTHIER G: **Characterization of a Toxin A-Negative, Toxin B-Positive Strain of *Clostridium difficile*.** *Infect Immun* 1992, **60**:4633–4639.

The authors examined the levels of toxic activity of the toxin B molecules produced by the novel isolate as well as a well-characterized strain. Differences were found in toxic activity as well as difference in restriction endonuclease fragments of the B genes in the two strains. Evidence that a portion of the A gene is present in the variant was also presented.

15. •• DEPITRE C, DELMEE M, AVESANI V, HARIDON RL, ROELS A, POPOFF M, CORTHIER G: **Serogroup F Strains of *Clostridium difficile* Produce Toxin B but Not Toxin A.** *J Med Microbiol* 1993, **38**:434–441.

Group F strains were characterized and found to produce toxin B, which seems to be more similar to *C. sordellii* lethal toxin than to the cytotoxin produced by prototype *C. difficile*. No toxin A activity was found.

16. RAMAMURTHY T, GARG S, SHARMA R, BHATTACHARYA SK, NAIR GB, SHIMADA T, TAKEDA T, KARASAWA T, KURAZANO H, PAL A, TAKEDA Y: **Emergence of Novel Strain of *Vibrio cholerae* with Epidemic Potential in Southern and Eastern India.** *Lancet* 1993, **341**:703–704.

17. ALBERT MJ, SIDDIQUE AK, ISLAM MS, FARUQUE ASG, ANSARUZZAMAN M, FARUQUE SM, SACK RB: **Large Outbreak of Clinical Cholera Due to *Vibrio cholerae* Non-O1 in Bangladesh.** *Lancet* 1993, **341**:704.

18. BHATTACHARYA MK, BHATTACHARYA SK, GARG S, SAHA PK, DUTTA D, NAIR GB, DEB BC, DAS KP.: **Outbreak of *Vibrio cholerae* Non-O1 in India and Bangladesh.** *Lancet* 1993, **341**:1346–1347.

19. SHIMADA T, NAIR GB, DEB BC, ALBERT MJ, SACK RB, TAKEDA Y: **Outbreak of *Vibrio cholerae* Non-O1 in India and Bangladesh [Letter].** *Lancet* 1993, **341**:1347.

20. • CDC: **Emerging Infectious Diseases. Imported Cholera Associated With a Newly Described Toxigenic *Vibrio cholerae* O139 Strain-California.** *MMWR Morb Mortal Wkly Rep* 1993, **42**:501–503.

The paper documents the first isolation of *V.cholerae* O139 in the United States and traces the epidemic underway in India and Bangladesh. This report mentions development of specific diagnostic antisera for recognition of the O139 serogroup of strains.

21. • WIDJOJOATMODJO MN, FLUIT AC, TORENSMA R, VERDONK GPHT, VERHOEF J: **The Magnetic Immunopolymerase Chain Reaction Assay for Direct Detection of Salmonellae in Fecal Samples.** *J Clin Microbiol* 1992. **30**:3195–3199.

The authors used immunomagnetic separation and PCR to detect *Salmonella* belonging to serogroups A to E in fecal samples. The magnetic beads were prepared using six separate monoclonal antibodies and pooled for use in the assay. The sensitivity of the assay was 10^5 CFU/mL of feces.

22. •• ISLAM D, LINDBERG AA: **Detection of *Shigella dysenteriae* Type 1 and *Shigella flexneri* in Feces by Immunomagnetic Isolation and Polymerase Chain Reaction.** *J Clin Microbiol* 1992, **30**:2801–2806.

The study describes a new assay which combines the isolation of shigellae from stool by reaction with antibody coated magnetic beads. DNA from the organisms is released by lysing the bacteria in boiling water followed by PCR amplification of a invasion-associated locus.

23. •• DE LEON R, MATSUI SM, BARIC RS, HERRMANN JE, BLACKLOW NR, GREENBERG HB, SOBSEY MD: **Detection of Norwalk Virus in Stool Specimens by Reverse Transcriptase-Polymerase Chain Reaction and Nonradioactive Oligoprobes.** *J Clin Microbiol* 1992, **30**:3151–3157.

The authors describe a sensitive and specific method of detection of Norwalk virus in stool sample. Their test approach involved use of spin-column chromatography to partially purify the virus from fecal debris.

24. • FIELDS PI, POPOVIC T, WACHSMUTH K, OLSVIK O: **Use of Polymerase Chain Reaction for Detection of Toxigenic *Vibrio cholerae* O1 Strains From the Latin American Cholera Epidemic.** *J Clin Microbiol* 1992, **30**:2118–2121.

Polymerase chain reaction amplification was used to detect a 564-bp fragment of the cholera toxin A subunit gene and thereby identify toxigenic *V. cholerae* O1 strains. One hundred-forty isolates were found to be toxigenic both by PCR and a routine ELISA . In addition, 100% specificity was found when 87 other well-characterized strains of *V. cholerae* and three other genera were tested.

25. •• OLSVIK O, WAHLBERG J, PETTERSON B, UHLEN M, POPOVIC T, WACHSMUTH IK, FIELDS PI: **Use of Automated Sequencing of Polymerase Chain Reaction-generated Amplicons to Identify Three Types of Cholera Toxin Subunit B in *Vibrio cholera* O1 Strains.** *J Clin Microbiol* 1993 **31**:22–25.

The authors sequenced the cholera toxin B subunit of 45 *V. cholerae* O1 strains isolated in 29 countries over 70 years. Three types of subunits were identified and were found to be consistent in strains isolated over long time periods. This technology has implications for vaccine development and diagnostic tests for cholera toxin.

26. •• OYOFO BA, THORNTON SA, BURR DH, TRUST TJ, PAVLOVSKIS OR, GUERRY P: **Specific Detection of *Campylobacter jejuni* and *Campylobacter coli* by Using Polymerase Chain Reaction.** *J Clin Microbiol* 1992, **30**:2613–2619.

The authors have developed the first sensitive PCR test for routine detection of thermophilic Campylobacter species. Primer pair for a conserved 5′ region of the gene (encoding one of the flagellin subunits) was used to amplify a 450-bp region by PCR. The assay could detect as little as 0.0062 pg of purified *C. coli* DNA. When human stool was tested, between 30 to 60 bacteria/PCR assay were detected.

27. • KWAGA J, IVERSEN JO, MISRA V: **Detection of Pathogenic *Yersinia enterocolitica* by Polymerase Chain Reaction and**

Digoxigenin-labeled Polynucleotide Probes. *J Clin Microbiol* 1992, **30**:2668–2673.

Accurate and rapid detection of pathogenic yersiniae was achieved using 19-base oligonucleotide primers to detect the *ail* (attachment invasion locus) gene conserved only in pathogenic strains. The target for amplification is found on the chromosome. Previous methods have targeted genetic sequences on a virulence plasmid and loss of the plasmid can lower detection frequencies. This method appears to have greater reliability.

28. • BOONDEEKHUN HE, GURTLER V, ODD ML, WILSON VA, MAYALL BC: **Detection of *Clostridium difficile* Enterotoxin Gene in Clinical Specimens by the Polymerase Chain Reaction.** *J Med Microbiol.* 1993, **38**:384–387.

The authors used a rapid DNA extraction using a Quiagen procedure followed by PCR amplification of the enterotoxin A gene. The procedure was completed within 3 hours.

Grace M. Thorne, PhD, Rapid Diagnostic Laboratory, Farley Building, Room 830, Children's Hospital, 300 Longwood Avenue, Boston, MA 02115, USA.

Small intestine

Editorial overview

Robin C. Spiller, MD

Queen's Medical Centre, University Hospital, Nottingham, UK

Current Opinion in Gastroenterology 1994, **10**:119–120

Water and electrolyte absorption and secretion

The ability to study the complexity of whole tissues without destroying their integrity is vital in building up a complete picture of intestinal function. Various attempts have been made to localize the site of chloride secretion using disruptive models that involve destroying the villi with hypertonic solutions. These studies have implied that secretion is mainly from the intestinal crypts. However, voltage scanning with micro-electrodes of an intact epithelium have been used recently to show that after allowing for the differences in surface area, the crypt and surface epithelia are equally involved in cyclic AMP–mediated chloride secretion in the rat distal colon. Other attempts to get closer to the pathologic situation are the recent use of cholera toxin to induce a secretory state in an intestine, which is used to test the efficiency of oral rehydration solutions. This model may be a better way of assessing such treatments than the previously used model which utilized a normal intestine.

There is much interest now in the inflammatory mediators that cause intestinal secretion and hence diarrhea. Isolated human derived crypt intestinal cells can be stimulated to secrete by contact with neutrophils. The active agent has recently been shown to be 5′ - AMP, which is apparently hydrolyzed to an adenosine that activates receptors on the apical membrane of the enterocyte.

As well as host-derived factors, bacterial toxins are undoubtedly important in colonic inflammation disease. One such toxin, endotoxin, has recently been shown to increase colonic permeability at doses that do not produce any obvious histologic defects. There is inhibition of water absorption in the colon, but not in the small bowel. Interestingly, the endotoxin had no effect on isolated cells implying that it works via intermediary factors such as inflammatory cells within the mucosa. The increased permeability that ensues may allow further ingress of bacterial products, which may produce a vicious circle of inflammation and increase permeability. The associated chloride secretion is probably a mechanism designed to wash out these inflammatory factors and induce diarrhea, thus terminating this vicious cycle.

Another group of toxins, the verotoxins, so called because of their toxicity to Vero cells in tissue culture, are produced by a group of *Escherichia coli* responsible for hemorrhagic enteritis. These toxins produce impaired sodium absorption and stimulate chloride secretion. Microscopically, this is associated with microvillus damage in the colon, but in animals infected with these organisms the small bowel is quite normal and its absorptive function unchanged.

It is clear that more detailed exploration of the interaction between bacterial toxins and colonic mucosa will throw light on the pathophysiology of the diarrhea in inflammatory bowel disease. The entire picture is likely to be extremely complex, involving both direct toxicity of bacterial products on epithelial cells as well as indirect effects via inflammatory cells and direct effects of bacterial toxins on mucosal nerves causing secondary changes in secretion. Detailed understanding of these complex interactions will allow targeting of specific therapies designed to minimize inflammation and its consequent diarrhea.

Pathophysiology and pharmacology of small intestinal motility

The initial excitement over the discovery of nitric oxide as a new neurotransmitter continues with the demonstration that nitric oxide solutions induce hyperpolarization and relaxation of human jejunal circular muscle. Furthermore, *in vitro* studies show that the nonadrenergic, noncholinergic inhibition induced by stimulating such preparations is attenuated by nitric oxide synthetase inhibitors. These developments are likely to be followed by the development of new pharmacologic agents acting via nitric oxide to modify motility in the not too distant future.

Likewise, there are numerous reports this year looking at indications and use of a number of novel prokinetics including cisapride, loxiglumide, and erythromycin and its derivatives. One erythromycin derivative, EM523, shows particular promise, being 18 times more potent than the native erythromycin, but without antibacterial effects. EM523 is capable of inducing migrating motor complexes (MMCs) within the human stomach at a dose as low as 0.5 mg intravenously. These

Abbreviation

MMC—migrating motor complex.

 ISBN 1-85922-607-8 ISSN 0267–1379

MMCs propagate well into the duodenum with an associated rise in plasma motilin, much more closely mimicking the normal MMC than those induced by erythromycin. This suggests that EM523 will be a much more effective prokinetic and we look forward to clinical trials with this drug.

The basic control of the MMC continues to be explored. The activity in phase 2 has now been shown to be stimulated by gas and luminal contents, a feature that makes teleologic sense if one of the functions of the MMC is to clear the small bowel of debris. Lack of detailed analysis of clinical problems has been a major weakness in previous motility research but this tendency is being addressed as more sophisticated techniques become available. Of particular interest is the elegant study from the Mayo Clinic in which a combination of scintigraphy and manometry with computer aided analysis of postprandial activity has allowed a detailed description of the functional problems in patients with symptoms after a partial gastrectomy with a Roux loop. The efferent Roux loop shows evidence of stasis and jejuno-gastric reflux in those patients with symptoms. This is associated with fewer propagated contractions in the postprandial period and elegantly explains much of their symptomatology.

Radiology of the small bowel

The abdomen with its mobile, hollow structures has usually been seen as a rather unfavorable area for conventional computed tomography assessment, but a number of recent papers have explored its utility in dealing with the abdomen. In particular, computed tomography appears to be useful in demonstrating closed loop obstruction and features of strangulation in patients with small bowel adhesions. Thickening of the bowel wall and engorgement of mesenteric vessels are helpful signs.

Another advance has been the use of Doppler ultrasound in diagnosing visceral ischemia, a condition which previously has required an arteriogram. A raised peak systolic velocity or absence of flow is able to predict with some accuracy clinically relevant stenoses in the celiac axis and the superior mesenteric artery. However, there is no doubt that the clinician wanting to take things further and perform vascular surgery on such patients would still require an arteriogram because of the superior definition that this gives. Doppler ultrasound is therefore a useful screening test for visceral ischemia.

The mobility of the bowel causes some difficulty when using scintigraphy to localize obscure gastrointestinal bleeding. Using substantial amounts of radiolabel, small amounts of blood loss can be detected by isotope appearing within the lumen. A recent study has shown that dynamic scintigraphy with pictures taken at 15-second intervals provides more accurate localization of bleeding source. Infrequent imaging either misses bleeding altogether or tends to indicate it is occurring in a region lower than it really is, as in many cases isotope is seen to rapidly move from its point of entry distally down the bowel, reflecting the laxative properties of blood. More sophisticated dynamic imaging allows a diagnosis in up to half the patients, depending on the precise series studied and are plainly a valuable addition to the assessment of these otherwise very difficult patients.

Surgery of the small intestine

The speed with which Crohn's disease relapses is often disappointing to those surgeons who feel they have removed the apparently discrete, radiologically visible lesions. However, several recent papers show that careful endoscopic assessment of the whole small bowel clearly demonstrates that the radiologically visible lesion is only the tip of the iceberg. In many cases, superficial erosions can be detected throughout the small bowel and plainly, removing the terminal ileum leaves many other lesions. Assessment of these lesions nonendoscopically would obviously be attractive and an important paper using the lactulose/mannitol permeability test suggests that those with evidence of deranged permeability are more likely to relapse. This is no doubt a noninvasive way of demonstrating multiple, radiologically invisible Crohn's ulcers throughout the small bowel.

Understanding the pathogenesis of Crohn's disease remains a very important area of research with much recent evidence focusing on the interaction between inflammatory mediators released in response to bacterial toxins. A recent study has drawn attention to the occurrence of axonal degeneration in Crohn's disease. A similar lesion has been observed after ileal pouch formation in patients who develop bacterially mediated pouchitis. This lesion is found in those in whom a colectomy has been performed both for ulcerative colitis and familial adenomatous polyposis, suggesting that it is not unique to Crohn's disease but may reflect the impact of chronic inflammation. Some of the possible mediators include proteins released from eosinophils which are capable of causing the axonal damage observed. Occult Crohn's disease may be a cause for pouch failure in patients operated on for what was initially thought to be ulcerative colitis. After the initial enthusiasm accompanying any new technique, there is now the opportunity to review large series (253 and 168) of patients showing improving results with increasing experience and a pouch failure rate varying between 30% and 10%.

Robin C. Spiller, MD, University Hospital, Queen's Medical Cent-re, Nottingham NG7 2 UH, UK.

A parable on the dangers of overclassification: can an enterocyte assume immune functions?

Editorial review

William F. Stenson, MD, and David H. Alpers, MD

Washington University School of Medicine, St. Louis, Missouri, USA

Enterocytes express proteins associated with immune functions when incubated with proinflammatory cytokines. They express major histocompatibility complex class II molecules associated with antigen presentation and increase the expression of the polymeric immunoglobulin receptor, which is involved in immunoglobulin A secretion. They also acquire the ability to synthesize and secrete acute-phase reactants and cytokines and to express enzymes (cyclooxygenase II and 12-lipoxygenase), involved in the synthesis of lipid mediators of inflammation. Finally, proinflammatory cytokines induce the synthesis of manganese superoxide dismutase, an enzyme that is not associated with an immune function in the enterocyte but rather with enterocyte self-defense against reactive oxygen species, products of immune activation from other cell types. These findings suggest that immune activation affects enterocytes by inducing the expression of genes associated with immune function, allowing the enterocytes to function as accessory immune cells.

Current Opinion in Gastroenterology 1994, **10**:121–124

Traditionally, the enterocyte monolayer is thought to serve as the barrier between the host and the contents of the intestinal lumen and it plays important roles in nutrient absorption and fluid and electrolyte absorption and secretion. However, there are many examples of cells which change phenotype under conditions of stress, such as inflammation. Because enterocytes are situated close to both intraepithelial lymphocytes and immune cells in the lamina propria, interactions between immune cells and enterocytes are beginning to be explored. A recent review has focused on the effects of products of the immune system on enterocyte function, particularly electrolyte absorption and secretion [1]. A series of studies have established that immune activation and infection can also affect enterocytes by inducing the expression of genes associated with immune function, allowing enterocytes to function as immune cells in the face of immune activation or infection. In this review, we will focus on this aspect of enterocyte interactions with the immune system, an aspect that might be overlooked by the traditional topic-oriented approach used in this series.

Major histocompatibility complex class II molecules serve to present peptide antigens to CD4+ helper T lymphocytes. The expression of class II antigens on monocytes, macrophages, and B lymphocytes is required for these cells to function as antigen-presenting cells. Over the past few years, normal and malignant nonlymphoid/monocytic cells have been described that are capable of expressing class II antigens in the setting of inflammation or interferon-γ. Enterocytes exposed to chronic inflammation in celiac sprue demonstrate class II antigen production (HLA-DQ), especially at villous tips [2].

In a recent study, the expression of class II antigen on human intestinal epithelial cells was assessed by immunohistochemistry [3]. The class II antigen HLA-DR was present in normal small bowel epithelial cells with diminished but present expression in the colon. HLA-DP staining was less prominent and HLA-DQ staining was absent. In inflammatory bowel disease, the expression of both HLA-DR and HLA-DP was increased but that of HLA-DQ remained absent. These findings suggest that major histocompatibility complex class II molecules can be induced by inflammatory mediators. This suggestion is supported by *in vitro* experiments, in which treatment of the human epithelial cell line T84 with interferon-γ induced the expression of HLA-DR but not HLA-DQ or HLA-DP.

Gut epithelial cells expressing class II antigens can act as stimulators in both autologous and allogeneic mixed

Abbreviations
12-HETE—12-*S*-hydroxy-eicosatetraenoic acid; **TNF**—tumor necrosis factor.

 ISBN 1-85922-607-8 ISSN 0267–1379

lymphocyte reactions. These cells are also capable of taking up the cellular antigen, tetanus toxoid, processing it, and presenting it to tetanus-primed T cells [4]. Thus, gut epithelial cells expressing class II antigens are capable of processing and presenting antigen in vitro. Whether or not these cells act as antigen presenting cells in intestinal inflammation in vivo is not clear.

Both interferon-γ and tumor necrosis factor (TNF)-α up-regulate the expression of secretory component, the receptor of polymeric immunoglobulin, on a human colonic carcinoma cell line (HT-29) [5,6]. The increase in expression of the polymeric immunoglobulin receptor is associated with a similar increase in the binding of polymeric immunoglobulin A to HT-29 cells treated with interferon-γ. Interferon-γ is produced by T cells during immune responses, whereas, TNF-α is produced by activated macrophages. These findings raise the possibility that activated macrophages and T cells may promote transport of immunoglobulin A into the intestinal lumen and, thereby, enhance the efferent limb of the secretory immune response.

During the host response to inflammation, there is a dramatic increase in the concentrations of "acute-phase" plasma proteins. Many of these acute-phase proteins are predominantly derived from the liver and their production can be elicited by incubating liver cells in tissue culture with cytokines such as interleukin-1, interleukin-6, TNF-α, or interferon-γ. However, acute-phase plasma proteins are also expressed in the human intestinal epithelial cell lines derived from colon cancers, Caco-2 and T-84 [7]. In these intestinal-like cell lines, their expression is induced and regulated by interleukin-1, interleukin-6, TNF-α, or interferon-γ, a pattern similar to that seen in hepatocytes.

Among the acute-phase proteins whose synthesis can be induced in intestinal epithelial cell lines are α-1-antitrypsin, α-1-antichymotrypsin, transferrin, and ceruloplasmin. These proteins have also been found in mature enterocytes. Intestinal epithelial cell lines can also be induced to synthesize the complement proteins factor B, C3, and C4 by incubation with cytokines [8]. These results indicate that there is a repertoire of acute-phase proteins expressed constitutively in intestinal-like epithelial cells and that the synthesis of these proteins is modulated by cytokines in a manner characteristic of the acute-phase response.

There is a specificity in the effects of the cytokines and the response of each target gene and that specificity is conserved from that of hepatic cells. It seems likely that the regulation of production by cytokines reflects events in the mature enterocytes and are not merely functions of the colonic tumor cells. The ability of cytokines to induce the synthesis of complement proteins in enterocytes is especially interesting in that diseases of intestinal inflammation such as ulcerative colitis are associated with the deposition of complement proteins in the inflamed tissue.

Epithelial cells have the capacity to express and secrete several cytokines constitutively or after stimulation with proinflammatory cytokines such as TNF-α or interleukin-1. Epithelial cells have been demonstrated to make transforming growth factor-β, interleukin-1, interleukin-6, and interleukin-8 [9–11]. An especially interesting finding is the demonstration that the intestinal epithelial cell line T84 secretes interleukin-8 in response to bacterial entry [12]. A variety of invasive bacteria, including those that remain inside phagosomal vacuoles, *eg*, *Salmonella* species, and those that enter the cytoplasm, *eg*, *Listeria* monocytogenes, stimulate this response. Increased interleukin-8 messenger RNA levels are detected within 90 minutes after infection. Neither bacterial lipopolysaccharide nor noninvasive bacteria, including *Escherichia coli*, induce an interleukin-8 response. interleukin-8 is a potent neutrophil chemotactic factor. Thus, these findings suggest that epithelial cells are a component of an early signaling system important in the activation of immune and inflammatory cells in the underlying mucosa following bacterial entry.

Human inflammatory bowel disease and other intestinal diseases marked by inflammation are associated with increased synthesis of prostaglandin E_2 and other cyclooxygenase products [13–15]. In patients with inflammatory bowel disease, eicosanoid synthesis has been assessed by rectal dialysis [13] and production by mucosal explants from surgical resections [14]. The preponderance of evidence suggests that most of the prostanoids present in intestinal inflammation are products of lamina propria inflammatory cells [15]; however, epithelial cells are also capable of producing prostaglandin E_2 and other eicosanoids.

For many years, it was thought that the only regulatory step in the production of prostanoids was the availability of arachidonic acid. Agents such as bradykinin that induce intestinal prostaglandin production act by stimulating cellular phospholipases that release arachidonic acid from membrane phospholipids. The released arachidonic acid is converted to prostanoids by cyclooxygenase.

Over the past few years, it has become clear that in many cell types there is more than one cyclooxygenase. Most mammalian cells contain cyclooxygenase I which is a constitutive enzyme. Some cells are also capable of expressing cyclooxygenase II, which is not expressed under basal conditions, but is expressed only when cells are stimulated with proinflammatory cytokines [16,17]. The human intestinal epithelial cell line Caco-2 can be induced to express cyclooxygenase II by incubation with TNF-α [18]. Thus, prostanoid production in human intestinal epithelial cells is controlled not only at the level of the availability of arachidonic acid, but also at the level of the synthesis of cyclooxygenase II.

Some cyclooxygenase products, including prostaglandin E_2, have proinflammatory effects, but in human inflammatory bowel disease, at least, prostaglandin E_2 production appears to be an immunomodulatory event that down-regulates the inflammatory response [19]. The evidence for this is that drugs, such as indomethacin, that selectively inhibit cyclooxygenase have no beneficial therapeutic effects in inflammatory bowel disease; in many patients these drugs exacerbate the severity of the disease. These findings raise the possibility that in intestinal inflammation the induction of cyclooxygenase II in intestinal epithelial cells serves to down-regulate the immune response.

Intestinal inflammation also affects the expression of lipoxygenase genes in the intestinal epithelium. One of several lipoxygenases found in mammalian tissues is 12-lipoxygenase, which catalyzes the conversion of arachidonic acid to the monohydroxyfatty acid 12-*S*-hydroxy-eicosatetraenoic acid (12-HETE). Increased 12-HETE synthesis by colonic tissue in patients with inflammatory bowel disease has been reported, but the cellular course of the 12-HETE-forming activity has not been established [14]. In normal human colonic tissue and in noninflamed colonic tissue from patients with ulcerative colitis and Crohn's disease, epithelial cells do not contain detectable 12-lipoxygenase antigen or exhibit significant 12-lipoxygenase activity. However, in inflamed colonic tissue from patients with ulcerative colitis and Crohn's disease, there is 12-lipoxygenase antigen in mucosal and glandular epithelial cells, as assessed by immunohistochemistry, and corresponding increases in 12-lipoxygenase activity, as assessed by incubating mucosa with exogenous arachidonic acid [20].

The increased levels of 12-lipoxygenase in epithelial cells in regions of the colon affected by inflammatory bowel disease and the absence of detectable 12-lipoxygenase in noninflamed areas of the same colons suggests that epithelial cell 12-lipoxygenase is induced by local mediators of inflammation and that epithelial cells may be the source of 12-HETE synthesis. In contrast to the established functional capacities of 5-lipoxygenase products (in particular, leukotriene B4), the biological roles of arachidonate 12-lipoxygenase products are less certain. The identification of high levels of 12-lipoxygenase in airway epithelial cells, vascular endothelial cells, and human keratinocytes has been related to the role of each of these cells types in host defense and to the localization of these cells at the boundary between host and environment. Thus, although we do not know the functional role of 12-lipoxygenase products in the inflamed intestine, there are data to suggest that they may be mediators of the inflammatory response.

Much of the damage to intestinal epithelial cells in inflammation is thought to be mediated by reactive oxygen species produced by activated neutrophils and macrophages. Superoxide and other reactive oxygen species damage enterocytes by oxidation and inactivation of enzymes, polysaccharide depolymerization, and DNA base modification. Damage also occurs by peroxidation of polyunsaturated lipids in the plasma membrane which then act as chemoattractants and perpetuate the inflammatory response. The ubiquitous nature of reactive oxygen species has required that all organisms develop intracellular and extracellular mechanisms for their detoxification. Among the intracellular defense mechanisms are manganese superoxide dismutase and copper/zinc superoxide dismutase. Superoxide dismutases catalyze the reaction of superoxide with hydrogen ions to yield hydrogen peroxide and oxygen. TNF-α, interleukin-1, and lipopolysaccharide are all involved in the induction of adhesion molecules on endothelial cells which results in the enhanced migration of leukocytes into the inflamed intestine. These same agents, incubated with the rat intestinal crypt-derived epithelial cell lines IEC-6 or IRD-98, induce in a marked increase in manganese superoxide dismutase, an enzyme which would protect the enterocytes from reactive oxygen species produced by activated leukocytes [21]. No changes were observed in the expression of copper/zinc superoxide dismutase.

These studies suggest that, in the face of inflammation, intestinal epithelial cells express proteins related to immune functions. The patterns of expression of enterocyte proteins in response to inflammation suggest important regulatory roles for certain proinflammatory cytokines. Interferon-γ induces both major histocompatibility complex class II antigen expression and the polymeric immunoglobulin receptor. The combination of interleukin-1 and interleukin-6 induces the expression of a wide range of acute-phase reactants. Thus, individual cytokines or combination of cytokines induce the expression of groups of genes which transform enterocytes into accessory immune cells. The production of interleukin-8 by T84 cells in response to bacterial entry is of particular interest in that it demonstrates that enterocytes can assume immune functions as a direct response to an invading pathogen without the mediation of proinflammatory cytokines produced by other cell types.

Inflammation clearly induces enterocytes to assume accessory immune functions. This raises the question as to whether this change in enterocyte phenotype results in up-regulation or down-regulation of the inflammatory response. Some of the functional changes induced in enterocytes by inflammatory cytokines and invading pathogens clearly up-regulate the inflammatory response. Interleukin-8 production up-regulates the inflammatory response by recruiting neutrophils into the site of infection. Enhanced expression of the polymeric immunoglobulin receptor up-regulates the immune response by facilitating the secretion of immunoglobulin A into the intestinal lumen. Expression of major histocompatibility complex class II antigens presumably allows enterocytes to present peptide antigens to $CD4^+$ T cells and thus is also probably part of the up-regulation of the immune and inflammatory responses. The induction of Cyclooxygenase II by TNF may either up-regulate or down-regulate the immune response depending on the effect of prostaglandin E_2 in this context, although as discussed above there is a suggestion that the primary effect of prostaglandin E_2 in intestinal inflammation is to down-regulate the immune response. Thus, the major functional effect of the phenotypic switch of enterocytes to accessory immune cells appears to be up-regulation of the immune response. However, it is unlikely that all the immune changes in enterocytes induced by inflammation have been uncovered and it may be that important down-regulatory events are yet to be revealed. Moreover, the array of immune proteins induced is a function of which cytokines are present and may vary among inflammatory disorders and even during the evolution of a single inflammatory process. Further understanding of the predicted response to anti-inflammatory agents in the intestine will need to take account of *all* mucosal cells, including immunocytes *and* enterocytes.

References

1. McKay DM, Perdue MH: **Intestinal Epithelial Function: The Case for Immunophysiological Regulation Cells and Mediators.** *Dig Dis Sci* 1993, **38**:1377–1388.
2. Scott H, Sollid LM, Fausa O, Brandtzaeg P, Thorsby E: **Expression of Major Histocompatibility Complex Class II Subregion Products by Jejunal Epithelium in Patients With Coeliac Disease.** *Scand J Gastro* 1987, **26**:563–573.
3. Mayer L, Eisenhardt D, Salomon P, Bauer W, Plous R, Piccinini L: **Expression of Class II Molecules on Intestinal Epithelial Cells in Humans: Differences Between Normal and Inflammatory Bowel Disease.** *Gastroenterology* 1991, **100**:3–12.
4. Mayer L, Shlein R: **Evidence for Function of Ia Molecules on Gut Epithelial Cells in Man.** *J Exp Med* 1987, **166**:1471–1483.
5. Sollid LM, Kvale D, Brandtzaeg P, Markussen G, Thorsby E: **Interferon-Gamma Enhances Expression of Secretory Component, the Epithelial Receptor for Polymeric Immunoglobulins.** *J Immunol* 1987, **138**:4303–4306.
6. Kvale D, Lovhaug D, Sollid LM, Brandtaeg P: **Tumor Necrosis Factor-Alpha Upregulates Expression of Secretory Component, the Epithelial Receptor for Polymeric Ig.** *J Immunol* 1988, **140**:3086–3089.
7. Molmenti EP, Zimbaras T, Perlmutter DH: **Evidence for an Acute Phase Response in Human Intestinal Epithelial Cells.** *J Biol Chem* 1993, **268**:14116–14124.
8. Andoh A, Fujiyama Y, Bamba T, Hosoda S: **Differential Cytokine Regulation of Complement C3, C4, and Factor B Synthesis in Human Intestinal Epithelial Cell Line, Caco-2.** *J Immunol* 1993, **151**:4239–4247.
9. Koyama SY, Podolsky DK: **Differential Expression of Transforming Growth Factors α and β in Rat Intestinal Epithelial Cells.** *J Clin Invest* 1989, **83**:1768–1773.
10. Radema SA, Vandeventer SJH, Cerami A: **Interleukin 1β is Expressed Predominantly by Enterocytes in Experimental Colitis.** *Gastroenterology* 1991, **100**:1180–1186.
11. Shirota K, LeDuy L, Yuan SY, Jothy S: **Interleukin-6 and its Receptor are Expressed in Human Intestinal Epithelial Cells.** *Virchows Archiv B Cell Pathol* 1990, **58**:303–308.
12. Eckmann L, Kagnoff MF, Fierer J: **Epithelial Cells Secrete the Chemokine Interleukin-8 in Response to Bacterial Entry.** *Inf and Immun* 1993, **61**:4569–4574.
13. Lauritsen K, Laursen LS, Bukhave K, Rask Madsen J.: **In Vivo Effects of Orally Administered Prednisolone on Prostaglandin and Leukotriene Production in Ulcerative Colitis.** *Gut* 1987, **28**:1095–1102.
14. Sharon P, Stenson W: **Enhanced Synthesis of Leukotriene B4 by Colonic Mucosa in Inflammatory Bowel Disease.** *Gastroenterology* 1984, **86**:453–463.
15. Zifroni A, Treves AJ, Sachar DB, Rachmilewitz D: **Prostanoid Synthesis by Cultured Intestinal Epithelial and Mononuclear Cells in Inflammatory Bowel Disease.** *Gut* 1983, **24**:659–664.
16. Raz A, Wyche A, Siegel N, Needleman P: **Regulation of Fibroblast Cyclooxygenase Synthesis by Interleukin-1.** *J Biol Chem* 1988, **203**:3022–3028.
17. Fu JY, Masferrer JL, Seibert K, Raz A, Needleman P: **The Induction and Suppression of Prostaglandin H2 Synthase (Cyclooxygenase) in Human Monocytes.** *J Biol Chem* 1990, **266**:16737–16740.
18. Stenson WF, Schloemann S, Griffin G: **Tumor Necrosis Factor Induces Cyclooxygenase and Enhances Prostaglandin Production in Caco-2 Cells.** *Gastroenterology* 1993, **104**:A783.
19. Stenson WF, MacDermott RP: **Inflammatory Bowel Disease.** In *Textbook of Gastroenterology.* Editor: T. Yamada. Lippincott, Philadelphia, 1991.
20. Shannon VR, Stenson WF, Holtzman MJ: **Induction of Epithelial Arachidonate 12-Lipoxygenase at Active Sites of Inflammatory Bowel Disease.** *Amer J Physiol* 1993, **264**:G104–G111.
21. Valentine JF, Nick HS: **Acute-Phase Induction of Manganese Superoxide Dismutase in Intestinal Epithelial Cell Lines.** *Gastroenterology* 1992, **103**:905–912.

William F. Stenson, MD, and David H. Alpers, MD, Division of Gastroenterology, Washington University School of Medicine, 660 South Euclid Avenue, St. Louis, MO 63110, USA.

Small intestine absorption and secretion

Charles M. Mansbach, II, MD

The University of Tennessee, Memphis, Tennessee, USA

Major advances have occurred in the study of intestinal physiology and biochemistry. A microsomal triglyceride transport protein has been described whose importance is highlighted in abetalipoproteinemics. These patients do not synthesize microsomal triglyceride transport protein and cannot transport triglycerides, but they do produce β lipoprotein. Circulating fatty acids were shown to enter the intestine, become esterified to triglyceride, and enter a pool in which chylomicron formation is selected against. Apolipoprotein A-IV was shown to be a physiologically important satiety factor. Intestinal alkaline phosphatase was transfected into Caco-2 cells that produced a surfactant-like particle. The ontology of complex lipid synthesis in Caco-2 cells as they matured at confluence was described. Aging was shown to be associated with a reduction in glucose transporters. Protein added to the diet was shown to increase peptidases at the level of transcription. A 14-kD protein appears to be important in intracellular bile-acid transport in the ileum. Sensitized rats responded to oral rechallenge by the specific antigen with an increase in intestinal permeability.

Current Opinion in Gastroenterology 1994, **10**:125–131

Lipids

Abetalipoproteinemia is a rare autosomal recessive disorder of lipid metabolism that has received considerable attention because of the lack of production of the β lipoprotein–containing major triacylglycerol transport lipoproteins, chylomicrons, and very low density lipoproteins (VLDLs) in these patients. Interest was peaked even more by the finding that restriction fragment length polymorphism excluded a mutated apolipoprotein β gene [1]. Wetterau *et al.* [2••] have provided a possible molecular basis for abetalipoproteinemia by finding that a microsomal triacylglycerol transfer protein is abnormally expressed in abetalipoproteinemics. In the first observation, microsomal triacylglycerol transfer protein activity, expressed as the ability to transport triacylglycerol from one membrane to another, was shown to be defective in specimens from intestinal biopsies of four patients. In the second observation, data from two of these patients were further analyzed and were demonstrated to have either a frame shift mutation caused by a cytosine deletion at base 215 or a nonsense mutation caused by a C to T mutation at base 1783 [3•]. These observations have major implications for the processing of triacylglycerol for transport, because both the liver (VLDL) and the intestine (chylomicrons) contain microsomal triacylglycerol transfer protein. We eagerly await knowledge of how this protein of predicted M_r 97 K functions in the complex area of lipoprotein assembly, in which the lipids are synthesized on the cytosolic leaflet of the microsome but the lipid-containing particles form in the microsomal lumen. Pharmacologic exploitation is also possible by inhibiting triacylglycerol transfer, thus causing reduced VLDL and chylomicron production.

The intestine is normally considered to process only dietary lipid. However, in rats that absorb large amounts of glyceryltrioleate the mucosa contains triacylglycerol-fatty acid other than oleate [4,5]. From where do the endogenous acyl groups come? The possibility that circulating fatty acid might contribute to the mucosal triacylglycerol-fatty acid pool was considered by Mansbach and Dowell [6••]. It was found that albumen-bound fatty acid did indeed enter the mucosa and was synthesized into triacylglycerol. It is interesting that the specific activity of the mucosal triacylglycerol-fatty acid was considerably greater than that of chylomicron triacylglycerol-fatty acid and moderately greater than VLDL triacylglycerol-fatty acid under steady state conditions (Fig. 1). These data indicate that there are at least two pools of triacylglycerol in the intestinal mucosa: one that is destined for export via chylomicron particles and the second by a nonlymphatic route, probably the portal vein [5].

Abbreviations
SLP—surfactant-like panicle; **VLDL**—very low density lipoprotein.

 ISBN 1-85922-607-8 ISSN 0267–1379

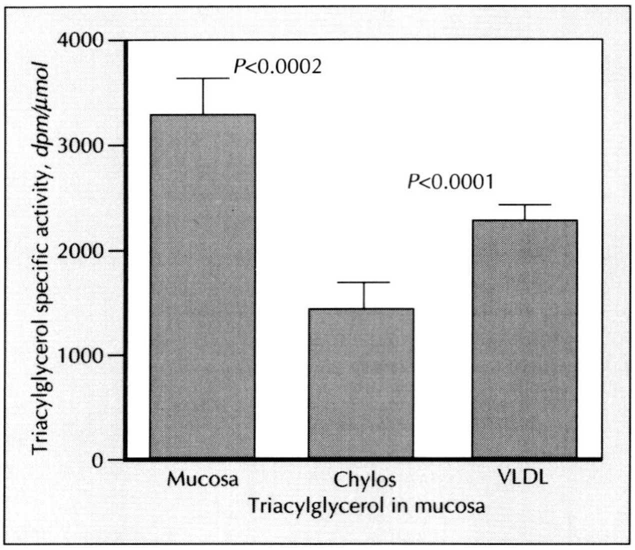

Fig. 1. Specific activity of triacylglycerol oleate in mucosa, chylomicrons (Chylos), and very low density lipoproteins (VLDL) after a 6-hour infusion intraduodenally with glycerol trioleate and intravenously with [^{3}H] oleate. Data are means ±SE of five experiments (*T-bars*). Significant differences between groups are indicated by *P* (paired *t* test) values. (*From* Mansbach and Dowell [6••]; with permission.)

Mansbach *et al.* [5] showed the portal vein to be a larger transport route for absorbed lipids than had previously been thought. Thirty-nine percent of dietary input was documented to be transported via the portal system. Because these lipids go directly to the liver, where they can either be oxidized, stored, or contribute to VLDL formation, physiological means were sought to reduce this flux. Both reducing the input load of lipid and including phosphatidylcholine (lecithin) in the glyceryltrioleate infusate were found to greatly decrease portal venous transport [7•]. This decreased lipid load to the liver would be expected to reduce VLDL production and its metabolic product, low-density lipoprotein, which is the major cholesterol transporter.

Recently, Fugimoto *et al.* [8••,9••] observed that apolipoprotein A-IV increased in the mesenteric lymph after a lipid meal. Interestingly, the authors also found that fatty lymph containing apolipoprotein A-IV or purified apolipoprotein A-IV, but not chylous lymph depleted of apolipoprotein A-IV by anti–apolipoprotein A-IV antibodies, suppressed food intake. These studies were extended to show that apolipoprotein A-IV infused into the third ventricle of rats caused food consumption to decline at concentrations that were obtainable in the cerebrospinal fluid postprandially [9••] (Fig. 2). Anti–apolipoprotein A-IV antibody placed in the third ventricle elicited a feeding response from the rats at a time when they normally do not feed. Apolipoprotein A-1 was without effect. These intriguing data suggest that the quality as well as the quantity of food eaten affects satiety, and that satiety may potentially be manipulated pharmacologically.

An important series of studies by DeSchryver-Kecskemeti *et al.* [10] has defined a surfactant-like particle (SLP) containing intestinal alkaline phosphatase that is secreted by rat jejunum. To develop a system to more clearly define a physiologic role for SLP, SLP production was determined in Caco-2 cells (a human colon carcinoma cell line that at confluence phenotypically resembles fetal human ileum) [11••]. Because only small amounts of SLP were found to be produced by these cells, Caco-2 cells were transfected with rat intestinal alkaline phosphatase, resulting not only in increases in the amount of intestinal alkaline phosphatase produced by these cells, but also in the amount of SLP produced. These striking results suggest that the overexpression of intestinal alkaline phosphatase can drive, in a yet-to-be-defined manner, the production of SLP. Although a physiologic role has not been defined for SLP, an association with lipid transport has been proposed. As Caco-2 cells transport absorbed triacylglycerol poorly, it will be of great interest to observe if triacylglycerol transport is improved by intestinal alkaline phosphatase transfection.

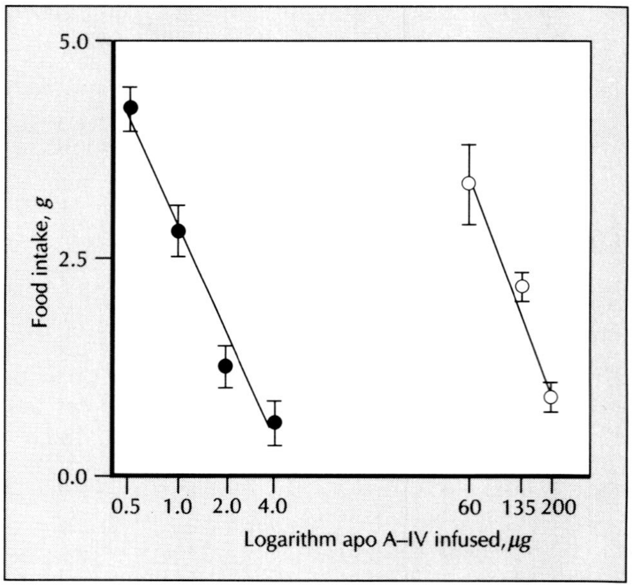

Fig. 2. The relationship between the suppression of food intake during the first 30 minutes of refeeding in 24-hour-fasted rats and the logarithm of the dose in micrograms of apolipoprotein (apo) A-IV infused either into the third ventricle (*closed circles*) or intravenously (*open circles*). Five animals were studied at each dose, and the values are expressed as mean±SE. Food intake diminished linearly with increasing amounts of apolipoprotein A-IV infused into the third ventricle ($y = -1.78 \log x + 2.84$, $r = 0.98$, $P < 0.01$). (*From* Fugimoto *et al.* [9••]; with permission.)

Caco-2 cells undergo differentiation as they become confluent. This fact was exploited by Trotter and Storch [12•] in investigating fatty-acid esterification as these cells undergo differentiation. They found that acyl-CoA synthetase activity increased and that the fatty acyl-CoAs produced were progressively incorporated into triacylglycerol as compared with phosphatidylcholine as the cells differentiated. These results paralleled the activities of diacylglycerol acyltransferase and choline phosphotransferase that control the fate of diacylglycerol, their common lipid precursor. The Caco-2 cell type was found not to express much monoacylglycerol acyltransferase activity, which is the primary route by which the intestine synthesizes triacylglycerol provided that there is enough monoacylglycerol as substrate. This lack of activity of an important enzyme may be related to the relatively undifferentiated state of Caco-2 cells, even at confluence, that has been compared to the level of a 12-day-old rat jejunum.

For many years it was thought that there were only two pathways of triacylglycerol synthesis in the intestine, *ie*, from phosphatidic acid and from sn-2 monoacylglycerol. Lehner and Kuksis [13•] now show that a third, acyl Co-A–independent, pathway exists that is a transacylase. The transacylase uses two sn-1,2(2,3) diacylglycerols, as substrate, resulting in triacylglycerol and sn-2-monoacylglycerol. The transacylase, located in the microsomal fraction, was purified to apparent homogeneity on nondenatured polyacrylamide gels, but two bands were noted on sodium dudecyl sulfate polyacrylamide gel electrophoresis, of 50 and 52 kD. The importance of this pathway to overall triacylglycerol synthesis in the intestine remains to be determined, but its presence requires that data be interpreted in light of these observations.

Carbohydrates

Some years ago it was shown that rats do not develop active sucrase-isomaltase until day 16 of life [14]. The study by Nanthakumar and Hemming [15•] was undertaken to determine if glucocorticoids could hasten the appearance of these enzymes, which are important to the terminal digestion of carbohydrates. If dexamethasone was given on day 9 after birth, by day 11 sucrose-isomaltase messenger RNA was clearly elevated and enzyme activity was present. This was due to premature gene activation. If dexamethasone was given at day 16, there was a hastening of sucrose-isomaltase activity toward the maximum due to a hastening of cryptal cells that expressed activity up the villus. Activity was not enhanced if dexamethasone was given on day 18. These studies form part of the puzzle of the control of maturation of the intestine.

It has long been known that glucocorticoids cause the precocious development of sucrase activity, along with other enzymes. Epidermal growth factor was shown by Foltzer-Jourdainne *et al.* [16•] to have similar, but not as potent, effects. Epidermal growth factor did potentiate the action of glucocorticoids, especially in the presence of sucrose. The action of epidermal growth factor was via a steroid-independent mechanism, as shown by adrenalectomy and the administration of an inhibitor of glucocorticoid activity (RU-38486). These studies suggest an interesting mechanism to enhance maturation of the intestine, without the detrimental effects of the glucocorticoids.

A potential reason for the enhanced maturation effect of epidermal growth factor is the further finding that epidermal growth factor increases the surface area of enterocyte brush-border membranes [17•]. The activity of an impermeant fluorophore in apical membranes of enterocytes was compared with that in unsealed erythrocyte ghosts. This effect was present within 10 minutes and was able to increase the surface area fourfold.

As rats age, their ability to absorb glucose declines. Ferraris *et al.* [18•] have shown that this decline is due to a reduced number of D glucose transporters in the intestine of aged rats. The apparent K_d, transporter turnover rate, and M_r of the transporter were all unchanged by age. Interestingly, uptake of several amino acids, folic acid, and nicotinamide did not decline with age. These studies suggest a possible contributor to the malnutrition seen in the elderly.

Peptides

The dietary regulation of intestinal brush-border hydrolases is complex, with multiple mechanisms of control. Little is known about peptide hydrolases. Suzuki *et al.* [19•] studied the regulation of two peptidases that hydrolyze prolyl containing peptides, angiotensin-converting enzyme and dipeptidyl peptidase IV, in rats on a high level of gelatin (high in prolyl residues, 50%) or three levels of casein. Both angiotensin-converting enzyme and dipeptidyl peptidase IV activities were increased in brush-border preparations from rats fed the high doses of casein or the gelatin at high doses. This was due to increased enzyme synthesis (as shown by Western blotting) and increased steady-state levels of messenger RNA (as shown by Northern analysis). In all cases the distal intestine had less activity than the proximal gut. These data are important to consider in poorly nourished individuals.

To better define the types of lysine transporters and as a first step toward their cloning, Harvey *et al.* [20•] injected purified intestinal poly (A)+ messenger RNA into *Xenopus laevis* oocytes. Functional expression showed that there were three different lysine transporters, one that was Na^+ dependent and two that were not. The Na^+-dependent one could be inhibited by leucine and alanine. One of the Na^+-independent transporters could be inhibited by leucine when Na^+ was present, but it was much less inhibited when no Na^+ was present. The third transporter was only inhibited by leucine when Na^+ was present. This important information will better allow functional cloning of the lysine transport systems.

The total brush-border absorptive capacity for three sugars and three amino acids was measured by Toloza and Diamond [21••] in the rat. The rate at which the rat pups gained weight was observed to have two peaks that coincided with peaks in intestinal growth and the ability to absorb glucose and proline. After weaning, proline uptake declined relative to glucose, reflecting the reduced need for bodily growth and decreasing protein intake compared with carbohydrates. Fructose uptake increased sharply with weaning, even if weaning was artificially delayed by feeding powdered milk. These data suggest that uptake capacities are coordinated with the needs of the whole animal, and that the weaning response is genetically built in rather than due to hormonal or other events occurring at weaning.

Peroxides

Lipid peroxides are potentially toxic dietary substances. Their absorption and lymphatic transport was studied by Aw and Williams [22•] in glutathione-depleted rats. Glutathione given exogenously with peroxidized lipids resulted in reduced lymphatic transport of the lipid peroxides as compared with in rats without glutathione. Studies in which inhibitors of glutathione uptake by the intestine were used showed that the expected improvement of lymphatic peroxidized lipid transport in response to intraluminal glutathione supplementation did not occur, suggesting that the reduction of the lipid peroxides occurs intracellularly. These studies suggest that glutathione, derived from vegetables, fruits, lean meats, and bile, is probably present in the intestinal lumen in concentrations that are effective in supplementing intracellular stores that prevent lipid peroxide absorption, provided that the concentration of peroxides does not exceed the intestines capacity to detoxify it.

Fatty acid hydroperoxides and H_2O_2 can be metabolized by two members of the selenium-dependent glutathione peroxidase family. Chu *et al.* [23•] show that a fourth peroxidase, GSHPx-GI, is present in the rat small intestine. It was previously known only by its complementary DNA, whose function was unknown. This cytosolic, tetrameric protein of 22-kD monomers is probably the major enzyme metabolizing H_2O_2 in the intestine, because the classic GSHPx-1 messenger RNA was not detectable.

Bile acids

Photoaffinity labeling has been effectively used by Lin *et al.* [24•] to study the transcellular transport of bile acids in rat ileum. These studies have revealed a 99-kD brush-border protein that is proposed to be the Na^+ -dependent active transporter for bile salts from the lumen. They further show that intracellular transport is facilitated by a 14-kD protein that has homology to gastropin and actin, and a 35-kD protein all found in the cytosol. A microsomal 20-kD protein was also labeled, but its role is uncertain. Finally, the bile salt is transferred to a 59-kD protein associated with the basolateral membrane and to an integral membrane 54-kD transporter. These studies show the complexity of bile acid transport even within the ileal cell. Further work more clearly defining the role of the intracellular transporters is awaited with considerable interest.

Mucins

Trefoil peptides are small peptides synthesized in goblet cells of both the small intestine and the colon. Intestinal trefoil peptides are proposed to stabilize the viscoelastic gel that mucins form at the apical portions of cells, which stabilizes the apical cell surface. As shown by Podolsky *et al.* [25•], the human intestinal trefoil peptide has a 70% homology to the rat, which is not surprising in view of the conservation of the P domain motif. *In situ* hybridization demonstrated that the peptides were synthesized exclusively in the small and large intestines. Of particular interest is the finding that intestinal trefoil peptides appears to be an early marker of goblet cell differentiation because intestinal trefoil peptides is expressed in cryptal cells prior to their being identifiable as goblet cells. Immunogold staining localized small amounts of intestinal trefoil peptides to the enterocyte, without identifiable specific messenger RNA being present. This finding suggests that the intestinal trefoil peptides was absorbed by apical-to-lateral transcytosis.

Ion absorption and secretion

Ileal neutral NaCl absorption is most often inhibited in diarrheal diseases. The ileal brush border transporter is made up of a Na^+/H^+ exchanger linked to a Cl^-/HCO^{3-} exchanger. Yun *et al.* [26•] explored the mechanism explaining the observation that glucocorticoids enhance NaCl absorption in the ileum. Methylprednisone increased steady-state levels of NHE-3 by four- to sixfold but not those of the other two exchangers, NHE-1 and NHE-2. In the glucocorticoid-deficient state, Na^+ absorption is impaired. The data suggest that NHE-3 is the major apical transporter of Na^+. Studies to determine whether or not enzyme protein is increased in response to glucocorticoid treatment are still awaited.

Electrogenic chloride secretion takes place in the cryptal epithelium of the intestine. Neutrophils invade these cells in response to luminal chemotactic factors, which creates the characteristic morphologic picture of inflammatory bowel disease. These neutrophils become activated and release a substance which, in turn, activates chloride secretion. Madera *et al.* [27••] have identified the secreted substance as 5′-adenosine by a variety of criteria. This substance is converted to adenosine by an ecto 5′ nucleotidase at the colonocyte surface. The adenosine is absorbed and drives chloride secretion. This may contribute to the diarrhea seen in inflammatory bowel disease.

The role of phosphatidic acid in chloride secretion was studied by Vajanaphanich *et al.* [28•] in T84 cell monolayers. Phosphatidic acid was found not to have a direct role in Cl– secretion itself, but it did potentiate the effect of carbachol in both increasing intracellular Ca^{2+} and Cl– secretion without altering AMP or GMP levels. Furthermore, it delayed Cl– secretion in response to vasoactive inhibitory peptide, but it enhanced the Cl– secretion driven by the heat stable toxin *Escherichia coli*. Thus, the effects of phosphatidic acid are dependent on the agonist.

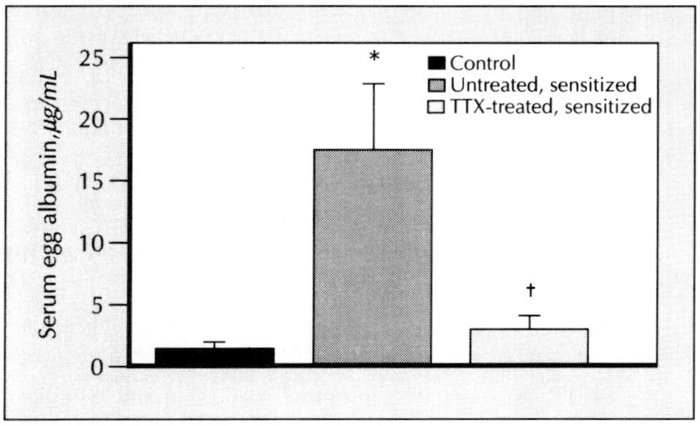

Fig. 3. Egg albumin levels in serum after antigen challenge in unsensitized control rats (*solid bar*, $n = 8$), untreated sensitized rats (*hatched bar*, $n = 11$), and tetrodotoxin (TTX)-treated sensitized rats (*cross hatched bars*, $n = 8$). T-bars represent means ± SE using maximum values obtained 1 to 3 hours after antigen challenge. Levels of immunoreactive egg albumin were increased in sensitized rats compared with controls (*asterisk* indicates $P < 0.005$) and decreased in TTX-treated compared with untreated sensitized rats (*dagger* indicates $P < 0.01$). (*From* Crowe *et al.* [29••]; with permission.)

Immunology, adaptive cytoprotection, and fatty acid binding protein

The effect of antigens on intestinal permeability has been studied by Crowe *et al.* [29••]. Remarkably, rats subcutaneously sensitized to egg albumin responded to rechallenge of antigen in the intestinal lumen with an increase in intestinal permeability within 15 minutes. This response is prior to any intestinal wall transit of the egg albumin. Bovine serum albumin had no effect. This resulted in a large (14-fold) increase in the amount of egg albumin (Stokes radius, 3.6 nm) present in the blood of the sensitized animals (Fig. 3). Mast cells were shown to degranulate in response to specific antigen challenge. Tetrodotoxin blunted these changes, indicating a neural component of these responses. These data are of considerable interest when considering the intestinal absorption of whole proteins to which an animal has been sensitized.

Adaptive cytoprotection is a phenomenon in which a low dose of an injurious agent ameliorates the injury caused by the subsequent administration of a larger dose of the same agent. Cepinskas *et al.* [30•] have shown that the prior administration of 10-mmol/L oleic acid lessened the injury to villus tip cells of rat intestine caused by 40-mmol/L oleate, as assessed morphologically. After recovery from 10-mmol/L oleate, an increase in the mucus layer overlying the villus tips was noted, and it served as a cytoprotective element when 40-mmol/L oleate was applied. Studies in Caco-2 cells showed that mucus was an important protective agent that was related to the thickness of the mucin layer, but that its protection broke down with time. These studies define a potentially important role for mucus in the intestine.

Intestinal fatty acid binding protein is a 12-kD cytosolic protein whose function remains unclear, but whose distribution is localized to the enterocytes of the intestine with predominance in the villus tips of the proximal intestine. Rottman and Gordon [31••] have used a fatty acid binding protein–human growth hormone fusion gene to probe what part of the gene is responsible for its expression in specific cell lines at different points of their differentiation. Nucleotides –103 to + 28 are able to direct expression of fatty acid binding protein in enterocytes in the correct geographic location. This sequence contains one copy of a 14-bp element which binds to two members of the steroid hormone receptor superfamily. On binding, the –103 to + 28 element is activated.

References and recommended reading

Papers of particular interest, published within the annual period of review, have been highlighted as:
- • Of special interest
- •• Of outstanding interest

1. TOLMUD PJ, LLOYD JR, MULLER DFR, COLLINS DR, SCOTT J, HUMPHRIES S: **Genetic Evidence From Two Families That Apolipoprotein B Gene Is Not Involved in Abetalipoproteinemia.** *J Clin Invest* 1988, **82**:1803–1806.

2. •• WETTERAU JR, AGGERBECK LP, BOVMA ME, EISENBERG C, MUNCK A, HERMIER M, SCHMITZ J, GARY G, RADER DJ, GREGG RE: **Absence of Microsomal Triglyceride Transport Protein in Individuals With Abetalipoproteinemia.** *Science* 1992, **258**:999–1001.

Evidence is presented that the microsomal triacylglycerol transfer protein is expressed abnormally in patients with abetalipoproteinemia. This protein may be crucial to normal neutral lipid transport because these patients have the gene for abetalipoprotein but cannot adequately transport neutral lipids.

3. • SHARP D, BLINDERMAN L, COMBS KA, KLENZIE B, RICCI B, WAGNER-SMITH K, GILL CM, TURCK CW, BOUMA ME, RADER DJ, *ET AL.*: **Cloning and Gene Defects in Microsomal Triglyceride Transfer Protein Associated With Abetalipoproteinemia.** *Nature* 1993, **365**:65–69.

The genetic defect in the microsomal triacylglycerol transfer protein is presented in two patients. One of these has a frame shift mutation and the other has a nonsense mutation.

4. PARLIER RD, FRASE S, MANSBACH CM II: **The Intraenterocyte Distribution of Absorbed Lipid and Effects of Phosphatidylcholine**. *Am J Physiol* 1989, **256**:G349–G355.

5. MANSBACH CM II, DOWELL RF, PRITCHETT D: **Portal Transport of Absorbed Lipids in Rats**. *Am J Physiol* 1991, **261**:G530–G538.

6. MANSBACH CM II, DOWELL RF: **Uptake and Metabolism of •• Circulating Fatty Acids by Rat Intestine**. *Am J Physiol* 1992, **262**:G927–G933.
Albumin-bound fatty acid was found to enter a mucosal neutral lipid pool that was selected against with respect to lymphatic triacylglycerol transport.

7. MANSBACH CM II, DOWELL RF: **Portal Transport of Long Acyl • Chain Lipids: Effect of Phosphatidylcholine and Low Infusion Rates**. *Am J Physiol* 1993, **264**:G1082–G1089.
The portal flux of fatty acids and triacylglycerols that was shown to be important in high-dose lipid infusions was considerably reduced when either phosphatidylcholine was added to a high rate of lipid infusion or the lipid infusion rate was reduced.

8. FUGIMOTO K, GARDELLA JA, TSO P: **Increased Apolipopro- •• tein A-IV in Rat Mesenteric Lymph After Lipid Meal Acts as a Physiological Signal for Saturation**. *Am J Physiol* 1993, **262**:G1002–G1006.
Apolipoprotein A-IV infused into the third ventricle of rats reduced food consumption. It is proposed that this lipoprotein is a postprandial satiety factor.

9. FUGIMOTO K, FUKAGAWA K, SAKETA T, TSO P: **Suppression •• of Food Intake by Apolipoprotein A-IV Is Mediated Through the Central Nervous System in Rats**. *J Clin Invest* 1993, **91**:1830–1833.
Apolipoprotein A-IV injected into the third ventricle in physiologic amounts reduced food intake.

10. DESCHRYVER-KECSKEMETI K, ELIAKIM R, CARROLL S, STENSON WF, MOXLEY MA, ALPERS DH: **Intestinal Surfactant-Like Material: A Novel Secretory Product of the Rat Enterocyte**. *J Clin Invest* 1989, **84**:1355–1361.

11. TIETZE CC, BECICH MJ, ENGLE M, STENSON WF, MAHMOOD •• A, ELIAKIM R, ALPERS DH: **Caco-2 Cell Transfection by Rat Intestinal Alkaline Phosphatase cDNA Increases Surfactant-Like Particles**. *Am J Physiol* 1992, **263**:G756–G766.
Intestinal alkaline phosphatase was transfected into a Caco-2 cell line, which caused the cell line to produce surfactant-like particles normally produced very sparingly in this cell line.

12. TROTTER P, STORCH J: **Fatty Acid Esterification During Differ- • entiation of the Human Intestinal Cell Line Caco-2**. *J Biol Chem* 1993, **268**:10017–10023.
The activity of neutral-lipid synthetic enzymes is explored during Caco-2 cell line differentiation.

13. LEHNER R, KUKSIS A: **Triacylglycerol Synthesis by an Sn-1,2 • (2,3)-Diacylglycerol Transacylase From Rat Intestinal Microsomes**. *J Biol Chem* 1993, **268**:8781–8786.
A novel pathway for triaglycerol synthesis is described, in which a transacylase produces one triacylglycerol and one monoacylglycerol from two diacylglycerols in the intestine.

14. HENNING SJ: **Postnatal Development: Coordination of Feeding, Digestion, and Metabolism**. *Am J Physiol* 1981, **4**:G199–G214.

15. NANTHAKUMAR NN, HEMMING SJ: **Ontogeny of Sucrase-Isoma- • ltase Gene Expression in Rat Intestine: Responsiveness to Glucocorticoids**. *Am J Physiol* 1993, **264**:G306–G311.
Glucocorticoids hasten the appearance of sucrase-isomaltase in rats, if given by the appropriate day after birth.

16. FOLTZER-JOURDAINNE C, GARAUD J-C, NSI-EMVO E, RAUL • P: **Epidermal Growth Factor and the Maturation of Intestinal Sucrase in Suckling Rats**. *Am J Physiol* 1993, **265**:G459–G466.
Epidermal growth factor is shown to hasten the maturation of intestinal sucrase in rats, and this action is less potent than the glucocorticoids.

17. HARDIN JA, BURET A, MEDDINGS JB, GALL DG: **Effect of Epi- • dermal Growth Factor on Enterocyte Brush-Border Surface Area**. *Am J Physiol* 1993, **264**:G312–G318.
Epidermal growth factor increases the surface area of the enterocyte brush border, thus increasing the absorptive surface area.

18. FERRARIS RP, HSIAO J, HERNANDEZ R, HIRAYAMA B: **Site Den- • sity of Mouse Intestinal Glucose Transporter Declines With Age**. *Am J Physiol* 1993, **264**:G285–G293.
Aged rats are shown to have a decreased number of glucose transporters.

19. SUZUKI S, ERICKSON R, SEDLMAYER S, CHANG S-K, IKEHARA Y, • KIM YS: **Dietary Regulation of Rat Intestinal Angiotensin-Converting Enzyme and Dipeptidyl Peptidase IV**. *Am J Physiol* 1993, **264**:G1153–G1159.
The dietary regulation of two peptidases that hydrolyze prolyl-containing peptides was studied and their increased activity was shown to be due to higher steady-state levels of messenger RNA.

20. HARVEY CM, MUZYKA WR, YAO SY-M, CHEESEMAN CI, YOUNG • JD: **Expression of Rat Intestinal L-Lysine Transport Systems in Isolated Oocytes of *Xenopus laevis***. *Am J Physiol* 1993, **265**:G99–G106.
Functional expression revealed the existence of three different lysine transporters.

21. TOLOZA EM, DIAMOND J: **Ontogenic Development of Nu- •• trient Transporters in Rat Intestine**. *Am J Physiol* 1993, **263**:G593–G604.
The weaning response in the intestine is shown to have a genetic basis rather than being hormonally based or related to dietary intake.

22. AW TY, WILLIAMS MW: **Intestinal Absorption and Lymphatic • Transport of Peroxidized Lipids in Rats: Effect of Exogenous GSH**. *Am J Physiol* 1992, **263**:G665–G672.
Intestinal repletion with glutathione reduces the amount of lipid peroxides.

23. CHU FF, DOROSHOW JH, ESWORTHY RS: **Expression, Char- • acterization, and Tissue Distribution of a New Cellular Selenium-Dependent Glutathione Peroxidase, GSPx-GJ**. *J Biol Chem* 1993, **268**:2571–2576.
A new glutathione peroxidase in the intestine is described that is likely to be the major metabolizer of H_2O_2 in the gut.

24. LIN MC, MULLADY E, WILSON FA: **Timed Photoaffinity Label- • ing and Characterization of Bile Acid Binding and Transport Proteins in Rat Ileum**. *Am J Physiol* 1993, **275**:G56–G62.
The proteins associated with the transcytosis of bile acids are identified by photoaffinity labeling.

25. PODOLSKY DK, LYNCH-DEVANEY K, STOW JL, OATES P, • MURGUE B, DEBEAUMONT M, SANDS BE, MAHIDA YR: **Identification of Human Intestinal Trefoil Factor: Goblet Cell-Specific Expression of a Peptide Targeted for Apical Secretion**. *J Biol Chem* 1993, **268**:6694–6702.
Trefoil peptides were shown to be synthesized only in the small and large intestine and to be early markers of goblet cell differentiation.

26. YUN CHC, GURUBHAGAVATULA S, LEVINE SA, MONTGOMERY JL, • BRANT SR, COHEN ME, CRAGOE EJ JR., POUYSSEGUR J, TSO C-M, DONOWIT M: **Glucocorticoid Stimulation of Ileal Na^+ Absorptive Cell Brush Border Na^+/H^+ Exchange and Association With an Increase in Message for NHE-3 and Epithelial Na^+/H^+ Exchange Isoform**. *J Biol Chem* 1993, **268**:206–211.
Glucocorticoids are shown to increase NaCl absorption in the ileum by increasing the amount of NHE-3.

27. MADARA JL, PATAPOFF TW, GILLECE-CASTRO B, COLGAN SP, •• PARKOS CA, DELP C, MRSNY RJ: **5′-Adensosine Monophosphate Is the Neutrophil-Derived Paracrine Factor That Elicits Chloride Secretion From T84 Intestinal Epithelial Cell Monolayers**. *J Clin Invest* 1993, **91**:2320–2325.
Neutrophils infiltrating the crystal cells are shown to produce 5′-adenosine that is hydrolyzed by an ecto 5′-nucleotidase, producing

adenosine, which in turn drives chloride transport and thus fluid secretion by the intestine.

28. VAJANAPHANICH M, KACHINTORN U, BARRETT KE, COHN JA,
• DHARMSATHAPHORN K, TRAYNOR-KAPLAN A: **Phosphatidic Acid Modulates C1-Secretion in T84 Cells: Varying Effects Depending on Mode of Stimulation.** *Am J Physiol* 1993, 264:C1210–C1218.

Phosphatidic acid is shown to have different effects on chloride secretion, depending on which agonist stimulates an intestine-like cell line.

29. CROWE SE, SODA K, STANISZ AM, PERDUE MH: **Intestinal Per-**
•• **meability in Allergic Rats: Nerve Involvement in Antigen-Induced Changes.** *Am J Physiol* 1993, 264:G617–G623.

Intestinally challenged rats presensitized to albumin increased egg albumin in the blood and were demonstrated to degranulate mast cells.

30. CEPINSKAS G, SPECIAN RD, KVIETYS PR: **Adaptive Cytoprotec-**
• **tion in the Small Intestine: Role of Mucus.** *Am J Physiol* 1993, 264:G921–G927.

Adaptive cytoprotection by oleate was shown to be due to an increase in mucus on the tips of the villi.

31. ROTTMAN JN, GORDON JI: **Comparison of the Patterns of Ex-**
•• **pression of Rat Intestinal Fatty Acid Binding Protein/Human Growth Hormone Fusion Genes in Cultured Intestinal Epithelial Cell Lines and in the Gut Epithelium of Transgenic Mice.** *J Biol Chem* 1993, 268:11994–12002.

Intestinal fatty acid binding protein is expressed geographically in the intestine due to a specific element in its DNA.

Charles M. Mansbach, II, MD, Department of Medicine, Division of Gastroenterology, University of Tennessee, Memphis, 951 Court Avenue, Room 555D, Memphis, TN 38163, USA.

Water and electrolyte absorption and secretion

Ian W. Booth, MSc, MD, FRCP, and Georgina K. Collington, PhD

Institute of Child Health, Birmingham, UK

Intestinal water and electrolyte transport mechanisms continue to be characterized in increasing depth. This review deals principally with the modulation of these processes. In particular, there is continuing interest in the effects of luminal contents on intestinal function in both normal and disease states. Various aspects of extrinsic and intrinsic neural control have been investigated by several groups whose findings are discussed.

Current Opinion in Gastroenterology 1994, **10**:132–137

Sodium-proton exchange

Electroneutral sodium chloride absorption by the small intestine is achieved by coupling Na^+/H^+ and HCO_3^-/Cl^- exchangers in the apical membrane of villus enterocytes. Yun *et al.* [1••] examined the role of Na^+/H^+ exchange in glucocorticoid-regulated sodium absorption by rabbit ileum. Pretreatment of animals with methylprednisolone stimulated Na^+ uptake across the brush border membrane, but only in the presence of a proton gradient. A corresponding increase in expression of messenger RNA encoding Na^+/H^+ exchanger NHE-3, but not NHE-1 or NHE-2, suggested the involvement of this isoform in Na^+ uptake across.

Abnormalities in Na^+/H^+ or HCO_3^-/Cl^- exchange have been associated with a number of diarrheal disorders. In a child with a mild form of congenital sodium-losing diarrhea, Fell *et al.* [2•] were able to show directly a partial defect in Na^+/H^+ exchange across the jejunal brush border membrane; glucose-coupled Na^+ transport was normal.

A number of isoforms of mammalian Na^+/H^+ exchanger have now been identified, localized, and assigned a physiologic role. Zamir *et al.* [3•] demonstrated a Na^+/H^+ antiport mechanism in human small intestinal basolateral membrane. The kinetic and amiloride sensitivity characteristics differed from the apical membrane exchanger. It has been suggested that basolateral Na^+/H^+ exchangers have a role in regulation of intracellular pH rather than sodium chloride uptake. The absence of a corresponding HCO_3^-/Cl^- antiport has been noted in a variety of tissues and species. Similarly, evidence for a basolateral Na^+/HCO_3^- cotransport system is varied but Zamir *et al.* discuss preliminary studies suggesting its presence in the human small intestine and speculate upon an involvement in pH regulation.

pH Regulation

Extracellular pH directly influences membrane transporters when a proton or bicarbonate gradient provides the driving force for their activity. In the apical membrane of rat duodenal enterocytes Brown *et al.* [4••] have characterized a Cl^- conductance, saturable at high chloride concentrations, which is potential driven but pH sensitive. In the absence of a transmembrane pH gradient, the apparent K_m for proton stimulation of this Cl^- uptake was 88 nmol/L (pH 7.05) with an apparent V_{max} of 5.5 nmol/mg/4 s. Sensitivity was localized to changes in extracellular pH. Having previously demonstrated the presence of Cl^-/HCO_3^- antiport in this membrane, the authors suggest a possible role for the proton-dependent conductance in recycling chloride to support exchanger activity, *ie*, bicarbonate secretion, when luminal microclimate pH is low.

To examine the influence of systemic acid-base variables on electrolyte and water transport in the human ileum *in vivo*, Eherer *et al.* [5•] used CO_2 breathing to induce respiratory acidosis in healthy volunteers. The small but significant changes in venous pH, pCO_2 and plasma HCO_3^- concentration had no effect upon net water, Na^+, K^+, or Cl^- absorption. However, in all subjects there was a rapid effect upon HCO_3^- transport, with increased net secretion or decreased net absorption.

Chloride transport

A resume of research that has given rise to the popular model of intestinal electrolyte secretion was provided recently by Michael Field [6••]. In this most entertaining review, the author included a personal account of work in this area and emphasized the impor-

Abbreviation

ANF—atrial natriuretic factor.

 ISBN 1-85922-607-8 ISSN 0267–1379

tance of adenosine 3′, 5′-cyclic monophosphate-activated Cl^- conductance. Although electrogenic Cl^- conductance and associated transport processes required for Cl^- secretion are now well characterized, their distribution between cells of the intestinal epithelium remains equivocal. Köckerling and Fromm [7•] stimulated Cl^- secretion in tissues from rat ileum and distal colon *in vitro* with various secretagogues. Changes in ion conductance were localized using an improved voltage scanning technique. Their observations prompted the authors to conclude that in both tissues studied, cyclic AMP-dependent Cl^- secretion occurred in cells present in crypts and on villi or surface epithelia.

There remains a necessity to identify the proteins responsible for chloride conductances in various tissues. Gabriel *et al.* [8•] presented the techniques they have used to successfully produce antibody in mice specific for proteins involved in chloride conductance demonstrated in porcine small intestinal brush border membrane. Chloride transport across the apical membrane of intestinal cells has been studied extensively whilst the pathways and mechanisms involved in basolateral transport are less well characterized. Using a vesicle preparation, Daher *et al.* [9•] investigated Cl^- transport in rat ileal basolateral membrane. In addition to an electrogenic conductance, which was insensitive to the Cl^- channel inhibitors anthracene-9-carboxylic acid and diphenylamine-2-carboxylate, chloride uptake was by bumetanide-sensitive cotransport with Na^+ and K^+. There was no evidence to indicate the presence of Cl^-/HCO_3^- or Na^+-coupled anion exchange mechanisms.

Modulators of water and electrolyte transport

Carbohydrates

There is continuing interest in determining the optimum composition of oral rehydration solutions for rehydration and maintenance of electrolyte balance in diarrheal diseases. Studies to date have been undertaken in a variety of model systems requiring extrapolation of the data to oral therapy in humans. The principal variables considered include osmolality, carbohydrate content, Na^+ concentration, and the glucose/Na^+ ratio.

Gisolfi *et al.* [10••] have used an *in vivo* segmental perfusion technique to examine the influence of qualitative and quantitative changes in perfusate carbohydrate on human small intestinal water and solute absorption. The solutions studied contained either glucose, sucrose, or seven- or three-unit glucose polymers (G7 and G3 respectively) at concentrations of 2%, 4%, 6%, or 8%. Osmolality was regulated, except in the 6% and 8% glucose solutions, by addition of sodium chloride. Net water absorption from solutions was improved by the inclusion of carbohydrate, irrespective of its nature, up to a concentration of 6% (Fig. 1). At the 8% level of inclusion, glucose or G3, but not sucrose or G7, produced substantial reductions in water absorption demonstrating the importance of carbohydrate choice at higher concentrations. Whilst net movement of water was unaffected by the glucose/Na^+ ratio, the authors demonstrated a relationship between glucose concentration and uptake that supported the hypothesis that glucose absorption at higher levels may involve mechanisms in addition to cotransport with Na^+.

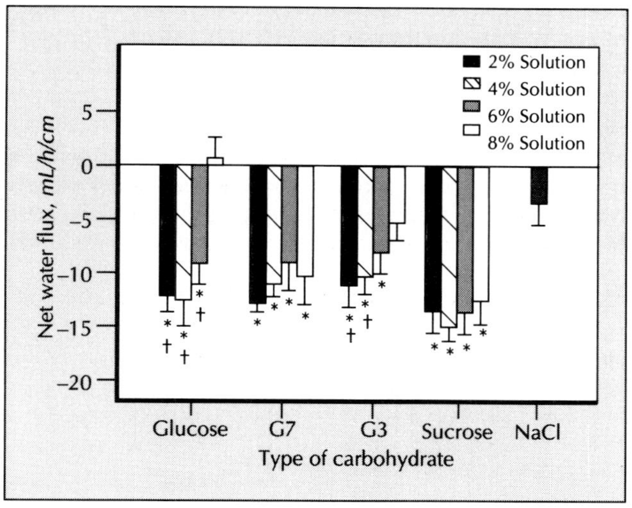

Fig. 1. Water flux in relation to carbohydrate concentration grouped by type (negative values indicate net absorption, positive values indicate net secretion). *Asterisk* indicates difference from control NaCl solution ($P < 0.05$). *Dagger* indicates difference from 8% solution of same carbohydrate type ($P < 0.05$). (*From* Gisolfi *et al.* [10 ••]; with permission.)

Rhoads *et al.* [11••] have used piglet jejunum *in vitro* to investigate the influence of L-glutamine on both intestinal electrolyte transport and tissue metabolism. The latter was assessed by measuring oxygen consumption. One crucial finding of this work was that although L-glutamine (>5 mmol/L, in the presence of mucosal or serosal glucose) or mucosal glucose increased electrogenic Na^+ uptake and raised tissue metabolism, only the amino acid stimulated electroneutral sodium chloride absorption. The authors present a model for L-glutamine stimulation of sodium chloride absorption, discuss the role of this amino acid in oxidative tissue metabolism and comment on its suitability for inclusion in oral rehydration solutions.

To evaluate the contribution of base or base precursor to oral rehyrdation solution performance, Elliott *et al.* [12•] employed an *in situ* perfusion of rat small intestine. This model system permitted study of responses in both normal and secreting tissue, the secretory state being induced by prior exposure to cholera toxin. The four oral rehydration solutions perfused enhanced water and sodium absorption but no further improvements were produced by addition of bicarbonate (30 mmol/L) or citrate (10 mmol/L) to the solutions studied.

Enteral feeding

Studies in fasted or hibernating animals have shown that prolonged withdrawal of enteral feeding alters intestinal morphology and enhances secretory capacity. Carey and Cooke [13•] have investigated this phenomenon further in the ground squirrel by creating a model that allows assessment of the direct effect of luminal contents. Animals underwent jejunal bypass or sham surgery, following which they remained active and feeding or were induced to hibernate. Ion transport studies were undertaken in Ussing chambers and results were adjusted to allow for mucosal structural differences. Tissues that had little or no exposure to luminal contents had improved short-circuit current responses to electrical stimulation of submucosal neurons, the presence of serosal carbachol, and the presence of mucosal alanine. These differences were evident in bypassed jejunum of actively feeding squirrels, suggesting direct influence of luminal contents.

Inflammatory agents

The impact of inflammatory mediators on intestinal structure and function is a particularly diverse topic. Therapeutic use may be limited by such effects and their involvement has been suggested in the pathophysiology of various diarrheal diseases. One mechanism involved in prostaglandin E stimulation of intestinal secretion has been considered by Pawlotsky *et al.* [14•] who examined the activity of adenylate cyclase in isolated guinea pig enterocytes. Prostaglandin E_2 activation of adenylate cyclase occurred in a dose-dependent manner, the magnitude of which was reduced by cholera toxin, and was inhibited by somatostatin. The prostaglandin E analogues, misoprostol and enprostil, were less effective activators of adenylate cyclase, leading the authors to remark that detrimental effects of prostaglandin administration may be reduced by judicious choice of analogue.

Ciancio *et al.* [15••] have used a rat model to investigate the effect on intestinal function of endotoxin, a lipopolysaccharide component of bacterial cell wall, which is known to stimulate inflammatory responses. Intravenous endotoxin administration had no effect upon saline absorption from small intestinal sites *in vivo* but markedly reduced uptake from the colon. Studies *in vitro* showed this decrease to be associated with an increased serosal to mucosal Na^+ flux. Endotoxin also increased colonic permeability to ^{3}H-inulin, but did not affect basal short-circuit current or conductance values. The authors consider intracellular signaling pathways that may be involved in these responses and discuss a likely role for endotoxin, possibly involving inflammatory agents, in development of the diarrhea frequently associated with inflammatory diseases.

Enterohemorrhagic *Escherichia coli* has been associated with diarrheal disease, in some cases involving extensive tissue damage. Li *et al.* [16•] have investigated enterohemorrhagic *E. coli* pathogenicity in the rabbit using a classical strain (EDL933) possessing recognized virulence properties of plasmid-encoded adhesion and verotoxin production. Infection with this organism had no effect on small intestinal structure and function but in the colon caused mucosal damage, reduced sodium chloride absorption, and increased Cl^- secretion. Other *E. coli* strains, possessing none or some of the virulence properties of EDL933, altered colonic transport to varying degrees. Neutrophil infiltration observed in infected colonic tissue prompted the authors to speculate upon a possible involvement of inflammatory mediators in enterohemorrhagic *E. coli* pathogenicity.

A neutrophil-derived secretagogue, which stimulated electrogenic Cl^- secretion from T84 intestinal cell monolayers, has recently been identified by Madara *et al.* [17••] as the ATP metabolite 5′-AMP. The authors propose a mechanism (Fig. 2) to describe how this mediator could be involved in the activation of secretory events producing diarrhea associated with inflammatory bowel disease.

Peptides

The peptide atrial natriuretic factor (ANF) has been shown to influence intestinal transport in a variety of species. Grotmol *et al.* [18•] have investigated the effect of ANF on human intestinal ion transport *in vitro.* In Ussing chamber studies with human colonic and ileal tissues, serosal application of ANF did not alter short-circuit current. Isotope flux studies revealed that ANF did not influence electroneutral Na^+ and Cl^- transport. ANF was found to enhance short-circuit current in porcine colon, a response apparently associated with electrogenic Cl^- secretion. Autoradiograph studies showed that specific binding sites for ANF are present in porcine colon, but are not evident in human distal colon.

Effects of the peptide sorbin on intestinal water and electrolyte transport have been investigated by Charpin *et al.* [19•] using *in situ* ligated duodenal loops in the rat. Responses and potency were compared with those obtained with various other intestinal peptides and synthetic C-terminal peptides of sorbin itself. Sorbin stimulated water, Na^+, and Cl^- absorption and, like angiotensin II, was active in the picomolar dose range. Unlike angiotensin, sorbin was found not to influence blood pressure. The shortest active site for synthetic sorbin peptides was the heptapeptide C-terminal end.

Neural control

Intestinal water and electrolyte transport processes are influenced by messengers originating from both intrinsic and extrinsic neurons. Kiyohara *et al.* [20•] have studied the influence of galanin, a 29-amino acid peptide with activity in intrinsic intestinal neurons, on ion transport by rat colon *in vitro.* Serosal addition of rat galanin produced a biphasic increase in short-circuit current that was dose dependent. This increase was associated with reductions in net Na^+ and net Cl^- absorp-

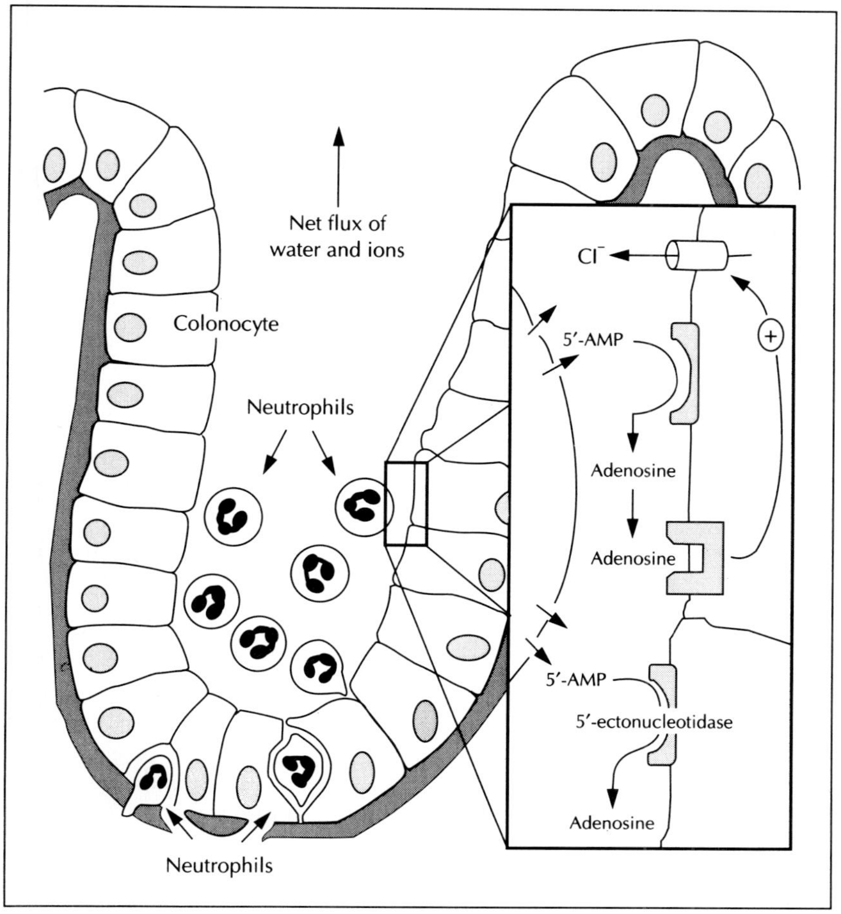

Fig. 2. Mechanism suggested for neutrophil stimulation of the secretory diarrhea associated with inflammatory bowel disorders. Neutrophils present in the crypt lumen produce the mediator 5′-AMP, subsequently converted to adenosine, which stimulates a secretory response. (*From* Madar *et al.*[17••]; with permission.)

tion. Galanin did not influence the short-circuit current generated by transmural electrical field stimulation. Their observations lead the authors to conclude that in the rat colon, galanin mediates secretion via noncholinergic nerves.

Hildebrand and Brown [21•] have presented evidence in porcine proximal jejunum to support the theory that effects of norepinephrine on active electrolyte transport are mediated by α_2-adrenoreceptors. Using chamber studies showed that serosal application of norepinephrine reduced short-circuit current with alterations in electrogenic transport varying according to basal condition. Norepinephrine inhibition of short-circuit current increases produced by electrical transmural stimulation, which were antagonized by α_2-receptor blockers, was mimicked by α_2-receptor agonists.

Because of their antisecretory activity, it is believed that α_2-receptor agonists may be of great therapeutic value. Valet *et al.* [22•] have used various α_2-receptor antagonists to provide evidence that the α_2-receptor expressed in human intestinal mucosa is of the α_{2A} subtype. Along the intestine, the receptor was found to be most concentrated in proximal colon. Within the mucosa, receptor expression was highest in crypt cells and localized to the basolateral membrane.

Chu *et al.* [23•] investigated the involvement of extrinsic and intrinsic neurons in control of water absorption *in vivo* from rat small intestine subject to a distension stimulus. Animals studied were intact or had undergone selective nerve transection. Two loops of intestine were isolated, the proximal loop was distended and net water absorption from the distal was determined by single-pass perfusion. With splanchnic nerves, intact distension of the intestine had no effect upon water absorption. Following splanchnectomy, but with vagal nerves intact, intestinal distension stimulated an increase in net water absorption. This effect was prevented by transection of vagal afferents. The authors also demonstrated, using an intracellular recording technique, that the increased water absorption was associated with a reduction in activity of vagal efferent neurons.

Small intestinal transplantation

There is continuing interest in the consequences of transplantation on structure and function of the small intestine. In particular, intestinal transplantation involves the transection of extrinsic nerves that influence water and electrolyte transport. Teitelbaum *et al.* [24••] have studied the absorptive capacity of transplanted intestine in a rat model. Jejunal water and Na^+ fluxes were determined *in vivo* 2, 4, 6, 8, and 10 days after transplant. Although both water and Na^+ fluxes were initially secretory, they became absorptive by days 8 and 6, respectively. The authors suggest that extrinsic denervation during intestinal transplant is associated with only a temporary reduction in the capacity of the jejunum to absorb water and Na^+.

References and recommended reading

Papers of particular interest, published within the annual period of review, have been highlighted as:

- • Of special interest
- •• Of outstanding interest

1. •• YUN CHC, GURUBHAGAVATULA S, LEVINE SA, MONTGOMERY JLM, BRANT SR, COHEN ME, CRAGOE EJ JR, POUYSSEGUR J, TSE CM, DONOWITZ M: **Glucocorticoid Stimulation of Ileal Na^+ Absorptive Cell Brush Border Na^+/H^+ Exchange and Association With an Increase in Message for NHE-3, an Epithelial Na^+/H^+ Exchanger Isoform.** *J Biol Chem* 1993, **268**:206–211.

Evidence that glucocorticoid-regulated Na^+ uptake across rabbit ileal villus brush border involves an effect on Na^+/H^+ exchange. Methylprednisolone treatment stimulated Na^+/H^+ exchange in parallel with increased NHE-3 message.

2. • FELL JM, MILLER MP, FINKEL Y, BOOTH IW: **Congenital Sodium Diarrhea With a Partial Defect in Jejunal Brush Border Membrane Sodium Transport, Normal Rectal Transport, and Resolving Diarrhea.** *J Pediatr Gastroenterol Nutr* 1992, **15**:112–116.

Direct evidence for a partial defect in Na^+/H^+ exchange in the jejunal brush border membrane of a child suffering from congenital sodium-losing diarrhea.

3. • ZAMIR Z, BARRY JA, RAMASWAMY K: **Sodium Transport in Human Intestinal Basolateral Membrane Vesicles.** *Gastroenterology* 1992, **103**:1817–1822.

An investigation of Na^+ transport in human small intestinal basolateral membrane vesicles. The characteristics of a distinct Na^+/H^+ exchange mechanism are described together with evidence for a minor Na^+ conductance pathway.

4. •• BROWN CDA, MCNICHOLAS CM, TURNBERG LA: **A Cl^- Conductance Sensitive to External PH in the Apical Membrane of Rat Duodenal Enterocytes.** *J Physiol* 1992, **456**:519–528.

The authors describe an electrogenic Cl^- conductance that is sensitive to extracellular pH and postulate upon the physiologic role of such a pathway if allosterically regulated by protons.

5. • EHERER AJ, PETRITSCH W, BERGER J, HINTERLEITNER T, CHARNEY AN, KREJS GJ: **Effects of Acute Respiratory Acidosis on Water and Electrolyte Transport in the Human Ileum.** *Eur J Clin Invest* 1993, **23**:206–210.

An investigation of the effects of systemic acid-base variables on water and electrolyte transport across the human ileum *in vivo* in which induction of acute respiratory acidosis produced a small but rapid and reversible effect on HCO_3^- transport.

6. •• FIELD M: **Intestinal Electrolyte Secretion. History of a Paradigm.** *Arch Surg* 1993, **128**:273–278.

A particularly interesting review given from a unique perspective.

7. • KÖCKERLING A, FROMM M: **Origin of cAMP-Dependent Cl^- Secretion From Both Crypts and Surface Epithelia of Rat Intestine.** *Am J Physiol* 1993, **264**:C1294–C1301.

A voltage scanning technique was used to determine the distribution of cyclic AMP-dependent Cl^- secretion in rat ileal and colonic epithelia.

8. • GABRIEL SE, RACETTE KJ, GASPAR KJ, FORSYTH GW: **Inhibition of Ileal Brush-Border Chloride Conductance by Specific Antibody.** *J Membr Biol* 1992, **129**:323–328.

Production of antibodies specific for proteins involved in the Cl^- conductance of porcine ileal brush border membrane.

9. • DAHER M, ACRA S, DYKES W, GHISHAN FK: **Chloride Transport Across Rat Ileal Basolateral Membrane Vesicles.** *Proc Soc Exp Biol Med* 1992, **201**:254–260.

The transport of chloride across rat ileal basolateral membrane is shown to occur by a bumetanide-sensitive $Na^+/K^+/2Cl^-$ cotransport mechanism and an electrogenic diffusion pathway.

10. •• GISOLFI CV, SUMMERS RW, SCHEDL HP, BLEILER TL: **Intestinal Water Absorption From Select Carbohydrate Solutions in Humans.** *J Appl Physiol* 1992, **73**:2142–2150.

An *in vivo* study providing considerable information about the effects of varying perfusate carbohydrate type and concentration on water and solute fluxes across human small intestine.

11. •• RHOADS JM, KEKU EO, WOODARD JP, BANGDIWALA SI, LECCE JG, GATZY JT: **L-Glutamine With D-Glucose Stimulates Oxidative Metabolism and NaCl Absorption in Piglet Jejunum.** *Am J Physiol* 1992, **263**:G960–G966.

A study into the influence of L-glutamine or D-glucose on small intestinal oxidative metabolism and ion transport prompting the authors to propose a model for L-glutamine-stimulated Na^+ and sodium chloride absorption.

12. • ELLIOTT EJ, WATSON AJM, WALKER-SMITH JA, FARTHING MJG: **Bicarbonate and Citrate in Oral Rehydration Therapy: Studies in a Model of Secretory Diarrhea.** *J Pediatr Gastroenterol Nutr* 1993, **16**:278–283.

A rat model for secretory diarrhea with *in situ* small intestinal perfusion is utilized in this investigation that provides evidence for the exclusion of base from oral rehydration solutions.

13. • CAREY HV, COOKE HJ: **Intestinal Secretion After Jejunal Bypass in the Ground Squirrel.** *Am J Physiol* 1992, **263**:R1209–R1214.

Provides evidence that luminal contents influence directly small intestinal secretory and absorptive function.

14. • PAWLOTSKY J-M, RUSZNIEWSKI P, REYL-DESMARS F, BOURGEOIS M, LEWIN MJM: **Effects of PGE_2, Misoprostol, and Enprostil on Guinea Pig Enterocyte Adenylate Cyclase.** *Dig Dis Sci* 1993, **38**:316–320.

A study in isolated enterocytes describing the activation of adenylate cyclase by prostaglandin E_2 and revealing that this may not be the principal mechanism involved in stimulation of intestinal hypersecretion by varying prostaglandin analogues.

15. •• CIANCIO MJ, VITIRITTI L, DHAR A, CHANG EB: **Endotoxin-Induced Alterations in Rat Colonic Water and Electrolyte Transport.** *Gastroenterology* 1992, **103**:1437–1443.

A study designed to investigate the possible involvement of endotoxin in development of secretory diarrhea such as that associated with inflammatory bowel diseases. Intravenous endotoxin reduced colonic but not small intestinal saline absorption *in vivo*.

16. • LI Z, BELL C, BURET A, ROBINS-BROWNE R, STIEL D, O'LOUGHLIN E: **The Effect of Enterohemorrhagic *Escherichia Coli* 0157:H7 on Intestinal Structure and Solute Transport in Rabbits.** *Gastroenterology* 1993, **104**:467–474.

The mucosal damage and abnormal transport caused by enterohemorrhagic *E. coli* infection in rabbits is confined to the colon. Studies involving various enterohemorrhagic *E. coli* strains reveals that their virulence is multifactorial.

17. •• MADAR TL, PATAPOFF TW, GILLECE-CASTRO B, COLGAN SP, PARKOS CA, DELP C, MRSNY RJ: **5′-Adenosine Monophosphate Is the Neutrophil-Derived Paracrine Factor That Elicits Chloride Secretion From T84 Intestinal Epithelial Cell Monolayers.** *J Clin Invest* 1993, **91**:2320–2325.

Secretagogue activity of purified neutrophil-derived secretagogue demonstrated using monolayers of the human intestinal cell line T84. Neutrophil-derived secretagogue, characterized by mass and Raman spectroscopic methods, was identified as 5′-AMP.

18. • GROTMOL T, RODNES JT, BUANES T, CHRISTENSEN G, LANDSVERK T: **Atrial Natriuretic Factor (ANF) Does Not Affect Ion Transport in Human Intestine but Does in Porcine Intestine.** *Acta Physiol Scand* 1993, **147**:417–429.

Atrial natriuretic factor is found not to influence electrolyte transport in human intestine. The lack of response is attributed to the absence of specific receptors for this peptide in tissues studied.

19. • CHARPIN G, CHIKH-ISSA AR, GUIGNARD H, JOURDAN G DUMAS C, PANSU D, DESCROIX-VAGNE M: **Effect of Sorbin on Duo-**

denal Absorption of Water and Electrolytes in the Rat. *Gastroenterology* 1992, **103**:1568–1573.
The intestinal peptide sorbin is shown to stimulate water and electrolyte absorption by rat duodenum *in situ*.

20. KIYOHARA T, OKUNO M, ISHIKAWA H, NAKANISHI T,
• SHINOMURA Y, YANAIHARA C, MATSUZAWA Y: **Galanin-Induced Alteration of Electrolyte Transport in the Rat Intestine**. *Am J Physiol* 1992, **263**:G502–G507.
Galanin is shown to influence electrolyte transport in rat colonic mucosa *in vitro*. Evidence suggests that this activity involves noncholinergic neural transmission.

21. HILDERBRAND KR, BROWN DR: **Norepinephrine and Alpha-2**
• **Adrenoreceptors Modulate Active Ion Transport in Porcine Small Intestine**. *J Pharmacol Exp Ther* 1992, **263**:510–519.
Demonstration *in vitro* of a relationship between norepinephrine and α-$_2$-adrenoreceptors furthers understanding of the regulation of small intestinal electrolyte transport by enteric neurons.

22. VALET P, SENARD J-M, DEVEDJIAN J-C, PLANAT V, SALOMON
• R, VOISIN T, DREAN G, COUVINEAU A, DAVIAUD D, DENIS C, LABURTHE M, PARIS H: **Characterization and Distribution of α_2-Adrenergic Receptors in the Human Intestinal Mucosa**. *J Clin Invest* 1993, **91**:2049–2057.
A comprehensive study *in vitro* classifying and describing the cellular and subcellular localization of α_2-adrenergic receptors along the human small intestine.

23. CHU X, ZHANG X, RENEHAN WE, BEIERWALTES WH, FOGEL
• R: **Intestinal Distension Alters Vagal Efferent Activity and Small Intestinal Transport In Vivo**. *Am J Physiol* 1993, **27**:G341–G350.
In the absence of sympathetic neural control, distension of the rat small intestine stimulated an increase in net water absorption. This response involved afferent and efferent vagal neurons.

24. TEITELBAUM DH, SONNINO RE, DUNAWAY DJ, STELLIN G,
•• HARMEL JR P: **Rat Jejunal Absorptive Function After Intestinal Transplantation**. *Dig Dis Sci* 1993, **38**:1099–1104.
Small intestinal transplantation in the rat produced only a short-term reduction in jejunal water and Na^+ absorptive capacity.

Ian W. Booth, MSc, MD, FRCP, and Georgina K. Collington, PhD, Institute of Child Health, Nuffield Building, Francis Road, Birmingham, B16 8ET, UK.

Circulation and mucosal injury

Eugene D. Jacobson, MD

University of Colorado Health Sciences Center, Denver, Colorado, USA

This review is concerned with major aspects of research on small bowel circulation. Of the hundreds of papers published in the past year dealing with intestinal vascular physiology, pathophysiology, and more clinical reports, only a small proportion fit into the scope of this section. The subtopics reviewed here include experimental intestinal ischemia-reperfusion injury (IRI), lung damage during IRI, immature gut ischemia, and neuroendocrine regulators of the mesenteric circulation. The importance of neutrophil adhesion, accumulation, and migration in IRI remains a popular object of laboratory investigation. The beneficial effects of local adenosine, prostaglandins, and nitric oxide in IRI have also been explored. Comparisons have been made of local neutrophil behavior versus that of recruited neutrophils in IRI. Plasma versus interstitial responses to lipid peroxidative systems have been delineated. The effect of IRI in the bowel on lung microcirculatory function has been investigated and pulmonary inflammatory responses show events that differ from intestinal counterparts. Similarly, neonatal bowel ischemia exhibits a unique pathophysiology. The range of endogenous mediators of intestinal circulatory change is growing and appears to encompass multiple neurotransmitters, paracrine, and endocrine agents. The breadth of investigative activity and the novelty of recent insights reflect the advances of research in an exciting arena.

Current Opinion in Gastroenterology 1994, **10**:138–142

Intestinal ischemia-reperfusion injury

Within this major subset of current investigation of the circulation of the gut, the search continues for identification of naturally occurring mediators of intestinal ischemia-reperfusion injury (IRI), as well as elucidation of its pathophysiologic processes. Small bowel ischemia is a more severe disorder than is colonic ischemia. Accordingly, mucosal underperfusion that provoked neutrophil infiltration in both the small intestine and the colon during the ischemic period caused less mucosal injury in the colon, was not ameliorated by allopurinol pretreatment, and was not damaged further during the reperfusion period [1•]. The sensitivity of rat small intestinal mucosa to reperfusion injury and to protection by allopurinol probably reflects its greater xanthine oxidase content.

Small bowel injury attributable to the reperfusion period supposedly results from increased availability of oxygen to tissue previously damaged by ischemia. Rat gut subjected previously to 30 minutes of blood flow interruption and reperfused with either venous blood or hemodiluted blood for 60 minutes (approximately 8 mL O_2/min per 100 g tissue) had significantly less histologic injury than ischemic gut reperfused for 1 hour with arterial blood containing approximately 12 mL O_2/min per 100 g tissue [2•]. These findings suggest the possibility of limiting oxygen delivery to ischemic bowel, at least for a short time, as part of managing recovery from the low flow state.

Intestinal ischemia-reperfusion injury was found to increase histamine release into the circulation and to decrease gut tissue diamine oxidase activity [3•]. Pretreatment with a diamine oxidase inhibitor increased the mortality rate of IRI, suggesting that locally released histamine mediates IRI effects. In related findings, topical ethanol induced rabbit jejunal plasma protein leakage via stimulating mast cell release of histamine [4•]. A cytoprotective prostaglandin attenuated vascular injury, presumably by antagonizing ethanol induced degranulation of mast cells.

A key early event in IRI is adherence of neutrophils to venular endothelium, and agents that combat chronic inflammation appear to inhibit neutrophil-endothelial cell adherence. Under *in vitro* conditions, methotrex-

Abbreviation

IRI—ischemia-reperfusion injury.

 ISBN 1-85922-607-8 ISSN 0267–1379

ate was effective against neutrophil adhesion induced by platelet-activating factor [5•]. Adenosine also inhibited granulocyte adhesion, and the antiadhesive action of methotrexate was blocked by an adenosine A_2 receptor antagonist and by adenosine deaminase. These results support the notion that adenosine A_2 receptors on neutrophils antagonize adhesion to the venular endothelium.

Is one neutrophil the same as another neutrophil in IRI? The roles of resident gut granulocytes and newly recruited neutrophils were compared in mediating IRI-induced increases in mucosal permeability of ^{51}Cr-EDTA from blood to lumen and decreases in the water absorptive capacity of the gut [6•]. Discrimination of neutrophil populations was performed in cat gut using a monoclonal antibody against the attachment molecule responsible for neutrophil migration into the interstitium. The mucosal water-absorptive defect appeared attributable to newly recruited neutrophils, whereas the resident gut granulocytes appeared to mediate the mucosal permeability change in IRI.

Although plasma and interstitial-lymphatic fluids are components of the extracellular space, they may not respond identically to a known stress. Thus, incubation of intestinal lymph with a peroxyl radical generating system produced lipid peroxidation and protein oxidation products, while reducing lymph sulfhydryl content [7•]. Lymphatic lipid peroxidative responses were inhibited by removal of apolipoprotein-B–containing lipoproteins. Exposure of plasma to the peroxyl generator produced similar protein oxidation products and reduced sulfhydryl content but failed to produce lipid peroxidation metabolites. Thus, plasma appears to be more resistant than the interstitial-lymphatic pools to lipid peroxidating radicals and has a different substrate for lipid peroxyl radicals.

In related investigations, eicosapentanoic acid and a specific platelet-activating factor antagonist attenuated two endotoxin-induced ileal events, namely neutrophil-endothelial cell adherence and the decline in microcirculatory erythrocyte velocity [8•]. Furthermore, the eicosanoid also attenuated the endotoxin-induced increase in ileal mucosal platelet-activating factor content. These findings more closely relate eicosanoid cytoprotective properties to microcirculatory mechanisms observed during IRI, endotoxemia, and other inflammatory events.

Lung damage during intestinal ischemia-reperfusion injury

Intestinal ischemia has been viewed by many investigators over the past half century as a critical common pathophysiologic event in various forms of acute circulatory collapse, septic shock, and multisystem organ failure. Leukostasis is considered to be an important early step in the evolution of IRI, as well as in adult respiratory distress syndrome following shock, sepsis, or trauma.

Ischemia-reperfusion injury provoked pulmonary ^{125}I-labeled albumin leakage, increased myeloperoxidase activity, and decreased ATP levels in the lung, as well as increased plasma leukotactic activity and xanthine oxidase activity [9•]. These IRI-induced rat lung and plasma abnormalities were prevented by feeding allopurinol- or a tungsten-enriched diet. Intravenously administered xanthine oxidase increased myeloperoxidase activities in the lung and plasma and increased plasma leukotaxis and xanthine oxidase activity. Xanthine oxidase antisera pretreatment attenuated IRI-induced increases in pulmonary myeloperoxidase, plasma leukotactic, and plasma xanthine oxidase activities but did not affect IRI-induced pulmonary albumin leak. These studies implicate circulating xanthine oxidase as the major contributor to pulmonary leukosequestration following IRI.

Pulmonary vascular leakage and leukosequestration plus plasma leukocytosis were demonstrated in IRI [10•]. Pretreatment with a monoclonal antibody to the neutrophil Mac-1 integrin (R 17 MAb) prevented the IRI-induced increase in pulmonary vascular permeability, but did not affect the increased pulmonary myeloperoxidase activity or the plasma leukocytosis after IRI. These studies implicate a neutrophil integrin in lung injury provoked by IRI and also raise questions about the importance of neutrophil accumulation in the pathogenesis of IRI-induced lung injury. In related studies, lung injury was documented by increases in endothelial permeability to ^{125}I-labeled albumin, myeloperoxidase activity, neutrophil superoxide production, and phospholipase A_2 activity [11•]. These aspects of pulmonary damage were prevented by quinacrine (a phospholipase A_2 inhibitor), suggesting that phospholipase A_2 stimulation is an early step in IRI-induced lung injury.

Ischemia-reperfusion injury, which increased gut myeloperoxidase activity and caused mucosal injury, also elevated serum complement and lung myeloperoxidase activities, gave evidence of endothelial cell injury, and increased lung vascular permeability to radiolabeled serum albumin [12••]. Pretreatment with a highly selective complement receptor inhibitor reduced the severity of all these abnormalities in the gut, lung, and the vasculature (except the increased lung myeloperoxidase activity), and also reduced the 5-day rat mortality to IRI by about half. Thus, complement appears to be a major mediator of both local intestinal and distant pulmonary responses to intestinal IRI. Again, the importance of neutrophil accumulation in the lung has to be questioned.

In another study of gut-lung interactions, monolayers of pulmonary artery endothelial cells were incubated with plasma samples from rats subjected to 90 and 120 minutes of intestinal ischemia without reperfusion [13•]. Endothelial ATP levels fell by nearly half after 4-hour incubation with such plasma but no significant cytotoxic injury was detected using the ^{51}Cr release assay. However, 24-hour survival of the cells was reduced from 100% with plasma from sham-operated rats to 40% (with plasma from the 90-minute ischemia group) and 0 (with plasma from the 120-minute ischemia group). Ischemic gut appears to release noncellular substances that injure pulmonary endothelial cells, again casting doubt on the central role of neutrophils in this phenomenon.

Postischemic injury to immature gut

The neonatal bowel is susceptible to life-threatening ischemic states and the neonatal gut appears to lack defense mechanisms that harness circulatory responses to changing metabolic need in the more mature intestine. Accordingly, in 3-day-old swine gut, it was found that there was no enhancement of pressure-flow autoregulation following either intra-arterial administration of 2,4-dinitrophenol or intraintestinal instillation of predigested swine milk [14•]. This behavior of the neonatal mesenteric circulation was in contrast to 35-day-old gut in which pressure decreases prompted more intense vasodilation in the face of increased oxygen need.

In weaning rat small bowel subjected to IRI with or without deferoxamine pretreatment, histopathologic consequences of experimental IRI in immature gut resembled findings in the human neonatal bowel in necrotizing enterocolitis [15•]. Thus, severe mucosal damage and necrosis occurred in both situations, despite a paucity of neutrophil infiltration. Pretreatment with the iron-chelating agent to inhibit metal catalysis of more reactive oxidants ameliorated mucosal histopathology and improved mortality profiles.

Neonatal rabbit gut subjected to systemic hypoxic insult exhibited reduced prostaglandin E_2 and elevated leukotriene B_4 levels without changes in the tissue content of several other endogenous eicosanoids [16•]. Mucosal histopathologic changes were mild. These findings suggest that an early neonatal gut response to hypoxia is a shift in eicosanoid metabolism toward increasing inflammatory and reducing cytoprotective mediators.

Neutroendocrine regulation

In recent years, evidence has accumulated to support the notion that intestinal blood flow is regulated physiologically by numerous neurotransmitters, immunological substances, paracrine agents, circulating chemicals, and metabolites (Fig. 1). Accordingly, in the *in vitro* guinea pig ileum, mechanical stimulation of the mucosa dilated submucosal arterioles precontracted with phenylephrine or prostaglandin $F_{2\alpha}$ [17•]. Tetrodotoxin or muscarinic receptor blockade inhibited this vasodilation in 60% of preparations, and the tetrodotoxin-insensitive vasodilation was inhibited by pretreatment with $5HT_3$ and histamine (H_1 and H_2) receptor antagonists and indomethacin.

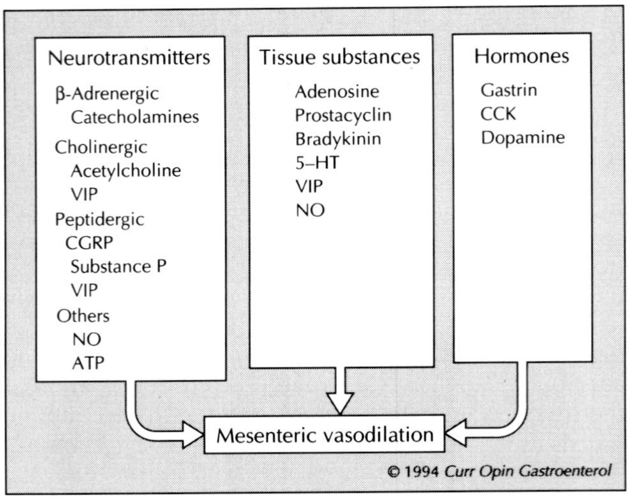

Fig. 1. Some endogenous vasodilator mediators in the gut. These agents may be neurocrine, paracrine, or endocrine substances.

In rat gut, perivascular splanchnic nerve stimulation under *in vivo* conditions evoked a vasoconstrictor response, whereas cessation of nerve stimulation was followed by a mesenteric hyperemia [18•]. Pretreatment with reserpine converted the nerve-stimulated constrictor response into a vasodilator response, the latter being abolished by capsaicin. Capsaicin, tetrodotoxin, and lidocaine also blocked the post–nerve stimulation hyperemia. These findings indicate the presence in perivascular splanchnic nerve trunks of both sympathetic vasoconstrictor and peptidergic vasodilator fibers.

In anesthetized sheep, splanchnic nerve stimulation prompted a transiently increased intestinal lymph flow, lymphatic contraction frequency, and arterial pressure without changing lymph protein concentration [19•]. Pretreatment with phentolamine inhibited these responses. α-Adrenergic receptors seem to mediate activation of a lymphatic pump without forming new lymph fluid.

Antagonists to α-adrenergic, angiotensin II, and vasopressin receptors were applied locally to first-, second-, and third-order rat mesenteric arterioles under *in vivo* microscopy [20••]. Phentolamine increased the diameter of third-order arterioles by nearly 15% and vasopressin antagonism increased the diameter of first-order arterioles by nearly 9% in normal rats, whereas in rats with chronic portal hypertension there was enhancement of vasopressin- and angiotensin II-antagonist effects on arteriolar diameters. α-Adrenergic and vasopressin receptors probably mediate most mesenteric arteriolar constriction under normal conditions.

In anesthetized dog gut, the hyperemia and increased oxygen consumption elicited by placement of nutrient in the gut lumen were abolished by pretreatment with adenosine deaminase and were enhanced by pretreatment with a blocker of adenosine reuptake [21•]. Both agents abolished the food-induced increase in oxygen uptake. Venous and lymphatic adenosine concentrations were increased by luminal food but not in the presence of adenosine deaminase.

Intra-arterial infusion of bradykinin increased rat mesenteric blood flow in a dose-dependent manner [22•]. This hyperemia was greatly inhibited by a bradykinin B_2-receptor subtype antagonist and by a nitric oxide synthase inhibitor, but not by a B_1 subtype antagonist nor by capsaicin. The B_2 subtype antagonist and the nitric oxide synthase inhibitor were ineffective against the mesenteric vasodilator effects of isoproterenol.

Nitric oxide is generated by several intestinal cell types that are vulnerable to IRI. The broad biologic range of nitric oxide actions has prompted investigation of its possible protective role in IRI [23•]. In the autoperfused feline small bowel, IRI provoked increased vascular and mucosal permeabilities to large molecules and water, which were dramatically augmented by L-NAME, a nitric oxide synthase inhibitor (Fig. 2). The exaggerated permeability changes caused by L-NAME were reversed by L-arginine (the substrate for nitric oxide synthesis). Histopathologic examination of post IRI mucosa revealed enhanced injury with L-NAME and protection with L-arginine. L-Arginine may be a potentially effective agent in clinical intestinal ischemia.

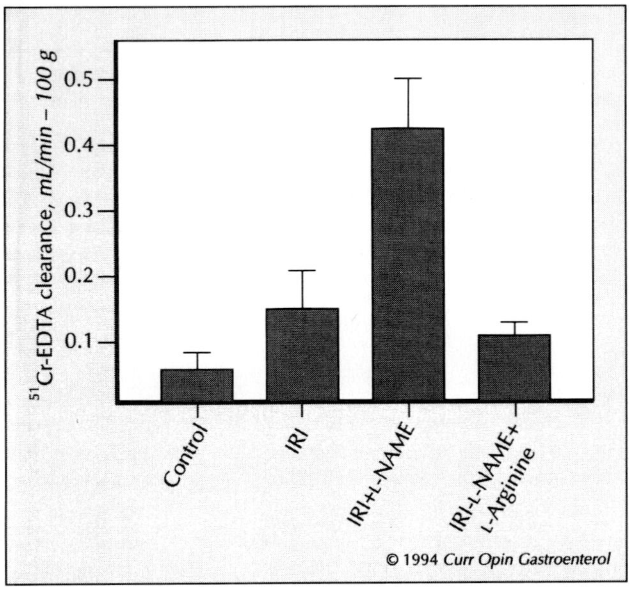

Fig. 2. Blood-to-lumen clearance of ^{51}Cr-EDTA in the gut was increased by ischemia-reperfusion injury (IRI), greatly enhanced by the combination of IRI and a nitric oxide synthase inhibitor, and antagonized by the substrate for nitric oxide.

References and recommended reading

Papers of particular interest, published within the annual period of review, have been highlighted as:
- • Of special interest
- •• Of outstanding interest

1. • Leung FW, Su KC, Passaro E, Guth PH: **Regional Differences in Gut Blood Flow and Mucosal Damage in Response to Ischemia and Reperfusion.** *Am J Physiol* 1992, **263**:G301–G305.

Iscehmia-reperfusion injury differed between small bowel and colonic mucosae, causing more severe injury yet being more responsive to allopurinol protection in the small intestine.

2. • Clark ET, Gewertz BL: **Limiting Oxygen Delivery Attenuates Intestinal Reperfusion Injury.** *J Surg Res* 1992, **53**:485–489.

Following intestinal ischemia, reperfusion with blood containing 33% less oxygen caused less histologic damage than reperfusion with arterial blood.

3. • Fujisaki J, Fujimoto K, Oohara A, Sakata T, Hirano M, Ohyama T, Iwakiri R, Yamaguchi M: **Roles of Histamine and Diamine Oxidase in Mucosa of Rat Small Intestine After Ischemia-Reperfusion.** *Dig Dis Sci* 1993, **38**:1195–1200.

Ischemia-reperfusion injury increased histamine release from gut mucosa, and a diamine oxidase inhibitor increased the mortality rate from IRI in a rat model.

4. • Dinda PK, Holitzner CA, Morris GP, Beck IT: **Ethanol-Induced Jejunal Microvascular and Morphological Injury in Relation to Histamine Release in Rabbits.** *Gastroenterology* 1993, **104**:361–368.

Ethanol perfusion of rabbit jejunum released histamine and prompted plasma protein leakage, both of which were attenuated by cytoprotective agents that stabilize mast cells.

5. • Asako H, Wolf RE, Granger DN: **Leukocyte Adherence in Rat Mesenteric Venules: Effects of Adenosine and Methotrexate.** *Gastroenterology* 1993, **104**:31–37.

The antiadhesive actions of methotrexate and adenosine on platelet-activating factor-induced neutrophil-endothelial interactions were blocked by adenosine deaminase and an adenosine A_2 receptor antagonist.

6. • Kubes P, Hunter J, Granger DN: **Ischemia/Reperfusion-Induced Feline Intestinal Dysfunction: Importance of Granulocyte Recruitment.** *Gastroenterology* 1992, **103**:807–812.

Resident interstitial neutrophils play a more important role in IRI-induced mucosal leakiness to macromolecules than do newly recruited neutrophils.

7. • Kurtel H, Granger DN, Tso P, Grisham MB: **Vulnerability of Intestinal Interstitial Fluid to Oxidant Stress.** *Am J Physiol* 1992, **263**:G573–G578.

A peroxyl radical generator produced lipid peroxidation products in intestinal lymph that depended on apo-B-containing lipoproteins but did not generate lipid peroxidation products in plasma.

8. • Miura S, Imaeda H, Shiozaki H, Kurose I, Fukumura D, Tashiro H, Serizawa H, Suematsu M, Sekizuka E, Tsuchiya M: **Attenuation of Endotoxin-Induced Intestinal Microcirculatory Damage by Eicosapentanoic Acid.** *Am J Physiol* 1993, **264**:G828–G834.

Eicosapentanoic acid and a platelet-activating factor antagonist attenuated endotoxin-induced neutrophil-endothelial adhesion and ischemia; the eicosanoid also antagonized the increased mucosal platelet-activating factor release.

9. • Terada LS, Dormish JJ, Shanley PF, Leff JA, Anderson BO, Repine JE: **Circulating Xanthine Oxidase Mediates Lung Neutrophil Sequestration After Intestinal Ischemia-Reperfusion.** *Am J Physiol* 1992, **263**:L394–L401.

Iscemia-reperfusion injury provoked pulmonary albumin leakage, increased myeloperoxidase and xanthine oxidase activities, and decreased ATP; most of these responses were prevented by an antiserum against xanthine oxidase.

10. • Hill J, Lindsay T, Rusche J, Valeri CR: **Mac-1 Antibody Reduces Liver and Lung Injury but Not Neutrophil Seues-**

tration After Intestinal Ischemia-Reperfusion. *Surgery* 1992, 112:166–172.
Monoclonal antibody to neutrophil Mac-1 integrin prevented IRI-induced increases in lung vascular permeability without preventing either the increased lung myeloperoxidase activity or plasma leukocytosis.

11. KOIKE K, MOORE EE, MOORE FA, CARL VS, PITMAN
• JM, BANERJEE A: **Phospholipase A_2 Inhibition Decouples Lung Injury From Gut Ischemia-Reperfusion.** *Surgery* 1992, 112:173–180.
Ischemia-reperfusion injury-induced lung injury was attenuated by a phospholipase A_2 inhibitor.

12. HILL J, LINDSAY TF, ORTIZ F, YEH CG, HECHTMAN HB, MOORE
•• FD, JR.: **Soluble Complement Receptor Type 1 Ameliorates the Local and Remote Organ Injury After Intestinal Ischemia-Reperfusion in the Rat.** *J Immunol* 1992, 149:1723–1728.
Treatment with a soluble complement receptor inhibitor reduced IRI-induced endothelial cell injury and pulmonary albumin leakage, but not lung myeloperoxidase activation.

13. GERKIN TM, WELLING TH, TURNAGE RH, RYAN US, GUICE
• KS, OLDHAM KT: **Pulmonary Endothelial Cell ATP Depletion Following Intestinal Ischemia.** *J Surg Res* 1992, 52:642–647.
Endothelial cell monolayers from the pulmonary artery were injured or killed by incubation with plasma from rats subjected to prolonged intestinal ischemia.

14 NOWICKI PT, MILLER CE: **Effect of Increased Tissue Oxygen**
• **Uptake on Autoregulation in Postnatal Intestine.** *Am J Physiol* 1992, 263:G690–G694.
The neonatal gut circulation (but not the more mature vasculature) was unable to vasodilate adequately in the face of a combined increased need for oxygen and a fall in driving pressure.

15. LELLI JL, JR., PRADHAN S, COBB LM: **Prevention of Postis-**
• **chemic Injury in Immature Intestine by Deferoxamine.** *J Surg Res* 1993, 54:34–38.
Deferoxamine ameliorated the histopathology and mortality rate of weaning rats subjected to IRI despite the lack of intestinal neutrophil infiltration in the immature ischemic gut.

16. DOLLBERG S, UDASSIN R, GINAT-ISRAELI T, WEIDENFELD J,
• BRANSKI D: **Eicosanoids in Hypoxic Insult to Neonatal Rabbit Bowel.** *J Pediatr Gastroenterol Nutr* 1992, 15:130–134.
Systemic hypoxia reduced prostaglandin E_2 and increased leukotriene B_4 levels in the neonatal gut, while provoking a mild mucosal histopathology.

17. VANNER S, JIANG M-M, SURPRENANT A: **Mucosal Stimulation**
• **Evokes Vasodilation by Neuronal and Nonneuronal Mechanisms.** *Am J Physiol* 1993, 264:G202–G212.
Mechanical stimulation of intestinal mucosa dilated submucosal arterioles by cholinergic and nonneuronal mechanisms, the latter involving $5HT_3$ and histamine receptors.

18. HOTTENSTEIN OD, REMAK G, JACOBSON ED: **Peptidergic**
• **Nerves Mediate Post-Nerve Stimulation Hyperemia in Rat Gut.** *Am J Physiol* 1992, 263:G29–G37.
Perivascular nerve stimulation evoked mesenteric vasoconstriction, and cessation of nerve stimulation elicited intestinal hyperemia; reserpine pretreatment converted the constriction into dilation, and capsaicin inhibited the post nerve stimulation hyperemia.

19. THORNBURY KD, HARTY HR, MCGEOWN JG, MCHALE NG:
• **Mesenteric Lymph Flow Responses to Splanchnic Nerve Stimulation in Sheep.** *Am J Physiol* 1993, 264:H604–H610.
α-Adrenergic receptors mediate increased lymph flow and lymphatic contraction frequency without forming additional lymph fluid.

20. JOH T, GRANGER DN, BENOIT JN: **Endogenous Vasoconstrictor**
•• **Tone in Intestine of Normal and Portal Hypertensive Rats.** *Am J Physiol* 1993, 264:H171–H177.
Normal mesenteric arteriolar constriction is mediated by αadrenergic and vasopressin receptors; in portal hypertension, angiotensin II and vasopressin receptors dominate constrictor tone.

21. SAWMILLER DR, CHOU CC: **Role of Adenosine in Postprandial**
• **and Reactive Hyperemia in Canine Jejunum.** *Am J Physiol* 1992, 263:G487–G493.
Intrajejunal nutrients increased blood flow, oxygen consumption, and the venous and lymphatic adenosine concentrations, all of which were prevented by adenosine deaminase.

22. BERGUER R, HOTTENSTEIN OD, PALEN TE, STEWART JM,
• JACOBSON ED: **Bradykinin Induced Mesenteric Vasodilation is Mediated by B2 Subtype Receptors and Nitric Oxide.** *Am J Physiol* 1993, 264:G492–G496.
Bradykinin increased mesenteric blood flow and the hyperemic response was attenuated by a B_2 receptor antagonist and by L-NAME but not by capsaicin or a B_1 blocker.

23. KUBES P: **Ischemia-Reperfusion in Feline Small Intestine: A**
• **Role for Nitric Oxide.** *Am J Physiol* 1993, 264:G143–G149.
Ischemia-reperfusion injury increased gut mucosal and vascular permeabilities and provoked histopathological injury; these defects were enhanced by L-NAME and reversed by L-arginine.

Eugene D. Jacobson, MD, Professor of Medicine and Physiology, University of Colorado Health Sciences Center, 4200 East Ninth Avenue, Box C-321, Denver, CO 80262, USA.

Diagnosis and management of small intestinal disease

Marc S. Levin, MD

Washington University School of Medicine, St. Louis, Missouri, USA

Topics relating to the diagnosis and medical management of small intestinal diseases include the use of the D-xylose hydrogen breath test in the clinical management of intestinal malabsorption, the measurement of unconjugated serum bile salts for diagnosing small intestinal bacterial overgrowth, identification of the etiology of abnormal lipid trafficking in patients with abetalipoproteinemia, evaluation of hypotonic oral rehydration solutions, the value of screening for celiac disease by detection of gliadin or endomysial antibodies, and recent advances in human small intestinal transplantation.

Current Opinion in Gastroenterology 1994, **10**:143–148

Although no novel diagnostic or therapeutic modalities of special value for small intestinal disorders were introduced in the past year, there were several noteworthy attempts to evaluate or modify existing procedures and therapies.

Small bowel enema

A retrospective review of the radiologic reports of small bowel enema (enteroclysis) examinations of 1465 patients from a single institution was used to estimate the sensitivity and specificity of this procedure [1•]. The reports were correlated with the subsequent clinical outcome, and where possible with findings at laparotomy (25% of cases). A sensitivity of 93.1% and a specificity of 96.9% were found, based on whether the small intestine was reported as normal or an abnormality was diagnosed to account for the patient's clinical presentation. The correct specific diagnosis was made in 67.5% of the examinations that were considered abnormal. The small bowel enema was reliable for the evaluation of the diagnosis of Crohn's disease and neoplasms, and for the localization of intestinal obstructions and other structural abnormalities. The sensitivity for the detection of celiac disease was at best 40%.

Although these data support the authors' conclusion that the small bowel enema is a dependable method, there is insufficient data to support their specific recommendation that it should be the routine barium examination for suspected disorders of the small intestine. Without a large prospective, randomized comparison of the small bowel follow-through series and the small bowel enema, there is insufficient data to reliably determine the relative costs and outcome benefits of the authors' recommended approach. Without such data, the increased expense and patient discomfort associated with the small bowel enema will discourage its use as the initial test unless the suspicion of small bowel disease is high.

D-Xylose hydrogen breath tests

Hydrogen (H_2) breath tests are based on the ability of bacteria to ferment carbohydrate substrates, such as glucose, xylose, and lactulose, producing H_2, which diffuses through the intestinal wall and is excreted through the lungs. Upper small intestinal absorptive efficiency is most frequently assessed by measuring the urinary excretion of an oral xylose load. Well-documented limitations of this test include the necessity for accurate urine collection, variability because of ascites or impaired renal function and sensitivity to hydration status [2]. Although H_2 breath tests are free of these limitations, the requirement for specialized equipment and the recognition that 3% to 25% of individuals are not colonized with H_2-producing bacterial flora [3–6] has limited their acceptance in clinical practice.

The potential usefulness of the H_2 breath test with D-xylose in clinical management of intestinal malabsorption was reassessed in 45 adults [7•]. Fifteen patients had proved malabsorption that was due to celiac disease in nine, and to lymphoma, Whipple's disease, or giardiasis in the remainder. Nine patients had small-bowel bacterial overgrowth secondary to either post-surgical sequelae or intestinal dysmotility. Twenty-one patients with irritable bowel syndrome and 21 healthy individuals served as controls. Following ingestion of 25 g of D-xylose, breath H_2 and 5-hour urinary excre-

Abbreviation

MTP—microsomal triglyceride transfer protein.

tion of D-xylose were compared. Modest increases in H_2 production were detected in healthy individuals and in patients with the irritable bowel syndrome. In contrast, the increase was of a much greater magnitude in the malabsorption group and there was little overlap between test and control groups (Fig. 1). The sensitivity and specificity of the breath test and the urinary D-xylose test were identical. Most patients who responded to treatment for malabsorption normalized their H_2 production, whereas nonresponders did not. In patients with bacterial overgrowth the sensitivity was poor, although the results were correlated with urinary D-xylose excretion. The presence of an early rise in H_2 excretion was specific for small bowel bacterial overgrowth.

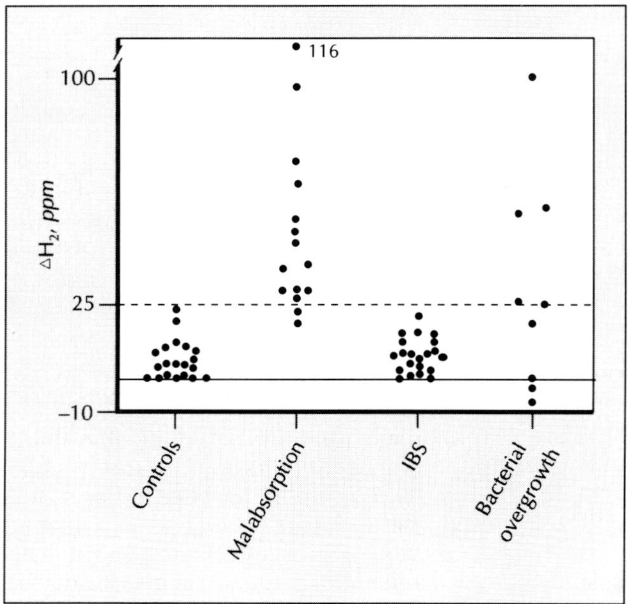

Fig. 1. Increase (Δ) in H_2 production after oral D-xylose in each patient included in the study. The *broken line* indicates the upper limit of normal range. In healthy controls H_2 production increased slightly. All but two patients with malabsorption had abnormally increased H_2 production. No difference was observed between patients with the irritable bowel syndrome (IBS) and healthy controls. In bacterial overgrowth, results were heterogeneous (although they correlated with the urinary excretion of D-xylose). (*From* Casellas *et al.* [7•]; with permission.)

This study confirms the usefulness of the breath H_2 D-xylose test for the detection of intestinal malabsorption in adult populations in whom non–H_2-producing flora are relatively uncommon. However, interpretation of a negative test will require the use of the standard urinary xylose excretion test or administration of lactulose to prove that a H_2-producing flora is in fact present. Based on these considerations, it would perhaps be best to recommend this as the initial test only for those individuals with renal insufficiency and other problems that can interfere with the interpretation of the standard urinary xylose excretion test.

Unconjugated serum bile salts and bacterial overgrowth

Quantitation of the aerobic and anaerobic small intestinal flora remains the "gold standard" for diagnosing bacterial overgrowth. This requires an invasive procedure and fastidious technique to obtain reliable data. The noninvasive [^{14}C]-xylose breath test has been reported to be a reliable and sensitive method by many, but not all, authors [2]. The observation that serum concentrations of unconjugated bile salts are increased in patients with small intestinal bacterial overgrowth [8–11] prompted a comparative study of the [^{14}C]-xylose breath test and the proportion of serum unconjugated bile salts in 36 patients with suspected bacterial overgrowth [12•]. After a 12-hour fast, venous blood was obtained, and a 1-g [^{14}C]-xylose breath test was performed. Serum concentrations of total and unconjugated cholic, chenodeoxycholic, and deoxycholic acids were determined with gas chromatography mass spectrometry.

The 22 patients with an abnormal breath test had on average a threefold increase in the proportion and amount of unconjugated bile salts. Total bile salts were not significantly different. The sensitivity and specificity of the blood test were 73% and 94%, respectively. The correlation coefficient between the [^{14}C]-xylose breath test and the proportion of unconjugated bile salts in peripheral blood was significant (r = 0.63, P<0.001).

Although, this study indicates that a relatively simple blood test is reasonably sensitive and specific when compared with the [^{14}C]-xylose breath test, it must be studied in a larger number of symptomatic patients with documented small intestinal bacterial overgrowth before its use can be considered in clinical practice. In addition, there are two important limitations of this method: the need for the presence of anaerobes in the colonizing small intestinal flora (to avoid false-negatives) and the need to eliminate patients with bile acid malabsorption (to avoid false-positives).

Evaluation of a hypotonic oral rehydration solution

Controversy exists regarding the optimal composition of glucose electrolyte oral rehydration solutions for the treatment of acute diarrhea. One of the goals of current research is the development of improved formulations that result in decreased stool volume and water loss while remaining effective for the treatment of dehydration. An additional goal is the avoidance of hypernatremia. Toward these ends, Hunt *et al.* [13•] have compared the efficacy of a hypotonic oral rehydration solution (sodium concentration 60 mmol/L, osmolality 240 mosm/kg) with those recommended by the World Health Organization (sodium 90 mmol/L, osmolality 331 mosm/kg) and the British National formulary (sodium 35 mmol/L, osmolality 310 mosm/kg).

Four perfusion models (normal human jejunum, normal rat small intestine, cholera toxin–treated secreting rat small intestine, and rotavirus-infected rat small intestine) were used for these studies.

The hypotonic oral rehydration solution promoted greater water absorption than the standard solutions in all four models, though statistical significance was not achieved in human jejunum. Sodium absorption with the experimental solution was adequate and it was less than or equal to absorption with the World Health Organization oral rehydration solution. Thus, these *in vitro* perfusion studies indicate that the hypotonic experimental solution may be more efficacious than standard oral rehydration formulations.

The conclusion of this study is consistent with a preliminary report of the clinical experience with the same formulation [14]. A Finnish open clinical trial compared a different hypotonic oral rehydration solution (total osmolality 224 mosm/L, Na^+ concentration 60 mmol/L) with an isotonic solution [15•]. Children given the hypotonic solution ($n = 103$) passed significantly fewer diarrhea stools, and their diarrhea and hospital stay were shorter than those of children given the isotonic oral rehydration solution ($n = 135$). Thus, these data also suggest that hypotonic oral rehydration solutions have clinical advantages over the standard solutions.

Abetalipoproteinemia

Abetalipoproteinemia is a recessive genetic disorder, that is characterized by absence of circulating apolipoprotein-B–containing lipoproteins, malabsorption of intestinal fat, and degenerative neurologic and retinal lesions [16••]. These abnormalities result from a defect in chylomicron and very low density lipoprotein assembly or secretion in the intestine and liver, respectively. Recent data have refuted the hypothesis that abetalipoproteinemia is due to a molecular defect in the apolipoprotein-B gene itself or to abnormal post-translational processing [16••]. A significant contribution to our understanding of the etiology of abetalipoproteinemia and of normal lipid processing was the discovery by Wetterau *et al.* [17••] that patients with abetalipoproteinemia are missing the 88-kD component of the heterodimeric microsomal triglyceride transfer protein (MTP). This protein is normally present in the lumen of microsomes isolated from the intestine and liver. The MTP complex mediates the transfer of cholesterol esters and triglycerides between membranes.

In the study by Wetterau *et al.* [17••], triglyceride transfer activity was assayed in intestinal biopsies from four patients with abetalipoproteinemia. Unafflicted controls and patients with two other disorders of chylomicron formation were included. In addition, immunblots prepared with intestinal homogenates were probed with affinity-purified MTP antibodies. In contrast to the controls, no triglyceride transfer activity and no immunodetectable MTP were detected in the abetalipoproteinemia patients. This study was the subject of an excellent commentary that focused on the mechanisms of triglyceride-rich particle assembly in healthy individuals and in patients with abetalipoproteinemia [18••].

Celiac disease

The pathogenesis of celiac disease appears to involve an interaction between HLA class II D gene products and the gliadin protein [19]. Markedly elevated levels of circulating gliadin-specific antibodies are common in patients with celiac disease. These antibodies can, however, be detected in the sera of healthy individuals as well. Circulating antibodies to reticulin and endomysial antibodies, which recognize antigens from the membrane of smooth muscle bundles, may also be present in patients with celiac disease. The role of these antibodies in the pathogenesis of celiac disease is not known.

Presently the "gold standard" for diagnosis of celiac disease is small intestinal biopsy. As of yet there is no alternative noninvasive method for diagnosing celiac disease, for monitoring the response to therapy, or for screening at-risk relatives of affected individuals. The latter task is important because of the increased risk of malignancy in patients with active or latent celiac disease. The value of screening for celiac disease by detection of gliadin [20•] or endomysial antibodies [21••] was the subject of two recent studies.

Corazza *et al.* [20•] screened 328 first-degree relatives of 128 adult celiac patients for the presence of antigliadin antibodies. Circulating antigliadin antibodies were detected in 21 subjects. Jejunal biopsies demonstrated subtotal villus atrophy in 13 patients. Although the remaining eight subjects had normal-appearing mucosa, morphometric evaluation showed a mean surface-to-volume ratio that, although in the normal range, was significantly lower than that of biopsied relatives and unrelated controls who were negative for antigliadin antibodies. Whereas this data suggests that the eight subjects with normal mucosa may have latent celiac disease, in the absence of long-term follow-up data, the possibility that some or all of them simply had a false-positive test result cannot be ruled out. Furthermore, it is not feasible to determine the false-negative rate because this would require subjecting asymptomatic relatives to small bowel biopsy. Given these limitations, it is fair to conclude that antigliadin antibody testing may be a useful screening test for diagnosing celiac disease in relatives of celiac patients. Because of the apparently high prevalence of false-positive tests, all patients with circulating antigliadin antibodies should undergo small intestinal biopsy.

Table 1. Sensitivity, specificity, and predictive values for antibody assays*

	Endomysial IgA	Antireticulin IgA	Antigliadin IgA	Antigliadin IgG
Sensitivity	100	91	91	76
Specificity	99	99	85	88
Positive predictive value	91	91	45	46
Negative predictive value	100	99	99	97

**From* Ferreira *et al.* [21••]; with permission.
Ig—immunoglobulin.

Ferreira *et al.* [21••] compared the sensitivities and specificities of circulating immunoglobulin A and immunoglobulin G antigliadin antibodies and immunoglobulin A antireticulin antibody with the endomysial antibody. A sum of 117 patients with adult celiac disease (21 untreated), 84 patients with inflammatory bowel disease, systemic lupus erythematosus, and rheumatoid arthritis (comprising the disease control group), 47 normal controls, and a miscellaneous group of 29 patients, who were selected because of a positive reticulin-staining pattern, were investigated.

Small bowel biopsies were obtained from many of the patients with celiac disease to correlate jejunal morphology with antibody titers. All of the patients with untreated celiac disease had villus atrophy and were endomysial antibody positive. Endomysial antibodies were also found in nearly half of patients on a nonstrict gluten-free diet. The only patient who was positive despite following a strict gluten-free diet had partial villous atrophy. The only false-positive results were in a patient with insulin dependent diabetes and another with thyroiditis. Neither of these patients consented to small intestinal biopsy to rule out celiac disease. Thus, the sensitivity and correlation with subtotal villous atrophy in the untreated patients was 100% (Table 1). The overall specificity and positive predictive value were 99% and 91%. By comparison, the sensitivity and specificity of the antigliadin antibody assays were considerably less (Table 1). These data support the authors' conclusion that the endomysial antibody is the superior test for the diagnosis of celiac disease. Before this recommendation can be accepted, these results will need to be verified in the clinical laboratories of additional institutions.

Small intestinal transplantation

Revillon *et al.* [22•] in Paris have provided a useful update and review of their experience with intestinal transplantation in children and in experimental models. The group at the University of Pittsburgh [23••,24•–27•] have productively continued their efforts to make small intestinal transplantation a feasible option for patients with severe short bowel syndrome. As documented in several short reports that appeared during the past year, they have made progress in the technical aspects, in the control of graft rejection, and in the assessment of graft rejection and function. For example, they have shown that biopsies obtained through an endoscope were useful for identifying rejection as a cause of graft damage [27•].

The Pittsburgh experience using FK506

Before the introduction of FK506, small bowel transplantation was rarely successful because of graft rejection and other complications. FK506 in combination with improved surgical techniques and refinements in graft monitoring have resulted in a marked improvement in graft survival, graft function, and patient survival. Of the nine recipients of an isolated small bowel intestinal graft, eight were alive and seven had functioning grafts at 8 to 15 months posttransplant. None of the patients with functioning grafts required parenteral nutrition. Thirteen of 17 recipients of combined liver and small intestinal grafts were alive at 5 to 30 months and 12 did not require parenteral nutrition. All of the patients that died were under 3 years old and only one had evidence of graft-versus-host disease. Sepsis resulting from technical complications was the cause of death in three patients and postoperative lymphoproliferative disease in the remaining patient. Abdominal multivisceral transplantation was performed in four patients. All were alive with functioning grafts at 3 to 15 months. In contrast to the pre-FK506 experience, these data suggest that isolated small intestinal transplantation is as effective as combination transplants. Thus, this procedure is preferred for patients with normal liver function without serious compromise of the celiac, mesenteric, or splanchnic circulation.

Although there has been great progress, it is clear that additional follow-up, refinement of postoperative management and research focused on augmenting the functional capacity of the transplanted intestine are critical for the further development of small intestinal transplantation as an effective therapeutic modality.

References and recommended reading

Papers of particular interest, published within the annual period of review, have been highlighted as:
- • Of special interest
- •• Of outstanding interest

1. • DIXON PM, ROULSTON ME, NOLAN DJ: **The Small Bowel Enema: A Ten Year Review.** *Clin Radiol* 1993, **47**:46–48.

A single institution retrospective study comparing clinical outcomes with the radiologic reports of small bowel enema (enteroclysis) examinations of 1465 patients. A sensitivity of 93.1% and a specificity of 96.9% was found, based on whether the small intestine was reported as normal or an abnormality was diagnosed to account for the patient's clinical presentation. The correct specific diagnosis was made in 67.5% of the examinations that were considered abnormal.

2. CRAIG RM, ATKINSON AJ JR: **D-Xylose Testing: A Review.** *Gastroenterology* 1988, **95**:223–231.

3. RAVICH WJ, BAYLESS TM, THOMAS M: **Fructose: Incomplete Intestinal Absorption in Humans.** *Gastroenterology* 1983, **84**:26–29.

4. BOND JH, LEVITT MD: **Use of Breath Hydrogen in the Study of Carbohydrate Absorption.** *Dig Dis* 1977, **22**:379–382.

5. GILAT T, BEN HUR H, GELMAN-MALACHI E, TERDIMAN R, PELED Y: **Alterations of the Colonic Flora and Their Effect on the Hydrogen Breath Test.** *Gut* 1978, **19**:602–605.

6. KING CE, TOSKES PP: **Comparison of the 1-Gram ^{14}C-Xylose, 10-Gram Lactulose-H_2, and 80-Gram Glucose-H_2 Breath Tests in Patients With Small Intestine Bacterial Overgrowth.** *Gastroenterology* 1986, **91**:1447–1451.

7. • CASELLAS F, CHICHARRO L, MALAGELADA JR: **Potential Usefulness of Hydrogen Breath Test With D-Xylose in Clinical Management of Intestinal Malabsorption.** *Dig Dis Sci* 1993, **38**:321–327.

Five-hour urinary D-xylose excretion was compared with breath H_2 excretion following administration of a standard 25-g dose of D-xylose to normal controls, controls with irritable bowel syndrome, or patients with documented malabsorption or small bowel bacterial overgrowth. The study clearly demonstrated the breath H_2 test with D-xylose is a useful and practical alternative to the standard urinary excretion test. However, the prevalence of non–H_2-producing colonizing flora was apparently low in this series. Unless the H_2 production phenotype of the resident flora is known, negative breath H_2 tests cannot be interpreted.

8. STELLARD R, SAUERBRUCH T, LUDERSCHMIDT CH, LEISNER B, PAUMGARTNER G: **Intestinal Involvement in Progressive Systemic Sclerosis Detected by Increased Unconjugated Serum Bile Acids.** *Gut* 1987, **28**:446–450.

9. MASCLEE A, TANGERMAN A, VAN SCHAIK A, VAN DER HOEK EW, VAN TONGEREN JHM: **Unconjugated Serum Bile Acids as Marker of Small Intestinal Bacterial Overgrowth.** *Eur J Clin Invest* 1989, **19**:384–389.

10. BOLT MJG, STELLARD F, SITRIN MD, PAUMGARTNER G: **Serum Unconjugated Bile Acids in Patients With Small Bowel Bacterial Overgrowth.** *Clin Chim Acta* 1989, **181**:87–102.

11. EINARSSON K, REIHNER E, EWERTH S, BJORKHEM I: **Serum Concentrations of Unconjugated and Conjugated Cholic Acid in Portal Venous and Systemic Venous Blood of Fasting Man.** *Scand J Clin Lab Invest* 1989, **49**:83–91.

12. • EINARSSON K, BERGSTROM M, EKLOF R, NORD CE, BJORKHEM I: **Comparison of the Proportion of Unconjugated to Total Serum Cholic Acid and the [14C]-Xylose Breath Test in Patients With Suspected Small Intestinal Bacterial Overgrowth.** *Scand J Clin Lab Invest* 1992, **52**:425–430.

The proportion of unconjugated to total cholic acid in fasting serum was significantly elevated in patients with suspected small intestinal bacterial overgrowth and an abnormal [^{14}C]-xylose breath test. The two tests were correlated (r= 0.63), suggesting that determination of the proportion of unconjugated to total cholic acid in peripheral venous blood may be a simple alternative for detection of bacterial contamination of the upper small intestine, provided the patients do not have bile acid malabsorption. Additional studies using patients with confirmation of small intestinal overgrowth by culture will be needed to reliably assess the potential of this diagnostic test.

13. • HUNT JB, THILLAINAYAGAM AV, SALIM AF, CARNABY S, ELLIOTT EJ, FARTHING MJ: **Water and Solute Absorption From a New Hypotonic Oral Rehydration Solution: Evaluation in Human and Animal Perfusion Models.** *Gut* 1992, **33**:1652–1659.

In attempt to improve oral rehydration therapy for the treatment of acute diarrheal disorders, four perfusion model systems were used to compare the efficacy of a hypotonic oral rehydration solution (sodium concentration 60 mmol/L, osmolality 240 mosm/kg) with those recommended by the World Health Organization (sodium 90 mmol/L, osmolality 331 mosm/kg) and the British National formulary (sodium 35 mmol/L, osmolality 310 mosm/kg). The hypotonic formula resulted in greater water absorption with adequate, but not excessive, sodium absorption.

14. CLEGHORN GJ, SHEPHERD RW, PATRICK MK, CHIN SE: **Comparison of Two Oral Rehydration Solutions in Children With Gastroenteritis in Australia.** *Clinical Therapeutics* 1990, **12** **Suppl A**:81–85.

15. • RAUTANEN T, EL-RADHI S, VESIKARI T: **Clinical Experience With a Hypotonic Oral Rehydration Solution in Acute Diarrhoea.** *Acta Paediatrica* 1993, **82**:52–54.

A hypotonic oral rehydration salts solution with total osmolality of 224 mosm/L was compared in an open clinical trial with an isotonic (osmolality 304 mosm/L) solution for the treatment of dehydration due to acute diarrhea. The hypotonic solution was more efficacious.

16. •• RADER DJ, BREWER HB JR: **Abetalipoproteinemia. New Insights Into Lipoprotein Assembly and Vitamin E Metabolism From a Rare Genetic Disease.** *JAMA* 1993, **270**:865–869.

Outstanding review discussing clinical and basic research aspects of abetalipoproteinemia.

17. •• WETTERAU JR, AGGERBECK LP, BOUMA ME, EISENBERG C, MUNCK A, HERMIER M, SCHMITZ J, GAY G, RADER DJ, GREGG RE: **Absence of Microsomal Triglyceride Transfer Protein in Individuals With Abetalipoproteinemia.** *Science* 1992, **258**:999–1001.

Breakthrough observation indicating that deficiency of a microsomal transfer protein may be the molecular etiology of abetalipoproteinemia.

18. •• HAMILTON RL, HAVEL RJ: **Is Microsomal Triglyceride Transfer Protein the Missing Link in Abetalipoproteinemia?** *Hepatology* 1993, **18**:460–463.

Commentary about Wetterau *et al.* (*Science* 1992, 258:999–1001) and outstanding review of the potential role of microsomal triglyceride transfer protein in lipoprotein particle assembly.

19. KAGNOFF MF: **Celiac Disease. A Gastrointestinal Disease With Environmental Genetic, and Immunologic Components.** *Gastroenterol Clin North Am* 1992, **21**:405–425

20. • CORAZZA G, VALENTINI RA, FRISONI M, VOLTA U, CORRAO G, BIANCHI FB, GASBARRINI G: **Gliadin Immune Reactivity Is Associated With Overt and Latent Enteropathy in Relatives of Celiac Patients.** *Gastroenterology* 1992, **103**:1517–1522 .

A total of 328 first-degree relatives of adult celiac patients were screened for the presence of antigliadin antibodies. Jejunal biopsies demonstrated subtotal villus atrophy in 13 of 21 positive patients. The remaining eight subjects had normal-appearing mucosa, although morphometric evaluation showed a mean surface-to-volume ratio significantly lower than negative controls. Whether these subjects are false-positives or have latent celiac disease will have a significant impact on the future use of this assay as a screening test.

21. •• FERREIRA M, DAVIES SL, BUTLER M, SCOTT D, CLARK M, KUMAR P: **Endomysial Antibody: Is It the Best Screening Test for Coeliac Disease?** *Gut* 1992, **33**:1633–1637.

Comparison of the sensitivities and specificities of circulating immunoglobulin A and immunoglobulin G antigliadin antibodies and immunoglobulin A antireticulin antibody with the endomysial antibody in 117 patients with treated or untreated celiac disease and normal controls and control patients a variety of inflammatory disorders. Based on superior sensitivity and specificity, the authors conclude that the endomysial antibody is superior to the other antibody tests for the diagnosis of celiac disease.

22. REVILLON Y, SARNACKI JS, GOULET O, BROUSSE N, RICOUR
•• C: **Intestinal Transplantation in the Child: Experimental and Clinical Studies.** *J Pediatr Surg* 1993, **28**:292–298.

The group at the University of Pittsburgh has productively continued its efforts to make small intestinal transplantation a feasible option for patients with severe short bowel syndrome. As documented in these short reports, they have made progress in the technical aspects, in the control of graft rejection, and in the assessment of graft rejection and function.

23. TODO S, TZAKIS A, ABU-ELMAGD K, REYES J, FURUKAWA H,
•• NOUR B, FUNG JJ, STARZL TE: **Clinical Intestinal Transplantation.** *Transplant Proc* 1993, **25**:2195–2197.

Follow-up of 30 transplant patients treated with FK 506 for posttransplant immunosuppression.

24. TZAKIS AG, REYES J, TODO S, NOUR B, SHAPIRO R, JORDAN
• M, MCCAULEY J, ARMITAGE J, FUNG JJ, STARZL TE: **Two-Year Experience With FK 506 in Pediatric Patients.** *Transplant Proc* 1993, **25**:619–621.

Reviews entire University of Pittsburgh transplant experience (liver, kidney, heart, lung, liver-small bowel, and small bowel) with FK 506 immunosuppression in children.

25. TODO S, TZAKIS A, REYES J, ABU-ELMAGD K, CASAVILLA A,
• FUNG JJ, STARZL TE: **Intestinal Transplantation in Humans Under FK 506.** *Transplant Proc* 1993, **25**:1198–1199.

Convincing demonstration that small bowel transplantation is feasibly with FK 506. Isolated small intestinal transplantation was not inferior to the results obtained from transplantation of combined grafts.

26. REYES J, TZAKIS AG, TODO S, NOUR B, CASAVILLA A, ABU-
• ELMAGD K, FUNG JJ, STARZL TE: **Nutritional Management of Intestinal Transplant Recipients.** *Transplant Proc* 1993, **25**:1200–1201.

Analysis intestinal function postintestinal transplant. Parameters including absorption, nutritional status, and graft motility and anatomy are discussed.

27. ABU-ELMAGD KM, TZAKIS A, TODO S, REYES J, FUNG J,
• NAKAMURA K, WRIGHT H, FURUKAWA H, DEMETRIS J, VAN THIEL DH, STARZL TE: **Monitoring and Treatment of Intestinal Allograft Rejection in Humans.** *Transplant Proc* 1993, **25**:1202–1203.

Description of the Pittusburgh experience with acute and chronic rejection and graft-versus-host disease. Acute rejection, which occurred in 21 of the 24 small bowel grafts, usually responded to an increase in basal FK 506 dose and a steroid bolus.

Marc S. Levin, MD, Department of Medicine, Division of Gastroenterology, Washington University School of Medicine, Box 8124, 660 South Euclid Avenue, St. Louis, MO 63110, USA.

Molecular and cell biology of the small intestine

David A. Brenner, MD*, and William J. Boyle, PhD†

*University of North Carolina, Chapel Hill, North Carolina, and †Amgen, Thousand Oaks, California, USA

The intestinal epithelium continues to be an excellent model system for studying regulation of gene expression during lineage commitment and differentiation. Recent studies have provided new insights into intestinal growth and adaptation and intestine-specific gene expression. The role of previously characterized growth factors, such as transforming growth factor-α, transforming growth factor-β, or growth hormone, has been investigated in the intestine. In addition, members of a newly described gene family called the trefoil peptides are being studied in the intestine and new insights into their functional significance are emerging.

Current Opinion in Gastroenterology 1994, **10**:149–155

Mechanisms of intestinal gene expression

The intestinal epithelium is a highly proliferative tissue that is constitutively renewed through adult life [1•]. It is generally felt that crypt stem cells give rise to rapidly proliferating progenitor cells capable of differentiating into one of four distinct lineages; enterocyte, goblet, enteroendocrine, and Paneth cells. There appears to be a dynamic equilibrium between crypt cell production and the senescence and exfoliation of highly differentiated epithelial cell types. The teleologic significance of constitutive renewal is not clear, but it might prevent the accumulation of mutations that could disrupt cell growth regulation. Normal intestinal epithelial growth regulation is thought to be regulated in part by soluble factors that stimulate mitogenesis, and in part by extracellular matrix proteins and adjacent mesenchyme-derived, pericryptal fibroblasts. The steps leading to terminally differentiated cell types from multipotent stem cells is not known, and specific markers identifying progenitor cell populations committed to various lineages have not been identified.

Studies using transgenic mice have demonstrated that the 5′ flanking sequences derived from various isoforms of fatty-acid binding protein genes contain *cis*-regulatory elements that control their expression [2•]. Recent studies have focused on using upstream sequences of the rat intestinal fatty-acid binding protein gene to direct a human growth hormone reporter [3•]. Nucleotides of −103 to +28 of the rat intestinal fatty-acid binding protein gene are sufficient to direct transgene expression in the appropriate cell lineage and crypt-villus compartment, as well as within the appropriate position along the cephalocaudal axis. In addition, the −103 to +28 promoter construct was expressed at high levels in Caco-2 cells, but not in epithelial cell lines derived from other tissues, suggesting that transcription factors in intestinal epithelia were required. Examination of the sequences within this promoter element indicated the presence of a 14-bp sequence previously shown to be binding sites for two members of the steroid hormone receptor superfamily, hepatocyte nuclear factor-4 and apolipoprotein regulatory protein-1 (Fig. 1). Cotransfection of the −103 to +28 reporter along with either hepatocyte nuclear factor-4 or apolipoprotein regulatory protein-1 expression vectors into CV-1 cells activated reporter expression, and suggests that the 14-bp repeat sequence of the rat intestinal fatty-acid binding protein gene upstream region responds to these two factors during enterocyte differentiation.

To address the normal regulation of villin gene expression during intestinal epithelial cell differentiation, a 2.0-kb 5′-flanking region of the human villin gene was linked to a luciferase reporter [4•]. The villin promoter-luciferase gene fusion was transfected into several epithelial cell types, and found only to be expressed in those cells that express the endogenous villin genes. When analyzed in HT-29 colon carcinoma cells, the reporter gene was dramatically up-regulated during terminal differentiation induced by galactose-containing medium. Further study using this *in vitro* model may help delineate the promoter elements involved.

The acute-phase response represents a dramatic change in host cell metabolism, particularly in the

Abbreviations

EGF—epidermal growth factor; **HITF**—human intestinal trefoil factor; **hSP**—human spasmolytic polypeptide; **pSP**—porcine spasmolytic polypeptide; **RITF**—rat intestinal trefoil factor; **TGF**—transforming growth factor.

 ISBN 1-85922-607-8 ISSN 0267–1379

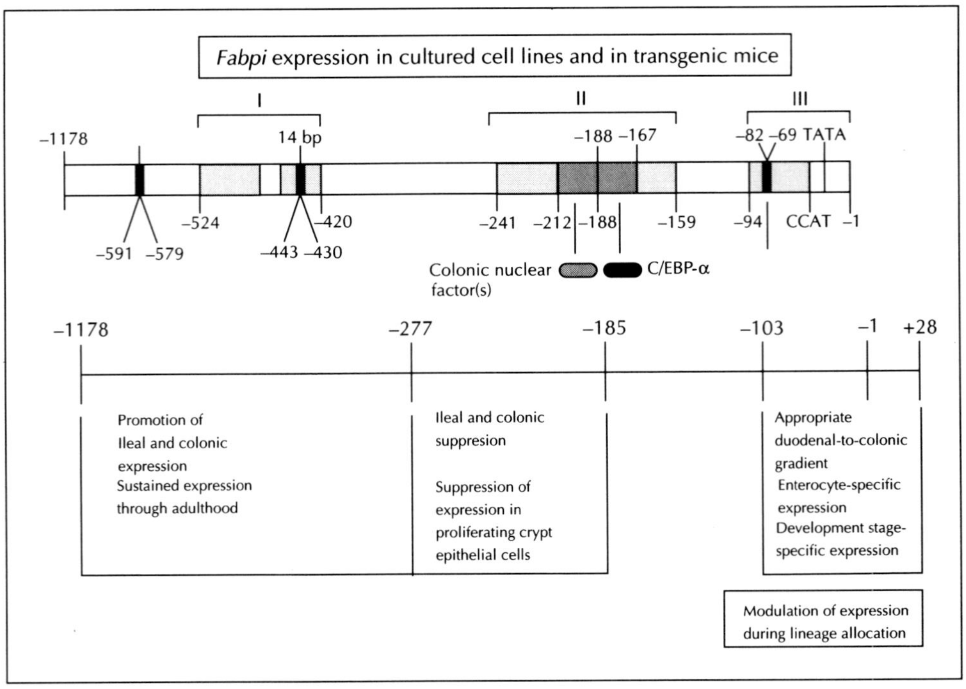

Fig. 1. I-FABP/hGH+3 DNAs characterized in transgenic mice and used for transfection of cultured primate epithelial cell lines. ARP—apolipoprotein regulatory protein; FABP—fatty-acid binding protein; HNF—hepatocyte nuclear factor. (*From* Rottman and Gordon [3•]; with permission.)

liver, in response to a systemic stress. Acute-phase proteins can be induced in hepatocytes *in vitro* by treatment with inflammatory cytokines such as interleukin-6, interleukin-1 and tumor necrosis factor-α. It has now been demonstrated that cultured intestinal epithelial cell lines are capable of a similar response to these cytokines [5]. Acute-phase proteins were induced at all stages of Caco-2 cell differentiation *in vitro*, suggesting that enterocytes derived from both the crypt and villus compartments were capable of responding. Caco-2 cells express receptors for both interleukin-1 and interleukin-6 at their apical and basolateral surface, while T84 cells express these receptors at only their basolateral surface.

Growth and adaptation

The nature and identity of the intestinal epithelial stem cell remains an enigma. Using transgenic and chimeric mice, several essential properties of stems cells have been illuminated as a paradigm for self-renewing and regenerating tissues [6•]. First, because crypt epithelium is monoclonal in nature, the stem cells must divide asymmetrically, producing a self-renewing stem cell and a progenitor cell committed to production of all differentiated cell types. Second, the daughter stem cell must have enormous proliferative capacity. Third, the stem cell must be functionally retained within the crypt niche and therefore have specific contacts with the lamina propria or other adjacent cells.

To help address the nature of intestinal epithelial differentiation, an *in vivo* system has been developed utilizing chimeric-transgenic mice [7••]. Embryonic stem cells transfected with a lineage and differentiation state-specific transgene were reimplanted into mouse blastocysts. The resulting offspring were chimeric with respect to intestinal crypt stem cells, and villus epithelium derived from adjacent crypts could be analyzed side-by-side. Thus, two monoclonal epithelial populations that differ only by the addition of a single transgene product and occupy identical positions along the cephalocaudal and crypt-to-villus axes can be compared.

Identification and characterization of crypt stem cells have been hampered by the lack of culture systems to expand intestinal epithelial lineages *in vitro*. Recently, attempts have been made to culture crypt cells that are derived from a transgenic mouse expressing a conditional form of SV40 large T antigen [8••]. At normal mouse body temperature the large T antigen is inactive, but upon culture at 39°C, large T antigen is activated and enables cells derived from various body tissues to grow in culture without the need for exogenous, or even unidentified, growth factors. Crypts isolated from young adult mice were dispersed and cultured at the permissive temperature. Resulting cell lines were maintained in liquid culture and expressed low levels of brush border enzymes. Upon shift to the nonpermissive temperature, cell growth ceases, suggesting that these cells have retained their ability to terminally differentiate.

Trefoil peptides

The trefoil peptides are a group of structurally related peptides containing a distinctive motif that harbors three disulfide bonds [9••]. The first member to be identified, pS2, was isolated as an estrogen-inducible transcript from a human breast carcinoma cell line, MCF-7. Other members of this rapidly growing family include porcine spasmolytic polypeptide (pSP), human spasmolytic polypeptide (hSP), and rat intestinal trefoil factor (RITF). The physiologic function of trefoil peptides is not clear, but the localization of trefoil peptides in normal and injured mucosa strongly suggests that they are of considerable functional importance. Trefoil peptides are present at the edges of healing ulcers, where a specialized ulcer-associated cell lineage appears that expresses high levels of various trefoil peptides (Fig. 2). Thus, at least some of the trefoil peptides help define histologically distinct regions of the mucosa and possibly mark specific cell types. pSP stimulates proliferation of a human colon cancer cell line *in vitro*, suggesting that trefoil peptides may be mitogenic for certain cell types.

A human homologue for RITF has been cloned from a normal human colon complementary DNA library by low stringency hybridization with RITF complementary DNA [10••]. The human protein, human intestinal trefoil factor (HITF) was found to be a 75-amino acid peptide that is approximately 70% homologous to RITF, and contains a conserved cysteine-rich internal domain present in all trefoil peptides. HITF is expressed predominantly in secretory vesicles of goblet cells, and is found coating the luminal surface of the mucosa. HITF expression was detected in HT-29 subclones expressing goblet cell markers, but not in differentiated Caco-2 cells. Trefoil peptide expression during intestinal adaptation has been studied by localization of pS2 and hSP expression in the ulceration-associated cell lineage and adjacent mucosa in Crohn's disease [11••]. pS2 and hSP are expressed in different locations with ductal cells adjacent to crypts. pS2 was also found to be expressed in secretory granules of goblet and enteroendocrine cells.

Growth factors

With the discovery of new growth factors and the technology to help determine their role in biological functions during development, there has been particular interest in identifying the factors that regulate growth and development of the mucosa and in evaluating their therapeutic potential. For example, factors that regulate growth of the small bowel mucosa could be useful for the treatment of short bowel syndrome because of the importance of adaptation of the mucosa to long-term patient survival [12]. Mucosal regeneration could also be a key force in avoiding morbidity associated with inflammation and ulceration. Because of the tremendous proliferative capacity of the intestinal epithelium, there is considerable interest in focusing on polypeptide growth factors receptors associated with oncogenesis [13•], including members of the epidermal growth factor (EGF), transforming growth factor (TGF)-α family, and their cognate receptors including EGF receptor, HER-2/Neu, and *erb*B-3. EGF and TGF-α are known to be mitogenic to intestinal epithelium. Examination of EGF and TGF-α messenger RNA expression during development of human fetal gut imply an important role [14•]. TGF-α messenger RNA was expressed at relatively high levels in the duodenum, whereas little or no EGF messenger RNA is normally expressed. In explanted jejunum, exogenous EGF increased TGF-α messenger RNA expression. Treatment of these same explants with exogenous TGF-α down-regulated endogenous TGF-α expression. EGF-induced TGF-α ex-

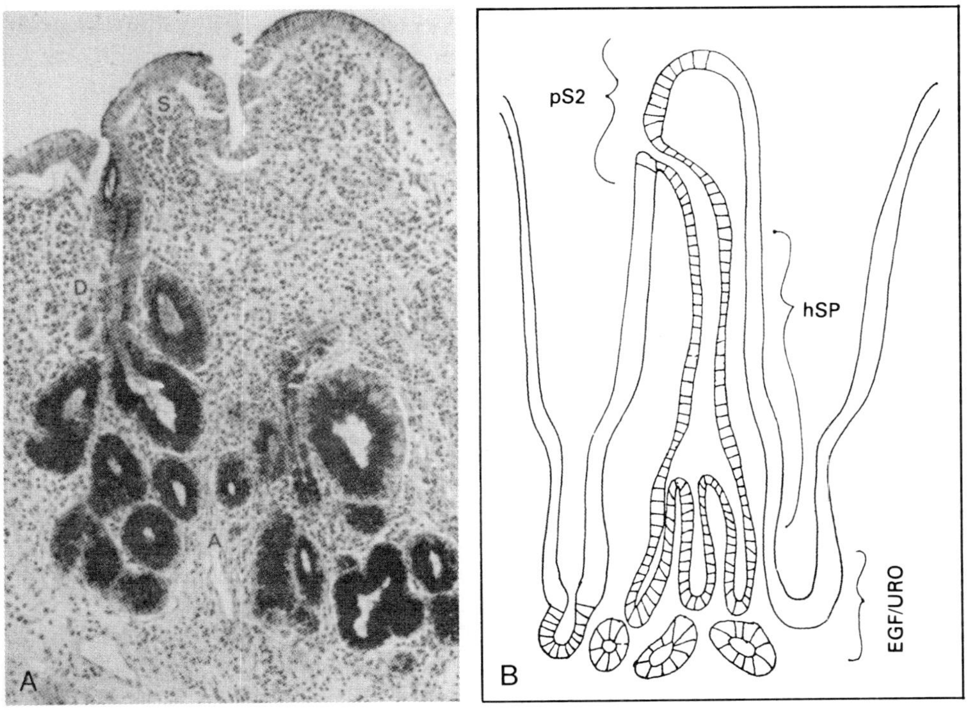

Fig. 2. A, Photomicrograph of the ulcer-associated cell lineage from a case of Crohn's disease showing the acini (A), the duct (D), and the surface cells (S) (original x 200). **B**, Ulcer-associated cell lineage with the secretory products of the several anatomic zones indicated. hSP—human spasmolytic polypeptide; EGF—epidermal growth factor; URO—urogastrone. (*From* Wright [9••]; with permission.)

pression resulted in the secretion of prepro-TGF-α, suggesting that further processing of the polypeptide is required to release active EGF receptor ligand.

Transgenic mice that overexpress bovine growth hormone show enhanced growth of the small intestinal mucosa [15•]. The trophic effects of long-term growth hormone treatment can be measured as a 50% to 100% increase in mucosal weight, particularly within the proximal bowel, and increased villus height. Increase in mucosal weight was not due to dietary intake. Interestingly, there is no observable increase in the proliferative capacity of intestinal epithelial precursors, suggesting that net increase in tissue weight was caused by the extended life span of these cells.

Transforming growth factor-β

Transforming growth factor-β can inhibit intestinal epithelial growth in culture and presumably functions to block proliferation *in vivo*. A recent study has reinvestigated the localization of TGF-β within the crypt and villus compartments of the small intestinal mucosa [16•]. Intestinal localization of TGF-β isoforms messenger RNA and protein indicates that three isoforms are expressed in the mucosa; TGF-β1, TGF-β2, and TGF-β3. Expression was most prominent at the villus tips, and no crypt expression was detected. This suggests that TGF-β may function to arrest crypt epithelial growth as cells migrate upward toward the villi. It is also possible that expression of TGF-β at this site is involved in maintaining the terminally differentiated phenotype of villus epithelium.

A further role for TGF-β in intestinal epithelial growth control was revealed by assaying its ability to regulate migration of rat intestinal epithelial cells across an artificial wound surface [17••]. Intestinal epithelial cell-6 cell monolayers were wounded *in vitro*, and the ability of cells to migrate and fill the wounded area was measured in the presence or absence of exogenous TGF-β. Although TGF-β inhibits cell proliferation, it stimulates the ability of intestinal epithelial cell-6 cells to migrate across and fill the wounded monolayer. This indicates that TGF-β may play an important role in reconstitution of the mucosa after injury *in vivo*.

Other gene products

Mucin

The mucosal surface is normally protected by a thick viscous gel, a critical component of which are mucous glycoproteins or mucins. Mucins have an internal tandem repeat core sequence that serves as a target for extensive O-linked glycosylation. However, little is known about the N- and C-terminal mucin peptide sequences that are not target for glycosylation and may play a role in mucin oligomerization important for mucous gel formation. The full-length complementary DNA for the MUC-2 gene product has recently been cloned and sequenced, revealing the primary structure of its core protein [18•]. An interesting cysteine-rich motif was identified at its N- and C-termini, which shared considerable homology with von Willebrand's factor. These regions are believed to be important for mucin protein crosslinking and oligomerization during formation of the protective mucous gel.

P-450

The mammalian intestinal epithelium produces cytochrome P-450–dependent monooxygenases capable of metabolizing luminal xenobiotics and rendering them inactive procarcinogens or converting them into potential mutagens. The P-450 enzyme systems known to be active in the intestinal mucosa include CYP1A1 (hydrocarbon-inducible), CYP2B1 (phenobarbital-inducible), and CYP3A (glutacorticoid-inducible). The presence of a particular P-450 system, as well as the type of xenobiotic present, influences the end product yielded from xenobiotic metabolism.

Expression of specific cytochrome P-450 genes along the intestinal crypt to villus axis has been studied to explain how xenobiotic metabolism occurs within the intestine *in vivo* [19••]. Using *in situ* hybridization, CYP1A1 and CYP2B1 messenger RNA was found to be constitutively expressed in villus epithelium, but not in crypts. Treatment with various xenobiotics induced CYP1A1 expression in both the crypt and villus epithelium, while CYP2B1 expression increased only within villus cells. Cytochrome P-450 reductase, a necessary component of all monooxygenase systems, was normally expressed only in villus cells, but could be induced in both crypt and villus compartments after dexamethsome treatment. This suggests that regulation of components of the P-450 system is complex, and can give rise to active monooxygenases in various compartments within the intestinal mucosa, depending on the presentation of luminal xenobiotics.

Regulation of brush border hydrolases

The differentiated enterocyte on the small intestinal villi contain brush border hydrolases required for terminal digestion of nutrients and have become model genes in which to study intestinal differentiation.

Sucrase-isomaltase

Sucrase and isomaltase, which are distinct enzymes that are synthesized as a single polypeptide from a single sucrase-isomaltase messenger RNA, rapidly rise to adult levels during the 3rd week of postnatal development. Because previous studies have demonstrated that glucocorticoids are potent regulators of sucrase activity in developing rat small intestine, a recent study [20•] investigated the molecular mechanism for this effect. This study demonstrated that both endogenous and exogenous glucocorticoids stimulated sucrase activity in parallel with increased sucrase-isomaltase messenger RNA levels. In the early phase of the developing intestine (postnatal day 10), glucocorticoids caused precocious appearance of both sucrase-isomaltase messenger RNA and sucrase activity; in a later phase (postnatal day 16), glucocorticoids accelerated epithelial cell kinetics resulting in the fast emergence of sucrase-isomaltase bearing enterocytes, and finally (postnatal day 18), there was a loss of responsiveness of sucrase-isomaltase to glucocorticoids. Increased sucrase-isomaltase activity is observed in the streptozocin-treated chronically diabetic rat. A study investigating the mechanism for this observation [21•] demonstrated increased sucrase activity with concomitant increased sucrase-isomaltase messenger RNA levels in the diabetic rat enterocytes. However, there was no difference in the rates of sucrase-isomaltase gene transcription between diabetic and control rats, implying adaptation through stabilization of sucrase-isomaltase messenger RNA.

Lactase-phlorzin hydrolase

Lactase-phlorzin hydrolase or lactase is critical for nursing when milk is the sole nutrient, but unnecessary after weaning. A recent study [22••] demonstrated that lactase messenger RNA and protein are located along the entire villus in the rat fetal intestine. In the newborn intestine, however, an entirely different pattern was demonstrated that persisted into adulthood. In later development, the crypt cells completely lacked lactase expression, the proximal villus cells had high lactase messenger RNA levels and the beginning of protein accumulation and the distal villus tip cells had decreased messenger RNA and maximum protein accumulation.

Dipeptidyl peptidase IV

The dipeptidyl peptidase IV, which cleaves aminoterminal dipeptides from polypeptides with either L-proline or L-alanine at the penultimate position, was demonstrated to be identical to CD26, a T-cell activation molecule. The relationship between these two disparate activities was recently investigated [23••,24•]. Jurkat T-cell lines were transfected with wild-type or mutant CD26 expression vectors that lacked dipeptidyl peptidase IV enzyme activity. Stimulation of these Jurkat cells demonstrated that the dipeptidyl peptidase IV activity of CD26 functions to augment the cellular responses of T cells to external stimuli mediated by CD26 or by independent receptor ligand interactions resulting in enhanced interleukin-2 production. The signal transduction pathway by which CD26 contributes to T-cell activation might be through adenosine deaminase, as adenosine deaminase and CD26 interact on the T-cell plasma membrane.

Gastrointestinal hormones

In the ileum, the enteroendocrine L cells synthesize the gastrointestinal hormones, enteroglucagon and peptide tyrosine tyrosine. Massive small bowel resection results in dramatic adaptation in the residual terminal ileum including increased enteroglucagon and peptide tyrosine tyrosine production, and increased polyamine synthesis. The administration of difluoromethylornithine, a specific inhibitor of ornithine decarboxylase, which is the rate-limiting enzyme in polyamine biosynthesis, blocks ileal adaptation after massive small bowel resection. To determine if the L-cell response of increased enteroglucagon and peptide tyrosine tyrosine messenger RNA was a primary response to massive small bowel resection or secondary to increased polyamine synthesis, ileal adaptation to massive small bowel resection was performed in the presence or absence of difluoromethylornithine [25•]. A decrease in both enteroglucagon and peptide tyrosine tyrosine messenger RNA levels after massive small bowel resection in the difluoromethylornithine-treated rats provided evidence that the L-cell response plays a secondary role following the induction of polyamine synthesis induction.

Many new gastrointestinal peptides have been recently characterized that cluster into families. The cloning of PEC-60 from the pig intestine [26•] enabled the analysis of its expression. PEC-60 has homology with pancreatic secretory trypsin inhibitor. PEC-60 messenger RNA is expressed at high levels in the duodenum with immunolocalization to the cytoplasm of goblet cells. In addition, PEC-60 is synthesized and secreted by peripheral monocytes indicating a potential role in the immune system.

During differentiation of intestinal cells along the crypt-villus axis, differences in responses to hormones reflects both the cell surface receptor and the associated signal transduction pathway. A recent study evaluated the intestinal expression of G proteins, which consist of heterotrimers composed of α, β, and γ subunits. This study [27••] demonstrated that G_s and G_i protein subunits undergo divergent expression during epithelial cell differentiation along the crypt villus axis with α_s subunit being more abundant in crypt cells and αi_2 and αi_3 more abundant in villus cells. The gradient of expression of the G protein subunits appear to be generated at the level of their messenger RNAs. Although G proteins may not be rate limiting in the transduction pathway of adenyl cyclase, these observations might explain why basal adenylcylase activity as well as vasoactive intestinal pepticle-stimulated cyclic AMP production is higher in crypt cells than villus cells.

Transporters

The sodium-dependent glucose cotransporter SGLT-1 is present in the brush border membrane of enterocytes in all vertebrates and related messenger RNAs are present in invertebrates [28•]. The activity of the sodium-glucose cotransporter is regulated by dietary substrate levels in many species. In the early postnatal period of all mammals, the primary dietary carbohydrate is lactose that is hydrolyzed to glucose and galactose. In nonruminant adults, including humans, other sources of dietary carbohydrate provide sugars. However, in ruminants, dietary carbohydrates are fermented and hexoses do not reach the small intestine. A recent study [29••] examined the SGLT-1 expression in ruminant sheep. During weaning in sheep, the activity of the sodium-glucose cotransporter falls dramatically while the level of SGLT-1 messenger RNA is essentially unchanged. Therefore, the regulation of SGLT-1 activity during sheep development is primarily controlled by posttranscriptional events. As discussed above, this mechanism appears to be analogous to the postnatal decline in lactase activity.

A family of complementary DNAs encode for facilitative glucose transporters referred to as Glut-1 through Glut-5. Previous studies have localized Glut-5 to the brush border membrane in normal human small intestine. A recent study [30•] demonstrated that Glut-5 is also expressed in CaCo-2 colon carcinoma cell line at both the messenger RNA and protein level and was appropriately localized on the brush border. The expression of Glut-5 increased with the passage number of the cell line and also with the differentiation process that occurs upon confluence of the cell. The physiologic role of Glut-5 was clear. However, by expressing Glut-5 in the xenopus oocyte, a detailed study of its substrate specificity and kinetic properties was possible [31••]. Glut-5 appears to selectively transport fructose and strong corroborative evidence indicates that fructose transport is its physiologic function.

References and recommended reading

Papers of particular interest, published within the annual period of review, have been highlighted as:
- • Of special interest
- •• Of outstanding interest

1. • PODOLSKY DK: **Regulation of Intestinal Epithelial Proliferation: A Few Answers, Many Questions.** *Am J Physiol* 1993, **264**:G179–G186.

Review of literature describing regulation of intestinal epithelial cell growth and differentiation.

2. • SIMON TC, ROTH KA, GORDON JI: **Use of Transgenic Mice to Map Cis-Acting Elements in the Liver Fatty Acid-Binding Protein Gene (FABPi) that Regulates its Cell Lineage-Specific, Differentiation-Dependent, and Spatial Patterns of Gene Expression in the Gut Epithelium and Liver Acinus.** *J Biol Chem* 1993, **268**:18345–18358.

Functional mapping of the FABPi promoter region in vitro and in vivo indicates it contains functional C/EBP-α binding sites.

3. • ROTTMAN JN, GORDON JI: **Comparison of the Patterns of Expression of Rat Intestinal Fatty Acid Binding Protein/Human Growth Hormone Fusion Genes in Cultured Intestinal Epithelial Cell Lines and in the Gut Epithelium of Transgenic Mice.** *J Biol Chem* 1993, **268**:11994–12002.

Functional mapping of fatty-acid binding protein gene promoter region *in vitro* and *in vivo* indicates it contains functional HNF-4 and ARP-1 binding sites.

4. • ROBIN S, SAHUQUILLO-MERINO C, LOUVARD D, PRINGAULT E: **Regulatory Sequences on the Human Villin Gene Trigger the Expression of a Reporter Gene in a Differentiating HT29 Intestinal Cell Line.** *J Biol Chem* 1993, **268**:11426–11434.

Identification of a cell culture systems useful for mapping the promoter elements of the human villin gene.

5. • MOLMENTI E, ZIAMBARAS T, PERLMUTTER DH: **Evidence for an Acute Phase Response in Human Intestinal Epithelial Cells.** *J Biol Chem* 1993, **268**:14116–14124.

Demonstrates that intestinal epithelial cells respond to inflammatory cytokines by rapidly synthesizing acute-phase proteins.

6. • GORDON JI, SCHMIDT GH, ROTH KA: **Studies of Intestinal Stem Cells Using Normal, Chimeric, and Transgenic Mice.** *FASEB* 1992, 6:3039–3050.

Review of literature describing the properties and characteristics of intestinal epithelial stem cells.

7. •• HERMISTRON ML, GREEN RP, GORDON JI: **Chimeric-Transgenic Mice Represent a Powerful Tool for Studying How the Proliferation and Differentiation Programs of Intestinal Epithelial Cell Lineages are Regulated.** *Proc Natl Acad Sci U S A* 1993, **90**:8866–8870.

Demonstrates the ability to generate chimeric mice expressing transgene in specific compartments of the intestinal mucosa, and discusses their ability in analyzing intestinal epithelial differentiation.

8. •• WHITEHEAD RH, VANEEDEN PE, NOBLE MD, ATALIOTIS P, JAT PS: **Establishment of Conditionally Immortalized Epithelial Cell Lines From Both Colon and Small Intestine of Adult H-2Kb-tsA58 Transgenic Mice.** *Proc Natl Acad Sci U S A* 1993, **90**:587–591.

Describes the use of transgenic mouse harboring a conditional oncogene to isolate and culture murine colonic crypt-derived epithelial cell lines with properties of normal, untransformed cells.

9. •• WRIGHT NA: **Trefoil Peptides and the Gut.** *Gut* 1993, **34**:577–579.

Review of literature describing the isolation and functional characterization of members of the trefoil peptide family.

10. •• PODOLSKY DK, LYNCH-DEVANEY K, STOW JL, OATES P, MURGUE B, DEBEAUMONT M, SANDS BE, MAHIDA YR: **Identification of Human Intestinal Trefoil Factor.** *J Biol Chem* 1993, **268**:6694–6702.

Identification of the human homologue for rat intestinal trefoil factor, and its characterization in goblet and enteroendocrine cells.

11. •• POULSOM R, CHINERY R, SARRAF C, LALANI E-N, STAMP G, ELIA G, WRIGHT N: **Trefoil Peptide Expression in Intestinal Adaptation and Renewal.** *Scand J Gastroenterol* 1992, **27**:17–28.

Analysis of the trefoil peptide pS2 expression in ulceration-associated cell lineage and in adjacent enteroendocrine goblet cells. A new human and rat intestinal trefoil peptide was identified and characterized.

12. • VANDERHOFF JA: **Regulatory Peptides and Intestinal Growth [Editorial].** *Gastroenterology* 1993, **104**:1205–1208.

Editorial discussing experimental application and therapeutic uses for factors active on intestinal epithelial cells.

13. • LEMOINE NR, LEUNG HY, GULLICK WJ: **Growth Factors in the Gastrointestinal Tract.** *Gut* 1992, **33**:1297–1300.

Review discussing the role of polypeptide growth factors and their receptors in controlling normal and abnormal proliferation in the gastrointestinal tract.

14. • MIETTINEN PJ: **Transforming Growth Factor-Alpha and Epidermal Growth Factor Expression in Human Fetal Gastrointestinal Tract.** *Pediatr Res* 1993, **33**:481–486.

Expression of EGF and TGF-α was measured during development of the fetal human intestine. EGF was shown to up-regulate TGF-α expression in explanted tissue placed in culture.

15. • ULSHEN MH, DOWLING RH, FULLER CR, ZIMMERMAN EM, LUND PK: **Enhanced Growth of Small Bowel in Transgenic Mice Overexpressing Bovine Growth Hormone.** *Gastroenterology* 1993, **104**:973–980.

Trophic effect of bovine growth hormone were demonstrated by transgenic expression in the mouse. Increased mass of intestine not due to dietary intake or increased cell proliferation, but believed to be due to prolonged epithelial cell life span.

16. BARNARD JA, WARWICK GJ, GOLD LI: **Localization of Transforming Growth Factor Beta Isoforms in the Normal Murine Small Intestine and Colon.** *Gastroenterology* 1993, **105**:67–73.
•

Further evidence is presented which suggests that TGF-β is expressed in villus epithelium, and that it plays a role in both decreasing cell proliferation and maintaining terminal differentiation.

17. CIACCI C, LIND SE, PODOLSKY DK: **Transforming Growth Factor Beta Regulation of Migration in Wounded Rat Intestinal Epithelial Monolayers.** *Gastroenterology* 1993, **105**:93–101.
••

TGF-β shown to induce migration of cultured rat intestinal epithelial cells across a artificial wound *in vitro*. Suggests a role for TGF-βduring regeneration of the mucosa following injury.

18. GUM JR, HICKS JW, TORIBARA NW, ROTHE E-M, LAGACE RE, KIM YS: **The Human MUC2 Intestinal Mucin Has Cysteine-Rich Subdomains Located Both Upstream and Downstream of its Central Repetitive Region.** *J Biol Chem* 1992, **267**:21375–21383.
•

Full length complementary DNA for the MUC-2 gene is characterized. N- and C-terminal regions are revealed that contain significant homology to von Willebrand's factor and are thought to play a functional role in mucous gel formation.

19. TRABER PG, WANG W, YU L: **Differential Regulation of Cytochrome P-450 Genes Along Rat Intestinal Crypt-Villus Axis.** *Am J Physiol* 1992, **263**:G215–G223.
••

Analysis of expression of various isoforms of P-450 monooxygenase along the crypt-villus axis in mouse small intestine before or after treatment with xenobiotic chemicals.

20. NANTHAKUMAR NN, HENNING SJ: **Ontogeny of Sucrase-Isomaltase Gene Expression in Rat Intestine: Responsiveness to Glucocorticoids.** *Am J Physiol* 1993, **264**:G306-G311.
•

Distinct phases of glucocorticoid effect on sucrase-isomaltase expression occur during development in the rat intestine.

21. HOFFMAN LR, CHANG EB: **Altered Regulation of Regional Sucrase-Isomaltase Expression in Diabetic Rat Intestine.** *Am J Physiol* 1992, **262**:G983–G989.
•

Increased sucrase-isomaltase in the diabetic rat intestine results from posttranscriptional regulation.

22. RINGS EHHM, DE BOER PAJ, MOORMAN AFM, VAN BEERS EH, DEKKER J, MONTGOMERY RK, GRAND RJ, BULLER HA: **Lactase Gene Expression During Early Development of Rat Small Intestine.** *Gastroenterology* 1992, **103**:1154–1161.
••

In situ hybridization for lactase messenger RNA with immunolocalization for lactase protein demonstrate a posttranscriptional regulation of lactase in fetal development.

23. TANAKA T, KAMEOKA J, YARON A, SCHLOSSMAN SF, MORIMOTO C: **The Costimulatory Activity of the CD26 Antigen Requires Dipeptidyl Peptidase IV Enzymatic Activity.** *Proc Natl Acad Sci U S A* 1993, **90**:4586–4590.
••

Demonstrates that CD26 requires its peptidase activity for maximal costimulatory effects on T cells.

24. KAMEOKA J, TANAKA T, NOJIMA Y, SCHLOSSMAN SF, MORIMOTO C: **Direct Association of Adenosine Deaminase With a T Cell Activation Antigen, CD26.** *Science* 1993, **261**:466–469.
•

Demonstrates that CD26 directly interacts with adenosine deaminase on the T-cell plasma membrane.

25. TAYLOR RG, BEVERIDGE DJ, FULLER PJ: **Expression of Ileal Glucagon and Peptide Tyrosine-Tyrosine Genes. Response to Inhibition of Polyamine Synthesis in the Presence of Massive Small-Bowel Resection.** *Biochem J* 1992, **286**:737–741.
•

Uses the model of massive small bowel resection to demonstrate that enteroglucagon and peptide tyrosine tyrosine expression occurs secondarily to polyamine biosynthesis.

26. METSIS M, CINTRA A, SOLFRINI V, ERNFORS P, BORTOLOTTI F, MORRASUTTI DG, OSTENSON C-G, EFENDIC S, AGERBERTH B, MUTT V, PERSSON H, FUXE K: **Molecular Cloning of PEC-60 and Expression of its mRNA and Peptide in the Gastrointestinal Tract and Immune System.** *J Biol Chem* 1992, **267**:19829–19832.
•

Describes a family of sodium-coupled cotransporters traced from bacteria to invertebrates to vertebrates.

27. COUVINEAU A, DARMOUL D, BLAIS A, ROUYER-FESSARD C, DAVIAUD D, VOISIN T, PARIS H, ROUOT B, LABURTHE M: **Gs and Gi Protein Subunits During Cell Differentiation in Intestinal Crypt-Villus Axis: Regulation at the mRNA Level.** *Am J Physiol* 1992, **262**:C1478–C1484.
••

Demonstrates that G_s and G_i can undergo divergent expression in the crypt-to-villus axis which is largely regulated at the level of messenger RNA expression.

28. PAJOR AM, HIRAYAMA BA, WRIGHT EM: **Molecular Biology Approaches to Comparative Study of Na+-Glucose Cotransport.** *Am J Physiol* 1992, **263**:R489–R495.
•

Describes a family of sodium-coupled cotransporters traced from bacteria to invertebrates to vertebrates.

29. FREEMAN TC, WOOD IS, SIRINATHSINGHJI DJS, BEECHEY RB, DYER J, SHIRAZI-BEECHEY SP: **The Expression of the Na+/Glucose Co-Transporter (SGLT1) Gene in Lamb Small Intestine During Postnatal Development.** *Biochim Biophys Acta* 1993, **1146**:203–212.
••

The regulation of SGLT-1 in ruminant lamb small intestine occurs at a posttranscriptional level during postnatal development, as demonstrated by an *in situ* hybridization study.

30. MAHRAOUI L, ROUSSET M, DUSSAULX E, DARMOUL D, ZWEIBAUM A, BROT-LAROCHE E: **Expression and Localization of GLUT-5 in Caco-2 Cells, Human Small Intestine, and Colon.** *Am J Physiol* 1992, **263**:G312–G318.
•

Demonstrates that Glut-5 expression is inducible in Caco-2 cells and its protein is appropriately expressed on the brush border.

31. BURANT CF, TAKEDA J, BROT-LAROCHE E, BELL GI, DAVIDSON NO: **Fructose Transporter in Human Spermatozoa and Small Intestine Is GLUT5.** *J Biol Chem* 1992, **267**:14523–14526.
••

Strong evidence that the physiologic role of the Glut-5 glucose transporter is actually to transport fructose.

David A. Brenner, MD, Center for Gastrointestinal Biology and Disease, University of North Carolina, Chapel Hill, NC, 27599-7080, USA.

William J. Boyle, PhD, Amgen, Thousand Oaks, CA, USA.

Pathophysiology and pharmacology of small intestinal motility

Robin D. Rothstein, MD, and Ann Ouyang, MD

University of Pennsylvania School of Medicine, Philadelphia, and Pennsylvania State University, Hershey, Pennsylvania, USA

Tremendous progress continues in the area of small bowel motility and pharmacology. Our understanding of small bowel motility has been further advanced over the past year with studies examining the role of various mediators of gastrointestinal physiology. Additional new evidence supports the role of nitric oxide as a key intracellular messenger for nonadrenergic, noncholinergic inhibition of the gastrointestinal tract. Our ability to more accurately define motor abnormalities of the small bowel has been expanded with new diagnostic techniques. There has also been greater delineation of the small bowel motility abnormalities that exist in a number of pathologic conditions. Our therapeutic options have increased as progress in pharmacologic therapy for small bowel dysmotility continues to be advanced.

Current Opinion in Gastroenterology 1994, **10**:156–162

Physiology

Mechanisms

Modulation of gastrointestinal motility appears to be a complex interaction involving various mediators acting at different levels between the central nervous system and the gastrointestinal tract. Neuropeptide Y, widely distributed in both the mammalian central nervous system and in the gut, causes a delay in small bowel transit of both solids and liquids [1•]. This effect appears to be mediated via a β-adrenergic pathway as propranolol, but not phentolamine, blocks the inhibitory effect of neuropeptide Y.

The importance of the role of 5-hydroxytryptamine (5HT) at 5-HT_3 receptors as a neurotransmitter in the enteric nervous system has been strengthened by recent work. Intra-arterial 5HT results in an ascending contraction in a loop of denervated jejunum in dogs. This effect is attenuated by tetrodotoxin, hexamethonium, and atropine. These data, along with studies showing that naloxone and nifedipine failed to alter this contraction, imply that the action of 5HT is mediated via a cholinergic pathway [2].

Studies of nitric oxide continue to support its role as a nonadrenergic, noncholinergic inhibitory neurotransmitter at various regions of the gastrointestinal tract. In both human and canine jejunum, circular muscle inhibition appears to be mediated via nonadrenergic, noncholinergic nerves, although the mechanism for this inhibition appears to be distinctly different in the two species [3••]. Nitric oxide evokes hyperpolarizing responses in both human and canine jejunum, but the rate of response in humans is slower and longer in duration than that noted in canine jejunum. In addition, the same concentration of nitric oxide caused a greater rate of change of voltage during hyperpolarization in the canine jejunum than in human jejunum. Support for a role of nitric oxide as a mediator in the gastrointestinal tract is also supported by the demonstration that enteric nerves in the canine ileum can generate nitric oxide from L-arginine, which can be endogenously supplied [4].

In conscious dogs with implanted electrodes on the small bowel, *N*-nitro-L-arginine, an inhibitor of nitric oxide synthase, reduces the periodicity of the migrating motor complex. In contrast, addition of arginine or

Abbreviation
5HT—5-hydroxytryptamine.

glycerin trinitrate, substrates of nitric oxide synthase, increases the interval between migrating motor complex and decreases spike activity [5].

Modulation of small bowel patterns

It is well established that there are distinct patterns of small bowel motility and that nutrients alter a fasting pattern to a fed state. Studies have now examined the effect of nonnutrients on small bowel motility. Noncaloric liquids and intraluminal gas effect the characteristics of the fasting state [6••]. Instillation of air leads to an increase in duration and amplitude of contractions of phase II in the duodenum. Conversely, removal of air from the upper gastrointestinal tract reduces these features.

Nonabsorbed nutrients have also been noted to affect phase II activity. Using oroileal perfusion catheters, the effect of ileal infusion of carbohydrates or lipids was assessed in healthy persons. Nonabsorbed nutrients abbreviate the duration of phase II [7].

The mechanism for release of motilin, a hormone that appears to regulate phase III of the migrating motor complex, has been examined. Using isolated canine intestinal cells, the effects of bombesin, morphine, erythromycin, cisapride, and cholecystokinin were determined. Although these agents are known stimulants for motilin release *in vivo*, there was no detectable effect *in vitro*. Carbachol did cause a dose-dependent release of motilin that was blocked by atropine, indicating the presence of muscarinic receptors [8••].

The response of motilin to both modified sham feeding and gastric balloon distention was determined in normal volunteers who underwent antroduodenal motility. Both forms of stimulation caused an increase in motilin levels, but only balloon distention evoked a premature phase III response, suggesting different pathways of motilin release (Fig. 1) [9•].

Stimulation of upper gastrointestinal motility in response to food has been divided into three phases: cephalic, gastric, and intestinal. The cephalic phase of antroduodenal motility appears to be under vagal control as atropine blocks the changes in motility. Sham feeding delays the appearance of phase III of the migrating motor complex that can be reversed by loxiglumide [10]. These data support evidence to suggest that the cephalic phase of antroduodenal motility is under cholinergic control and that cholecystokinin is an important mediator of sham feeding.

Studies of transit

Determination of transit of the gastrointestinal tract is important in the evaluation of patients with suspected motility disturbances, in differentiating gastric and small bowel disorders, and in evaluating therapeutic responses. Basile *et al.* [11] described a novel method of measuring transit throughout the gastrointestinal tract. By following an orally ingested magnetized marker and using a biomagnetic superconducting instrument, the spatial location of the marker could

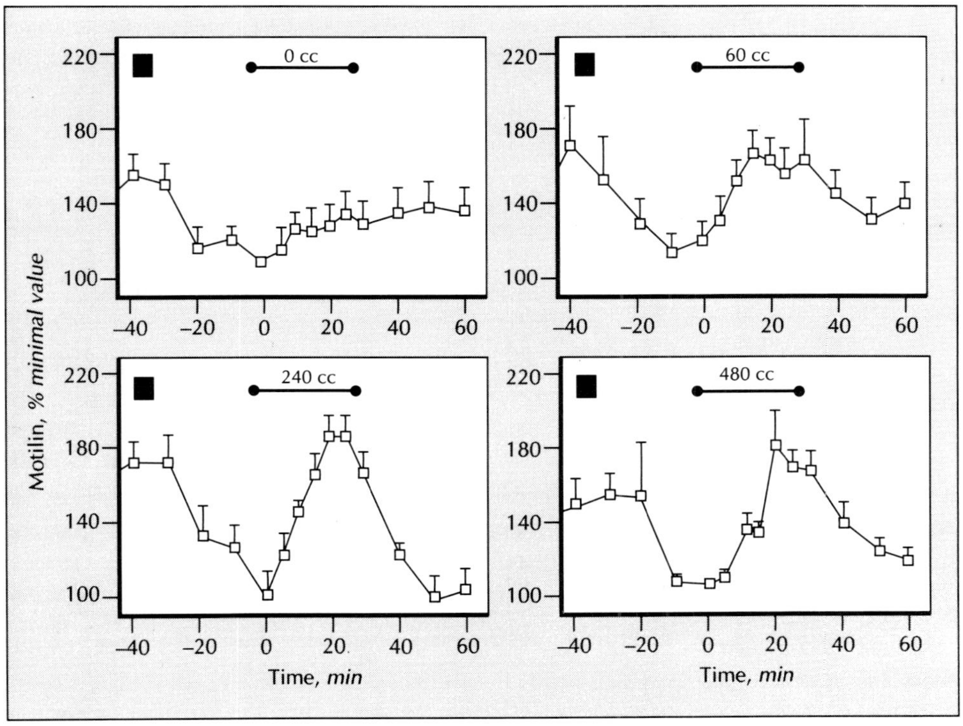

Fig. 1. Mean plasma motilin concentrations (expressed as percent of lowest value measured during the basal migrating motor complex) in subjects submitted to gastric distention with ballons filled with 0, 60, 240, or 480 cc of air. Distention was done 30 minutes after phase III (*solid block*) was seen migrating from the antrum to the duodenum. Five subjects in each group. (*From* Boivin *et al.* [9•]; with permission.)

be determined. Oroanal time and orocecal and colonic transit time could be safely, noninvasively, and accurately recorded.

An alternative approach to assess gastrointestinal transit was set forth by Ohe and Camilleri [12]. Patients first ingested a methacrylate-coated capsule of ^{111}In-labeled polystyrene pellets. Once the capsule was emptied from the stomach, the patient ingested a breakfast labeled with ^{99m}Tc polystyrene pellets in cooked eggs. A regular lunch was eaten after 4 hours and dinner in 8 hours. Using this technique, images could be obtained throughout a 24-hour period to determine gastric, small bowel, and colonic emptying.

Motility in pathologic conditions

Unfortunately, motility disturbances are frequently associated with a number of underlying medical problems. Small bowel motility may be impaired in patients with adhesions, including those who are asymptomatic. Small bowel transit time as assessed by hydrogen breath testing is increased from a median of 110 minutes to 140 minutes in asymptomatic patients with adhesions [13]. Orocecal time is also delayed by cigarette smoking, possibly mediated by nicotine [14]. Peritonitis also appears to adversely affect small bowel motility. Phase III activity is not affected, but phase II activity is diminished [15].

Patients who have undergone a Roux-en-Y gastrojejunostomy often have postprocedure symptoms. Using nuclear scintigraphy, stasis in the Roux limb has been noted to be more common in symptomatic patients. Stasis of the Roux limb is independent of vagotomy (Fig. 2) [16••]. Intestinal motility of the Roux limb has been found to be reduced. There are fewer clustered contractions and diminished migration of clustered waves compared with the jejunal activity in normal subjects. There is no relationship between gastric emptying rates and Roux-en-Y stasis [17••].

Chronic portal hypertension may also affect small bowel motility. In rats with portal hypertension induced by portal vein constriction, small bowel motility has been analyzed using an implanted catheter and measuring transit of radioactive chromium. The frequency of the migrating motor complex is decreased and phase III amplitude and frequency is diminished in the distal small bowel, but transit was not affected [18••].

Cirrhosis appears to alter small bowel motility. In 16 patients with cirrhosis, two had absence of the migrating motor complex. In the remaining 14, there was prolongation of the duration of the migrating motor complex cycle, primarily due to lengthening of phase II. These alterations could not be explained by bacterial overgrowth as patients with cirrhosis with and without evidence of bacterial overgrowth have similar findings. In addition, these alterations in motility are not affected by therapy with tetracycline [19].

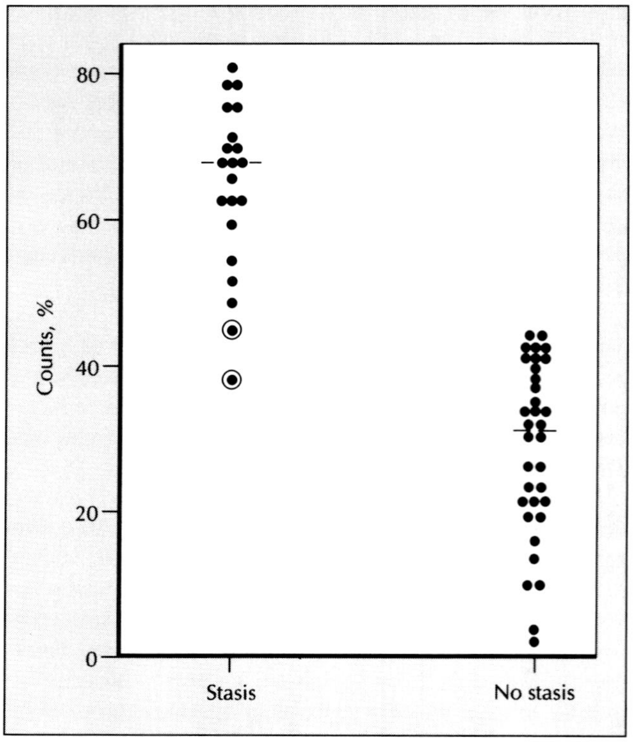

Fig. 2. Counts in the Roux limb at 60 minutes as a percentage of those emptied from the gastric remnant in 60 minutes, for 21 patients with Roux limb stasis and 34 without, as assessed visually. *Bars* represent medians. *Concentric circles* represent patients with a period of reflux from the Roux limb to the gastric remnant just before the 60th minute. (*From* Van der Mijle [16••]; with permission.)

Motility abnormalities of the small intestine occur in patients with symptomatic progressive systemic sclerosis. As expected, changes in motility are more apparent in symptomatic patients. In a group of asymptomatic patients with scleroderma, there is no difference in small intestinal transit time of cellulose or plastic particles compared with a group of normal, healthy subjects [20].

Ischemia or low perfusion state appears to have a deleterious effect on small bowel motility. When nonocclusive mesenteric ischemia is induced in piglets, small bowel motility is affected. The periodicity of the migrating motor complex is prolonged and the velocity of propagation is diminished with ischemia. Phase III was not affected. Reversal of ischemia leads to normalization of the small bowel pattern [21••].

Motility of both the ileum and the ileal reservoir has been studied in patients following proctocolectomy and ileal anal pullthroughs with variously designed pouches. In a review by Pescatori [22], the author outlines the motility studies that have been previously performed in patients with ileoanal anastomosis. Propulsive waves are propagated from the reservoir to the efferent limb in response to distention and are associated with a sensation of urgency. Studies of the small bowel proximal to the reservoir demonstrate discrete ileal clustered contractions, reminiscent of the electrical pattern noted in small bowel obstruction [22].

Severe obesity results in altered patterns of motility. Although there are no changes in the duration of the total migrating motor complex or of its phases, plasma motilin levels are reduced compared with subjects of normal weight [23•]. The potential implications of these findings remain unclear.

Pharmacology

There has been continued advancement in the pharmacology of the small bowel in the past year with inroads into the therapy of small bowel motor abnormalities. Cisapride, a well-studied promotility agent, has recently been approved for treatment of gastroesophageal reflux disease. Cisapride has also been shown to affect small bowel motility. In normal, healthy subjects, cisapride increases the amplitude of contractions during phase II and increases the percentage of migrating motor complexes that are distally propagated. Cisapride has no effect on the duration of the migrating motor complex cycle, including the duration of phase II, the frequency of phase II contractions, or the velocity of phase III [24].

In disorders of small bowel motility, cisapride improves small bowel function. In patients with quadriplegia who have delayed small bowel transit, cisapride normalizes the orocecal time [25]. Cisapride also improves small bowel motility in some children with pseudoobstruction. Overall, those children with intact migrating motor complexes on antroduodenal manometry and those with normal small bowel diameter on barium studies are most likely to benefit from cisapride [26].

An alternative prokinetic agent, erythromycin, has been used to affect small bowel motility. In dogs, erythromycin results in giant retrograde contractions and increases duodenal motor activity. This effect is attenuated by hexamethonium and atropine, implicating that the mechanism of action of erythromycin is via a ganglionic cholinergic pathway [27••].

In human studies, erythromycin induces a migrating motor complex that is similar to a spontaneous migrating motor complex in that it is associated with a rise in motilin levels. However, drug-induced migrating motor complexes have a diminished amplitude of contraction in the duodenum compared with spontaneous migrating motor complexes [28•]. Despite its promotility effect, erythromycin does not appear to have a role in reducing the period of postoperative ileus [29]. An erythromycin derivative, EM523L, has a promising future as a motilin agent, as it induces migrating motor complexes with an associated increase in plasma motilin concentrations in normal subjects [30•].

Other drugs have demonstrated a beneficial effect on small bowel motility. Acarbose and miglitol, α-glucosidase inhibitors that impair starch and sucrose digestion, abbreviate orocecal transit. It has been postulated that as these agents cause carbohydrate malabsorption, the colon receives an increased load of carbohydrate that is available as bacterial substrates. The metabolites of bacterial fermentation stimulate small intestinal peristalsis and small bowel transit is decreased [31•].

Interleukin-1β appears to affect small intestinal motility by a centrally mediated mechanism. When interleukin-1β is administered by the intracerebroventricular route to fed rats, there is disruption of the fed state and return of the migrating motor complex. In contrast, a tenfold higher dose of interleukin-1β administered peripherally has minimal effect on small bowel motility [32••]. Indomethacin antagonizes the effect of interleukin-1β and decreases the response of the small bowel to interleukin-1β. Indomethacin alone increases postprandial small bowel activity. The mechanism of action of interleukin-1β remains unclear. The effect of interleukin-1β may be due to inhibition of gastric acid or possibly the release of prostaglandin E. The specific prostaglandin E antagonist, SC 19220, ablates the effects of interleukin-1β, but alone has no effect on small bowel motility.

Ketorolac, a nonsteroidal anti-inflammatory medication that is administered parenterally, may be useful in patients with prolonged ileus. In initial studies in rats, ketorolac improves small bowel transit in postoperative rats with a more rapid return of the migrating motor complex than rats treated with saline [33•]. Similarly, misoprostol, a prostaglandin E1 analogue, results in accelerated small bowel transit by suppressing bowel activity [34•].

Substantive work has been performed in the area of inhibiting small bowel motility, which has been key in the treatment of various types of diarrhea, especially in patients with diabetes mellitus. Nifedipine, as determined by hydrogen breath test, has been shown to delay orocecal transit [35]. In the rat model, the calcium channel antagonists, nifedipine and nimodipine, inhibit spontaneous migrating motor complexes. In contrast, diltiazem and verapamil had no effect [36•]. Phenylephrine, an α_1-adrenergic agonist, also delays orocecal time and appears to reduce the amplitude of contraction in the duodenum. Frequency of contractions is unaffected [37•].

Extensive research on the effects of octreotide has established its profound effect on small bowel motility. The effect of this drug is complex and is dependent on a myriad of factors, including route of administration and dose [38]. Infusion of octreotide reduces the periodicity of the migrating motor complex and stimulates nonprogated phase III patterns. Octreotide has been used in a number of pathologic conditions. Patients with diabetes mellitus and diarrhea experience a reduction in stool weight and frequency and an increase in mouth-to-cecum time [39]. Octreotide may also have a role in reducing the period of postoperative ileus. Dogs with surgically induced ileus experienced a more rapid return of small bowel function. Octreotide was given in two doses and routes, 1.5 μg/kg/h subcutaneously or 0.83 μg/kg/h intravenously. Although small bowel transit improved, the higher dose of octreotide delayed gastric emptying [40•]. Despite promising work with octreotide, its mechanism of action remains less well established.

Pharmacology studies have also examined agents that have subsequently been demonstrated to have little or no effect on the small bowel. Olestra is a mixture of nonabsorbable sucrose and fatty acids. As duodenal fatty acids are felt to be important in suppressing gastric motility, the effect of olestra which is not hydrolyzed was hypothesized to be negligible. In a group of normal volunteers, gastric, small bowel, and colonic transit, as determined by nuclear scintigraphy, was unchanged after ingestion of a fatty meal with up to 30 g of olestra in a 45-g fat meal [41•].

Postlaparotomy ileus has also been studied in the rat model. Using selective α-adrenergic drugs in the rat, it has been shown that the selective α-agonist medetomidin delays small bowel transit and that this effect was reversed by the α_2-antagonist, atipamezole. However, atipamezole did not affect small bowel transit when used alone but did reverse surgically induced ileus [42••].

Conclusions

Our knowledge of small bowel pathophysiology and pharmacology has been expanding at an ever increasing rate. New information from ongoing studies will further advance our understanding of small bowel disease and broaden the range of pharmacologic interventions.

References and recommended reading

Papers of particular interest, published within the annual period of review, have been highlighted as:
- • Of special interest
- •• Of outstanding interest

1. • MATSUDA M, AONO M, MORGIA M, OKUMA M: **Centrally Administered Neuropeptide Y (NPY) Inhibits Gastric Emptying and Intestinal Transit in the Rat.** *Dig Dis Sci* 1993, **38**:845–850.

Neuropeptide Y, when administered centrally, impairs gastric and small bowel transit. Both propranolol and carbachol block the action of neuropeptide Y.

2. MIZUTANI M, NEYA T, NAKAYAMA S: **Ascending Contraction Mediated by 5-Hydroxytamine3 Receptors in Canine Small Intestine.** *Am J Physiol* 1992, **263**:G306–G311.

3. •• STARK ME, BAUER AJ, SARR MG, SZURSZEWSKI JH: **Nitric Oxide Mediates Inhibitory Input in Human and Canine Jejunum.** *Gastroenterology* 1993, **104**:398–409.

Nitric oxide inhibits mechanical activity and causes a hyperpolarization in canine and human jejunum. However, synthase inhibitors appear to have different effects in both species, suggesting different mechanisms of action for nitric oxide.

4. • KOSTKA P, JANG E, WATSON EGT, STEWART JL, DANIEL EE: **Nitric Oxide in the Autonomic Nervous System of Canine Ileum.** *J Pharmacol Exp Ther* 1993, **264**:234–239.

5. MACZKA M, THOR P, LORENS K, KONTUREK SJ: **Nitric Oxide Inhibits the Myoelectric Activity of the Small Intestine in Dogs.** *J Physiol Pharmacol* 1993, **44**:31–42.

6. •• SMITH D, WALDRON B, CAMPBELL FC: **Response of Migrating Motor Complex to Variation of Fasting Intraluminal Content.** *Am J Physiol* 1992, **263**:G533–G537.

The effect of intraluminal contents on the migrating motor complex was studied in a normal, healthy host. Aspiration of gas from the proximal small bowel decreased phase II amplitude and duration in the duodenum. After gas was instilled into the stomach, phase II amplitude and duration was increased in the duodenum and the jejunum.

7. LAYER P, SCHLESINGER T, GROGER G, GOEBELL H: **Modulation of Human Periodic Interdigestive Gastrointestinal Motor and Pancreatic Function by the Ileum.** *Pancreas* 1993, **8**:426–432.

8. •• POITRAS P, DUMONT A, CUBER JC, TRUDEL L: **Cholinergic Regulation of Motilin Release from Isolated Canine Intestinal Cells.** *Peptides* 1993, **14**:207–213.

Using isolated canine intestinal cells, carbachol was noted to stimulate motilin release in a dose-dependent fashion and its effect was abolished by atropine.

9. • BOIVIN M, BRADETTER M, RAYMOND MC, RIBERDY-POITRAS M, POITRAS P: **Mechanisms for Postprandial Release of Motilin in Humans.** *Dig Dis Sci* 1992, **37**:1562–1568.

Modified sham feeding and gastric stimulation with air-filled balloons are stimulants for motilin release. Only the latter causes initiation of a premature phase III from the stomach.

10. KATSCHINSKI M, DAHMEN G, REISHAGEN M, BEGLINGER C, KOOP H, NUSTEDE R, ADLER G: **Cephalic Stimulation of Gastrointestinal Secretory and Motor Responses in Humans.** *Gastroenterology* 1992, **103**:383–391.

11. BASILE M, NERI M, CARRIERO A, CASCIARDI S, COMANI S, DEL GRATTA C, DIDONATO L, DILUZIO S, MACRI MA, PASQUARELLI A, PIZZELLA V, ROMANI GL: **Measurement of Segmental Transit Through the Gut in Man.** *Dig Dis Sci* 1993, 37:1537–1543.

12. VON DER OHE M, CAMAILLERI M: **Measurement of Small Bowel and Colonic Transit: Indications and Methods.** *Mayo Clin Proc* 1992, 67:1169–1179.

13. SCOTT-COOMBES DM, VIPOND MN, THOMPSON JN: **Small Bowel Transit Time in Patients with Intra-abdominal Adhesions.** *Br J Surg* 1992, 79:1076.

14. SCOTT AM, KELLOW JE, ECKERSLEY GM, NOLAN JM, JONES MP: **Cigarette Smoking and Nicotine Delay Postprandial Mouth-Cecum Transit Time.** *Dig Dis Sci* 1992, 37:1544–1547.

15. FRANTZIDES CT, MATHIAS C, LUDWIG KA, EDMISTON CE, CONDON RE: **Small Bowel Myoelectric Activity in Peritonitis.** *Am J Surg* 1993, 165:681–685.

16. •• VAN DER MIJLE HCJ, BEEKHUIS H, BLEICHRODT RP, KLEIBERKER JH: **Transit Disorders of the Gastric Remnant and Roux Limb After Roux-en-Y Gastrojejunostomy: Relation to Symptomatology and Vagotomy.** *Br J Surg* 1993, 80:60–64.

Stasis of the Roux limb is common after Roux-en-Y gastrojejunostomy and occurs more often in symptomatic patients. Although vagotomy is associated with delayed gastric emptying, it does not seem to affect emptying of the Roux limb.

17. •• MIEDEMA BW, KELLY KA, CAMILLERI M, HANSON RB, ZINSMEISTER AR, O'CONNOR MK, BROWN ML: **Human Gastric and Jejunal Transit and Motility After Roux Gastrojejunostomy.** *Gastroenterology* 1992, 103:1133–1143.

Motility abnormalities were examined in patients after Roux gastrojejunostomy. Roux transit is abnormally slow in the Roux limb and reflux from the Roux limb into the gastric remnant is a frequent problem.

18. •• STEWART JJ, BATTARBEE HD, FARRAR GE, BETZING KW: **Intestinal Myoelectrical Activity and Transit Time in Chronic Portal Hypertension.** *Am J Physiol* 1992, 263:G474–G479.

The effects of surgically induced portal hypertension were studied in adult rats. Transit time, as measured by movement of radioactive chromium, was delayed with portal hypertension. Using a chronically implanted catheter, the amplitude of phase III of the migrating motor complex was reduced as well as its occurrence.

19. CHESTA J, DEFILIPPI C, DEFILIPPI C: **Abnormalities in Proximal Small Bowel Motility in Patients with Cirrhosis.** *Hepatology* 1993, 17:828–832.

20. MADSEN JL, HENDEL L, MADSEN JL, HENDEIL L: **Gastrointestinal Transit Times of Radiolabeled Meal in Progressive Systemic Sclerosis.** *Dig Dis Sci* 1992, 37:1404–1408.

21. •• HEBRA A, BROWN MF, MCGEEHIN K, BROUSSARD D, ROSS AJ III: **The Effects of Ischemia and Reperfusion on Intestinal Motility.** *J Pediatr Surg* 1993, 28:262–366.

Nonocclusive mesenteric ischemia in piglets is associated with an increase in cycling time and velocity of migrating motor complexes, but not a change in phase III.

22. PESCATORI M: **The Results of Pouch Surgery After Ileo-anal Anastomosis for Inflammatory Bowel Disease: The Manometric Assessment of Pouch Continence and Its Reservoir Function.** *World J Surg* 1992, 16:872–879.

23. • PIERAAMICO O, MALFERTHEINER P, NELSON DK, GLASBRENNER B, DITSCHUNEIT H: **Interdigestive Gastroduodenal Motilin and Cycling of Putative Regulatory Hormones in Severe Obesity.** *Scand J Gastroenterol* 1992, 27:538–544.

Obese subjects had no significant differences in the duration of the total migrating motor complex or its phases. Gastric phase III activity did occur less often in obese subjects and plasma motilin levels were decreased during phase I, II, and III.

24. BENSON MJ, CASTILLO FD, DEEKS JJ, WINGATE DL: **Assessment by Prolonged Ambulatory Manometry of the Effect of Oral Cisapride on Proximal Small Bowel Inter-Digestive Motility.** *Dig Dis Sci* 1992, 37:1569–1575.

25. RAJENDRAN SK, REISER JR, BAUMAN W, ZHANG RL, GORDON SK, KORSTEN MA: **Gastrointestinal Transit After Spinal Cord Injury: Effect of Cisapride.** *Am J Gastroenterol* 1992, 87:1614–1617.

26. HYMAN PE, DILORENZO C, MCADAMS L, FLORES AF, TOMOMASA T, GARVEY TQ III: **Predicting the Clinical Response to Cisapride in Children with Chronic Intestinal Pseudo-Obstruction.** *Am J Gastroenterol* 1993, 88:832–836.

27. •• HOLLE GE, STEINBACH E, FORTH W: **Effects of Erythromycin in the Dog Upper Gastrointestinal Tract.** *Am J Physiol* 1992, 263:G52–G59.

The effects of erythromycin infusion on the proximal gastrointestinal tract of dogs were examined using implanted strain gauges. An increase in motility was noted with erythromycin and a majority of animals had giant retrograde contractions with the onset of vomiting.

28. • KAWAMURA O, SEKIGUCHI T, KUSANO M, NISHIOKA T, ITOH Z: **Effect of Erythromycin on Interdigestive Gastrointestinal Contractile Activity and Plasma Motilin Concentration in Humans.** *Dig Dis Sci* 1993, 38:870–876.

The effects of erythromycin in healthy subjects were studied. Erythromycin induced interdigestive migrating contractions at doses equal or greater than 0.375 mg/kg. Doses of erythromycin greater than 0.375 mg/kg caused phase III-like activity, but these contractions did not migrate completely to the duodenum.

29. BONACINI M, QUIASON S, REYNOLDS M, GADDIS M, PEMBERTON B, SMITH O: **Effect of Intravenous Erythromycin on Postoperative Ileus.** *Am J Gastroenterol* 1993, 88:208–211.

30. • KAWAMURA O, SEKIGUCHI T, ITOH Z, OMURA S: **Effect of Erythromycin Derivative EM 5231 on Human Interdigestive Gastrointestinal Tract.** *Dig Dis Sci* 1993, 38:1026–1031.

The effect of the erythromycin derivative, EM 5231, in doses ranging from 500 to 2000 µg was examined in normal subjects. EM 5231 caused a rise in plasma motilin levels and induced interdigestive migrating contractions forming in the stomach.

31. • LADAS SD, FRYDA A, PAPADOPOULOS RAAPTIS SA: **Effects of Alpha-Glucosidase Inhibitors on Mouth to Caecum Transit Times in Humans.** *Gut* 1992, 33:1246–1248.

Acarbose and miglitol are α-glucosidase inhibitors that have been used in control of hyperglycemia in patients with diabetes mellitus. Both agents have been shown to decrease the orocecal time.

32. •• FARGEAS MJ, FIORAMONTI J, BUENO L: **Central Action of Interleukin 1β on Intestinal Motility in Rats: Mediation by Two Mechanisms.** *Gastroenterology* 1993, 104:377–383.

Intracerebroventricular, but not peripheral administration of interleukin 1 in rats, stimulated small bowel motility. This effect was reduced by indomethacin.

33. • KELLEY MC, HOCKING MP, MARCHAND SD, SNINSKY CA: **Ketorolac Prevents Postoperative Small Intestinal Ileus.** *Am J Surg* 1993, 165:107–112.

Ketorolac, a nonsteroidal anti-inflammatory drug that can be administered parenterally, had been shown to reduce the delay in the return of the migrating motor complex in a rat model of postoperative ileus.

34. • SOFFER EE, LAUNSPACH J: **Effect of Misoprostol on Postprandial Intestinal Motility and Orocecal Transit Time in Humans.** *Dig Dis Sci* 1993, 38:851–855.

The effect of misoprostol, at doses ranging from 200 to 800 µg, compared with placebo was studied in normal volunteers. Misoprostol, especially at higher doses, blocked the fed phase and diminished the orocecal time.

35. Chiarioni G, Scattolini C, Bonfante F, Brentegani MT, Santini I: **Effect of Nifedipine on Mouth-to-Cecum Transit of Liquid Meal in Normal Subjects.** *Dig Dis Sci* 1993, 38:1022–1025.

36. Thollander M, Hellstrom PM, Svensson TH: **Dihydropyridine Calcium Channel Antagonists Disrupt Migrating Myoelectric Complexes and Counteract Intestinal Disorders Associated With Morphine Withdrawal Diarrhea.** *Scand J Gastroenterol* 1993, 28:137–144.
•
Both nifedipine and nimodipine, dihydropyridine calcium channel antagonists, inhibited the occurrence of migrating motor complexes in rats, but nimodipine did not affect the fasting pattern in normal, healthy human subjects. In morphine-dependent rats, both agents blocked the effect of naloxone-induced diarrhea.

37. McIntyre AS, Thompson DG, Burnham WR, Walker E: **The Effect of Alpha-1-Adrenoreceptor Agonist and Antagonist Administration on Human Upper Gastrointestinal Transit and Motility.** *Aliment Pharmacol Ther* 1992, 6:415–426.
•
Phenylephrine, an α_1-agonist, prolonged the orocecal time in normal volunteers. Thymoxamine, an α_1-antagonist, obliterated this effect, but alone it did not affect orocecal time.

38. Gyr KE, Meier R: **Pharmacodynamic Effects of Sandostatin in the Gastrointestinal Tract.** *Metabolism* 1992, 41:17–21.

39. Mourad FH, Gorard D, Thillainayagam AV, Colin-Jones D, Farthing MJG: **Effective Treatment of Diabetic Diarrhoea with Somatostatin Analogue, Octreotide.** *Gut* 1992, 33:1578–1580.

40. Cullen JJ, Eagon C, Dozois EJ, Kelly KA: **Treatment of Acute Postoperative Ileus with Octreotide.** *Am J Surg* 1993, 165:113–120.
•
Electrical activity was recorded from small bowel and gastric serosal electrodes in dogs. After an ileus was induced by celiotomy and intestinal abrasion, dogs received different doses of octreotide or placebo. Octreotide 1.5 µg/kg/8h subcutaneously or 0.83 µg/kg/h reduced the period of ileus, compared with placebo. Gastric emptying was delayed with the larger dose of octreotide.

41. Aggarwal A, Camilleri M, Phillips SF, Schlagheck T, Brown ML, Thomforde GM: **Olestra, a Nondigestible, Nonabsorbable Fat: Effects on Gastrointestinal and Colonic Transit.** *Dig Dis Sci* 1993, 38:1009–1114.
•
Olestra, at doses up to 30 g in a 45-g fat meal, did not appear to affect small bowel or colonic transit as measured by dual gamma camera scintigraphy.

42. Tanila H, Kauppila T, Taira T: **Inhibition of Intestinal Motility and Reversal of Postlaparotomy Ileus by Selective Alpha 2-Adrenergic Drugs in the Rat.** *Gastroenterology* 1993, 104:819–824.
••
Atipamezole, an α_2-antagonist, partially reversed narcotic-induced small bowel hypomotility and completely reversed laparotomy-induced ileus in the rat.

Robin D. Rothstein, MD, University of Pennsylvania School of Medicine, Hospital of the University of Pennsylvania, Gastroenterology Division, 8 Gates Bldg., 3400 Spruce Street, Philadelphia, PA 19104, USA.

Ann Ouyang, MD, Gastroenterology Division, Department of Medicine, The Milton S. Hershey Medical Center, The Pennsylvania State University, 500 University Drive, P.O. Box 850, Hershey, PA 17033, USA.

Radiology of the small intestine

Philip Shorvon, MA, MB BS, MRCP, FRCR, and Gabrielle Lamb, MA, MB BS, MRCP

Central Middlesex Hospital NHS Trust, London, UK

This review outlines the recent contributions to the literature in the investigation of alterations of small intestinal blood flow. In particular, Doppler studies of the celiac axis and superior mesenteric artery have been validated and barium and cross-sectional imaging appearances have been described in different clinical scenarios. The value of computed tomography in small bowel obstruction has been recognized to be in those with high-grade obstruction who are being considered for conservative treatment. Further evidence of the role of angiography in unexplained gastrointestinal bleeding is presented and the use of computed tomography in detecting small bowel damage in blunt trauma is emphasized. Several papers attest to the superiority of enteroclysis over conventional follow-up examinations in the investigation of small bowel neoplasms and inflammatory disease, although the evidence remains uncontrolled.

Current Opinion in Gastroenterology 1994, **10**:163–170

Alterations of small bowel blood flow

Disturbances of small bowel blood flow generally can be categorized into acute or chronic arterial ischemia, acute venous occlusion, or chronic venous thrombosis, which usually results from concurrent portal thrombosis or as a consequence of a hypercoagulopathy. A further condition labeled *chronic nonischemic disturbance of superior mesenteric venous blood flow* and its small bowel enema appearances have been described [1•]. A total of 11 patients between 1 and 29 years old all presented with recurrent rectal bleeding and episodic anemia. Small bowel enemas were performed using barium single contrast and air-barium double contrast after a variety of nondiagnostic tests. Diffuse intramural edema extending from the proximal jejunum to the distal ileum were documented, being most pronounced in the transitional segment between the jejunum and ileum. An important feature were compressible nodules between 3 and 7 mm in diameter, which were ascribed to varices. There was no dilation of bowel or increase in intraluminal fluid and there was normal separation of bowel loops.

Following angiography and laparotomy, the etiology was termed idiopathic in three patients and attributed to super mesenteric vein compression by bands in two, abnormal arterial arcades in two, localized lymphoma in three, and microthrombi in mesenteric border veins from an ileal hemangioma in the last patient. Although it might be argued whether a discrete entity was investigated, this is an interesting report of a heterogenous condition in children and young adults in which the cardinal feature is recurrent hemorrhage from small bowel varices [1•].

Doppler duplex studies of chronic arterial ischemia

Important additions to the debate on the value of Doppler duplex scanning in the detection of superior mesenteric artery (SMA) and celiac axis stenoses have been reported. In the largest study [2••], 100 patients were studied prospectively and findings at Doppler duplex scanning were compared with a lateral aortogram taken within 2 weeks. From the authors own previous data, a fasting peak systolic velocity of more than 200 cm/s or no flow in the celiac axis, and a velocity over 275 cm/s or absence of flow in the SMA predicted a 70% or greater stenosis. Using these criteria, a high accuracy in predicting a 70% or greater stenosis was achieved particularly for the SMA (Table 1). End diastolic velocity was less reliable than peak systolic velocity. The authors pointed out that other ultrasound and Doppler criteria such as the enlargement of the inferior mesenteric artery, retrograde and turbulent flow in the hepatic artery, and postprandial effects on flow may increase the accuracy of these techniques but have not been systematically studied.

A smaller retrospective study [3] was less conclusive. In addition to the peak systolic velocity, peak and end diastolic velocities and the ratio between the peak di-

Abbreviation

SMA—superior mesenteric artery.

ISBN 1-85922-607-8 ISSN 0267–1379

Table 1. Sensitivity, specificity, positive predictive value, and negative predictive value of Doppler duplex scanning in detecting 70% or more stenosis in the celiac artery or superior mesenteric artery*

	Visualization, %	Sensitivity, %	Specificity, %	PPV, %	NPV, %
Celiac artery	83	87	80	63	94
Superior mesenteric artery	93	92	96	80	99

*From Moneta *et al.* [2••]; with permission.
NPV—negative predictive value; PPV—positive predictive value.

astolic velocities in the SMA and aorta (the peak diastolic ratio) were correlated with the lateral aortogram. A 50% stenosis was used as the cut-off point for significance. The peak diastolic ratio was shown to produce the best correlation but only achieved significance for the celiac axis and not the SMA. This study was clearly at variance with the first study, but, as the authors pointed out, prospective studies are more reliable. Furthermore, no comparative peak systolic velocity data were published.

A further prospective study of 38 patients [4••] who underwent Doppler duplex scanning and lateral aortography was reported. Most of the patients were suspected of having chronic mesenteric ischemia or mesenteric involvement by an aortic aneurysm. This group reported absolute Doppler frequency rather than estimated velocities.

Using a peak systolic frequency of 4.5 kHz for the SMA and of 4.0 kHz for the celiac axis, a 50% or more stenosis was predicted in the SMA with a sensitivity of 96%, specificity of 92%, positive predictive value of 96%, and negative predictive value of 92%. For the celiac axis, the figures were 100%, 88%, 97%, and 100% respectively. In addition, they demonstrated excellent correlations between the degree of stenosis in the vessels and the concomitant peak systolic frequency for stenoses greater than 50% (r values 0.89 and 0.86 for the SMA and celiac axis, respectively) (Fig. 1). They demonstrated that end diastolic frequency data did not add to accuracy.

The larger studies support the contention that Doppler duplex scanning studies are accurate in the assessment of celiac axis and SMA stenoses, but warn they can only be used for screening. At present the jury must remain out as to which are the most useful criteria to adhere to and, as with all Doppler work, whether such excellent results will apply to units without specific interest in this field.

Computed tomography in acute mesenteric venous obstruction

Computed tomography was performed in four patients with intestinal infarction secondary to mesenteric venous thrombosis who had undergone laparotomy within 6 hours [5]. The fresh thrombus was of high density within the vessel on unenhanced scan, and appeared as a low density with a sharply defined enhancing venous wall during dynamic computed tomography. The authors noted that the bowel wall thickening accompanying the thrombosis ranged from 1.3 to 1.6 cm (beyond that normally seen in arterial occlusion) with alternating layers of high and low intensity within the wall corresponding to layers of hemorrhage and edema (Fig. 2). Mesenteric edema was present in all cases. The authors believe that this constellation of findings is highly suggestive of this rare diagnosis.

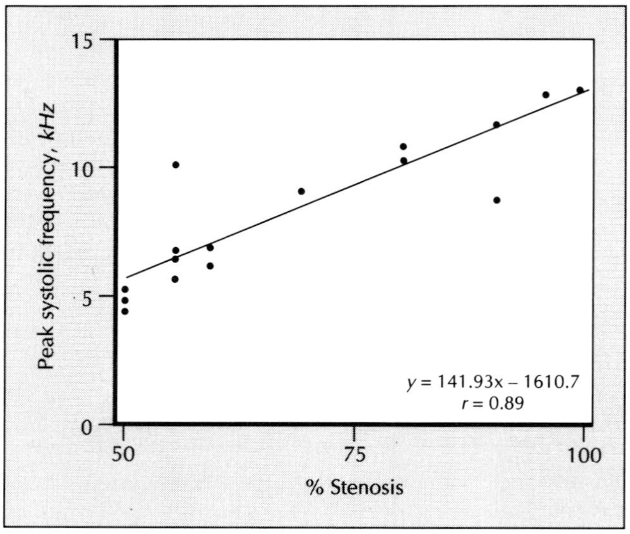

Fig. 1. Linear regression analysis of Doppler peak systolic frequency in the superior mesenteric artery plotted against the degree of stenosis estimated from the lateral aortogram. (*From* Harward *et al.* [4••]; with permission.)

Other modalities of arterial ischemia

Iida *et al.* [6••] retrospectively reviewed 13 patients with small bowel ischemia who underwent either a standard small bowel meal or a modified intubated small bowel barium study using air contrast. The patients all had a subacute form of ischemia akin to the better recognized ischemic colitis. No patient progressed to small bowel necrosis and eight patients underwent laparotomy between 1 and 34 days after the barium study. An etiology for the ischemia was found in one patient only (occluded SMA). Nine of the patients had a "stricturing" form and four had a "transient" form.

This study showed that involvement tended to be confined to a small segment of small bowel, that thumbprinting or fold thickening was common, and that double contrast studies demonstrated small ulcers in three patients. In contradistinction to ischemic colitis, longitudinal ulceration, sacculation, or eccentric deformity were rare. Tubular strictures that produced proximal dilatation were seen. The contours of the strictures were often irregular and this was correlated with the

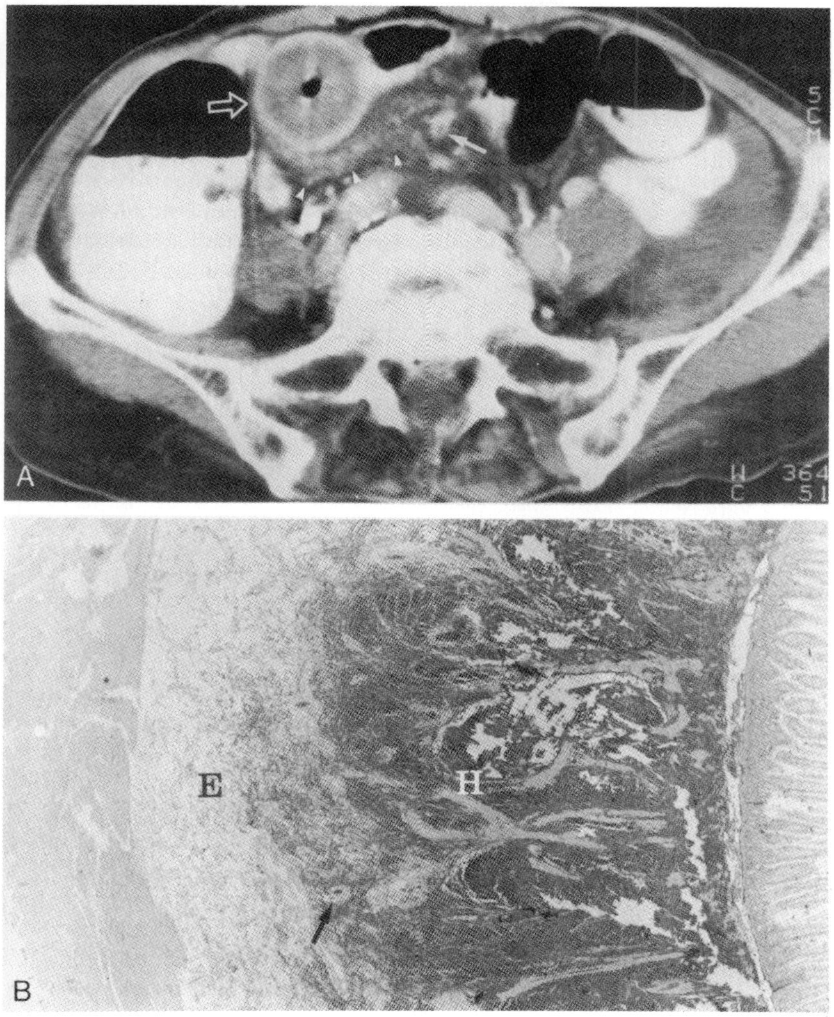

Fig. 2. A, Contrast-enhanced computed tomography shows marked thickening of jejunal wall with alternating layers of high and low density and peripheral enhancement. Super mesenteric vein branches have thrombus (*closed arrow*) and there is mesenteric edema (*arrowheads*). **B**, Histology of resected specimen shows hemorrhage (H) and edema (E) and thrombus in submucosal veins (*arrow*). (*From* Kim *et al.* [5]; with permission.)

pathologic specimens and shown to be due to shallow ulcerations and granulation tissue. The authors believed that the radiographic findings reflected the clinical course and pathologic findings, but this should be viewed with some caution as the diagnosis was only presumptive in a significant proportion of patients [6••].

Finally, Bloom *et al.* [7] remind us that gas in the bowel wall can be seen by ultrasound as a bright ring and in the correct clinical setting is almost diagnostic for necrosis.

Small bowel obstruction

In recent years there have been a number of articles encouraging the use of computed tomography in small bowel obstruction, but many involved only patients with high-grade obstruction as opposed to the clinically more problematic low-grade obstruction. Maglinte *et al* [8••] attempted to evaluate this further by retrospectively studying 55 patients who underwent both abdominal computed tomography and enteroclysis for suspected small bowel obstruction, using the enteroclysis findings as their standard of reference for analysis. The final diagnosis was verified by notes review and pathology reports. A total of 46 of 55 patients were found to have small bowel obstruction; 25 had low-grade and 21 had high-grade partial obstruction. All the latter were confirmed by surgery, whereas only 17 of the low-grade obstructions had such confirmation. Computed tomography identified 29 of 46 (63%) patients with obstruction and seven of nine without. Computed tomography diagnosed 17 of 21 (81%) in high-grade obstruction, but only 12 of 25 (48%) in low-grade obstruction. Computed tomography detected the six patients who had tumor-related small bowel obstruction and the series also confirmed that failure to visualize a mass at the site of obstruction accurately implies an adhesion obstruction. The authors argue that whereas computed tomography has little place in obvious obstruction that requires surgery, it should be performed if a trial of nonsurgical treatment is being contemplated so that unsuspected bowel strangulations, herniae, and tumors may be diagnosed. Computed tomography has little place in the diagnosis of low-grade obstruction.

Ha *et al.* [9] examined the ability of computed tomography in bowel obstruction to detect early strangulation. All patients were at risk of adhesions. They showed that the presence of serrations at the beak-like luminal narrowing as well as bowel wall thickening of over 6 mm only occurred in patients subsequently shown to have strangulation. Mesenteric vascular engorgement and edema were also suggestive but not specific.

Balthazar *et al.* [10•] reviewed retrospectively 19 patients having laparotomy-proven closed-loop obstruction who had undergone abdominal computed tomography within 40 hours of operation. All patients had computed tomography evidence of small bowel obstruction and 15 of 19 had computed tomography signs of closed loop obstruction, including fluid-filled, U-shaped loop of bowel, engorged mesenteric vessels stretched towards a point of obstruction, and a variety of other minor signs. Signs of strangulation were seen in 10 of 16 patients with ischemic bowel at operation.

There are many faults with this study [11], but it demonstrates the use of computed tomography as the first step in identifying a potentially life-threatening situation in patients being treated conservatively for obstruction. Conversely, two papers [12,13•] suggest a very conservative approach can be taken towards small bowel obstruction. The first [12] suggests that if 100 mL of Gastrografin (Schering Health Care, West Sussex, UK) is administered and seen in the colon on a 4-hour film, then no surgery is necessary. There have been criticisms of the use of Gastrografin because of possible fluid shifts and the danger of pulmonary edema if aspirated. The second paper [13•] advocates up to 5 days conservative treatment in those patients presenting with small bowel obstruction and a history of previous abdominal operation. This, too, has been criticized particularly for being an uncontrolled study and for the increased risk of bowel strangulation posed by this conservative treatment.

Gastrointestinal hemorrhage

It is now well-established that endoscopy should be the first line in the investigation of acute and chronic gastrointestinal hemorrhage. A more difficult investigative problem is endoscopy negative bleeding. Whitaker and Gregson [14•] reviewed the role of angiography in 46 patients with overt and nine patients with chronic nonvariceal gastrointestinal bleeding referred during an 8-year period. In the first group, 59% of technically successful studies were true-positives with 10 cases of active bleeding and 19 patients with vascular abnormalities not actively bleeding, giving a sensitivity for localization of 64% and an accuracy of 63%. The small bowel was the source of pathology in over 20% of cases. The accuracy of angiography was markedly higher in those patients investigated within 24 hours of admission (92%) and in those who were thought clinically to be actively bleeding (74%). This study confirmed the view that mesenteric angiography should be performed where initial hematologic and endoscopic investigations are negative, preferably within 6 hours of presentation.

The other key modality in investigating obscure upper gastrointestinal bleeding is radionuclide scintigraphy. This has the advantage of its ability to detect lower rates of bleeding (0.05 to 0.1 mL/min).

Ohri *et al.* [15•] reported their experience of 49 patients who underwent ^{99m}Tc-labeled autologous erythrocyte scans for gastrointestinal bleeding. All patients had been previously investigated with endoscopy and 40 also had angiography. This study from a tertiary referral center had a high incidence of small bowel pathology, with more than 90% having upper gastrointestinal sources of hemorrhage.

Although scintigraphy proved to be the most useful single investigation for localizing bleeding, it was less sensitive than in other published series. Localization was thought to be more difficult in the upper gastrointestinal tract because of the faster transit and the irritant effect of blood in the bowel lumen causing increased peristalsis, resulting in a bleeding site distal to the true source. Angiography and scintigraphy in conjunction allowed localization of bleeding in 45% compared with 33% for scintigraphy alone [15•]. The use of cinematic scintigraphy techniques as used by Ohri *et al.* [15•] is thought to be superior to conventional static imaging and this was confirmed by a prospective study of 52 patients [16•] who underwent radionuclide scintigraphy using ^{99m}Tc-labeled autologous erythrocytes. All patients were studied within 4 hours of presentation with cine techniques comprising a radionuclide angiogram (3 frames/s over 60 seconds) followed by 15-second images for 15 minutes (total of 60 images) and repeated until four sequences had been obtained. A retrospective comparison with static imaging methods showed that cinematic display improved detection or localization in 38% of patients. The largest errors in static display interpretation were in distinguishing small bowel versus large bowel bleeding, and both antegrade and retrograde movement in the gastrointestinal tract were observed. Cine scintigraphic methods appear to be the most accurate for localizing gastrointestinal hemorrhage, particularly in episodic bleeding difficult to detect by angiography.

Blunt trauma

The role of computed tomography in detecting injuries to solid viscera from blunt trauma is well documented. The identification of bowel and mesenteric injuries at an early stage in blunt trauma cases is also essential, as there is increased morbidity and mortality associated with diagnostic delay. Small bowel perforations may have subtle or no clinical signs. The sensitivity of computed tomography in such injuries has been subject to much review in the past with discrepant results. The generally accepted scanning technique involves the use of oral, water-soluble contrast agents, administered nasogastrically, if necessary, with intravenous dynamic contrast enhancement. It is necessary to view the scans with a large window width to detect small amounts of air. This is emphasized in a pictorial review by Nghiem *et al* [17•] who detailed the important computed tomography signs:

1) *Pneumoperitoneum.* Very small quantities of air can be reliably detected by computed tomography and it is fairly specific for perforation (if no diagnostic lavage has been performed). Computed tomography is not sensitive, however, as fluid-filled small bowel can perforate without pneumoperitoneum.

2) *Free intra-abdominal fluid.* Fluid between bowel loops indicates injury of the small bowel or mesentery. Low attenuation fluid (< 20 henrys) is suggestive of small bowel perforation. High attenuation fluid (> 25 H) suggests hemoperitoneum.

3) *Bowel wall thickening.* This thickening indicates intramural hematoma from bówel laceration. Intense enhancement of the bowel is another recognized sign of injury.

4) *Mesenteric hematoma.* The presence of hematoma in the mesentery should raise the suspicion of mesenteric vascular damage or bowel perforation. Jejunal and ileal injuries most commonly occur at points of attachment such as the ligament of Treitz, with perforation occurring usually on the antimesenteric border.

Mirvis *et al.* [18•] prospectively studied the accuracy of computed tomography in diagnosing bowel rupture following blunt trauma in 16 patients (17 scans) who subsequently all had surgical confirmation. Thirteen of 19 ruptures in the 16 patients occurred in the small bowel. In 15 of 17 scans there were prospective findings suggestive or diagnostic of bowel rupture and retrospective analysis revealed findings in all 17 scans. In many cases the findings were subtle, requiring detailed examination of the scans, and it was felt that the use of oral contrast was important.

Small bowel tumors

Small bowel tumors are rare and most studies are anecdotal or uncontrolled. A retrospective review [19] of 40 malignant tumors seen in one Japanese institution over a period of 14 years has been reported. This included 19 adenocarcinomas, 12 lymphomas, eight leiomyosarcomas, and only one carcinoid. Barium studies detected 20 of 24 in which they were performed. Computed tomography and ultrasonography were less sensitive for jejunal (17% and 31%, respectively) than duodenal (100% and 50%) or ileal (70% and 73%) tumors. Six of seven lymphomas had positive gallium scans. All five patients with ileal tumors were detected by angiography but only two were able to be diagnosed by barium studies. Unfortunately, there is a paucity of details on methodology and protocols for the various imaging methods to know the general relevance of their results.

A study of 18 patients with problematic benign tumors [20•] diagnosed over a period of 7 years by single contrast enteroclysis reported that the average time from symptoms to diagnosis was 16 months (range 1 month to 7 years). Most of the tumors were leiomyomas, adenomas, and hamartomas. The authors claimed a high degree of preoperative differentiation of these entities by enteroclysis, although they frequently missed ulceration. Though strongly in favor of their technique for diagnosis, as only cases subsequently proven by surgery were included, we have no idea of the false-negative rate or overall accuracy of the technique. A careful study of the ultrasound appearances of 27 small bowel tumors [21•] showed that locating the position of the tumor in the bowel wall and assessing echogenicity and compressibility allowed a high degree of accuracy in differentiating the tumors. The painstaking technique, in which patients drank 500 mL of water and were scanned every 10 to 15 minutes over 1 hour, was impractical for most, but did aid localization.

Inflammatory diseases

Crohn's disease

One of the most important indications for small bowel barium studies is suspected Crohn's disease. There is still debate as to the best method of study because it is not ethical to perform both a small bowel meal and enteroclysis on each patient. An important contribution [22••] to this debate reported a minimum 2-year follow-up after barium-methylcellulose double-contrast enteroclysis on 138 patients with suspected Crohn's disease. Only one false-positive and no false-negative examinations with a sensitivity of 100% and specificity of 98.3% were claimed. These results should be interpreted in the knowledge that there was a high prevalence of Crohn's disease in the study group and an unnamed proportion had suffered previous episodes of Crohn's disease. Another review [23•] of enteroclysis (single contrast) of 1465 patients (not confined to Crohn's disease) is also reported. Once again a high sensitivity (93%) and specificity (97%) was demonstrated, although like many such studies it lacks independent confirmation of findings in a significant proportion of patients.

Eosinophilic gastroenteritis

Two reports [24,25] discussed the value of imaging in this rare condition. The disease tends to affect one of three layers: the mucosa, muscularis propria, or subserosa. To some extent the ultrasound appearances can reflect this by which ultrasonic layer is thickened and the presence of ascites in subserosal disease, although the value of cross-sectional imaging is mostly in detecting nonspecific wall thickening and in the follow-up of patients on steroid treatment.

Intestinal anisakiasis

Intestinal anisakiasis is likely to become more common in the West with increasing consumption of raw fish [26••]. Patients often present with acute abdominal pain. Barium studies are nonspecific showing segmental narrowing with a "thumbprinted" or "saw-tooth" pattern to the mucosa. Visualization of the worm is unusual. Ultrasound can be extremely helpful by demonstrating segmental bowel wall thickening with some adjacent localized ascites, which if aspirated is shown to be rich in eosinophils (Fig. 3).

Pediatrics

The importance of the relative position of the superior mesenteric vein to the artery was emphasized in a review of ultrasound examinations of 337 children [27••]. The position could be determined in 74% and in five of these the super mesenteric vein was located to the left of the artery. All of these patients were subsequently shown to have intestinal malrotation. In the four patients with the vein ventral to the artery, only one had malrotation. Of the vast majority of patients with the vein to the right of the artery, only 15% underwent a barium study and none of these showed malrotation. This study confirms the usefulness of this sign and suggests the relationship should be specifically sought in ultrasound examinations of children.

A case report [28] of ileocecitis caused by *Escherichia coli* O157:H7 diagnosed by ultrasonography in an 8-year-old boy adds this organism to the list of causes of inflammation in this area and demonstrates the usefulness of ultrasonography in excluding appendicitis. Some patients with Henoch-Schonlein purpura present with gastrointestinal symptoms before skin lesions appear [29]. The majority of such patients are reported to have characteristic echogenic thickening of the duodenal wall, often with enlargement of the lumen, and the authors believe this may prove useful in early diagnosis.

Other reports

An expert overview [30•] of the clinical, pathologic, and radiologic features of diseases producing small bowel malabsorption emphasizes the value of enteroclysis in those who need barium studies. The problems of diagnosing seven cases of midgut volvulus in young adults is reported [31]. The computed tomography "whirl" sign or the barium "corkscrew" sign can be useful in subacute cases, but three of the patients presented with severe ischemia or infarction requiring immediate laparotomy. A case report [32] of heterotopic pancreatic tissue of the ileum causing gastrointestinal bleeding reminds us that this condition is included in the list of polypoid small bowel lesions.

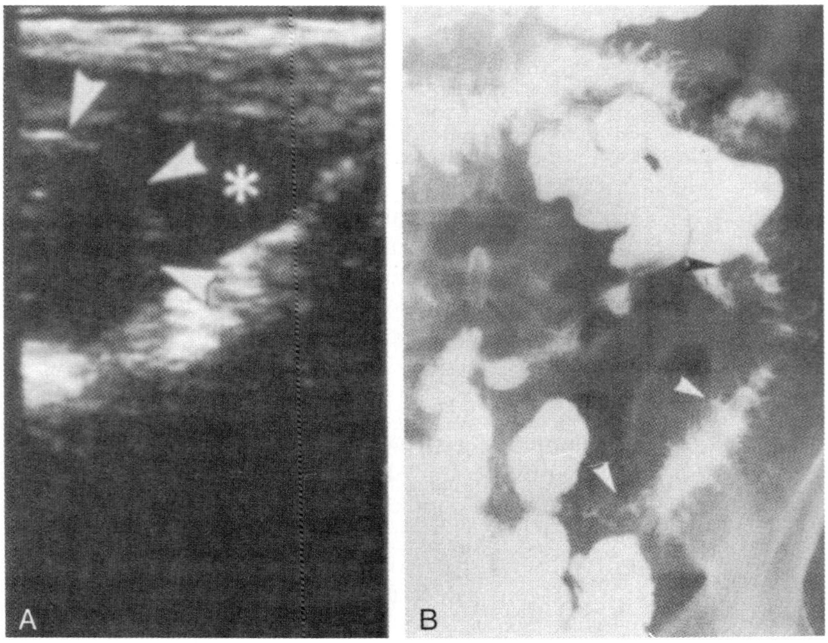

Fig. 3. A, Ultrasound scan reveals thickened ileum (*arrowheads*) with adjacent ascitic fluid (*asterisk*). The fluid was rich in eosinophils. **B**, Barium study shows long edematous loop with luminal narrowing (*arrowheads*). (*From* Shirahama *et al.* [26••]; with permission.)

References and recommended reading

Papers of particular interest, published within the annual period of review, have been highlighted as:

- • Of special interest
- •• Of outstanding interest

1. • BOVERIE JH, COUNET D, MEUNIER P, DONDELINGER RF: **Small Bowel Enema and Diagnosis of Chronic Nonischemic Disturbance of Superior Mesenteric Venous Blood Flow.** *Abdom Imaging* 1993, **18**:265–270.

Slightly confusing but interesting description of new entity characterized by intermittent small bowel bleeding and anemia in young people from varices best visualized by small bowel enema examination.

2. •• MONETA GL, LEE RW, YEAGER RA, TAYLOR LM, PORTER JM: **Mesenteric Duplex Scanning: A Blinded Prospective Study.** *J Vasc Surg* 1993, **17**:79–86.

Strong evidence in a study of 100 patients that mesenteric duplex scanning should prove a useful screening examination to detect superior mesenteric and celiac axis stenosis in patients with clinical suspicion of chronic intestinal ischemia.

3. HEALY D A, NEUMYER MM, ATNIP RG, THIELE BL: **Evaluation of Celiac and Mesenteric Vascular Disease With Duplex Ultrasonography.** *J Ultrasound Med* 1992, **11**:481–485.

4. •• HARWARD TRS, SMITH S, SEEGER JM: **Detection of Celiac and Superior Mesenteric Artery Occlusive Disease With Use of Abdominal Duplex Scanning.** *J Vasc Surg* 1993, **17**:738–745.

In a study of 38 patients, peak systolic frequency detected at Doppler duplex examination correlated well with the degree of stenosis in the celiac and superior mesenteric arteries.

5. KIM JY, HA HK, BYUN JY, LEE JM, YONG BK, KIM IC, LEE JY, PARK WS, SHINN KS: **Intestinal Infarction Secondary to Mesenteric Venous Thrombosis: CT-Pathologic Correlation.** *J Comput Assist Tomogr* 1993, **17**:382–385.

6. •• IIDA M, MATSUI T, YAO T, IWASHITA A, SAKAMOTO K, FUCHIGAMI T, YAO T, FUJISHIMA M: **Radiographic Features in Ischemic Jejunoileitis: Serial Changes and Comparison With Pathologic Findings.** *Gastrointest Radiol* 1992, **17**:327–332.

This outlines the features of a disorder akin to ischemic colitis but occurring in the small bowel.

7. BLOOM RA, CRACIUN E, LEBENSART PD, LEVY P, BAR ZIV J: **The Ultrasound Appearance of Intramural Bowel Gas: The Bright Ring Appearance and the Effervescent Bowel. A Report of Three Cases.** *Br J Radiol* 1992, **65**:585–588.

8. •• MAGLINTE DT, GAGE SN, HARMON BH, KELVIN FM, HAGE JP, CHUA GT, NG AC, GRAFFIS RF, CHERNISH SM: **Obstruction of the Small Intestine: Accuracy and Role of CT in Diagnosis.** *Radiology* 1993, **188**:61–64.

A sane and careful study of the accuracy of computed tomography in small bowel obstruction using enteroclysis as the gold standard.

9. HA HK, PARK CH, KIM SK, CHUN CS, KIM IC, LEE HK, SHINN KS, BAHK YW: **CT Analysis of Intestinal Obstruction Due to Adhesions: Early Detection of Strangulation.** *J Comput Assist Tomogr* 1993, **17**:386–389.

10. • BALTHAZAR EJ, BIRNBAUM BA, MEGIBOW AJ, GORDON RB, WHELAN CA, HULNICK DH: **Closed-Loop and Strangulating Intestinal Obstruction: CT Signs.** *Radiology* 1992, **185**:769–775.

Study showing that computed tomography is promising in picking up closed-loop and strangulating intestinal obstruction. The study is retrospective and uncontrolled and therefore the ability of computed tomography to diagnose this situation is unproven.

11. WILLS JS: **Closed-Loop and Strangulating Obstruction of the Small Intestine: A New Twist.** *Radiology* 1992, **185**:635–636.

12. JOYCE WP, DELANEY PV, GOREY TF, FITZPATRICK JM: **The Value of Water-Soluble Contrast Radiology in the Management of Acute Small Bowel Obstruction.** *Ann R Coll Surg Engl* 1992, **74**:422–425.

13. • SEROR D, FEIGIN E, SZOLD A, ALLWEIS TM, CARMON M, NISSAN S, FREUND HR: **How Conservatively Can Post-Operative Small Bowel Obstruction Be Treated?** *Am J Surg* 1993, **165**:121–126.

This paper challenges the dictum that acute intestinal obstruction should be treated by early operation. A conservative approach in obstruction secondary to adhesion is proposed but heavily criticized in the discussion at the end of the paper.

14. • WHITAKER SC, GREGSON RHS: **The Role of Angiography in the Investigation of Acute or Chronic Gastrointestinal Haemorrhage.** *Clin Radiol* 1993, **47**:382–388.

A review of experience of angiography and gastrointestinal bleeding from Nottingham confirms its value.

15. • OHRI SK, DESA LA, LEE H, PATEL T, JACKSON J, LAVENDER JP, SPENCER J: **Value of Scintigraphic Localization of Obscure Gastrointestinal Bleeding.** *J R Coll Surg Edinb* 1992, **37**:328–332.

Technetium-99m–labeled red blood cell scanning was found to be the most useful form of localization in patients with obscure gastrointestinal bleeding.

16. • MAURER AH, RODMAN MS, VITTI RA, REVEZ G, KREVSKY B: **Gastrointestinal Bleeding: Improved Localization With Cine Scintigraphy.** *Radiology* 1992, **185**:187–192.

This study demonstrates improved accuracy for technetium-labeled erythrocyte scanning when performed with cinematic acquisition.

17. • NGHIEM HV, JEFFREY RB, MINDELZUN RE: **CT of Blunt Trauma to the Bowel and Mesentery.** *Am J Radiol* 1993, **160**:53–58.

A pictorial essay series. This is an elegant contribution to the value of computed tomography of blunt trauma to the bowel and mesentery.

18. • MIRVIS SE, GENS DR, SHANMUGANATHAN K: **Rupture of the Bowel After Blunt Abdominal Trauma: Diagnosis With CT.** *Am J Radiol* 1992, **159**:1217–1221.

Study confirming that computed tomography is fairly accurate in diagnosing bowel trauma, but the signs are often quite subtle.

19. KUSUMOTO H, TAKAHASHI I, YOSHIDA M, MAEHARA Y, WATANABE A, OSHIRO T, SUGIMACHI K: **Primary Malignant Tumours of the Small Intestine: Analysis of 40 Japanese Patients.** *J Surg Oncol* 1992, **50**:139–143.

20. • GOURTSOYIANNIS NC, BAYS D, PAPAIOANNOU N, THEOTOKAS J, BAROUXIS G, KARABELAS T: **Benign Tumours of the Small Intestine: Pre-operation Evaluation With a Barium Infusion Technique.** *Eur J Radiol* 1993, **16**:115–125.

A large series of benign small bowel intestine tumors from one of the foremost proponents of the single contrast enteroclysis technique. Some elegant radiologic pathologic correlations are presented.

21. • BIN W, JIANGUO L, BAOWEI D: **The Sonographic Appearances of Small Bowel Tumours.** *Clin Radiol* 1992, **46**:30–33.

A study suggesting that if a bowel-related mass is detected on ultrasound, a small bowel waterload should be given to aid its diagnosis and localization.

22. •• MAGLINTE DD, CHERNISH SM, KELVIN FM, O'CONNOR KW, HAGE JP: **Crohn Disease of the Small Intestine: Accuracy and Relevance of Enteroclysis.** *Radiology* 1992, **184**:541–545.

A study suggesting the extraordinary accuracy (99%!) for enteroclysis in diagnosing Crohn's disease of the small intestine. The study is probably somewhat bias by the high prevalence of Crohn's disease in the population and the exclusion of Crohn's disease in barium-negative patients by follow-up alone.

23. • DIXON PM, ROULSTON ME, NOLAN DJ: **The Small Bowel Enema: A Ten Year Review.** *Clin Radiol* 1993, **4**:46–48.

Almost 1500 patients over 10 years who underwent enteroclysis by the single contrast method are reviewed. The technique was felt to be very accurate, although the true number of false-negative examinations is always difficult to ascertain.

24. TUNCALI K, ERZEN C, GURMEN N, TUZUNER N, ULUSOY NB: **Eosinophilic Gastroenteropathy: Ultrasonographic Features and the Role of Ultrasonography in Follow-up.** *J Clin Ultrasound* 1992, **20**:475–478.

25. LEE C-M, CHANGCHIEN C-S, CHEN P-C, LIN D-Y, SHEEN I-S, WANG C-S, TAI D-I, SHEEN-CHEN S-M, CHEN W-J,

WU C-S: **Eosinophilic Gastroenteritis: 10 Years Experience.** *Am J Gastroenterol* 1993, **88**:70–74.

26. SHIRAHAMA M, KOGA T, ISHIBASHI H, UCHIDA S, OHTA Y,
•• SHIMODA Y: **Intestinal Aniskiasis: US in Diagnosis.** *Radiology* 1992, **185**:789–793.

Good descriptive article on a condition that may become more common in the West.

27. WEINBERGER E, WINTERS WD, LIDDELL RM, ROSENBAUM DM,
•• KRAUTER D: **Sonographic Diagnosis of Intestinal Malrotation in Infants: Importance of the Relative Positions of the Superior Mesenteric Vein and Artery.** *AJR Am J Roentgenol* 1992, **159**:825–828.

A large study confirming the value of this sign in detecting intestinal malrotation.

28. TARR PI, WEINBERGER E, HATCH EI, CHRISTIE DL: **Bacterial Ileocecitis Caused by Escherichia Coli O157:H7.** *J Pediatr Gastroenterol Nutr* 1992, **14**:261–263.

29. KAGIMOTO S: **Duodenal Findings on Ultrasound in Children With Schonlein-Henoch Purpura and Gastrointestinal Symptoms.** *J Pediatr Gastroenterol Nutr* 1993, **16**:178–182.

30. RUBESIN SE, RUBIN RA, HERLINGER H: **Small Bowel Malabsorp-**
• **tion: Clinical and Radiologic Perspectives.** *Radiology* 1992, **184**:297–305.

An expert and well-illustrated state-of-the-art lecture.

31. FUKUYA T, BROWN BP, LU CC: **Midgut Volvulus as a Complication of Intestinal Malrotation in Adults.** *Dig Dis Sci* 1993, **38**:438–444.

32. TANIGAWA K, YAMASHITA S, TEZUKA H, MORITA S, OHTSUBO T, MAEDA R: **Diagnostic Difficulty in a Case of Heterotopic Pancreatic Tissue of the Ileum.** *Am J Gastroenterol* 1993, **88**:451–453.

Philip Shorvon MA, MB BS, MRCP, FRCR, and Gabrielle Lamb MA, MB BS, MRCP, Department of Radiology, Central Middlesex Hospital NHS Trust, Acton Lane, London NW10 7NS, UK.

Pathology of the small intestine

Katherine DeSchryver, MD

St. Louis, Missouri, USA

This year's literature further dissected the different components of the gut wall layer by layer, and the mind-boggling complexities of the system are continuing to slowly emerge. The review of general concepts is followed by a review of the literature on inflammatory and infectious diseases and tumors, both lymphoid and epithelial.

Current Opinion in Gastroenterology 1994, **10**:171–175

General concepts

It is theorized that the enterocyte may have multiple secretory functions and possibly immunologic functions in addition to its already well-known absorptive role. So-called inflammatory cells are thought to have and increasingly proven to have physiologic trophic roles for epithelium. Atrophy of the villi with an inappropriately low mitotic activity is found in gut epithelial cells following depletion of CD4 but not CD8 lymphocytes. Attention to this phenomenon initially focused on patients with AIDS-associated diarrhea with no identifiable pathogenic organisms [1••]. It is also seen, however, in some cases of intractable diarrhea of infancy. Whether lack of trophic cytokines or the gut autoantibodies identified (GECA) or a combination of their interactions is involved, is as yet unclear. Whether cytokines elaborated by enterocytes contribute to the state of basal activation in monocytes or lymphocytes is a possibility also being explored.

Another player that might be destined to become important in the innumerable and as yet poorly understood inflammatory conditions is the pericrypt fibroblast mesenchymal cell. A recent review article [2•] reexamines its possible role, together with intraepithelial lymphocytes in the disposition of effete epithelial cells. Autophagocytosis or apoptosis of enterocyte basal portions is the mode of operation, as gleaned from experimental data. This process, leaving in place the uppermost portion of the enterocyte without a nucleus but with the tight junctions intact, protects from a possible momentary breach in the barrier system. Whether a similar mechanism is operative in the human gut is yet unknown. Such a mechanism certainly does exist in human cylindrical epithelia at multiple organ sites, as ciliated pinched-off, anucleated upper portions of epithelial cells are a well-known pitfall in diagnostic cytology. Occurrence of such cellular mechanisms imply a way for self-recognition in tandem with self-limited auto-destruction. Carrhiorhectic nuclei and phagocytosed nuclear debris within the area of a thickened subepithelial basement membrane are commonly seen in patients with a variety of low-grade but clearly inflammatory conditions. The clinical significance, if any, is as yet unclear, as is the relationship to the above described phenomenon. The pericrypt fibroblast might be a facultative lamina propria histiocyte in some of these conditions. It may also be the intermediary link between inflammatory cells and signal multiplier-modulator phenomena, analogous to renal inflammation [3].

The presence of axonal necrosis by ultrastructure within the superficial and deep myenteric plexus is known to be highly associated with Crohn's disease. It now has been reported [4••] in continent ileal pouches with pouchitis, a high percentage with positive bacterial cultures. Pouchitis is now felt to share clinical similarities with Crohn's disease, even though the pouches may have been constructed for chronic ulcerative colitis or familial polyposis coli. This interesting and important paper by the original authors of this observation in Crohn's disease begs the question of possible shared pathogenesis in the two conditions, based on the similarity of morphologies and clinical characteristics. These observations are particularly timely in light of the resurgence of the mycobacterial hypothesis in the etiology of Crohn's disease that has recently been given added support by new methodologic approaches using molecular biology.

Along with the topic of possible primary nerve damage in Crohn's disease, the expression of major histocompatibility complex class II antigens by myenteric plexus was reexamined [5•]. The intensity of positive staining on glial cells correlated with the enhanced epithelial expression of these glycoproteins during inflammatory activity.

A sporadic case of multiple and protracted episodes of pseudoobstruction is described [6•] in a patient with what proved to be absence of an α-actin isoform and attendant functional defect. The patient was without a diagnosis for years, as the morphology of the smooth muscle was essentially unremarkable on routine sections. Immunohistochemistry, however, for

 ISBN 1-85922-607-8 ISSN 0267–1379

smooth muscle α-actin was nonreactive. Although the work-up of this case was very sophisticated and not available to routine laboratories using conventionally processed material, awareness of this diagnostic possibility will promote better recognition for these patients' needs in terms of specialized procedures.

Inflammatory changes, exclusive of inflammatory bowel disease

Nonsteroidal anti-inflammatory drug–associated disease

Nonsteroidal agent–associated disease has attracted much attention again this year. The highlights of a number of reports are, that in addition to "diaphragm disease" and recurrent stricturing ulcers in the small bowel, nonsteroidal anti-inflammatory drugs are also the likely agents involved in an unknown number of nonspecific enterocolitides and ulcers (Table 1). The prevalence is widespread; indeed, long-term use of these agents might be causing symptoms in about 70% of patients.

Table 1. Spectrum of nonsteroidal anti-inflammatory drug–associated disease*

	Small bowel	Colon
Normal intestine	Perforation	Eosinophilic colitis
	Massive bleeding	Pseudomembranous colitis
	Broad-based strictures	Collagenous colitis
	Diaphragm-like strictures	Ulcers
		Colitis
	Recurrent ulcers	
	Enteropathy	
Effect on preexisting disease	Relapse of IBD	Relapse of IBD
		Complications diverticular disease
		Appendicitis

*Adapted from Bjarnason *et al.* [7•]: with permission.
Both small bowel and colon are listed, as combinations of these are possible in any patient at any given time.
IBD—inflammatory bowel disease.

Celiac disease and related diagnostic quandaries

The differential diagnosis of active duodenitis ought to include celiac disease, as this diagnosis is increasingly made on endoscopic biopsies. A very interesting article [8••] focuses attention on how classic histologic features of active duodenitis with polymorphonuclears, usually attributed to peptic disease in the duodenum, in fact represented cases of celiac disease. Intraepithelial lymphocytes were present in each, further reinforcing the notion of constellations of diagnostic features to arrive at the correct identification of disease processes.

The problem of cases of collagenous colitis diagnosed by morphologic and clinical criteria, in fact corresponding to celiac disease, is repeatedly present in the literature [9••]. The recommendation is made to obtain a small bowel biopsy in every patient with the diagnosis of collagenous colitis. Collagenous colitis, however, is reported to have multiple other possible associations. Lymphocytic colitis seems to be a heterogenous group of disorders as well. Approximately 30% of apparent sprue patients will have colon biopsies that fulfill diagnostic criteria for lymphocytic colitis. Some of these will respond to gluten withdrawal at both sites; others, morphologically indistinguishable, will not. These issues await further clarifications.

Vasculitis

Vasculitis, in a general sense, is increasingly recognized as a cause of nonspecific ulcers and hemorrhage in gastrointestinal disease. Not uncommonly, small intestinal presentation is the first or only manifestation of the patient's disease. The reports are individual cases, partially listed in Table 2, including such disparate entities as Buerger's disease [10•], polyarteritis nodosa [11•], leukocytoclastic vasculitis, familial free protein S deficiency with mesenteric venous thrombosis, and ileo-cecal tuberculosis. These possibilities need to be kept in mind when interpreting biopsies with an unusual constellation of clinical, endoscopic, and so-called nonspecific morphologic findings.

Table 2. Partial differential diagnosis of small intestinal diseases with a vasculitic component.

Vasculitides	
Thromboangiitis obliterans	Gastrointestinal disease 2 y prior to clinical peripheral vasculitis
Polyarteritis nodosa	With or without hepatitis B
Leukocytoclastic vasculitis	Without Henoch-Schonlein purpura
	Possibly with mixed cryoglobulinemia
	Sepis
	Lupus or lupus anticoagulant syndrome
	Rheumatoid arthritis
Inherited metabolic disease of coagulation proteins	Protein S deficiency
Unknown etiology	Crohn's disease
Infectious	Tuberculosis
	Cytomegalovirus

Infectious etiologies

Pneumocystis carinii

The most surprising "new" infectious agent said to involve the gastrointestinal tract is *Pneumocystis carinii* [12••]. The morphologic hallmark is the frothy exudate with cysts that can be highlighted with silver stains. The distribution of the telltale exudates might be within lamina propria, with or without any surrounding inflammatory changes, or even intravascularly. Although these reports were in AIDS patients on prophylactic treatment for the lung disease, this fungus might well appear in other circumstances as a pathogen.

Cytomegalovirus

Further attention was drawn to the well known difficulty [13•] of recognizing early cytomegalovirus inclusions in gastrointestinal biopsies. These are atypical and do not fulfill set morphologic criteria, but are important to recognize, so that treatment may be attempted. *In situ* hybridization with commercial probes works well and is technically easy, aiding in diagnosis.

Histoplasma

Cases of histoplasmosis [14•] presenting as malabsorption or protein-losing enteropathy are reported. Awareness of this fact is important in making the diagnosis, as endoscopically ulcers may not be present, and random biopsy is instrumental in identifying the lesion.

Tumors

Lymphocytes and their tumors

The literature of lymphomas of the gastrointestinal tracts is as convoluted as any T-cell nucleus ever described! There is abundant clinical evidence that lymphomas of the gastrointestinal tract are different in some regards from nodal lymphomas. These differences are thought to stem from the privileged sequestered nature of the mucosa-associated lymphoid system and its lymphocytes. Lymphomas are the most common malignant tumors of the small intestine.

A study of 119 cases of small intestinal lymphomas has shown that 66% were B-cell and 34% were T-cell tumors [15••]. Within B cell tumors, 62% were high grade lesions and only 20% had the low grade MALT associated phenotype. T-cell tumors accounted for the worst prognostic group, as 83% were high grade and 50% were enteropathy associated.

Another article [16•] reports on 27 patients and subdivides "peripheral T-cell lymphomas of the intestine" into three categories: enteropathy associated, enteropathy associated-like, and without enteropathy. A high recurrence rate and multifocality characterized the enteropathy-associated group.

Finally, now that we had rested peacefully with the knowledge that gastrointestinal lymphomas do not express the peptide product of the bcl-2 protooncogene, we have an in-depth study [17••] demonstrating that follicular lymphomas, although rare, do exist in the gastrointestinal tract. The discussion of the paper briefly reviews the controversies trying to distinguish between neoplastic cells simply colonizing reactive centers, imparting a falsely follicular appearance to the lesion versus a true neoplasm of centrocytes still differentiated enough to evoke the follicular architecture. At any rate, these tumors are most common in the terminal ileum, and the bcl-2 protooncogene product is most useful in immunohistochemical studies distinguishing follicular lymphomas from lymphoid hyperplasia, especially on a small sample: the bcl-2 oncogene product is absent from germinal centers.

Although the majority of malignancies associated with inflammatory bowel disease are carcinomas, malignant lymphomas is known to be a possible complication of both ulcerative colitis and Crohn's disease. A case report [18] reminds us of this rare occurrence, with a review of the literature as it pertains to Crohn's disease.

Epithelial tumors and their precursors

Nonpenetrance and late appearance of polyps was recently described for the first time in families with familial polyposis coli and Gardner syndrome [19••]. The identification of such occurrences although uncommon, might affect our clinical reasoning: could a patient with late onset but multiple gastrointestinal lesions and a family history of colon cancer represent a bearer of the faulty gene with incomplete penetrance? Might this be more common than we now know? Could some now considered sporadic small intestinal malignancies be part of a form fruste of Gardner syndrome? At this time there are no answers to such questions, but the report in *Gut* is certainly most provocative.

In patients with familial polyposis coli and Gardner syndrome, upper gastrointestinal proliferative lesions are increasingly recognized as the source of malignancy after the colonic lesions have been preventively resected. Duodenal and periampullary adenomatous or dysplastic proliferative lesions are the precursors, with or without a visible polypoid lesion on endoscopy. Such gastroduodenal polyposis was recently reported [20•] to have *ras* mutations within the lesions. The *ras* family of genes have a putative role in cellular signal transduction. The *ras* proteins acquire transforming activity, when amino acids are substituted at one of a few specific sites, as a result of point mutations in the gene. These investigations have important diagnostic and prognostic potential as tumorigenesis is increasingly better understood at the molecular level.

Other conditions of the small intestine that predispose to epithelial malignancy include long-standing Crohn's disease. This topic is controversial, but there is increasing consensus that dysplasia is present and can be mapped in surveillance studies, similar to the practice in longstanding ulcerative colitis. These evaluations also include DNA ploidy analysis and search for mutated forms of the *p53* gene product on the biopsies.

References and recommended reading

Papers of particular interest, published within the annual period of review, have been highlighted as:

- • Of special interest
- •• Of outstanding interest

1. •• Martin-Villa JM, Camblor S, Costa R, Arnaiz-Villena A: **Gut Epithelial Cell Autoantibodies in AIDS Pathogenesis.** *The Lancet* 1993, **342**:342–380.

Seventy-one percent of 100 cases of HIV infected patients without advanced disease were found to have gut epithelial autoantibodies. Depletion of CD4 positive lymphocytes was striking among intraepithelial lymphocytes and lamina propria lymphocytes, as was the inappropriately low mitotic count and attendant villous atrophy. Whereas this observation is important from a clinical point of view, it also highlights the many yet unanswered questions about complex epithelial-immune phenomenon in the gut.

2. • CROITORU K, RIDDELL RH: **Reduce, Reuse and Recycle: Shedding Light on Shedding Cells.** *Gastroenterology* 1993, **105**:1243–1250.

Review article about "stromal" cells along the basement membrane focusing on the mechanisms involved in disposing of effete epithelial cells. Considerations involve subepithelial macrophages, the pericrypt (myo)fibroblast as a "stem cell," and other thought-provoking concepts.

3. OKEGAWA T, JONAS PE, DESCHRYVER K, KAWASAKI A, NEEDLEMAN P: **Metabolic and Cellular Alterations Underlying the Exaggerated Renal Prostaglandin and Thromboxane Synthesis: Inflammatory Response Involving Fibroblasts and Mononuclear Cells.** *J Clin Invest* 1983, **71**:81–90.

4. •• DVORAK AM, ONDERDONK AB, MCLEOD RS, MONAHAN-EARLEY RA, CULLEN J, ANTONIOLI DA, BLAIR JE, MORGAN ES, CISNEROS RL, ESTRELLA P, COHEN Z, SILEN W: **Axonal Necrosis of Enteric Autonomic Nerves in Continent Ileal Pouches; Possible Implications for Pathogenesis of Crohn's Disease.** *Ann Surg* 1993, **217**:260–271.

Ileal pouches constructed during resection for ulcerative colitis or familial polyposis coli are small bowel mucosal segments with a 10% to 45% risk of developing clinically significant inflammation (pouchitis), resembling Crohn's disease. 114 cases represented the present study group of replicate biopsies for ultrastructure and microbiology. 53% of Crohn's disease control subjects previously reported to have nerve damage of axonal necrosis within myenteric plexus, had the lesion in the current study. It occurred in 42% of pouches, regardless whether constructed for ulcerative colitis or familial polyposis coli, particularly in those with clinically significant inflammation and positive bacterial cultures. Interesting parallels are hypothesized between pathogenesis of pouchitis and Crohn's disease.

5. • GEBOES K, RUTGEERTS P, ECTORS N, MEBIS J, PENNINCKX F, VANTRAPPEN G, DESMET VJ: **Major Histocompatibility Class II Expression on the Small Intestinal Nervous System in Crohn's Disease.** *Gastroenterology* 1992, **103**:439–447.

This paper reexamines the pathologic and possibly etiologic importance of class II antigen expression on the supporting cells of the myenteric plexus, as it may be relevant to inflammatory bowel disease. Whether the plexus is a primary actor-target in Crohn's disease or a bystander is not resolved by this approach. Glial cells of the plexus nevertheless seem to be involved, possibly also in antigen presentation.

6. • SMITH VV, LAKE BD, KAMM MA, NICHOLLS RJ: **Intestinal Pseudo-Obstruction With Deficient Smooth Muscle α-Actin.** *Histopathology* 1992, **21**:535–542.

The use of specific antibodies to isoforms of contractile proteins may have an important role in the diagnosis of unexplained recurrent episodes of small intestinal pseudoobstruction.

7. • BJARNASON I, HAYLLAR J, MACPHERSON AJ, RUSSELL AS: **Side Effects of Nonsteroidal Anti-Inflammatory Drugs on the Small and Large Intestine in Humans.** *Gastroenterology* 1993, **104**:1832–1847.

Review article of side effects and the postulated pathogenetic mechanisms in nonsteroidal anti-inflammatory drugs, with extensive bibliography.

8. •• JEFFERS MD, HOURIHANE DO'B: **Coeliac Disease With Histological Features of Peptic Duodenitis: Value of Assessment of Intraepithelial Lymphocytes.** *J Clin Pathol* 1993, **46**:420–424.

The jejunal biopsy for ruling out celiac disease is now mostly replaced by endoscopic biopsies of second duodenum. Morphologic features were reevaluated for specificity. Gastric metaplasia and significant polymorphonuclear infiltrates, usually taken as evidence for peptic disease in the duodenum, were seen in four of 13 cases of celiac disease. Intraepithelial lymphocytes were the additional morphologic discriminant for this diagnosis.

9. •• ARMES J, GEE DC, MACRAE FA, SCHROEDER W, BHATHAL PS: **Collagenous Colitis: Jejunal and Colorectal Pathology.** *Gut* 1992,

Ten patients with collagenous colitis also had had small intestinal biopsies. Features of celiac disease were found in 4. The authors' conclusion is that a small bowel biopsy is warranted in patients with collagenous colitis to find cases of treatable celiac disease.

10. • BROIDE E, SCAPA E, PEER A, WITZ E, ABRAMOWICH D, ESHCHAR J: **Buerger's Diseases Presenting as Small Bowel Ischemia.** *Gastroenterology* 1993, **104**:1192–1195.

Thromboangiitis obliterans presented in a 20-year-old male with acute small bowel ischemia, two years before peripheral vascular disease became symptomatic. Morphologically, the mesenteric vascular changes on the resection specimens were unexpected at this location, but classical for the disease entity.

11. • WILLIAMS DH, KRATKA CD, BONAFEDE JP, KATON RM: **Polyarteritis Nodosa of the Gastrointestinal Tract With Endoscopically Documented Duodenal and Jejunal Ulceration.** *Gastrointest Endosc* 1992, **38**:501–503.

First case report of deep serpiginous necrotic duodenal and jejunal ulcers due to vasculitis identified by endoscopy. Such cases may now therefore come to biopsy. Gastrointestinal involvement occurs in about 50% cases of polyarteritis nodosa, with the gastrointestinal involvement being the initial or the only manifestation of the disease in 36%.

12. •• DIETERICH DT, LEW EA, BACON DJ, PEARLMAN KI, SCHOLES JV: **Gastrointestinal Pneumocystosis in HIV- Infected Patients on Aerosolized Pentaminidine: Report of Five Cases and Literature Review.** *Am J Gastroenterol* 1992, **87**:1763–1770.

Five patients with AIDS are reported to have gastrointestinal pneumocystosis following aerosolized pentamidine prophylaxis. The paper illustrates *P. carinii* cysts in dilated mucosal capillaries and interstitially in the lamina propria. Gomori's methenamine silver stain is helpful in diagnosis. Tissue reaction is variable, often none in the duodenal and colonic biopsies illustrated (liver showed granulomatous inflammation).

13. • SCHWARTZ DA, WILCOX CM: **Atypical Cytomegalovirus Inclusions in Gastrointestinal Biopsy Specimens From Patients With the Acquired Immunodeficiency Syndrome. Diagnostic Role of In-Situ Nucleic Acid Hybridization.** *Hum Pathol* 1992, **23**:1019–1026.

Cytomegalovirus infection of the gastrointestinal tract is a common cause of morbidity in the AIDS syndrome complex. This paper highlights the well known diagnostic difficulty with the commonly atypical morphology of the inclusions, which do not fulfill the established minimum criteria, and have previously been well described from the lung. *In situ* hybridization with commercial probes is important in making the diagnosis.

14. • ORCHARD JL: **Malabsorption Due to Gastrointestinal Histoplasmosis.** *Am J Med* 1992, **93**:237–238.

Histoplasmosis-associated gastrointestinal disease has recently been reported to be sometimes present in unexpected ways. Patients with malabsorption or protein losing enteropathy of unknown etiology had no ulcers on endoscopy, with random biopsies yielding the diagnosis. In another case, inflammatory pseudopolypoid lesions were present.

15. •• DOMIZIO P, OWEN RA, SHEPHER NA, TALBOT IC, NORTON AJ: **Primary Lymphoma of the Small Intestine. A Clinicopathologic Study of 119 Cases.** *Am J Surg Pathol* 1993, **17**:429–442.

The authors review 119 cases of small bowel lymphoma with a peak incidence in the seventh decade. Two thirds of the patients are men. A total of 66% proved to be B-cell tumors, with two thirds high-grade diffuse lesions. Only 20% were low-grade mucosa-associated lymphoid type tumors. B-cell lymphomas tended to be annular or polypoid lesions distally (terminal ileum). T-cell lymphomas represented about 34% of all lymphomas and tended to present as multifocal ulcerated plaque-like lesions or strictures proximally, associated about half of the time with enteropathy. Eighty-three percent were high grade with a poor prognosis. Reagents to subtype B and T cells were found to work reliably in paraffin tissues.

16. Chott A, Dragosics B, Radaszkiewicz T: **Peripheral T**
• **Cell Lymphomas of the Intestine.** *Am J Pathol* 1992, **141**:1361–1371.

Twenty-seven cases of T-cell lymphoma of the intestine were reviewed. The authors' conclusion is that the neoplastic T cells are mucosa derived. Why the designation of peripheral T cell? This reviewer found this most confusing.

17. LeBrun DP, Kamel OW, Cleary ML, Dorfman RF, Warnke
•• RA: **Follicular Lymphomas of the Gastrointestinal Tract. Pathologic Features in 31 Cases and bcl-2 Oncogenic Protein Expression.** *Am J Pathol* 1992, **140**:1327–1335.

Thirty-one cases of follicular lymphomas of the gastrointestinal tract were reviewed. A female preponderance was striking, in contrast to the male predominance for diffuse lymphomas of the gastrointestinal tract. Five cases had the endoscopic and gross appearance of multiple polypoid lesions, consistent with multiple lymphomatous polyposis. Others in the small intestine presented with obstruction.

18. Perosio PM, Brooks JJ, Saul SH, Haller DG: **Primary In-**
• **testinal Lymphoma in Crohn's Disease: Minute Tumor With a Fatal Outcome.** *Am J Gastroenterol* 1992, **87**:894–898.

This case report reviews and tabulates the literature on this rare complication of long-standing Crohn's disease, which also has been reported in longstanding ulcerative colitis.

19. Evans DGR, Guy SP, Thakker N, Armstrong JG, Dodd
•• C, Davies DR, Babbs C, Clancy T, Warnes T, Sloan P, Taylor TV, Harris R: **Non-Penetrance and Late Appearance of Polyps in Families With Familial Adenomatous Polyposis.** *Gut* 1993, **34**:1389–1394.

The authors followed 30 families in the North West of England with Familial adenomatous polyposis. They reported three families with late onset of polyps and an individual with nonpenetrance at age 59. Although such patients so far reported are rare, the concept and its implications are important.

20. Odze RD, Quinn PS, Terrault NA, Vivona AA, Ward MA,
• Cohen Z, Gallinger S: **Advanced Gastroduodenal Polyposis With Ras Mutations in a Patient With Familial Adenomatous Polyposis.** *Hum Pathol* 1993, **24**:442–448.

Upper gastrointestinal proliferative lesions are increasingly recognized in patients with familial polyposis coli and Gardner syndrome to be the source of malignancy after the colonic lesions have been preventively resected, with duodenal and periampullary adenomatous proliferative lesions being the precursors. Using the polymerase chain reaction with mismatced primers, a k-*ras* codon 12 mutation was detected within the periampullary adenoma in areas of severe dysplasia.

Katherine DeSchryver, MD, Department of Surgical Pathology, 450 North New Ballas Road, Suite 156, St. Louis, MO 63141, USA.

Surgery of the small bowel

Devinder Kumar, PhD, FRCS

Queen Elizabeth Hospital, Birmingham, UK

During the past year, developments in laparoscopic surgery of the small intestine, management of enterocutaneous fistulas, patterns of recurrence following resection for Crohn's disease, long-term results of restorative proctocolectomy, and small bowel transplantation received considerable attention in the literature. The diagnostic and therapeutic potential of laparoscopic surgery has been fully explored. Patterns of recurrence following resection for Crohn's disease have been described. Two series have reported long-term results of ileal pouch–anal anastomosis with a special reference to pouch failure. Nontransplant surgical options for management of the short bowel syndrome have also been discussed. A new technique for combined hepatic-intestinal retrieval has been described and the results of intestinal transplantation in composite visceral grafts compared with those of intestinal grafts only.

Current Opinion in Gastroenterology 1994, **10**:176–182

Laparoscopy

Laparoscopy has long been used by gynecologists to diagnose and treat pelvic disease. More recently the diagnostic and therapeutic potential of laparoscopic surgery has been fully explored by general surgeons. Procedures such as laparoscopic cholecystectomy, antireflux surgery, appendicectomy, and laparoscopic hernia repair have been well established as safe and widely acceptable. Many conventional operations are being replaced by laparoscopic procedures because of the rapid recovery of the patient and avoidance of major surgery. Similarly, the indications for laparoscopy as a diagnostic tool are steadily increasing. Ogbana *et al.* [1•] used laparoscopy in patients with acute abdomen and improved the diagnostic accuracy and significantly reduced the rate of unnecessary laparotomies from 14% to 6%. Attwood *et al.* [2] described an approach to small bowel dissection using laparoscopic assisted mobilization and exteriorization. In three patients they were able to avoid narcotic analgesia and postoperative paralytic ileus. Two other studies [3,4] described laparoscopic jejunostomies. One study used T fasteners as retractors and anchors to secure the jejunum to the abdominal wall and the other study used conventional silk sutures to secure the jejunum to the abdominal wall.

Crohn's disease

Recurrence of symptoms following resection for Crohn's disease is common. Intestinal permeability is increased in patients with Crohn's disease but it is not known whether the increased permeability precedes relapse. Wyatt *et al.* [5••] measured intestinal permeability in 72 patients with quiescent Crohn's disease using the Lactulose/Mannitol test. They found that the permeability index was significantly higher in patients than in controls (Fig. 1), and, more importantly, patients who had a higher permeability had a significantly higher incidence of relapse of Crohn's disease within 1 year of the test ($P<0.001$) (Fig. 2). These are important data as they may help to select patients suitable for maintenance therapy for Crohn's disease following resection.

In another study, May *et al.* [6•] studied intestinal permeability using the Lactulose-Mannitol test in patients with Crohn's disease and their first degree relatives. Permeability in relatives was found to be similar to that in the control group but a subpopulation had abnormally high permeability in the absence of clinical manifestation of Crohn's disease. To investigate the pattern of anastomotic recurrence of Crohn's disease after ileocolic resection, 11 patients underwent colonoileoscopy

[7••]. Ileal inflammation occurred soon after surgery in eight patients and was more severe within 1 to 3 cm above the ileocolic anastomosis than that seen 5 cm above the anastomosis. The postanastomotic colonic mucosa showed no inflammatory changes. In another study [8], 86 patients with Crohn's disease undergoing ileocolic resection were randomly assigned to receive either an end-to-end or side-to-end anastomosis. In patients with an end-to-end anastomosis, there were 10 ileal recurrences and all of these involved distal ileum in the preanastomotic location. In the end-to-side anastomosis group, there were 11 recurrences but none of these patients had recurrence in the blind ileal pouch. This study concluded that the fecal stream and reflux of colonic contents may be an important factor in determining the pattern of ileal recurrence.

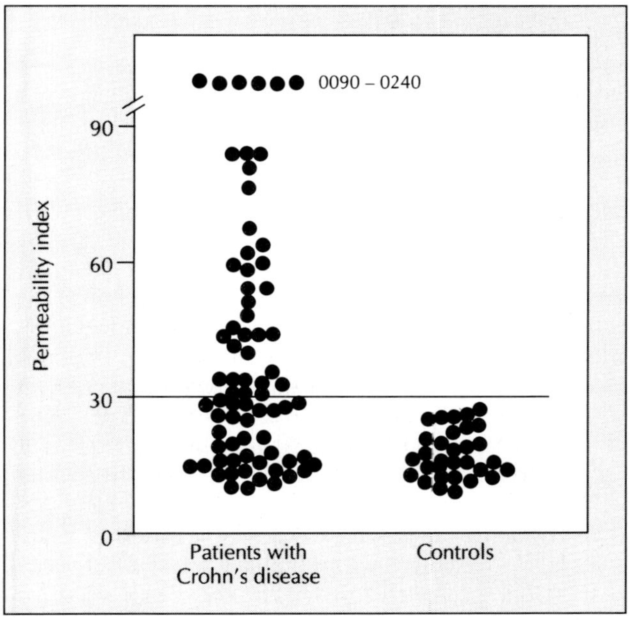

Fig. 1. Permeability index in patients with Crohn's disease (n = 72) and controls (n = 30). (*From* Wyatt *et al.* [5••]; with permission.)

At laparotomy, Crohn's lesions are sought by inspection and palpation of the small bowel and in some cases passage of a balloon through the small bowel to search for small bowel stenosis. However, these techniques often fail to diagnose diseased areas in all patients. To investigate the feasibility of perioperative endoscopy of the whole small bowel in Crohn's disease, Lescut *et al.* [9•] studied 20 patients undergoing surgery for Crohn's disease. They were able to identify Crohn's lesions scattered over the whole small intestine in 13 of the 20 cases. These included aphthoid ulceration, superficial ulceration, mucosal edema, erythema, pseudopolyps, deep ulceration, ulcerative stenosis, and nonulcerative stenosis. Patients with multiple strictures due to Crohn's disease of the small bowel are often treated with strictureplasty in order to conserve the small bowel. Fazio *et al.* [10•] have reported a 3-year median follow-up result in 116 patients with obstructive Crohn's disease undergoing 452 strictureplasties. In this group, the rates of restricture and new stricture formation were 2.8% and 24% respectively. Of the total patient group, 15% needed reoperation for obstructive symptoms.

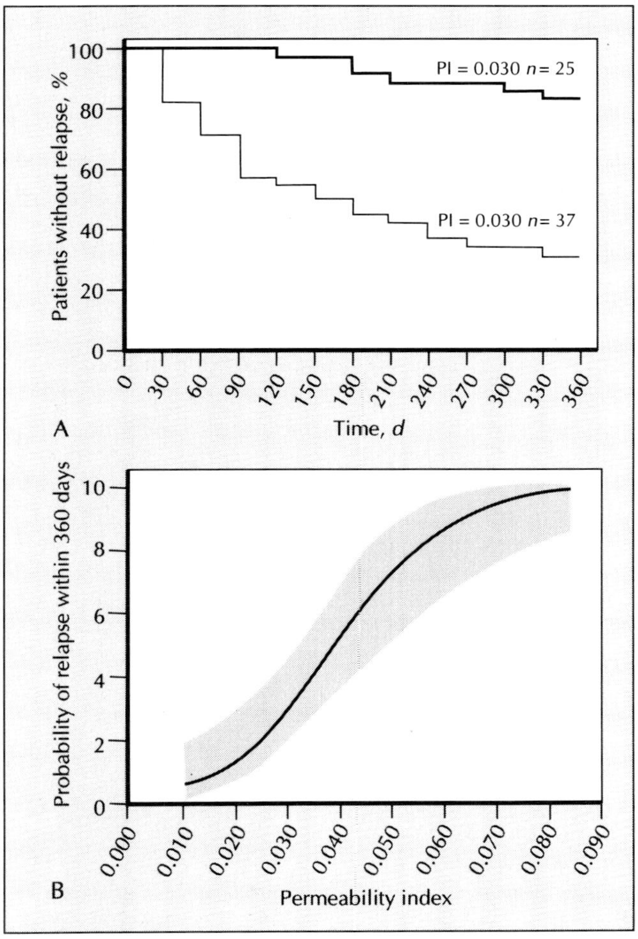

Fig. 2. **A**, Percentage of patients without a relapse over 1 year. **B**, Probability of a relapse within 1 year. The shaded area represents the 95% confidential interval. PI—permeability index. (*From* Wyatt *et al.* [5••]; with permission.)

Another study looked at the risk factors for the development of small bowel cancer in Crohn's disease [11••]. Suspected risk factors include surgically excluded small bowel loops, chronic fistulous disease, long duration of unresected disease, and male sex. This study failed to confirm any of these risk factors but identified three alternative risk factors in a case-controlled study: proximal small bowel disease, 6 mercaptopurine use, and hazardous occupations known to be associated with an increased risk of colorectal cancer. These are important observations because some of the risk factors identified are preventable and may lead to a reduced incidence of malignant change in Crohn's disease.

Enterocutaneous fistula

Enterocutaneous fistula complicated by local or systemic sepsis or bacteremia and cancer are difficult clinical problem to manage. Most of these patients require operative intervention. Although there are some known predictive factors for spontaneous closure, spontaneous closure is not predictable with any degree of confidence. To look for predictors of spontaneous closure with enterocutaneous fistulas, Kuvshinoff *et al.* [12] studied 79 patients with 116 fistulas. Parameters such as fistula output, number of blood transfusions, presence of sepsis and metabolic parameters including serum transferrin retinol-binding protein, thyroxin-binding prealbumin, and serum albumin were investigated. None of the other parameters except serum transferrin were predictive of spontaneous closure. The authors concluded that turnover proteins, particularly serum transferrin, might be useful in predicting which patients with enterocutaneous fistulas should undergo surgery despite anatomic criteria favorable for spontaneous closure.

In a 5-year retrospective review of 28 patients with low output enterocutaneous fistulas, Borison *et al.* [13] studied the outcome of early surgical and nonsurgical treatment. Six patients had early operative intervention, whereas the remaining 22 patients were treated medically. Four of the 22 patients in the conservative group received parenteral somatostatin analogue. All patients in the surgical group resumed normal gastrointestinal function within 2 weeks. Of the 22 medically treated patients, three of the four who received somatostatin analogue were healed of their fistulas within 2 weeks. Fistulas healed in only two of the other medically treated patients. The authors concluded that early surgery or the use of somatostatin analogue should be considered in the treatment of patients with low output intestinal fistulas.

In another study [14], two patients received octreotide acetate for the treatment of postoperative enterocutaneous fistulas. One was a high output fistula and the other one was a low output fistula. Octreotide was given subcutaneously, 50 to 100 μg every 8 hours. A significant reduction in fistula output was noted only after three doses of octreotide. Both fistulas closed promptly after nine doses of octreotide, but the high-output fistula recurred 2 days later. This fistula eventually closed spontaneously 1 month later. Octreotide does appear to be a useful adjunct to the conventional treatment of enterocutaneous fistulas. It may help to reduce the fistula output and therefore aid in spontaneous closure.

Ileal pouch–anal anastomosis

Restorative proctocolectomy is now established as the operation of choice for ulcerative colitis; however, the long-term function of various pouch designs has yet to be established. Complications such as pouchitis remain a major clinical problem and efforts are being made to study the pattern of physiology of pouchitis. At the same time, new pouch designs continue to be investigated with a view to improving pouch function. A combination of an upper triplicate and a lower duplicate ileal pouch has been described [15]. This two-chamber pouch model is supposed to delay pouch filling because of the bigger diameter of the proximal chamber. The functional result of this pouch remains to be evaluated. Penna *et al.* [16] studied the effects of previous subtotal colectomy with ileostomy on the outcome of ileal J-pouch anal anastomosis in patients with acute ulcerative colitis. They concluded that a previous subtotal colectomy did not compromise the results of later ileal pouch–anal anastomosis. Furthermore, it did not increase the morbidity of subsequent ileal pouch–anal anastomosis and was associated with more rapid functional recovery.

In another study, short- and long-lateral ileal reservoirs in a canine preparation were evaluated to determine the optimal reservoir size and configuration [17•]. It was found that short-lateral isoperistaltic reservoirs emptied more effectively than long reservoirs. Harms *et al.* [18] reported long-term assessment of W ileal reservoirs after proctocolectomy for ulcerative colitis and familial polyposis in 109 patients. They found that 24-hour stool frequency decreased and pouch compliance increased in both groups between 2 months and 1 year. There was no significant change in either parameter after 1 year. Only 10% of the patients experienced occasional minor leakage at night. There was no loss of reservoir reported in this series. In another study [19], pouch function after proctocolectomy and ileal J-pouch anal anastomosis was assessed at 1 and 5 years in 41 patients with familial adenomatous polyposis. Unlike the previous study, the mean stool frequency per 24 hours and the mean nocturnal stool frequency decreased significantly between 1 and 5 years. At 5 years, only one patient was following a strict diet and two patients need antidiarrheal medication. They concluded that the function of ileal pouch–anal anastomosis continued to improve over time in patients with familial adenomatous polyposis.

Following restorative proctocolectomy, gross continence is reasonably well preserved. However, leakage of mucus or small amounts of feces classed as minor episodes of incontinence is common and some patients suffer from skin soreness and need to wear protective pads. Hallgren *et al.* [20] studied the possible role of the autonomic nervous system in sphincter impairment after restorative proctocolectomy. They performed preoperative manometry in 12 patients undergoing endoanal proctectomy and a hand-sewn pouch-anal anastomosis and in another 12 who had a proctectomy from above with a stapled ileal pouch–anal anastomosis. In both groups, the division of the superior rectal artery reduced the median resting anal pressure. Complete rectal mobilization to the pelvic floor decreased resting pressure by an additional 22%. Irrespective of the operative technique used, after completion of anastomosis, a further decline in median pressure could be demonstrated. They concluded that the autonomic nervous supply to the anal sphincter mechanism might be the major cause for this reduction in the resting anal pressure [20].

Comparing the complications after a stapled and hand-sewn J-pouch ileoanal anastomosis, Wettergren *et al.* [21] reported that there was a significantly higher rate of anastomotic stenosis in the hand sewn group and that patients who developed anastomotic breakdown lost significantly more blood during operation. Overall, the stapled anastomosis was shown to give better results compared with the hand-sewn procedure. In a study to determine the predictive factors for postoperative complications and outcome after ileal pouch–anal anastomosis in patients with ulcerative colitis and primary sclerosing cholangitis, 40 patients were assessed [22•]. It was found that immediate postoperative and remote ileoanal anastomosis–related complications were high in this group of patients, but they appeared to be related directly to the severity of liver disease. This study suggested that in patients with ulcerative colitis and primary sclerosing cholangitis, ileal pouch–anal anastomosis is a safe option.

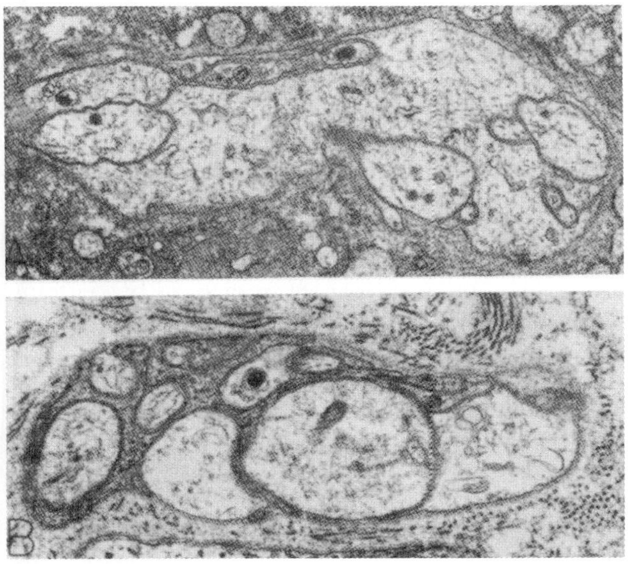

Fig. 3. Axonal necrosis in culture-positive ulcerative colitis pouchitis (*A*, original × 18,000) and FP pouchitis (*B*, original × 17,000) biopsies. (*From* Dvorak *et al.* [23••]; with permission.)

Axonal necrosis was first described in samples of small intestine obtained from patients with Crohn's disease. Patients who develop pouchitis following restorative proctocolectomy also show evidence of axonal necrosis in pouch biopsies. To study the possible implications for pathogenesis of Crohn's disease, Dvorak *et al.* [23••] evaluated replicate biopsies from 114 samples of human intestine. Biopsies from ileum, colon, conventional ileostomy, or continent pouches were obtained from patients with ulcerative colitis, Crohn's disease, or familial polyposis. The ultrastructural diagnosis of damaged enteric nerves was based on previously published criteria for axonal necrosis. They found that the highest incidence of axonal necrosis was present in Crohn's disease control biopsies. Axonal necrosis also occurred in more ulcerative colitis and familial polyposis biopsies that had positive bacterial cultures than in those that did not (Fig. 3). A total of 42% of the biopsies from pouches that were found to be inflamed by clinical criteria also showed axonal necrosis (Fig. 4). Control patients with ulcerative colitis and familial polyposis had significantly less nerve damage than pouch biopsies in the presence of positive cultures or inflammation. This study concluded that the association of damaged nerves and invasive bacteria in pouchitis may suggest machinistic similarities for the pathogenesis of Crohn's disease and has provided further support to the hypothesis that the ileoanal pouch may be an excellent model for the study of the pathogenesis of Crohn's disease.

Two papers audited long-term results to examine patterns of pouch failure and other associated complications. In one study [24••], 253 patients underwent ileal pouch–anal anastomosis over a 10-year period and 25 of them experienced pouch failure. The most common cause of pouch failure in this series was a poor functional result seen in 28% of the patients. In 13 patients, unsuspected Crohn's disease became manifest and resulted in perianal sepsis or pouch fistulas leading to pouch failure. Pouchitis accounted for four of 25 failures but patients with pouchitis were not found to be at higher risk for pouch failure than those who did not have pouchitis. Pelvic sepsis was another significant indicator of pouch failure and was seen in five patients.

In the second study [25], the results of 168 restorative proctocolectomies were audited. In this series, morbidity from pelvic sepsis accounted for 12% of the patients, ileoanal stricture occurred in 15%, and pouch-related fistulas occurred in 16%. Pouch excision for pouch failure occurred in 30% of the first 50 patients but only in 4% of the last 68 patients. As in the first study, unidentified Crohn's disease was a significant factor in pouch failure. As the results of long-term audit of restorative proctocolectomy are being presented from various centers, it is becoming clear that although the operation of ileal pouch–anal anastomosis is a major advance over a panproctocolectomy, it still has a number of significant problems that remain to be addressed. It has to be said, however, that with increasing experience, the results are improving.

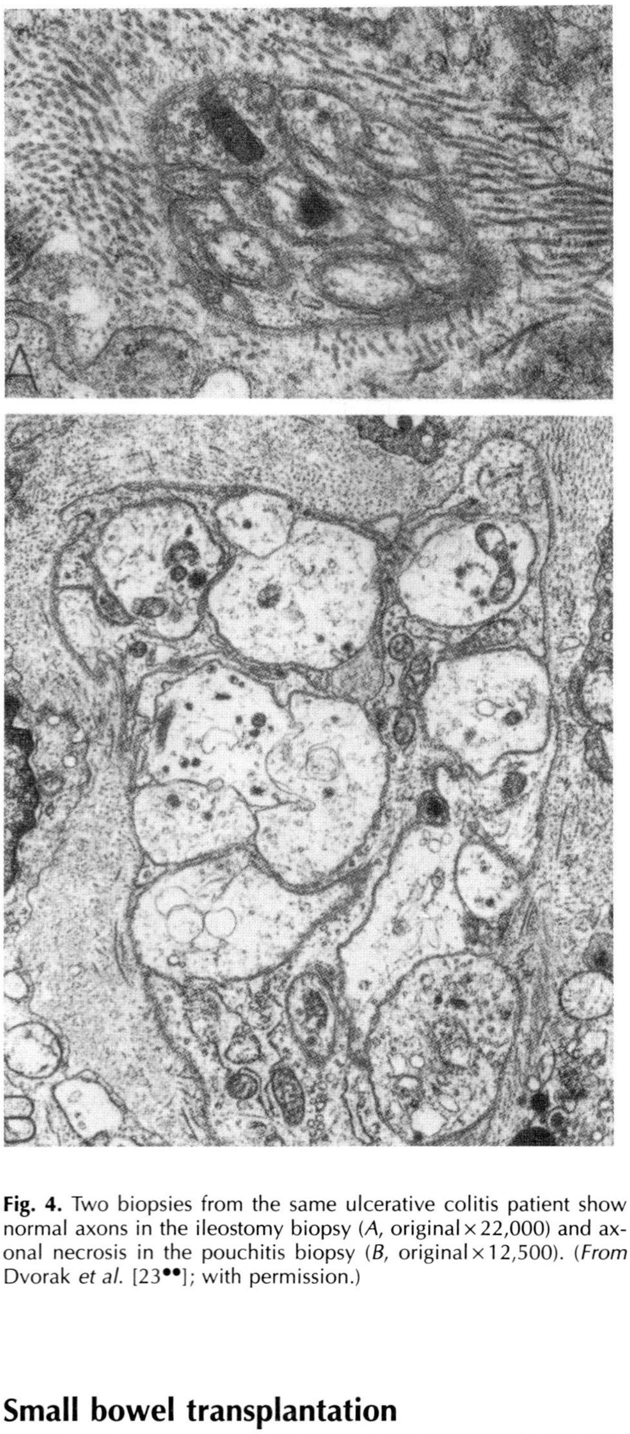

Fig. 4. Two biopsies from the same ulcerative colitis patient show normal axons in the ileostomy biopsy (*A*, original × 22,000) and axonal necrosis in the pouchitis biopsy (*B*, original × 12,500). (*From* Dvorak *et al.* [23••]; with permission.)

Small bowel transplantation

The debate over indications for small bowel transplantation continues. Patients with short bowel syndrome are faced with problems that are a direct result of rapid intestinal transit, decreased mucosal surface area, ineffective peristalsis and reduced intestinal length. In a very well written review, the non-transplant surgical options for management of the short bowel syndrome are discussed [26••]. The authors review the role of pharmaceutical agents in slowing intestinal transit, surgical construction of intestinal valves, the use of reversed intestinal segments, recirculating intestinal loops, colonic interposition, reversed electrical intersonal pacing, tapering, and intestinal lengthening. In addition, they also stress the importance of carefully measuring and documenting the entire length of bowel, and of inspecting the gallbladder for stones and strongly recommend a cholecystectomy in a young patient with gallstones. The indications for various surgical options are clearly outlined.

In another study [27], the authors report the case of a baby who underwent massive small bowel resection along with resection of the cecum and part of the ascending colon because of intestinal malrotation with volvulus. The total length of the residual small intestine was 11 cm and was composed of the duodenum and a small part of the jejunum. The patient was managed with parenteral nutrition until the age of 4 months when oral supplements were included. At 8 months, the patient had an episode of septicemia after a catheter infection; at this stage the catheter was removed, the patient was maintained on an oral diet, and 1 month later the patient had to be supported by parenteral nutrition. With intensive supportive measures, the patient continued to thrive. Although this is an isolated case report, it does question the minimum length of small bowel required for survival.

Ingham Clark *et al.* [28] have looked at the other end of the spectrum to identify potential candidates for small bowel transplantation. They investigated one region in the United Kingdom and defined potential recipients as those with irreversible small intestinal failure, including those treated with permanent parenteral nutrition. They were able to identify 10 patients as possible recipients. When this data was extrapolated to national figures on the incidence of irreversible small intestinal failure it was suggested that each year up to 20 new adult patients in the United Kingdom alone might benefit from small bowel transplantation.

Casavilla *et al.* [29] reported their results with an en-block liver-small bowel cadaveric graft in seven children and one adult. All grafts functioned immediately and all but one of the recipient patients recovered. The small bowel absorptive function was slow to return, but the integrity of the bacterial intestinal barrier did not appear to be disrupted. They also described the technique for combined hepatic intestinal retrieval. The same group in another study [30•] compared intestinal transplantation in composite visceral grafts with intestinal grafts only. Eight patients had intestine in continuity with the liver, eight patients received the intestine only, and one patient received a multivisceral graft that included the liver, stomach, and pancreas. All patients except for one liver-intestine recipient were reported to be alive after 1 to 2 months following transplantation. In this series the convalescence of the eight patients receiving intestine only was faster and more trouble free than after liver-intestine or multivisceral transplantation. There was no greater difficulty in the control of rejection in the intestine only group.

References and recommended reading

Papers of particular interest, published within the annual period of review, have been highlighted as:
- • Of special interest
- •• Of outstanding interest

1. • OGBONNA BC, OBEKPA PO, MOMOH JT, OBAFUNWA JO, NWANA EJ: **Laparoscopy in Developing Countries in the Management of Patients With an Acute Abdomen.** *Br J Surg* 1992, 79:964–966.

This is an important paper that highlights the value of laparoscopy in the management of patients admitted with severe pain in the abdomen.

2. ATTWOOD SEA, KELLY I, O'CONNELL PR, CORRIGAN T: **Laparoscopic Mobilisation and Exteriorization for Minimally Invasive Small Bowel Resection.** *Br J Surg* 1993, **80**:225.

3. QUAN-YANG DUH, WAY LAWRENCE W: **Laparoscopic Jejunostomy Using T-Fasteners as Retractors and Anchors.** *Arch Surg* 1993, 128:105–108

4. MORRIS JB, MULLEN JL, YU JC, ROSATO EF: **Laparoscopic-Guided Jejunostomy.** *Surgery* 1992, **112**:96–99.

5. •• WYATT J, VOGELSANG H, HUBL W, WALDHOER T, LOCHS H: **Intestinal Permeability and the Prediction of Relapse in Crohn's Disease.** *Lancet* 1993, **341**:1437–1439.

This interesting paper investigates whether intestinal permeability predicts relapse in Crohn's disease. Significantly more patients with raised permeability index had relapses than those with normal index.

6. • MAY GR, SUTHERLAND LR, MEDDINGS JB: **Is Small Intestine Permeability Really Increased in Relatives of Patients With Crohn's Disease.** *Gastroenterology* 1993, **104**:1627–1632.

This paper, too, examines intestinal permeability in relatives of patients with Crohn's disease. It shows that increased intestinal permeability in a small proportion of individuals had high risk of developing Crohn's disease may precede clinical manifestations of Crohn's disease.

7. •• SMEDH K, OLAISON G, SJODAHL R: **Initiation of Anastomotic Recurrence of Crohn's Disease After Ileocolic Resection.** *Scand J Gastroenterol* 1992, **27**:691–694.

The pattern of anastomotic recurrence of Crohn's disease after resection is reported. It indicates that recurrent inflammation after ileocolic resection in Crohn's disease is initiated close to the anastomosis in the neoterminal ileum.

8. CAMERON JL, HAMILTON SR, COLEMAN J, SITZMAN JV, BAYLESS TM: **Patterns of Ileal Recurrence in Crohn's Disease.** *Ann Surg* 1992, **215**:546–552.

9. • LESCUT D, VANCO D, BONNIERE P, LECOMTE-HOUCKE M, QUANDALLE P, WURTZ A, COLOMBEL JF, DELMOTTE JS, PARIS JC, CORTOT A: **Perioperative Endoscopy of the Whole Small Bowel in Crohn's Disease.** *Gut* 1993, **34**:647–649.

This paper describes the value of peri-operative endoscopy in identifying lesions that are not visible or palpable at laparotomy.

10. • FAZIO VW, TJANDRA JJ, LAVERY IC, CHURCH JM, MILSOM JW, OAKLEY JR: **Long Term Follow Up of Strictureplasty in Crohn's Disease.** *Dis Colon Rectum* 1993; **36**:355–361.

This interesting paper shows that strictureplasties in Crohn's disease is a safe and satisfactory operation and the rate of restricturing after a median follow-up of 3 years is relatively low.

11. •• LASHNER BA: **Risk Factors for Small Bowel Cancer in Crohn's Disease.** *Dig Dis Sci* 1992, **37**:1179–1184.

This important paper investigates risk factors for the development of small bowel cancer in Crohn's disease. The presence of disease in the proximal small bowel, use of 6 mercaptopurines and hazardous occupations were all identified as potential risk factors.

12. KUVSHINOFF BW, BRODISH RJ, MCFADDEN DW, FISCHER JE: **Serum Transferrin as a Prognostic Indicator of Spontaneous Closure and Mortality in Gastrointestinal Cutaneous Fistulas.** *Ann Surg* 1993, **217**:615–623.

13. BORISON DI, BLOOM AD, PRITCHARD TJ: **Treatment of Enterocutaneous and Colocutaneous Fistulas With Early Surgery or Somatostatin Analog.** *Dis Colon Rectum* 1992, **35**:635–639.

14. CHEN R-J, FANG J-F, CHEN M-F: **Octreotide in the Management of Postoperative Enterocutaneous Fistulas and Stress Ulcer Bleeding.** *Am J Gastroenterol* 1992, **87**:1212–1215.

15. GOES RN, FAGUNDES JJ, COY CS, AMARAL CA, PERES MA, MEDEIROS RR: **The Two Chamber Ileal Pelvic Reservoir - An Alternative Design.** *Dis Colon Rectum* 1993, **36**:403–404.

16. PENNA C, DAUDE F, PARC R, TIRET E, FRILEUX P, HANNOUN L, NORDLINGER B, LEVY E: **Previous Subtotal Colectomy With Ileostomy and Sigmoidostomy Improves the Morbidity and Early Functional Results After Ileal Pouch-Anal Anastomosis in Ulcerative Colitis.** *Dis Colon Rectum* 1993, **36**:343–348.

17. • STELZNER M, FONKALSRUD EW: **Functional Changes Associated With Short and Long Lateral Ileal Reservoirs in a Canine Model.** *Dis Colon Rectum* 1993, **36**:266–272.

This interesting paper compares the functional changes associated with short and long lateral ileal reservoirs. It was found that short lateral isoperistaltic reservoirs emptied more effectively than long reservoirs. These observations are likely to influence the planning of pouch designs.

18. HARMS BA, ANDERSON AB, STARLING JR: **The W Ileal Reservoir: Long-Term Assessment After Proctocolectomy for Ulcerative Colitis and Familial Polyposis.** *Surgery* 1992, **112**:638–648.

19. PENNA C, TIRET E, KARTHEUSER A, HANNOUN L, NORDLINGER B, PARC R: **Function of Ileal J Pouch-Anal Anastomosis in Patients With Familial Adenomatous Polyposis.** *Br J Surg* 1993, **80**:765–767.

20. HALLGREN T, FASTH S, DELBRO D, NORDGREN S, ORESLAND T, HULTEN L: **Possible Role of the Autonomic Nervous System in Sphincter Impairment After Restorative Proctocolectomy.** *Br J Surg* **80**:631–635.

21. WETTERGREN A, GYRTRUP HJ, GROSMANN E, SVENDSEN LB, HJORTRUP A, STADIL F, KIRKEGAARD P: **Complications After J-Pouch Ileoanal Anastomosis: Stapled Compared With Hand-sewn Anastomosis.** *Eur J Surg* 1993, **159**:121–124.

22. • KARTHEUSER AH, DOZOIS RR, WIESNER RH, LARUSSO NF, ILSTRUP DM, SCHLECK CD: **Complications and Risk Factors After Ileal Pouch-Anal Anastomosis for Ulcerative Colitis Associated With Primary Sclerosing Cholangitis.** *Ann Surg* **217**:314–320.

Ulcerative colitis is occasionally complicated by primary sclerosing cholangitis. This paper evaluates the complications and risk factors after ileal pouch–anal anastomosis in such patients. It is concluded that ileal pouch–anal anastomosis is a safe procedure in patients with ulcerative colitis associated with primary sclerosing cholangitis.

23. •• DVORAK AM, ONDERDONK AB, MCLEOD RS, MONAHAN-EARLEY RA, CULLEN J, ANTONIOLI DA, BLAIR JE, MORGAN ES, CISNEROS RL, ESTRELLA P: **Axonal Necrosis of Enteric Autonomic Nerves in Continent Ileal Pouches.** *Ann Surg* 1993, **217**:266–271.

This is an important paper which looks axonal necrosis of enteric nerves in ileal pouches. The finding that axonal necrosis is commonly found in pouches that are clinically inflamed and have positive bacterial cultures suggests possible similarities in the pathogenesis of Crohn's disease and pouchitis.

24. •• GEMLO BT, WONG D, ROTHENBERGE DA, GOLDERBERGE SM: **Ileal Pouch-Anal Anastomosis.** *Arch Surg* 1992, **127**:784–787.

Pouch failure occurs in approximately 5% to 10% of all ileal pouch–anal anastomosis. This paper outlines the factors and mechanisms involved that lead to pouch failure and pouch excision.

25. KEIGHLEY MRB, GROBLER S, BAIN I: **An Audit of Restorative Proctocolectomy**. *Gut* 1993, 34:680–684.

26. WARNER BW, CHAET MS: **Nontransplant Surgical Options for**
•• **Management of the Short Bowel Syndrome**. *J Pediatr Gastroenterol Nutr* 1993, 17:1–12.

This is an excellent review that discusses the non-transplant surgical options for the management of the short bowel syndrome. An algorithm has been proposed for the management of the short bowel syndrome.

27. IACONO G, CARROCCIO A, MONTALTO G, CAVATAIO F, LOCASCIO M, NOTARBATOLO A: **Extreme Short Bowel Syndrome: A Casae for Reviewing the Guidelines for Predicting Survival**. *J Pediatr Gastroenterol Nutr* 1993, 16:216–219.

28. INGHAM CLARK CL, LEAR PA, WOOD S, LENNARD-JONES JE, WOOD RF: **Potential Candidates for Small Bowel Transplantation**. *Br J Surg* 1992, 79:676–679.

29. CASAVILLA A, SELBY R, ABU-ELMAGD K, TZAKIS A, TODO S, REYES J, FUNG J, STARZL TE: **Logistics and Technique for Combined Hepatic-Intestinal Retrieval**. *Ann Surg* 1992, 216:605–609.

30. TODO S, TZAKIS AG, ABU-ELMAGD K, REYES J, NAKAMURA
• K, CASAVILLA A, SELBY R, NOUR BM, WRIGHT H, FUNG JJ: **Intestinal Transplantation in Composite Visceral Grafts or Alone**. *Ann Surg* 1992, 216:223–234.

This paper compares the results of intestinal transplantation in composite visceral grafts to those of intestinal grafts only. The convalescence of intestinal only grafts was faster and more trouble-free than that of the liver-intestine grafts.

Devinder Kumar, PhD, FRCS, Queen Elizabeth Hospital, The University of Birmingham, Edgbaston, Birmingham B12 2TH, UK.

New developments in the enteric nervous system

Michael D. Gershon, MD, and Paul R. Wade, PhD

Columbia University College of Physicians and Surgeons, New York, New York, USA

Research on the enteric nervous system is important because the mechanism by which the motility of the bowel is locally controlled is still not understood and because this research is critical in developing effective therapies for functional bowel disease. Although the behaviors regulated by the enteric nervous system cannot yet be explained in terms of the activity of single cells, it should soon be possible to do so. Considerable progress has been made in determining the function of particular types of enteric neurons, including sensory neurons of the submucosal plexus, motor neurons, and interneurons of the myenteric plexus. Uncertainty persists as to the nature of the myenteric neuron classified electrophysiologically as type 2/AH and morphologically as Dogiel type II. These cells may act as sensory neurons, as interneurons, or both. Nitric oxide has clearly been established to play a critical role as an intrinsic inhibitory neurotransmitter, as has ATP and vasoactive intestinal peptide, although neurons, smooth muscle, and interstitial cells of Cajal may each be both sources nitric oxide and the targets of its action. Interstitial cells appear to play roles as both as pacemaker cells for the circular muscle and in transmitting neural signals to smooth muscle cells. Although one cannot yet map the components of an enteric microcircuit, it should soon be possible to do so.

Current Opinion in Gastroenterology 1994, **10**:183–192

The rapid escalation of scientific interest in the enteric nervous system (ENS) that was noted when this subject was reviewed this past year [1••] has continued. That review should be consulted by readers who are not familiar with the historical path of research on the ENS; the current article will focus on recent developments and on subjects that can be said to have reached maturity during the past year. The ability of the ENS to mediate reflex activity in the absence of input from the central nervous system [2–4] remains a primary drive motivating research in enteric neurobiology. Unfortunately, the behaviors regulated by the ENS are sufficiently complicated that the microcircuits responsible for its function have not yet been elucidated.

In the past, the most popular topics selected for investigation have reflected technologic advances, adapting to the bowel progress made in other areas. As a result, scientific papers have tended to cluster around "hot" subjects. For example, the ENS emerged from a long period of relative neglect when it became possible to identify the putative or established neurotransmitters in particular neurons and to study the projections of these chemically identified cells in the wall of the gut [1••,5,6]. Advances in this area, extremely rapid at one time, have now slowed and attention has tended to become concentrated on individual transmitter candidates for which new investigational tools have become available. Two examples are nitric oxide and serotonin, two substances that are likely to be as important to the function of the bowel as they are to the brain.

The realization that the ENS contains primary afferent neurons prompted attempts to identify these cells. One such cell has been found in the submucosal plexus [7] and a strong argument has emerged suggesting that sensory neurons are also present in the myenteric plexus [8]; these putative primary afferent cells have been classified physiologically as type 2/AH and morphologically as Dogiel type II neurons. Despite this argument, the function of the type 2/AH-Dogiel type II neuron still remains to be established, a mystery

Abbreviations

ENS—enteric nervous system; **EPSP**—excitatory postsynaptic potential; **ICC**—interstitial cells of Cajal; **IJP**—inhibitory junction potential; **VIP**—vasoactive intestinal peptide.

 ISBN 1-85922-607-8 ISSN 0267–1379

that has focused a great deal of attention on this cell type. Technique-driven research on the ENS still occurs; however, sufficient progress has been made in characterizing the ENS, that it is becoming possible to define the roles of particular substances and cells in the physiology of the bowel.

Classification of myenteric neurons

Electrophysiologic recording with sharp microelectrodes has been used to classify myenteric neurons. Most investigators have agreed that there are at least two classes, type 1/S and type 2/AH, although they have differed as to the criteria used in cellular identification [1••]. The inward current of the action potential in type 1/S cells is primarily carried by Na^+; therefore, there is no Ca^{2+} shoulder on the falling phase of the action potential and action potentials are abolished by tetrodotoxin. In contrast, Ca^{2+} carries a significant portion of the inward current of the action potential in type 2/AH neurons, which thus displays a distinct Ca^{2+} shoulder on the falling phase and persists in the presence of tetrodotoxin. Another major difference between the two cell types is that type 2/AH, but not type 1/S neurons, display a marked Ca^{2+}-activated potassium ion conductance that contributes both to the resting potential of these cells and to an after-spike hyperpolarizing potential. Other purported differences between types 1/S and 2/AH neurons, such as the restriction of synaptic input to the type 1/S cell, have been used, but are invalid.

In general, most type 1/S neurons in the small intestine have a Dogiel type I morphology (many short-paddle shaped dendrites and a single long process), whereas most type 2/AH neurons are Dogiel type II cells (several long processes extending from a large smooth cell body). In the guinea pig small bowel, but not that of other species or in other regions of the gut, about 80% of Dogiel type II neurons contain calbindin, which has thus been used as an immunocytochemical marker for these cells [9]. Clearly, the calbindin marker is of limited usefulness. It is applicable only in the guinea pig small intestine and, even there, it fails to detect a significant fraction of type 2/AH neurons.

Type 2/AH neurons

A relatively simple scheme that relates the electrophysiologic classification of myenteric neurons to function has been proposed (Fig. 1). This idea considers that all of the type 2/AH cells are primary sensory neurons [10••], whereas type 1/S neurons are either motor neurons or interneurons [11•]. The evidence favoring a sensory role for type 2/AH cells is based on deductions from studies of their projections [12,13] and an inference drawn from the observation that few of these cells are excited when reflexes are evoked in the bowel [8,14]. One difficulty in interpreting these data comes from the limitations of the marker, calbindin immunoreactivity, which has been utilized in some studies to identify type 2/AH neurons [15,16]. Because calbindin is not present in all type 2/AH neurons, it is not clear that the projections of those cells that lack the marker are identical to those that do contain it. The major difficulty with the hypothesis, however, is that all of the evidence suggesting that type 2/AH neurons are sensory is indirect and deductive. As yet, there has been no study that has succeeded in demonstrating that sensory stimulation of the small intestine activates type 2/AH neurons without an intervening synapse.

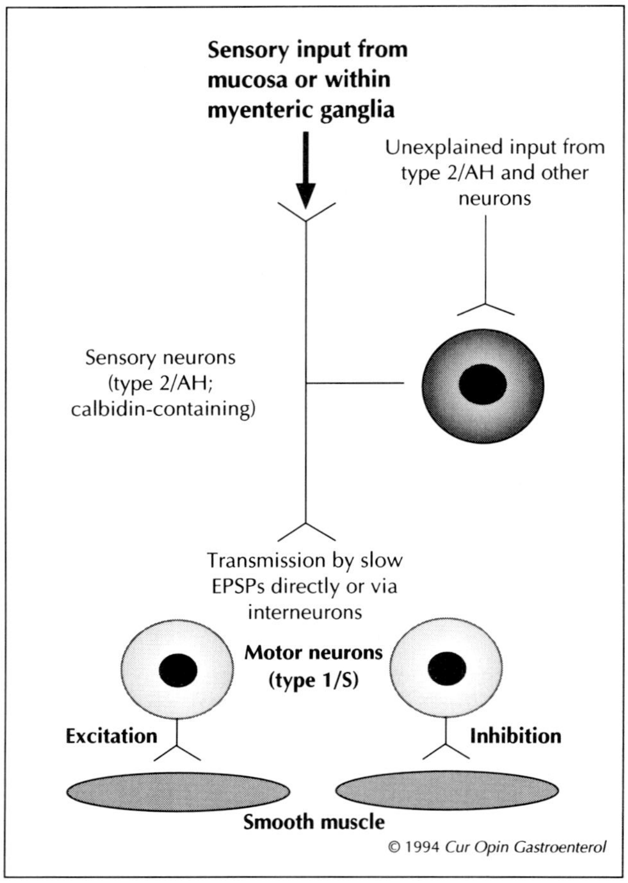

Fig. 1. A diagram showing one hypothesis proposed to explain the arrangement and function of type 2/AH neurons of the myenteric plexus. These cells are considered to be sensory neurons. They transmit via slow excitatory postsynaptic potentials (EPSPs). In contrast to vertebrate sensory neurons in other locations, type 2/AH neurons receive synaptic inputs that may be fast or slow EPSPs. The function of this innervation of a neuron that is presumed to be a primary afferent is unexplained. Because type 2/AH neurons innervate other neurons of the same type, at least some of these cells are interneurons. Targets of type 2/AH neurons include motor neurons and interneurons. The presumed sensory input to these cells (if it is not via an intermediary synapse) is proposed to arrive both from within myenteric ganglia and from the mucosa, to which at least some of these cells project.

In contrast to the submucosal neurons that become active (detected by visualizing the expression of Fos, the protein encoded by the *c-fos* protooncogene) in response to distention of the mucosa, the activation of myenteric neurons by mucosal distention is completely blocked by hexamethonium [7]. The effect of hexamethonium suggests that the myenteric plexus receives cholinergic projections from submucosal sensory cells, which have also been found to contain substance P. Reflexes in the myenteric plexus, however, can be elicited by stimuli that do not involve the mucosa [8,14,17]. The existence of these reflexes suggests that sensory neurons may be present in the myenteric, as well as the submucosal plexus. On the other hand, dissociation of the myenteric and submucosal plexuses diminishes the peristaltic reflex and increases the threshold for the response [17]; moreover, it has recently been demonstrated that intraluminal administration of 0.1% glutaraldehyde or a low Na^+ solution will inhibit the peristaltic reflex without interfering with contractions of the longitudinal muscle evoked by direct stimulation of motor neurons [18••]. These observations suggest that stretch or distention receptors are located in the mucosa of the small intestine and that these receptors are critical for evoking the peristaltic reflex. Actually, this new evidence demonstrating that the peristaltic reflex is mucosa dependent, confirms much earlier work that showed that the reflex is abolished by anesthetizing or asphyxiating the mucosa [19–21].

However important mucosal receptors and submucosal sensory neurons may be in mediating the peristaltic reflex, it is not the only reflex mediated by the ENS. Myenteric sensory neurons may be responsible for detecting sensory stimuli that impinge on the bowel from the serosal surface [8]; nevertheless, myenteric sensory neurons cannot be identified by deduction alone. The direct demonstration that type 2/AH or other neurons of the myenteric plexus are activated nonsynaptically by sensory stimulation, is needed to confirm that such neurons are indeed primary afferent cells.

The problem posed to the sensory neuron hypothesis that type 2/AH neurons are innervated, despite their presumed role as sensory cells, has been met in the past by ignoring or denigrating it. Type 2/AH neurons were originally believed to receive no synaptic input [22]. After the cells were shown to respond to synaptic activation [23–26] and to be covered with synapses [25], the input was said to be restricted to slow excitatory postsynaptic potentials (EPSPs) [9]. After it was shown that type 2/AH neurons exhibit fast [27], as well as slow EPSPs, the significance of the fast input in type 2/AH neurons was diminished by noting that the amplitude of the fast EPSPs in these cells is much smaller than that of fast EPSPs in type 1/S neurons [9,10••]. The nature of the type 2/AH cell, however, makes it impossible to draw functional conclusions from comparisons of the amplitude of their fast EPSPs with those of type 1/S cells, because the size of the fast EPSP in type 2/AH neurons must be activity-dependent. In resting type 2/AH neurons, the recorded amplitude of EPSPs would be low because of the large Ca^{2+}-activated K^+ conductance, which is a defining characteristic of these cells; essentially, fast EPSPs are short circuited by the low input resistance of the membrane of type 2/AH neurons. When type 2/AH neurons receive slow synaptic excitation, however, the Ca^{2+}-activated K^+ conductance is inhibited; therefore, the cells become far more excitable and the amplitude of fast EPSPs should be much greater [28].

It seems clear that both of the physiologic classes of myenteric neuron are well innervated (Fig. 1); thus, if either is a sensory neuron, myenteric sensory neurons would have to be different from other vertebrate sensory neurons, which are not innervated cells. Synapses on type 2/AH cells might be active in modulating their receptivity (if they are sensory) or they may enable a single type 2/AH neuron to function in two capacities. An innervated type 2/AH neuron might be able to both respond directly to sensory stimuli and act as an interneuron.

The properties of the type 2/AH cell underlie the hypothesis that it functions as an interneuron, instead of, or in addition to, its role as a sensory cell (Fig. 2). In fact, the above discussion of the amplitude of fast EPSPs is relevant in this regard. The low amplitude fast inputs to type 2/AH neurons would be unlikely to drive the cells, which are relatively inexcitable (under resting conditions) and do not fire repetitively because of their Ca^{2+}-activated K^+ conductance [23,29]. When the cells receive a slow EPSP, however, and the Ca^{2+}-activated K^+ conductance is inhibited, the excitability of the neurons increases [26,28]. The presence or absence of slow synaptic input, therefore, would permit type 2/AH neurons to act as gates, regulating the flow of excitation within the myenteric plexus [30•].

Most type 2/AH neurons are short cells that project in the circumferential direction [12]; they may thus regulate the spread of excitation around the bowel [30•]. This concept envisions the long descending- and ascending-type 1/S cells to be the projection cells of the myenteric plexus, responsible both for the long range conduction of signals within the plexus and for the innervation of smooth muscle (Fig. 2). Most of the motor neurons and some of the long interneurons, in fact, have been demonstrated to be Dogiel type I in shape [31–34].

Very recently, the technologic feat of recording simultaneously from two myenteric neurons, separated by a circumferential distance of 100 to 200 μm, has been accomplished [10••]. In this study, type 2/AH neurons were driven by injecting depolarizing current pulses through an intracellular recording microelectrode and responses were detected in type 1/S or type 2/AH recipients. Of 79 pairs of cells that were simultaneously impaled, responses to stimulation of the type 2/AH neuron were obtained in 20 recipients. Unfortunately, no direct evidence that these responses were monosynaptic was reported; however, if one assumes that the responses recorded in the recipient neurons

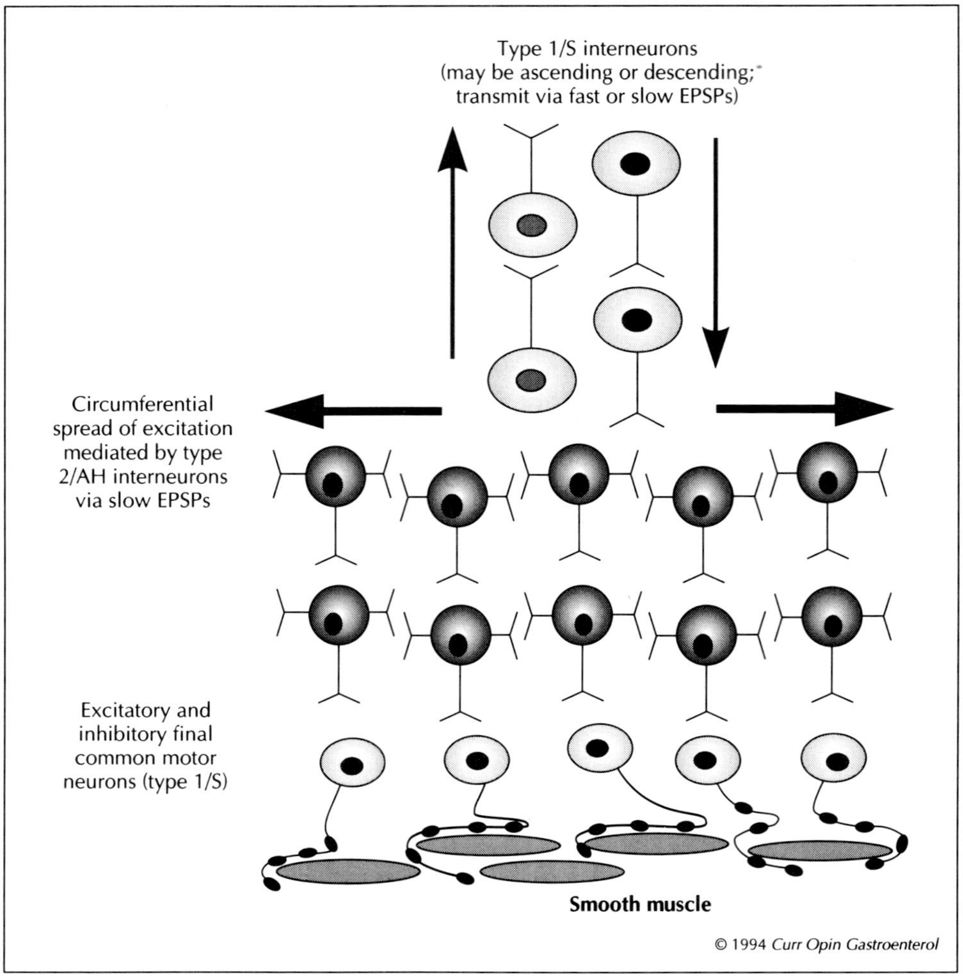

Fig. 2. An alternative hypothesis proposed to explain the arrangement and function of type 2/AH neurons of the myenteric plexus. In this case, the cells are considered to be interneurons that are responsible for the circumferential spread of excitation around the bowel. Slow excitatory postsynaptic potentials (EPSPs) in these cells enable them to act as gates regulating the spread of excitation. Type 1/S interneurons are responsible for the conduction of excitation in the ascending or descending directions. Motor neurons, like the long-projecting interneurons, are proposed to be type 1/S cells. Sensory input is not indicated and is not encompassed by this hypothesis; however, it could arise from either primary afferent neurons, which are known to exist in the submucosal plexus, or from the sensory neurons that are thought also to be present in the myenteric plexus.

were transmitted by synapses of the stimulated type 2/AH neurons, the results are interesting and important. Of the recipients, 17 were classified as type 1/S cells and three were classified as type 2/AH. Every one of responses in the recipient cells of either class was a slow EPSP. These observations indicate that type 2/AH neurons transmit by slow EPSPs. That finding, in turn, establishes that neurotransmission mediated entirely by slow EPSPs can occur in the ENS. The observations also demonstrate that type 2/AH neurons innervate both type 1/S and type 2/AH follower cells. The results do not rule out the idea that type 2/AH neurons are primary afferent neurons, but they do establish without doubt that at least some are interneurons. Those type 2/AH neurons that are excited by input from other type 2/AH neurons are, by definition, interneurons (Figs. 1 and 2).

Markers in enteric microcircuit studies

Synaptic connections between neurons in the ENS have been very difficult to study. One problem is that the morphologic appearance of connections is often misleading. For example, in the studies discussed above, in which simultaneous recordings were obtained from pairs of myenteric neurons, the driver and recipient neurons were injected with neurobiotin so that they could later be identified and studied morphologically [10••]. This study revealed the presence of a significant proportion of neuron pairs that appeared to be connected morphologically, but in fact were not connected physiologically. In part, this paradoxic situation arises from the fact that synaptic gaps are impossible to discern with a light microscope. One cannot determine whether or not a glial process is present between what appears to be a nerve terminal and what one assumes is the follower cell. For this reason, synaptic connectivity must be demonstrated physiologically, and if it is to be supported morphologically, electron microscopic evidence must be obtained. Even electron microscopy, however, is problematic unless specific markers can be used to identify cells and processes as members of a functional class of neuron.

Calbindin immunoreactivity is an example of such a class-specific marker [16]. If used only to identify processes that are likely to be those of Dogiel type II neurons in the myenteric plexus of the guinea pig ileum, this marker is valuable. When equated with the entire set of type 2/AH neurons, even in the guinea pig ileum, the marker is invalid and potentially misleading because it fails to demonstrate the entire set of the cells it is used to identify.

Calbindin-immunoreactive synapses are found on many non–calbindin-containing neurons in the myenteric plexus, but few are found on other calbindin-immunoreactive cells. This observation has been accepted as evidence in support of the hypothesis that type 2/AH neurons are sensory in function. The relative scarcity of calbindin immunoreactive terminals on calbindin immunoreactive neurons has been taken to mean that type 2/AH neurons probably do not innervate other type 2/AH neurons [15,16]. If they did, they would have to be to be considered to be interneurons. That deduction, however, has recently been demonstrated to be wrong; as noted above, type 2/AH neurons do innervate other type 2/AH cells [10••]. This new observation serves to demonstrate how misleading deductive arguments can be when they are based on the presumed universality of cell markers.

Another example of a presumed functional marker is γ-amino butyric acid (GABA) immunoreactivity [35]. This marker is said to reveal cells that provide inputs to muscle, but not to other neurons of the myenteric plexus. An additional marker is nitric oxide synthase, which is identical to NADPH diaphorase [36], and thus can be investigated immunocytochemically, by demonstrating nitric oxide synthase immunoreactivity [37,38,39•] or histochemically, by demonstrating NADPH activity [40]. Nitric oxide synthase-NADPH diaphorase is thought to provide a marker for descending interneurons and motor neurons of the guinea pig small intestine [37]. Although persuasive evidence exists that favors the idea that nitric oxide serves as an inhibitory transmitter to smooth muscle [41–46,47•,48,49], the subject has recently become complicated. These complications are discussed later. Again, caution must be exercised before one reads function into the immunocytochemical demonstration of a marker, even at the ultrastructural level.

A recent marker that has been related to functional classes of enteric neuron is calretinin, which is a Ca^{2+}-binding protein like calbindin [33]. Calretinin is thought to mark small Dogiel type I cells that are longitudinal muscle motor neurons and medium sized Dogiel type I cells that function as ascending interneurons. The calretinin immunoreactive neurons have been investigated in detail [11•].

The calretinin-immunoreactive motor neurons are reported to make up about 20% of the neurons of the myenteric plexus, whereas the calretinin-immunoreactive ascending interneurons constitute an additional 5%. There is also a small population of filamentous calretinin-immunoreactive neurons that do not fit easily into one of the Dogiel classes. The motor neurons were observed to project into the tertiary plexus that ramifies over the surface of the longitudinal muscle at a considerable distance from ganglia and is thought to be the morphologic representation of the motor innervation of this muscle layer [50•]. The interneurons formed baskets around their follower cells in myenteric ganglia. The data suggest that calretinin-immunoreactive interneurons form long chains of interconnected cells that ascend in the myenteric plexus.

The calretinin-immunoreactive interneurons are suggested to provide as many as one-third of the inputs received by the calretinin-immunoreactive motor neurons to the longitudinal muscle. The remaining two thirds of the inputs to motor neurons are likely to be local, as they persist when lesions are made in the myenteric plexus above and below the site examined. Because Dogiel type II neurons are short, one might guess that the remaining inputs to motor neurons arise from such cells. The function of the remaining inputs has not been studied; however, a speculative argument has been presented that these inputs must be sensory because they are deduced to arise from Dogiel type II cells. That argument proceeds from the assumptions, discussed above, that Dogiel type II cells (shape classification) are all type 2/AH cells (electrophysiologic classification), which are all sensory in function. As these assumptions are not supported by any direct evidence, the function of the inputs to calretinin-immunoreactive motor neurons will have to be experimentally determined in the future.

Targets of enteric neurons

The most common method for determining the morphologic properties of functionally identified enteric neurons is to record from the cells and to inject them with a tracer for later visual examination [25,51,52]. Relatively small numbers of cells can be examined in this way in any given preparation. Another method is to use a functional parameter that can be evaluated histochemically or immunocytochemically. Examples of methods that have successfully been used for this purpose include the demonstration of cytochrome oxidase activity [53–55] and the immunoreactivity of Fos, the protein encoded by the *c-fos* protooncogene [7,56].

More recently, a very interesting approach of this type, the demonstration of cyclic GMP immunoreactivity, has been used to identify the targets of nitric oxide in the guinea pig small intestine [57••]. Nitric oxide activates soluble guanyl cyclase and thus increases the levels of cyclic GMP in its follower cells [58]. The intensity of cyclic GMP immunostaining thus reflects the activation of guanyl cyclase. If cells are immunostained after they have been incubated with a nitric oxide donor such as sodium nitroprusside, the potential targets of nitric oxide can be identified. In these experiments, however, it is good to bear in mind that nitric oxide will have access to all cells that are capable of responding to it; the set of cells revealed by the technique is thus potentially larger than the set of cells that actually do respond to nitric oxide released under physiologic circumstances. Which cells respond physiologically to endogenous nitric oxide will be determined both by the ability of cells to respond and by the diffusion of nitric oxide from its sources in the tissue.

Targets of nitric oxide–neurons

The anatomic location of the cells upon which nitric oxide acts is important because general agreement is lacking as to exactly how the motility of the bowel is affected by nitric oxide. As noted earlier, considerable evidence suggests that nitric oxide is an inhibitory neurotransmitter to intestinal smooth muscle. Two distinct inhibitory (hyperpolarizing) responses, however, have been identified in the guinea pig ileum and taenia coli [59,60]. These have been called fast and slow inhibitory junction potentials (IJPs) and have been postulated to be mediated by vasoactive intestinal peptide (VIP) and ATP [61,62]. If nitric oxide is, as postulated, *the* final common mediator of inhibitory innervation to intestinal smooth muscle [49], then what are the roles played by VIP and ATP? ATP, in particular, has a long history of well-documented involvement in the inhibitory innervation of the gut [63]. New data now suggest that in the circular muscle of the guinea pig, nitric oxide is not the transmitter of fast IJPs, which are mediated by ATP, but is involved in the mediation of slow IJPs, which result from the combined effects of nitric oxide and VIP acting in series [64••]. The slow IJP is normally masked by simultaneous depolarization due to the concomitant secretion of substance P induced by VIP.

Whether smooth muscle cells themselves are the targets of inhibitory nerves is not clear. An alternative idea is that the recipients of the inhibitory innervation are interstitial cells of Cajal (ICCs) [65–71], which transmit the effects of this innervation to circular smooth muscle cells by way of gap junctions [71–73]. Stimulation of intrinsic nerves or administration of nitric oxide increases the levels of cyclic GMP in ICCs [74•] and ICCs respond to stimulation by several different neurotransmitters [75•,76••]. It has even been suggested that the primary transmitter released by intrinsic inhibitory neurons is not nitric oxide or ATP, but VIP, which causes nitric oxide to be produced and released from the smooth muscle [77•,78••,79•]. The smooth muscle–derived nitric oxide is thought to induce smooth muscle relaxation and to cause further release of VIP from nerves. Within the myenteric plexus, the effects of nitric oxide has been found to be inhibitory and presynaptic [80]. In morphologic studies when the gut was exposed to the nitric oxide donor, sodium nitroprusside, cyclic GMP immunoreactivity was found to be increased in subsets of neurons in both the submucosal and the myenteric plexuses in both small intestine and colon [57••]. These neurons in the ileum comprised about 2% of myenteric neurons and about 40% of submucosal neurons. The cyclic GMP-immunoreactive neurons contained VIP immunoreactivity, but they did not display nitric oxide synthase. ICCs found beneath the serosa and variable numbers of ICCs at the inner surface of the circular muscle as well as both longitudinal aid circular smooth muscle cells exhibited increases in cyclic GMP. These studies thus indicate that nitric oxide could act at a number of possible sites in the bowel wall. Because cyclic GMP is induced in both ICCs and smooth muscle, the data are compatible with either (or both) serving as the target of nitric oxide. Further work is needed to rule the hypothesis that smooth muscle is both source and target of nitric oxide in or out.

Interstitial cells and motility

The possibility that ICCs may be targets or sources of nitric oxide is attractive, because considerable evidence has accumulated that suggests that these cells are pacemakers responsible for slow waves in the intestinal muscle. Pacemaker-rich domains of the bowel musculature have been shown to be particularly rich in ICCs [81]. ICCs form networks along the submucosal and myenteric surfaces of the circular muscle layer [72,82•,83,84••,85] and on septae [86], where pacemaker activity is generated. If ICCs are mechanically cut away from the submucosal boundary of the circular muscle, the slow waves disappear [73,81]. Rhodamine 123 accumulates in ICCs and its uptake is associated with the loss of pacemaker activity [83]. Recently, ICCs have been isolated and their electrical properties have been demonstrated to be those of pacemakers; that is, they are excitable cells [87] that exhibit spontaneous depolarizations and oscillations in their internal Ca^{2+} [75•], and exhibit a low threshold Ca^{2+} current [88••]. If ICCs are pacemakers responsible for slow waves, as seems likely, then they would make strategic targets for neurally-released nitric oxide. If they are also sources of nitric oxide, then they might very effectively amplify the action of nitric oxide on the muscle layer and enhance its action as an inhibitory transmitter [76••]. In either case, the function of ICCs in the physiology of the bowel is becoming increasingly prominent as a subject of investigation. Among the remaining enigmatic features of these cells is their embryologic origin. Whether ICCs are derived, like the neurons and glia of the ENS, from the neural crest [89•], or like the muscle from mesoderm remains to be ascertained.

Future directions

It is always difficult to predict the future, especially of research, which by its nature is the exploration of the unknown. Still, it seems clear that current directions will lead to rapid identification of the components of enteric microcircuits and to their mapping. An explanation of how the central nervous system interacts with the local circuits of the ENS should soon be explained.

The sensory receptors that give rise to enteric reflexes are likely to be discovered. Transmitters will continue to be an active research front. Clearly, the role of nitric oxide will soon be definitively established; moreover, the recent explosion of research on subtypes of serotonin receptors in the central nervous system will be extended to the bowel. Finally, it seems likely that the rapid advance in basic knowledge about the ENS will find application to understanding the pathophysiology of the highly prevalent but poorly comprehended functional diseases of the bowel.

References and recommended reading

Papers of particular interest, published within the annual period of review, have been highlighted as:

• Of special interest
•• Of outstanding interest

1. GERSHON MD, WADE PR: **Enteric Nervous System.** *Curr Opin*
•• *Gastroenterol* 1993, **9**:246–253.

This is a relatively comprehensive review of the subject. It covers the background of the research on enteric microcircuits involved in the mediation of the peristaltic reflex and the organization of the ENS. The current review assumes a knowledge of much of the material covered in this publication.

2. BAYLISS WM, STARLING EH: **The Movements and Innervation of the Small Intestine.** *J Physiol (Lond)* 1899, **24**:99–143.

3. TRENDELENBURG P: **Physiologische Und Pharmakologische Versuche Über Die Dünndarm Peristaltick.** *Naunyn-Schmiedebergs Arch Exp Pathol Pharmakol* 1917, **81**:55–129.

4. GERSHON MD: **The Enteric Nervous System: Neurotransmitters and Neuromodulators.** *Curr Opin Neurol Neurosurg* 1990, **3**:517–522.

5. FURNESS JB, BORNSTEIN JC, MURPHY R, POMPOLO S: **Roles of Peptides in Transmission in the Enteric Nervous System.** *Trends Neurosci* 1992, **15**:66–71.

6. GERSHON MD, KIRCHGESSNER AL, WADE PR: **Functional Anatomy of the Enteric Nervous System.** In *Physiology of the Gastrointestinal Tract.* Third Edition, vol 1. Edited by Johnson LR. New York: Raven Press; 1994, in press.

7. KIRCHGESSNER AL, TAMIR H, GERSHON MD: **Identification and Stimulation by Serotonin of Intrinsic Sensory Neurons of the Submucosal Plexus of the Guinea Pig Gut: Activity-Induced Expression of Fos Immunoreactivity.** *J Neurosci* 1992, **12**:235–249.

8. SMITH TK, BORNSTEIN JC, FURNESS JB: **Convergence of Reflex Pathways Excited by Distension and Mechanical Stimulation of the Mucosa Onto the Same Myenteric Neurons of the Guinea Pig Small Intestine.** *J Neurosci* 1992, **12**:1502–1510.

9. IYER V, BORNSTEIN JC, COSTA M, FURNESS JB, TAKAHASHI Y, IWANAGA T: **Electrophysiology of Guinea-Pig Myenteric Neurons Correlated With Immunoreactivity for Calcium Binding Proteins.** *J Auton Nerv Syst* 1988, **22**:141–150.

10. KUNZE WA, FURNESS JB, BORNSTEIN JC: **Simultaneous Intracel-**
•• **lular Recordings From Enteric Neurons Reveal That Myenteric AH Neurons Transmit Via Slow Excitatory Postsynaptic Potentials.** *Neuroscience* 1993, **55**:685–694.

This is a well-written paper that presents one of the current hypotheses concerning the function of type 2/AH neurons. Although the authors understandably favor their own ideas, the work is a technological tour de force and is also very important in showing how type 2/AH neurons transmit signals to their follower neurons.

11. POMPOLO S, FURNESS JB: **Origins of Synaptic Inputs to Cal-**
• **retinin Immunoreactive Neurons in the Guinea-Pig Small Intestine.** *J Neurocytol* 1993, **22**:531–546.

This is a comprehensive work that nicely traces the inputs received by interneurons and motor neurons in the ENS.

12. BORNSTEIN JC, HENDRIKS R, FURNESS JB, TRUSSELL DC: **Ramifications of the Axons of AH-Neurons Injected With the Intracellular Marker Biocytin in the Myenteric Plexus of the Guinea Pig Small Intestine.** *J Comp Neurol* 1991, **314**:437–451.

13. SONG Z-M, BROOKES SJH, COSTA M: **Identification of Myenteric Neurons Which Project to the Mucosa of the Guinea-Pig Small Intestine.** *Neurosci Lett* 1991, **129**:294–298.

14. BORNSTEIN JC, FURNESS JB, SMITH TK, TRUSSELL DC: **Synaptic Responses Evoked by Mechanical Stimulation of the Mucosa in Morphologically Characterized Myenteric Neurons of the Guinea Pig Ileum.** *J Neurosci* 1991, **11**:505–518.

15. FURNESS JB, TRUSSELL DC, POMPOLO S, BORNSTEIN JC, SMITH TK: **Calbindin Neurons of the Guinea-Pig Small Intestine: Quantitative Analysis of Their Numbers and Projections.** *Cell Tissue Res* 1990, **260**:261–272.

16. POMPOLO S, FURNESS JB: **Ultrastructure and Synaptic Relationships of Calbindin-Reactive, Dogiel Type II Neurons, in the Myenteric Ganglia of Guinea-Pig Small Intestine.** *J Neurocytol* 1988, **17**:771–782.

17. TSUJI S, ANGLADE P, OZAKI T, SAZI T, YOKOYAMA S: **Peristaltic Movement Evoked in Intestinal Tube Devoid of Mucosa and Submucosa.** *Jpn J Physiol* 1992, **42**:363–375.

18. SUZUKI N, GOMI Y: **Evidence That Stretch Receptors for**
•• **Peristalsis are Located in the Mucosal Layer of the Guinea Pig Ileum.** *Jpn J Pharmacol* 1992, **60**:261–267.

This is an important paper that confirms the importance of the mucosa in the mediation of the peristaltic reflex. The significance of the mucosa was documented long ago; however, the role played by receptors in this layer has been questioned. This publication definitively shows that the earlier reports of sensory receptors that initiate the peristaltic reflex being present in the mucosa were correct.

19. BÜLBRING E, CREMA A: **Observations Concerning the Action of 5-Hydroxytryptamine on the Peristaltic Reflex.** *Br J Pharmacol* 1958, **13**:444–457.

20. BÜLBRING E, LIN RCY: **The Effect of Intraluminal Application of 5-Hydroxytryptamine and 5-Hydroxytryptophan on Peristalsis, the Local Production of 5-Hydroxytryptamine and Its Release in Relation to Intraluminal Pressure and Propulsive Activity.** *J Physiol (Lond)* 1958, **140**:381–407.

21. BÜLBRING E, LIN RCY, SCHOFIELD G: **An Investigation of the Peristaltic Reflex in Relation to Anatomical Observations.** *Q J Exp Physiol* 1958, **43**:26–37.

22. HIRST GDS, HOLMAN ME, SPENCE I: **Two Types of Neurons in the Myenteric Plexus of Duodenum in the Guinea-Pig.** *J Physiol (Lond)* 1974, **236**:303–326.

23. WOOD JD, MAYER CJ: **Intracellular Study of Electrical Activity of Auerbach's Plexus in Guinea-Pig Small Intestine.** *Pflugers Arch* 1978, **338**:247–256.

24. WOOD JD, MAYER CJ: **Serotonergic Activation of Tonic-Type Enteric Neurons in Guinea Pig Small Bowel.** *J Neurophysiol* 1979, **422**:582–593.

25. ERDE SM, SHERMAN D, GERSHON MD: **Morphology and Serotonergic Innervation of Physiologically Identified Cells of the Guinea Pig's Myenteric Plexus.** *J Neurosci* 1985, **5**:617–633.

26. JOHNSON SM, KATAYAMA Y, NORTH RA: **Slow Synaptic Potentials in Neurons of the Myenteric Plexus.** *J Physiol (Lond)* 1980, **301**:505–516.

27. GRAFE P, WOOD JD, MAYER CJ: **Fast Excitatory Postsynaptic Potentials in AH(Type 2) Neurons of Guinea-Pig Myenteric Plexus.** *Brain Res* 1979, **163**:349–352.

28. GRAFE P, MAYER CJ, WOOD JD: **Synaptic Modulation of Calcium-Dependent Potassium Conductance in Myenteric Neurones in the Guinea-Pig.** *J Physiol (Lond)* 1980, **305**:235–248.

29. HIRST GDS, JOHNSON SM, VAN HELDEN DF: **The Slow Calcium-Dependent Potassium Current in a Myenteric Neurone of the Guinea-Pig Ileum.** *J Physiol* 1985, **361**:315–337.

30. WOOD JD: **Functions of AH/Dogiel II and S/Dogiel I Neurons**
• **in the Enteric Microcircuits.** In *Advances in the Innervation of the Gastrointestinal Tract,* Edited by Holle GE, Wood JD. New York: Elsevier Science Publishers BV; 1992:125–145.

This is an elegant review that presents the hypothesis that type 2/AH neurons are interneurons.

31. BROOKES SJH, COSTA M: **Identification of Enteric Motor Neurones Which Innervate the Circular Muscle of the Guinea Pig Small Intestine.** *Neurosci Lett* 1990, **118**:227–230.

32. BROOKES SJH, STEELE PA, COSTA M: **Identification and Immunohistochemistry of Cholinergic and Non-Cholinergic Circular Muscle Motor Neurons in the Guinea-Pig Small Intestine.** *Neuroscience* 1991, **42**:863–878.

33. BROOKES. SHJ, STEELE PA, COSTA M: **Calretinin Immunoreactivity in Cholinergic Motor Neurones, Interneurones and Vasomotor Neurones in the Guinea-Pig Small Intestine.** *Cell Tiss Res* 1991, **263**:471–481.

34. BROOKES SJH, SONG Z-M, STEELE A, COSTA M: **Identification of Motor Neurons to the Longitudinal Muscle of the Guinea Pig Ileum.** *Gastroenterology* 1992, **103**:961–973.

35. POMPOLO S, FURNESS JB: **Ultrastructure and Synaptology of Neurons Immunoreactive for Gamma-Aminobutyric Acid in the Myenteric Plexus of the Guinea Pig Small Intestine.** *J Neurocytol* 1990, **19**:539–549.

36. DAWSON TM, BREDT DS, FOTUHI M, HWANG PM, SNYDER SH: **Nitric Oxide Synthase and Neuronal NADPH Diaphorase are Identical in Brain and Peripheral Tissue.** *Proc Natl Acad Sci U S A* 1991, **88**:7797–7801.

37. LLEWELLYN-SMITH IJ, SONG Z-M, COSTA M, BREDT DS, SNYDER SH: **Ultrastructural Localization of Nitric Oxide Synthase Immunoreactivity in Guinea-Pig Enteric Neurons.** *Brain Res* 1992, **577**:337–342.

38. COSTA M, FURNESS JB, POMPOLO S, BROOKES SJH, BORNSTEIN JC, BREDT DS, SNYDER SH: **Projections and Chemical Coding of Neurons With Immunoreactivity for Nitric Oxide Synthase in the Guinea-Pig Small Intestine.** *Neurosci Lett* 1992, **148**:121–125.

39. SAFFREY MJ, HASSALL CJS, HOYLE CHV, BELAL A, MOSS J,
• SCHMIDT HHHW, FÖRSTERMANN U, MURAD F, BURNSTOCK G: **Colocalization of Nitric Oxide Synthase and NADPH-Diaphorase in Cultured Myenteric Neurones.** *NeuroReport* 1993, **3**:333–336.

This paper demonstrates conclusively that neurons that contain nitric oxide synthase are intrinsic to the bowel and is one of several that confirm that nitric oxide synthase is coexpressed with NADPH diaphorase.

40. YOUNG HM, FURNESS JB, SHUTTLEWORTH CWR, BREDT DS, SNYDER SH: **Colocalization of Nitric Oxide Synthase Immunoreactivity and NADPH Diaphorase Staining in Neurons of the Guinea-Pig Intestine.** *Histochemistry* 1992, **97**:375–378.

41. BOECKXSTAENS GE, PELCKMANS PA, BULT H, DE MAN JG, HERMAN AG, VAN MAERCKE YM: **Evidence for Nitric Oxide as Mediator of Non-Adrenergic, Non-Cholinergic Relaxation Induced by ATP and GABA in the Canine Gut.** *Br J Pharmacol* 1991, **102**:434–438.

42. BOECKXSTAENS GE, PELCKMANS PA, BOGERS JJ, BULT H, DE MAN JG, OOSTERBOSCH L, HERMAN AG, VAN MAERCKE YM: **Release of Nitric Oxide Upon Stimulation of Nonadrenergic Noncholinergic Nerves in the Rat Gastric Fundus.** *J Pharmacol Exp Ther* 1991, **256**:441–447.

43. BULT H, BOECKXSTAENS GE, PELCKMANS PA, JORDAENS FH, VAN MAERCKE YM, HERMAN AG: **Nitric Oxide as an Inhibitory Non-Adrenergic Non-Cholinergic Neurotransmitter.** *Nature* 1990, **345**:346–347.

44. DALZIEL HH, THORNBURY KD, WARD SM, SANDERS KM: **Involvement of Nitric Oxide Synthetic Pathway in Inhibitory Junction Potentials in Canin Proximal Colon.** *Am J Physiol* 1991, **260**:G789–G792.

45. THORNBURY KD, WARD SM, DALZIEL HH, CARL A, WESTFALL DP, SANDERS KM: **Nitric Oxide and Nitrosocysteine Mimic Nonadrensergic, Noncholinergic Hyperpolarization in Canine Proximal Colon.** *Am J Physiol* 1991, **261**:G553–G557.

46. WARD SM, DALZIEL HH, THORNBURY KD, WESTFALL DP, SANDERS KM: **Nonadrenergic, Noncholinergic Inhibition and Rebound Excitation in Canine Colon Depend on Nitric Oxide.** *Am J Physiol* 1992, **262**:G237–G243.

47. STARK ME, BAUER AJ, SARR MG, SZURSZEWSKI JH: **Nitric Oxide**
• **Mediated Inhibitory Input in Human and Canine Jejunum.** *Gastroenterology* 1993, **104**:398–409.

This is an important paper in that it confirms that nitric oxide is likely to be physiologically important in inhibiting motility in human as well as in canine bowel.

48. STARK ME, BAUER AJ, SZURSZEWSKI JH: **Effect of Nitric Oxide on Circular Muscle of the Canine Small Intestine.** *J Physiol (Lond)* 1991, **444**:743–761.

49. CHRISTINCK F, JURY J, CAYABYAB F, DANIEL EE: **Nitric Oxide May Be the Final Mediator of Nonadrenergic, Noncholinergic Inhibitory Junction Potentials in the Gut.** *Can J Physiol Pharmacol* 1991, **69**:1448–1458.

50. LLEWELLYN-SMITH IJ, COSTA M, FURNESS JB, BORNSTEIN JC:
• **Structure of the Tertiary Component of the Myenteric Plexus in the Guinea-Pig Small Intestine.** *Cell Tissue Res* 1993, **272**:509–516.

This very nice manuscript describes the structure of the tertiary plexus and helps to establish that this structure provides a motor innervation to the longitudinal muscle.

51. BORNSTEIN JD, FURNESS JB: **Correlated Electrophysiological and Histochemical Studies of Submucous Neurons and Their Contribution to Understanding Enteric Neural Circuits.** *J Auton Nerv Syst* 1988, **25**:1–13.

52. BORNSTEIN JC, COSTA M, FURNESS JB, LEES GM: **Electrophysiological and Enkephalin Immunoreactivity of Identified Myenteric Plexus Neurones of Guinea-Pig Small Intestine.** *J Physiol (Lond)* 1984, **351**:313–325.

53. WONG-RILEY MTT: **Cytochrome Oxidase: An Endogenous Metabolic Marker for Neuronal Activity.** *Trends Neurosci* 1989, **12**:94–101.

54. Mawe GM, Gershon MD: **Functional Heterogeneity in the Myenteric Plexus: Demonstration Using Cytochrome Oxidase as a Verified Cytochemical Probe of the Activity of Individual Enteric Neurons.** *J Comp Neurol* 1986, **249**:381–391.

55. Kirchgessner AL, Mawe GM, Gershon MD: **Evaluation of the Activity of Chemically Identified Enteric Neurons Through the Histochemical Detection of Cytochrome Oxidase.** *J Comp Neurol* 1990, **301**:1–14.

56. Morgan J, Curran T: **Stimulus-Transcription Coupling in the Nervous System: Involvement of the Inducible Proto-Oncogenes *Fos* and *Jun*.** *Annu Rev Neurosci* 1991, **14**:421–451.

57. •• Young HM, McConalogue K, Furness JB, De Vente J: **Nitric Oxide Targets in the Guinea-Pig Intestine Identified by Induction of Cyclic GMP Immunoreactivity.** *Neuroscience* 1993, **55**:583–596.

This study is a very important advance. It adapts a new method to the bowel and morphologically locates the potential targets of nitric oxide in the bowel. The authors present and document their data very well.

58. Ignarro LJ: **Biological Actions and Properties of Endothelium-Derived Nitric Oxide Formed and Released From Artery and Vein.** *Circ Res* 1989, **65**:1–21.

59. Niel JP, Bywater RAR, Taylor GS: **Apamin-Resistant Post-Stimulus Hyperpolarization in the Circular Muscle of Guinea Pig Ileum.** *J Auton Nerv Syst* 1983, 9:565–569.

60. Bywater RA, Taylor GS: **Non-Cholinergic Excitatory and Inhibitory Junction Potentials in the Circular Muscle of the Guinea-Pig Ileum.** *J Physiol (Lond)* 1986, **374**:153–164.

61. Crist JR, He XD, Goyal RK: **Both ATP and the Peptide VIP are Inhibitory Neurotransmitters in Guinea Pig Ileum Circular Muscle.** *J Physiol (Lond)* 1992, **447**:119–131.

62. Crist JR, Xue DH, Goyal RK: **The Nature of Noncholinergic Membrane Potential Responses to Transmural Stimulation in Guinea Pig Ileum.** *Gastroenterology* 1991, **100**:1006–1015.

63. Burnstock G: **Purinergic Nerves.** *Pharmacol Rev* 1981, **24**:509–581.

64. •• He XD, Goyal RK: **Nitric Oxide Involvement in the Peptide VIP-Associated Inhibitory Junction Potential in the Guinea-Pig Ileum.** *J Physiol (Lond)* 1993, **461**:485–499.

This is a comprehensive study that clearly documents the existence of two types of IJPs in the enteric musculature. The authors also demonstrate the relative roles played by three putative mediators in each IJP: ATP, VIP, and nitric oxide.

65. Christensen J: **A Commentary on the Morphological Identification of Interstitial Cells of Cajal in the Gut.** *J Auton Nerv Syst* 1992, **37**:75–88.

66. Christensen J, Rick GA, Lowe LS: **Distributions of Interstitial Cell of Cajal in Stomach and Colon of Cat, Dog, Ferret, Opossum, Rat, Guinea Pig, and Rabbit.** *J Auton Nerv Syst* 1992, **37**:47–56.

67. Faussone-Pellegrini MS: **Comparative Study of Interstitial Cells of Cajal.** *Acta Anat* 1987, **130**:109–126.

68. Thuneberg L: **Interstitial Cells of Cajal: Intestinal Pacemaker Cells?** *Adv Anat Embryol Cell Biol* 1982, **71**:1–130.

69. Thuneberg L: **Interstitial Cells of Cajal.** In *The Gastrointestinal System.* Part 1, vol 1. Edited by Wood JD. Bethesda, MD. American Physiological Society; 1989:349–386.

70. Prosser CL, Holzwarth MA, Barr L: **Immunocytochemistry of the Interstitial Cells of Cajal in the Rat Intestine.** *J Auton Nerv Syst* 1989, **27**:17–25.

71. Cajal SR: **Sur Les Ganglions et Plexus Nerveux de L'Intestin.** *C R Soc Biol (Paris)* 1893, **45**:217–223.

72. Berezin I, Huizinga JD, Daniel EE: **Interstitial Cells of Cajal in the Canine Colon: A Special Communication Network at the Inner Bordser of the Circular Muscle.** *J Comp Neurol* 1988, **273**:42–51.

73. Liu LWC, Daniel EE, Huizinga JD: **Excitability of Canine Colon Circular Muscle Disconnected From the Network of Interstitial Cells of Cajal.** *Can J Physiol Pharmacol* 1992, **70**:289–295.

74. • Shuttleworth CW, Sanders KM, Keef KD: **Inhibition of Nitric Oxide Synthesis Reveals Non-Cholinergic Excitatory Neurotransmission in the Canine Proximal Colon.** *Br J Pharmacol* 1993, **109**:739–747.

This paper contributes to knowledge of the role of nitric oxide and of the interaction between excitatory and inhibitory neurotransmitters to smooth muscle.

75. • Publicover NG, Horowitz NN, Sanders KM: **Calcium Oscillations in Freshly Dispersed and Cultured Interstitial Cells From Canine Colon.** *Am J Physiol* 1992, **262**:C589–C597.

This is an elegant study that establishes that interstitial cells are a distinct cell type and provides strong data in support of the hypothesis that they play a role as pacemaker cells.

76. •• Publicover NG, Hammond EM, Sanders KM: **Amplification of Nitric Oxide Signaling by Interstitial Cells Isolated From Canine Colon.** *Proc Natl Acad Sci U S A* 1993, **90**:2087–2091.

This paper provides an important insight into the potential role played by interstitial cells in the mediation of the effects of nitric oxide (and thus the inhibitory innervation) on enteric motility.

77. • Grider JR, Murthy KS, Jin J-G, Makhlouf GM: **Stimulation of Nitric Oxide From Muscle Cells by VIP: Prejunctional Enhancement of VIP Release.** *Am J Physiol* 1992, **25**:G774–G778.

This paper should be read together with the paper below that followed it. The two papers clearly present a novel view of the secretion and ultimate effects of nitric oxide on the bowel.

78. •• Grider JR: **Interplay of VIP and Nitric Oxide in Regulation of the Descending Relaxation Phase of Peristalsis.** *Am J Physiol* 1993, **264**:G334–G340.

79. • Grider JR, Jin J-G: **Vasoactive Intestinal Peptide Release and L-Citrulline Production From Isolated Ganglia of the Myenteric Plexus: Evidence for Regulation of Vasoactive Intestinal Peptide Release by Nitric Oxide.** *Neuroscience* 1993, **54**:521–526.

This paper is one of a series that provide support for the authors' novel hypothesis that smooth muscle secretes nitric oxide and that nitric oxide releases VIP.

80. Tamura K, Schemann M, Wood JD: **Action of Nitric Oxide in the Microcircuits of the Guinea Pig Small Intestinal Myenteric Plexus.** *Soc Neurosci Abst* 1992, **18**, part 1:915.

81. Smith TK, Reed JB, Sanders KM: **Origin and Propagation of Electrical Slow Waves in Circular Muscle of Canine Proximal Colon.** *Am J Physiol* 1987, **252**:C215–C224.

82. • Liu LWC, Thuneberg L, Daniel EE, Huizinga JD: **Selective Accumulation of Methylene Blue by Interstitial Cells of Cajal in Canine Colon.** *Am J Physiol* 1993, **264**:G64–G73.

This is a useful and careful demonstration of interstitial cells of Cajal by vital staining.

83. Ward SM, Burke EP, Sanders KM: **Use of Rhodamine 123 to Label and Lesion Interstitial Cells of Cajal in Canine Colonic Circular Muscle.** *Anat Embryol* 1990, **182**:215–224.

84. XUE C, WARD SM, SHUTTLEWORTH CW, SANDERS KM: **Identification of Interstitial Cells in Canine Proximal Colon Using NADH Diaphorase Histochemistry**. *Histochemistry* 1993, **99**:373–384.
•• This is an important observation that supports the idea that interstitial cells amplify the signal to muscle provided by neurally released nitric oxide by acting as a supplementary source of nitric oxide.

85. WARD SM, KELLER RG, SANDERS KM: **Structure and Organization of Electrical Activity of Canine Distal Colon**. *Am J Physiol* 1991, **260**:G724–G735.

86. WARD SM, SANDERS KM: **Pacemaker Activity in Septal Structures of Canine Colonic Circular Muscle**. *Am J Physiol* 1990, **259**:G264–G273.

87. LANGTON P, WARD SM, CARL A, NORELL MA, SANDERS KM: **Spontaneous Electrical Activity of Interstitial Cells of Cajal Isolated From Canine Proximal Colon**. *Proc Nat Acad Sci U S A* 1989, **86**:7280–7284.

88. LEE HK, SANDERS KM: **Comparison of Ionic Currents From Interstitial Cells and Smooth Muscle Cells of Canine Colon**. *J Physiol* 1993, **460**:135–152.
•• This is an elegant paper that supports the idea that interstitial cells are a distinct cell type, with pacemaker activity.

89. GERSHON MD, CHALAZONITIS A, ROTHMAN TP: **From Neural Crest to Bowel: Development of the Enteric Nervous System**. *J Neurobiol* 1993, **24**:199–214.
• This is a comprehensive review of the development of the ENS.

Michael D. Gershon, MD, and Paul R. Wade, PhD, Department of Anatomy and Cell Biology, Columbia University College of Physicians and Surgeons, New York, NY 10032, USA.

Effects of dietary components on cellular elements and metabolism

Richard E. Goldstein, MD*†, and Paul J. Flakoll, PhD*

*Vanderbilt University and †The Veterans Administration Medical Center, Nashville, Tennessee, USA

This article reviews recent work by investigators examining modifications in lipid and protein intake and their subsequent effects on various measured parameters. Structured triglycerides were demonstrated to decrease plasma high-density lipoprotein cholesterol and positively effect the muscle fractional synthetic rate. In addition, structured triglycerides modify the plasma membrane lipid composition, the effects of which are yet to be determined. Several additional studies have produced encouraging results in patients with hepatic dysfunction. Another recent report suggests a possible relationship between low levels of the (ω-3) fatty acid, docosahexaenoic acid, and encephalopathy in cirrhotic patients. Additionally, there continues to be active research into specific individual amino acid (glutamine, arginine), dipeptide, ketoacid, and nucleotide supplementation and their effects on muscle fractional synthetic rates and intestinal mucosal viability.

Current Opinion in Gastroenterology 1994, **10**:193–198

Over the past year a variety of reports have been published that explore the effects of protein, protein fragments, and lipids on various parameters of metabolism. This review will focus on some of these reports that deal with research into areas that are of particular interest. Some of these investigations could be considered preliminary but may yield considerable rewards in the future.

Structured lipids

Triglycerides constructed with both medium-chain and very long chain fatty acids are referred to as structured lipids and have been the subject of recent interest. The potential for altering properties among these fatty acids with regard to absorption and incorporation into circulating lipoprotein lipids has stimulated their research. In the study by Swift *et al.* [1], changes in plasma lipids and lipoproteins were assessed in 10 healthy male subjects after 6 days of oral dietary modification, one arm of which contained structured lipid supplementation. High-density lipoprotein cholesterol was decreased 14% by the structured lipid enhanced diet. The lipid composition of lipoproteins were unaltered by the structured lipid diet.

Structured lipids were also studied by Mendez *et al.* [2••]. In this study, the short-term effect of a 3-day infusion of three total parenteral nutrition solutions, each with a different lipid source (one with structured lipids incorporating fish oil and medium-chain triglycerides, a similar physical mix of medium-chain triglycerides and fish oil, or long-chain triglycerides) was assessed in a rat cancer model. Medium-chain triglycerides can be made rapidly available to tissue and may be preferentially oxidized compared with long-chain triglycerides. They also do not provide linoleic acid for the arachidonic pathway and thus may alter prostaglandin synthesis. The results demonstrated that, whereas tumor growth was the slowest in the structured lipid group, the muscle fractional synthetic rate was restored by structured lipids in the tumor-bearing group. The au-

Abbreviation

SAMe—*S*-adenosyl-L-methionine.

 ISBN 1-85922-607-8 ISSN 0267–1379

thors also speculate that the (ω-3) fatty acids in the structured lipids could potentially decrease arachidonic acid in tumor leading to alterations in prostaglandin production, a possible mechanism for the relative inhibition of tumor growth. Further investigation in this field is certainly warranted.

Pironi *et al.* [3•] evaluated the effect of a linoleic acid based structural enteral lipid formula versus an oleic acid based structural enteral lipid formula on plasma erythrocyte membrane phospholipid fatty acid pattern, neutrophil superoxide anion generation, and eicosanoid production. The linoleic acid formula had a high linoleic/α-linolenic acid ratio compared with the oleic acid formula. The study was based on the theory that linoleic and α-linolenic acids modify the activity of the immune system by effecting membrane fluidity (permeability, membrane receptors, and enzyme function) and by regulating the production of eicosanoids. The study was performed on adult males undergoing laryngectomy. The results demonstrated significant differences between the two groups in plasma and erythrocyte membrane phospholipid fatty acids after 14 days of treatment. The monounsaturated fatty acid content of erythrocytes decreased in the linoleic acid group, theoretically increasing membrane susceptibility to peroxidative damage and changing membrane fluidity. In addition, the linoleic acid group had greater neutrophil superoxide anion generation, potentially allowing for greater free radical damage. Thus, these results suggest that changes in structured lipids can alter membrane characteristics.

Changes in plasma and erythrocyte fatty acids brought about by the administration of structured lipids were also detected by Adams *et al.* [4]. Patients received enteral nutrition with either a formula containing structured triglycerides enriched with the longer chain (ω-3) fatty acids, eicosapentaenoic acid and docosahexaenoic acid, or a formula enriched with linoleic acid. The group that received structured lipids with (ω-3) fatty acids had a decreased ratio of arachidonic acid to eicosapentaenoic acid in plasma and decreased linoleic acid in the erythrocytes. Thus, structured triglyceride administration appears to be a mechanism that can alter the lipid content of membranes. Whether the consequences of these changes are metabolically significant remains to be determined.

Lipids and heart disease

The effect of dietary fats on plasma lipid concentrations and the risk of heart disease continues to be an area of interest. In particular, trans-fatty acids, a major source of which are margarine and spreads, have come under scrutiny. Troisi *et al.* [5] collected dietary intake data from 985 men over a 3-year period and correlated this data with measured serum lipids. They concluded that trans-fatty acid intake was directly related to total serum and low-density lipoprotein cholesterol and inversely related to high-density lipoprotein cholesterol. Trans-fatty acid intake positively correlated with the ratios of total to high-density lipoprotein cholesterol. Based on previously published data, the authors estimated that results from their study corresponded to a 27% increase in the risk of myocardial infarction. However, outcome was not assessed in this study [5].

In another study looking at trans-fatty acids, Mensink *et al.* [6] examined the effects of dietary fatty acid composition on serum lipoprotein[a]. Lipoprotein[a] is a macromolecular complex, made up of apolipoprotein B, cholesterol, other proteins, and a protein called apolipoprotein[a]. Subjects with elevated lipoprotein[a] levels may be at increased risk of coronary heart disease. In this study, after subjects consumed a control diet high in saturated fatty acids, they were assigned to diets replaced with monounsaturates and polyunsaturates or polyunsaturates alone. In another experiment, fat in the diet was increased with either oleic acid or trans-monounsaturated fatty acids. Plasma levels of lipoprotein[a] doubled on the trans-fatty acid diet. These results indicate that trans-fatty acids can elevate serum lipoprotein[a] levels and suggest a role for dietary modification.

Metabolism, nutritional support, and liver failure

There continues to be great interest in the relationship between nutritional factors and hepatic function, particularly in those patients with hepatic failure. Patients with liver cirrhosis are felt to have an impaired transsulphuration pathway in which there is a defective metabolic step at the site of *S*-adenosyl-L-methionine (SAMe) formation from methionine. SAMe serves as the methyl donor in methylation reactions. In addition, decreased SAMe utilization might result in decreased formation of secondary sulphur containing amino acids.

In a study designed to evaluate the effects of exogenous SAMe administration on plasma concentrations of several metabolites of the transsulphuration pathway in patients with cirrhosis, Marchesini *et al.* [7••] administered SAMe or placebo intravenously and orally to two groups of cirrhotic patients. The SAMe treatment increased plasma levels of taurine and cystine without increasing plasma levels of methionine, suggesting that exogenous SAMe was taken up by hepatocytes and metabolized via the transsulphuration pathway. The authors cite data in the literature relating taurine deficiency with decreased bile secretion and SAMe deficiency with decreased de novo biosynthesis of choline, a potential nutrient in malnourished patients with cirrhosis [7••].

With the increased interest in lipid composition, a recent report from Cabre *et al.* [8••] raised an interesting issue. They compared the fatty acid composition and distribution in various plasma fractions in normal humans as well as cirrhotic patients with and without hepatic encephalopathy. The most significant findings were a decrease in total (ω-6) polyunsaturated fatty acid plasma levels in patients with cirrhosis and a selective decrease in plasma arachidonic acid and docosahexaenoic acid levels in those patients with cirrhosis and hepatic encephalopathy. The fact that docosahexaenoic acid is the most abundant fatty acid in phospholipids of neuronal membranes and in the rods of the retina suggests the possibility that a causative relationship may exit between the decrease in this fatty acid and neuronal dysfunction.

Alterations in the fat metabolism of cirrhotic patients were the focus of two other studies. Riggio *et al.* [9] used indirect calorimetry to assess energy expenditure and oxidation rates of carbohydrate, fat, and protein metabolism before and 3 hours after a mixed meal in stable cirrhotic and control patients. The primary finding was that fat oxidation was increased in both the postprandial and postabsorptive periods, suggesting an increased reliance on fatty acids for fuel. The authors indicate that this finding is at odds with a few other studies in the literature.

Gonzalez *et al.* [10] looked at the relationship between the nutritional status of cirrhotic patients and the levels of various plasma lipids. They determined that decreases in plasma cholesterol and linoleic, dihomo-γ-linolenic, and arachidonic acid levels were related to the degree of protein-energy malnutrition. They reported significant differences in (ω-6) polyunsaturated fatty acids in plasma, plasma phospholipids, and plasma cholesterol esters. There was also a decrease in the (ω-3) polyunsaturated fatty acid docosahexaenoic acid. Thus, with long-chain polyunsaturated fatty acids playing key roles in membrane structure, these studies raise the question of whether dietary modification can increase the level of certain fatty acids in plasma and membranes and whether such modification will have beneficial effects on the morbidity and mortality of patients suffering from cirrhosis or hepatitis.

There have also been several reports exploring the combined use of nutritional supplementation in combination with the anabolic steroid oxandrolone in patients with hepatic dysfunction. An anabolic steroid has the theoretic advantage of promoting both protein synthesis and appetite. In a Veterans Administration Cooperative Study, Mendenhall *et al.* [11•] investigated oral nutritional support with and without oxandrolone in moderate and severely malnourished patients with alcoholic hepatitis. Treatment consisted of placebo or oxandrolone for 30 inpatient and 60 outpatient days, accompanied by a high-caloric, high-protein food supplement (Hepatic Aid II, McGaw, Irvine, CA) enriched with branched-chain amino acids. The primary endpoint was survival at 60 days. Those patients with moderate protein-calorie malnutrition in the treatment arm had a 9.4% 30-day mortality versus a 20.9% mortality in the placebo arm. This difference in mortality was also significant at 6 months (20.3% mortality versus 37.3% mortality). There was no difference in survival in the patients with severe protein-calorie malnutrition. Missing from this study was a treatment arm aimed specifically at addressing the effects of oxandrolone alone.

In another recent report, Bonkovsky *et al.* [12] studied patients with alcoholic cirrhosis randomized into 1) a balanced oral diet, 2) a balanced oral diet plus oxandrolone, 3) peripheral total parenteral nutrition used to supplement an oral diet, and 4) peripheral total parenteral nutrition plus an oral diet plus oxandrolone. Leucine metabolism was assess with ^{15}N, 1-^{13}C-L-leucine before and after 3 weeks of treatment. Total protein and caloric intake were different in the four groups. The results did not demonstrate any positive effect as assessed by changes in leucine metabolism. However, nitrogen balance was improved by the addition of peripheral total parenteral nutrition. The only specific effect of oxandrolone appeared to be an isolated increase in the plasma prealbumin level. Additional well-controlled studies are probably indicated to further investigate both enteral and parenteral nutrition and the use of anabolic steroids in patients with hepatitis or cirrhosis. At present, however, evidence for a positive effect of anabolic steroids in the setting of liver failure is weak.

Amino acids, ketoacids, and nucleotides

The importance of dietary amino acids continues to be carefully studied. Preed and Garlick [13••] published a particularly interesting manuscript in which they demonstrated that the 6-hour infusion of mixed amino acids (N 15 mg/h), glucose, or branched chain amino acids to rats increased skeletal muscle protein fractional synthetic rates and riboneucleic acid activity by 50%, 25%, and 20%, respectively. However, this was significantly below that of fed animals. Interestingly, glucose added to the mixed amino acid infusion resulted in no additional stimulation of skeletal muscle protein synthesis.

Clinical interest for the use of the ketoacids of amino acids persists, particularly during states of excessive plasma nitrogen accumulation. The ketoanalogues of amino acids were found to maintain nutrition in uremic rats, provided that basal protein in the diet was greater than 50% of minimal requirements [14]. These data add to the list of publications demonstrating the potential benefits of ketoacids.

In a model of intestinal atrophy induced by starvation, rats were administered either chow, a standard total parenteral nutrition solution (16% glucose, 2.8% fat, and 4.25% standard amino acids), or the same total parenteral nutrition solution enriched with 1.5% glutamine for 7 days [15]. Whereas the chow diet restored normal intestinal anatomy and function, the standard total parenteral nutrition solution did not improve these variables. The addition of glutamine to the solution improved the recovery from intestinal atrophy, but not to the degree of the oral diet group.

In rats that were fasted for 3 days and then refed for 7 days with an oral diet containing either ornithine α-ketoglutarate, glutamine, or casein, the main effect of ornithine α-ketoglutarate was seen in the viscera with a normalization of most amino acid pools in the small bowel and liver [16]. The main effect of glutamine was observed in the muscle, with a normalization of glutamine and leucine pools. Therefore, ornithine α-ketoglutarate and glutamine may act in different target tissues, splanchnic areas, and muscle, respectively.

Glutamine supplementation improved structure and function in a rat model of total parenteral nutrition and small bowel transplantation [17]. Rats undergoing transplantation of the small intestine were administered either intravenous glutamine, intravenous nonessential amino acids, glutamine into the graft, or nonessential amino acids into the graft. Infusion of glutamine increased mucosal villus height, surface area, weight, and glucose absorption when compared with controls. Beneficial effects of glutamine were not different between intravenous and graft administration.

One of the problems associated with glutamine infusion is the chemical stability of glutamine. For this reason, interest in the use of glutamine dipeptides has flourished. Infusions of either glutamine or glutamine-dipeptide solutions in dogs increased serum glutamine concentrations and enhanced glutamine uptake in the hindlimb [18]. After a 50% intestinal resection, both glutamine and glutamine dipeptide solutions resulted in increased serum glutamine concentrations, nitrogen balance, intestinal mucosal thickness, and villi area. Similarly, after an 85% bowel resection, rats were infused with either a standard amino acid solution, twofold standard amino acids, or the standard amino acid solution plus 2% alanyl-glutamine for 1 week [19]. Mucosal wet weight, protein, RNA, DNA, villi height, and maltase and sucrase activities were greater in the group given glutamine, suggesting that adaptation of the remaining intestine after resection can be promoted by administration of alanyl-glutamine–enriched total parenteral nutrition.

Although glutamine supplementation has received the greatest share of publication, interest in the use of arginine and RNA nucleotides has increased, particularly owing to their potential for enhancing immune and gastrointestinal function. This potential for immunomodulation and enteral hyperalimentation has been nicely reviewed by McClave *et al.* [20•] this past year. Several reports have demonstrated that dietary arginine improves resistance to infection, but the mechanisms involved are not well defined. Balb/c mice were fed with a defined diet, alone or the same diet supplemented with 2% arginine, or 4% glycine, or standard laboratory chow [21]. Survival after cecal ligation and puncture was 56% in the arginine-supplemented group versus 28% in the nonsupplemented group and 20% in the chow group. Survival after gavage with *Escherichia coli* and a 20% burn injury was 100% in the arginine-supplemented group versus 50% in both the glycine-supplemented and chow groups and 35% in the nonsupplemented group. Translocation to the liver and spleen was not decreased by arginine, suggesting that the effect was on the immune system rather that on mucosal integrity. In the animals receiving the arginine-supplemented diet, the nitric oxide inhibitor, *N*-nitro-L-arginine, reversed the beneficial effects of arginine, suggesting that arginine-nitric oxide pathway is important in arginine's effects.

In the clinical setting, after oncologic surgery, patients received either a standard enteral diet or a diet supplemented with arginine, RNA, and (ω-3) fatty acids [22••]. Nitrogen balance was improved with the supplemented diet. In addition, infectious and wound complications occurred less often (11% vs 37%) and mean length of stay in the hospital was shorter (15.8 ± 5.1 vs 20.2 ± 9.4 days) for the supplemented group. In another clinical study [23] with renal failure patients requiring long-term total parenteral nutrition therapy, supplemental arginine and ornithine had beneficial effects on ammonia toxicity.

The potential benefits for the use of nucleotides were examined in a well-designed study by Iijima *et al.* [24•]. Rats were given total parenteral nutrition that was either standard, nucleoside- and nucleotide-enriched, glutamine-alone enriched, or glutamine-, nucleoside-, and nucleotide-enriched. It was observed that the supplementation of nucleotides prevented atrophic changes in the intestinal mucosal more effectively than did the supplementation of glutamine. In addition, combining glutamine and the nucleotides enhanced the development of brush border enzymes.

Conclusions

The modification of dietary lipids has become an intense field of research. The use of structured lipids has become a mechanism to bring about changes in the lipid composition of membranes. What remains to be explored are the metabolic consequences of these modifications. With the recent encouraging results of dietary supplementation in patients with liver dysfunction, several adjuvant modalities to enhance the nutrition in this patient population are in the early stages of exploration. The use of supplemental amino acids, dipeptides, and nucleotides remains a very active field of research with exciting potential.

References and recommended reading

Papers of particular interest, published within the annual period of review, have been highlighted as:

- • Of special interest
- •• Of outstanding interest

1. SWIFT LL, HILL JO, PETERS JC, GREEN HL: **Plasma Lipids and Lipoproteins During 6 d of Maintenance Feeding With Long-Chain, Medium-Chain, and Mixed-Chain Triglycerides.** *Am J Clin Nutr* 1992, 56:881–886.

2. •• MENDEZ B, RA LING P, ISTFAN NW, BABAYAN VK, BISTRIAN BR: **Effects of Different Lipid Sources in Total Parenteral Nutrition on Whole Body Protein Kinetics and Tumor Growth.** *JPEN J Parenter Enteral Nutr* 1992, 16:545–551.

This interesting study examined the effects of structural triglycerides on muscle fractional synthetic rate and tumor growth. It will definitely form the basis for future investigations.

3. • PIRONI L, BELLUZZI A, GIONCHETTI P, RUGGERI E, BOSCHI S, GUARNIERI C, CALICETI U, CENACCHI V, BARBARA L, MIGLIOLI M: **Possible Role of Structural Lipids in Artificial Nutrition: Comparison of a Linoleic Acid-Based With an Oleic Acid-Based Enteral Formula in Humans.** *Clin Nutr* 1993, 12(Suppl 1):S91–S96.

This study looked at the ability of structural triglycerides to alter erythrocyte membrane phospholipid fatty acid pattern. The results demonstrate that structured triglycerides can alter membrane composition.

4. ADAMS S, YEH YY, JENSEN GL: **Changes in Plasma and Erythrocyte Fatty Acids in Patients Fed Enteral Formulas Containing Different Fats.** *JPEN J Parenter Enteral Nutr* 1993, 17:30–34.

5. TROISI R, WILLETT WC, WEISS ST: **Trans-Fatty Acid Intake in Relation to Serum Lipid Concentrations in Adult Men.** *Am J Clin Nutr* 1992, 56:1019–1024.

6. MENSINK RP, ZOCK PL, KATAN MB, HORNSTRA G: **Effect of Dietary Cis and Trans Fatty Acids on Serum Lipoprotein[a] Levels in Humans.** *J Lipid Res* 1992, 33:1493–1501.

7. •• MARCHESINI G, BUGIANESI E, BIANCHI G, FABBRI A, MARCHI E, ZOLI M, PISI E: **Effect of S-Adenosyl-L-Methionine Administration on Plasma Levels of Sulphur-Containing Amino Acids in Patients with Liver Cirrhosis.** *Clin Nutr* 1992, 11:303–308.

This very interesting study was designed to investigate whether SAMe can modify the levels of certain plasma amino acids. It is based on the theory that cirrhotic patients have an impaired transsulphuration pathway. The results suggest SAMe can be taken up by the hepatocyte and metabolized via this pathway increasing the plasma levels of taurine and cystine.

8. •• CABRE E, PERIAGO JL, GONZALEZ J, GONZALEZ-HUIX F, ABAD-LACRUZ A, GIL A, SANCHEZ-MEDINA F, ESTEVE-COMAS M, FERNANDEZ-BANARES F, PLANAS R, GASSULL MA: **Plasma Polyunsaturated Fatty Acids in Liver Cirrhosis With or Without Chronic Hepatic Encephalopathy: A Preliminary Study.** *JPEN J Parenter Enteral Nutr* 1992, 16:359–363.

The central finding of this study is that cirrhotic patients with encephalopathy had decreased levels of docosahexaenoic acid. As this fatty acid is a major component of neuronal membranes, the possibility of a cause and effect relationship is raised.

9. RIGGIO O, MERLI M, ROMITI A, PINTO G, FANELLA R, ATTILI AF, CAPOCACCIA L: **Early Postprandial Energy Expenditure and Macronutrient Use After a Mixed Meal in Cirrhotic Patients.** *JPEN J Parenter Enteral Nutr* 1992, 16:445–450.

10. GONZALEZ J, PERIAGO JL, GIL A, CABRE E, ABAD-LACRUZ A, GASSLL MA, SANCHEZ DE MEDINA F: **Malnutrition-Related Polyunsaturated Fatty Acid Changes in Plasma Lipid Fractions of Cirrhotic Patients.** *Metabolism* 1992, 41:954–960.

11. • MENDENHALL CL, MORITZ TE, ROSELLE GA, MORGAN TR, NEMCHAUSKY BA, TAMBURRO CH, SCHIFF ER, MCCLAIN CJ, MARSANO LS, ALLEN JI, SAMANTA A, WEESNER RE, HENDERSON W, GARTSIDE P, CHEN TS, FRENCH SW, CHEDID A, VETERANS AFFAIRS COOPERATIVE STUDY GROUP 275: **A Study of Oral Nutritional Support with Oxandrolone in Malnourished Patients with Alcoholic Hepatitis: Results of a Department of Veterans Affairs Cooperative Study.** *Hepatology* 1992, 17:564–576.

This study investigated the use of enteral nutritional support and the anabolic steroid, oxandrolone, in patients with alcoholic hepatitis. Although the effect of oxandrolone alone was not investigated, the study demonstrated a decrease in mortality with aggressive nutritional support.

12. BONKOVSKY HL, SINGH RH, JAFRI IH, FIELLIN DA, SMITH GS, SIMON D, COTSONIS GA, SLAKER DP: **A Randomized, Controlled Trial of Treatment of Alcoholic Hepatitis with Parenteral Nutrition and Oxandrolone. II. Short-Term Effects on Nitrogen Metabolism, Metabolic Balance, and Nutrition.** *Am J Gastroenterol* 1991, 86:1209–1218.

13. •• PREED VR, GARLICK PJ: **Response of Muscle Protein Synthesis to Parenteral Administration of Amino Acid Mixtures in Growing Rats.** *JPEN J Parenter Enteral Nutr* 1993, 17:113–118.

This study looked at the effects of amino acid mixtures on skeletal muscle protein fractional synthetic rates.

14. MANIAR S, LAOUARI D, BURTIN M, PARVY PR KLEINKNECHT C: **Nutritional Effects of Feeding a Ketoanalogue Mixture in Growing and Adult Uremic Rats.** *Am J Clin Nutr* 1992, 56:1025–1033.

15. INOUE Y, GRANT JP, SNYDER PJ: **Effect of Glutamine-Supplemented Total Parenteral Nutrition on Recovery of the Small Intestine After Starvation Atrophy.** *JPEN J Parenter Enteral Nutr* 1993, 17:165–170.

16. ZIEGLER F, COUDRAYLUCAS C, JARDEL A, LASNIER E, LEBOUCHER J, EKINDJIAN OG, CYNOBER L: **Ornithine α-Ketoglutarate and Glutamine Supplementation During Refeeding of Food-Deprived Rats.** *JPEN J Parenter Enteral Nutr* 1992, 16:505–510.

17. FRANKEL WL, WEI Z, AFONSO J, KLURFELD DM, DON SH, LAITIN E, DEATON D, FURTH EE, PIETRA GG, NAJI A, ROMBEAU JL: **Glutamine Enhancement of Structure and Function in Transplanted Small Intestine in the Rat.** *JPEN J Parenter Enteral Nutr* 1993, 17:47–55.

18. JIANG ZM, WANG LJ, QI Y, LIU TH,, QIU MR, YANG NF, WILMORE DW: **Comparison of Parenteral Nutrition Supplemented With L-Glutamine or Glutamine Dipeptides.** *JPEN J Parenter Enteral Nutr* 1993, 17:142–144.

19. TAMADA H, NEZU R, MATSUO Y, IMAMURA I, TAKAGI Y, OKADA A: **Alanyl Glutamine-Enriched Total Parenteral Nutrition Re-**

stores Intestinal Adaptation After Either Proximal or Distal Massive Resection in Rats. *JPEN J Parenter Enteral Nutr* 1993, 17:236–242.

20. McClave SA, Lowen CC, Snider HL: **Immunonutrition and**
• **Enteral Hyperalimentation of Critically Ill Patients [Review].** *Dig Dis Sci* 1992, 37:1153–1161.

A good review of arginine and RNA nucleotides and their applications to nutrition.

21. Gianotti L, Alexander JW, Pyles T, Fukushima R: **Arginine-Supplemented Diets Improve Survival in Gut-Derived Sepsis and Peritonitis by Modulation of Bacterial Clearance - The Role of Nitric Oxide.** *Ann Surg* 1993, 217:644–654.

22. Daly JM, Lieberman MD, Goldfine J, Show J, Weintraub
•• F, Rosato EF, Lavin P: **Enteral Nutrition with Supplemental Arginine, RNA, and Omega-3 Fatty Acids in Patients After Operation—Immunologic, Metabolic, and Clinical Outcome.** *Surgery* 1992, 112:56-57.

An excellent study investigating the use of arginine, RNA, and (ω-3) fatty acids as a dietary supplement in patients undergoing oncologic surgery. Nitrogen balance, infections, and wound complications were all improved in the group receiving this modified diet.

23. Nakasaki H, Katayama T, Yokoyama S, Tajima T, Mitomi T, Tsuda M, Suga T, Fujii K: **Complication of Parenteral Nutrition Composed of Essential Amino Acids and Histidine in Adults with Renal Failure.** *JPEN J Parenter Enteral Nutr* 1993, 17:86–90.

24. Iijima S, Tsujinaka T, Kido Y, Hayashida Y, Ishida H,
• Homma T, Yokoyama H, Mori T: **Intravenous Administration of Nucleosides and a Nucleotide Mixture Diminished Intestinal Mucosal Atrophy Induced by Total Parenteral Nutrition.** *JPEN J Parenter Enteral Nutr* 1993, 17:265–270.

A well-designed study aimed at investigating the use of nucleosides and nucleotides on the intestinal mucosa in rats. Nucleotides prevented intestinal mucosal changes more effectively than did glutamine.

Richard E. Goldstein, MD, AA-2219 Medical Center North, Vanderbilt University, Nashville, Tennessee 37232-2739, USA.

Paul J. Flakoll, PhD, 750 MRB, Vanderbilt University, Nashville, Tennessee 37232-0615, USA.

Nutrition in the prevention and treatment of cancer

David Heber, MD, PhD

University of California at Los Angeles School of Medicine, Los Angeles, California, USA

A combination of epidemiologic evidence, animal studies, and intervention trials provides evidence supporting the hypothesis that Western diets and lifestyle contribute to common forms of cancer including breast, colon, and prostate cancer. Antioxidants including vitamin E, ascorbic acid, and β-carotene and other micronutrients may have protective effects and may act as antipromoters of carcinogenesis. Rapid advances in research may lead to further advances that will reduce the incidence of these common forms of cancer and complement advances in the understanding of the molecular basis of cancer by elucidating the influence of nutrition on carcinogenesis. The complexity of the relationship between nutrition and lifestyle to common gastrointestinal cancers including colorectal and gastric cancers is rapidly advancing. General recommendations can be made based on the available evidence to encourage patients to reduce their risk of developing cancer through dietary modification, including increased intake of fruits and vegetables, high-fiber cereals and grains, and antioxidant micronutrients, while reducing the intake of fat and salted, pickled, and smoked foods.

Current Opinion in Gastroenterology 1994, **10**:199–202

There has been a great deal of research in the areas of nutrition and cancer prevention as well as in the treatment of the malnourished cancer patient during the past year. The major emphasis of this review is on gastrointestinal cancers, especially colorectal cancer, in which genetic advances are being complemented by the rapid growth of nutritional knowledge that will provide preventive strategies for patients at risk and the general population. Recent advances in nutrition and the prevention of other forms of cancer and the treatment of the malnourished cancer patient are covered more briefly, but other reviews [1•,2••] are suggested that direct the reader to further sources of information.

Colorectal cancer

There is a great deal of information on the role of nutrition in colorectal cancer etiology and progression drawn from epidemiologic and animal investigations. New data on the role of nutritional factors in colon cancer complement the emerging body of information on both the genetic basis of familial colorectal cancer and the understanding of the progression of colonic hyperproliferation to adenomatous and carcinomatous changes (not covered in this review). In addition to specific nutrients in the diet, other nutritional and physiologic factors including obesity, energy intake, alcohol abuse, parity, and physical activity may affect the risk of developing colorectal cancer [3]. Among the specific dietary factors are dietary fiber, vegetables, fat, and folate deficiency.

Colorectal adenomas are a reasonable precursor lesion to study for clues as to the risk of developing colorectal cancer, because most of these cancers develop on adenomatous polyps. In an epidemiologic investigation of the risk of developing colorectal adenomas, Sandler *et al.* [4] used a case-control design to compare 236 patients having histologically proven adenomas with 406 control subjects ascertained at colonoscopy without adenomas. In this study, smoking was not associated with increased risk of colorectal polyps, but alcohol was a significant risk factor for men but not women. In men, the highest tertile of beer consumers were six times as likely to develop colorectal adenomas than nondrinkers. In this study population, beer drinking was a risk factor. Animal studies can do much both to elucidate potential hypotheses raised in epidemiologic studies and to help develop intermediate markers for human intervention trials.

A great deal of interest has developed in the use of intermediate markers related to dysregulation of cellular proliferation rates (CPR) in colonic epithelial biopsy

Abbreviation

CPR—cellular proliferation rates.

© 1994 Current Science ISBN 1-85922-607-8 ISSN 0267–1379

scrapings obtained at colonoscopy. It has been proposed that conditions that increase CPR also potentiate carcinogenesis. A report that a decrease in protein kinase C was observed in colonic adenomas raised the possibility that this enzyme could also be an intermediate marker for colonic carcinogenesis.

Craven and DeRubertis [5] compared tritiated thymidine incorporation that measured CPR, total protein kinase C, subcellular distribution of protein kinase C, and protein kinase C isoenzyme masses in fasted, fasted-refed, and ad libitum-fed rats. Tritiated thymidine incorporation as expected was decreased in fasted compared with fasted-refed or ad libitum fed rats. However, there was no correlation of changes in tritiated thymidine with any of the aspects of protein kinase C measured. Despite an 11-fold increase in DNA synthesis, no changes in protein kinase C activity were noted. These results failed to support a role for protein kinase C as an intermediate marker of CPR.

Barsoum *et al.* [6] investigated the interaction of dietary calcium and small bowel resection on CPR and colon carcinogenesis in rats using rectal instillation of 1,2-dimethylhydrazine to induce cancers. They confirmed that increasing dietary calcium reduced both CPR and colorectal cancer induction. A 70% small bowel resection led to marked increases in CPR that could also be reduced by dietary calcium. In the groups treated with both calcium and surgical resection, there was no reduction in colorectal tumor incidence. The authors suggest that this finding sheds doubt on the concept of CPR as an intermediate marker, but in examining their results, it is evident that resection is a very potent stimulus to increasing CPR and that calcium only reduced CPR partially to levels still higher than those in the group treated with calcium but not surgical resection.

Although it is generally regarded that increased dietary fiber is beneficial in preventing colorectal cancer, insightful investigations by Boffa *et al.* [7••] have shed new light on the conundrum of observed increases in cellular proliferation with dietary fiber supplementation in carcinogen-treated rats. They observed the effects of increasing amounts of wheat bran fiber (0%, 5%, 10%, and 20% by weight) on CPR. Fiber is composed of soluble and insoluble fractions. The insoluble fraction decreases intestinal transit time and increases stool bulk by being indigestible, whereas soluble fibers are fermented by bacteria and increase stool weight by promoting bacterial multiplication. Short-chain fatty acids are products of soluble fiber fermentation, which is thought to increase CPR. In particular, butyric acid has been proposed to act in this way as well as other molecular and cellular mechanisms reviewed in this paper. It was found that butyric acid levels and CPR were high with the 0% fiber diet without an obvious endogenous source of production of the butyrate. A 5% fiber diet decreased CPR, but as fiber was increased to 10% and 20%, there was an increase in butyrate levels and CPR. These results suggest that moderate fiber diets may reduce colorectal cancer risk, but that diets with excessive fiber may increase colorectal cancer risk.

In a separate study of this important area, McIntyre *et al.* [8] studied butyrate production and protection from large bowel cancer in 1,2-dimethylhydrazine-treated groups fed 5% guar gum, oat bran, or wheat bran fiber in addition to the 5% or 10% pure cellulose found in the control diets. In this study, increasing butyrate found with increased fermentable fiber correlated with reduced tumor formation. However, the higher amounts of added fiber studied by Boffa *et al.* [7••] were not examined in this study.

Because human diets contain multiple nutrients, it is possible that nutrient-nutrient interactions are also important in prevention of colon carcinogenesis. Alink *et al.* [9] attempted to recreate the human diet and look for interactions. They studied five groups of rats treated with dimethylhydrazine receiving a control diet, a fruit and vegetable diet, a human diet of raw meat, raw eggs, and bread, a human diet of fried and baked meat, eggs, and bread, and a diet combining fruits and vegetables with the fried and baked human diet. The diet containing fruits and vegetables resulted in a lower tumor yield compared with the control animal diet. No differences were found between the animal diet and the control and heat-processed human diets. However, the addition of fruits and vegetables to the heat-processed human diet increased the incidence of tumors. This study will need to be repeated with additional study groups before any conclusion can be reached on its implications for human colon cancer prevention through diet.

The situation in the human colon is further complicated by the presence of different bacterial populations. Using an ingenious magnetically recoverable capsule, Rumney *et al.* [10] studied the effects of human bacterial flora compared with germ-free colonic lumens *in vivo* following various diets on the production of DNA adducting and cross-linking substances. The activity of cecal nitrate reductase, an enzyme involved in nitrosamine formation, was highest in beef fed animals, whereas trapping of cross-linking agents was highest in the high-fiber–fed animals.

Dietary selenium has been shown to be associated with a number of cancers, but Reddy *et al.* [11] examined the chemopreventive effect of 40% and 80% of the maximum tolerated dose of a novel organic form of selenium. They found inhibition at both the initiation and postinitiation phases of colon carcinogenesis associated with changes in prostaglandins and glutathione peroxidase, which may provide clues for the design of future mechanistic studies.

Vitamin E deficiency is associated with steatorrhea of more than 9 months' duration resulting from different causes, including celiac sprue and chronic pancreatitis. These latter conditions are also associated with an increased incidence of colon cancer as is a rare disorder resulting from vitamin E deficiency called brown bowel syndrome. Although there have been only 80 cases of brown bowel syndrome, Reynaert *et al.* [12•] present a case study and suggest a possible relationship between observed colorectal cancer and vitamin E deficiency, because epidemiologic studies have found that vitamin E levels are lower in patients with colonic polyps or cancer. They suggest that vitamin E status be reviewed in patients with gastrointestinal disease and that supplementation be carried out as potential preventive therapy.

Gastric cancer

Despite a decrease in the incidence of gastric cancer in the United States, gastric cancer remains a major problem in many parts of the world. In Spain, gastric cancer is the third most common cancer in men and women, and a recent case-control study conducted in Barcelona suggested that a high intake of salted, smoked, and pickled foods was associated with a high risk of gastric cancer [13]. There was a negative association with the intake of citrus fruits and raw green vegetables, but not with the intake of vegetables in general. Similarly, among the 15 fruits studied, only citrus fruits were associated with a decreased risk. The leading theory for the cause of gastric cancer implicates a chronic atrophic gastritis and the formation of free radicals and nitrosamines. Dietary sources of vitamin C, such as citrus fruits and antioxidants and folate, such as raw green vegetables, may counteract nitrosamine formation and free-radical action to inhibit gastric cancer development.

Many studies have found a clear association between salted foods and nitrites with stomach cancer, and the decrease in the incidence of this cancer in the United States has been attributed to the wide availability of refrigeration as an alternative to salting and pickling. However, in the Kashmir region of India, large amounts of salted tea are consumed (average, four cups per day; range, two to 14 cups per day). There is a high incidence of esophagitis in this region, and the consumption of this salted tea has been associated with increased esophageal and gastric cancer. Kumar *et al.* [14•] identified the formation of caffeine-derived *N*-nitroso compounds. Although the carcinogenicity of these substances is under study in rats, this is the first time that caffeine has been shown to lead to nitrosated compounds, and it is interesting to consider the possibility that tea leaves boiled under alkaline conditions can form mutagenic substances. This may explain some of the epidemiologic associations between tea drinking and esophageal cancer.

Conclusions

There is an emerging body of evidence drawn from a combination of epidemiologic and animal studies as well as from many different disciplines, suggesting strong associations between nutrition and cancers of the gastrointestinal tract. In particular, the evidence reviewed on colorectal cancer points to many potentially exciting areas of intervention for colon cancer prevention. This work is complementary to work on the molecular and genetic etiologies of colorectal cancer. As with other forms of cancer, this cancer is polygenically inherited and environmentally influenced. Only a minority of individuals developing colorectal cancer can be shown to have a strong familial predisposition, but virtually all colorectal cancer patients demonstrate the genetic lesions characteristic of cancer cells. Therefore, the complex set of events in the colonic lumen including the interactions of various nutrients, micronutrients, bacterial flora, fiber, calcium, and aspects of both physiologic and cellular function determines the risk of any given individual to develop this common form of cancer.

The work reviewed may seem to be a patchwork at this time, but a pattern of promotion of cancer by high-fat, high-meat, low-calcium, low-fiber, low-antioxidant diets is emerging. The ultimate proof of these many varied hypotheses using the limited number of established models available (*eg*, the 1,2-dimethylhydrazine-treated rat) and the limited numbers of high-risk populations will necessarily lead to the formulation of a series of dietary recommendations based on prudence and the available information. As a result of careful examination of the available scientific data, The American Cancer Society, the National Cancer Institute of the National Institutes of Health, and other governmental bodies have recommended that the general population limit the use of smoked, pickled, and salted foods, avoid excess alcohol consumption, limit dietary fat intake, and increase the intake of fruits, vegetables, cereals, and grains. As physicians treating patients at risk of gastrointestinal malignancies including colorectal cancer and gastric cancer, it is incumbent on gastroenterologists and other clinicians to see that these patients do no less.

References and recommended reading

Papers of particular interest, published within the annual period of review, have been highlighted as:
- • Of special interest
- •• Of outstanding interest

1. STATLAND BE: **Nutrition and Cancer.** *Clin Chem* 1992,
• **38**:1587–1594.

This is a good recent review of general nutritional factors that are important in preventing common forms of cancer.

2. BOZZETTI F: **Nutritional Support in the Adult Cancer Patient.**
•• *Clin Nutr* 1992, **11**:167–179.

This is an excellent recent review of the nutritional issues involved in the treatment of the malnourished cancer patient. In particular, issues related to the appropriate use of total parenteral and enteral nutrition are covered. Because a significant number of patients with colorectal and other gastrointestinal cancers present with weight loss this review will be of interest to clinicians.

3. LEVIN B: **Nutrition and Colorectal Cancer.** *Cancer* 1992, 70:1723–1726.

4. SANDLER RS, LYLES CM, MCAULIFFE C, WOOSLEY JT, KUPPER LL: **Cigarette Smoking, Alcohol, and the Risk of Colorectal Adenomas.** *Gastroenterology* 1993, 104:1445–1451.

5. CRAVEN PA, DERUBERTIS FR: **Alterations in Protein Kinase C System of Colonic Epithelium During Fasting-Refeeding.** *Dig Dis Sci* 1992, 37:1162–1169.

6. BARSOUM GH, THOMPSON H, NEOPTOLEMOS JP, KEIGHLEY MRB: **Dietary Calcium Does Not Reduce Experimental Colorectal Carcinogenesis After Small Bowel Resection Despite Reducing Cellular Proliferation.** *Gut* 1992, 33:1515–1520.

7. •• BOFFA LC, LUPTON JR, MARIANI MR, CEPPI M, NEWMARK HL, SCALMATI A, LIPKIN M: **Modulation of Colonic Epithelial Cell Proliferation, Histone Acetylation, and Luminal Short Chain Fatty Acids by Variation of Dietary Fiber (Wheat Bran) in Rats.** *Cancer Res* 1992, 52:5906–5912.

There has been a long-standing controversy regarding the role of fiber in preventing colorectal cancer; this role is largely based on rat studies in which fermentable fibers have been shown to increase cellular proliferation rates. This study demonstrates that moderate amounts of wheat bran fiber reduce cellular proliferation, whereas excessive amounts may increase cellular proliferation. This provides a major new direction for investigations relevant to the prevention of colon cancer in humans.

8. MCINTYRE A, GIBSON PR, YOUNG GP: **Butyrate Production From Dietary Fibre and Protection Against Large Bowel Cancer in a Rat Model.** *Gut* 1993, 34:386–391.

9. ALINK GM, KUIPER HA, HOLLANDERS VMH, KOEMAN JH: **Effects of Heat Processing and of Vegetables and Fruit in Human Diets on 1,2 Dimethylhydrazine-induced Colon Carcinogenesis in Rats.** *Carcinogenesis* 1993, 14:519–524.

10. RUMNEY CJ, ROWLAND IR, COUTTS TM, RANDERATH K, REDDY R, SHAH AB, ELLUL A, O'NEILL IK: **Effects of Risk-Associated Human Dietary Macrocomponents on Processes Related to Carcinogenesis in Human-Flora-Associated (HFA) Rats.** *Carcinogenesis* 1993, 14:79–84.

11. REDDY BS, RIVENSON A, KULKARNI N, UPADHYAYA P, EL-BAYOUMY K: **Chemoprevention of Colon Carcinogenesis by the Synthetic Organoselenium Compound 1,4-Phenylbis(methylene)selenocyanate.** *Cancer Res* 1992, 52:5635–5640.

12. • REYNAERT H, DEBEUCKELAERE S, DE WAELE B, MEYSMAN M, GOOSSENS A, DEVIS G: **The Brown Bowel Syndrome and Gastrointestinal Carcinoma.** *J Clin Gastroenterol* 1993, 16:48–51.

The description of this rare disease is thought-provoking in raising issues related to the possibility that vitamin E may be important in colorectal cancer prevention.

13. RAMON JM, SERRA L, CERDO C, OROMI J: **Dietary Factors and Gastric Cancer Risk.** *Cancer* 1993, 71:1731–1735.

14. • KUMAR R, MENDE P, WACKER CD, SPIEGELHALDER B, PREUSMANN R, SIDDIQI M: **Caffeine-derived N-nitroso Compounds-I: Nitrosatable Precursors From Caffeine and Their Potential Relevance in the Etiology of Oesophageal and Gastric Cancers in Kashmir, India.** *Carcinogenesis* 1992, 13:2179–2182.

This report is the first to demonstrate formation of a mutagenic nitrosated compound from caffeine and may have significance for other studies of the role of teas in the etiology of esophageal and gastric cancers.

David Heber, MD, PhD, Professor of Medicine, Chief, Division of Clinical Nutrition, and Director, UCLA Clinical Nutrition Research Unit, Department of Medicine, University of California at Los Angeles School of Medicine, 1000 Veteran Ave., Room AI-57, Los Angeles, CA 90024-1742, USA.

Nutrition and multiple organ dysfunction syndrome

Gretchen M. Ahrendt, MD, and Adrian Barbul, MD

Sinai Hospital and the Johns Hopkins Medical Institutions, Baltimore, Maryland, USA

Multiple organ dysfunction syndrome (MODS) is seen with increasing frequency in intensive care units as a result of our ability to support single-organ systems and prolong survival in patients with severe illness. One hypothesis of MODS is that altered intestinal permeability during periods of stress allows translocation of bacteria and endotoxin to sterile tissues, thereby initiating this inflammatory process. Nutritional therapy aims to maintain gastrointestinal structure and function to prevent translocation and allow absorption and metabolism of nutrients. Organ-specific nutrient therapy for the gut includes supplementation of either enteral or parenteral formulas with glutamine, arginine, specific fatty acids, and fiber. Ideally, these nutrients would provide stimulus to the gut mucosa to preserve important immune and barrier function as well as modulate the host's immune response to limit cytokine toxicity.

Current Opinion in Gastroenterology 1994, **10**:203–209

Multiple organ dysfunction syndrome (MODS) describes the clinical complex of pulmonary, hepatic, intestinal, renal, hematologic, and often cardiac failure seen in critically ill patients. The hallmark of the syndrome is that organs remote from the initial injury or primary disease process are affected, often in a predictable order [1••]. The mortality ranges between 70% and 100% [2••] and MODS remains a leading cause of death among intensive care unit patients.

Multiple organ failure can ensue from a variety of insults including infection, shock, trauma, burns, or major inflammatory processes such as severe pancreatitis [1••]. Interestingly, increased gastrointestinal permeability and bacterial translocation have been observed to occur after these same inciting events [3•,4–6,7•–9•]. The gastrointestinal tract, once thought to be quiescent during states of critical illness, is now understood to have important immunologic and barrier functions in addition to its traditional role in nutrient absorption [10]. The changes observed in small intestinal structure and function that occur during critical illness are summarized in Table 1. The observation that many patients dying of multiple organ dysfunction have bacteremias with enteric organisms without a septic focus centered attention on the role of the gut in the pathogenesis of MODS [11].

Table 1. Effects of critical illness on the small intestine*

Circulation	↑ Mesenteric vascular resistance
	↓ Mesenteric blood flow
Structure	Mucosal and submucosal edema
	Mucosal hemorrhage
	Disruption of intraepithelial tight junctions
Function	
Extraction from messenteric circulation	↓ Oxygen
	↓ Glutamine
	↓ Glucose
Metabolic activity	↓ Utilization of glucose and glutamine
	↓ Mucosal enzyme activity
Barrier	↑ Intestinal permeability to hydrophilic probes
	↑ Bacterial translocation

**Adapted from* Gardiner and Barbul [56]; with permission.

An intact functioning intestinal mucosa prevents the adherence of bacteria and endotoxin and their penetration to sterile organs and tissues. Any direct physical disruption of the gut mucosa, as may occur with ischemia or atrophy, will facilitate translocation. In addition, alterations in the normal intestinal microflora allowing overgrowth of certain organisms or impaired host immune defenses will facilitate translocation [12]. Critically ill patients taking antibiotics or antacids, and nothing orally satisfy several of these criteria, setting the stage for gut-derived sepsis. Current treatment of

Abbreviations

MODS—multiple organ dysfunction syndrome; **PUFA**—polyunsaturated fatty acid; **TPN**—total parenteral nutrition.

 ISBN 1-85922-607-8 ISSN 0267–1379

these patients usually requires individual organ support once failure is already manifested. Dietary interventions aimed at prevention of this syndrome would be desirable.

The "gut hypothesis" (Fig. 1) assumes that intestinal permeability has been altered to allow passage of bacteria or endotoxin to mesenteric lymph nodes. There is a plethora of data, both in animals and humans, demonstrating increased intestinal permeability after burn injury, endotoxin administration, trauma, and shock [3•,4–6,7•,8•,9]. An association between intestinal permeability and systemic infection in burn patients has been shown by several investigators [6,13]. A recent study by Roumen *et al.* [8•] in trauma patients and patients with hemorrhagic shock showed that intestinal permeability was increased without relation to septic complications. Increased permeability did not correlate with the severity of injury or shock or with subsequent infectious complications, adult respiratory distress syndrome, or multiple organ failure. Unfortunately, sample sizes were small in this study but the results emphasize that altered permeability is not the only factor in developing MODS. The current hypotheses of the pathophysiology of multiple organ failure have been thoroughly reviewed by Deitch [11].

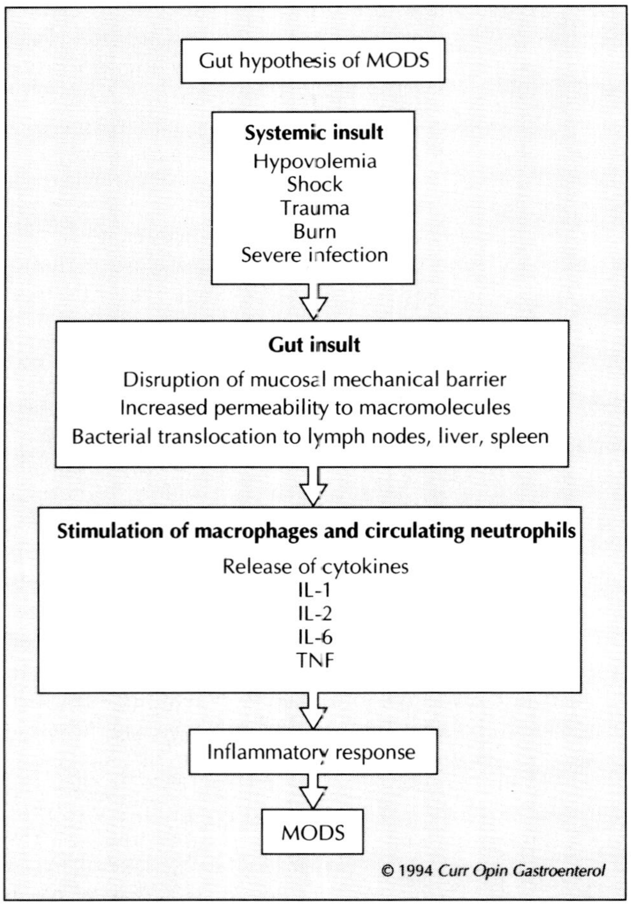

Fig. 1. Paradigm for the gut hypothesis of multiple organ dysfunction syndrome (MODS). IL—interleukin; TNF—tumor necrosis factor.

It is important to bear in mind that nutritional therapy aimed at the prevention and treatment of MODS must not only maintain gut integrity but also influence the host's immune system. Translocated, intestinally derived bacteria or endotoxin stimulate macrophages, lymphocytes, endothelial cells, and neutrophils to release cytokines, prostanoids, and reactive oxygen and nitrogen metabolites, which initiates a systemic inflammatory response [2••]. These substances are the final common pathway toward MODS and are the result of the host's own immune response. Furthermore, the microcirculatory effects of these mediators may result in gut ischemia that worsens the intestinal mucosal barrier and facilitates further translocation, thus creating a vicious cycle.

Enteral versus parenteral nutrition

The goal of nutritional support in patients with MODS is to prevent the lethal consequences of the progression of MODS while the inciting factors are identified and treated. Not only is the composition of nutrient formulas important but the route of delivery is known to have important implications for gut mucosal barrier function. Total parenteral nutrition (TPN), often used as a first line of nutritional support, may in fact be deleterious and contribute to the worsening of gut barrier dysfunction. TPN promotes intestinal mucosal atrophy [14••,15•] and has immunosuppressive effects on neutrophil and lymphocyte function and serum microbicidal activity [16••]. Also, TPN decreases brush-border amino acid and glucose transport activity [17••]. Diamine oxidase levels decrease with parenteral nutrition, reflecting the intestinal hypoplasia that occurs [18]. Parenteral feeding of trauma patients may contribute to septic morbidity when compared with enteral feeding [19].

Animal studies have demonstrated bacterial translocation in parenterally fed rats as well as animals fed TPN solution enterally [20]. A recent study in rats suggests that gut atrophy, bacterial translocation, and permeability to macromolecules are not necessarily related [14••]. In this study, TPN induced mucosal atrophy and increased permeability to lactulose but did not result in more bacterial translocation compared with chow-fed or combined enterally and parenterally fed animals. It may be that TPN primes the small intestine for a "second hit" and any additional insult tips the balance toward translocation. Spitz *et al.* [16••] propose that TPN's lack of gastrointestinal stimulation may be its most deleterious side effect and may alter host survival during critical illness.

Enteral feeding remains the most reliable mechanism of maintaining gut integrity and should be initiated early whenever possible [21]. Although it may not always be possible to deliver all nutrients enterally, there is evidence that the presence of luminal nutrients is important for intestinal mucosal metabolism and for maintenance of intestinal barrier function.

Role of specific nutrients

Glutamine

Current research focuses on specific nutrient supplementation that may attenuate mucosal atrophy and thereby prevent translocation. Glutamine has received the most attention. Glutamine, a nonessential amino acid, is not added to standard TPN formulas because of its instability during storage. During critical illness several organs have a high demand for glutamine to support cellular metabolism and function. Glutamine is the primary fuel for the enterocyte as well as other rapidly replicating cell populations including lymphocytes [22]. Glutamine requirements appear to increase markedly during catabolic states [23,24] and despite increased release of glutamine from skeletal muscle and the lung, circulating plasma levels of this amino acid fall [25]. This may create a relative state of glutamine deficiency for the demands of a stimulated immune system as well as the intestinal mucosa. In addition, gut glutamine uptake is diminished in septic patients and brush-border transport of glutamine is decreased in septic rats [26]. Impaired gut glutamine usage during critical illness is associated with structural damage to gut mucosa [27]. The intestinal mucosa is a dynamic structure that undergoes continuous sloughing and renewal necessitating a constant fuel source. Any insult that results in a higher rate of cell loss than cell renewal will necessarily impair mucosal integrity and function [28].

There is ample literature documenting that glutamine-supplemented TPN is important for gut immune function [29], maintains both B- and T-cell populations in gut lamina propria [30], and is involved in secretory IgA synthesis [31••]. Glutamine-supplemented TPN administered to rats 7 days prior to intraperitoneal *Escherichia coli* challenge improves survival compared with rats receiving standard TPN [32•]. Glutamine-supplemented TPN can improve the recovery of the small intestine from starvation atrophy as measured by intestinal mucosal weight, mucosal nitrogen content, villous height, mucosal thickness, and mucosal disaccharidase activities [33•]. Glutamine-supplemented TPN improved survival in rats after cecal ligation and puncture; it also improves nitrogen balance, and increases intestinal mucosal thickness, DNA, and protein content [34•].

Studies in humans have shown that parenteral glutamine prevents intracellular glutamine decline and improves nitrogen balance after elective abdominal surgery [35]. Bone marrow transplant recipients show a decrease in incidence of infection when given TPN supplemented with glutamine [36]. In a recent study, the addition of glutamine dipeptide to standard TPN formula preserved mucosal structure and prevented the deterioration in gut permeability observed in patients on standard TPN [37••]. The experimental data in both animals and humans suggest that during catabolic states, glutamine becomes an essential amino acid and parenteral or enteral supplementation is beneficial for both gut barrier function and immune defense.

Arginine

Arginine is known to be immunostimulatory [38–40], but its role is gut-derived sepsis has only recently been studied. With the discovery of NO (nitric oxide) as an important endogenous vasodilator, arginine has become the focus of more active interest. Arginine has been shown *in vitro* to be necessary for stimulated macrophages to perform cytotoxic effector mechanisms [41]. NO is produced by the conversion of arginine to citrulline; this pathway is thought to be the primary defense mechanism for killing of intracellular organisms by macrophages [41,42]. Gionotti *et al.* [43••] investigated the effects of diets enriched with arginine on the resistance of mice to bacterial peritonitis following cecal ligation and puncture and on the susceptibility of burned animals to gut-origin sepsis. Arginine supplementation of the standard enteral diet improved survival in mice that had undergone cecal ligation and puncture or gavage with *E. coli* and burn injury. Treatment of mice with the NO inhibitor *N*-ω-nitro-L-arginine reversed the beneficial effects of arginine on immune defenses [43••]. Importantly, these authors observed bacterial translocation to systemic organs in all groups studied. They postulated that the increased survival seen in arginine-fed animals was caused by improved ability of the host to kill translocated organisms in the mesenteric lymph nodes and the spleen.

Lipids

Dietary fat can potentially influence the immune system by altering the fatty acid composition of membrane phospholipids. Eicosanoids are metabolites of arachidonic acid, an ω6-polyunsaturated fatty acid (PUFA), and include prostaglandins, thromboxane, and leukotrienes [2••]. Certain arachidonic acid metabolites have been associated with immunosuppression, inhibiting lymphocyte proliferation, cytokine secretion, and macrophage activity [44••]. Theoretically, by manipulating the lipid content of nutrient formulas, metabolism of inflammatory cells can be altered in favor of host survival [44••]. Current TPN solutions provide ω6-PUFA, which increases arachidonic acid production and may have proinflammatory effects. Research in guinea pigs shows that feeding with ω3-PUFA (found in fish oils) improves survival after endotoxin challenge [45]. Eicosapentanoic acid is a competitive inhibitor of cyclooxygenase and thereby limits production of inflammatory eicosanoids. Similar benefits in response to endotoxin have been observed with cyclooxygenase inhibitors [46]. Eicosapentanoic acid replaces arachidonic acid in cell membranes and has been shown to reduce interleukin-1 and tumor necrosis factor production in stimulated monocytes *in vitro* [47]. Oral supplementation with ω3-PUFA significantly decreased production of interleukin 1β, tumor necrosis factor, and interleukin-6 in healthy women. This was associated with a significant decrease in the arachidonic acid to eicosapentanoic acid plasma ratio [48••], which implies that dietary modification of lipids can have an impact on cell membrane composition and in turn eicosanoid production. Lymphocyte proliferation is also reduced with ω3-PUFA, which may compromise cell-mediated immunity. Because cytokines mediate both health and disease, any dietary intervention will affect the full spectrum of cytokine-mediated events [48••]; this must be considered carefully before instituting nutritional therapy.

Prostaglandins may also have direct effects on intestinal structure. Oral prostaglandin E_2 given to parenterally fed rats potently attenuated the intestinal atrophy associated with parenteral feeding with improvement in mucosal weight, DNA content, and protein content. Importantly, no differences in the incidence or magnitude of bacterial translocation between rats receiving prostaglandin E_2 and those on standard TPN were observed [49•]. These results suggest that the preservation of mucosal structure is not all that is required to prevent bacterial translocation. The authors did not examine changes in intestinal flora or immune responses of the different groups, which could account for the persistent translocation.

In addition to the noted effects on the immune system, different lipid substrates may influence intestinal morphology and thus alter gut barrier function. Enterally administered medium-chain triglycerides have been shown to increase mucosal mass, protein content, and increase villus length and crypt depth in the proximal small intestine compared with enteral feeding of long-chain triglycerides. Medium-chain triglycerides also stimulate crypt cell renewal [50•]. Although enterocytes prefer glutamine as a fuel source, colonocytes utilize 2-, 3-, and 4-carbon short-chain fatty acids. Short-chain fatty acids are produced in the cecum and colon by bacterial fermentation of dietary fiber. The presence of short-chain fatty acids in the lumen may be important for regulating cell turnover and water absorption. Colonic infusion of short-chain fatty acids has been shown to have trophic effects on colonic mucosa [51].

Fiber

Provision of fiber and bulking agents in enteral diets has been used in attempts to normalize bowel function and minimize diarrhea; however, the effects on gut structure and function are not well defined. There is evidence that the soluble fibers pectin and guar have trophic effects on the small intestine after small bowel resection [52]. Psyllium fiber supplementation of a defined enteral diet in rats prevents loss of small bowel mass, but does not maintain jejunal mucosal thickness. In addition, fiber supplementation does not alter the incidence of spontaneous bacterial translocation of *E. coli* to mesenteric lymph nodes nor does it improve survival after endotoxin challenge [53].

In contrast, Spaeth *et al.* [54] found that the administration of cellulose fiber or kaolin, both bulk-forming agents, but not citrus-pectin (fully fermentable nonresidue fiber), prevents the bacterial translocation induced by oral administration of TPN in mice. The authors ascribed these effects to the ability of bulk-forming agents to prevent the TPN-induced changes in intestinal microflora because neither the dietary fibers nor the bulk-forming agent prevented the oral TPN–induced loss of ileal mucosal protein. Haskel *et al.* [3•] had similar results with cellulose fiber reducing the incidence of bacterial translocation in mice fed TPN orally, and found that fiber reduced cecal total anaerobic and gram-negative enteric population levels compared with the nonfiber-diet animals. Bulk-forming properties appear to be more important than fermentability in preventing translocation. The exact mechanism remains to be elucidated.

Nucleosides

Intestinal mucosal cells are constantly undergoing turnover and therefore require a continuous source of purines and pyrimidines. Glutamine, known to be an important intestinal fuel source, is also a source of nitrogen for *de novo* synthesis of nucleosides. However, in severe stress or MODS, liver synthetic capacity may be impaired, and it is attractive to postulate that dietary supplementation with nucleosides or nucleotides may prevent intestinal mucosal atrophy [15•]. Iijima *et al.* [15•] studied the effects of standard TPN, TPN supplemented with nucleosides, TPN plus glutamine, and TPN supplemented with both. Supplementation with nucleosides prevented the intestinal mucosal atrophic changes induced by TPN more effectively than glutamine supplementation. In addition, the number of crypt cells actively proliferating increased in the nucleoside- and combined-supplement groups compared with control groups [15•].

A recent prospective randomized trial attempted to evaluate the immunologic, metabolic, and clinical effects of an enteral diet supplemented with arginine, ω3-fatty acids, and RNA in patients undergoing major abdominal surgery for upper gastrointestinal malignancies [55••]. Improved lymphocyte responsiveness and decreased infections and wound complications occurred in the supplemented group. The decrease in postoperative morbidity resulted in a significantly decreased length of hospitalization. Unfortunately, the diets in this study were not isonitrogenous and the supplemented group had a significantly greater mean daily nitrogen balance than the standard group. Further clinical trials employing isocaloric, isonitrogenous diets with supplementation are warranted.

Conclusions

Multiple organ dysfunction syndrome carries a poor prognosis and with it a high cost of care for critically ill patients. Although the details of the pathophysiology are still being elucidated, there is substantial evidence that the gastrointestinal tract plays a role in the inflammatory response that can lead to multiple organ dysfunction. The potential ability to modulate this response through immunonutrition is an important area of basic research. Nutritional support in MODS should achieve several goals: 1) provide adequate calories and protein to prevent catabolism and loss of lean body mass and meet requirements for tissue healing and repair, 2) provide stimulus to the gut mucosa to preserve the important immune and barrier functions, and 3) modulate the host's immune response to downregulate cytokine toxicity.

References and recommended reading

Papers of particular interest, published within the annual period of review, have been highlighted as:

• Of special interest
•• Of outstanding interest

1. DEITCH EA: **Multiple Organ Failure.** *Adv Surg* 1993,
•• **26**:333–356.
Excellent discussion of the current hypotheses of multiple organ dysfunction: occult focus of infection, impaired oxygen delivery, gut failure, and reticuloendothelial system failure. Therapeutic options and organ-specific therapy are discussed.

2. CIPOLLE MD, PASQUALLE MD, CERRA FB: **Secondary Organ**
•• **Dysfunction: From Clinical Perspectives to Molecular Mediators.** *Circ Shock* 1993, 9:261–298.
Excellent review clarifying the terminology of sepsis, infection, systemic inflammatory response, and MODS. Current understanding of the molecular mediators of MODS including cytokines, eicosanoids, reactive oxygen and nitrogen metabolites are discussed.

3. HASKEL Y, XU D, LU Q, DEITCH E: **Elemental Diet-Induced**
• **Bacterial Translocation Can Be Hormonally Modulated.** *Ann Surg* 1993, **217**:634–643.
An elemental diet will increase bacterial translocation from the intestine, and this can be reversed by insoluble fiber or the hormone bombesin. Somatostatin reverses the beneficial effects of fiber.

4. O'DWYER ST, MICHIE HR, ZIEGLER TR, REVHAUG A, SMITH RJ, WILMORE DW: **A Single Dose of Endotoxin Increases Intestinal Permeability in Healthy Humans.** *Arch Surg* 1988, **123**:1459–1464.

5. DEITCH EA, BERG R, SPECIAN R: **Endotoxin Promotes the Translocation of Bacteria From the Gut.** *Arch Surg* 1987, **122**:185–190.

6. ZIEGLER TR, SMITH RJ, O'DWYER ST, DEMLING RH, WILMORE DW: **Increased Intestinal Permeability Associated With Infection in Burn Patients.** *Arch Surg* 1988, **123**:1313–1319.

7. RYAN CM, YARMUSH ML, BURKE JF, TOMPKINS RG: **Increased**
• **Gut Permeability Early After Burns Correlates With the Extent of Burn Injury.** *Crit Care Med* 1992, **20**:1508–1512.
In humans with at least 20% body surface–area burns, the percentage of polyethylene glycol 3350 excreted in the urine correlates with the percentage of body surface area burned.

8. ROUMEN RMH, HENDRIKS T, WEVERS RA, GORIS JA: **Intestinal**
• **Permeability After Severe Trauma and Hemorrhagic Shock Is Increased Without Relation to Septic Complications.** *Arch Surg* 1993, **128**:453–457.
A recent human study of intestinal permeability in patients following trauma or hemorrhagic shock. Intestinal permeability, reflected by lactulose to mannitol ratio, was increased in both groups compared with control groups. However, the degree of permeability did not correlate with injury severity score, APACHE II score, shock score, or plasma lactate levels. Endotoxemia was only demonstrated before the measurement of increased permeability.

9. BRATHWAITE CEM, ROSS SE, NAGELE R, MURE AJ, O'MALLEY
• KF, GARCIA-PEREZ FA: **Bacterial Translocation Occurs in Humans After Traumatic Injury: Evidence Using Immunofluorescence.** *J Trauma* 1993, **34**:586–590.
An elegant study documenting bacterial translocation after traumatic injury by demonstrating *E. coli* β-galactosidase in the cytoplasm of macrophages obtained from mesenteric lymph nodes. The study was flawed by lack of a suitable control group.

10. BAUE AE: **The Role of the Gut in the Development of Multiple Organ Dysfunction in Cardiothoracic Patients.** *Ann Thorac Surg* 1993, **55**:822–829.

11. DEITCH EA: **Multiple Organ Failure: Pathophysiology and Potential Future Therapy.** *Ann Surg* 1992, **216**:117–134.

12. DEITCH EA: **The Role of Intestinal Barrier Function and Bacterial Translocation in the Development of Systemic Infection and Multiple Organ Failure.** *Arch Surg* 1990, **125**:403–404.

13. JONES WG, MINEI JP, BARBER AE, RAYBURN JL, FAHEY TJ, SHIRES GT III, SHIRES GT: **Bacterial Translocation and Intestinal Atrophy After Thermal Injury and Burn Wound Sepsis.** *Ann Surg* 1990, **211**:399–405.

14. ILLIG KA, RYAN CK, HARDY DJ, RHODES J, LOCKE W, SAX HC:
•• **Total Parenteral Nutrition-Induced Changes in Gut Mucosal Function: Atrophy Alone is Not the Issue.** *Surgery* 1992, **112**:631–637.
Rats receiving TPN developed gut atrophy and increased permeability to lactulose but not bacterial translocation. The authors suggest that gut-origin sepsis during TPN may be caused by increased escape of macromolecules from the gut; bacterial translocation may be the end result rather than the primary cause of septic episodes.

15. IIJIMA S, TSUJINAKA T, KIDO Y, HAYASHIDA Y, ISHIDA H,
• HOMMA T, YOKOHAMA H, MORI T: **Intravenous Administration of Nucleosides and a Nucleotide Mixture Diminished Intestinal Mucosal Atrophy Induced by Total Parenteral Nutrition.** *JPEN J Parenter Enteral Nutr* 1993, **17**:265–270.
Intravenous administration of inosine, guanosine 5-monophosphate, cytidine, uridine, and thymidine with TPN prevents the intestinal mucosal atrophy associated with TPN, and this trophic effect is more potent than low-dose glutamine supplementation. Enterocyte proliferation is also enhanced.

16. SPITZ J, GANDHI S, HECHT G, ALVERDY J: **The Effects of Total**
•• **Parenteral Nutrition on Gastrointestinal Function.** *Clin Nutr* 1993, **12(Suppl 1)**:S33–S37.
The authors discuss the importance of enteral stimulation for activation of the neuroendocrine immune axis of the gut.

17. INOUE Y, ESPAT J, FROHNAPPLE DJ, EPSTEIN H, COPELAND EM,
•• SOUBA WW: **Effect of Total Parenteral Nutrition on Amino Acid and Glucose Transport by the Human Small Intestine.** *Ann Surg* 1993, **217**:604–614.
This study examined the effects of 7 days of TPN and bowel rest on amino acid and glucose transport in the human small intestine in healthy, well-nourished patients. Brush-border membrane vesicle uptake of glucose, leucine, arginine, alanine, and methyl amino isobutyric acid were significantly decreased. Transport of glutamine was not affected in this model.

18. THOMPSON JS, VAUGHAN WP, FORST CF, JACOBS DL, WEEKLY JS, RIKKERS LF: **The Effect of the Route of Nutrient Delivery on Gut Structure and Diamine Oxidase Levels.** *JPEN J Parenter Enteral Nutr* 1987, **11**:28–32.

19. Kudsk KA, Croce MA, Fabian TC, Minard G, Tolley EA, Poret A, Kuhl MR, Brown RO: **Enteral Versus Parenteral Feeding.** *Ann Surg* 1992, **215**:503–513.

20. Alverdy JC, Aoys E, Moss GS: **Total Parenteral Nutrition Promotes Bacterial Translocation From the Gut.** *Surgery* 1988, **144**:185–190.

21. Jenkins M, Gottschlich M, Alexander JW, Warden CD: **Effect of Immediate Enteral Feeding on the Hypermetabolic Response Following Severe Burn Injury.** *JPEN J Parenter Enteral Nutr* 1989, **13**:12S.

22. Ziegler TR, Smith RJ, Byrne TA, Wilmore DW: **Potential Role of Glutamine Supplementation in Nutrition Support.** *Clin Nutr* 1993, **12**:S82–S90.

23. Souba WW: **Glutamine: A Key Substrate for the Splanchnic Bed.** *Ann Rev Nutr* 1991, **11**:285–308.

24. Smith RJ: **Glutamine Metabolism and its Physiologic Importance.** *JPEN J Parenter Enteral Nutr* 1990, **14**:40S–44S.

25. Souba WW, Austgen TR: **Interorgan Glutamine Flow Following Surgery and Infection.** *JPEN J Parenter Enteral Nutr* 1990, **14**:90S–93S.

26. Salloum RM, Copeland EM, Souba WW: **Brush Border Transport of Glutamine and Other Substrates During Sepsis and Endotoxemia.** *Ann Surg* 1991, **213**:401–410.

27. Souba WW, Herskowitz K, Austgen TR, Chen MK, Salloum RH: **Glutamine Nutrition: Theoretical Considerations and Therapeutic Impact.** *JPEN J Parenter Enteral Nutr* 1990, **14(Suppl 5)**:237S–243S.

28. Jackson WD, Grand RJ: **The Human Intestinal Response to Enteral Nutrients: A Review.** *J Am Coll Nutr* 1991, **10**:500–509.

29. Burke DJ, Alverdy JC, Aoys E, Moss GS: **Glutamine-Supplemented Total Parenteral Nutrition Improves Gut Immune Function.** *Arch Surg* 1989, **124**:1396–1399.

30. Klimberg VS, Salloum RM, Kasper M, Plumley DA, Dolson DJ, Hautamaki RD, Mendenhall WR, Bova FC, Bland KI, Copeland EM, Souba WW: **Oral Glutamine Accelerated Healing of the Small Intestine and Improves Outcome After Whole Abdominal Radiation.** *Arch Surg* 1990, **125**:1040–1045.

31. •• Alverdy JA, Aoys E, Weiss-Carrington P, Burke DA: **The Effect of Glutamine-Enriched TPN on Gut Immune Cellularity.** *J Surg Res* 1992, **52**:34–38.

Standard parenteral diets result in significant decreases in biliary secretory IgA and IgA^+ plasma cells in the gut lamina propria and a marked depletion of $CD4^+$ and $CD8^+$ lymphocytes compared with chow-fed rats. Addition of glutamine to the standard TPN maintained both B- and T-cell populations.

32. • Inoue Y, Grant JP, Snyder PJ: **Effect of Glutamine-Supplemented Intravenous Nutrition on Survival After *Escherichia Coli*-Induced Peritonitis.** *JPEN J Parenter Enteral Nutr* 1993, **17**:41–46.

Additional data supporting glutamine supplementation of TPN.

33. • Inoue Y, Grant JP, Snyder PJ: **Effect of Glutamine-Supplemented Total Parenteral Nutrition on Recovery of the Small Intestine After Starvation Atrophy.** *JPEN J Parenter Enteral Nutr* 1993, **17**:165–170.

Starvation-induced intestinal mucosal atrophy (reflected in mucosal nitrogen losses, decreased villus height, and mucosal thickness), can be attenuated by the addition of glutamine to TPN solutions but recovery back to normal is not achieved.

34. • Ardawi MSM: **Effect of Glutamine-Supplemented Total Parenteral Nutrition on the Small Bowel of Septic Rats.** *Clin Nutr* 1992, **11**:207–215.

The effects of glutamine-supplemented TPN on jejunal weight, protein content, villus height, crypt depth, and overall survival in rats made septic by cecal ligation and puncture were studied. Glutamine improved all indices of small bowel morphology, nitrogen balance, and survival.

35. Hammarquist F, Wernerman J, Ali R, von der Decken A, Vinnars E: **Addition of Glutamine to Total Parenteral Nutrition After Elective Abdominal Surgery Spares Free Glutamine in Muscle, Counteracts the Fall in Muscle Protein Synthesis, and Improves Nitrogen Balance.** *Ann Surg* 1989, **209**:455–461.

36. Ziegler TR, Young LS, Benfell K, Scheltinga M, Hortos K, Bye R, Morrow FD, Jacobs DO, Smith RJ, Atin JE, Wilmore DW: **Clinical and Metabolic Efficacy of Glutamine Supplemented Parenteral Nutrition After Bone Marrow Transplant.** *Ann Intern Med* 1992, **116**:821–828.

37. •• van der Hulst RRWJ, van Kreel BK, von Meyenfeldt MF, Brummer RM, Arends JW, Deutz NEP, Soeters PB: **Glutamine and the Preservation of Gut Integrity.** *Lancet* 1993, **334**:1363–1365.

A randomized trial of patients with inflammatory bowel disease or malignancy to determine the effect of glutamine-supplemented TPN on gut function. Intestinal permeability was unchanged in the glutamine-supplemented group but increased in the standard TPN group. Villus height was normal in the glutamine group but showed a small but significant decrease in the standard group.

38. Barbul A, Wasserkrug HL, Yoshimura N, Tao R, Efron G: **High Arginine Levels in Inteavenous Hyperalimentation Abrogate Post-Injury Immune Suppression.** *J Surg Res* 1984, **36**:620–624.

39. Barbul A, Wasserkrug HL, Seifter E: **Immunostimulatory Effects of Arginine in Normal and Injured Rats.** *J Surg Res* 1980, **29**:228–235.

40. Kirk SJ, Regan MC, Wasserkrug HL, Sodeyama M, Barbul A: **Arginine Enhances T Cell Responses in Athymic Nude Mice.** *JPEN J Parenter Enteral Nutr* 1992, **16**:429–432.

41. Hibbs JB, Taintor RR, Vavrin Z: **Macrophage Cytotoxicity: Role for L-Arginine Deiminase and Imino Nitrogen Oxidation to Nitrate.** *Science* 1987, **235**:473–476.

42. Moncada S, Higgs EA: **Endogenous Nitric Oxide: Physiology, Pathology and Clinical Relevance.** *Eur J Clin Invest* 1991, **21**:361–374.

43. •• Gianotti L, Alexander JW, Pyles T, Fukushima R: **Arginine-Supplemented Diets Improve Survival in Gut-Derived Sepsis and Peritonitis by Modulating Bacterial Clearance.** *Ann Surg* 1993, **217**:644–654.

Arginine supplementation of a defined enteral diet enhanced the ability to kill translocated organisms in mice subjected to cecal ligation and puncture or gavage with *E. coli* and burn injury. Treatment with the NO inhibitor Nω-nitro-L-arginine reversed the benefits of arginine. The benefits of arginine may be mediated by enhanced bactericidal mechanisms via the arginine-NO pathway.

44. •• Blackburn GL: **Nutrition and Inflammatory Events: Highly Unsaturated Fatty Acids (ω-3 vs ω-6) in Surgical Injury.** *Proc Soc Exp Biol Med* 1992, **200**:183–188.

Manipulation of macrophage eicosanoid production with ω3-PUFA may reduce the cellular immune response by competitive inhibition of cyclooxygenase.

45. Mascioli EA, Iwasa Y, Trimbo S, Leader L, Bistrian BR, Blackburn GL: **Endotoxin Challenge After Menhaden Oil Diet: Effects on Survival of Guinea Pigs.** *Am J Clin Nutr* 1989, **49**:277–282.

46. Wise WC, Cook JA, Ellert, Halushka PV: **Ibuprofen Improves Survival From Endotoxic Shock in the Rat.** *J Pharmacol Exp Ther* 1980, **215**:160–164.

47. Billiar TR, Bankey PE, Svingen BA, Curran RD, West MA, Holman RT, Simmons RL, Cerra FB: **Fatty Acid Intake and Kupffer Cell Function: Fish Oil Alters Eicosanoid and Monokine Production to Endotoxin Stimulation.** *Surgery* 1988, **104**:343–349.

48. MEYDANI SN: **Modulation of Cytokine Production by Dietary**
•• **Polyunsaturated Fatty Acids.** *Proc Soc Exp Biol Med* 1992, **200**:189–193.

The synthesis and biologic function of cytokines can be modified by ω3-PUFA. These changes may be partially mediated via changes in the formation of arachidonic acid– and eicosapentanoic acid–derived metabolites.

49. HELTON WS: **Oral Prostaglandin E_2 Prevents Gut Atrophy**
• **During Intravenous Feeding but Not Bacterial Translocation.** *Arch Surg* 1993, **128**:178–184.

Oral supplementation with prostaglandin E_2 maintains intestinal structure during parenteral feeding but does not prevent bacterial translocation. The authors suggest that translocation is related to factors other than gut atrophy.

50. GALLUSER M, DREYFUSS H, GOSSE F, GUEROLD B,
• KACHELHOFFER J, DOFFOEL M, RAUL F: **Comparison of Different Lipid Substrates on Intestinal Adaptation in the Rat.** *Gut* 1993, **34**:1069–1074.

Enteral elemental diets containing medium-chain triglycerides increase intestinal mucosal mass and exert trophic effects on small bowel mucosa.

51. KRIPKE SA, FOX AD, BERMAN JM, SETTLE RG, ROMBEAU JL: **Stimulation of Intestinal Mucosal Growth With Intracolonic Infusion of Short Chain Fatty Acids.** *JPEN J Parenter Enteral Nutr* 1989, **13**:109–116.

52. KORUDA MJ, ROLANDELLI RH, SETTLE RG, SAUL SH, ROMBEAU JL: **The Effect of a Pectin-Supplemented Elemental Diet in Intestinal Adaptation to Massive Small Bowel Resection.** *JPEN J Parenter Enteral Nutr* 1986, **10**:343–350.

53. BARBER AE, JONES WG, MINEI JP, FAHEY TJ, MOLDAWER LL, RAYBURN JL, FISCHER E, KEOGH CV, SHIRES GT, LOWRY SF: **Glutamine or Fiber Supplementation of a Defined Formula Diet: Impact on Bacterial Translocation, Tissue Composition, and Response to Endotoxin.** *JPEN J Parenter Enteral Nutr* 1990, **14**:335–343.

54. SPAETH G, SPECIAN RD, BERG RD, DEITCH EA: **Bulk Prevents Bacterial Translocation Induced by the Oral Administration of Total Parenteral Nutrition Solution.** *JPEN J Parenter Enteral Nutr* 1990, **14**:442–447.

55. DALY JM, LIEBERMAN MD, GOLDFINE J, SHOU J, WEINTRAUB
•• F, ROSATO EF, LAVIN P: **Enteral Nutrition With Supplemental Arginine, RNA, and Omega-3-Fatty Acids in Patients After Operation: Immunologic, Metabolic, and Clinical Outcome.** *Surgery* 1992, **112**:56–67.

A recent clinical trial evaluating the benefits of an enteral diet supplemented with arginine, ω3 fatty acids, and RNA. Although clinical characteristics were similar between groups as were mean caloric intakes, nitrogen intake and balance were significantly greater in the supplemented group. Infections, wound complications, and length of hospitalization were significantly reduced in the supplemented group. Whether these benefits were due to the supplementary nutrients or improved nitrogen balance is unclear.

56. GARDINER K, BARBUL A: **Intestinal Amino Acid Absorption During Sepsis.** *JPEN J Parenter Enteral Nutr* 1993, **17**:277–283.

Gretchen M. Ahrendt, MD, and Adrian Barbul, MD, Department of Surgery, Sinai Hospital and the Johns Hopkins Medical Institutions, 2401 West Belvedere, Baltimore, MD 21215, USA.

Nutritional support in the pediatric intensive care unit

John R. Wesley, MD

Mayo Medical Center, Rochester, Minnesota, USA

The effect of malnutrition on critically ill infants in the intensive care unit includes dysfunction of most organ systems, made worse by organ immaturity and reduced intrinsic energy stores. The current review focuses on the medical and surgical literature from the past 18 months, including select overview articles, studies on infant stress, metabolic indices, and the effect of nutrition on postoperative mortality in surgical infants. Gastrointestinal priming and early enteral feeding are receiving increased emphasis, and a number of studies on the composition and physiology of nutrition support have highlighted the small margin for error in the neonatal age group, focusing on several specific vital nutrients such as vitamin A, thiamine, iron, and intravenous lipids. Updates on safety, sepsis, and vascular access are also reviewed, as are the studies on the long-term effects and complications of nutritional support, including hepatobiliary function, gut mucosal barriers to bacterial translocation, and total parental nutrition–related bone disease.

Current Opinion in Gastroenterology 1994, **10**:210–217

Effect of malnutrition on critical illness

Premature infants in the intensive care unit are difficult to nourish because of their high nutrient requirements, their complex medical needs, and the technical difficulties encountered in delivering nutrients. Moreover, malnutrition in critical illness, unlike simple starvation, results in the dysfunction of most organ systems. Because of immature organ systems and reduced energy stores in critically ill neonatal patients, malnutrition is an important determinant of outcome. This review will focus on the medical and surgical literature of the past 18 months concerning the present status of nutritional support in the neonatal period, its long-term implications, and its complications.

Three recent reviews [1••,2••,3] cover the challenging field of nutritional support of the neonatal and pediatric patient, ranging from interventional schemes based on experimental studies of the metabolism of starvation, stress, and shock to the practical considerations of establishing daily caloric budgets and providing reliable enteral and parenteral access and metabolic monitoring. *Nutrient Metabolism in Relation to the Systemic Stress Response* [1••] focuses on the specific metabolic effects of starvation and stress in the early pediatric age group, covering the functional consequences of malnutrition, the importance of efficient protein utilization for lean body mass accrual, effective means of estimating and providing for energy requirements, and the necessity of keeping a careful metabolic inventory and replacement plan for vitamins, minerals, and trace elements essential to the healing and recovery process. Although most of the extensive investigations into the hormonal and metabolic response to stress over the past 100 years have been carried out in the adult, recent attention by pediatric investigators to the often different physiology of the newborn infant and young child have covered important hormonal and metabolic responses to operative stress in the human neonate.

Wesley and Coran [2••] review the indications and limitations of parenteral nutrition, emphasizing that, although total parenteral nutrition (TPN) is an accepted practice and a potentially lifesaving therapy for pediatric patients who cannot be fed through the gastrointestinal tract, it is associated with the risk of serious metabolic, mechanical, and infectious complications. Well-defined indications for parenteral nutrition are spelled out, with careful attention given to nutritional assessment and fluid, electrolyte, vitamin, trace element, and caloric requirements. In order to achieve protein sparing with lean body mass accretion, total calories should be administered so that the nonprotein calorie to gram-nitrogen ratio is in the range of 150:1 to 250:1. Although short-term supplemental nutritional support can be administered through a peripheral vein, long-term TPN is best delivered by central venous access, either with temporary or permanent central ve-

Abbreviations

PEM—protein energy malnutrition; **TPN**—total parenteral nutrition.

 ISBN 1-85922-607-8 ISSN 0267–1379

nous access devices. Most importantly, recent experience has demonstrated that parenteral and enteral nutrition should be initiated and monitored in accordance with well-established protocols. The lowest complication rate and highest cost-effectiveness are achieved by an interdisciplinary team that includes one or more nurses, dietitians, pharmacists, and physicians.

Murray Pollack, in an excellent review of nutritional support of children in the intensive care unit, emphasizes the relationship of critical illness to malnutrition (Fig. 1) [3]. Protein energy malnutrition (PEM) occurs very early in the course of critical illness. A 6-month prospective study, assessing the nutritional status of all medical and surgical patients in a pediatric intensive care unit showed that the prevalence of acute PEM was 19% and chronic PEM was 18%. Significant somatic protein depletions and fat depletions were 21% and 14%, respectively. Children at highest risk for nutritional depletion were those less than 2 years of age and surgical patients of all ages. Pollack further emphasizes that infants and children are more likely than adults to develop PEM with critical illness for the following reasons:

1) Children have greater caloric requirements per unit weight than adults

2) Major metabolic organs (brain, heart, kidney, liver) make up 16% to 17% of body weight in children versus 5% to 6% in adults, and a child's brain consumes about 60% of basal energy requirement versus 20% in an adult

3) Children have lower caloric reserves than adults, especially infants under 1 year. Fat represents about 1% of a premature infant's weight; 16% of a full-term infant's weight, and 20% of the weight of a 1-year-old child

4) Many infants and children have decreased caloric intake leading up to critical illness, resulting in depletion of their nutritional reserves

5) Severe chronic disease leading to hospitalization are often associated with PEM

Other physiologic consequences of protein-calorie malnutrition in the neonate include dysfunction of their respiratory, cardiovascular, and immune systems, hypovolemia, gastrointestinal mucosal atrophy, decreased gastrointestinal motility, malabsorption, decreased pancreatic and hepatic function, bacterial overgrowth, and decreased erythropoietin and bone marrow stem cell function leading to anemia.

Two additional review articles are of practical use to the clinician caring for pediatric patients in an intensive care unit environment. Chwals [4••] reviews several subjects not included in other reviews, including nutrition assessment employing bioelectric impedance analysis, injury severity scores in pediatrics, and hormonal supplementation as a means of increasing the efficiency of nutritional support during injury states. *The Efficacy and Safety of Total Parenteral Nutrition* [5•] reviews the experimental evidence and clinical documentation that supports the use of TPN in selected pediatric patients. The cost and ethical issues are also briefly reviewed.

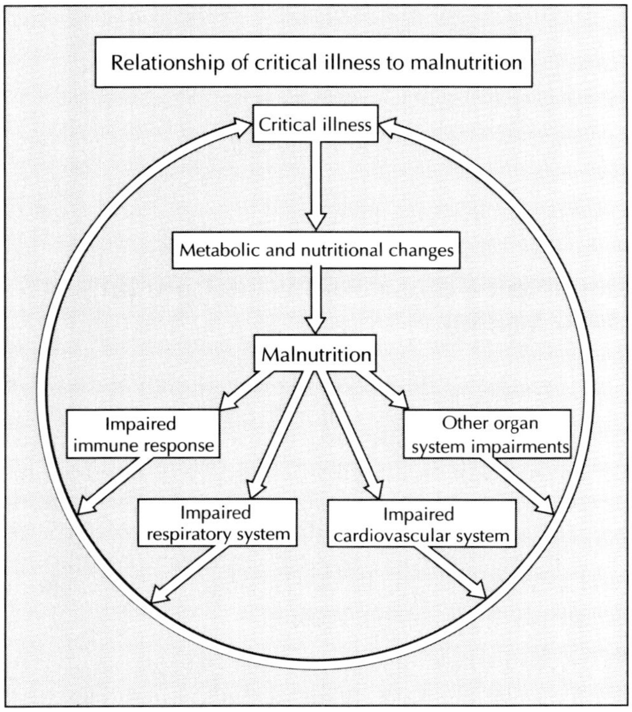

Fig. 1. Relationship of critical illness to malnutrition. (*From* Pollak [3]; with permission.)

Stress, metabolic indices, and postoperative mortality in surgical infants

Chwals *et al.* [6•] studied the metabolic response to acute injury in 41 surgical infants (average age at time of study, 47 days) and demonstrated a significant relationship between metabolic indices and clinical outcome, especially mortality. Measuring serum C-reactive protein levels and serum prealbumin levels, the authors found that infants with more depressed prealbumin levels before surgery had a high risk of dying within 30 days of surgery, suggesting that metabolic stress changes due to preoperative disease–induced injury have outcome significance independent of surgical trauma. Infants with the highest mortality risk were those whose serum prealbumin concentrations remained low beyond postoperative day 4, indicating ongoing acute injury catabolism with failure of the liver to revert back to constituitive protein synthesis. This study concluded that serial determinations of stress-associated changes in acute-phase serum protein levels have at least three important clinical implications:

1) Stratification of injury severity based on the intensity and duration of the acute metabolic stress response to the injury insult

2) Assessment of the efficacy of treatment, such as the adequate control of sepsis, during the postoperative period

3) As a marker for the return to anabolic metabolism, which is important in the proper timing of increased protein-calorie administration to keep up with increased growth requirements as acute stress metabolism resolves

Importance of gastrointestinal priming and early feeding

Neonatologists often delay the use of enteral nutrition in premature infants for fear of precipitating necrotizing enterocolitis. More recent studies, however, have found that lack of enteral feeding may result in an absence of the natural stimulus for growth of the intestinal mucosa, as well as diminished production of intestinal mucus, which acts as a barrier to bacterial translocation. Moreover, these natural stimuli are thought to be provided by enteral feeding.

In a prospective randomized trial, Meetze *et al.* [7••] showed that high-risk infants weighing less than 1250 g and receiving TPN with a background drip of enteral nutrition (n = 19) do better than infants receiving TPN alone (n = 21). Although there was no significant difference in weight gain at the end of the study, this so-called "gastrointestinal priming" improved later tolerance to feedings, accelerated the rise in serum gastrin during the first weeks of life, and did not increase the risk of necrotizing enterocolitis and other feeding complications when compared with TPN alone. Based on earlier experimental animal investigations, the authors believe that the higher serum gastrin levels play an important role in improved tolerance to enteral feeding in human infants because of the trophic effects of gastrin on the immature stomach, pancreas, and jejunum. This study supports the growing clinical practice in a number of neonatal intensive care units of starting a background drip of elemental formula or breast milk at 1 to 2 cc/h by nasogastric or nasoduodenal feeding tube as soon as practicable in order to improve the local nutrition of the enterocyte. Clinical and experimental evidence indicates a reduction in bacterial translocation and stimulation of growth of the gastrointestinal tract, particularly by the trophic factors contained in breast milk.

Blondheim *et al.* [8•], in an important study from the University of Pennsylvania, compared the effects of intermittent and continuous feedings on pulmonary function in 24 very low birth weight neonates at 2 to 4 weeks of age. All infants had a previous diagnosis of respiratory distress syndrome but no subsequent diagnosis of bronchopulmonary dysplasia. Twelve infants were randomly assigned to intermittent and 12 to continuous feedings; these infants had a similar birth weight, gestational age, study age, and baseline lung function. After intermittent feeding, however, there was a significant decrease in tidal volume (38%), minute ventilation (44%), and dynamic compliance (28%), with an accompanying increase in pulmonary resistance by 100%. In comparison, the pulmonary function data remained stable and unchanged after continuous feedings. This study demonstrated that intermittent feedings of very low birth weight infants can lead to airflow and respiratory instability and exacerbate a tendency toward respiratory distress. The effects appear to be dependent on the rate that feedings are administered; a slower pace of feeding may be more advantageous for infants prone to respiratory distress.

In a series of related studies, Berseth *et al.* [9–11] used low-compliance, continuous perfusion manometry to investigate the gastric, enteral, and duodenal motility of full-term and premature infants, adding to our understanding of the physiology of early motility and enabling earlier and safer enteral feedings. In a prospective randomized study involving 27 preterm infants, Berseth [12•] demonstrated that early feeding of preterm infants leads to an earlier establishment of full oral nutrition, fewer days of feeding intolerance, and shorter hospital stays. She found that minimal feedings could be safely administered to preterm infants and resulted in the same maturation patterns of motor activity as seen in older infants who had received full oral feedings. Early feeding enhanced the postnatal increase in serum gastrin and gastric inhibitory peptide levels as well as neurotensin and peptide YY. An increase in serum levels of these peptides parallels the improved manometrics in the growing neonate, and may be usable as markers of intestinal maturation [12•].

A similar study by Shulman and Kanarek [13] showed that enteral nutrition in very low birth weight infants is associated with a relative increase in peripheral motilin and gastrin concentrations, compared with parenterally fed infants. The net observed effect was a reduction in small-intestinal transit time. An increase in levels of motilin was observed in very low birth weight infants receiving enteral feedings over 22 days and was comparable to that in premature infants of greater gestational age. The authors concluded that early initiation of enteral feeding in very low birth weight infants results in increased blood gastrin and motilin concentrations and equivalent levels of insulin and insulin-like growth factor-1 compared with those of TPN fed infants. Although the clinical condition of the infant may also influence hormonal responses, these measurements likely reflect early metabolic, and physiologic adaptation to postnatal enteral nutrition.

Composition and physiology of nutrition support

Ongoing studies by a number of investigators in the composition and physiology of nutrition support in the premature infant have emphasized the small margin for error in this age group and have focused on several specific vital nutrients. In an important study comparing early versus delayed vitamin A supplementation in very low birth weight infants, Robbins and Fletcher [14••] focused on the function of vitamin A as a mediator of cell differentiation and repair in the lung. Low birth-weight infants (< 2000 g) have been shown to be vitamin A deficient, as evidenced by low serum vitamin A levels and low serum retinal-binding protein levels. Low vitamin A concentrations in the liver were found in infants of less than 1500 g birth weight who died within 24 hours of birth compared with term infants or older children. Infants with bronchopulmonary dysplasia had lower serum vitamin A levels in the first month of life compared with similar size infants of less than 32 weeks gestation who did not develop this disease.

The study by Robbins and Fletcher [14••] involved administering vitamin A to deficient infants in a systematic fashion to further test the hypothesis that vitamin A supplementation given to a very diverse group of very low birth weight infants at risk for bronchopulmonary dysplasia might reduce the incidence of chronic lung disease. Group I received late (10 to 14 days postnatal) initiation of supplementation versus group II, which received early supplementation (2 to 4 days postnatal). The incidence of oxygen support at 28 days was similar in both groups, although in group II there was a trend toward less vigorous ventilatory support. X^3 analysis showed that a significantly smaller proportion of infants in group II had bronchopulmonary dysplasia at 36 weeks gestation than in group I. Length of neonatal intensive care unit stay was significantly reduced in group II from 81 to 60 days. The authors emphasize that appropriate monitoring and supplementation of vitamin A levels in the low birth-weight premature infant is essential.

Two recent investigations have emphasized the importance of recognizing how rapidly thiamine deficiency, which is often lethal, can occur in infants and children. Barrett *et al.* [15] point out that the clinical presentation of the deficiency may be more florid in children receiving parenteral glucose when excess pyruvate is converted into lactate. The diagnosis should be considered in children on TPN who present with an unexpected encephalopathic illness. Parenteral thiamine, 250 mg every 6 hours, should be started and continued for 2 days while waiting for the results of red cell transketolase activation studies, a sensitive measure of thiamine deficiency. Seear *et al.* [16] unexpectedly uncovered findings of Wernicke encephalopathy (thiamine deficiency) at autopsy in three children who died after prolonged enteral feedings. They prospectively investigated the vitamin B status of three groups of children, 27 patients fed entirely by nasogastric tubes for 6 months or more, 80 infants and children admitted to a pediatric intensive care unit for 2 weeks or longer, and six children receiving intensive chemotherapy. Thiamine deficiency was detected in 10 of the 80 patients receiving intensive care, and four of six patients receiving chemotherapy, prompting the investigators to conclude that this potentially fatal, but treatable disease, can occur in malnourished patients of any age and is probably underdiagnosed among chronically ill children. They recommend an enteral thiamine dose of 0.5 mg/kg/d for high-risk children.

The intake of iron during TPN has been established on the basis of the bioavailability of orally administrated iron, resulting in a generally accepted recommendation of TPN-iron intake of 100 µg/kg/d, corresponding to 10% of the recommended oral intake. Hariz *et al.* [17•] evaluated the iron status of 30 children aged 1 to 18 years receiving TPN for an average of 43 months with iron intakes of 100 µg/kg/d [17•]. Iron status was assessed by measuring the serum iron and ferritin levels and the transferrin saturation coefficient as a function of iron intake. Twelve children had serum ferritin levels greater than 300 ng/mL (the upper limit of normal), and eight had levels greater than 800 ng/mL. The serum ferritin level and the transferrin saturation coefficient were positively correlated ($r = 0.81$; $P < 0.01$). The serum ferritin level was also positively correlated with TPN duration and with the total iron intake ($r = 0.68$; $P < 0.01$). Thirteen liver biopsy specimens were also obtained, of which six showed signs of iron deposition. The authors concluded that there is a risk of iron overload in children receiving 100 µg/kg/d by TPN, indicating that the intake of iron should be reduced.

Premature newborn infants have metabolic evidence of essential fatty acid deficiency as early as 5 to 8 days postpartum and, when they cannot be fed enterally, lipid infusion is considered an essential clinical requirement. Salas-Salvado *et al.* [18••], in an excellent study from the University of Barcelona, compared the effects of varying the proportion of energy administration as carbohydrates and fats within a range normally applicable in clinical practice in 26 newborn infants divided into three groups. The energy substrate utilization, gas exchange, and protein metabolism were measured comparing three different isocaloric, isonitrogenous TPN solutions in which only the proportions of calories derived from fat and glucose were varied. Maximum fat oxidation was observed in group C receiving 2 g/kg/d, in which energy delivered by fat represented 40% of total calories. This group was more energy efficient than group A (18% fat) or group B (29% fat). Despite the differences in carbon dioxide production (highest in group A), arteriocapillary PCO_2 was not effected, indicating that adequate pulmonary compensation occurred during the low-fat, high carbohydrate regimen. Although arteriocapillary PO_2 was significantly lower during the high-fat regimen ($P<0.05$), protein retention was significantly enhanced. Protein oxidation was significantly greater in group A (1.14±0.32 g/kg/d), than in group B (0.70±0.21 g/kg/d) or group C (0.78±−0.28 g/kg/d). Energy expenditure in groups A and B were significantly higher than in group C. The higher fat infusion in group C was accompanied by slight changes in the plasma lipid profile, which may indicate possible adverse effects of long-term lipid infusion. Patients in this study had neither sepsis nor infection, and only five were studied 6 to 10 days after surgery. Overall, the results indicate that the addition of more calories as fat emulsion significantly reduces protein oxidation while significantly enhancing protein retention. High-glucose TPN regimens, therefore, should not be advocated, as they result in decreased protein retention and increased energy expenditure.

Another important study of intravenously administered lipids by Haumont *et al.* [19•] demonstrated that the use of a 20% rather than a 10% fat emulsion allows for efficient triglyceride clearance in low birth-weight neonates, even in higher triglyceride intake levels of up to 4 g/kg/d. This is due to the presence of lipoprotein x-like particles in the low density lipoprotein fraction of the 10% emulsion, which are not present in the 20% solution. The net result is safer administration of lipids at a level greater than 2 g triglycerides/kg/d to low birth-weight infants.

Safety, sepsis, and vascular access

The high-tech evolution of increasingly more sophisticated and sensitive pumps and monitoring devices in the neonatal intensive care unit continues at a rapid rate, improving the level of care obtainable for sick neonates, while at the same time driving up the daily cost. It is always refreshing to encounter simple techniques for improved monitoring with less risk and reduced cost. Such a study is reported by Greenberg *et al.* [20•], using real-time portable ultrasonography to examine the pylorus of infants in the intensive care unit for confirmation of feeding tube placement. The technique is rapid and easy in the neonatal population because of the small size of the patients and the small fluid volume needed to visualize the pylorus. Eight of 26 tubes located by ultrasonography were not able to be localized by radiography. Demonstrated advantages over radiography included bedside real-time placement, enhanced ability to locate the tube relative to the pylorus, no exposure to ionizing radiation, and the capacity to detect transpyloric reflux. This technique has the potential for greater ease of application and reduced cost in neonatal and pediatric intensive care units in which an ultrasound machine is readily available.

Further cost savings can be obtained by reducing the frequency and extent of biochemical monitoring of infants on TPN in the intensive care unit. Puntis *et al.* [21], in a study involving 30 consecutive patients on parenteral nutrition, demonstrated that electrolyte disturbance most commonly occurs before starting parenteral nutrition and that subsequent biochemical abnormalities are generally found only in patients with clinically obvious fluid and electrolyte losses. Traditional protocols for biochemical surveillance during parenteral nutrition error on the side of caution and often suggest frequent and comprehensive blood and urine tests. Once intensive care unit patients are stabilized, this is both expensive and unnecessary. Puntis *et al.* justify and advocate a much simpler monitoring regimen with less frequent biochemical surveillance, which is more cost effective without sacrificing safety.

At Osaka University Medical School, Inoue *et al.* [22] have developed a new technique that markedly reduced catheter-related sepsis during parenteral nutrition. This consists of an "I" system that combines the advantages of a rubber diaphragm with the security of a Luer-Lok (Becton-Dickinson, Rutherford, NJ, USA), and, when used in place of the standard Luer-Lok connecter in a prospective study involving 230 patients, resulted in a significantly lower incidence of catheter-related sepsis (1.89% per catheter) compared with a control group (12.1% per catheter). Furthermore, the average duration of use of each catheter was significantly longer in the study group than in the control group. The discussion of this paper provides a good overview of the important problem of catheter sepsis in the pediatric intensive care unit.

Klein and Shahrivar [23] confirmed the efficacy of percutaneous silastic central venous catheters in 35 neonates studied prospectively in a neonatal intensive care unit with the average duration of catheterization 32±18.2 SD days; 19 patients (56%) had lines in place for more than 30 days. Five patients had mechanical complications (15%) and four cases of bacteremia were identified, representing 3.7 infections per 1000 days of catheter use. Two patients required catheter removal to clear the bacteremia, and two were successfully treated by administration of antibiotic therapy through the central catheter. Placement of a percutaneous subclavian central silastic line obviates a cut-down and further simplifies the total care of sick neonates while reducing the costs.

The entire subject of long-term central venous access devices is reviewed in a new and extremely useful journal, *Seminars in Pediatric Surgery* [25••]. Totally implantable venous access systems have been successfully used for long-term infusion of chemotherapeutic agents, antibiotics, blood products, and total parenteral nutrition in infants and children accompanied by decreased complication rates, improved patient comfort, and increased cost-effectiveness. The recent introduction of permanent peripheral central venous catheters has further decreased the expense and complication rate of long-term venous access in infants and children. The evolution of new catheter materials and the accumulated expertise in finding alternative venous access sites (common fascial, deep inferior epigastric, lumbar, and azygos veins) have helped minimize mechanical and septic complications and have increased the safety of even the most difficult venous access procedures [24•].

Long-term effects and complications

Any discussion of the long-term effects and complications of nutrition support in sick neonates must inevitably include the hepatobiliary system. The importance of and frustrations with the topic are reflected in a number of excellent reviews that have appeared over the past 10 years. The most recent and comprehensive is provided by Quigley *et al.* [24•]. He emphasizes that it is often difficult to extricate the effects of TPN on hepatobiliary function from the many other hepatotoxic factors that may occur in these sick neonates. Considerable evidence supports a role for caloric excess in TPN solutions as the pathogenesis of steatosis in older children and young adults. However, a loss of enteric stimulation, and not TPN per se, may be the primary factor in the development of cholestasis, biliary sludge, and gallstones in neonates and young infants. The predilection of infants to TPN-related cholestasis may be based on the relative immaturity of the neonatal liver and biliary excretory system. In the majority of young patients receiving TPN, enzyme elevations are usually mild and often transient. Most series report either a fall or normalization of these elevated enzyme levels despite continuance of TPN. In cases where mild elevation persists, normalization usually occurs when the TPN is stopped. Reports of severe hepatic complications of TPN have generally been confined to low birth-weight premature infants, and infants with severe short bowel syndrome. The precise incidence of hepatic dysfunction in this age group remains to be fully defined, and has varied from as low as 7.4% to as high as 84%.

In addition to the adverse effects of sepsis on TPN-associated liver failure, Quigley *et al.* [24•] reviewed the role of peroxidase free-radical damage caused by TPN-related deficiencies of vitamin E and selenium, and the ameliorating role of taurine. Recent studies suggest that TPN may decrease the natural barrier to bacteria by reducing intestinal mucous production and impairing local immunity. Translocation of bacteria across the gut wall is promoted in animal studies by both oral and intravenous administration of TPN solutions and prevented by the addition of fiber. TPN-related translocation is thought to be mediated both by structural change in the intestinal mucosa and by the development of small intestinal bacterial overgrowth. Fiber supplementation inhibits the latter. In addition, the administration of glutamine appears to have a protective effect against TPN-related hepatic dysfunction through an effect on gut immunity. Glutamine enrichment of TPN solutions has been shown not only to attenuate TPN-associated gut hypoplasia, but also to prevent TPN depletion of gut lamina propia plasma cells, which produce immunoglobulin A. Quigley also reviews the detrimental effects of cholestatic metabolites caused by the degradation of tryptophan in TPN solutions contaminated by sodium bisulfite and the toxic effect of aluminum. Recommendations for prevention of TPN-related liver injury include 1) avoidance of excess caloric loads by accurate measurement and prediction of energy requirements, 2) cycling of TPN during the day, 3) early resumption of oral intake, and 4) avoidance of excessive amino acid loads. Whereas the administration of phenobarbital has been advocated by some clinicians to reduce neonatal cholestasis, its beneficial effect has not been consistent.

Another important complication of long-term TPN is reviewed by Koo [26•]: parenteral nutrition–related bone disease. Koo emphasizes that our incomplete understanding of the pathogenesis of parenteral nutrition–related bone disease is complicated by the effect of underlying illnesses, therapeutic interventions, and preexisting nutrition deficiencies before the initiation of parenteral nutrition therapy. The typical radiographic manifestations in infants include osteopenia, fractures, and the bowing characteristic of rickets. Although the prevalence of nutrition-related bone disease associated with parenteral nutrition is unknown, infants with the lowest gestational ages and birth weights tend to develop bone disease after a much shorter period of parenteral nutrition support compared with older children and adults. Paradoxically, the effects of underlying illnesses and associated nutritional deficiencies, including disturbed mineral homeostasis and low bone mineral content, may become more prominent as the general nutritional status of the infant improves. For example, nutritional rickets tends to develop during the period of postnatal "catch-up" growth during recovery from serious illness.

Koo [26•] emphasizes the complex interrelation of various nutrients such as calcium, phosphorus, and vitamin D in their effects on bone mineralization, and that this increases the difficulty in defining the role of a single nutrient in the development of bone disease. Of the many factors that are important in the development of parenteral nutrition–related bone disease, however, some factors, such as increased mineral requirement, are unique to growing infants whereas other factors, such as aluminum toxicity, may be common to both adult and pediatric populations. Nonnutritional factors, including long-term use of potent loop diuretics and altered acid-base status, can affect urine mineral loss, cell metabolism, and bone mineralization, particularly in small, premature infants. Other investigators, such as Prestridge *et al.* [27], have studied the effect of parenteral calcium and phosphorus therapy on mineral retention and bone mineral content in very low birth weight infants, and concur, along with Koo [26•], that failure to provide adequate calcium and phosphorus is critical in the development of nutrition-related bone disease. Current evidence indicates that the cause of parenteral nutrition–related bone disease is multifactoral, and the prevention of parenteral nutrition–related bone disease is under continued investigation for the exact sequence of pathogenic events.

References and recommended reading

Papers of particular interest, published within the annual period of review, have been highlighted as:

- • Of special interest
- •• Of outstanding interest

1. WESLEY JR: **Nutrient Metabolism in Relation to the Systemic Stress Response**. In *Pediatric Critical Care*. Edited by Fuhrsman BP, Zimmerman JJ. St. Louis: Mosby-Year Book; 1992:755–774.
••

This chapter reviews the altered metabolic (nutrient) equilibrium of critical illness in infants and children, including a discussion of the fuel conservation of starvation, the neuroendocrine response to stress, the functional consequences of malnutrition, as evidenced by altered hepatic secretory protein output, secondary immunodeficiency, altered skeletal muscle function, and altered organ function. Also emphasized and reviewed is the importance of estimating and providing for energy requirements, the necessity for keeping a careful metabolic inventory and replacement plan for vitamins, minerals, and trace elements essential to the healing and recovering process, and a discussion of the advantages and limitations of specialized nutrition support of the critically ill child.

2. WESLEY JR, CORAN AG: **Intravenous Nutrition for the Pediatric Patient**. *Semin Pediatr Surg* 1992, **1**:212–230.
••

This is a "how to do it" review of the indications for parenteral nutrition in the critically ill infant, focusing on nutrition requirements, estimation of energy requirements, the administration and composition of daily parenteral nutrition, technical, septic, and metabolic complications of TPN and a discussion of home parenteral nutrition.

3. POLLAK MM: **Nutritional Support in the Intensive Care Unit**. In *Textbook of Pediatric Nutrition, 2nd edn*. Edited by Suskind RM, Suskind LL. Philadelphia: WB Saunders; 1989:1118–1125.

4. CHWALS WJ: **Metabolism and Nutritional Frontiers in Pediatric Surgical Patients**. *Pediatr Surg* 1992, 72:1237–1266.
••

This is an excellent and concise review of the current status of nutritional support in the pediatric age group, including new areas of investigation into cytokines, bacterial translocation, glutamine, peptide growth factors, growth hormone supplementation, and nutritional immunomodulation with ω-3 fatty acids, nucleotides, and arginine.

5. WESLEY JR: **Efficacy and Safety of Total Parenteral Nutrition**. *Mayo Clin Proc* 1992, 67:671–675.
•

This is a review of selected studies that document and justify the use of TPN in selected pediatric patients.

6. CHWALS WJ, FERNANDEZ ME, JAMIE AC, CHARLES BJ: **Relationship of Metabolic Indexes to Postoperative Mortality in Surgical Infants**. *J Pediatr Surg* 1993, **28**:819–822.
•

This study measures the cytokine (tumor necrosis factor), acute-phase protein (C-reactive protein), and visceral protein (prealbumin) responses to acute metabolic stress in 41 infants. The results suggest an increased risk of poor outcome if metabolic stress has not abated by the fourth postoperative day and is one of the first studies to illustrate this significant relationship.

7. MEETZE WH, VALENTINE C, MCGUIGAN JE, CONLON M, SACKS N, NEU J: **Gastrointestinal Priming Prior to Full Enteral Nutrition in Very Low Birth Weight Infants**. *J Pediatr Gastroenterol Nutr* 1992, **15**:163–170.
••

This is an important paper demonstrating that high-risk infants requiring TPN and given a background drip of enteral nutrition have fewer septic complications and recover gastrointestinal function faster than infants receiving TPN alone.

8. BLONDHEIM O, ABBASI S, FOX WW, BHUTANI VK: **Effect of Enteral Gavage Feeding Rate on Pulmonary Functions of Very Low Birth Weight Infants**. *J Pediatr* 1993, **122**:751–755.
•

This is an important study demonstrating that low birth-weight infants at 2 to 4 weeks of age receiving continuous feedings maintain better pulmonary function and have less respiratory distress than infants receiving intermittent bolus feedings.

9. BERSETH CL, ITTMANN PI: **Antral and Duodenal Motor Responses to Duodenal Feeding in Preterm and Term Infants**. *J Pediatr Gastroenterol Nutr* 1992, **14**:182–186.

10. BERSETH CL, MCCOY HH: **Birth Asphyxia Alters Neonatal Intestinal Motility in Term Neonates**. *Pediatrics* 1992, 90:669–673.

11. BERSETH CL, NORDYKE CK: **Manometry Can Predict Feeding Readiness in Preterm Infants**. *Gastroenterology* 1992, **103**:1523–1528.

12. BERSETH CL: **Effect of Early Feeding on Maturation of the Preterm Infant's Small Intestine**. *J Pediatr* 1992, **120**:947–953.
•

This is an important prospective randomized study demonstrating that early feeding of preterm infants leads to earlier establishment of full oral nutrition, fewer days of feeding intolerance, and shorter hospital stays.

13. SHULMAN DI, KANAREK K: **Gastrin, Motilin, Insulin, and Insulin-Like Growth Factor-I Concentrations in Very-Low-Birth-Weight Infants Receiving Enteral or Parenteral Nutrition**. *JPEN J Parenter Enteral Nutr* 1993, 17:130–133.

14. ROBBINS ST, FLETCHER AB: **Early vs Delayed Vitamin A Supplementation in Very-Low-Birth-Weight Infants**. *JPEN J Parenter Enteral Nutr* 1993, 17:220–225.
••

Tests the hypothesis that vitamin A administration in a systematic fashion to a very diverse group of very low birth weight infants at risk for BPD might reduce the incidence of chronic lung disease. Infants so treated trend toward requiring less vigorous ventilatory support and show significantly less BPD at 36 weeks gestation than infants not receiving vitamin A supplementation.

15. BARRETT TG, FORSYTH JM, NATHAVITHARANA KA, BOOTH IW: **Potentially Lethal Thiamine Deficiency Complicating Parenteral Nutrition in Children**. *Lancet* 1993, **341**:901.

16. SEEAR M, LOCKITCH G, JACOBSON B, QUIGLEY G, MACNAB A: **Thiamine, Riboflavin, and Pyridoxine Deficiencies in a Population of Critically Ill Children**. *J Pediatr* 1992, **121**:533–538.

17. HARIZ MB, GOULET O, DE POTTER S, GIROT R, RAMBAUD C. COLOMB V, CORRIOL O, RICOUR C: **Iron Overload in Children Receiving Prolonged Parenteral Nutrition**. *J Pediatr* 1993, 123:238–241.
•

Commonly accepted doses for administering iron with TPN may result in chronically elevated serum iron and ferratin levels, deposition of iron in the liver, and iron toxicity. The routine parenteral iron intake in children receiving TPN should be reduced.

18. SALAS-SALVADO J, MOLINA J, FIGUERAS J, MASSO J: **Effect of the Quality of Infused Energy on Substrate Utilization in the Newborn Receiving Total Parenteral Nutrition**. *Pediatr Res* 1993, 33:112–117.
••

This important and well done study compares the energy substrate utilization, gas exchange, and protein metabolism in three matched groups of newborn infants receiving three different isocaloric, isonitrogenous TPN solutions in which only the proportions of calories derived from fat and glucose were varied. Although arterial capillary PO_2 was lower during the high-fat regimen, TPN regimens containing between 29% and 40% of calories as fat emulsion result in enhanced protein retention.

19. HAUMONT D, RICHELLE M, DECKELBAUM RJ, COUSSAERT E, CAPRENTIER YA: **Effect of Liposomal Content of Lipid Emulsions on Plasma Lipid Concentrations in Low Birth Weight**
•

Infants Receiving Parenteral Nutrition. *J Pediatr* 1992, **121**:759–763.
The use of 20% rather than 10% fat emulsion allows for more efficient triglyceride clearance, even at a higher triglyceride intake. This difference is interpreted in part to a lipoprotein X-like particle together with an increase in intermediate-density lipoprotein fraction in infants who receive 10% emulsion.

20. • GREENBERG M, BEJAR R, ASSER S: **Confirmation of Transpyloric Feeding Tube Placement by Ultrasonography**. *J Pediatr* 1993, **122**:413–415.
This is a comparison of ultrasonography with radiography for placement and confirmation of transpyloric feeding tubes, demonstrating the greater ease, less radiation, and "real time" advantages of ultrasound in the pediatric intensive care unit.

21. PUNTIS JWL, HALL SK, GREEN A, SMITH DE, WALL PA, BOOTH IW: **Biochemical Stability During Parenteral Nutrition in Children**. *Clin Nutr* 1993, **12**:153–159.

22. INOUE Y, NEZU R, MATSUDA H, FUJII M, NAKAI S, WASA M, TAKAGI Y, OKADA A: **Prevention of Catheter-Related Sepsis During Parenteral Nutrition: Effect of a New Connection Device**. *JPEN J Parenter Enteral Nutr* 1992, **16**:581–585.

23. KLEIN JF, SHAHRIVAR F: **Use of Percutaneous Silastic Central Venous Catheters in Neonates and the Management of Infectious Complications**. *Am J Perinatol* 1992, **9**:261–264.

24. • QUIGLEY EM, MARSH MN, SHAFFER JL, MARKIN RS: **Hepatobiliary Complications of Total Parenteral Nutrition**. *Gastroenterology* 1993, **104**:286–301.
This is an excellent and comprehensive review and is highly recommended for those taking care of both infants and older children.

25. •• WESLEY JR: **Permanent Central Venous Access Devices**. *Semin Pediatr Surg* 1992, **1**:118–201.
This is a comprehensive review of not only the many venous access devices available but techniques of insertion and alternative insertion sites to be considered when the standard sites have been exhausted.

26. • KOO WWK: **Parenteral Nutrition-Related Bone Disease**. *JPEN J Parenter Enteral Nutr* 1992, **16**:386–394.
This is an excellent review of an important problem in the pediatric age group by a highly regarded current investigator in pediatric TPN-related bone disease.

27. PRESTRIDGE LL, SCHANLER BJ, SHULMAN RJ, BURNS PA, LAINE LL: **Effect of Parenteral Calcium and Phosphorus Therapy on Mineral Retention and Bone Mineral Content in Very Low Birth Weight Infants**. *J Pediatr* 1993, **122**:761–768.

John R. Wesley, MD, Pediatric Surgery, 5301 F Street, Suite 216, Sacramento, CA 95819, USA.

Nutrition in HIV infection

Kathleen Mulligan, PhD*‡, and Carl Grunfeld, MD, PhD†‡

*San Francisco General Hospital, †Department of Veterans Affairs Medical Center, and ‡University of California, San Francisco, California, USA

Body wasting, characterized by loss of body cell mass, is a frequent accompaniment to infection with HIV and is a factor in survival itself. Periods of rapid weight loss are typically associated with episodes of secondary infection. Chronic weight loss is usually the result of gastrointestinal disorders. Increased rates of resting energy expenditure and alterations in lipid, protein, and carbohydrate metabolism have been noted in persons with HIV infection. However, no statistical association has been demonstrated between these alterations and the wasting syndrome. Therapies that increase energy intake can increase body weight but do not consistently restore body cell mass. Treatment with recombinant human growth hormone has increased body weight, nitrogen retention, and lean body mass in patients with the wasting syndrome. If these promising results can be sustained during long-term therapy, anabolic agents such as recombinant human growth hormone may be effective in reversing or forestalling HIV-associated wasting.

Current Opinion in Gastorenterology 1994, **10**:218–226

Body wasting is a frequent and potentially devastating accompaniment to infection with HIV. Wasting can impair functional performance, immune function, and quality of life. In many patients infected with HIV, death occurs when body cell mass (BCM) is depleted below a level that is critical to sustain life [1], implying that death in these patients may be due to malnutrition per se, rather than the direct effects of infection and malignancy.

The demonstrated associations between loss of body weight or BCM and survival imply that maintenance or restoration of weight or BCM could prolong life in HIV-infected persons [1]. Thus, considerable effort has been directed to the search for effective anabolic therapies. Evaluation of their efficacy has shed further light on the mechanisms underlying HIV-associated wasting.

Energy balance in HIV infection

Maintenance of energy balance is achieved when energy intake matches expenditure. However, without precise quantification of changes in body composition, simple examination of the external components of the energy balance equation provides an unsatisfactory framework for evaluation of the processes underlying the wasting syndrome. For example, increases in resting energy expenditure (REE) averaging from 8% to greater than 30% have been extensively demonstrated in patients on all points along the spectrum of HIV infection [2–4,5•,6••].

Although REE is not increased in every HIV-infected person [7,8], hypermetabolism is a common hallmark of HIV infection and has been hypothesized to contribute to HIV-associated weight loss. Mathematical analysis, however, demonstrates that hypermetabolism alone cannot explain the magnitude of loss of body weight [2–4] or specific loss of BCM in HIV infection. Increases in REE have been noted in HIV-infected patients with stable or changing weight. There was no correlation between REE and weight change in these patients [4]. In addition, it is theoretically possible to compensate for relatively modest increases in REE by increasing energy intake [9••]. However, as will be discussed later, increasing energy and macronutrient intake does not necessarily restore BCM [10,11,12•,13,14].

Rapid weight loss was found in HIV-infected patients with secondary infection who have significant anorexia [4]. Short-term weight change in these patients correlated with caloric intake. Although hypermetabolism per se does not drive weight loss, it certainly contributes to weight loss in combination with anorexia.

Abbreviations
BCM—body cell mass; **REE**—resting energy expenditure.

 ISBN 1-85922-607-8 ISSN 0267–1379

Healthy subjects who decrease energy intake have decreased rates of REE [15]. In contrast, in HIV infection, particularly during episodes of secondary infection when energy intake is reduced, REE remains elevated [4] or increases further [5•]. Thus, the combined energy deficit resulting from anorexia and hypermetabolism accelerates weight loss [4,5•].

Characterizing patterns of weight loss

Mechanistic studies first indicated that rapid weight loss was associated with secondary infection [4]. Now, in the 8th year after "slim disease" was first described [16], prospective analysis of changes in weight and associated manifestations of HIV infection has demonstrated statistical associations between the patterns of weight loss and clinical events.

Macallan *et al.* [17••] examined weight changes over periods ranging from 9 to 49 months in 30 men with AIDS-defining conditions (Fig. 1). Episodes of acute weight loss (>4 kg in <4 months) were associated primarily with nongastrointestinal systemic infections such as *pneumocystis carinii* pneumonia [17••]. Such infections had previously been associated with significant decreases in energy intake [4]. On the other hand, chronic weight loss events (>4 kg occurring over >4 months) were most often associated with gastrointestinal disease and presumed malabsorption, a frequent complication of HIV infection [18,19]. Significantly, periods of weight stability were noted in 43% of the individuals studied, and episodes of weight gain (>4 kg) were recorded in the majority of patients, typically occurring during recovery from infections such as *pneumocystis carinii* pneumonia. These results demonstrate that weight loss is not necessarily a steadily progressive phenomenon in persons with HIV infection. Nonetheless, it should be emphasized that there was a pronounced net decline in median weight from 74.5 to 56.0 kg during the long period of study, indicative of failure to fully regain weight lost during episodes of secondary infection or malabsorption.

The results reported by Macallan *et al.* [17••] underscore the utility of carefully recorded weight data in regular medical care of HIV-infected persons [20••]. Examination of body weight alone, however, does not adequately describe the effects of HIV infection on body composition. Studies using total body potassium counting and isotope dilution techniques have documented a disproportionate depletion of BCM and intracellular fluid volumes in persons with HIV infection [21,22•]. It has also been reported that some persons with HIV infection fail to fully replenish these compartments during periods of clinical stability [21] and nutritional therapy [10]. It is possible that changes in body composition may begin in the early stages of HIV infection. Ott *et al.* [23•] reported reductions in BCM and increases in extracellular fluid volumes, estimated by bioelectrical impedance analysis, in a group of otherwise asymptomatic HIV-positive men whose body weight and body mass index matched HIV-negative controls.

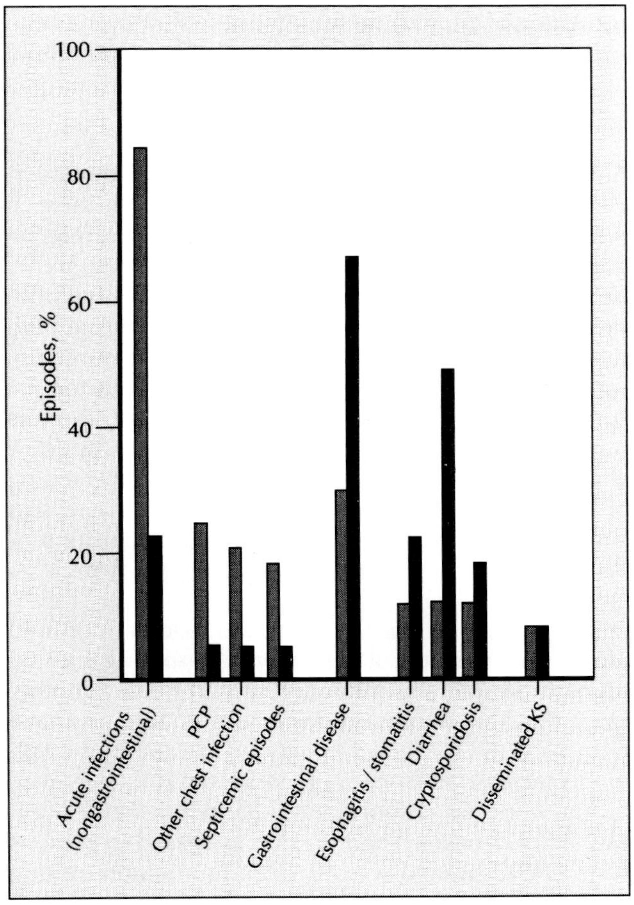

Fig. 1. Clinical features associated with episodes of acute weight loss in less than 4 months (*lightly shaded bars*) compared with episodes of chronic weight loss in 4 months or more (*darkly shaded bars*). Acute infections and gastrointestinal disease are subdivided into major categories. Several weight-loss episodes were associated with more than one clinical event. KS—Kaposi's sarcoma; PCP—*Pneumocystis carinii* pneumonia. (*From* Macallan *et al.* [17••]; with permission).

Metabolic alterations in HIV infection

The metabolic alterations described in the following paragraphs could contribute to loss of BCM in HIV infection if the result is net redirection of substrates in ways that are metabolically inappropriate. However, it should be noted that the statistical association between these alterations and wasting has not been demonstrated. Furthermore, the biochemical mediators and teleologic significance of these alterations remain to be adequately described.

Alterations in lipid metabolism

HIV infection is associated with strikingly elevated plasma triglyceride concentrations [24,25]. Associated alterations in lipid metabolism that have been documented in persons with HIV infection include decreased lipoprotein lipase activity and triglyceride clearance [25], increased plasma free–fatty acid concentrations [25], and increased rates of *de novo* hepatic lipogenesis [26••]. There have also been reports of tendencies to increased rates of whole-body lipolysis [6••,27] and nonoxidative lipid disposal [6••].

Although one recent report suggested a correlation between triglyceride levels and survival [28], there is no statistical association between hypertriglyceridemia and wasting [24]. Because hypertriglyceridemia occurs late in HIV infection (predominantly at CD4 lymphocyte counts less than 200), it occurs in patients at high risk for other adverse events. No data have been presented that hypertriglyceridemia is a risk factor for survival independent of CD4 counts. In fact, there is no evidence that hypertriglyceridemia per se or other changes in lipid metabolism are harmful in the setting of HIV infection. Instead, it has been speculated that some changes in lipid metabolism might actually represent an appropriate response to infection [9••].

Because increased mobilization and oxidation of lipid are well-recognized adaptive protein-sparing mechanisms in simple starvation [29], it had been hypothesized that the disproportionate loss of lean tissue in persons with HIV infection may be the result of a failure to increase reliance on lipid as fuel [11]. However, recent work has demonstrated that whole body lipolysis is not decreased and may be increased in persons with HIV-associated wasting [6••]. In addition, resting lipid oxidation rates are greater in HIV-positive persons than HIV-negative controls [3,30]. Thus, it appears that the use of lipid oxidation to spare protein continues to function appropriately to some degree during HIV infection.

Alterations in protein metabolism

Whole-body protein turnover typically increases during acute infection and trauma [31] and decreases during episodes of negative energy balance [32]. As both of these clinical conditions may occur in the course of HIV infection, it is not surprising that protein turnover has been reported to be decreased [33] and increased [34•] in HIV-positive persons.

Alterations in carbohydrate metabolism

Insulin-mediated glucose uptake was increased [30], while non–insulin-mediated glucose uptake was unaffected [35•] in studies of groups of clinically stable HIV-positive patients. The authors of these studies point out that this result distinguishes the metabolic effects of HIV infection from other catabolic states, which are characterized by insulin resistance [30,35•].

There have been reports of slight increases in hepatic glucose production [6••,30,35•] and nonoxidative glucose disposal [6••,30] in HIV-positive persons, although differences between HIV-positive persons and HIV-negative controls did not generally achieve levels of statistical significance. Hepatic glucose production and glucose cycling were unaffected or lower in the same patients in whom protein turnover was decreased [33].

Futile cycling and hypermetabolism

Increased rates of substrate flux present the possibility of increased recycling or futile cycling of these substrates with an accompanying waste of energy. An increase in energy required by these cycles when measured under fasting conditions would be reflected in increased REE. Recently, it has been demonstrated that the quantitative contribution of futile cycling of lipid to increased REE in HIV-positive patients with weight loss is trivial, accounting for less than 5% of observed increases in REE [6••].

Increases in cycling or nonoxidative disposal of glucose [6••] and amino acids (should recycling of amino acids be reported), might account for a more significant portion of the increase in REE. As noted earlier, however, hypermetabolism alone does not drive HIV-associated wasting. Certainly the additional energy expended in futile cycling under fasting conditions is not a quantitatively significant factor in the wasting syndrome.

Biochemical mediators of metabolic alterations

HIV-associated alterations in triglyceride metabolism, especially hypertriglyceridemia, slowed triglyceride clearance, and increased *de novo* hepatic lipogenesis, correlate with elevated circulating levels of interferon-α [24,25,26••]. Antiretroviral therapy of previously untreated subjects with advanced HIV infection leads to improvement in both interferon-α and triglyceride levels [36].

A role for cytokines such as tumor necrosis factor, interleukin-1, and interferon-α in the wasting that accompanies infection has been postulated [9••,37,38]. However, there are no studies to date that adequately link any cytokine with wasting per se.

There are no data linking hormonal abnormalities to wasting in HIV infection. As seen in the euthyroid-sick syndrome, acutely ill patients with AIDS have decreased levels of 3,3′,5-triiodothyronine [39•]. In stable patients, the levels are closer to normal.

Therapies for weight loss

Body weight and total body potassium increased in a cohort of patients who were successfully treated with ganciclovir for disseminated cytomegalovirus infection [40]. Likewise, body weight increased in another group following initiation of therapy with azidothymidine [41]. The strong association between recovery from systemic illness and episodes of weight gain [17••] reinforces the importance of aggressive medical care in preservation or restoration of body weight. Strategies more specifically targeted to restoration of body weight and BCM include increased energy and macronutrient intake by hyperalimentation or appetite stimulation, hormonal anabolic agents, and exercise.

Increased energy and macronutrient intake

Nutritional supplementation and hyperalimentation

Supplementation by enteral [42] and parenteral [10,43, 44] routes has increased body weight in some patients with HIV-associated wasting. Accompanying increases in total body potassium were noted in patients with decreased nutrient intake associated with eating disorders [42] or malabsorption [10]. On the other hand, a group of patients with systemic infections but no malabsorptive disorders gained weight and fat but lost total body potassium while receiving total parenteral nutrition [10]. Increases in fat rather than lean tissue during hyperalimentation have also been reported in patients with cancer [45,46] and sepsis [47].

The efficacy and tolerability of specific oral dietary supplements or modifications, including elemental formulas, structured lipids, and low-fat diets are currently under investigation.

Appetite stimulants

Increases in energy intake and body weight have been reported in HIV-positive patients with weight loss who participated in trials of megestrol acetate [11,13,14] and dronabinol, an active ingredient in marijuana [12•]. On the basis of reported increases in body weight, the Food and Drug Administration has approved both of these agents for treatment of weight loss in HIV infection. As with hyperalimentation, however, results of studies with dronabinol in HIV-positive patients [12•] and megestrol acetate in patients with HIV infection [14] and cancer cachexia [48•] suggest that the majority of the weight gained was fat. Side effects include impotence with megestrol acetate [13] and psychoactive effects of dronabinol [12•].

This apparent failure of strictly nutritional remedies to consistently restore lean tissue suggests that in at least some HIV-infected individuals, metabolic alterations either specifically promote nitrogen wasting or at least prevent repletion of lean tissue during periods of presumably adequate energy intake. Although HIV-infected persons have the capability of increasing their reliance on fat as a fuel [3,6••,30] and there may be nothing intrinsically wrong with increasing body fat, there is no correlation between body fat content and survival [1]. Thus, the search for effective therapies for the wasting syndrome includes investigation of specific protein anabolic agents and methods for reversing the metabolic abnormalities that may contribute to wasting.

Hormonal anabolic agents

Growth hormone

In a metabolic ward-based study, treatment with recombinant human growth hormone (0.1 mg/kg/d) produced prompt and progressive increases in body weight in HIV-positive men with an average weight loss of 19% [6••]. Weight gain averaged 2.0 ± 0.3 kg over 7 days of treatment. Urinary nitrogen excretion decreased by 4.0 ± 0.2 g/d. Protein oxidation decreased, while protein-sparing lipid oxidation increased significantly. Of note, average nitrogen retention in the HIV-positive patients was similar to that of weight-stable HIV-negative controls, demonstrating that persons with significant HIV-associated weight loss are capable of gaining not only weight, but also replenishing lean tissue in response to treatment with recombinant human growth hormone (Fig. 2). No untoward effects were noted during short-term recombinant human growth hormone treatment, although modest increases in fasting plasma glucose, insulin, and triglyceride levels were observed [6••].

Increases in body weight, lean body mass, strength, and endurance have also been reported in a small group of HIV-positive patients who received recombinant human growth hormone (5 mg every other day) for 3 months [49•]. The efficacy and safety of chronic recombinant human growth hormone treatment are being evaluated in placebo-controlled multicenter trials.

Plasma levels of insulin-like growth factor-I increased significantly in HIV-positive and HIV-negative subjects during treatment with recombinant human growth hormone [6••,49•]. Exogenous insulin-like growth factor-I reduces protein losses in other catabolic states [50–52] and may be similarly effective in treating HIV-associated wasting.

Anabolic steroids

Although there is considerable anecdotal evidence of use of anabolic steroids, there are limited published data on their efficacy in reversing HIV-associated weight loss. One recent case report [53•] detailed increases in body weight of 1.6 to 4.1 kg, increased muscle strength, and improved general sense of well-being in three HIV-positive men with weight loss who

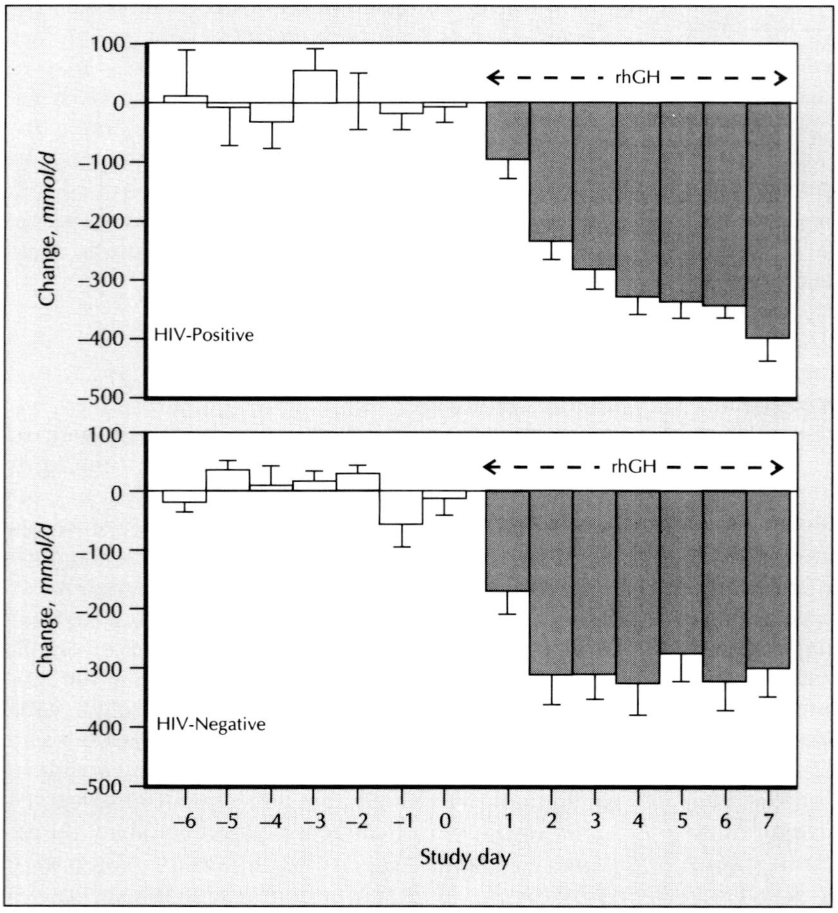

Fig. 2. Urinary nitrogen excretion before and during recombinant human growth hormone (rhGH) treatment, expressed as the difference between daily and mean baseline values. Retention of nitrogen during 7 days of recombinant human growth hormone treatment averaged 4.0 ±0.2 and 4.0 ±0.6 g/d in HIV-positive and HIV-negative subjects, respectively. (*From* Mulligan *et al.* [6••]; with permission.)

were given stanozolol, an oral testosterone derivative, for periods ranging from 1 to 2.5 months. Controlled clinical trials are under way.

Exercise

A group of HIV-positive men who underwent a course of progressive resistance training during recovery from *pneumocystis carinii* pneumonia were reported to experience increases in upper and lower body strength and body weight, when compared with a control (nonexercise) group who experienced decreases in these parameters during a comparable recovery period [54]. No data on the effect of exercise on the overall clinical outcome or recovery from *pneumocystis carinii* pneumonia were reported, however. Resistance training does increase muscle protein synthesis in healthy persons with decreased muscle mass due to aging [55] and, thus, might also be useful in persons with HIV-associated muscle wasting.

Moderate exercise has been shown to increase fitness level with no apparent acceleration in the decline in indices of immune function in persons with early and advanced HIV infection [56•,57•]. However, adherence to exercise protocols is limited [57•]. Overall, moderate exercise in persons who are motivated and can tolerate it may play a role in maintaining or potentially replenishing muscle mass.

Conclusions

Identification of the mechanisms underlying HIV-associated metabolic alterations and determination of the relationship between these alterations and the wasting syndrome will greatly enhance efforts to appropriately target anabolic strategies. Certainly, increasing energy and macronutrient intake in persons whose wasting is attributable primarily to malabsorptive disorders is an obvious first step. It seems apparent, however, that increasing energy intake will not effectively restore lean tissue in many HIV-infected persons with the wasting syndrome. Early data on the effectiveness of hormonal anabolic agents are promising. However, it is not yet known if the increases in body weight and lean tissue can be sustained during long-term therapy or whether survival will ultimately be improved.

As the emphasis in medical care has shifted from treatment to prevention of opportunistic infections such as *pneumocystis carinii* pneumonia, cytomegalovirus, and *mycobacterium avium* complex, perhaps it is appropriate to also consider the concept of prophylaxis, rather than reversal, of the wasting syndrome. On a simplistic level, there have been reports of apparently deliberate increases in body weight, presumably associated with increases in energy intake, in selected populations at risk for [58•] or known to be in the early stages of HIV infection [58•,59]. These populations might be those in which moderate exercise might be most effective, as well. More significantly, however, the evidence that changes in body composition and some metabolic alterations occur early in the course of HIV infection [3,23•,26••] suggests that intervention at this stage might help to at least forestall the wasting syndrome. It is possible that prevention of the wasting syndrome may ultimately be linked to prevention of progression of HIV infection or debility.

Acknowledgments

Supported in part by grants from the National Institutes of Health (DK-40990, DK-45833), the Research Service of the Department of Veterans Affairs, and the University of California Universitywide AIDS Research Program (R90SF211, 91RCC86-SF).

References and recommended reading

Papers of particular interest, published within the annual period of review, have been highlighted as:
• Of special interest
•• Of outstanding interest

1. KOTLER DP, TIERNEY AR, WANG J, PIERSON RN JR: **Magnitude of Body-Cell-Mass Depletion and the Timing of Death From Wasting in AIDS.** *Am J Clin Nutr* 1989, **50**:444–447.

2. MELCHIOR J-C, SALMON D, RIGAUD D, LEPORT C, BOUVET E, DETRUCHIS P, VILDE J-L, VACHON F, COULAND J-P, APFELBAUM M: **Resting Energy Expenditure is Increased in Stable, Malnourished HIV-Infected Patients.** *Am J Clin Nutr* 1991, **53**:437–441.

3. HOMMES MJT, ROMIJN JA, ENDERT E, SAUERWEIN HP: **Resting Energy Expenditure and Substrate Oxidation in Human Immunodeficiency Virus (HIV)-Infected Asymptomatic Men: HIV Affects Host Metabolism in the Early Asymptomatic Stage.** *Am J Clin Nutr* 1991, **54**:311–315.

4. GRUNFELD C, PANG M, SHIMIZU L, SHIGENAGA JK, JENSEN P, FEINGOLD KR: **Resting Energy Expenditure, Caloric Intake and Short-Term Weight Change in Human Immunodeficiency Virus Infection and the Acquired Immunodeficiency Syndrome.** *Am J Clin Nutr* 1992, **55**:455–460.

5. • MELCHIOR J-C, RAGUIN G, BOULIER A, BOUVET E, RIGAUD D, MATHERON S, CASALINO E, VILDE J-L, VACHON F, COULAND J-P, APFELBAUM M: **Resting Energy Expenditure in Human Immunodeficiency Virus-Infected Patients: Comparison Between Patients With and Without Secondary Infections.** *Am J Clin Nutr* 1993, **57**:614–619.

Hypermetabolism has been extensively documented in patients with HIV infection. This paper reports a further increase in REE in patients with secondary infections. Rates of REE in two groups of HIV-positive patients with prior weight loss of more than 10% of pre-illness weight were compared with those of HIV-negative controls. REE was 11% greater than control in clinically stable HIV-positive patients and 34% greater in those with secondary infections. The authors suggest that an elevation in REE of this magnitude may accelerate rate of weight loss during secondary infection.

6. •• MULLIGAN K, GRUNFELD C, HELLERSTEIN MK, NEESE RA, SCHAMBELAN M: **Anabolic Effects of Recombinant Human Growth Hormone in Patients With Wasting Associated With Human Immunodeficiency Virus Infection.** *J Clin Endocrinol Metab* 1993, 77:956–962.

Short-term treatment with recombinant human growth hormone resulted in significant weight gain, nitrogen retention, and increases in lipid oxidation in both HIV-positive men who had lost an average of 19% of pre-illness weight and HIV-negative controls. Although nutritional therapies have produced weight gain in persons with HIV infection, they do not consistently restore lean body mass as they would in otherwise healthy persons recovering illness or starvation. In contrast, treatment with recombinant human growth hormone prompted similar protein anabolic and other metabolic responses in HIV-positive and HIV-negative subjects, demonstrating that HIV-positive persons have the metabolic capability of replenishing lean tissue. In HIV-positive patients, recombinant human growth hormone achieved its protein anabolic effect without reversal of metabolic alterations such as increased rates of REE, *de novo* hepatic lipogenesis, and nonoxidative glucose and lipid disposal.

7. KOTLER DP, TIERNEY AR, BRENNER SK, COUTURE S, WANG J, PIERSON RN JR: **Preservation of Short-Term Energy Balance in Clinically Stable Patients With AIDS.** *Am J Clin Nutr* 1990, **51**:7–13.

8. SUTTMANN U, OCKENGA J, HOOGESTRAAT L, SELBERG O, DEICHER H, MULLER MJ: **Resting Energy Expenditure and Weight Loss in Human Immunodeficiency Virus-Infected Patients.** *Metabolism* 1993, **42**:1173–1179.

9. •• GRUNFELD C, FEINGOLD KR: **Metabolic Disturbances and Wasting in the Acquired Immunodeficiency Syndrome.** *N Engl J Med* 1992, **327**:329–337.

A detailed review of the metabolic alterations and their potential relationship to wasting in AIDS. The complex role of cytokines in wasting and hypertriglyceridemia is explored in detail, as are the effects of HIV infection on each component of the energy balance equation.

10. KOTLER DP, TIERNEY AR, CULPEPPER-MORGAN JA, WANG J, PIERSON RN JR: **Effect of Home Total Parenteral Nutrition on Body Composition in Patients With Acquired Immunodeficiency Syndrome.** *JPEN J Parenter Enteral Nutr* 1990, **14**:454-458.

11. HELLERSTEIN MK, KAHN J, MUDIE H, VITERI F: **Current Approach to the Treatment of Human Immunodeficiency Virus-Associated Weight Loss: Pathophysiologic Considerations and Emerging Management Strategies.** *Semin Oncol* 1990, **17**(suppl 9):17–33.

12. • STRUWE M, KAEMPFER SH, GEIGER CJ, PAVIA AT, PLASSE TF, SHEPARD KV, RIES K, EVANS TG: **Effect of Dronabinol on Nutritional Status in HIV Infection.** *Ann Pharmacother* 1993, 27:827–831.

The effects of dronabinol, an active ingredient in marijuana and known appetite stimulant, on food intake and body composition in patients with HIV-associated weight loss were evaluated in a randomized, double-blind, placebo-controlled, crossover trial. Only five of 12 patients who enrolled completed the protocol. Energy intake and body weight tended to increase during dronabinol treatment. Percent body fat, estimated by anthropometry, increased and symptom distress decreased significantly with dronabinol. Side effects included mood alteration, inability to operate a motor vehicle, and sedation. The authors acknowledge that it is unlikely that this study was truly blinded, because the side effects of dronabinol were quite apparent.

13. SUMMERBELL CD, YOUL M, MCDONALD V, CATALAN J, GAZZARD BG: **Megestrol Acetate vs Cyproheptadine in the Treatment of Weight Loss Associated With HIV Infection.** *Int J STD AIDS* 1992, **3**:278–280.

14. VON ROENN JH, ROTH EL, CRAIG R: **HIV-Related Cachexia: Potential Mechanisms and Treatment.** *Oncology* 1992, **49**(Suppl 2):50–54.

15. APFELBAUM M, BOSTSARRCN J, LUCATIS D: **Effect of Caloric Restriction and Excessive Caloric Intake on Energy Expenditure.** *Am J Clin Nutr* 1971, **24**:1405–1409.

16. SERWADDA D, MUGERWA RD, SEWANKAMBO NK, LWEGABA A, CARSWELL JW, KIRYA GB, BAYLEY AC, DOWNING RG, TEDDER RS, CLAYDEN SA, WEISS RA, DALGLEISCH AG: **Slim Disease: A New Disease in Uganda and Its Association With HTLV-III Infection.** *Lancet* 1985, **ii**:849–852.

17. •• MACALLAN DC, NOBLE C, BALDWIN C, FOSKETT M, MCMANUS T, GRIFFIN GE: **Prospective Analysis of Patterns of Weight Change in Stage IV HIV Infection.** *Am J Clin Nutr* 1993, **58**:417–424.

This systematic analysis of weight data collected prospectively demonstrates significant associations between rate of weight loss and underlying causes. Rapid weight loss is suggestive of secondary infection. A slower rate of weight loss suggests gastrointestinal disease. During periods of study, which ranged from 9-49 months, there were also periods of weight stability and episodes of weight gain.

18. MILLER TL, ORAV EJ, MARTIN WR, COOPER ER, MCINTOSH K, WINTER HS: **Malnutrition and Carbohydrate Malabsorption in Children With Vertically Transmitted Human Immunodeficiency Virus 1 Infection.** *Gastroenterology* 1991, **100**:1296–1302.

19. HARRIMAN GR, SMITH PD, MCDONALD KH, CECIL HF, KOENIG S, LACK EE, LANE HC, FAUCI AS: **Vitamin B_{12} Malabsorption in Patients With the Acquired Immunodeficiency Syndrome.** *Arch Intern Med* 1989, **149**:2039–2041.

20. •• GRUNFELD C, FEINGOLD KR **Body Weight as Essential Data in the Management of Patients With Human Immunodeficiency Virus Infection and the Acquired Immunodeficiency Syndrome.** *Am J Clin Nutr* 1993, **58**:317–318.

This editorial, published in conjunction with the paper of Macallan *et al.* (*Am J Clin Nutr* 1993, 58:417–424) points out that a measurement as simple as body weight, when systematically obtained and plotted, can be a valuable clinical tool. Just as growth data are plotted in children and used to anticipate a variety of disorders, changes in weight patterns of HIV-positive patients could serve as an early warning system that could facilitate prompt diagnosis and treatment of AIDS-related disorders.

21. KOTLER DP, WANG J, PIERSON RN JR: **Body Composition Studies in Patients With the Acquired Immunodeficiency Syndrome.** *Am J Clin Nutr* 1985, **42**:1255–1265.

22. • WANG J, KOTLER DP, RUSSELL M, BURASTERO S, MAZARIEGOS M, THORNTON J, DILMANIAN FA, PIERSON RN JR: **Body-Fat Measurement in Patients With Acquired Immunodeficiency Syndrome: Which Method Should Be Used?** *Am J Clin Nutr* 1992, **56**:963–967.

The pattern of disproportionate loss of lean tissue in patients with AIDS alters many of the assumptions underlying traditional methods for estimating body fat and may make those methods inappropriate for use in patients with AIDS. When several whole-body methods for measuring body composition were compared in men with AIDS, total body water by tritium dilution and dual-photon absorptiometry were found to yield the most reliable estimates of fat, when compared with the reference method, *in vivo* neutron activation. The authors point out, however, that total body water is a major component of the *in vivo* neuton activation method, so it is not altogether surprising to find a high degree of concordance between the two methods. Total body potassium may overestimate fat in men with HIV disease. Bioelectrical impedance analysis and traditional anthropometry also provide less accurate estimates of body fat in this population. These two latter methods have been used in many studies of body composition in HIV-patients.

23. • OTT M, LEMBCKE B, FISCHER H, JAGER R, POLAT H, GEIER H, RECH M, STASZESWKI S, HELM EB, CASPARY WF: **Early Changes of Body Composition in Human Immunodeficiency Virus-Infected Patients: Tetrapolar Body Impedance Analysis Indicates Significant Malnutrition.** *Am J Clin Nutr* 1993, **57**:15–19.

Decreased body cell mass and increased extracellular mass, estimated by bioelectrical impedance analysis, were reported in groups of HIV-positive men at all points along the spectrum of HIV infection. Notably, differences in these compartments were noted even in a group of asymptomatic men whose body mass index matched that of HIV-negative controls.

24. GRUNFELD C, KOTLER DP, HAMADEH R, TIERNEY A, WANG J, PIERSON RN JR: **Hypertriglyceridemia in the Acquired Immunodeficiency Syndrome.** *Am J Med* 1989, **86**:27–31.

25. GRUNFELD C, PANG M, DOERRLER W, SHIGENAGA JK, JENSEN P, FEINGOLD KR: **Lipids, Lipoproteins, Triglyceride Clearance, and Cytokines in Human Immunodeficiency Virus Infection and the Acquired Immunodeficiency Syndrome.** *J Clin Endocrinol Metab* 1992, **74**:1045–1052.

26. •• HELLERSTEIN MK, GRUNFELD C, WU K, CHRISTIANSEN M, KAEMPFER S, KLETKE C, SHACKLETON CHL: **Increased De Novo Hepatic Lipogenesis in Human Immunodeficiency Virus Infection.** *J Clin Endocrinol Metab* 1993, **76**:559–565.

De novo hepatic lipogenesis, or synthesis of fat from nonlipid precursors, was found to be greater than normal in HIV-positive persons with significant weight loss, as well as those in the early, asymptomatic, stages of infection. Rates of *de novo* hepatic lipogenesis in patients with weight loss were three- to four-fold greater than those in controls and could represent an inappropriate redirection of substrate. Such redirection could contribute to the wasting syndrome. The finding of increased *de novo* hepatic lipogenesis in the clinically asymptomatic stages of infection suggests that there are early effects of HIV on intermediary metabolism. The increase in fasting *de novo* hepatic lipogenesis correlated with circulating interferon-α levels.

27. HOMMES MJT, ROMIJN JA, ENDERT E, EEFTINCK-SCHATTENKERK JKM, SAUERWEIN HP: **Basel Fuel Homeostasis in Symptomatic Human Immunodeficiency Virus Infection.** *Clin Sci* 1991, **80**:359–365.

28. GONZALEZ-CLEMENTE JM, MIRO JM, NAVARRO MP, ZAMORA L, VILARDELL E: **High Triglyceride Levels as a Predictor of Mortality in AIDS Patients.** *AIDS* 1993, **7**:1022–1023.

29. RUNCIE J, HILDITCH TE: **Energy Provision, Tissue Utilization, and Weight Loss in Prolonged Starvation.** *Br Med J* 1974, **2**:352–356.

30. HOMMES MJT, ROMIJN JA, ENDERT E, EEFTINCK-SCHATTENKERK JKM, SAUERWEIN HP: **Insulin Sensitivity and Insulin Clearance in Human Immunodeficiency Virus-Infected Men.** *Metabolism* 1991, **40**:651–656.

31. RENNIE MJ: **Muscle Protein Turnover and the Wasting Due to Injury and Disease.** *Br Med Bull* 1985, **41**:257–264.

32. WATERLOW JC: **Metabolic Adaptation to Low Intakes of Energy and Protein.** *Ann Rev Nutr* 1986, **6**:495–526.

33. STEIN TP, NUTINSKY C, CONDOLUCI D, SCHLUTER MD, LESKIW MJ: **Protein and Energy Substrate Metabolism in AIDS Patients.** *Metabolism* 1990, **39**:876–881.

34. • MACALLAN DC, GRIFFIN GD: **Metabolic Disturbances in AIDS.** *N Engl J Med* 1992, **327**:1530–1531.

This letter to the editor describes elevated rates of protein turnover in men with AIDS. The authors point out that such elevations are consistent with increased protein turnover noted during infection and trauma, conditions that are typically also associated with a hypermetabolic state.

35. • HEYLIGENBERG R, ROMIJN JA, HOMMES MJT, ENDERT E, EEFTINCK-SCHATTENKERK JKM, SAUERWEIN HP: **Non-Insulin-Mediated Glucose Uptake in Human Immunodeficiency Virus-Infected Men.** *Clin Sci* 1993, **84**:209–216.

To determine whether an increase in insulin-mediated glucose uptake in men with HIV infection was attributable to increased rates of non–insulin-mediated glucose uptake, rates of glucose uptake were measured during a hyperglycemic, insulinopenic clamp. Under these conditions, there were no differences between HIV-positive patients and controls in glucose uptake. Thus, the mechanism and metabolic significance of increased insulin sensitivity in HIV-positive men remain to be determined.

36. MILDVAN D, MACHADO SG, WILETS I, GROSSBERG SE: **Endogenous Interferon and Triglyceride Concentrations to Assess Response to Zidovudine in AIDS and Advanced AIDS-Related Complex.** *Lancet* 1992, 339:453–456.

37. BEUTLER B: **The Presence of Cachectin/Tumor Necrosis Factor in Human Disease States.** *Am J Med* 1988, **85**:287–288.

38. TRACEY KJ, CERAMI A: **The Role of Cachectin/Tumor Necrosis Factor in AIDS.** *Cancer Cells* 1989, 1:62–63.

39. • GRUNFELD C, PANG M, DOERRLER W, JENSEN P, SHIMIZU L, FEINGOLD KR, CAVALIERI RR: **Indices of Thyroid Function and Weight Loss in Human Immunodeficiency Virus Infection and the Acquired Immunodeficiency Syndrome.** *Metabolism* 1993, **42**:1270–1276.

Thyroid hormone levels were compared in men at various stages of HIV infection. Asymptomatic, weight-stable patients maintained normal levels of 3, 3′, 5-triiodothyronine (T_3). Levels of T_3 were decreased by 19% in weight stable patients with AIDS. In patients with AIDS and active secondary infection, in whom there were significant short-term weight loss and anorexia, there was a 45% decrease in T_3 levels. This latter finding is consistent with the "euthyroid-sick syndrome."

40. KOTLER DP, TIERNEY AR, ALTILIO D, WANG J, PIERSON RN: **Body Mass Repletion During Ganciclovir Treatment of Cytomegalovirus Infections in Patients With Acquired Immunodeficiency Syndrome.** *Arch Intern Med* 1989, **149**:901–905.

41. YARCHOAN R, KLECKER RW, WEINHOLD KJ, LYERLY HK, GELMANN E, BLUM RM, SHERER GM, MITSUYA H, COLLINS JM, MYERS CE, MARKHAM PD, DURACK DT, LEHRMAN SN, BARRY DW, FISCHL MA, GALLO RC, BOLOGNESI DP, BRODER S: **Administration of 3'-Azido-3'Deoxythimidine, an Inhibitor of HTLV-III/LAV Replication, to Patients With AIDS or AIDS-Related Complex.** *Lancet* 1986, i:575–580.

42. KOTLER DP, TIERNEY AR, FERRARO R, CUFF P, WANG J, PIERSON RN JR, HEYMSFIELD SB: **Enteral Alimentation and Repletion of Body Cell Mass in Malnourished Patients With Acquired Immunodeficiency Syndrome.** *Am J Clin Nutr* 1991, 53:149–154.

43. SINGER P, ROTHKOPF MM, KVETAN V, KIRVELA O, GAARE J, ASKANAZI J: **Risks and Benefits of Home Parenteral Nutrition in the Acquired Immunodeficiency Syndrome.** *JPEN J Parenter Enteral Nutr* 1991, **15**:75–79.

44. SINGER P, RUBINSTEIN A, ASKANAZI J, CALVELLI T, LAZARUS T, KIRVELA O, KATZ DP: **Clinical and Immunologic Effects of Lipid-Based Parenteral Nutrition in AIDS.** *JPEN J Parenter Enteral Nutr* 1992, **16**:165–167.

45. COHN SH, VARTSKY D, VASWANI AN, SAWITSKY A, RAI K, GARTENHAUS W, YASUMURA S, ELLIS KJ: **Changes in Body Composition of Cancer Patients Following Combined Nutritional Support.** *Nutr Cancer* 1982, 4:107–119.

46. SHIKE M, RUSSELL DMCR, DETSKY AS, HARRISON JE, MCNEILL KG, SHEPHERD FA, FELD R, EVANS WK, JEEJEEBHOY KN: **Changes in Body Composition in Patients With Small Cell Lung Cancer. The Effect of Total Parenteral Nutrition as an Adjunct to Chemotherapy.** *Ann Intern Med* 1984, 101:303–309.

47. STREAT SJ, BEDDOE AH, HILL GL: **Aggressive Nutritional Support Does Not Prevent Protein Loss Despite Fat Gain in Septic Intensive Care Patients.** *J Trauma* 1987, **27**:262–266.

48. • LOPRINZI CL, SCHAID DJ, DOSE AM, BURNHAM NL, JENSEN MD: **Body-Composition Changes in Patients Who Gain Weight While Receiving Megestrol Acetate.** *J Clin Oncol* 1993, **11**:152–154.

Using dual-energy x-ray absorptiometry to estimate fat and fat-free mass and tritiated water to estimate total body water, the authors evaluated changes in body composition in patients with cancer who gained weight with megestrol acetate. Dual energy x-ray absorptiometry is a safer, more accurate variant of dual-photon absorptiometry, which was one of the methods recommended by Wang *et al.* (*Am J Clin Nutr* 1992, 56:963–967) for use in patients with AIDS. Increases in body weight averaged 5.9 kg during the treatment periods, which ranged from 5 weeks to 8 months. Greater than 75% of the weight gained, however, was fat. Moreover, the hydration of fat-free mass increased by 4%, suggesting that a portion of the modest increase in fat-free mass was additional extracellular water, rather than body cell mass. Although this study was not conducted in patients with HIV infection, it is included in this review because it is the first study of appetite stimulants that reports changes in body fat estimated independently of changes in fat-free mass, which could be affected significantly by changes in body water content.

49. • KRENTZ AJ, KOSTER FT, CRIST DM, FINN K, JOHNSON LZ, BOYLE PJ, SCHADE DS: **Anthropometric, Metabolic, and Immunological Effects of Recombinant Human Growth Hormone in AIDS and AIDS-Related Complex.** *J AIDS* 1993, 6:245–251.

The effects of pharmacologic and physiologic treatment with recombinant human growth hormone were evaluated over 3 months in seven catabolic HIV-positive patients. The four patients who received pharmacologic doses experienced significant weight gain. Increases in lean body mass and decreases in fat mass, estimated by bioelectrical impedance analysis, were reported in this group. Muscle power and endurance tended to increase, suggesting that the increases in lean tissue might improve functional capacity. These results and those of Mulligan *et al.* (*J Clin Endocrinol Metab* 1993, 77:956–962) suggest that recombinant human growth hormone has a therapeutic advantage over strictly nutritional approaches and may be an effective means of restoring lean tissue and improving functional capacity in patients with the wasting syndrome.

50. CLEMMONS DR, SMITH-BANKS A, UNDERWOOD LE: **Reversal of Diet-Induced Catabolism by Infusion of Recombinant Insulin-Like Growth Factor-I in Humans.** *J Clin Endocrinol Metab* 1992, 75:234–238.

51. DOUGLAS RG, GLUCKMAN PD, BALL K, BREIER B, SHAW JHF: **The Effects of Infusion of Insulinlike Growth Factor (IGF) I, IGF-II, and Insulin on Glucose and Protein Metabolism in Fasted Lambs.** *J Clin Invest* 1991, **88**:614–622.

52. KUPFER AR, UNDERWOOD LE, BAXTER RC, CLEMMONS DR: **Enhancement of the Anabolic Effects of Growth Hormone and Insulin-Like Growth Factor I by Use of Both Agents Simultaneously.** *J Clin Invest* 1993, 91:391–396.

53. • BERGER JR, PALL L, WINFIELD D: **Effect of Anabolic Steroids on HIV-Related Wasting Myopathy.** *South Med J* 1993, 86:865–866.

This case report contains the only information published thus far in the scientific literature on the effects of anabolic steroids in persons with HIV-associated weight loss. Three men who had lost at least 10% of pre-illness weight were given stanozolol, an oral testosterone derivative, for periods ranging from 1 to 2.5 months. All three men experienced increases in weight, muscle strength, and "sense of well-being."

54. SPENCE DW, GALANTINO MLA, MOSSBERG KA, ZIMMERMAN SO: **Progressive Resistance Exercise: Effect on Muscle Function and Anthropometry of a Select AIDS Population.** *Arch Phys Med Rehabil* 1990, **71**:644–648.

55. YARASHESKI KE, ZACHWIEJA JJ, BIER DM: **Acute Effects of Resistance Exercise on Muscle Protein Synthesis Rate in Young and Elderly Men and Women.** *Am J Physiol* 1993, **265**:E210–E214.

56. • RIGSBY LW, DISHMAN RK, JACKSON AW, MACLEAN GS, RAVEN PB: **Effects of Exercise Training on Men Seropositive for the Human Immunodeficiency Virus-1.** *Med Sci Sports Exerc* 1992, **24**:6–12.

HIV-positive men showed significant improvements in cardiovascular and neuromuscular responses to exercise following a 12-week training program that included exercise designed to improve both aerobic fitness (heart rate, time to exhaustion) and strength (chest press and leg extension). A control group of HIV-positive men assigned to receive counseling during a comparable period showed no change in these variables. Exercise had no significant effect on lymphocyte counts.

57. • MACARTHUR RD, LEVINE SD, BIRK TJ: **Supervised Exercise Training Improves Cardiopulmonary Ritness in HIV-Infected Persons.** *Med Sci Sports Exerc* 1993, **25**:684–688.

Significant improvements in maximal oxygen consumption, heart rate, and rating of perceived exertion were noted in a group of HIV-positive patients who completed a 24-week exercise program. However, only six of 32 patients who enrolled in the study actually completed the program. Thus, it appears that although exercise in HIV-positive individuals can improve fitness level and should no doubt be encouraged, the ability to adhere to a regular exercise program might ultimately limit its utility.

58. • HOOVER DR, GRAHAM NMH, PALENICEK JG, BACELLAR H, SAAH AJ: **Weight Changes in HIV-I Seropositive and Seronegative Homosexual Men.** *Nutr Res* 1992, **12**:297–305.

This paper describes weight changes in a cohort of 1153 homosexual and bisexual men studied semiannually over a 6-year period. In 86 patients who underwent seroconversion during the study, weight increased progressively prior to seroconversion, declined at the time of seroconversion, and then rebounded to greater than prestudy levels. In the HIV-positive men, weight loss began 12 to 18 months before progression to a formal diagnosis of AIDS, and the rate of weight loss accelerated during this period.

59. SMITH J, BIRMINGHAM CL: **HIV Seropositivity and Deliberate Weight Gain.** *N Engl J Med* 1990, **322**:1089–1090.

Kathleen Mulligan, PhD, Division of Endocrinology, Building 100, Room 286, San Francisco General Hospital, 1001 Potrero Avenue, San Francisco, CA 94110, USA.

Carl Grunfeld, MD, PhD, Metabolism Section (111F), Department of Veterans Affairs, 4150 Clement Street, San Francisco, CA 94121, USA.

Long-term hyperalimentation

Margaret Malone, MSc, PhD, and Lyn Howard, MB, FRCP

Albany College of Pharmacy, and Albany Medical Center, Albany, New York, USA

During this review period, outcome data relating to long-term home parenteral nutrition (HPN) were reported in both adult and pediatric patients from the United States and Europe. Several diagnostic categories including inflammatory bowel disease, radiation enteritis, cancer, hyperemesis gravidarum, and pediatrics were discussed and issues pertaining to complications associated with long-term therapy for, in particular, metabolic bone disease and liver disease were reviewed. Choline and taurine supplements have been demonstrated to reverse hepatic steatosis, while catheter-related sepsis continues to be reported and appears to be more prevalent in pediatric patients and the immunocompromised. However, conflicting data were published regarding the HPN complication rate in patients with AIDS. Several case reports described serious complications associated with thiamine deficiency in patients not receiving vitamin supplements. Future developments in long-term HPN should address the role of new substrates such as alternative fat sources, including medium-chain triglycerides, structured lipids, and fish oils and the requirement for and provision of conditionally essential nutrients, *eg*, glutamine, arginine, taurine, choline, and *S*-adenosyl-*L*-methionine. In particular, health care reform and limited resources will drive the demand for objective outcome data especially in patients with a short-term prognosis.

Current Opinion in Gastroenterology 1994, **10**:227–234

Incidence, indications, and outcomes

Specialized nutrition support accounts for 1% of the total health care budget in the United States. Of this amount, about 20% is expended in the nonhospital setting. The approximate number of home parenteral nutrition (HPN) Medicare patients and the overall cost between 1989 and 1992 is presented in Figure 1 [1•]. During this 4-year period, the number of patients and dollars spent more than doubled. It has been estimated that the use of HPN in the US Medicare population is about 100 per million of Medicare-eligible beneficiaries. As 26% of the HPN patients reported to the North American Home Parenteral and Enteral Nutrition (HPEN) Patient Registry have Medicare as their primary payer, this suggests there were approximately 40,000 HPN patients in the United States in 1992. Data from the United Kingdom and Ireland HPN Patient Registry indicate that HPN is used in two to five per million of their population. The difference between US and UK utilization is principally that the UK physicians rarely initiate this therapy in patients with a short-term outcome or in the terminal stages of their disease [2•,3]. A similar restraint is true in Europe, Canada, and Australia [4].

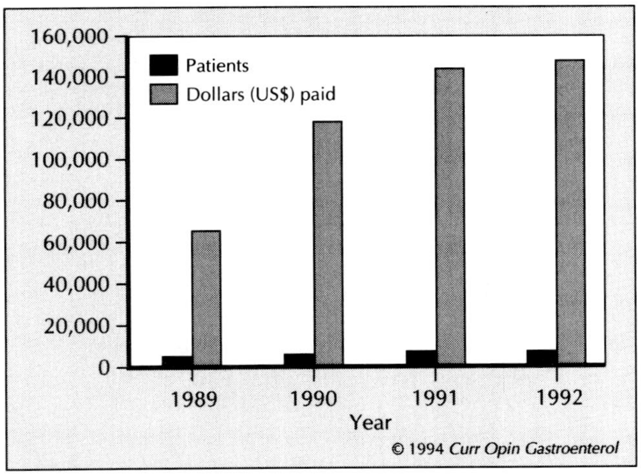

Fig. 1. Estimate of the number of home parenteral nutrition Medicare patients and the dollars paid between 1989 and 1992.

There is evidence that in the United States, HPN therapy is being used increasingly in patients with a more short-term clinical outcome. The 37 programs that have consistently reported their data to the North American

Abbreviations

HPEN—home parenteral and enteral nutrition; **HPN**—home parenteral nutrition; **TPN**—total parenteral nutrition.

© 1994 Current Science ISBN 1-85922-607-8 ISSN 0267–1379

HPEN Registry have experienced an annual increase in new patients of around 5%; 90% of this increase was accounted for by patients with an active cancer diagnosis. The percentage of new patients with Crohn's disease and short bowel syndrome has decreased but their absolute numbers have remained relatively constant.

Figure 2 illustrates the current distribution of the 5393 HPN patients reported to the North American registry within different diagnostic groups. The seven principal diagnoses accounting for 77% of HPN cases were active cancer, Crohn's disease, ischemic bowel disease, motility disorders, radiation enteritis, AIDS, and congenital bowel disease.

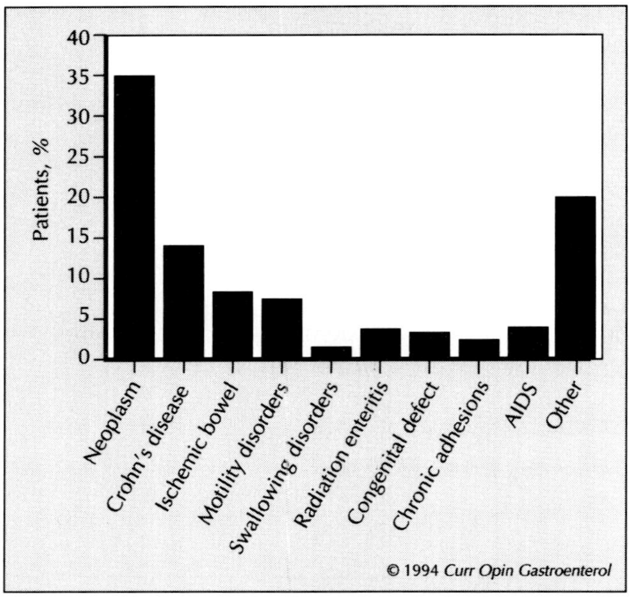

Fig. 2. Distribution of 5393 home parenteral nutrition patients reported to the North American HPEN Registry within different diagnostic groups.

The outcome of HPEN patients reported to the North American registry in the major diagnostic groups is presented in Table 1 [4]. Patients with Crohn's disease continue to act as the "gold standard" for HPN therapy. Patients with ischemic bowel disease, motility disorders, radiation enteritis, and congenital bowel disease also have a good long-term outcome. Patients with active cancer or AIDS have a shorter, more pessimistic prognosis. The data suggests that the outcome of HPEN therapy is primarily related to the underlying disease state rather than the parenteral nutrition support.

Studies in the major diagnostic groups

Inflammatory bowel disease

There were several reviews of the use of nutritional therapy in inflammatory bowel disease in adult [5–7] and pediatric patients [8–10]. Nutritional repletion rather than bowel rest per se seems to be the major role of nutritional support in patients with active inflammatory bowel disease. There is limited data suggesting that fish oils and steroid sparing may be beneficial in patients with ulcerative colitis but not in those with Crohn's disease [5]. Although high-dose steroids have been shown to induce faster and longer remissions than nutritional support using a tube enteral defined formula diet or parenteral nutrition alone, in patients requiring surgery or children with growth failure, the nutritional approach and avoidance of steroids may still be the preferred therapeutic option [6].

In pediatric patients, growth failure and delayed maturation occurs in 85% of prepubertal patients with Crohn's disease and 6% to 12% of patients with ulcerative colitis. This can be significantly reversed by the provision of aggressive nutritional support [8]. Rannem *et al.* [11] reported a prospective study in which selenium status was evaluated in 66 consecutive outpatients with Crohn's disease. Fourteen patients were receiving parenteral nutrition. None of the patients were receiving oral or intravenous selenium supplements. They observed that 27 of the 66 patients had reduced concentrations of selenium and glutathione peroxidase in plasma and erythrocytes. Selenium deficiency was strongly correlated with a small bowel resection of greater than 200 cm. Whilst no clinical signs of depletion were apparent, these investigators felt that patients with a small bowel resection of greater than 200 cm should be considered candidates for selenium supplementation.

Abrams *et al.* [12] described a case report of a patient with short bowel syndrome in whom selenium deficiency developed after 3 years of total parenteral nutrition (TPN) without selenium supplements. The patient did not show any cardiac or muscle changes commonly associated with selenium depletion but had white nail beds, which returned to normal after supplementation.

Radiation enteritis

Data from the North American HPEN Registry described 205 patients with radition enteritis. These patients had a 90% per annum survival rate on HPN therapy, 20% resumed oral intake, and 50% were completely rehabilitated. Silvain *et al.* [13], in contrast, reported a somewhat less optimistic outcome in a much smaller study population of 31 patients with severe radiation enteritis treated with HPN for a median follow-up period of 2.5 years. Oral feeding was resumed in 11 patients after a range of 6 to 142 months. Eighteen patients died, primarily because of their underlying disease. The probability of radiation enteritis recurrence, defined as intestinal disease requiring admission to hospital, was 34% at 1 year and 47% at 2 years. The 5-year survival rate was 36%. The authors concluded that whereas HPN maintained the patients nutritional status and deferred surgery in some cases, the underlying radiation enteritis remained associated with a poor outcome in patients with severe disease.

Table 1. Description of clinical outcome of home parenteral nutrition in seven diagnostic categories*

Diagnosis	1-Year survival rate, %	Therapy status (1st annual follow-up)	Complications, *n/y*	Rehabilitation over 2 y, %†
Crohn's disease	95	About 1/2 stayed on HPN 1/2 resumed oral intake	1 due to HPN (0.5 sepsis), 1.5 due to non HPN	70, 25, 5
Ischemic bowel	90	The majority stayed on HPN; only 1/6 resumed full oral intake	1 due to HPN (0.5 sepsis 1.5 due to non HPN	30, 50, 20
Motility disorder	90	The majority stayed on HPN; only 1/4 resumed full oral intake	2 due to HPN (1sepsis), 1 due to non HPN	35, 50, 15
Radiation enteritis	85	The majority stayed on HPN; only 1/6 resumed full oral intake	1 due to HPN (0.5 sepsis), 1 due to non HPN	40, 50, 10
Congenital bowel	90	1/2 stayed on HPN; 1/3 resumed full oral intake	2.5 due to HPN (0.5 sepsis), 1.5 due to non HPN	60, 35, 5
Neoplasm	25	1/2 stayed on HPN; 1/2 resumed full oral intake	1 due to HPN (0.5 sepsis), 4 due to non HPN	20, 40, 40
AIDS	0	No survivors	1 due to HPN (0.5 sepsis), 3.5 due to non HPN	5, 40, 55

**Data from* Howard *et al.* [31].
†Complete, partial, minimal.
HPN—home parenteral nutrition

Cancer

The clinical outcomes of 2968 HPEN patients with cancer reported to the North American HPEN Registry were reviewed [1•]. This is currently the largest single diagnostic group starting HPEN. The mean survival time is 6 months, but 25% live beyond 1 year and 20% resume oral nutrition. The outcome is better for childhood malignancies, hematologic malignancies, and small bowel or liver cancer, possibly owing to more effective treatment for these tumor types. However, these particular gastrointestinal malignancies represent only a small proportion of the overall HPN cancer population. The primary tumor sites of patients who received HPN are presented in Table 2. Although adult active cancer patients did not have a greater HPN-related rehospitalization rate than other diagnostic groups, they had much more frequent readmissions because of their underlying disease.

It has been suggested that patients receiving aggressive chemotherapy [14] and those cancer patients with major weight loss before surgery benefit from nutritional support [15]. A meta-analysis of the available data suggested TPN may be associated with greater morbidity due to infectious complications and that even noncatheter infections are increased. The meta-analysis findings have been used as the basis for the American Society for Parenteral and Enteral Nutrition guidelines on nutritional support in cancer patients [16]. However, the interpretation of the meta-analysis data has been questioned in an extensive review of nutritional support in cancer patients. It was pointed out that the number of patients included in the meta-analysis was small and the range of cancer diagnoses was very wide. Furthermore, not all of the subjects were malnourished. In 20% of these patients, nutritional status was not assessed, 16% of patients had good nutritional status, and of the rest only half of the patients were malnourished [17•]. Wasting in cancer patients appears to relate to a range of tumor-induced metabolic disturbances, involving cytokines and appetite-inhibiting peptides. Under these circumstances, nutritional support may not effectively redress the wasting but does expose the patient to the risks associated with parenteral nutrition.

Hyperemesis gravidarum

Hyperemesis gravidarum can be defined as intractable nausea and vomiting during pregnancy, so severe as to necessitate hospitalization. Many of these patients can be successfully managed as outpatients using intravenous fluid and electrolytes and where necessary, parenteral nutrition [18]. The theories of the etiology and pathophysiology of this disorder have been reviewed [19•]. Alternative methods of nutritional support including use of the enteral route were reported [20, 21]. Greenspoon *et al.* [22] discussed their experience of three women with hyperemesis gravidarum who received TPN via a peripherally inserted central catheter for 28, 32, and 137 days respectively. No problems were experienced, leading the authors to advocate this route of administration instead of conventional central venous access.

Table 2. Primary tumor sites of 2772 cancer patients reported to the North American Home Parenterial and Enteral Nutrition Registry between between 1985 and 1990*

Site	Patients, %
Genitourinary	20.4
Large bowel	17.0
Hematological	13.8
Pancreas	8.0
Stomach	8.0
Oropharynx/esophagus	5.7
Central nervous system	4.1
Breast	3.1
Liver	2.6
Lung	2.3
Small bowel	1.9
Other	6.6

**Data from* Howard *et al.* [31].

Pediatrics

Data from the North American HPEN Registry [4] reviewed the outcome of 385 children aged 0 to 15 years. When compared with adults with the same diagnosis, the children had a similar 2-year survival rate on HPN. The frequency of complications resulting in rehospitalization was the same in children and adults with Crohn's disease or cystic fibrosis. HPN children with active cancer tended to be younger than those with Crohn's disease or cystic fibrosis and experienced a 50% greater sepsis rate, compared with adults with cancer.

De Potter *et al.* [23] reported the outcome of 156 children enrolled in their HPN program in France from 1981 to 1990. Their age at discharge was 3 to 24 months (n=80), 2 to 10 years (n=39), and 10 to 18 years (n=37). The principal diagnoses were short bowel syndrome (n=64), Crohn's disease (n=24), pseudoobstruction (n=29), intractable diarrhea (n=8), and immune deficiency (n=13). A total of 30% were exclusively on HPN while the rest had some oral or tube enteral intake. The mean duration of HPN was 615 days (range 30 to 3532 days). Twenty-nine patients died but only three deaths were HPN related: one due to cirrhosis and two due to catheter-related sepsis. Catheter-related complications included occlusion (n=10), dislodgment (n=9), and sepsis (n=105). With regard to the functional capacity of these patients, 86% achieved normal growth, 89% were regularly attending school, 91% took part in physical activities, and 50% were able to go on family vacations.

Prior to discharge, patients and their parents were trained for a 3-week period in TPN administration techniques. In contrast, the current HPN training time covered by US health insurance agencies is only 5 days, although in practice patients are often hospitalized for a longer duration owing to their underlying illness.

The same group described the successful use of a mixed 50% medium-chain triglyceride and 50% long-chain triglyceride emulsion over a 6-month period in 12 children (age range 1.5 to 17 years) receiving HPN [24]. The only significant ($P<0.05$) changes when compared with the previous baseline values, following the administration of long-chain triglyceride emulsions, were an increase in apolipoproteins A-I and A-II and a decrease in gamma-glutamyl transferase on the structured lipid. They advocated the use of a medium-chain triglyceride/long-chain triglyceride emulsions in long-term TPN, given its metabolic advantages relative to standard long-chain triglyceride emulsions.

Complications associated with parenteral nutrition

Complications due to short bowel syndrome

Two separate reviews provided an update on the adaptation process in short bowel syndrome and methods of management including intestinal lengthening procedures and transplantation [25•,26]. Transplantation may be an option for some patients and may involve bowel and liver transplants if the patient has combined intestinal and liver failure. It has particular future significance for young patients running out of venous access. At the present time, however, 5-year outcome transplant data is unavailable and thus for stable long-term patients, HPN still appears to be the preferred option [27].

Drug administration in patients with short bowel syndrome is a common practical therapeutic problem and limited data are available regarding drug bioavailability studies in this population. McFadden *et al.* [28•] provided a useful review of the literature and alternative routes of medication administration for short bowel syndrome patients.

Thompson [29] reported the clinical course of 53 adult patients with short bowel syndrome to determine the morbidity and likelihood of reoperation. Mesenteric vascular disease (n=23) and complications associated with malignancy or irradiation (n=18) were the most frequent causes of resection. Early reoperation, prior to discharge, was necessary in nine patients. Thirty-eight patients were eventually discharged, of whom 20 required a later abdominal procedure. Cholelithiasis developed in six out of 28 patients at risk for this problem. It was suggested that prophylactic cholecystectomy should be considered because of the high incidence of cholelithiasis associated with short bowel syndrome. Gastric hypersecretion in short bowel syndrome is a common but usually transient phenomenon; however, nine patients developed clinical symptoms of peptic ulceration.

Nightingale *et al.* [30] compared 46 patients having less than 200 cm of jejunum and no colon with 38 patients having similar jejunal lengths in continuity with the colon. All patients without a colon and less than 85 cm of jejunum, and all those with a colon but less than 45 cm of jejunum, required long-term parenteral nutrition. Most of the patients without a colon, not requiring TPN, nonetheless needed oral electrolyte replacement. Four patients with 85 cm of jejunum and a colon did not require fluid and electrolytes. None of the patients without a colon developed renal stones compared with nine of 38 with a colon. Both groups had an equally high prevalence (44%) of gallstones.

Georgeson and Breaux [10] reviewed the outcome of 52 neonatal patients requiring long-term hyperalimentation primarily as a consequence of necrotizing enterocolitis. The mean duration of HPN was 16.6 months and 39 patients were successfully weaned from it. The authors concluded that the absence of the ileocecal valve prolonged the duration of HPN but did not influence the overall outcome in terms of successful weaning from the therapy.

Infectious complications

Data from the large North American HPEN Registry [31] reported a yearly incidence of infection-related hospital readmissions of 0.53 for catheter-related sepsis and 0.04 for infection localized to the tunnel or exit site. Similar data was reported from the UK and Ireland HPN registry [2]; there were 97 episodes of catheter-related sepsis in 221 patients with an overall incidence of 0.47 episodes per annum. Herfindal *et al.* [32] reported retrospective data from 56 HPN patients. HPN was used for a mean duration of 1.02 years (range 7.3 days to 4.33 years), giving a cumulative total of 20,805 catheter days. There were 18 episodes of exit site infection and eight episodes of catheter-related septicemia. The overall incidence of infectious episodes was 0.46 per annum. The risk of developing catheter-related septicemia was significantly higher ($P<0.03$) for patients receiving long-term therapy and young patients. Burnes *et al.* [33] reported a 3-year analysis of their experience with 63 patients receiving HPN. The overall mortality was low (5% per year), but 73% required readmission to the hospital during the 3-year period for a mean duration of 10.6 days, primarily for suspected catheter-related sepsis. The most commonly isolated bacteria was *Staphylococcus epidermis.* Eight patients had fungemias of which six were due to *Candida albicans.*

Mukau *et al.* [34] described their experience in the management of 127 patients requiring long-term venous access for HPN or antibiotics, of whom 56 had AIDS. Catheter-related sepsis was higher in patients with AIDS and those receiving HPN. *Staphylococcus aureus* was the most common infecting pathogen and only 14 catheters (37.8%) were salvaged using antibiotic therapy. The authors suggested that because AIDS patients are susceptible to infection owing to their immunocompromised status, catheter-related sepsis should be treated by line removal and antibiotics.

Others have reported a complication rate of 0.43 per 100 catheter days in 47 AIDS patients with implanted central venous access devices (Port-A-Cath Pharmacia, Uppsala, Sweden) [35]. Only five of these patients were receiving HPN. There were 16 infectious complications in nine patients (0.13 per 100 catheter days). Three were puncture site infections, one was a tunnel infection, six were due to primary catheter-related sepsis, and six were due to secondary septicemia from another source. Three of the six infected devices were successfully treated with antibiotics without requiring removal. The authors attributed their relatively low infectious complication rate, when compared with other similar series, to limited use of the device including no blood sampling, no transfusions, and the maximum use of a single needle for 24 hours [35].

Cardiovascular and hematologic complications

Naidoo *et al.* [36] reported three cases of cardiovascular complications leading to congestive cardiac failure following the administration of parenteral nutrition containing standard vitamin supplements for at least 1 month. In one case, persistent vomiting caused by intestinal obstruction led to the development of thiamine deficiency and beriberi. Recurrent catheter tip sepsis causing the development of thrombosis and endocarditis were implicated in the other two cases. The authors recommended that patients should receive a loading dose of 100 mg of thiamine at the initiation of parenteral nutrition, especially alcoholic patients and those with protracted gastrointestinal disease. There was another report of thiamine deficiency in three patients who received prolonged parenteral nutrition without any vitamin supplements. These three patients developed fatal acute hemorrhagic encephalopathy [37].

Sola *et al.* [38] described their 6-year experience with 22 Infuse-A-Ports (Infusaid Corp., Sharon, MA, USA) in 15 cystic fibrosis patients. The overall complication rate was low, one in 1483 catheter days. However, the incidence of major thrombotic events was sufficiently high, three of 22 catheters (13.6%), that a policy of administering low-dose aspirin therapy (80 mg/d) was instituted in all patients without liver disease or other risks for bleeding complications.

Metabolic bone disease

The incidence and pathogenesis of bone disease associated with long-term parenteral nutrition was extensively reviewed [39••]. The difficulties of establishing the cause of metabolic bone disease in parenteral nutrition patients is due to the multifactorial nature of the disease. The complex interrelationship of parenteral calcium, phosphorus, and vitamin D has not been clearly elucidated. In the past, a link between aluminum content of casein hydrolysates and metabolic bone disease was established. Although these solutions are no longer used, aluminum remains a significant contaminant of some components of the parenteral nutrition solutions, particularly the mineral additives such as calcium gluconate and phosphate salts. The role of aluminum in the pathogenesis of bone disease requires further study, especially in pediatric patients and those with impaired renal function.

Renal impairment

Buchman *et al.* [40] reported a prospective evaluation of the renal function of 33 long-term parenteral nutrition patients. They concluded that long-term TPN is associated with a marked decrease in both glomerular filtration rate and tubular function. The observed decline could not be entirely explained on the basis of nutritional status, age, duration of TPN, the protein load, exposure to nephrotoxic drugs, or the frequency of infectious episodes.

Hepatic dysfunction

The hepatobiliary complications associated with total parenteral nutrition were comprehensively reviewed [41••]. The authors concluded that there is considerable evidence to support the role of excessive caloric provision, especially when administered as carbohydrate in the pathogenesis of steatosis. However, loss of enteric stimulation rather than TPN per se may be the critical determinant in the development of cholestasis, biliary sludge, and gallstones.

Buchman *et al.* [42] reported an evaluation of choline status and its relationship to hepatocyte damage in 41 HPN patients treated for 5.5 ± 4.7 years. Plasma-free choline was low in 33 of 41 subjects whereas phospholipid-bound choline was normal in 34/41 patients. They found that there was a significant correlation ($P<0.02$) between low free-plasma choline and elevations in serum aminotransferases; however, there was no correlation with phospholipid-bound choline. They concluded that choline deficiency was prevalent in this patient group and that the lipid emulsion they received as a source of phospholipid choline was inadequate to correct this deficiency. The same workers reported the reversal of TPN-associated hepatic steatosis in four long-term HPN patients using an intravenous choline supplement added to the TPN, 1 to 4 g/d for 6 weeks [43]. Fifteen of their HPN patients who had a low plasma choline were randomly assigned to receive oral lecithin 40 g/d or placebo for 6 weeks [44]. Lecithin supplementation increased plasma free choline by 53.4% ± 15.4%. In the placebo group, levels had decreased by 25.4% ±7.1% at 6 weeks. Patients in the lecithin-treated group showed a significant and progressive reduction in hepatic fat as assessed by computed tomography. The authors concluded that hepatic steatosis may be caused by a deficiency of plasma-free choline, which they suggest is a conditionally essential nutrient in this population. Taurine deficiency has also been implicated in the etiology of cholestasis associated with parenteral nutrition [45,46].

Mechanical complications

Complications associated with cyclical parenteral nutrition were reviewed [47]. The yearly reported frequency of catheter occlusion in European centers was 0.18 and 0.32. Catheter migration was reported 0.11 to 0.12 times per year. Problems with clotting were more common with external catheters whereas skin erosion was a greater issue with implanted devices. In the North American HPEN Patient Registry, mechanical complications were 0.10 to 0.15 per year and twice as common in patients with congenital bowel disorders.

Conclusions

Recent data from large groups of HPN patients followed by registries in the United States and the United Kingdom confirm good long-term functional rehabilitation when the primary disease causing the bowel failure is relatively stable. Medicare data point to a major expansion of this expensive therapy in the United States between 1989 and 1992, such that it is now used in 100 patients per million of the eligible Medicare population. This is 20 to 50 times higher than the utilization in other medically advanced countries. This difference appears to reflect the growing US use of HPN in short-term clinical situations such as unresectable cancer and AIDS patients. In other countries, HPN is seldom instituted in terminally ill patients. The average life expectancy of an active cancer patient who starts HPN is 6 months. The benefit of HPN versus simple hydration in this setting has not been properly evaluated, from either a quality of life or clinical outcome standpoint.

Catheter-related sepsis is the most common HPN complication and occurs on average once every 2 years in both the US and UK registry series. Death in HPN-treated patients is invariably due to the underlying disease and is not HPN-therapy related. In Crohn's disease patients receiving HPN, the mortality is 4% per year and only one in 10 of these deaths is therapy related. In active cancer patients where the 6-month mortality is 50%, only one in 100 of these deaths is therapy related. There are several other key issues that remain to be addressed in the area of long-term hyperalimentation. Significant advances have been made in the provision of nutrition support via the enteral route [48]. Better guidelines concerning which HPN patients can successfully switch to HEN are needed. Conversely, intestinal transplant and bowel lengthening procedures are showing some promising results especially using alternative immunosuppressive agents such as FK 506 [49,50]. It will be important to establish which HPN patients are good transplant candidates. Finally, the significance of certain conditionally essential nutrients such as parenteral glutamine [51–53], arginine [54], carnitine [55], *S*-adenosyl-L-methionine [56], taurine, and choline must be more clearly defined.

References and recommended reading

Papers of particular interest, published within the annual period of review, have been highlighted as:
• Of special interest
•• Of outstanding interest

1. • HOWARD L: **Home Parenteral and Enteral Nutrition in Cancer Patients.** *Cancer Suppl* 1993, **72**:3531–3541.
This is the most recent and largest available review of the outcome of HPEN cancer patients.

2. • O'HANRAHAN T, IRVING MH: **The Role of Home Parenteral Nutrition in the Mangement of Intestinal Failure: Report of 400 Cases.** *Clin Nutr* 1992, **11**:331–336.
Retrospective review of the outcome of HPN patients in Britain.

3. ELIA M: **Artificial Nutritional Support in Clinical Practice in Britain.** *J R Coll Physicians Lond* 1993, **27**:8–15.

4. HOWARD L, ALGER S, MICHALEK A, HEAPHEY L, AFTAHI S, JOHNSTON KR: **Home Parenteral Nutrition.** In *Parenteral Nutrition* edn. 2. Edited by Rombeau JL, Caldwell MD. Philadelphia: WB Saunders; 1993:814–839.

5. WILLIAMS CN: **Special Issues in Nutritional Therapy of Inflammatory Bowel Disease.** *Can J Gastroenterol* 1993, **7**:196–199.

6. GREENBERG GR: **Nutrition Support in Inflammatory Bowel Disease: Current Status and Future Directions.** *Scand J Gastroenterol* 1992, **27 (Suppl 192)** :117–122.

7. STOKES MA: **Crohn's Disease and Nutrition.** *Br J Surg* 1992, **79**:391–394.

8. SUTTON MM: **Nutritional Needs of Children With Inflammatory Bowel Disease.** *Compr Ther* 1992, **18**:21–25.

9. NOUSIA-ARVANITAKIS S, ANGELOPOULOU-SAKADAMI N, METROLIOU K: **Complications Associated With Total Parenteral Nutrition in Infants With Short Bowel Syndrome.** *Hepato gastroenterology* 1992, **39**:169–172.

10. GEORGESON KE, BREAUX CW: **Outcome and Intestinal Adaptation in Neonatal Short Bowel Syndrome.** *J Pediatr Surg* 1991, **27**:344–350.

11. RANNEM T, LADEFOGED K, HYLANDER E, HEGNHOJ J, JARNUM S: **Selenium Status in Patients With Crohn's Disease.** *Am J Clin Nutr* 1992, **56**:933–937.

12. ABRAMS CK, SIRAM SM, GALSIM, C, JOHNSON-HAMILTON H, MUNFORD FL, MEZGHEBE H: **Selenium Deficiency in Long Term Total Parenteral Nutrition.** *Nutr Clin Pract* 1992, **7**:175–178.

13. SILVAIN C, BESSON I, INGRAND P, BEAU P, FORT E, MATUCHANSKY C, CARRETIER M, MORICHEAU-BEAUCHANT M: **Long Term Outcome of Severe Radiation Enteritis Treated by Total Parenteral Nutrition.** *Dig Dis Sci* 1992, **37**:1065–1071.

14. IGNOFFO RJ: **Parenteral Nutrition Support in Patients With Cancer.** *Pharmacotherapy* 1992, **12**:353–357.

15. DALY JM, REDMOND HP, GALLAGHER H: **Perioperative Nutrition in Cancer Patients.** *JPEN J Parenter Enteral Nutr* 1992, **16**:100s–105s.

16. ASPEN BOARD OF DIRECTORS: **Nutrition Support for Adults With Specific Diseases and Conditions: Cancer.** *JPEN J Parenter Enteral Nutr* 1993, **17**:12–13SA.

17. • BOZZETTI F: **Nutritional Support in the Adult Cancer Patient.** *Clin Nutr* 1992, **11**:167–179.
An excellent comprehensive review of the available data evaluating the role of TPN and enteral nutrition in cancer patients.

18. CHARLIN V, BORGHESI L, HASBUN J, VON MULENBROCK R, MORENO MI: **Parenteral Nutrition in Hyperemesis Gravidarum.** *Nutrition* 1993, **9**:29–32.

19. • ABELL TL, RIELY CA: **Hyperemesis Gravidarum** *Gastroenterol Clin North Am* 1992, **21**:835–849.
A comprehensive review of the etiology and pathophysiology of hyperemesis gravidarum and associated metabolic derangements.

20. BOYCE RA: **Enteral Nutrition in Hyperemesis Gravidarum: A New Development.** *J Am Diet Assoc* 1992, **92**:733–736.

21. GULLEY RM, VANDER PLEOG N, GULLEY JM: **Treatment of Hyperemesis Gravidarum With Nasogastric Feeding.** *Nutr Clin Practice* 1993, **8**:33–35.

22. GREENSPOON JS, ROSEN DJD, AULT M: **Use of the Peripherally Inserted Central Catheter for Parenteral Nutrition During Pregnancy.** *Obstet Gynecol* 1993, **81**:831–834.

23. DE POTTER S, GOULET O, LAMOR M, CORRIOL O, COLOMB V, SADOUN E, RICOUR C: **263 Patient-Years of Home Parenteral Nutrition in Children.** *Transplant Proc* 1992, **24**:1056–1057.

24. GOULET O, POSTAIRE M, DE POTTER S, BOYA I, JOUNAIAUX AM, BEREZIAT G, RICOUR C: **Medium Chain Triglycerides and Long Term Parenteral Nutrition in Children.** *Nutrition* 1992, **8**:333–337.

25. • VANDERHOOF JA, LANGNAS AN, PINCH LW, THOMPSON JS, KAUFMAN SS: **Short Bowel Syndrome.** *J Pediatr Gastroenterol Nutr* 1992, **14**:359–370.
Review of the adaptation process in short bowel syndrome, the effects of specific nutrients, clinical management, and chronic complications, and the role of surgery.

26. NIGHTINGALE JMD, LENNARD-JONES JE: **The Short Bowel Syndrome.** *Dig Dis* 1993, **11**:12–31.

27. HIYAMA DT: **The Current Role of Small Bowel Transplantation in Intestinal Failure.** *Nutr Clin Practice* 1993, **8**:5–11.

28. • MCFADDEN MA, DELEGGE MH, KIRBY DF: **Medication Delivery in the Short Bowel Syndrome.** *JPEN J Parenter Enteral Nutr* 1993, **17**:180–186.
This review provides extensive lists of alternative methods of administering commonly prescribed drugs. Very limited data are available regarding the pharmacokinetics of drugs in the short bowel syndrome patient.

29. THOMPSON JS: **Reoperation in Patients With the Short Bowel Syndrome.** *Am J Surg* 1992, **164**:453–457.

30. NIGHTINGALE JMD, LENNARD-JONES JE, GERTNER DJ, WOOD SR, BARTRAM CI: **Colonic Preservation Reduces the Need for Parenteral Therapy, Increases the Incidence of Renal Stones, but Does not Change High Prevalence of Gall Stones in Patients With Short Bowel Syndrome.** *Gut* 1992, **3**:1493–1497.

31. HOWARD L, HEAPHEY L, FLEMING CR, LININGER L, STEIGER E: **Four Years of North American Registry Home Parenteral Nutrition Outcome Data and Their Implications for Patient Management.** *JPEN J Parenter Enteral Nutr* 1991, **15**:384–393.

32. HERFINDAL ET, BERNSTEIN LR, WONG AF, HOGUE VW, DARBINIAN JA: **Complications of Home Parenteral Nutrition.** *Clin Pharm* 1992, **11**:543–548.

33. BURNES JU, O'KEEFE SJD, FLEMING R, DEVINE RM, BERKNER S, HERRICK L: **Home Parenteral Nutrition: A 3 Year Analysis of Clinical and Laboratory Monitoring.** *JPEN J Parenter Enteral Nutr* 1992, **16**:327–332.

34. MUKAU L, TALAMINI MA, SITZMAN JV, BURNS RC, MCGUIRE ME: **Long Term Central Venous Access vs Other Home Therapies: Complications in Patients With Acquired Immunodeficiency Syndrome.** *JPEN J Parenter Enteral Nutr* 1992, **16**:455–459.

35. VAN DER PIJL H, FRISSEN PHJ: **Experience With a Totally Implantable Venous Access Device (Port-A-Cath) Patients With AIDS.** *AIDS* 1992, **6**:709–713.

36. NAIDOO DP, SINGH B, HAFFEJEE A: **Cardiovascular Complications of Parenteral Nutrition.** *Postgrad Med J* 1992, **68**:629–633.

37. VORTMEYER AO, HAGEL C, LAAS R: **Hemorrhagic Thiamine Deficient Encephalopathy Following Prolonged Parenteral Nutrition.** *J Neurol Neurosurg Psychiatry.* 1992, **55**:826–829.

38. SOLA JE, STONE MM, WISE B, COLOMBANI PM: **Atypical Thrombotic and Septic Complications of Totally Implantable Venous Access Devices in Patients With Cystic Fibrosis.** *Pediatr Pulmonol* 1992, **14**:239–242.

39. •• KOO WWK: **Parenteral Nutrition Related Bone Disease.** *JPEN J Parenter Enteral Nutr* 1992, **16**:386–394.
Excellent comprehensive review of the pathogenesis of bone disease including the role of calcium, phosphorus, vitamin D, aluminum, and micronutrients.

40. BUCHMAN AL, MOUKARZEL A, AMENT ME, GORNBEIN J, GOODSON B, CARLSON C, HAWKINS RA: **Serious Renal Impairment is Associated With Long Term Parenteral Nutrition.** *JPEN J Parenter Enteral Nutr* 1993, **17**:438–444.

41. •• QUIGLEY EMM, MARSH MN, SHAFFER JL, MARKIN RS: **Hepatobiliary Complications of Total Parenteral Nutrition.** *Gastroenterology* 1993, **104**:286–301.
Excellent review of the relationships between various hepatobiliary disorders and the administration of TPN, in particular, the role of TPN in their pathogenesis.

42. BUCHMAN AL, MOUKARZEL A, JENDEN DJ, ROCH M, RICE K, AMENT ME: **Low Plasma Free Choline Is Prevalent in Patients Receiving Long Term Parenteral Nutrition and Is Associated With Hepatic Aminotransferase Abnormalities.** *Clin Nutr* 1993, **12**:33–37.

43. BUCHMAN AL, DUBIN M, MOUKARZEL AA, JENDEN D, ROCH M, RICE K, GORNBEIN J, AMENT ME: **Choline Deficiency Causes TPN-Associated Hepatic Steatosis in Man and Is Reversed by Choline Supplemented TPN.** *Gastroenterology* 1993, **104**:A881.

44. BUCHMAN AL, DUBIN M, JENDEN D, MOUKARZEL A, ROCH MH, RICE K, GORNBEIN J, AMENT ME, ECKHERT CD: **Lecithin Increases Plasma Free Choline and Decreases Hepatic Steatosis in Long Term Total Parenteral Nutrition Patients.** *Gastroenterology* 1992, **102**:1363–1370.

45. HOWARD D, THOMPSON DF: **Taurine: An Essential Amino Acid to Prevent Cholestasis in Neonates?** *Ann Pharmacother* 1992, **26**:1390–1392.

46. DESAI TK, REDDY J, KINZIE JL, EHRINPREIS MN: **Taurine Supplementation and Cholestasis During Bone Marrow Transplantation.** *Gastroenterology* 1993, **104**:A616.

47. MATUCHANSKY C, MESSING B, JEEJEEBHOY KN, BEAU P, BELIAH M, ALLARD JP: **Cyclical Parenteral Nutrition.** *Lancet* 1992, **340**:588–592.

48. BASKIN WN: **Advances in Enteral Nutrition Techniques.** *Am J Gastroenterol* 1992, **11**:1547–1553.

49. TODO S, TZAKIS A, REYES J, ABU-ELMAGD, CASAVILLA A, FUNG JJ, STARZL.: **Intestinal Transplant in Humans Under FK 506.** *Transplant Proc* 1993, **25**:1198–1199.

50. TODO S, TZAKIS AG, ABU-ELMAGD K, REYES J, NAKAMURA K, CASAVILLA A, SELBY R, NOUR BM, WRIGHT H, FUNG JJ, DEMETRIS AJ, VAN THIEL DH, STARZL TE: **Intestinal Transplantation in Composite Visceral Grafts or Alone.** *Ann Surg* 1992, **216**:223–234.

51. VAN DER HULST RRW, VAN KREEL BK, VON MEYENFELDT MF, BRUMMER RJM, ARENDS JW, DEUTZ NEP, SOETERS PB: **Glutamine and the Preservation of Gut Integrity.** *Lancet* 1993, **341**:1363–1365.

52. PLATELL C, MCCAULEY R, MCCULLOCH R, HALL J: **The Influence of Parenteral Glutamine and Branched Chain Amino Acids on Total Parenteral Nutrition- Induced Atrophy of the Gut.** *JPEN J Parenter Enteral Nutr* 1993, **17**:348–354.

53. POWELL-TUCK J: **Glutamine, Parenteral Feeding and Intestinal Nutrition.** *Lancet* 1993, **342**:451–452.

54. DALY JM, LIEBERMAN MD, GOLDFINE J, SHOU J, WEINTRAUB F, ROSATO EF, LAVIN P: **Enteral Nutrition With Supplemental RNA, and Omega-3 Fatty Acids in Patients After Operation: Immunologic, Metabolic and Clinical Outcome.** *Surgery* 1992, **112**:56–67.

55. BUCHMAN AL, VINTERS HV, DIETHELM S, AMENT ME, VERITY MA: **Late Onset Primary Systemic Carnitine Deficiency Exacerbated by Carnitine-Free Parenteral Nutrition.** *Clin Nutr* 1992, **11**:368–372.

56. OSMAN E, OWEN JS, BURROUGHS AK: **Review Article: S-Adenosyl L-Methionine A New Therapeutic Agent in Liver Disease?** *Aliment Pharmacol Ther* 1993, **7**:21–28.

Margaret Malone, MSc, PhD, Associate Professor, Department of Pharmacy Practice, Albany College of Pharmacy, 106 New Scotland Avenue, Albany, NY 12208, USA.

Lyn Howard, MB, FRCP, Professor of Medicine, Head of Division of Clinical Nutrition, Albany Medical Center, New Scotland Avenue, Albany, NY 12208, USA.

Liver

Editorial review

Norman Gitlin, MD, and Johan Fevery, MD, PhD

School of Medicine, Emory University, Atlanta, Georgia, USA, and University Hospital Gasthuisberg, Leuven, Belgium

Current Opinion in Gastroenterology 1994, **10**:235–236

Another interesting and challenging year has passed. Hepatology continues to make inroads into a number of independent conditions; our understanding of the pathogenesis and management of previously obscure entities has been the basis of the spectacular advances in hepatology over the past decade. We extend a very sincere thank you to our contributors for their outstanding overviews. Our endeavor to reflect a spectrum of international opinions is noted by the names and countries of our authors. Clearly, the approach meets with the approval of our readership and it is reflected in our growing number of subscribers.

The correlation between the presence of a specific mutation of the tumor suppressor gene, p53, and exposure to large amounts of aflatoxin points to an association between environment and cancer. The additional association between chronic hepatitis C infection and hepatocellular cancer has been compelling. The interaction between hepatitis B and hepatitis C infections and the carcinogenic role of alcohol remain to be clarified.

The challenge to identify an effective therapy against hepatocellular cancer has spawned a number of novel approaches. The use of intrahepatic ablation of small neoplasms by means of alcohol injections has produced encouraging results, albeit in select cases. The search continues for more effective chemotherapy agents. Prophylaxis against a number of recognizable etiologic agents (*eg*, hepatitis B virus, hepatitis C virus, alfatoxins, iron overload, and thorotrast) remains a prime focus.

Hepatitis C virus continues to be an enigma. The initial acute infection is complicated by a chronic course in almost 80% of cases. The natural history of chronic hepatitis attributed to hepatitis C virus is extremely variable. Infection-causing hepatitis in many patient smolders on for decades without the development of cirrhosis or hepatic decompensation. Other patients, especially males 60 years of age or older, appear to rapidly progress to cirrhosis and the ramifications of portal hypertension. The factors governing the outcome of an acute infection with hepatitis C virus are unclear, however, the host's immune status appears to be important. The role of the patient's age, alcoholism, and the size of the initial viral inoculum (blood transfusion or needle stick) may be important.

The past year has seen sobering developments relating to new forms of drug therapy for chronic hepatitis due to hepatitis B virus infection. The experience regarding a nucleoside analogue fluoro-iodo-arabinofuranosyl-uracil indicate the hazards to all concerned when embarking on pilot studies with novel preparations.

Experience with the transjugular intrahepatic portosystemic shunt procedure for variceal bleeding has tempered the initial enthusiasm for this procedure. Clearer indications, contraindications, and an awareness of the natural history of transjugular intrahepatic portosystemic shunt procedure have enabled a more selective use of this valuable tool. Its role in the management of severe ascites or pulmonary hydrothorax is unclear.

The attempt to revise the nomenclature for chronic hepatitis is timely and appropriate. However, it is a herculean task beset with obstacles. Its best chance of success rests with a gradual, logical change rather than an abrupt *fait accompli*.

The importance of the production of the different cytokines during hepatic inflammation and regeneration is of considerable interest. The recognition of a hepatocytic factor "hepitoin," which may activate Ito cells, and the recognition of "injurin," which may induce hepatic growth factor, indicates that this research may provide critical input to our understanding of the development of cirrhosis or hepatic regeneration. A role has been postulated for interleukin-1 and interleukin-6 (both are involved in the induction of the acute-phase response) in the sequelae of alcoholic liver disease. The similarity of clinical features in the acute-phase response and alcoholic hepatitis suggests a parallel pathogenesis.

Viral hepatitis A is not considered a serious disease and does not progress to chronic inflammation or cirrhosis, yet fulminant hepatic failure can occur. However, the disease is poorly tolerated in patients over 60 years of age. The advent of a safe and effective vaccine is a welcome addition to the prophylactic arsenal against viral hepatitis.

 ISBN 1-85922-608-6 ISSN 0267–1379

The development of an artificial hepatic support system for the temporary management of fulminant hepatic failure or acute hepatic failure superimposed on established cirrhosis is an important advance in the treatment of these entities, both of which carry a very high mortality rate. Artificial hepatic support systems can maintain a patient temporarily until either hepatic regeneration or hepatic transplantation occurs. An expanded role for those systems is envisioned.

Further development of molecular medicine will help to delineate the pathogenesis of diseases and the function of various proteins. Indeed, the "knock-out" procedures to eliminate a gene coding for a given protein, can teach us a lot about the functions of that protein as well as feedback and compensatory systems involved when the given protein is defective.

Future research will continue to expand our understanding and treatment of liver diseases.

Norman Gitlin, MD, Division of Digestive Diseases, Emory University School of Medicine, Drawer AL, Atlanta, GA 30322, USA.

Johan Fevery, MD, PhD, University Hospital Gasthuisberg, v.s. Gasthuisberg, Herestraat 49, 3200, Leuven, Belgium.

Recent developments in viral hepatitis

Elias I. Fanous, Jr, MD, and Luis A. Balart, MD

Louisiana State University Medical Center, New Orleans, Louisiana, USA

Our understanding of viral hepatitis becomes greater with time. The ubiquitous hepatitis A virus could soon become obsolete with advances in the development of new vaccines. Hepatitis B is well characterized by its serologic markers and the potential role of the polymerase chain reaction. Its presentation and prognosis can be influenced by the development of cirrhosis, concurrent immunocompromised states, and age. The transmission, diagnosis, and long-term prognosis of chronic hepatitis C is becoming less cryptic and more defined with the help of more sensitive and specific testing methods and continued patient follow-up. Close associations to hepatitis C are being established with many other disease states. Hepatitis D and its relationship to hepatitis B are defined. Finally, an overview of the developing characterization of hepatitis E is also presented.

Current Opinion in Gastroenterology 1994, **10**:237–242

Hepatitis A

Hepatitis A virus (HAV) is responsible for one third of the clinical cases of hepatitis in the United States. It may have a protracted or relapsing course, trigger autoimmune hepatitis, or rarely result in fulminant hepatic failure. Classically, the mode of transmission is fecal-oral, but rarely blood-borne transmission has been noted. Studies using polymerase chain reaction (PCR) show that viremia in HAV infection lasts longer than has previously been thought (up to 7 days after clinical onset), causing concern of possible transmission with blood [1]. Currently, the standard recommendation for pre- and post-exposure prophylaxis is passive immunization with immune globulin. Active immunization would benefit those at highest risk including travelers, health care workers (especially those in pediatrics and nursing homes [2]), food handlers, sewage workers, child care center workers, institutionalized persons, illicit drug users, and homosexuals. Inactivated purified HAV vaccine has been tested and is well tolerated. A single dose is highly protective against clinically apparent HAV, but it is unlikely that one dose will be enough to afford long-lasting protection [3]. One of the most effective vaccines appears to be an inactivated HAV coupled to immunopotentiating reconstituted influenza virosomes, resulting in high antibody titers for up to 1 year after immunization [4].

Hepatitis B

Hepatitis B virus (HBV) is a hepadnavirus composed of surface (envelope), core, and e antigens. The entire genome has been cloned. It is most prevalent in developing countries of Asia, Africa, and the Pacific Islands where it is spread vertically and horizontally. In low prevalence areas, transmission is through sexual contact or intravenous drug abuse. Other high-risk groups include homosexual men, transfusion recipients, dialysis patients, health care personnel, and institutionalized persons. The risk of persistent HBV infection is inversely related to the age of a child, with neonates developing chronic infection up to 90% of the time. Worldwide over 250,000 people die annually from HBV-associated disease. In countries with vertical transmission, the risk of developing hepatocellular carcinoma is more than 200 times that of controls [5]. Hepatitis B surface antigen (HBsAg) has been identified in virtually all body secretions, but transmission has been documented only with saliva or semen.

Transmission

Vertical transmission of HBV is most likely to occur in the third trimester (at the time of birth rather than *in utero*), and more so if mothers are hepatitis B e antigen (HBeAg)-positive. Passive transfer of maternal core antibodies can occur. Combined passive-ac-

Abbreviations

HAV—hepatitis A virus; **HBeAg**—hepatitis B e antigen; **HBsAg**—hepatitis B surface antigen; **HBV**—hepatitis B virus; **HCV**—hepatitis C virus; **HDV**—hepatitis D virus; **HEV**—hepatitis E virus; **PCR**—polymerase chain reaction.

 ISBN 1-85922-608-6 ISSN 0267–1379

tive immunoprophylaxis is recommended shortly after birth [6]. HBV infection has also been associated with finger-stick devices [7]. Among adults, sexual transmission seems to be the most common mode [8,9].

Diagnosis

In acute, self-limited infection, anti–hepatitis B core (immunoglobulin M and immunoglobulin G) appears first with (HBsAg) and HBeAg identified 2 to 4 weeks before onset of symptoms. Core immunoglobulin M becomes undetectable by 6 months. In some patients with chronic HBV, concurrent hepatitis B surface antibody may be present, representing low-titer Ab directed at a heterotypic subdeterminant of HBsAg having no clinical significance. The lag time between loss of HBsAg and appearance of hepatitis B antibody is referred to as the window period where anti-HBc may be the only serologic marker of infection. Core Ab is a common screening marker and if present as the only marker could represent one of four entities: resolved prior infection (without hepatitis B antigen), current infection with loss of surface antigen, the window period of resolution, or a false-positive test result. A total of 90% to 95% of persons with acute HBV recover, whereas 5% to 10% develop persistent infection, and 1% develop fulminant hepatitis with up to an 80% mortality. HBeAg is associated with infectivity and correlates with the presence of HBV DNA. However, in the Mediterranean and Far East regions, some mutant strains of HBV have been found that do not secrete HBeAg and yet are associated with severe chronic hepatitis [10].

The PCR allows viral DNA to be amplified and sequenced. No two HBV are genetically identical and significant mutations exist, like the subgroup of patients that do not secrete HBeAg (precore mutant). The same variant can also cause a different clinical picture in another host, which may be related to the degree of interferon production and immunologic response to HBV antigen by the host. PCR has its potential limitations at present. For instance, HBV DNA can be detected at low levels by PCR for months despite absence of replication; therefore, positive PCR may not always be indicative of viral replication [11]. Its use should be focused on three scenarios: detection of viral replication in HBsAg-positive, HBeAg-positive patients with active liver disease despite negative spot tests for HBV DNA, evaluation of HBsAg-negative patients with liver disease, and follow-up of HBV infection in liver transplant patients. In the future, PCR may be more useful with quantification techniques, decreased price, and increased availability. This would allow for follow-up of antiviral treatment and screening blood donations [12].

Prognosis

Cirrhosis is the leading cause of nonmalignant mortality in the United States. However, death rates have declined 26% since 1973. This seems to be related to advances in medical management as well as socioeconomic and population changes [13]. In one study HBsAg-positive patients with cirrhosis had survival rates of 92%, 79%, and 71% at 1, 3, and 5 years, respectively. Age, bilirubin level, and ascites were significant variables related to survival. Patients defined as decompensated (ascites, jaundice, portosystemic encephalopathy, and variceal bleeding) had a greatly decreased 5-year survival (14% vs 84%). HBeAg was a negative prognostic factor in those with cirrhosis and conversion to HBeAb was associated with a 55% decrease in mortality [14•]. Based on these findings, one might consider more aggressive modalities such as liver transplant in those with decompensated cirrhosis and antiviral prescriptions in those with e antigen-positive cirrhosis.

Immune compromise

HIV infection seems to add a twist to HBV infection. A history of HBV exposure is apparent in 80% to 95% of HIV patients, but carrier states exist in only 10% to 15%. However, carrier states are higher if HIV or AIDS exist prior to HBV exposure [15]. HIV patients have higher levels of HBV DNA and a greater incidence of HBeAg positivity but less severe hepatitis on histology and lower aminotransferase levels. In HIV-infected patients, reports of fulminant HBV are extremely rare in the absence of concurrent hepatitis D virus (HDV). HBV vaccine tends to be effective in only 35% to 56% of HIV-infected individuals and other immunocompromised states versus 85% to 95% in controls [15]. When HIV patients develop frank AIDS, they tend to have a higher prevalence of HBsAg and hepatitis B core antibody than non-AIDS HIV patients [16•]. This may be a result of a failing immune system's inability to keep the HBV in check.

Prevention

Hepatitis B virus seems to behave differently in children; 90% of children are asymptomatic and 1% to 3% of infections occur before the age of 5. Current prevention includes universal HBsAg screening in all pregnant women and integration of HBV vaccine into childhood immunization schedules [9]. Poor correlation exists between unregistered prenatal patients with illicit drug use and HBsAg-positivity. This data would not support empiric HBV prophylaxis for neonates born to mothers without prenatal care in certain populations. However, currently the American College of Gynecology and the Centers for Disease Control recommend universal screening because of favorable cost-benefit profiles [17].

Hepatitis C

Hepatitis C virus (HCV) seems to have highly diverse genomic sequences around the world with two serologically distinct core antigen subtypes that may represent clinical variations [18,19]. Patients with HCV predominantly complain of fatigue, abdominal pain, and jaundice, with 25% being asymptomatic. Physical findings include a palpable liver, spiders, and splenomegaly [20••].

Transmission

Horizontal transmission of HCV has been related to transfusion of blood products, intravenous drug abuse, sexual intercourse, transplantation, and tattooing [21]. Many recent studies have shown that the sexual transmission of HCV seems to be very infrequent [21–23]. A 5.4% transmission of HCV (proven by identifying homologous HCV RNA) predominantly to the spouse through sexual intercourse, saliva, or other intimate contact has been reported [24]. Among patients in a venereal clinic, the primary mode of transmission was via intravenous drug abuse [22].

Previous studies have shown that renal transplant recipients are at high risk of becoming PCR positive, but may not produce anti-HCV or have abnormal liver function tests. A more recent study showed no detection of HCV by PCR or second-generation enzyme-immunoassay in 143 transplanted patients [25]. This might theoretically reflect a low level of viremia, a strain with low infectivity, or be a result of organ preservation techniques. This may support the immunopathic versus cytopathic nature of HCV. The majority of transplant recipients seem to acquire HCV before or during transplantation [26].

Needlestick accidents pose a varying rate of transmission, from 0% in 81 Spanish patients followed for 12 months by radioimmunoblot assay II [27] up to as high as 10% in other studies using detection by PCR [28,29]. This rate is lower than that of HBV (7% to 30%) [30] but is higher than HIV (0.5%) [31]. The resultant hepatitis seems to be mild, transient, and less likely to evolve into a chronic hepatitis [28,29]. This may reflect a low virus load or different HCV strains. There is no evidence to date to support the use of antiviral therapy for acute exposures.

Institutionalized patients seem to have a lower prevalence of HCV in contrast to HBV. In a study of 113 previously institutionalized out-patients in New York, none were HCV positive, but 21% were HBsAb-positive and 2.7% were HBsAg-positive. Other previous studies have shown a 5% to 11% prevalence of HCV in in-patients but higher rates of HBsAg (up to 20%) [32]. This difference may reflect more out-patient care, HBV immunization, or the infrequency of sexual transmission in HCV.

Older conflicting studies have suggested that body fluids of patients with chronic HCV rarely, if ever, contain detectable HCV RNA [33], but more recent studies show that HCV RNA has been detected in the saliva of pregnant HCV-positive patients (but not in breast milk) [34] and in the saliva of the majority of HCV-positive patients [35]. However, to date no clear-cut cases of saliva transmission of HCV have been noted.

Vertical transmission of HCV seems to be very infrequent, with a transmission rate of zero of 24 at 1 year in one study [36], and one of 21 in another (using PCR) [37]. Nevertheless, passive transfer of maternal HCV antibody can be detected transiently in neonates and usually does not denote infection. Neonates are capable of mounting antibodies to HCV as they do with vaccines [35]. If the mother is coinfected with HIV, the transmission rate may be significantly increased with 11 of 25 positive by PCR in one study [24,36,38]. Coinfection of HIV with HCV may theoretically stimulate viral replication or increase infectivity. This is questioned, however, by one study with no transmission by PCR in eight HIV-confirmed mothers with PCR-positive HCV [35]. This brings up the question of false positivity (contaminant) versus false negativity with the use of PCR. Heparin and prolonged freezing of samples seem to interfere with the PCR assay and may lead to false-negatives [39].

Diagnosis

The diagnosis of HCV infection can be made earlier now. PCR can detect HCV RNA as early as 1 to 3 weeks from clinical onset. First-generation enzyme immunoassays were unreliable but second-generation enzyme immunoassay is more sensitive and specific, allowing earlier detection, and correlating closely to PCR [40]. Second-generation enzyme immunosorbent assay was even more sensitive than radioimmunoblot assay up until 21 weeks [41]. The presence of HCV RNA correlates with alanine aminotransferase level but not with age, sex, or aspartate aminotransferase level [42]. In immunocompromised patients (*eg*, hemodialysis patients), HCV infection may not be detected by conventional anti-HCV testing (second-generation enzyme immunoassay) or abnormal liver function tests (up to 66% had normal liver function tests) [39,41]. With the advent of PCR, it seems that more patients have detectable levels of RNA than antibody. This may reflect a decreased immunopathic effect with immunosuppression. Despite this, prolonged presence of HCV RNA may not always be associated with liver damage. In addition, HCV antibody may be present with a negative PCR [43,44]. This could be explained by intermittent replication with intervening clearance [45]. Viremia without liver or lab abnormality might be the result of a nonvirulent strain, tolerance, or viral replication at a different organ site [42]. HCV has been found in the liver of patients with chronic HCV when searched for by reverse transcriptase PCR and in peripheral blood mononuclear cells [46,47]. It appears very possible that other tissues may harbor this virus.

Disease associations

Hepatitis C virus has been associated with cryoglobulinemia, membranous glomerulonephritis, autoimmune hepatitis, porphyria cutanea tarda, sicca syndrome, Sjogren's, aplastic anemia [48], polyarteritis nodosa, and Waldenstrom's macroglobulinemia. Up to 79% of patients with nonfamilial type porphyria cutanea tarda were found to be HCV positive and have biopsy proven liver disease, whereas none of the familial type had HCV infection. HCV may unmask the underlying uroporphyrinogen decarboxylase defect or patients with porphyria cutanea tarda may in some way be more susceptible to HCV infection [49,50]. Numerous studies have linked HCV and HBV with cryoglobulinemia types II, III, and essential mixed cryoglobulinemia, but recently HCV seems to be more implicated (up to 84% by PCR in type II) [51]. HCV RNA has been detected in both serum and cryoprecipitate in these patients [52,53•,54]. A large number of false-positive second-generation enzyme immunoassays have been found in RNA-positive patients with type II cryoglobulinemia [55]. Abnormal liver biopsies correlated with PCR positivity [50,54]. Treatment with interferon-α seemed to decrease or eliminate cryoglobulins and the vasculitis [53•,56,57]. Recent studies have also associated HCV with membranoproliferative glomerulonephritis (confirmed with kidney biopsies) [50,58,59]. Up to 27% of these patients had trace to 2+ proteinuria with normal creatinine, which seemed to improve after interferon therapy [50].

Chronic HCV can mimic type 1 or 2 autoimmune hepatitis and must be considered in those unresponsive to immunosuppression [60]. Patients can be divided into two groups: true autoimmune patients with high titers of anti–liver-kidney microsomes (young females) and negative radioimmunoblot assay or those with HCV hepatitis with low titers of anti–liver-kidney microsomes (older males). Anti–liver-kidney microsomes can also be seen in drug-induced hepatitis and HDV [61].

Prognosis

Longer term prognosis in HCV infection is not yet well defined. One study of 568 patients over 18 years showed survival curves similar to two other control groups without liver disease unless there was concomitant ethanol use (71% of deaths related to liver disease). Compared with the control groups, there was only a small but statistically significant increase in deaths due to liver disease [62]. Despite this, HCV infection seems to persist indefinitely and long-term progression to cirrhosis does not seem to be unusual. In one study of HCV-positive patients, 37% had cirrhosis, with 20% progressing to cirrhosis on re-biopsy after 5 years (increasing age correlating with more severe liver disease) [20••]. Another study of 135 coronary bypass–related HCV-positive patients followed for up to 13 years showed chronicity in 70%, with 32% progressing to cirrhosis, and 4.8% dying from liver-related disease (only one hepatocellular carcinoma) [63]. Chronic HCV infection may also predispose to development of hepatocellular carcinoma. A recent meta-analysis of 1930 patients with hepatocellular carcinoma found anti-HCV positivity in 47%, which was comparable to those with HBV infection [64]. HCV replication has been found in hepatocellular carcinoma cells [65], but the exact relationship has not been determined.

Hepatitis D

Hepatitis D virus is a defective RNA virus requiring the presence of HBV. It coexists in three scenarios: acute HBV and HDV coinfection, acute HDV in an HBV carrier, and chronic HBV with chronic HDV. HBV replication can occur with a chronic HDV state. Exacerbations of disease in B and D patients may be secondary to either HBV or HDV reactivation. HCV does not seem to be related to HDV. New strains or mutations of HDV infecting new hepatocytes are also known to occur. Therefore, HDV patients during their course may have stable or reactivation courses. Late in the course replication of either B or D may exist without evidence of hepatocellular damage [66]. Tests for HDV include both immunoglobulin M or immunoglobulin G anti-HDV. Anti-HDV is likely, but not yet proven to provide protection in the event of subsequent HDV exposures [67].

Hepatitis E

Hepatitis E virus (HEV) is transmitted via the fecal-oral route, being ultimately related to contaminated water sources. The diagnosis is now based on serologic evidence of anti-HEV to immunoglobulin M. Detection of the immunoglobulin A class has also been noted in outbreaks [68]. Data suggest that immunoglobulin G against HEV persists for long periods of time [69]. No endemic US contacts have been noted as yet, but outbreaks in India, Africa, central Asia, Soviet republics, Afghanistan, Bangladesh, Borneo, Burma, China, India, Mexico, Mongolia, Nepal, Pakistan, and several Middle-Eastern countries have been confirmed.

The incubation period of HEV ranges from 2 to 9 weeks with a mean of 45 days. It seems to infect persons in the range of 15 to 40 years of age. It is known to cause a 15% to 20% fatality rate in pregnant women in the third trimester. Chronic liver disease or persistent viremia have not been observed [70•]. One should suspect it in travelers negative for hepatitis A, B, or C. A detailed exposure history is helpful in the diagnosis (*eg*, ingestion of ice, non-bottled water, or uncooked food) and all cases should be reported [71].

References and recommended reading

Papers of particular interest, published within the annual period of review, have been highlighted as:

- • Of special interest
- •• Of outstanding interest

1. Yotsuyanagi H, Shiro I, Kazuhiko K, Kiyomi Y, Kunihiko H, Kiyoshi K: **Duration of Viremia in Human Hepatitis A Viral Infection as Determined by Polymerase Chain Reaction.** *J Med Virol* 1993, **40**:35–38.

2. Van Damme P, Cramm M, van der Auwera JC, Meheus A: **Hepatitis A Vaccination for Health Care Workers.** *BMJ* 1993, **306**:1615.

3. Sjogren MH: **Acute Hepatitis A: An Endangered Species.** *Hepatology* 1993, **17**:519–520.

4. Gluck R, Mischler R, Brantschen S, *et al.*: **Hepatitis A Vaccines: Past, Present and Future.** *Gastroenterology* 1993, **105**:943–946.

5. Perrilo RP: **Hepatitis B: Transmission and Natural History.** *Gut* 1993, **34**:S48-S49.

6. Beasley RP, Hwang LY, Lee GC, *et al.*: **Prevention of Perinatally Transmitted Hepatitis B Virus Infection With Hepatitis B Immune Globulin and Hepatitis B Vaccine.** *Lancet* 1983, **2**:1099.

7. Marcus DL, Lordi PF Jr: **Transmission of Hepatitis B Virus Associated With a Finger-Stick Device.** *N Engl J Med* 1993, **328**:969.

8. Hou MC, Wu JC, Juo BIT, Sheng WY, Chen TZ, Lee SD, Lo KJ: **The Heterosexual Transmission as the Most Common Route of Hepatitis B Virus Infection Among Adults in Taiwan: The Importance of Extending Vaccination to Susceptible Adults.** *J Infect Dis* 1993, **167**:938–941.

9. Alter MJ: **Community Acquired Viral Hepatitis B and C in the United States.** *Gut* 1993, **34**:S17–S19.

10. Brown JL, Carman WF, Thomas HC: **The Clinical Significance of Molecular Variation Within the Hepatitis B Virus Genome.** *Hepatology* 1992, **15**:144–148.

11. Lazizi Y, Pilot J: **Delayed Clearance of HBV-DNA Detected by PCR in the Absence of Viral Replication.** *J Med Virol* 1993, 39:208–213.

12. Brechot C: **Polymerase Chain Reaction for the Diagnosis of Viral Hepatitis B and C.** *Gut* 1993, **34**:S39–S44.

13. Everhart JE, Hoofnagle JH: **Hepatitis B-Related End-Stage Liver Disease [Editorial].** *Gastroenterology* 1992, **103**:1692–1694.

14. • de Jongh FE, Janssesen HLA, de Man RA, Hop WCI, Schlam SW, van Blankenstein M: **Survival and Prognostic Indicators in Hepatitis B Surface Antigen-Positive Cirrhosis of the Liver.** *Gastroenterology* 1992, **103**:1630–1635.

Hepatitis B surface antigen–positive patients with cirrhosis had decreasing survivals at 1-, 3-, and 5-year follow up, and even less when defined as decompensated or eAg positive. Recommendations are made for liver transplant versus interferon treatment.

15. Lichtenstein DR, Makadon HJ, Chopra S: **Fulminant Hepatitis B and Delta Virus Coinfection in AIDS.** *Am J Gastroenterol* 1992, **87**:1643–1647.

16. • Scharmchmidt BF, Held MJ, Hollander HH, Read AE, Lavine JE, Veereman G, Meguire RF, Thaler MM: **Hepatitis-B in Patients With HIV Infection: Relationship to AIDS and Patient Survival.** *Ann Intern Med* 1992, **117**:837–838.

AIDS patients had a statistically significant higher prevalence of HBsAg and HBcAb versus non-AIDS HIV-positive patients.

17. Dankner WM, Dixon SD, Lane TA, Moore T: **Hepatitis-B in a Prenatal Population.** *JAMA* 1993, **269**:589–590.

18. Machida A, Ohuma H, Tsuda F, Munekala E, Tnaka T, Akahane Y, Okamoto H, Mishiro S: **Two Distinct Subtypes of Hepatitis C Virus Defined by Antibodies Directed to the Putative Core Protein.** *Hepatology* 1992, 16:886–891.

19. Overby LR: **Hepatitis C: Looking at a Virus That Hasn't Been Seen.** *Gut* 1993, **34**:S6–S9.

20. •• Merican I, Sherlock S, Mcintyre N, Dusheiko GM: **Clinical, Biochemical and Histological Features in 102 Patients with Chronic Hepatitis C Virus Infection.** *Q J Med* 1993, **86**:119–125.

This article describes well the clinical presentations and physical findings of 102 chronic hepatitis C patients with liver biopsies upon entry and at 4- to 5-year follow-up.

21. Ko YC, Ho MS, Chiang TA, Chang SJ, Chang PY: **Tattooing as a Risk of Hepatitis C Virus Infection.** *J Med Virol* 1992, **38**:288–291.

22. Weinstock HS, Bolan G, Reingold AL, Polish LB: **Hepatitis C Virus Infection Among Patients Attending a Clinic for Sexually Transmitted Diseases.** *JAMA* 1993, **269**:392–394.

23. Osmond DH, Padian NS, Sheppard HW, Glass S, Shiboski SC, Reingold A: **Risk Factors for Hepatitis C Virus Seropositivity in Heterosexual Couples.** *JAMA* 1993, **269**:361–365.

24. Kao JH, Chen PJ, Yang PM, Lai MY, Sheu JC, Wang TH, Chem DS: **Intrafamilial Transmission of Hepatitis-C Virus: The Important Role of Infections Between Spouses.** *J Infect Dis* 1992, **166**:900–903.

25. Vincenti F, Lake J, Wright T, Kuo G, Weber P, Stempel C: **Nontransmission of Hepatitis C From Cadaver Kidney Donors to Transplant Recipients.** *Transplantation* 1993, **55**:674–675.

26. Chan T-M, Lok ASF, Cheng IKP, Chan RT: **A Prospective Study of Hepatitis C Virus Infection Among Renal Transplant Recipients.** *Gastroenterology* 1993, **104**:862–868.

27. Hernandez ME, Bruguera M, Puyuelo T, Barrero JM, Tapias JMS, Rodes J: **Risk of Needle Stick Injuries in the Transmission of Hepatitis C Virus in Hospital Personnel.** *J Hepatol* 1992, **16**:45–58.

28. Schiff ER: **Hepatitis C Among Health Care Providers: Risk Factors and Possible Prophylaxis [Editorial].** *Hepatology* 1992, **16**:1300–1301.

29. Mitsui T, Iwano K, Masuko K, Yamazaki C, Okamoto H, Tsuda F, Tanaka T, Mishiro S: **Hepatitis C Virus Infection in Medical Personnel After Needlestick Accident.** *Hepatology* 1992, **16**:1109–1114.

30. Occupational Safety and Health Administration: **Occupational Exposure to Bloodborne Pathogens: Proposed Rule and Notice of Hearing.** *Federal Register* 1989, **54**:23042–23139.

31. Levinson WM, Womser GP, Forseter G, Calmann M, Obrien TA: **Hepatitis-C Virus Seroprevalence in the Developmentally Disabled.** *Arch Intern Med* 1992, **152**:2309–2311.

32. Esteban JI, Lopez-Talavera JC, Genesca J, Madoz P, Viladomil L, Muniz E, Martin-Vega C, Rosell M, Allende H, Vidal X, *et al.*: **High Rate of Infectivity and Liver Disease in Blood Donors With Antibodies to Hepatitis C Virus.** *Ann Intern Med* 1991, **115**:443–449.

33. Marcus R, the CDC Cooperative Needlestick Surveillance Group: **Surveillance of Health Care Workers Exposed to Blood From Patients Infected with the Human Immunodeficiency Virus.** *N Engl J Med* 1988, **319**:1118–1123.

34. Ogasawara S, Kage M, Kosai K, Shimamatsu K, Kojiro M: **Hepatitis C Virus RNA in Saliva and Breastmilk of Hepatitis C Carrier Mothers.** *Lancet* 1993, **341**:561.

35. Couzigou P, Richard L, Dumas F, Shouler L, Fleury H: **Detection of HCV-RNA in Saliva of Patients With Chronic Hepatitis C.** *Gut* 1993, **34**:S59–S60.

36. Reinus JF, Leikin EL, Alter HJ, Cheung L, Shindo M, Jett B, Piazza S, Shih JWK: **Failure to Detect Vertical Transmission of Hepatitis C Virus.** *Ann Intern Med* 1992, **117**:881–886.

37. Wejstal R, Widell A, Mansson AS, Hemodsson S, Norkraus G: **Mother-to-Infant Transmission of Hepatitis C Virus.** *Ann Intern Med* 1992, **117**:887–890.

38. Bach N, Bodenheimer HC: **Transmission of Hepatitis C: Sexual, Vertical or Exclusively Blood-Borne.** *Hepatology* 1992, **16**:1497–1499.

39. Koff RS: **The Low Efficiency of Maternal-Neonatal Transmission of Hepatitis C Virus: How Certain Are We [Editorial].** *Ann Intern Med* 1992, **117**:967–969.

40. Chan TM, Lok ASF, Heng IKP, Chan RT: **Prevalence of Hepatitis C Virus Infection in Hemodialysis Patients: A Longitudinal Study Comparing the Results of RNA and Antibody Assays.** *Hepatology* 1993, **1**:5–8.

41. Hou MC, Wu JC, Kuo BIT, Sheng WY, Chen TZ, Lee SD, Lo KJ: **Heterosexual Transmission as the Most Common Route of Acute Hepatitis-B Virus Infection Among Adults in Taiwan: The Importance of Extending Vaccination to Susceptible Adults.** *J Infect Dis* 1993, 67:938–941.

42. Puoti M, Zonaro A, Ravaggi A, Marin MG, Castlenuovo F, Cariani E: **Hepatitis C Virus RNA and Antibody Response in the Clinical Course of Acute Hepatitis C Virus Infection.** *Hepatology* 1992, **16**:877–881.

43. Sakamoto N, Enomoto N, Maruno F, Sato C: **Prevalence of Hepatitis C Virus Infection Among Long-Term Hemodialysis Patients: Detection of Hepatitis C Virus RNA in Plasma.** *J Med Virol* 1993, **39**:11–15.

44. Brillanti S, Foli M, Gaiani S, Masci C, Miglioli M, Barbara L: **Persistent Hepatitis C Viraemia Without Liver Disease.** *Lancet* 1993, **341**:464.

45. Alter MJ, Margolis HS, Krawczynski K, Judson FN, Mares A, Alexander WJ, Hu PY, Miller JK, Gerber MA, Sampliner RE, *et al.*: **The Natural History of Community-Acquired Hepatitis C in the United States.** *N Engl J Med* 1992, **327**:1899–1905.

46. Balart L, Perrillo R, Roddenberry J, Regenstein F, Shim KS, Shieh YS, Taylor B, Dash S, Gerber MA: **Hepatitis C RNA in Liver of Chronic Hepatitis C Patients Before and After Interferon Alpha Treatment.** *Gastroenterology* 1993, **104**:1472–1477.

47. Bouffard P, Hayashi PH, Acevedo R, Levy N, Zeldis JB: **Hepatitis C Virus Is Detected in a Monocyte/Macrophage Subpopulation of Peripheral Blood Mononuclear Cells of Infected Patients.** *J Infect Dis* 1992, **166**:1276–1280.

48. Bachwich D, Dienstag J: **Aplastic Anemia and Hepatitis C: Molecular Biology Exonerates Another Suspect.** *Hepatology* 1993, **17**:340–342.

49. Fargion S, Piperno A, Cappellini MD, Sampietro M, Francansani AL, Romano R, Caldarelli R, Marcelli R, Vecchi L, Fiorelli G: **Hepatitis C Virus and Porphyria Cutanea Tarda: Evidence of a Strong Association.** *Hepatology* 1992, **16**:1322–1326.

50. Herrero C, Vicente A, Bruguera M, Ercilla MG, Barrera JM, Vidal J, Teres J, Mascaro JM, Rodes J: **Is Hepatitis C Virus Infection a Trigger of Porphyria Cutanea Tarda?** *Lancet* 1993, **341**:788–789.

51. Bloch KJ: **Cryoglobulinemia and Hepatitis C Virus [Editorial].** *N Engl J Med* 1992, **327**:1521–1522.

52. Harle JR, Disdier P, Dussol B, Bolla G, Casanova P, Weiller PJ: **Membranoproliferative Glomerulonephritis and Hepatitis C Infection.** *Lancet* 1993, **341**:904.

53. • Misiani R, Bellavita P, Fenili D, Boreli G, Marchesi D, Massazza M, Vendramin G, Comotti B, Tanzi E, Scudeller G, Zanetti A: **Hepatitis C Virus Infection in Patients With Essential Mixed Cryoglobulinemia.** *Ann Intern Med* 1992, **117**:573–577.

A study of 19 patients with cryoglobulinemia tested for the presence of HCV by second-generation enzyme immunosorbent assay and PCR shows a strong association between the two entities. Also notes possible therapeutic implication of interferon-α.

54. Roth D, Fernandez JA, Babischkin S, Demattos A, Buck BE, Quan S, Olson L, Burke GW, Nery JR, Esquenazi V, Schiff ER, Miller J: **Detection of Hepatitis C Virus Infection Among Cadaver Organ Donors: Evidence for Low Transmission of Disease.** *Ann Intern Med* 1992, **117**:470–475.

55. Agnello V, Chung RT, Kaplan LM: **A Role for Hepatitis C Virus in Type II Cryoglobulinemia.** *N Engl J Med* 1992, **327**:1490–1495.

56. Pecherebertschi A, Perrin L, Desaussure P, Widmann JJ, Giostra E, Schifferli JA: **Hepatitis C: A Possible Etiology for Cryoglobulinemia Type II.** *Clin Exp Immunol* 1992, **89**:419–422.

57. Cacoub P, Lunel F, Musset L, Opolon P, Piette JC: **Hepatitis C Virus and Cryoglobulinemia.** *N Engl J Med* 1993, **328**:1121–1122.

58. Doutrelepont J-M, Adler M, Willems M, Durez P, Yap SH: **Hepatitis C Infection and Membranoproliferative Glomerulonephritis.** *Lancet* 1993, **341**:317.

59. Johnson RJ, Gretch DR, Yamabe H, Hart J, Bacchi CE, Hartwell P, Couser WG, Corey L, Wener MH, Alpers CE, *et al.*: **Membranoproliferative Glomerulonephritis Associated With Hepatitis C Virus Infection.** *N Engl J Med* 1993, **328**:465–470.

60. Pawlotsky J-M, Deforges L, Bretagne S, Andre C, Metreau J-M, Thiers V, Zafrani E-S, Goosens M, Duval J, Mavier J-P, Dhumeaux D: **Hepatitis C Virus Infection Can Mimic Type 1 (Antinuclear Antibody Positive) Autoimmune Chronic Active Hepatitis.** *Gut* 1993, **34**:S66–S68.

61. Lunel F, Abuaf N, Franguel L, Grippon P, Perrin M, Lecoz Y, Valla D, Borotto E, Yamamoto AM, Huraux JM, Opolon P, Homberg JC: **Liver/Kidney Microsome Antibody Type I and Hepatitis C Virus Infection.** *Hepatology* 1992, **16**:630–636.

62. Seeff LB, Buskell-Bales Z, Wright EC, Durako SJ, Alter HJ, Iber FL, Hollinger FB, Gitnick G, Knodell RG, Perrillo RP, *et al.*: **Long-Term Mortality After Transfusion-Associated Non-A, Non-B Hepatitis.** *N Engl J Med* 1992, **327**:1906–1911.

63. Tremolada F, Casarin C, Alberti A, Drago C, Tagger A, Ribero MI, Realdi G: **Long Term Follow-up of Non-A, Non-B (Type-C) Post-Transfusion Hepatitis.** *J Hepatol* 1992, **16**:273–281.

64. Resnick RH, Koff R: **Hepatitis C-Related Hepatocellular Carcinoma.** *Arch Intern Med* 1993, **153**:1672–1677.

65. Gerber M: **Relation of Hepatitis C Virus to Hepatocellular Carcinoma.** *J Hepatol* 1993, **17**:S108–S111.

66. Ackerman Z, Valinluck B, Mchutchison JG, Eedeker AG, Govindarajan S: **Spontaneous Exacerbation of Disease Activity in Patients With Chronic Delta-Hepatitis Infection: The Role of Hepatitis-B, Hepatitis-C or Hepatitis-D.** *Hepatology* 1992, **16**:625–629.

67. Mishra L, Seeff LB: **Viral Hepatitis, Hepatitis-A Through Hepatitis-E, Complicating Pregnancy.** *Gastroenterol Clin North Am* 1992, **21**:873–887.

68. Chau KH, Dawson GJ, Bile KM, Magnius LO, Sjogren MH, Mushawar IK: **Detection of IgA Class Antibody to Hepatitis E Virus in Serum Samples From Patients with Hepatitis E Virus Infection.** *J Med Virol* 1993, **40**:334–338.

69. Khuroo MS, Kamili S, Dar MY, Moecklii R, Jameel S: **Hepatitis E and Long-Term Antibody Status [Letter].** *Lancet* 1993, **341**:1355.

70. • Krawczynski K: **Hepatitis E.** *Hepatology* 1993, **17**: 932–941.

A good overview on the current knowledge of HEV.

71. Herrera JL, Hill S, Shaw J, Fleenor M, Bader T, Wolfe MS: **Hepatitis-E Among United States Travelers, 1989-1992, (Reprinted from MMWR, Vol 42, Pg. 1-4, 1993).** *JAMA* 1993, **269**:845–846.

Elias I. Fanous, Jr., MD, and Luis A. Balart, MD, Louisiana State University Medical Center, Department of Gastroenterology, 2820 Napoleon Avenue #700, New Orleans, LA 70115, USA.

Treatment of chronic hepatitis

Professor Dame Sheila Sherlock

Royal Free Hospital, London, UK

Chronic hepatitis is classified etiologically. The autoimmune type predominantly affects genetically predisposed females. It is classified according to the pattern of circulating autoantibodies. Long-term corticosteroid therapy is usually successful. Associations between antibodies to liver-kidney microsomes and the hepatitis C virus can cause diagnostic difficulties. Antiviral treatment of chronic hepatitis B and C is aimed at controlling symptoms and abnormal biochemistry and particularly the progression to cirrhosis and liver cancer. Interferon-α is usually employed but there is no consensus concerning the best regimen. Patients who have developed cirrhosis rarely respond. Hepatitis C is particularly liable to relapse after apparently successful treatment. Serum hepatitis C viral RNA should be used to predict response and monitor progress. Alternative therapies such as thymosin for hepatitis B virus and ribavirin for hepatitis C virus are being evaluated. Some nucleoside analogues such as FIAU (fluoro-iodo-arabino-furanosyl-uracil) have had disastrous results in clinical trials.

Current Opinion in Gastroenterology 1994, **10**:243–248

Chronic hepatitis is a chronic inflammatory disease of the liver lasting longer than 6 months. Common clinical, biochemical, and hepatic histologic features can be associated with more than one etiologic agent. Three main types have been identified. One is associated with continuing hepatitis B virus (HBV) infection, another is related to chronic hepatitis C virus (HCV) infection, and the third is termed *autoimmune*, because of the association with positive serum autoantibodies. Identical clinical functional and morphologic features may be found associated with some drug reactions. A classification based on liver biopsy histology into chronic persistent and chronic active types has been largely abandoned and emphasis is placed on recognizing the etiology of the various types [1••].

Autoimmune chronic active hepatitis

Autoimmune chronic active hepatitis predominantly affects genetically predisposed females. It is characterized by hyperglobulinemia, histologic evidence of severe inflammatory liver disease, and the presence of various circulating autoantibodies. There is a satisfactory response to corticosteroid therapy, although this usually has to be continued on a long-term basis, even for life. The circulating autoantibodies vary [2•]. The most usual is antinuclear antibody together with anti–smooth muscle (actin) and the disease is termed *autoimmune chronic active hepatitis type 1*.

Autoimmune hepatitis type II usually affects children and is associated with antibodies to liver-kidney microsomes (LKM)-1. Antibodies to soluble liver antigen may also be found but do not define a distinct group of patients with autoimmune hepatitis [3•]. Attempts to identify the target antigens triggering off the autoantibody response have largely failed. However, an association has been found between the HCV and a positive antibody test for LKM-1 [4•]. This subgroup of patients has been termed *autoimmune chronic active hepatitis type IIB*. The association might be related to shared antigenic sites between chronic HCV infection and LKM-1 autoimmune chronic active hepatitis, although detailed analysis has shown the sites to differ [5•]. Nevertheless, the finding of autoantibodies in the patient who is anti HCV- and HCV RNA–positive can lead to difficulties in deciding the appropriate treatment, whether immunosuppressive (corticosteroids), to which genuine chronic autoimmune patients will respond, or antiviral (interferon), to which those infected with HCV infec-

Abbreviations

HBeAg—hepatitis B e antigen; **HBsAG**—hepatitis B surface antigen; **HBV**—hepatitis B virus; **HCV**—hepatitis C virus; **LKM**—liver-kidney microsomes.

 ISBN 1-85922-608-6 ISSN 0267–1379

tion may derive benefit. In doubtful cases, it is advisable to start with prednisolone, and if this fails, revert to antivirals.

Chronic hepatitis B virus infection

The aims of antiviral therapy in chronic HBV and chronic HCV infection, unfortunately, are rarely achieved [6•]. Viral markers of infectivity may be cleared from the serum, but they often persist in the liver and in extra-hepatic sites. Symptoms may increase because of the side-effects of antiviral drugs. Inflammation may be reduced in the liver, but this is difficult to prove short of serial liver biopsies. Serum transaminase levels may fall, but these can bear little relationship to viral markers. It is hoped that the progression to cirrhosis and hepatocellular carcinoma will be delayed, but there are no long-term follow-ups to support this view.

The chances of successful antiviral therapy depend on the immunologic status of the patient. The neonate, infected in the perinatal period, is immunologically tolerant and likely to develop persistent HBV infection. The adult, when infected with HBV, is less likely to develop chronic liver disease, but once present, the disease is likely to be progressive and active with marked viremia. Finally, in the third stage, the viral genome has integrated with the host and the disease becomes quiescent, but cirrhosis is often present and hepatocellular cancer is a possible complication. There are considerable differences in the time intervals between these various stages, both in the child and in the adult. This differs in different parts of the world. Asians are particularly likely to have a prolonged stage of viremia with immunologic tolerance, a positive circulating e antigen, and high HBV DNA levels. Europeans typically have a long asymptomatic period where e antibody is negative, biochemical tests are normal, and the risk for hepatocellular cancer may be reduced [7•]. At any stage, the disease may reactivate.

Viral persistence is probably related to a specific failure of T cells to recognize HBV antigens [8••]. Interferons would be expected to be most effective in the stage of immune clearance when it would potentiate the individuals' own efforts at eliminating infected hepatocytes. In addition, interferon may promote interferon-γ and tumor necrosis factor-α production, which would amplify the destruction of liver cells. However, this could be a double-edged weapon and might lead to severe liver necrosis and be dangerous in those with decompensated liver disease.

Recommendations for the correct therapeutic regimen are varied and there is no consensus of opinion [9••]. Interferon is used only in patients with replicating virus as shown by a positive serum hepatitis B e antigen (HBeAg) and HBV DNA and, if necessary, by the presence of hepatitis B core antigen in hepatocytes shown by liver biopsy. The treatment protocol approved by the Food and Drug Administration of the United States is a 16-week course of 5 million units interferon-α daily or 10 million units three times per week. This is a larger dose than is usually prescribed in Europe and has many side-effects; there are many treatment dropouts.

Interferon treatment is undoubtedly effective. A recent meta-analysis of 15 controlled studies of interferon used for HBeAg-positive patients showed a fourfold increase in loss of hepatitis B surface antigen (HBsAg) in those treated and a threefold loss of HBeAg (Table 1) [10••]. A total of 40% to 50% of the treated patients lost e antigen and HBV DNA within 12 months. In a Japanese study, 3 million U interferon-α given intravenously once a week for 6 months seemed to give the same results as the traditional daily or three times a week regimen, and side-effects were few [11•]. Small amounts of interferon can be given cautiously to those with decompensated HBV disease but monitoring should be close as side-effects, including infections, can be marked and the patient may deteriorate [12••]. It is possible that interferon simply hastens the seroconversion from an HBeAg-positive active stage to a quiescent HBeAb-positive one and that this would have been achieved anyway with the passage of time. In a follow-up, approximately three times after the loss of HBeAg, the percentage reactivation and loss of HBsAg was similar whether or not the patient had received antiviral treatment or was untreated (Table 2) [13••].

Table 1. Interferon therapy for hepatitis B e–positive hepatitis B virus*

	Loss, %	
	HBsAg	HbeAg
Interferon	7.8	33
Spontaneous	1.8	12

*Data from Wong *et al.* [10••].
HBeAg—hepatitis B e antigen; HBsAg—hepatitis B surface antigen.

Therapeutic efficacy is difficult to monitor. Serum transaminase levels are crude indicators, repeated liver biopsy must necessarily be limited. A late flare-up in serum transaminase levels after 2 to 3 months' treatment implies immunologic lysis of virally laden cells and, hence, successful treatment. Loss of serum HBeAg can be unreliable, because viral DNA may persist in the liver when the HBeAg is negative [14•]. A new enzyme immunoassay has been devised to measure HBeAg concentration and may be useful for predicting response to treatment [15•].

Table 2. Follow-up to chronic heptatitis B virus after hepatitis B e antigen loss*

Patients	Follow-up, *y*	Reactivated, %	HBsAg loss, %
Treated with antivirals (*n* = 49)	2.8	16	28
Untreated (*n* = 19)	3.5	21	31

*From Marcellin *et al.* [13••]; with permission.
HBsAg—hepatitis B surface antigen.

In general, the results of interferon therapy have been unsatisfactory. Alternative measures must be considered. Patients selected for treatment have usually failed interferon and thus the disease may be more advanced and the patient cirrhotic. Results would not be expected to be as good as for interferon. HIV and HBV replicate by way of an RNA intermediate that requires reverse transcriptase activity. It is not surprising therefore, that nucleoside analogues used to treat HIV infection have been tried in HBV sufferers.

2′, 3′, Dideoxyinosine (DDI) is given orally to treat patients with HIV infection. It inhibits HBV in ducks but in clinical trials had no effect on human HBV replication [16•].

Fluoro-iodo-arabino-furanosyl-uracil (FIAU) is a pyrimidine analogue and inhibits HBV DNA replication. Preliminary trials were promising, but long-term controlled trials gave disastrous results. Severe side-effects included lactic acidosis, mitochondrial dysfunction, and even death; the trials were terminated.

Lamivudine is an oral nucleoside analogue of 2-deoxy-3-thiacytidine and is active against human and duck HBV replication *in vitro*. In a randomized placebo-controlled multicenter trial, it suppressed HBV DNA in a dose-dependent fashion [17•]. Transaminase levels were stable. Unfortunately, there was a rebound when the drug was stopped. Side-effects included headache, nausea, and fatigue. In view of these, further testing will have to be considered with extreme caution. In fact, the fluoro-iodo-arabino-furanosyl-uracil experience will certainly reduce future trials of nucleosides in HBV infection, which are likely to be undertaken extremely cautiously, if at all.

Combination therapy has proved disappointing. Levamisole had no additive effect when combined with interferon-α in the treatment of HBeAg-positive chronic hepatitis [18•]. Interferon combined with zidovudine in a randomized placebo-controlled trial was associated with considerable side-effects [19•].

Hepatitis delta virus is a defective RNA virus that requires the help of HBV to cause infection. It largely affects drug abusers and in Southern Europe has followed the use of unsterile needles and syringes for medicinal purposes. It is decreasing with large scale vaccination against HBV. A small proportion of cases respond to high doses of interferon, but relapses are usual, and the drug has to be continued long-term [20••].

Chronic hepatitis C virus

Chronic HCV is an indolent disease, often symptomless and extending over many years (Fig. 1). In a follow-up of chronic posttransfusion hepatitis patients, the disease was usually a biochemical and histologic one [21•]. If hepatic failure occurred, it was usually only after 10 or more years of disease. Before that time, many infected patients die from other diseases. This prolonged course makes it difficult to select patients for antiviral treatment. There is no consensus. In general, a preliminary liver biopsy is indicated. Cirrhosis makes therapy unlikely to succeed and minor disease makes it unnecessary. Symptoms and serum transaminase levels are taken into account. The diagnosis of chronic HCV is usually made by finding a positive second-generation recombinant immunoblot assay II that detects antibodies to viral antigens. It would be more satisfactory to measure the actual viral antigen (HCV RNA), but this is difficult because only small amounts circulate. A polymerase chain reaction is necessary, a technique that can be unreliable. In a recent survey, sera were tested for HCV polymerase chain reaction in 31 laboratories using coded sera, and only five (16%) performed faultlessly on the entire panel of samples [22•]. Reports of the presence of HCV RNA should be interpreted with care until reliable HCV-RNA detection becomes widely available.

A new quantitative method is branched DNA signal amplification. This is simpler to perform, and has a sensitivity of 72% [23••]. Patients who acquired HCV infection by blood transfusion had a higher viremia than health workers, and intravenous drug abusers. Patients with a sustained complete response to interferon-α therapy had lower pretreatment viremia levels [24••]. High viremia levels were related to active inflammation in the liver biopsy. This technique is increasingly being used to monitor antiviral treatment. At present however, serum transaminase levels are the usual mode of assessment. Patients responding show a prompt (within 2 months) return to normal levels.

The standard regimen is 3 million units interferon-α three times a week for 26 weeks. With this dose, side-effects are mild. Response is 40% to 50%, but 50% of those responding relapse when the treatment is stopped. Modification of the regimen seems to have little effect on the result. Increasing the duration of ther-

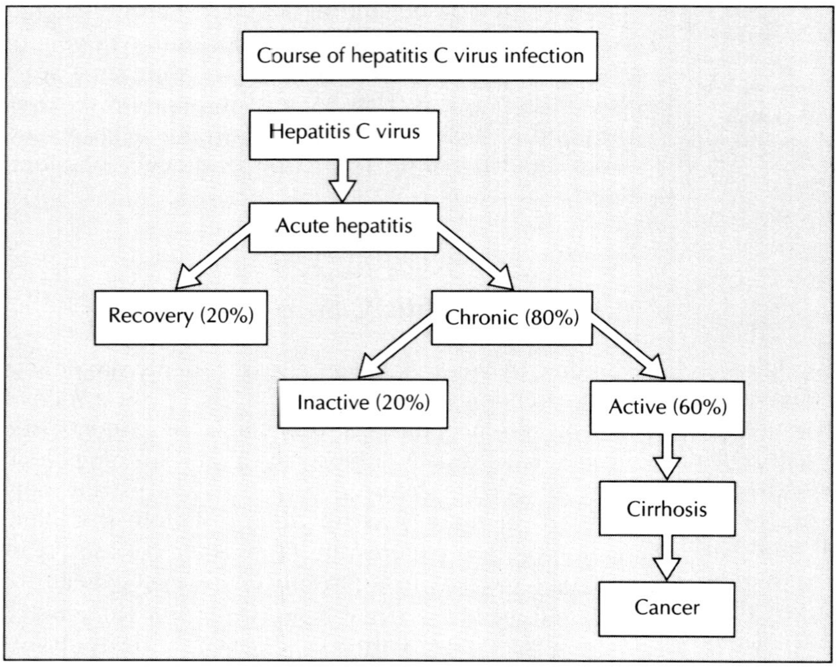

Fig. 1. The natural history of hepatitis C virus from infection to recovery or to chronicity.

apy may be useful. Using low doses of lymphoblastoid interferon for 1 year in a controlled trial, 40% showed a long-standing remission [25••]. Others have found that 48 weeks' therapy is better than 24 [26•]. Lymphoblastoid interferon diminishes inflammation and fibrosis, and procollagen type III amino peptide falls in those with a long-standing response [25••]. Responders show disappearance of HCV RNA from liver tissue but this does not exclude the possibility of relapse [27•]. Snap frozen liver tissue gives a fall in hepatic HCV antigen in responders and this becomes undetectable in those responding long-term [28•].

Sustained remissions are unusual and were seen in only six of 10 interferon-treated patients followed for 3 to 6 years [29•]. In assessing pretreatment, the responses show that one of the most important factors is underlying cirrhosis. Others include a high-gamma GT and obesity [30•]. Serum HCV RNA is the strongest predictor of a sustained response [24••]. It is more important than the HCV subtype [31•]. In a pilot study, large doses of interferon were given to nine chronic HCV patients, who were also asymptomatic for HIV type I, and five had a complete response [32•].

Ribavirin has a broad spectrum of activity against RNA and DNA viruses, including the flavi virus family. It is being used for those who relapse or fail to respond to interferon, or where interferon is contraindicated because of thrombocytopenia or cirrhosis. It may also be useful long-term to maintain viral suppression. The advantages are oral administration and few side-effects. Transaminase and HCV RNA levels decrease significantly, but values usually rebound when the drug is stopped [33•]. In a randomized, double-blind, placebo-controlled trial of ribavirin therapy for chronic hepatitis C, the serum transaminases fell and the hepatic histology improved, but serum HCV RNA was unchanged [33•].

The present position of therapy for chronic HCV infection is unsatisfactory. The response rate and the relapses are unacceptable for both interferon and ribavirin and both are costly drugs. They will continue to be used only because some patients do, in fact, respond and until more effective drugs, or combinations, become available.

References and recommended reading

Papers of particular interest, published within the annual period of review, have been highlighted as:

- • Of special interest
- •• Of outstanding interest

1. •• Maddrey WC: **Chronic Hepatitis.** *Dis Mon* 1993, **39**: 53–126.
A very full and up-to-date account of chronic hepatitis.

2. • Maddrey WC: **How Many Types of Autoimmune Hepatitis Are There?** *Gastroenterology* 1993, **105**:1571–1574.
An editorial covering the subtypes of autoimmune hepatitis and their relationship to HCV.

3. • Czaja AJ, Carpenter HA, Manns MP: **Antibodies to Soluble Liver Antigen, P450 II D6, and Mitochondrial Complexes in Chronic Hepatitis.** *Gastroenterology* 1993, **105**:1522–1528.
Antibodies to soluble liver antigen do not define a distinct subgroup of patients with autoimmune hepatitis.

4. • Bianchi FB: **Autoimmume Hepatitis: The Lesson of the Discovery of Hepatitis C Virus.** *J Hepatol* 1993, **18**:273–275.

Leading article that discusses the dilemma of deciding treatment in patients with chronic liver disease who have HCV RNA and autoantibodies.

5. Yamamoto AM, Cresteil D, Homberg G, Alvarez F: **Characterization of Anti-Liver-Kidney Microsome Antibody (Anti-LKMI) From Hepatitis Virus-Positive and -Negative Sera.** *Gastroenterology* 1993, **104**:1762–1769.
•
The antigenic sites recognized by anti-HCV-positive sera differ from those recognized by sera from patients with autoimmune hepatitis.

6. Sherlock S: **Strategies for Treating Chronic Hepatitis B and Chronic Hepatitis C Infections.** *L'Internista* 1993, 3:139–143.
•
An up-to-date review of the aims of treating chronic HBV and HCV infection.

7. De Franchis R, Meucci G, Vecchi M, Tatarella M, Colombo M, Del Ninno E, Rumi MG, Donato MF, Ronchi G: **The Natural History of Asymptomatic Hepatitis B Surface Antigen Carriers.** *Ann Intern Med* 1993, **118**:191–194.
•
An Italian paper emphasizing the good prognosis for HBeAg-negative patients. The risk for hepatocellular carcinoma is low.

8. Lau JYN, Wright TL: **Molecular Virology and Pathogenesis of Hepatitis B.** *Lancet* 1993, **342**:1335–1340.
••
Compulsory reading. A well-illustrated review of the molecular biology of the HBV and its relationship to chronicity.

9. Wright TL, Lau JYN: **Clinical Aspects of Hepatitis B Virus Infection.** *Lancet* 1993, **342**:1340–1344.
••
A very full review, well tabulated. The problem of liver transplant and HBV reinfection is discussed.

10. Wong DKH, Cheung AM, O'Rourke K, Naylor CD, Detsky AS, Heathcote J: **Effect of Alpha-Interferon in Patients With Hepatitis B e Antigen-Positive Chronic Hepatitis B: A Meta-Analysis.** *Ann Intern Med* 1993, **119**:312–323.
••
A total of 33% HBeAg-positive patients lost HBeAg within 1 year of starting interferon treatment compared with 12% spontaneous seroconversions.

11. Kagawa T, Morizante T, Saito H, Kagawa T, Morizane T, Saito H, Tsunematsu S, Tada S, Kumagai N, Tsuchimoto K, Sugiura H, Mukai M, Tsuchiya M: **A Pilot Study of Long-Term Weekly Interferon-Alpha Administration for Chronic Hepatitis B.** *Am J Gastroenterol* 1993, **88**:212–216.
•
Weekly intravenous interferon for 6 months gave results as good as the three times a week regimen and with fewer side effects.

12. Hoofnagle JH, Di Bisceglie AM, Waggoner JG, Park Y: **Interferon Alfa for Patients With Clinically Apparent Cirrhosis Due to Chronic HBV.** *Gastroenterology* 1993, **104**:1116–1121.
••
Cirrhotic patients may be treated with interferon, but dose must be reduced, clinical observations must be close, and infections may develop.

13. Marcellin P, Boyer N, Loriot MA, Degott C, Erlinger S, Benhamou JP: **Long-Term Outcome After Spontaneous or Therapeutically Induced Loss of HBeAg in Patients With Chronic Hepatitis B [Abstract].** *J Hepatol* 1993, **18**:S24.
••
Follow-up 3 years after loss of HBsAg or HBeAg showed no difference in those treated with antivirals compared with those seroconverting spontaneously.

14. Fong T-L, Di Bisceglie AM, Gerber MA, Waggoner JG, Hoofnagle JH: **Persistence of Hepatitis B Virus DNA in the Liver After Loss of HBsAg in Chronic Hepatitis B.** *Hepatology* 1993, **18**:1313–1318.
•
Low levels of HBV DNA, determined by PCR may persist in the liver after loss of HBsAg.

15. Perrillo R, Mimms L, Schechtman K, Robbins D, Campbell C: **Monitoring of Antiviral Therapy With Quantitative Elevation of HBeAg: A Comparison With HBV DNA Testing.** *Hepatology* 1993, **18**:1306–1312.
•
A microparticle capture enzyme immunoassay (Mx) can be used simply to quantitate HBeAg and so assess the effects of treatment.

16. Fried MW, Korenman JC, Di Bisceglie AM, Park Y, Waggoner JG, Mitsuya H, Hartman HR, Yarchoan R, Broder S, Hoofnagle JH: **A Pilot Study of 2′, 3′-Dideoxyinosine for the Treatment of Chronic Hepatitis B.** *Hepatology* 1992, **16**:861–864.
•
Treatment with 2′, 3′-dideoxyinosine had no appreciable effect on viral replication in patients with chronic hepatitis B.

17. Tyrrell DJ, Mitchell MC, DeMan RA, Schalm SW, Main J, Thomas HC, Fevery J, Nevens F, Beranek P, Vicary C: **Phase II Trial of Lamivudine for Chronic Hepatitis B.** *Hepatology* 1993, **18**:113A.
•
Multicenter trial of a nucleoside analogue that reduces HBV DNA. Side-effects are worrying. A further assessment is necessary.

18. Fattovich G, Guistina G, Brollo L, Guido M, Pontisso P, Noventa F, Alberti A: **Therapy for Chronic Hepatitis B With Lymphoblastoid Interferon-Alpha and Levamisole.** *Hepatology* 1992, **16**:1115–1119.
•
Levamisole had no additive effects when combined with inteferon-α.

19. Janssen HLA, Berk L, Heijtink RA, Tenkate FJW, Schalm SW: **Interferon-Alpha and Zidovudine Combination Therapy for Chronic Hepatitis B: Results of a Randomized, Placebo-Controlled Trial.** *Hepatology* 1993, **17**:383–388.
•
This combination induced considerable side-effects and cannot be recommended.

20. Hadziyannis SJ, Taylor JM, Bonino F: *Hepatitis Delta Virus: Molecular Biology, Pathogenesis and Clinical Aspects.* New York: Wiley-Liss; 1993.
••
The proceedings of an international symposium on hepatitis delta virus held in 1992 on the Greek island of Rhodes. Everything you want to know about hepatitis delta virus.

21. Koretz RL, Abbey H, Coleman E, Gitnick G: **Non-A, Non-B Post-Transfusion Hepatitis. Looking Back in the Second Decade.** *Ann Intern Med* 1993, **119**:110–115.
•
Follow-up of patients showed few had symptoms and the disease was biochemical and histologic. Hepatic failure is seen 10 or more years after the acute episode.

22. Zaaijer HL, Cuypers HTM, Reesink HW, Winkel IN, Gerken G, Lelie PN: **Reliability of Polymerase Chain Reaction for Detection of Hepatitis C Virus.** *Lancet* 1993, **341**:722–724.
•
Samples for detecting HCV RNA by polymerase chain reaction often gave unreliable results in different laboratories.

23. Lau JYN, Davis GL, Kniffen J, Qian K-P, Urdea J, Chan CS, Mizokami M, Neuwald PD, Wilber JC: **Significance of Serum Hepatitis C Virus RNA Levels in Chronic Hepatitis C.** *Lancet* 1993, **341**:1501–1504.
••
Introduces the b DNA amplification method of measuring serum HCV RNA, which is relatively simple and can be used to follow treatment.

24. Hagiwara H, Hayashi N, Mita E, Takehara T, Kasahara A, Fusamoto H, Kamada T: **Quantitative Analysis of Hepatitis C Virus RNA in Serum During Inteferon Alpha Therapy.** *Gastroenterology* 1993, **104**:877–883.
••
The titer of HCV RNA is the most important factor influencing the successful response to interferon treatment.

25. Castilla A, Camps-Bansell J, Civeira M-P, Prieto J: **Lymphoblastoid Alpha-Interferon for Chronic Hepatitis C: a Randomized Controlled Study.** *Amer J Gastroenterol* 1993, **88**:233–239.
••
Inflammation and fibrogenesis decreased and 40% of patients treated had a long-standing remission.

26. Saracco G, Rosina F, Abate ML, Chiandussi L, Gallo G, Cerutti E, Dinapoli A, *et al.*: **Long-Term Follow-Up of Pa-**
•

tients With Chronic Hepatitis Treated With Different Doses of Interferon-Alpha 2B. *Hepatology* 1993, **18**:1300–1305.
Four responders to interferon had a normal liver biopsy 2 years after stopping therapy. Three were negative for serum HCV RNA.

27. • Balart LA, Perillo R, Roddenberry J, Regenstein F, Shim K-S, Shieh YSC, Taylor B, Dash S, Gerber MA: **Hepatitis C RNA in Liver of Chronic Hepatitis C Patients Before and After Interferon Alfa Treatment.** *Gastroenterology* 1993, **104**:1472–1477.
Hepatitis C virus RNA disappeared from liver tissue in 10 of 11 responders. Unfortunately, five relapsed.

28. • Di Bisceglie AM, Hoofnagle JH, Krawczynski K: **Changes in Hepatitis C Virus Antigen in Liver With Antiviral Therapy.** *Gastroenterology* 1993, **105**:858–862.
Hepatic C virus staining in liver biopsy specimens may be useful in predicting and monitoring the response to antiviral therapy.

29. • Shindo M, DiBisceglie AM, Hoofnagle JH: **Long-Term Follow-up of Patients With Chronic Hepatitis C Treated With Alpha-Interferon.** *Hepatology* 1992, **15**:1013–1026.
Only six of 10 treated with interferon and followed for 3 to 6 years had a sustained remission.

30. • Camps J, Chrostomo S, Garcia-Granero M, Piezu-Boj JI, Civira MP, Prieto J: **Prediction of the Response of Chronic Hepatitis C to Interferon Alfa: a Statistical Analysis of Pretreatment Variables.** *Gut* 1993, **34**:1714–1717.
Eighteen baseline variables were present in 100 patients with chronic hepatitis C treated with a 12-month course of interferon alfa. Only three variables were independently predictive of response: low gamma GT, absence of obesity, and absence of cirrhosis.

31. • Kobayashi Y, Watanabe S, Konishi M, Yokoi M, Kakehashi R, Kaito M, Kondo M: **Quantitation and Typing of Serum Hepatitis C Virus in Patients With Chronic Hepatitis C Treated With Interferon-Beta.** *Hepatology* 1993, **18**:1319–1325.
Pretreatment serum level of HCV RNA is a more important predictor of outcome of interferon therapy than virus genotype.

32. • Marriott E, Navas S, del Rossero J, Garcia S, Castillo I, Quiroga JA, Carreno V: **Treatment With Recombinant Alpha-Interferon of Chronic Hepatitis C in Anti-HIV-Positive Patients.** *J Med Virol* 1993, **40**:107–111.
Asymptomatic HIV and anti-HCV patients were treated with large doses of interferon-α for 9 months. Five of nine patients had a complete response.

33. • Di Bisceglie AM, Fried MO, Swain MG, Bergasa NV, Yurdaydin C, Simpson LH, Sallie R, Conieevaram H, Kleiner D, Park Y, Hoofnagle JH: **Randomized Double-Blind, Placebo-Controlled Trial of Ribavirin Therapy for Chronic Hepatitis C.** *Hepatology* 1993, **18**:93A.
Serum transaminases fell and hepatic histology improved, but serum HCV RNA was unchanged.

Professor Dame Sheila Sherlock, Department of Medicine, Royal Free Hospital, Pond Street, Hampstead, London NW3 2QG, United Kingdom.

Pathology of the liver

Jay H. Lefkowitch, MD

College of Physicians and Surgeons of Columbia University, New York, New York, USA

Immunohistochemistry provided new perspectives on diagnostic problems in liver pathology in 1993, including the use of a monoclonal antibody, hepatocyte paraffin 1, to stain normal and malignant hepatocytes. Several experimental models investigated programmed cell death (apoptosis). After decades of use, the nomenclature of chronic hepatitis (chronic persistent, chronic lobular, and chronic active hepatitis) will undergo revision. An association between primary sclerosing cholangitis and Hodgkin's disease is reported and HIV-1 is identified by *in situ* hybridization in Kupffer cells and hepatocytes. Pathologic studies in liver transplantation have highlighted the cytopathic injury seen in the fibrosing cholestatic hepatitis associated with recurrent hepatitis B infection.

Current Opinion in Gastroenterology 1994, **10**:249–256

Pathobiology and special techniques

Pathologists facing the diagnostic problem of identifying the primary site of a metastatic tumor may entertain hepatocellular carcinoma as a candidate, but have had little success with special stains and immunohistochemistry. However, a new monoclonal antibody, hepatocyte paraffin 1 (Hep Par 1) has been developed from formalin-fixed liver tissue and provides fairly specific staining of fetal, adult, and malignant liver tissue (Fig. 1) [1••]. Immunohistochemical stains for proliferating cell nuclear antigen can demonstrate proliferation of hepatocytes in chronic hepatitis [2•] and may be applied to fine-needle aspiration cytology for differentiating normal and regenerating liver from hepatocellular carcinoma [3•].

Pit cells (large granular lymphocytes) of the liver can be fractionated into high-density and low-density types [4•]. The extracellular matrix of the liver, consisting of collagens and noncollagenous glycoproteins, has been extensively mapped out [5••,6••]. The mechanisms by which apoptosis (programmed cell death) develops were studied after a single exposure to transforming growth factor (TGF)-β1 and with modulations in protein synthesis, calcium, and protein kinase C activity in cultured hepatocytes treated with vinblastine or colchicine [7•,8•].

Viral hepatitis

Investigation of autopsy tissues from patients with chronic hepatitis B provides an explanation for the high recurrence rate after liver transplantation: a host of extrahepatic tissues contain HBV nucleic acid sequences and proteins, including lymph nodes, kidney, colon, stomach, and periadrenal ganglia [9••]. The Pekin duck was sought as a model of hepatocarcinogenesis after exposure to aflatoxin B_1, but proved disappointing [10•]. Aflatoxin produced reactive bile ductules and fatty change, but these regressed later and were not followed by hepatocellular carcinoma.

Effects of interferon therapy on expression of intercellular adhesion molecule (ICAM)-1 [11•] and intracytoplasmic hepatitis C virus (HCV) antigen [12•] were studied. Patients who responded to interferon showed down-regulation of ICAM-1 on hepatocytes and substantial loss of stainable HCV antigen. Change is in the offing with regard to the standard nomenclature of chronic hepatitis. The shortcomings of terms such as chronic persistent, chronic lobular, and chronic active hepatitis have been pointed out [13••,14••] and a new terminology based primarily on etiology (Fig. 2) with systems for grading necroinflammatory activity and staging of fibrosis or cirrhosis are in development. Additional histologic studies characterized bile duct damage, portal lymphoid follicles and aggregates and steatosis as important HCV lesions [15••,16••] and an elegant immunohistochemical study showed that the portal lymphoid follicles actually represent the full complement of lymph node follicle B, T, and dendritic cells in miniature [17••]. The cholestatic lesions of hepatitis E virus (HEV) infection were discussed in a major review of the topic [18••].

Abbreviations

HBV—hepatitis B virus; **HCV**—hepatitis C virus; **HEV**—hepatitis E virus; **ICAM**—intercellular adhesion molecule; **PBC**—primary biliary cirrhosis; **PSC**—primary sclerosing cholangitis; **TGF**—transforming growth factor.

 ISBN 1-85922-608-6 ISSN 0267–1379

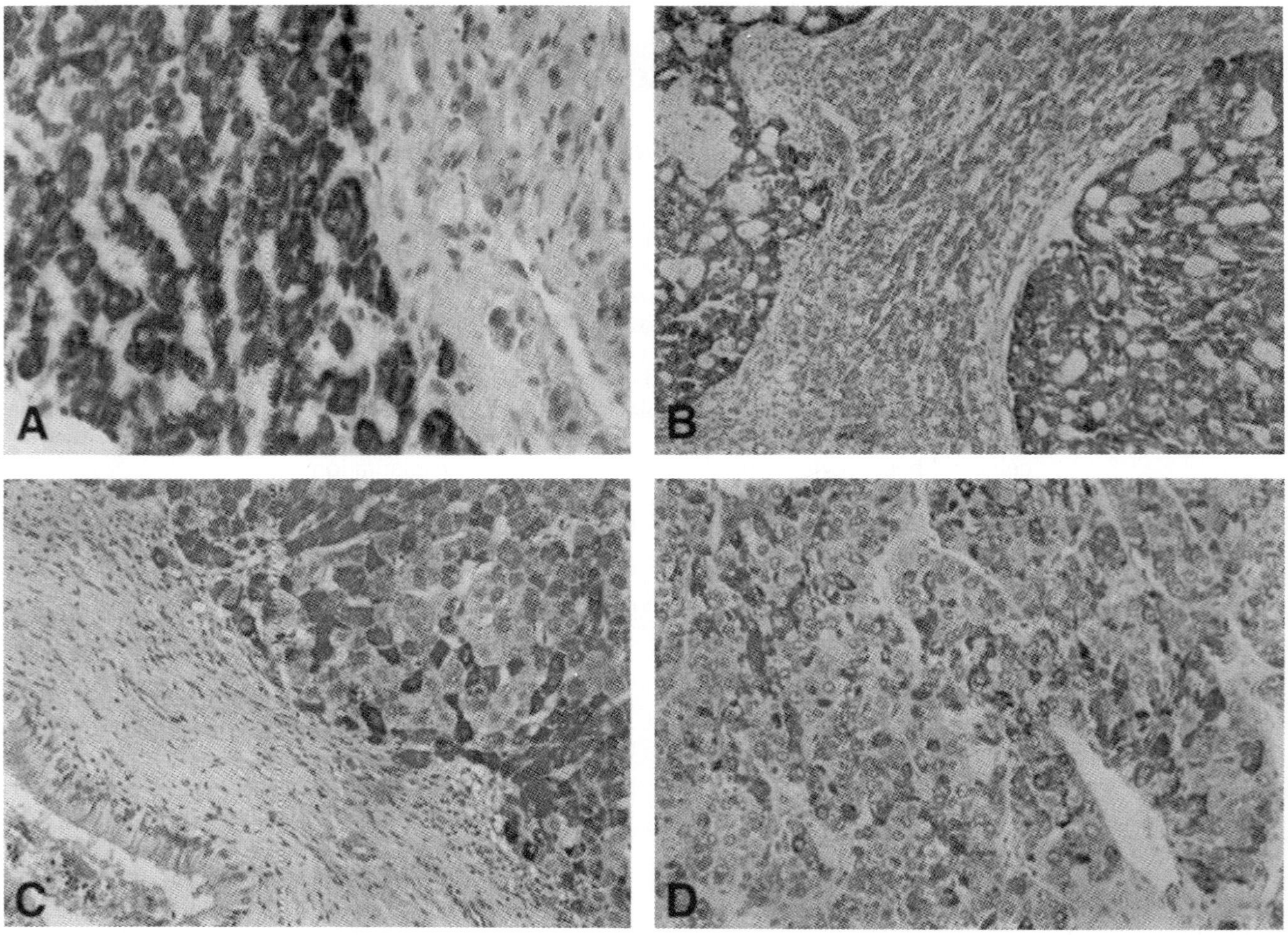

Fig. 1. A, Original screening slide. Hep Par 1–positive hepatocytes adjacent to nonstaining neuroendocrine tumor (original magnification, x 400). **B**, Moderately differentiated hepatocellular molecules strongly Hep Par 1 positive. Intervening liver with compression (original magnification, x 100). **C**, Cirrhotic liver with heterogenous Hep Par 1–positivity. Bile ducts are Hep Par 1 negative (original magnification, x 200). **D**, Positive Hep Par 1 staining in hepatocellular carcinoma (original magnification, x 200). (*From* Wennerberg *et al.* [1••]; with permission.)

Biliary tract disease

The liver in primary biliary cirrhosis (PBC) shows prominent eosinophil infiltrates around damaged bile ducts and vessels [19•] and frequently has intra-acinar foci of necrosis and inflammation [20•]. PBC portal infiltrates include CD4 lymphocytes [21•], but patterns of mixed B and T cells or B-cell–predominant infiltrates are also seen [22•]. A form of steroid-responsive autoimmune hepatitis with the cholestatic biochemistry and bile duct lesions of PBC was designated *autoimmune cholangiopathy* [23•]. The expression of heat-shock protein on duct epithelium in primary sclerosing cholangitis (PSC) and PBC may play a role in immunologic duct damage [24•]. Proliferation of bile ductules was recognized as an important histologic component of alcoholic liver disease [25•] and in many conditions with ductular proliferation these structures express parathyroid hormone-related peptide [26•]. Laboratory studies of cholestasis in bile duct–ligated rats showed activation of sinusoidal macrophages and periportal perisinusoidal cells, the latter implicated in progression to portal/periportal fibrosis [27•]. Hodgkin's disease is now among the many conditions seen in association with PSC [28•].

Metabolic and systemic diseases

Severe neonatal liver disease associated with mitochondrial cytopathy results in microvesicular steatosis with ultrastructural mitochondrial alterations [29•] and should be considered in patients with liver failure and lactic acidosis. Bile acid therapy can markedly improve liver histology in certain rare inborn errors of bile acid metabolism [30•].

Hepatic pathology in several systemic diseases was studied. Giant cell arteritis may be associated with fibrin-ring granulomas in the liver [31•]. Liver biopsy provided diagnostic information in nearly 17% of cases of fever of unknown origin [32•] and chronic hepatitis, nodular regenerative hyperplasia, and drug hepatitis were found in biopsies of patients with collagen-vascular diseases [33•]. A study of human hepatic in-

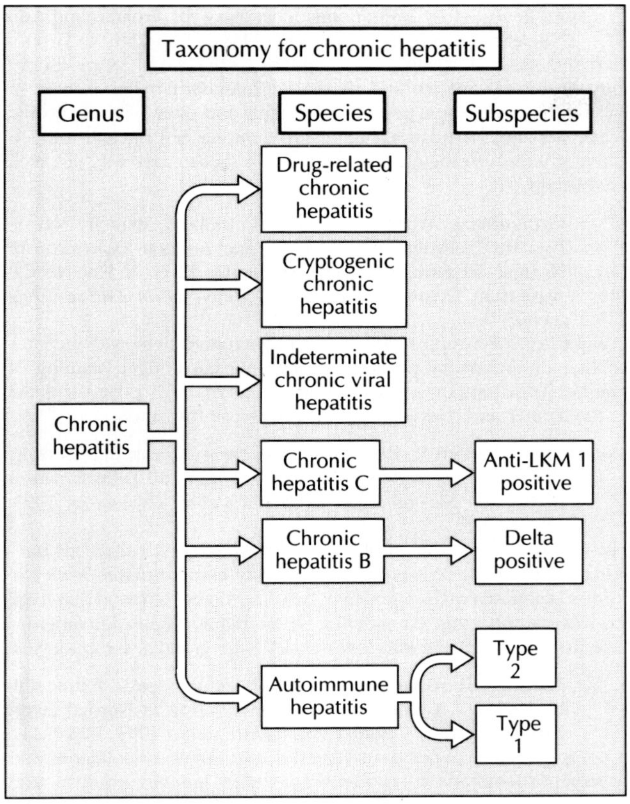

Fig. 2. Taxonomy for chronic hepatitis. (*Adapted from* Czaja [13••]; with permission.)

farction stressed the importance of portal vein obstruction [34••].

Liver involvement in AIDS may be related to direct infection by HIV-1, though the number of infected Kupffer cells and hepatocytes appears to be small [35••]. Hepatic amyloidosis [36•] and unexplained severe steatosis [37•] may cause hepatomegaly in AIDS or HIV-1 infection. Microsporidal agents such as *Enterocytozoon bieneusi* are important in AIDS cholangitis [38•,39••]. HCV infection is widely prevalent as a cause of chronic hepatitis in patients with porphyria cutanea tarda [40•].

Nodules and neoplasms

Several unusual tumors came to attention, including the biliary adenofibroma [41•], which resembles fibroadenomas of the breast, and inflammatory pseudotumors [42•–44•], which are reactive lesions composed of plasma cells and other leukocytes in a dense spindle cell–rich collagen matrix. Primary lymphomas of the liver were reviewed [45••]. Several cases of Hodgkin's disease presenting with intrahepatic cholestasis and bile duct paucity were postulated to be due to the effects of tumor cytokine secretion [46•]. An interesting case of liver cell adenoma progressing to carcinoma over 19 years of follow up was described [47].

Immunohistochemical staining for very late activation integrins is useful in differentiating hepatocellular carcinoma (very late activation-α1 positive) from cholangiocarcinoma (very late activation-β4 positive) [48•]. Mutations of the p53 gene, now widely studied in colon carcinomas and many other neoplasms, were examined in hepatocellular carcinoma. Nuclear staining for p53 proteins were found in more Asian than non-Asian hepatocellular carcinomas, and occasional cells showed cytoplasmic staining [49•] (Fig. 3). There was no difference in staining between hepatitis B virus (HBV)-positive and -negative Asian cases, suggesting that factors other than HBV, such as aflatoxin, may be involved in the pathogenesis of these cases. Ongoing work on adenomatous hyperplasia (macroregenerative nodules) was reviewed [50••] and special characteristics were described [51•,52•]. The higher prevalence of aneuploidy in type 2 macroregenerative nodules was taken as evidence of their premalignant nature [53•].

Transplantation

After liver transplantation, problems of graft dysfunction may be caused by primary dysfunction, preservation injury, acute and chronic rejection, intercurrent disease, and recurrence of the original disease. Among the factors linked to primary dysfunction is fatty change in the donor liver [54•]; routine donor liver biopsies help eliminate this problem. Adherence of platelets to damaged endothelium following cold ischemia may contribute to injury [55•]. ICAMs mediate the development of endotheliitis and inflammation in cellular rejection [56•,57••]. Current terminology used to define hepatic allograft rejection was presented in a paper from the Mayo Clinic [58••].

Posttransplant liver biopsies with features of biliary obstruction may be due to systemic infections [59•] and immunohistochemical staining of cytomegalovirus antigens may help to diagnose that infection early [60•]. There are a number of causes of late allograft dysfunction [61•], including rejection vasculopathy [62••], which may involve veins as well as arteries. Recurrent HBV infection in the graft may evolve to cirrhosis within a year [63•], produce chronic hepatitis [64•], or lead to excessive HBV transcription with cytopathic change manifested as fibrosing cholestatic hepatitis [65••], even in patients infected with HBV precore mutant [66•]. The state of HBV replication influences the morphology of recurrent hepatitis D virus infection in transplant livers [67•]. Polymerase chain reaction is useful in documenting HCV infection of allografts [68•]. PBC recurs in transplanted livers, as evidenced by granulomatous bile duct lesions [69•,70•]. The outcome of transplants for hepatocellular carcinoma is related to the size and number of lesions [71•].

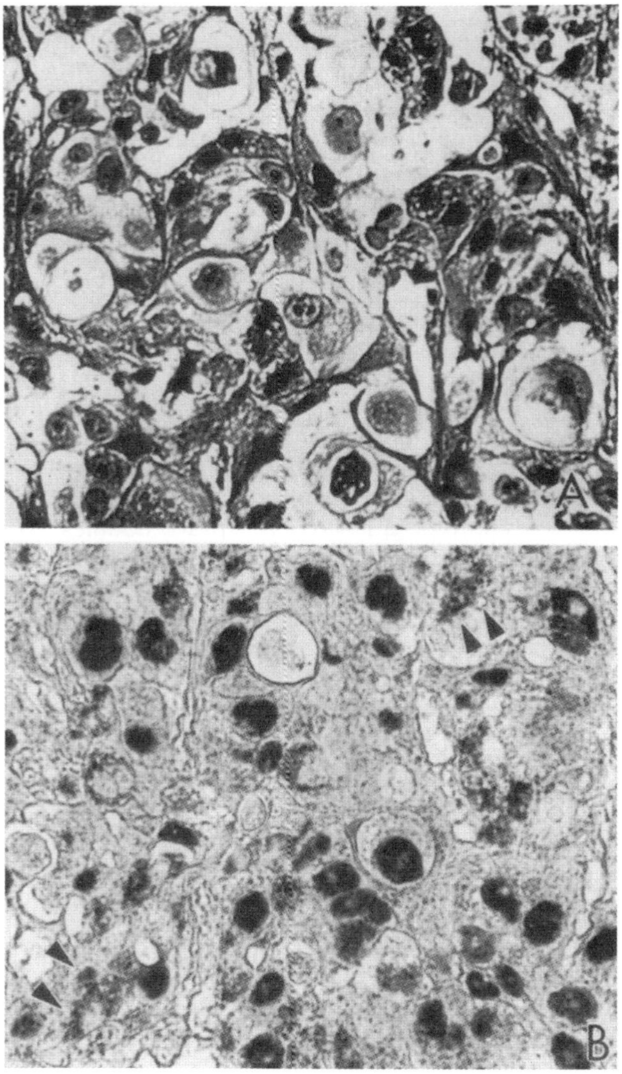

Fig. 3. Moderately differentiated hepatocellular carcinoma showing nuclear staining for p53 antigen in most tumor cells. Cytoplasmic staining is also seen in occasional cells (arrowheads). (Original magnification, x 200). (*From* Choi *et al.* [49•]; with permission.)

References and recommended reading

Papers of particular interest, published within the annual period of review, have been highlighted as:

- • Of special interest
- •• Of outstanding interest]

1. •• Wennerberg AE, Nalesnik MA, Coleman WB: **Hepatocyte Paraffin 1: A Monoclonal Antibody That Reacts With Hepatocytes and Can Be Used for Differential Diagnosis of Hepatic Tumors.** *Am J Pathol* 1993, **143**:1050–1054.

A new monoclonal antibody, Hep Par 1, was produced against an immunogen derived from 10% neutral, formalin-fixed hepatocytes from a failed allograft liver. The antibody stains fetal and adult hepatocytes as well as hepatocellular carcinomas (including the fibrolamellar variant), with granular or ring-like staining. Among the cases examined, several poorly differentiated gastric carcinomas and normal small intestinal mucosa also showed strong staining.

2. • Nakamura T, Hayama M, Sakai T, Hotchi M, Tanaka E: **Proliferative Activity of Hepatocytes in Chronic Viral Hepatitis As Revealed By Immunohistochemistry for Proliferating Cell Nuclear Antigen.** *Hum Pathol* 1993, **24**:750–753.

Sixty-five cases of chronic viral hepatitis were stained for proliferating cell nuclear antigen and showed differential labeling indices of 3.0% or less in chronic persistent hepatitis and over 3.5% in chronic active hepatitis. A relationship of proliferating cell nuclear antigen labeling with histologic activity indices in these cases was not well established.

3. • Ojanguren I, Ariza A, Llatjos M, Castella E, Mate JL, Navas-Palacios JJ: **Proliferating Cell Nuclear Antigen Expression in Normal, Regenerative, and Neoplastic Liver: a Fine-Needle Aspiration Cytology and Biopsy Study.** *Hum Pathol* 1993, **24**:905–908.

Comparison of samples of normal, regenerative liver with hepatocellular carcinoma by proliferating cell nuclear antigen staining of fine-needle aspiration samples showed less than 5% positive nuclei in the former and over 15% positive nuclei in the latter.

4. • Vanderkerken K, Bouwens L, De Neve W, van den Berg K, Baekeland M, Delens N, Wisse E: **Origin and Differentiation of Hepatic Natural Killer Cells (Pit Cells).** *Hepatology* 1993, **18**:919–925.

The sinusoidal population of natural killer cells (pit cells) was fractionated into high-density and low-density compartments, with the former being asialo-GM1-positive. Labeling studies showed that large granular lymphocytes marginating within hepatic sinusoids differentiate from high-density into low-density large granular lymphocytes.

5. •• Martinez-Hernandez A, Amenta PS: **The Hepatic Extracellular Matrix. I. Components and Distribution in Normal Liver.** *Virchows Arch A Pathol Anat Histopathol* 1993, **423**:1–11.

A comprehensive paper discussing the distribution of collagens and basement membrane components (including laminin, entactin, and heparan sulfate proteoglycan) in normal liver. This multireferenced work has fine conceptual diagrams and schematics of the hepatic extracellular matrix constituents. Matrix alterations in hepatic embryology and development are also discussed.

6. •• Martinez-Hernandez A, Amenta PS: **The Hepatic Extracellular Matrix. II. Ontogenesis, Regneration and Cirrhosis.** *Virchows Arch A Pathol Anat Histopathol* 1993, **423**:77–84.

A companion paper to part I, in which changes in the hepatic matrix system in regeneration and cirrhosis are discussed and illustrated.

7. • Oberhammer F, Bursch W, Tiefenbacher R, Fröschl G, Pavelka M, Purchio T, Schulte-Hermann R: **Apoptosis Is Induced by Transforming Growth Factor-β1 Within 5 Hours in Regressing Liver Without Significant Fragmentation of the DNA.** *Hepatology* 1993, **18**:1238–1246.

Wistar rats treated with a single intravenous injection of mature TGF-β1 augmented apoptosis ninefold. Chromatin condensation within apoptotic bodies was shown not to be due to *in vivo* digestion of the DNA.

8. • Tsukidate K, Yamamoto K, Snyder JW, Farber JL: **Microtubule Antagonists Activate Programmed Cell Death (Apoptosis) in Cultured Rat Hepatocytes.** *Am J Pathol* 1993, **143**:918–925.

Cell death of cultured rat hepatocytes treated with vinblastine or colchicine was prevented by inhibiting protein synthesis and removing calcium from the culture medium. A third requirement for programmed killing was protein kinase C activity. This model supports the development of apoptosis without necessary fragmentation of internucleosomal DNA.

9. •• Mason A, Wick M, White H, Perrillo R: **Hepatitis B Virus Replication in Diverse Cell Types During Chronic Hepatitis B Virus Infection.** *Hepatology* 1993, **18**:781–789.

Extrahepatic autopsy tissues of four patients with chronic HBV infection were examined by *in situ* hybridization and immunohistochemical staining for HBV surface and core antigens. HBV was detected in lymph nodes, spleen, bone marrow, kidney, skin, colon, stomach, testes and periadrenal ganglia. The authors postulate that phenomena such as vasculitis, glomerulonephritis, neuropathy, and dermatitis in patients with chronic HBV infection may be related to the presence of HBV in these respective tissues.

10. Seawright AA, Snowden RT, Olusola Olubuyide I, Riley J,
• Judah DJ, Neal GE: **A Comparison of the Effects of Aflatoxin B1 on the Livers of Rats and Duck Hepatitis B Virus-Infected and Noninfected Ducks.** *Hepatology* 1993, **18**:188–197.

A comparison of aflatoxin toxicity and carcinogenesis between the hepatitis virus–infected Pekin duck and the aflatoxin B–sensitive F344 rat. After aflatoxin dosing in ducks, bile ductular hyperplasia, lymphoid nodules, inflammation, and steatosis developed, but later regresssed, with no tumor development. In contrast, at 52 weeks, hepatocellular carcinoma was found in all treated rats.

11. Garcia-Monzon C, Garcia-Buey L, Garcia-Sanchez A, Pajares
• JM, Moreno-Otero R: **Down-Regulation of Intercellular Adhesion Molecule 1 on Hepatocytes in Viral Chronic Hepatitis Treated With Interferon Alpha-2b.** *Gastroenterology* 1993, **105**:462–469.

Biopsies from 12 patients with chronic hepatitis B and 14 patients with chronic hepatitis C were studied immunohistochemically for ICAM-1 and leukocyte function–associated antigen-3 before and after interferon therapy. Interferon responders in both groups showed down-regulation of both molecules, whereas expression did not change in nonresponders.

12. Di Bisceglie AM, Hoofnagle JH, Krawczynski K: **Changes in**
• **Hepatitis C Virus Antigen in Liver With Antiviral Therapy.** *Gastroenterology* 1993, **105**:858–862.

Liver biopsies from 35 patients with hepatitis C infection were studied by immunohistochemistry for hepatitis C virus antigen staining before and after interferon and ribavirin therapy. A total of 86% of the patients showed initial HCV antigen staining (although not correlated to either serum aminotransferase levels, hepatic histology or serum HCV RNA). Responders to interferon showed significant reduction in stainable HCV antigen in posttherapy biopsies, as compared with nonresponders.

13. Czaja AJ: **Chronic Active Hepatitis: The Challenge for a New**
•• **Nomenclature.** *Ann Intern Med* 1993, **119**:510–517.

The author reviews the etiologic, pathologic, and serologic distinctions among causes of chronic hepatitis and highlights problems with the current classification system. A new classification should be based on etiologic agent or the major pathogenic mechanism.

14. Ludwig J: **The Nomenclature of Chronic Active Hepatitis:**
•• **an Obituary.** *Gastroenterology* 1993, **105**:274–278.

A position paper advocating abandoning the terms chronic persistent, chronic lobular, and chronic active hepatitis for an etiologic terminology. The methods of formulating a diagnosis from liver biopsies using etiology, grading of necroinflammatory activity, and staging of fibrosis or cirrhosis are examined.

15. Kobayashi K, Hashimoto E, Ludwig J, Hisamitsu T, Obata
•• H: **Liver Biopsy Features of Acute Hepatitis C Compared With Hepatitis A, B, and Non-A, Non-B, Non-C.** *Liver* 1993, **13**:69–73.

Specific histologic features in 85 biopsies from patients with acute hepatitis A, B, C, and non-A, non-B, non-C were compared. Portal lymphoid aggregates, bile-duct lesions, and sinusoidal inflammation were common and reliable features of acute HCV infection.

16. Lefkowitch JH, Schiff ER, Davis GL, Perrillo RP, Lindsay K,
•• Bodenheimer HC, Balart LA, Ortego TJ, Payne J, Dienstag JL, Gibas A, Jacobson IM, Tamburro CH, Carey W, O'Brien C, Sampliner R, van Thiel DH, Feit D, Albrecht J, Meschievitz C, Sanghvi B, Vaughan RD, The Hepatitis Interventional Therapy Group: **Pathological Diagnosis of Chronic Hepatitis C: A Multicenter Comparative Study With Chronic Hepatitis B.** *Gastroenterology* 1993, **104**:595–603.

Two multicenter trials of interferon therapy for chronic hepatitis B and C, were the basis for review of HCV histologic features. Bile-duct damage, portal lymphoid follicles or aggregates, and large droplet steatosis were found to be useful parameters of HCV infection. Mallory body–like material was also found in hepatocytes of patients with chronic HCV infection.

17. Mosnier J-F, Degott C, Marcellin P, Hénin D, Erlinger S,
•• Benhamou J-P: **The Intraportal Lymphoid Nodule and Its Environment in Chronic Active Hepatitis C: an Immunohistochemical Study.** *Hepatology* 1993, **17**:366–371.

An elegant immunohistochemical analysis of the components of portal tract lymphoid follicles in chronic hepatitis C and autoimmune hepatitis shows these to be functional follicles that stimulate effector T cells and B cells. The components identified included activated B cells in germinal centers surrounded by a follicular dendritic cell network, a mantle zone of B cells and a peripheral T cell zone comprising CD4-, CD8-, and a few CD25-positive T cells.

18. Krawczynski K: **Hepatitis E.** *Hepatology* 1993, **17**:
•• 932–941.

A comprehensive review, with 69 references, of the epidemiologic, pathologic, and clinical features of HEV infection.

19. Terasaki S, Nakanuma Y, Yamazaki M, Unoura M:
• **Eosinophilic Infiltration of the Liver in Primary Biliary Cirrhosis: a Morphological Study.** *Hepatology* 1993, **17**:206–212.

Large numbers of eosinophils were found in 29% of PBC specimens, compared to 4% of specimens from patients with chronic viral hepatitis. The eosinophils of PBC are oriented around damaged bile ducts, around portal vein branches, and at the margins of portal tracts. In chronic viral hepatitis, the eosinophils were diffusely scattered throughout the portal tracts.

20. Nakanuma Y: **Necroinflammatory Changes in Hepatic Lob-**
• **ules in Primary Biliary Cirrhosis With Less Well-Defined Cholestatic Changes.** *Hum Pathol* 1993, **24**:378–383.

Zonal necrosis, acidophilic bodies, swollen Kupffer cells with transition to epithelioid macrophages, sinusoidal activated T lymphocytes, and epithelioid granulomas may be seen in early, noncholestatic PBC. These intra-acinar changes may be correlated with elevated serum glutamic oxaloacetic transaminase levels.

21. Hashimoto E, Lindor KD, Homburger HA, Dickson ER, Czaja
• AJ, Wiesner RH, Ludwig J: **Immunohistochemical Characterization of Hepatic Lymphocytes in Primary Biliary Cirrhosis in Comparison With Primary Sclerosing Cholangitis and Autoimmune Chronic Active Hepatitis.** *Mayo Clin Proc* 1993, **68**:1049–1055.

Immune cell infiltrates were compared in 20 patients with PBC, 19 with PSC, and 11 with autoimmune chronic active hepatitis. PBC portal infiltrates featured more CD4 than CD8 cells, whereas piecemeal necrosis in PBC showed mostly CD8 cells. The portal infiltrates in autoimmune chronic hepatitis were similar. In contrast, natural killer cells were twice as common in PSC as in PBC.

22. Nakanuma Y: **Distribution of B Lymphocytes in Nonsuppu-**
• **rative Cholangitis in Primary Biliary Cirrhosis.** *Hepatology* 1993, **18**:570–575.

An immunohistochemical study defining the portal infiltrates in PBC as activated T-cell predominant, mixed T cell and B cell, or B-cell predominant. Whereas other papers have recognized the CD8 T-lymphocyte nature of PBC infiltrates, the author focuses on the role of B-cells and humoral immunity in this disease.

23. Ben-Ari Z, Dhillon AP, Sherlock S: **Autoimmune Cholan-**
• **giopathy: Part of the Spectrum of Autoimmune Chronic Active Hepatitis.** *Hepatology* 1993, **18**:10–15.

Four patients are described in whom serum biochemistry (elevated alkaline phosphatase levels) and bile-duct lesions on liver biopsy consistent with PBC coexisted with serum antinuclear and anti-actin (but no antimitochondrial) antibodies and a clinical response to corticosteroids. These were evidently a subgroup of patients with autoimmune chronic active hepatitis who displayed cholestatic serum biochemistry and bile-duct damage.

24. Broomé U, Scheynius A, Hultcrantz R: **Induced Expression**
• **of Heat-Shock Protein on Biliary Epithelium in Patients With Primary Sclerosing Cholangitis and Primary Cirrhosis.** *Hepatology* 1993, **18**:298–303.

Monoclonal antibody ML30 to 65-kD heat-shock protein of mycobacterium and a monoclonal antibody against human leukocyte antigen-DR–stained bile-duct epithelium in PBC and PSC biopsies. The role of heat-shock proteins in autoimmune diseases such as juvenile arthritis may be involved in the pathogenesis of duct damage in PBC and PSC.

25. Ray MB, Mendenhall CL, French SW, Gartside PS, Veterans
• Administration Cooperative Study Group: **Bile Duct Changes in Alcoholic Liver Disease.** *Liver* 1993, **13**:36–45.

Cytokeratin staining of bile ductules demonstrate their proliferation in the fibrosis and cirrhosis of alcoholic liver disease. These structures are also important components of alcoholic piecemeal necrosis.

26. • Roskams T, Campos RV, Drucker DJ, Desmet VJ: **Reactive Human Bile Ductules Express Parathyroid Hormone-Related Peptide**. *Histopathology* 1993, **23**:11–19.

The immunohistochemical identification of parathyroid hormone-related peptide in reactive bile ductular cells in cholestasis, regenerating liver, PBC, PSC, and focal nodular hyperplasia suggests that the peptide may participate in an autocrine growth regulatory loop.

27. • Hines JE, Johnson SJ, Burt AD: **In Vivo Responses of Macrophages and Perisinusoidal Cells to Cholestatic Liver Injury**. *Am J Pathol* 1993, **142**:511–518.

Common bile duct-ligated Wistar rats were used as an intriguing model of nonparenchymal cell (Kupffer cell–perisinusoidal cell) reactivity in the process of portal and periportal fibrosis. Immunohistochemical staining demonstrated a peak macrophage proliferation at 3 days after ligation, whereas smooth muscle actin–positive perisinusoidal cells (transitional to myofibroblast-like cells) peaked at day 21. These responses were similar to those seen after toxin-induced hepatocyte necrosis.

28. • Man KM, Drejet A, Keeffe EB, Garcia-Kennedy R, Imperial JC, Esquivel CO: **Primary Sclerosing Cholangitis and Hodgkin's Disease**. *Hepatology* 1993, **18**:1127–1131.

Three patients are presented in whom PSC was diagnosed years prior to the development of Hodgkin's disease. They presented for liver transplantation due to advanced biliary cirrhosis.

29. • Bioulac-Sage P, Parrot-Roulaud F, Mazat JP, Lamireau T, Coquet M, Sandler B, Demarquez JL, Cormier V, Munnich A, Carré M, Balabaud C: **Fatal Neonatal Liver Failure and Mitochondrial Cytopathy (Oxidative Phosphorylation Deficiency): a Light and Electron Microscopic Study of the Liver**. *Hepatology* 1993, **18**:839–846.

Ten cases of mitochondrial respiratory chain defects associated with neonatal liver failure and hyperlactacidemia are presented. Microvesicular steatosis and widespread cholestasis were the major histopathology features, and abnormal mitochondria with few or no cristae and granular fluffy matrices were seen ultrastructurally.

30. • Daughtery CC, Setchell KDR, Heubi JE, Balistreri WF: **Resolution of Liver Biopsy Alterations in Three Siblings With Bile Acid Treatment of an Inborn Error of Bile Acid Metabolism (4-3-Oxosteroid 5β-Reductase Deficiency**. *Hepatology* 1993, **18**:1096–1101.

Cholestatic liver disease with giant-cell transformation in male twins and their brother, all with an inborn error of bile acid synthesis, was followed morphologically with serial liver biopsies during the course of bile acid therapy. Resolution of cholestasis, giant-cells and ultrastructural abnormalities of bile canaliculi occurred after therapy.

31. • De Bayser L, Roblot R, Ramassamy A, Silvain C, Levillain P, Becq-Giraudon B: **Hepatic Fibrin-Ring Granulomas in Giant Cell Arteritis**. *Gastroenterology* 1993, **105**:272–273.

A brief case report of a patient with giant cell arteritis, fever, and a liver biopsy with fibrin-ring granulomas. Other causes of this type of granuloma are discussed.

32. • Holtz T, Moseley RH, Scheiman JM: **Liver Biopsy in Fever of Unknown Origin. A Reappraisal**. *J Clin Gastroenterol* 1993, **17**:29–32.

Of 24 patients investigated by liver biopsy in the workup of fever of unknown origin, four (16.7%) showed diagnostic lesions (histoplasmosis and tuberculosis).

33. • Keshavarzian A, Rentsch R, Hodgson HJF: **Clinical Implications of Liver Biopsy Findings in Collagen-Vascular Disorders**. *J Clin Gastroenterol* 1993, **17**:219–226.

Liver biopsies of 46 patients with various collagen vascular diseases demonstrated drug-induced liver disease in 17%, chronic liver disease in 24%, and lesions of polyarteritis nodosa in three cases.

34. •• Saegusa M, Takano Y, Okudaira M: **Human Hepatic Infarction: Histopathological and Postmortem Angiological Studies**. *Lancet* 1993, **13**:239–245.

This helpful study demonstrates the role of portal vein occlusion in hepatic infarctions and characterizes the pathological features in 20 cases. "Congestive" and "anemic" regions of infarcted tissue are illustrated and the effects of postmortem embolization studies are described.

35. •• Housset C, Lamas E, Courgnaud V, Boucher O, Girard P-M, Marche C, Brechot C: **Presence of HIV-1 in Human Parenchymal and Non-Parenchymal Liver Cells In Vivo**. *J Hepatol* 1993, **19**:252–258.

An important paper studying HIV-1 DNA by PCR and HIV-1 RNA by *in situ* hybridization in eight of 13 patients who were positive for anti–HIV-1 antibody. In the eight positive cases, polymerase chain reaction hybridization signals were weak (*ie*, only limited numbers of cells were infected). *In situ* hybridization showed approximately 1 to 10 labeled cells per tissue section, most of which appeared to be Kupffer cells, with three cases showing positivity in putative hepatocytes.

36. • Osick LA, Lee T-P, Pedemonte MB, Jacob L, Chauhan P, Navarro C, Comer GM: **Hepatic Amyloidosis in Intravenous Drug Abusers and AIDS Patients**. *J Hepatol* 1993, **19**:79–84.

Sixteen patients with intravenous and subcutaneous cocaine and heroin use and chronic skin ulceration were found to have amyloidosis on liver biopsy or at autopsy. Vascular and parenchymal amyloid were present; amyloidosis was diagnosed prior to death in only five of the 16 patients.

37. • Freiman JP, Helfert KE, Hamrell MR, Stein DS: **Hepatomegaly With Severe Steatosis in HIV-Seropositive Patients**. *AIDS* 1993, **7**:379–385.

Eight cases of severe steatosis (six fatal) in HIV-positive patients without AIDS were retrieved via the AIDS Clinical Trials Group Adverse Reactions and the Food and Drug Administration's Spontaneous Report databases. Zidovudine is postulated as a potential cause.

38. • Bouche H, Housst C, Dumont J-L, Carnot F, Menu Y, Aveline B, Belghiti J, Boboc B, Erlinger S, Berthelot P, Pol S: **AIDS-Related Cholangitis: Diagnostic Features and Course in 15 Patients**. *J Hepatol* 1993, **17**:34–39.

Cryptosporidia (57%), cytomegalovirus (28%), and microsporidia (7%) were the associated infections in 15 AIDS patients investigated for cholangitis. Endoscopic retrograde cholangiopancreatography is important in evaluating AIDS patients with cholangitis or cholestasis, particularly because of the high frequency of papillary stenosis.

39. •• Pol S, Romana CA, Richard S, Amouyal P, Desportes-Livage I, Carnot F, Pays J-F, Berthelot P: **Microsporidia Infection in Patients With the Human Immunodeficiency Virus and Unexplained Cholangitis**. *N Engl J Med* 1993, **328**:95–99.

Eight patients with unexplained AIDS-related cholangitis were shown to have biliary tract microsporidiosis (*E. bieneusi*). Duodenal biopsy specimens, bile samples, common bile duct smear, gallbladder epithelium, and ductal biliary cells on liver biopsy were all sites where *E. bieneusi* could be demonstrated.

40. • Decastro M, Sanchez J, Herrera JF, Chaves A, Duran R, Garcia-Buey L, Garcia-Monzon C, Sequi J, Moreno-Otero R: **Hepatitis C Virus Antibodies and Liver Disease in Patients With Porphyria Cutanea Tarda**. *Hepatology* 1993, **17**:551–557.

The high frequency of antibodies to HCV (62%) and histologic features consistent with chronic HCV infection in patients with porphyria cutaneau tarda imply an important contribution of chronic viral injury to liver disease in these patients.

41. • Tsui WMS, Loo KT, Chow LTC, Tse CCH: **Biliary Adenofibroma. A Heretofore Unrecognized Benign Biliary Tumor of the Liver**. *Am J Surg Pathol* 1993, **17**:186–192.

A 7-cm tumor composed of tubulo-cystic biliary structures containing bile is described. Although somewhat resembling the much smaller von Meyenburg complex (microhamartoma), this rare tumor most closely resembles the fibroadenoma of the breast.

42. • Shek TWH, Ng IOL, Chan KW: **Inflammatory Pseudotumor of the Liver. Report of Four Cases and Review of the Literature**. *Am J Surg Pathol* 1993, **17**:231–238.

Four cases of inflammatory pseudotumor are described, along with a review of the literature. The immunocytes within the tumor are polyclonal, and the accompanying spindle cells express vimentin.

43. • Lyons TJ, Benbow EW, Taylor PM, McCloy R: **Inflammatory Pseudotumor of the Liver: Antecedent Causes and Clinical Experience.** *J Hepatol* 1993, **19**:273–278.

A case report, complicating Caroli's disease, with a review of 45 other reported cases. The histologic features, clinical presentation, liver test results and radiography are discussed.

44. • Nakajima T, Sugano I, Matsuzaki O, Nagao K, Kondo Y, Miyazaki M, Konno A, Shimura T: **Hepatic Inflammatory Lesions Manifested As a Pseudotumor. Report of Two Cases With Different Characteristics.** *Arch Pathol Lab Med* 1993, **117**:157–159.

Two cases are described, one an inflammatory pseudotumor, the other a necrotizing granuloma. The authors suggest a relationship between cholangitis and the development of the pseudotumor.

45. •• Zafrani ES, Gaulard P: **Primary Lymphoma of the Liver.** *Liver* 1993, **13**:57–61.

A review of the presentations, including liver failure, of primary hepatic lymphomas, most of which are B cell neoplasms.

46. • Hubscher SG, Lumley MA, Elias E: **Vanishing Bile Duct Syndrome: a Possible Mechanism for Intrahepatic Cholestasis in Hodgkin's Lymphoma.** *Hepatology* 1993, **17**:70–77.

This report describes and illustrates three cases of Hodgkin's disease associated with severe intrahepatic cholestasis. In seven of 10 liver biopsies obtained within 30 weeks of the onset of jaundice, portal tracts showed loss of bile ducts. More than 1 year later, three biopsies showed portal fibrosis, ductular proliferation and deposits of copper-binding protein. The authors postulate that cytokine release from tumor cells may be responsible for ductopenia.

47. Janes CH, McGill LB, Ludwig J, Krom RAF: **Liver Cell Adenoma at the Age of 3 Years and Transplantation 19 Years Later After Development of Carcinoma: a Case Report.** *Hepatology* 1993, **17**:583–585.

48. • Volpes R, Van Den Oord JJ, Desmet VJ: **Integrins As Differential Cell Lineage Markers of Primary Liver Tumors.** *Am J Pathol* 1993, **142**:1483–1492.

A study demonstrating the practical value of immunostaining for integrin subtypes in the histologic diagnosis of hepatocellular carcinoma versus cholangiocarcinoma. Very late activation integrin-α1 was present in hepatocellular carcinoma, but not in cholangiocarcinma. Very late activation integrin-β4 was present in cholangiocarcinoma, but not in hepatocellular carcinoma. Neural cell adhesion molecule was present in proliferating bile ductules but in neither of the two malignant tumors.

49. • Choi SW, Hytiroglou P, Geller SA, Kim SM, Chung KW, Park DH, Theise ND, Thung SN: **The Expression of p53 Antigen in Primary Malignant Epithelial Tumors of the Liver: an Immunohistochemical Study.** *Liver* 1993, **13**:172–176.

The p53 antigen was identified in 31.6% of Asian hepatocellular carcinomas in contrast to 6.7% of hepatocellular carcinomas in non-Asians. In addition to nuclear staining, a novel identification of cytoplasmic staining is reported. The authors discuss the point mutation of p53 involving codon 249 and geographic differences in its expression.

50. •• Nakanuma Y, Terada T, Ueda K, Terasaki S, Nonomura A, Matusui O: **Adenomatous Hyperplasia of the Liver As a Precancerous Lesion.** *Liver* 1993, **13**:1–9.

A well-references review of the pathologic characteristics, clinical features, radiology, and immunohistochemistry of macroregenerative nodules (adenomatous hyperplasia).

51. • Terada T, Ueda K, Nakanuma Y: **Histopathological and Morphometric Analysis of Atypical Adenomatous Hyperplasia of Human Cirrhotic Livers.** *Virchows Archiv A Pathol Anat Histopathol* 1993, **422**:381–388.

From a review of the 49 nodules of atypical adenomatous hyperplasia, the authors describe histologic features (increased nuclear density, iron resistance, reduced reticulin, clear cell change, sinusoidal dilatation, and abnormal arteries) that distinguish malignant or equivocal nodules from nonmalignant adenomatous hyperplasia.

52. • Terada T, Kitani S, Ueda K, Nakanuma Y, Kitagawa K, Masuda S: **Adenomatous Hyperplasia of the Liver Resembling Focal Nodular Hyperplasia in Patients With Chronic Liver Disease.** *Virchows Archiv A Pathol Anat Histopathol* 1993, **422**:247–252.

Two cases of adenomatous hyperplasia with central scarring, resembling focal nodular hyperplasia, are discussed with regard to the mechanisms of vascular change that may have produced this variation.

53. • Orsatti G, Theise ND, Thung SN, Paronetto F: **DNA Image Cytometric Analysis of Macroregenerative Nodules (Adenomatous Hyperplasia) of the Liver: Evidence in Support of Their Preneoplastic Nature.** *Hepatology* 1993, **17**:621–627.

The association of aneuploid peaks with type 2 (atypical) macroregenerative nodules is evidence favoring the premalignant potential of these lesions.

54. • Ploeg RJ, D'Alessandro AM, Knechtle SJ, Stegall JD, Pirsch JD, Hoffmann RM, Sasaki T, Sollinger HW, Belzer FO, Kalayoglu M: **Risk Factors for Primary Dysfunction After Liver Transplantation–a Multivariate Analysis.** *Transplantation* 1993, **55**:807–813.

Univariate and multivariate analyses of donor and recipient factors associated with primary dysfunction (including primary nonfunction and initial poor function). In addition to older donor age (over 49 years) and prolonged cold ischemic time, fatty change in donor liver biopsies was associated with a higher incidence of primary graft dysfunction.

55. • Cywes R, Packham MA, Tietze L, Sanabria JR, Harvey PRC, Phillips MJ, Strasberg SM: **Role of Platelets in Hepatic Allograft Preservation Injury in the Rat.** *Hepatology* 1993, **18**:635–647.

Wistar rat livers exposed to cold ischemia in University of Wisconsin solution, reperfusion, warming before reperfusion and either unactivated or activated platelets were examined to determine platelet dynamics. Platelets in the circulation dropped and were found ultrastructurally to adhere to sinusoidal endothelium or its remnants; adherent platelets showed evidence of degranulation. Rewarming before reperfusion and activation of platelets increased adherence.

56. • Bacchi CE, Marsh CL, Perkins JD, Carithers RL, McVicar JP, Hudkins KL, Benjamin CD, Harland JM, Lobb R, Alpers CE: **Expression of Vascular Cell Adhesion Molecule (VCAM-1) in Liver and Pancreas Allograft Rejection.** *Am J Pathol* 1993, **142**:579–591.

An immunohistochemical study demonstrating staining of endothelium for vascular cell adhesion molecule–1 in arteries, veins and sinusoids in rejecting liver allograft endotheliitis. A subpopulation of dendritic cells also showed positive vascular cell adhesion molecule–1 staining.

57. •• Steinhoff G, Behrend M, Schrader B, Pichlmayr R: **Intercellular Immune Adhesion Molecules in Human Liver Transplants: Overview on Expression Patterns of Leukocyte Receptor and Ligand Molecules.** *Hepatology* 1993, **18**:440–453.

A superb examination of the role of integrin, immunoglobulin and selectin families in mediating transplant rejection and other inflammatory conditions. Of particular interest is a schematic representation of the inflammatory cascade in portal and sinusoidal compartments, broken into four steps: physiologic intravascular rolling, endothelial activation with reversible adhesion, leukocyte activation with irreversible firm adhesion, and transendothelial migration and tissue infiltration.

58. •• Wiesner RH, Ludwig J, Krom RAF, Hay JE, Van Hoek B: **Hepatic Allograft Rejection: New Developments in Terminology, Diagnosis, Prevention, and Treatment.** *Mayo Clin Proc* 1993, **68**:69–79.

Comprehensive guidelines are discussed for the characterization of cellular and ductopenic rejection in liver transplantation.

59. • Rubin R, Munoz SJ, Moritz M: **Rejection-Independent Cholangitis and Cirrhosis Following Orthotopic Liver Transplantation.** *Hum Pathol* 1993, **24**:996–1002

Fourteen patients whose liver biopsies showed biliary obstructive portal features after transplantation were evaluated; nine had normal cholangiograms. The obstructive histologic picture was related to systemic infections in 10 patients. In addition to obtaining cholangiograms to exclude obstruction, the serum alkaline phosphatase level in such cases may be disproportionately low compared with that seen in obstruction.

60. Theise ND, Conn M, Thung SN: **Localization of Cytomegalovirus Antigens in Liver Allografts Over Time.** *Hum Pathol* 1993, **24**:103–108.
•

An immunohistochemical study using monoclonal antibodies to immediate early and early antigens of cytomegalovirus demonstrated that graft infection probably begins in sinusoidal endothelium and that infection can be sensitively detected earlier than in routine hematoxylin and eosin-stained sections.

61. Rubin R, Munoz SJ: **Clinicopathologic Features of Late Hepatic Dysfunction in Orthotopic Liver Transplants.** *Hum Pathol* 1993, **24**:643–651.
•

Twelve patients with late hepatic dysfunction after transplantation showed a variety of etiologies, including fulminant hepatitis, ductopenia and rejection arteriopathy. Liver biopsy plays a helpful role in documenting some of these complications.

62. Liu G, Butany J, Wanless IR, Cameron R, Greig P, Levy G: **The Vascular Pathology of Human Hepatic Allografts.** *Hum Pathol* 1993, **24**:182–188.
••

A study of 20 unselected liver allografts and transplant vasculopathy involving arteries as well as portal and hepatic veins. The predominant changes include foam cell lesions, myointimal thickening, and fibrocellular lesions.

63. Harrison RF, Davies MH, Goldin RD, Hubscher SG: **Recurrent Hepatitis B in Liver Allografts: a Distinctive Form of Rapidly Developing Cirrhosis.** *Histopathology* 1993, **23**:21–28.
•

Among 14 patients with recurent HBV infection in their liver allografts, three evolved from fibrosing cholestatic hepatitis to cirrhosis within 12 to 23 months after transplant.

64. Walker N, Apel R, Kerlin P, Horn M, Tinniswood R, Lynch S, Strong R: **Hepatitis B Virus Infection in Liver Allografts.** *Am J Surg Pathol* 1993, **17**:666–677.
•

Six cases of recurrent HBV infection of liver allografts demonstrated a spectrum of pathologic lesions, including fibrosing cholestatic hepatitis, chronic active hepatitis, cirrhosis, and minimal changes.

65. Mason AL, Wick M, White HM, Benner KG, Lee RG, Regenstein F, Riely CA, Bain VG, Campbell C, Perrillo RP: **Increased Hepatocyte Expression of Hepatitis B Virus Transcription in Patients With Features of Fibrosing Cholestatic Hepatitis.** *Gastroenterology* 1993, **105**:237–244.
••

Strong HBV RNA hybridization signals were observed in 11 of 12 biopsies showing fibrosing cholestatic hepatitis due to recurrent HBV infection in liver allografts. Enhanced viral transcription appears to be linked to cytopathic viral damage in this syndrome.

66. Fang JWS, Tung FYT, Davis GL, Dolson DJ, Van Thiel LDH, Lau JYN: **Fibrosing Cholestatic Hepatitis in a Transplant Recipient With Hepatitis B Virus Precore Mutant.** *Gastroenterology* 1993, **105**:901–904.
•

A case report demonstrating that reinfection of graft livers with HBV precore mutants can occur and lead to fibrosing cholestatic hepatitis, despite the absence of hepatitic hepatitis B e antigen.

67. David E, Rahier J, Pucci A, Camby P, Scevens M, Salizzoni M, Otte JB, Galmarini D, Marinucci G, Ottobrelli A, Marzano A, Smedile A, Fabiano A, Mollo F, Verme G, Rizzetto M: **Recurrence of Hepatitis D (Delta) in Liver Translants: Histopathological Aspects.** *Gastroenterology* 1993, **104**:1122–1128.
•

Active inflammatory lesions in hepatitis D virus–infected liver transplants develop when there is active HBV replication, as evidenced by staining for intranuclear HBV core antigen. Without active HBV replications, parenchymal changes are primarily cytopathic, with positive staining for intranuclear delta antigen.

68. Thung SN, Shim K-S, Shieh C, Schwartz M, Theise N, Borcich A, Katz E, Miller C, Gerber MA: **Hepatitis C in Liver Allografts.** *Arch Pathol Lab Med* 1993, **117**:145–149.
•

A study demonstrating the usefulness of polymerase chain reaction for detection of HCV recurrent or intercurrent infection in liver allografts.

69. Hubscher SG, Elias E, Buckels JAC, Meayer AD, McMaster P, Neuberger JM: **Primary Biliary Cirrhosis. Histological Evidence of Disease Recurrence After Liver Transplantation.** *J Hepatol* 1993, **18**:173–184.
•

One hundred seventy-two biopsies from 83 patients transplanted for PBC were examined for histologic evidence of recurrent disease. In 16 biopsies, there were features including portal granulomas and bile duct damage, which provided evidence that PBC can recur after transplantation.

70. Wong PYN, Portmann B, O'Grady JG, Devlin JJ, Hegarty JE, Tan K-C, Williams R: **Recurrence of Primary Biliary Cirrhosis After Liver Transplantation Following FK506-Based Immunosuppression.** *J Hepatol* 1993, **17**:284–287.
•

Two patients on FK506 immunosuppresion after liver transplantation for PBC developed bile duct destruction with a portal granulomatous reaction indicative of recurrent PBC.

71. McPeake JR, O'Grady JG, Zaman S, Portmann B, Wright DGD, Tan KC, Calne RY, Williams R: **Liver Transplantation for Primary Hepatocellular Carcinoma: Tumor Size and Number Determine Outcome.** *J Hepatol* 1993, **18**:226–234.
•

A study analyzing 87 patients transplanted for hepatocellular carcinoma. Single lesions less than 4 cm did not recur, whereas there was recurrence in 40% of patients in whom the lesions were 4 to 8 cm. Multifocal lesions or size over 8 cm resulted in recurrence in 78%.

Jay H. Lefkowitch, MD, Department of Pathology, College of Physicians and Surgeons, PH 15 West, 630 West 168th Street, New York, NY 10032, USA.

Immunopathogenesis of autoimmune hepatobiliary diseases

Bradley L. Freilich, MD, Ke-Qin Hu, MD, and John M. Vierling, MD

Cedars-Sinai Medical Center, University of California at Los Angeles, Los Angeles, California, USA

Immunologic mechanisms have been proposed in the pathogenesis of the putative autoimmune hepatobiliary diseases: primary biliary cirrhosis, autoimmune hepatitis, and primary sclerosing cholangitis. Advances in our understanding of the human immune response have led to an appreciation of the complexity of interactions that initiate, perpetuate, and regulate autoimmunity. This appreciation has catalyzed the rapid pace of investigation into the immunogenetics of disease susceptibility, identification of B-cell and T-cell antigenic epitopes involved in autoantibody production, functional analyses of T cells from both peripheral blood and the inflamed livers of patients, and the immunologic mechanisms of hepatocellular necrosis and bile duct injury. Although specific immunologic mechanisms of hepatobiliary injury remain poorly defined, continued studies are likely to provide the insights necessary to devise new diagnostic and therapeutic approaches.

Current Opinion in Gastroenterology 1994, **10**:257–268

Immunopathogenic mechanisms in liver diseases

Immunologic mechanisms have been implicated in the primary pathogenesis of several hepatobiliary diseases [1••,2••]. The immunopathogenic mechanisms range from responses against infectious agents such as hepatitis B virus (HBV) to reactions against autoantigens in autoimmune hepatitis, primary biliary cirrhosis (PBC), and primary sclerosing cholangitis (PSC). During the review period, there has been continued progress in understanding the mammalian immune response, the role of adhesion molecules and cytokines, the triggering events that initiate autoimmunity, immunogenetic predisposition to liver diseases, and the antigen specificity of autoantibodies. The precise immunologic mechanisms, however, that ultimately mediate hepatobiliary injury remain poorly defined [1••,2••].

Knowledge of allogeneic reactions that mediate graft versus host disease after bone marrow transplantation or blood transfusion and mediate rejection of transplanted livers has also increased. These topics have been recently reviewed elsewhere [3•,4•] and are beyond the scope of this article.

Mammalian immune response

The mammalian immune response can be subdivided into afferent and efferent limbs (Fig. 1). The principal events of the afferent limb are the processing and presentation of peptide antigenic epitopes in the binding grooves of class I and II major histocompatibility complex (MHC) molecules to the T-cell receptors (TCRs) of CD4 (helper) T cells and CD8 (cytotoxic) T cells. Activation of CD4 T cells is particularly crucial because their production of potent cytokines is a prerequisite for the proliferation and maturation of the cellular immune response and the production of antibodies in the humoral immune response.

Activation of CD4 T cells requires presentation of peptide antigen in the antigen-binding grooves of class II MHC molecules, the appropriate TCR repertoire for recognition of the specific antigen, augmentation by interaction of CD4 molecules with self class II MHC molecules on the antigen-presenting cell and intercellular binding of adhesion molecules to their counter-receptors (Table 1). Activation involving only these elements, however, results in clonal energy rather than maturation of the effector elements of the immune response [5•,6••]. Developmental effector functions re-

Abbreviations

ANCA—antineturophilic cytoplasmic antibody; **CTL**—cytotoxic T lymphocyte; **HBV**—hepatitis B virus; **HCV**—hepatitis C virus; **LKM**—liver-kidney microsomal; **MHC**—major histocompatibility complex; **PBC**—primary biliary cirrhosis; **PSC**—primary sclerosing cholangitis; **TCR**—T-cell receptor; **TNF**—tumor necrosis factor.

 ISBN 1-85922-608-6 ISSN 0267–1379

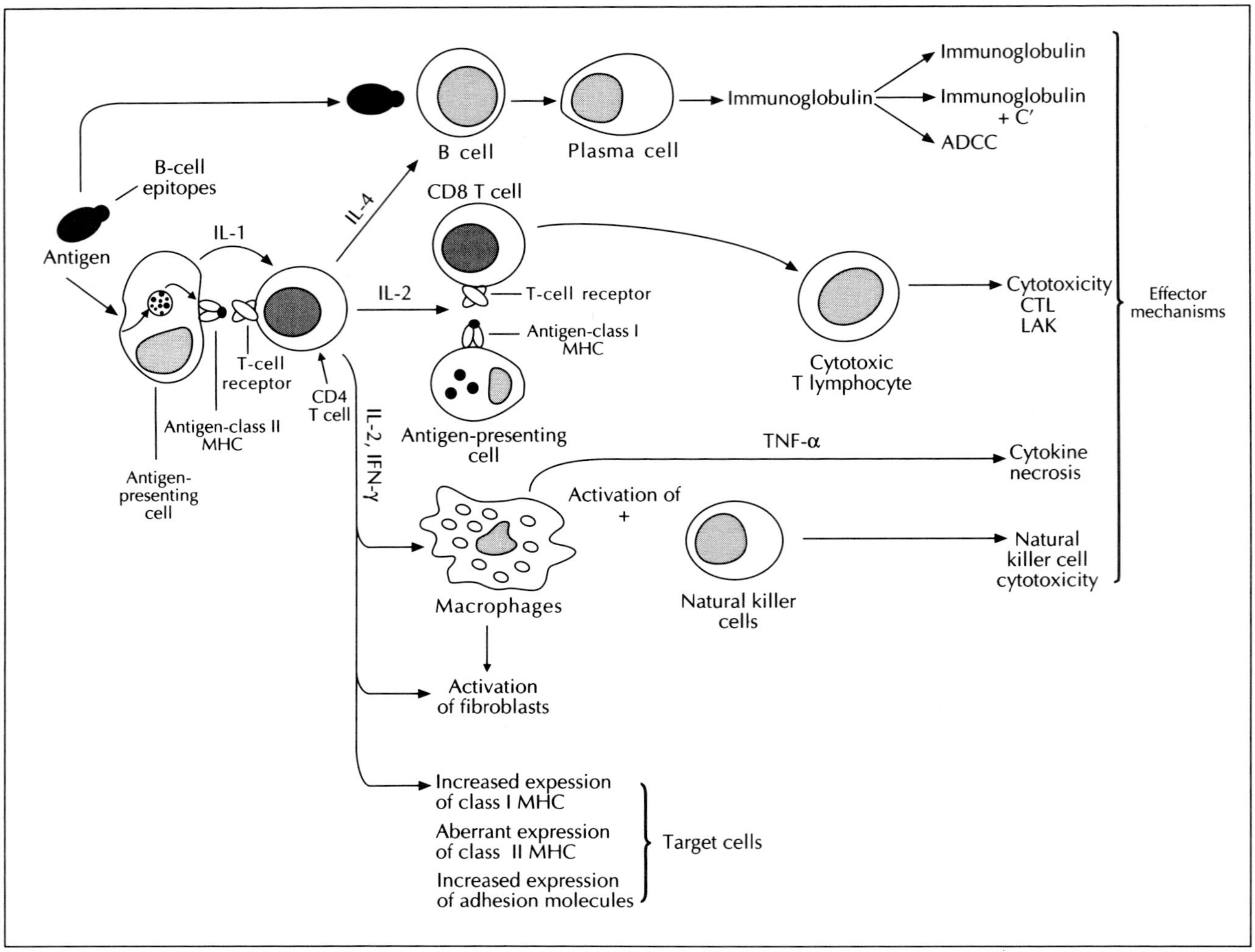

Fig. 1. The immune response can be subdivided into afferent and efferent limbs. The afferent limb involves activation of T cells through antigen processing and presentation. The efferent limb involves the proliferation and maturation of effector mechanisms of cellular and humoral immunity. Antigen activation of CD4 and CD8 T cells in the absence of costimulatory signals results in clonal anergy of the T cells, and aborts the development of the efferent response. Cytokines play crucial role by regulating the magnitude and duration of the immune response, the trafficking of cells, the localization of inflammation and the gene expression and metabolism of target cells. ADCC—antibody-dependent cellular cytotoxicity; C′—complement; CTL—cytotoxic T lymphocytes; IFN—interferon; Ig—immunoglobulin; IL—interleukin; LAK—lymphokine-activated killer cells; MHC—major histocompatibility complex; TNF—tumor necrosis factor. (*From* Hu and Vierling [1••]; with permission.)

quires both TCR activation and costimulatory or second signals. Costimulatory signaling results from the binding of ligand molecules (B7-1, B7-2) present on antigen-presenting cells with their complementary receptors on the T-cell surface (CD28 and its homologue CTLA-4) [5•,6••–8••].

Similar events are required for the activation and maturation of effector mechanisms of CD8 T cells except that antigen is presented in the antigen-binding grooves of class I MHC molecules and activation is augmented by CD8. Activation of TCR with costimulatory signaling results in the proliferation and differentiation of functional CD4 and CD8 T cells and immunoglobulin-secreting B cells.

Cytokines control both the development and modulation of this entire sequence of events [1••,2••]. In addition to the generation of effector mechanisms of target cell injury (Fig. 1), cytokines have potent effects on the expression of adhesion molecules by hepatocytes, biliary epithelial cells, and hepatic endothelial cells. Moreover, cytokines stimulate metabolic changes that alter cellular homeostasis (*eg*, the acute-phase response of hepatocytes to inflammation).

Autoimmunity as a cause of hepatobiliary diseases

Autoimmunity can develop when dysfunction of the host's normal ability to maintain tolerance to self-antigens occurs [1••,2••]. Three mechanisms are responsible for development and maintenance of tolerance to self-antigens: 1) elimination in the thymus of the TCR repertoire reactive to self-antigens (clonal deletion); 2) inactivation of T cells following interactions TCR with antigens in the absence of co-stimulatory signaling (clonal anergy), and 3) suppression of autoreac-

Table 1. Adhesion molecules and the liver

Receptor	Counter-receptor (Ligand)	Immunologic effects
LFA-1	ICAM-1, ICAM-2	T cell and APC interactions T cell and target cell interactions
CD2	LFA-3	T cell and APC interactions T cell and target cell interactions
VLA integrins	Addressins	Leukocyte migration
	INCAM-1	Adhesion to endothelial cells
	Laminin, fibronectin, collagen	Adhesion to extracellular matrix
ELAM-1	Leukocyte adhesion molecules	Adhesion of granulocytes and lymphocytes to endothelial cells
CD62	Leukocyte adhesion molecules	Adhesion of granulocytes and monocytes to endothelial cells in procoagulant state

APC—antigen-presenting cell; ELAM-1—endothelial leukocyte adhesion molecule-1; LFA—leukocyte function antigen; ICAM—intercellular adhesion molecule; INCAM-1—inducible cell adhesion molecule-1; VLA—very late activation (a misnomer).

tive T cells. Loss of self-tolerance and development of autoimmunity may involve immunogenetic, immunologic, and environmental factors. The immunogenetic factors include class I and II HLA alleles capable of binding autoantigens and a TCR repertoire capable of recognizing autoantigens. Immunologic factors include the presence of autoreactive T cells (due to a failure of clonal deletion, clonal anergy, or suppressor mechanisms) and processing and presentation of autoantigens. Environmental exposures may incite autoimmune reactions by molecular mimicry between peptide antigens of infectious agents and autoantigens, induction of autoantigenic cytochrome P-450 isoenzymes, or nonspecific inflammatory induction of hepatobiliary antigen presentation and expression of adhesion molecules [1••,2••].

Primary biliary cirrhosis

Immunogenetics

Previous observations indicating an association between the HLA haplotype DR8 and PBC in patients with European ancestry have been confirmed in the United Kingdom by analysis using polymerase chain reaction and restriction length polymorphism [9]. The relative risk of PBC with DR8 was 2.0 to 3.3. Moreover, the DR8 haplotype was associated with higher bilirubin levels, indicative of a worse prognosis [10]. Using the same technique, an increased frequency of HLA-B8, HLA-DR3, DRw52, DQw2, but not DR3, was also observed in Swedish patients [11]. Previous immunogenetic studies in Japanese patients demonstrated an HLA haplotype association with DR7 rather than DR8 [12]. Recent Japanese studies using polymerase chain reaction and restriction-length polymorphism demonstrated an increased frequency of DQ3 and DPB1* 0501 with a leucine substitution at amino acid position 35 [13]. Thus, differences exist in the immunogenetic association with PBC among different ethnic groups.

Autoantibodies

Extensive progress has been made in our understanding of antimitochondrial antibodies in PBC. The antimitochondrial antibodies specific for PBC react primarily with the E-2 subunits of the 2-oxoacid dehydrogenase complex. E-2 subunits (dihydrolipoamide acetyltransferase) are present in the pyruvate dehydrogenase complex, the branched chain ketodehydrogenase complex, and the oxoglutarate dehydrogenase complex of the 2-oxoacid dehydrogenase pathways [2••]. Using fluorescence *in situ* hybridization, the gene for dihydrolipoamide acetyltransferase has been mapped to human chromosome 11, band q23.1 [14].

A major conformational epitope of E-2 is the lipoic acid binding domain [15••]. A synthetic peptide conjugated with lipoic acid was able to detect 85% of serum samples from PBC patients positive for antimitochondrial antibodies and showed no false-positive reactions with antimitochondrial antibody–negative control sera [16••]. Commercially available 2-oxoacid dehydrogenase enzyme complexes have been successfully used for immunoblotting and have employed specificity for detection of PBC-specific antimitochondrial antibodies [17•]. Although immunoblotting was less sensitive than standard tissue section immunofluorescence, the specificity was superior (positive predictive value of 86%). The antimitochondrial antibodies of PBC patients reacted with four specific peptides on immunoblots: pyruvate dehydrogenase-E2 (74 kD), pyruvate dehydrogenase X (51 kD), branched-chain ketodehydrogenase-E2 (52 kD), and an unknown antigenic peptide of 43 kD. Some of the antimitochondrial antibodies cross-reacted with peptides containing similar epitopes, and different sera with the same immunoblotting pattern contain antibodies with different antigenic specificities [18•]. A flow cytometric immunoassay using pyruvate dehydrogenase enzyme complex as antigen demonstrated a sensitivity rate of 94% and a specificity of 100% for detection of antimitochondrial antibodies in PBC [19]. This was corroborated using the conventional antimitochondrial antibody assay and immunoblotting.

Analysis of the binding specificity of antimitochondrial antibody using an enzyme immunoassay revealed genetic and geographic variability [20•]. In North American PBC patients, 95% of sera reacted to the pyruvate dehydrogenase complex-E2 moiety, compared with only 65% of Japanese patients' sera.

Confocal microscopy of the bile ducts of patients with PBC demonstrated dense localization of an E2-like antigen to the submembranous cytoplasm of the apical domain of biliary epithelial cells [21••]. This localization of antigen was not observed in bile ducts of normal or diseased controls. Discordant results of the binding of monoclonal antibodies that react with conformational epitopes of E2 led to the speculation that immunoglobulin G and immunoglobulin A antimitochondrial antibodies may be reacting with a neoantigen (autoantigen?) that shares cross-reactive epitopes with the pyruvate dehydrogenase complex E2. The expression of E2 on the surface membrane of viable biliary epithelial cells and hepatocytes isolated from the livers of PBC patients has been detected [22•,23]. It was not, however, observed in control biliary epithelial cells. The data from these studies suggest a possible pathogenetic role for antimitochondrial antibodies binding to either E2 or cross-reactive antigens expressed on the surface membrane of biliary epithelial cells. It is attractive to speculate that a neoantigen that possesses epitopes cross-reactive with PBC-specific antimitochondrial antibodies would also have additional epitopes recognized by the TCR of infiltrating T cells mediating nonsuppurative destructive cholangitis.

Circulating B cells from patients with PBC that secrete antimitochondrial antibodies *in vitro* were shown to be maximally stimulated [24]. This finding indicates that a specific subset of antigen-stimulated B cells produce antimitochondrial antibodies, rather than polyclonal B cell populations. B-cell predominance in some portal infiltrates associated with nonsuppurative destructive cholangitis and B-cell infiltration of the biliary epitopes were also observed [25]. These findings suggested that humoral immunity may be directly involved in the effector mechanisms of nonsuppurative destructive cholangitis.

The possibility that production of antimitochondrial antibodies results from molecular mimicry remains an intriguing hypothesis. Previous studies demonstrated that antimitochondrial antibodies from patients with PBC reacted against the M2 antigen components of rough forms of *Escherichia coli* [26•], membrane fragments from mycobacteria [27•], and lower plants, such as algae, fungi, and ferns [28•]. Antimitochondrial antibodies specific for M2 are also formed in patients suffering from mycobacterium tuberculosis but not other bacterial infections including *E. coli* [27•]. These data suggest that the molecular mimicry of these highly conserved M2 epitopes could stimulate antimitochondrial antibodies production in immunogenetically susceptible patients. A corollary of this hypothesis is that patients who develop PBC lack either a component of natural immunity or tolerance to mitochondrial antigens.

Although it is well established that a familial predisposition to PBC exists, recent studies failed to identify an increased frequency of autoantibodies to 2-oxoacid dehydrogenase complex enzymes or naturally occurring antimitochondrial antibodies in asymptomatic relatives of patients with PBC [29•].

A recent study indicated that expression of anion exchanger genes in PBC patients was abnormal [30]. This defect could result in intensified cholestasis, exocrine gland dysfunction, and abnormal immune responses.

Recent studies assessed the possibility that the antimitochondrial antibodies of patients with PBC also react against the E3 constituent of the 2-oxoacid dehydrogenase complex [31]. The frequency of anti-E3 antibodies in PBC did not differ significantly from that in normal controls. Moreover, purified anti-E3 was not cross-reactive with other antigenic epitopic components of the 2-oxoacid dehydrogenase complex and did not react with the E3 subunits of either *E. coli* or yeast. These data argue against the hypothesis that reactions against the E3 constituents of bacteria or yeast initiate PBC.

The significance of previous data indicating variation in the specificities of antimitochondrial antibodies in patients with PBC were recently questioned. Studies indicating that disease severity and prognosis of PBC were related to the binding specificity of antimitochondrial antibodies to M4 and M9 antigens were not confirmed by two independent studies [32•,33•]. These investigators did not detect disease-specific reactivity against the purported M4 and M9 antigens (epitopes on the enzymes glycogen phosphorylase and sulfite oxidase, respectively).

In contrast to earlier reports, a study of antinuclear antibodies that react in a multiple nuclear dot pattern demonstrated that this pattern was not specific for PBC [34]. Although the immunoglobulin G3 subclass of antimitochondrial antibodies was significantly increased in the PBC patients compared with controls, they had a lower affinity for the nuclear antigens than did other immunoglobulin G subclasses.

T cells and cytokines

Previous studies of T-cell lines and clones derived from the liver biopsies of patients with PBC demonstrated reactivity to 2-oxoacid dehydrogenase complex antigens in the presence of autologous antigen-presenting cells and cytotoxic function in assays of lectin-mediated cellular cytotoxicity [2••]. Because nonsuppurative destructive cholangitis is characterized by T-cell infiltration of the bile duct epithelia and necrosis of biliary epithelial cells, T cells appear to play a direct role in bile duct destruction. In addition, the presence of T cells in the periportal inflammatory infiltrates in PBC also suggests that they are directly involved in hepatocellular necrosis. Despite these putative roles of cytotoxic T lymphocytes (CTLs) in hepatobiliary necrosis, CTLs reactive against antigens expressed by biliary epithelial cells or hepatocytes have not been identified.

Splenic cells obtained from patients with advanced PBC exhibited cytotoxicity against autologous biliary epithelial cells, and the majority of cytotoxic cells were CD8 T cells [35]. In contrast, cytotoxicity against autologous biliary epithelial cells was absent in patients without PBC. T-cell clones derived from the liver biopsies of patients with PBC were established that reacted specifically to bovine pyruvate dehydrogenase complex, a purified E2 subunit and a crude preparation of human liver mitoplasts prepared by removing the outer membrane of mitochondria [36••]. Reactive T-cell clones were CD4 T cells, and HLA class II restriction was observed. Similar reactivity was absent using hepatic T-cell clones obtained from the biopsies of either patients with a variety of other inflammatory liver diseases or normal controls [37]. A non-M2 protein (B1) in the bile of PBC patients stimulated proliferation of PBC peripheral lymphocytes *in vitro* [38]. This protein was postulated to be an immunologic cofactor in the development of PBC.

A defect in T-cell suppressor mechanisms has been postulated to promote autoimmune reactions in PBC. A recent study detected suppressor T-cell impairment in 39% of healthy first-degree relatives of patients with PBC, indicating a possible immunogenetic association [39]. However, there was no correlation between the degree of suppressor cell dysfunction and HLA haplotypes. Shedding of the CD8 antigen from CD8 T cells was recently proposed as a mechanism of suppressor cell dysfunction [40].

Two independent studies [41,42] confirmed prior observations that T cells from the livers or peripheral blood of patients with PBC secrete decreased levels of cytokines *in vitro.* In the first [41], spontaneous secretion of tumor necrosis factor (TNF)-α was significantly reduced in comparison with either healthy controls or patients with PSC. Lipopolysaccharide-stimulated TNF-α production by T cells from PBC patients was also lower than that of PSC patients. Both spontaneous and lipopolysaccharide-stimulated production of interleukin-1 by monocytes was comparable for control patients and patients with either PBC or PSC. Cytokine production by T cells, however, was not correlated with histologic activity, total bilirubin, Child's Pugh classification, or the presence of chronic ulcerative colitis. In the second study, T cells cultured from either percutaneous liver biopsies or the peripheral blood synthesized reduced amounts of TNF-α, TNF-β, and interferon-γ. Reduced TNF-β synthesis was more profound in patients with early histologic stages. Analysis of messenger RNAs indicated that decreased TNF-β levels were related to a defect in transcription of interleukin-2.

Diminished cytokine production by T cells from patients with PBC may be related to the recently identified deficiency of the proliferative response of T cells to the interleukin-2–dependent pathway [43]. Overall, the relationship between diminished cytokine production by T cells in PBC and mechanisms of immunopathogenesis remains unknown.

Other studies

Spontaneous occurrence of nonsuppurative destructive cholangitis was recently reported in senescent mice [44]. The lymphocytes infiltrating the biliary epithelia were CD8 T cells, and immunoelectron microscopy demonstrated contact junctions between the T cells and biliary epithelial cells, reminiscent of those observed in PBC. The mechanisms responsible for emergence of T cell reactivity were not defined, but loss of self-tolerance with aging is a likely explanation.

A recent study of the prevalence of anti-hepatitis C virus (HCV) antibodies in PBC indicated that most anti-HCV reactions were false-positive results due to elevated levels of circulating immunoglobulin G [45•,46•]. Furthermore, anti-HCV positivity was not correlated with either clinical features, the disease course, or life expectancy.

Classically, 90% to 95% of patients with PBC have antimitochondrial antibodies, whereas 5% to 10% of PBC patients are antimitochondrial antibody–negative. The antimitochondrial antibody–negative subgroup is characterized by circulating antinuclear antibodies or smooth muscle antibodies. These differential patterns of autoantibodies led to the speculation that antimitochondrial antibody–negative PBC may be a distinct disease, variously referred to as autoimmune cholangiopathy or autoimmune cholangitis [47]. Current data indicate that antimitochondrial antibody–positive and –negative patients are similar with respect to gender ratios, age, duration of disease, natural history, and histopathology [2••,47]. Thus, it remains unclear whether antimitochondrial antibody–negative PBC constitutes a separate disease. Identification of the precise immunopathogenic mechanisms of nonsuppurative destructive cholangitis in each subgroup will be required to answer this question because none of the autoantibodies appear to mediate tissue injury.

Portal inflammatory infiltrates in PBC contain not only T cells and B cells but also variable proportions of granulocytes, including eosinophils. A recent histopathologic study documented a significant increase in portal eosinophils in PBC compared with chronic viral hepatitis [48]. The degree of eosinophil infiltration was significantly correlated with the magnitude of inflammation and was more prominent in prefibrotic histologic stages of the disease. Presumably, the accumulation of eosinophils is related to chemotactic cytokines, adhesion receptors, and a local milieu containing interleukin-5. The role of eosinophils in the pathogenesis of nonsuppurative destructive cholangitis remains unclear. However, portal eosinophils are a characteristic of features of hepatic allograft rejection, which also involves nonsuppurative destructive cholangitis [49].

Orthotopic liver transplantation remains the only curative therapy for patients with advanced PBC. During prolonged postoperative follow-up, several patients developed recurrence of PBC in the allograft [50••,51]. Recurrence was associated with increased titers of antimitochondrial antibodies bile ductal proliferation and portal granulomas. The latter helped to distinguish recurrent PBC from either the bile duct destruction of refractory rejection or the rare occurrence of chronic graft versus host disease following liver transplantation. Further studies of patients with recurrent disease should provide important insights into the mechanisms of immunopathogenesis, especially with respect to effector T-cell mechanisms and their postulated self-HLA restriction. Because HLA matching is not performed between donor and recipient in liver transplantation, identity at any HLA-locus occurs only by chance.

Autoimmune hepatitis

Type 1

Patients with autoimmune hepatitis may be subdivided into three groups on the basis of the specificity of circulating autoantibodies (Table 2). Type I autoimmune hepatitis is associated with antinuclear antibody or SMA that react specifically with actin. Previous studies of patients of European ancestry indicated age-related differences in the HLA haplotype associations with type I autoimmune hepatitis. Younger patients were associated with the HLA haplotype A1, B8, DR3. In patients with type 1 autoimmune hepatitis who were DR3-negative, an independent association with DR4 was detected and the DR4-positive patients were significantly older [2]. These HLA haplotype differences may contribute to the bimodal distribution of the age of onset of type 1 autoimmune hepatitis by altering susceptibility to triggering stimuli with advancing age. A recent study of Japanese patients using polymerase chain reaction and restriction-length polymorphism confirmed an association of HLA haplotypes DR4 and B54 with type 1 autoimmune hepatitis in this ethnic group [52,53]. In addition, new associations with DR53 and DQ4 were observed. Type 1 autoimmune hepatitis was associated with the DR4 haplotype in 89% of patients. Among DR4-negative patients, there was a statistically significant independent association with DR2. The data also indicated that the amino acid at position 13 (Arg on DR2 and His on DR4) may contribute to susceptibility for type 1 autoimmune hepatitis among Japanese. These data, which parallel the observation in patients of European ancestry, underscore the role of immunogenetic susceptibility in type 1 autoimmune hepatitis and ethnic differences in HLA association.

The relationship between type 1 autoimmune hepatitis and HCV infection remains intriguing because it implies complicity between viral infection and autoimmune reactivity. In addition to false-positive tests for anti-HCV, patients with type 1 autoimmune hepatitis and true-positive anti-HCV (confirmed by recombinant immunoblot assay or polymerase chain reaction) have been recently recognized [2••]. In contrast, an American study of type 1 autoimmune hepatitis patients found a 4% prevalence of anti-HCV by second-generation enzyme immunoassay and none were confirmed by recombinant immunoblot assay 2 [54•]. Compared with a group of patients with typical chronic hepatitis C infection, patients with type 1 autoimmune hepatitis characteristically had titers of antinuclear antibody and SMA greater than the ratio of 1:80 and a statistically significant association with the HLA haplotype B8 and DR3. The mechanisms responsible for production of low titers of antinuclear antibody or SMA in patients with HCV infection remain undefined, and a role for autoimmune reactions in hepatocellular necrosis is speculative. A small number of patients with features of type 1 autoimmune hepatitis and HCV detected by polymerase chain reaction were reported who failed to respond to immunosuppressive therapy [55•]. In these patients, a viral rather than autoimmune mechanism of pathogenesis would be suspected.

Type 2

Type 2 autoimmune hepatitis is associated with anti-liver-kidney microsomal (LKM1) antibodies [2••]. Anti-LKM 1 antibodies react with cytochrome p450 IID6 as

Table 2. Autoantibodies in autoimmune liver diseases and hepatitis C infection

	Autoantibodies										Anti-HCV	
Disease	ANA	SMA	LKM1	SLA	AMA	ASGP-r	LP	LC	GOR	pANCA	EIA	RIBA
Autoimmune hepatitis												
Type 1	+	+	–	–	±*	+	–	–	–	+	±†	±
Type 2	–	–	+	–	–	–	±	±	–	–	±	±
Type 3	–	–	–	+	–	–	±	–	–	–	–	–
Primary biliary cirrhosis	±	±	–	–	+	±	–	?	–	+	–	–
Autoimmune cholangitis	+	–	–	–	–	?	–	?	–	?	–	–
Primary sclerosing cholangitis	+	–	–	–	–	–	–	?	–	+	–	–
Chronic hepatitis C	±	±	+	–	–	–	–	–	+	–	+	+

*Epitope specificity remains undefined; not M2 (E-2 of 2-oxoacid dehydrogenase multienzyme complex).
†Approximately 50% false-positive results.
AMA—antimitochondrial antibodies (E2 in primary biliary cirrhosis); ANA—antinuclear antibodies; ASGP-r—anti-asialoglycoprotein receptor antibodies; EIA—enzyme immunoassay; GOR—anti-GOR (nuclear antigen); HCV—hepatitis C virus; LC—anti-liver cytosol antigen type 1 (antigens undefined); LKM1—anti-liver-kidney microsomal (cytochrome P450IID6 and other epitopes) antibodies; LP—anti-liver pancreas (antigens undefined) antibodies; pANCA—perinuclear staining pattern of antineutrophil cytoplasmic antibodies (antigens undefined); RIBA—recombinant immunoblot assay; SLA—anti-soluble liver antigen (cytokeratins 8 and 18) antibodies; SMA—anti-smooth muscle (actin) antibodies; +, present; –, absent; ±, occasionally present; ?, reactivity undefined.

well as other microsomal epitopes. Previous epitope mapping showed that anti-LKM1 binding sites shared homology with peptides from salmonella species, human T lymphocytotropic viruses 1 and 2, herpes simplex virus, and hepatitis C virus (HCV) [56].

The association of type 2 autoimmune hepatitis and HCV infection led to a proposed subclassification: type 2a defined as anti-LKM1 positive and anti-HCV negative and type 2b, defined as anti-LKM1 positive and anti-HCV positive. Several reports have validated the observation that a substantial proportion of patients with LKM and chronic active hepatitis are associated with bona fide HCV infection, based on the presence of HCV-specific antibodies or detection of HCV RNA by polymerase chain reaction [2••,57,58•,59•]. These patients are predominantly males and are generally older than the classic young female patients with type 2 autoimmune hepatitis. Among more classic patients with type 2 autoimmune hepatitis, anti-HCV tests were negative and HCV RNA was undetectable. Classic type 2 autoimmune hepatitis patients were also more likely to be symptomatic and jaundiced at presentation [60]. Disparate results have been reported regarding the prevalence of anti-LKM1 antibodies among randomly selected patients with anti-HCV positivity. One group reported a prevalence of 3.2% whereas another found no anti-LKM1 antibodies [57,61•].

Among American patients with autoimmune hepatitis of any type, 19% were found to be anti-HCV positive by enzyme immunoassays 1 and 2 [62•]. Only one patient had HCV infection (confirmed by recombinant immunoblot assay 2 and HCV RNA polymerase chain reaction); this patient had anti-LKM1 antibodies and did not respond to immunosuppression. The remaining anti-HCV positive patients were recombinant immunoblot assay 2 negative, and all responded to immunosuppressive therapy. Similar findings have also been reported for patients in the United States [63] and the United Kingdom [59].

Whereas 59% of Italian patients with autoimmune hepatitis have been found to have true-positive anti-HCV (confirmed by recombinant immunoblot assay), only the recombinant immunoblot assay-negative patients responded to corticosteroids [64].

In general, autoantibodies (*eg*, antinuclear antibodies, SMA, and anti-LKM1) occur frequently in patients with HCV infection. Their clinical significance and their relation to induction or perpetuation of immunopathogenic mechanisms of hepatocellular injury remain undefined.

The principle antigenic epitopes of cytochrome P450IID6 lie between amino acid positions 254 and 271 [65]. Anti-cytochrome P450IID6 antibodies were used as reagents to detect the presence of cytochrome P450 epitopes expressed on the plasma membrane of human hepatocytes [66•]. These data suggested that anti-LKM1 antibodies might directly participate in antibody mediated mechanisms of hepatocellular necrosis type 2 in autoimmune hepatitis. Another study, however, failed to detect plasma membrane expression of cytochrome P450 epitopes [67•]. Immunoblot assays using recombinant cytochrome P450IID6 proteins (reported to be more sensitive and specific than traditional immunofluorescent methods) showed that the antigenic specificity differs between patients with classical type 2 autoimmune hepatitis and patients with HCV markers [68]. In the latter group, anti-LKM1 antibodies appeared to react against discontinuous or conformational epitopes.

Hepatic T cells in patients with type 2 autoimmune hepatitis have been analyzed at the clonal level [69]. CD4 T cells proliferated in response to recombinant human cytochrome P450IID6 antigen in an HLA class II–restricted manner. CD8 and CD4 T cell clones demonstrated cytotoxicity against both autologous and allogeneic Epstein Barr virus transformed B cells. Five clones were cytotoxic for autologous but not for allogeneic B cell lines, indicating HLA1 class I restriction.

The association between autoantibody production and viral hepatitis is well established. It is unclear whether the autoimmune responses (presumably instigated by viral hepatitis) and the resulting tissue necrosis include autoimmune effector mechanisms capable of perpetuating or worsening chronic hepatitis. In patients with anti-LKM1 and HCV infection, it appears that HCV triggers production of a nonpathogenic autoimmune response, because the clinical course and response to therapy are indicative of chronic hepatitis C rather than type 2 autoimmune hepatitis. Another example of this phenomenon is development of autoantibodies to the pentadecapeptide GOR, during HCV infections [70•]. A recent American series reported a prevalence of 50% among patients with chronic hepatitis C, but there was no correlation between the presence of anti-GOR and response to interferon therapy [71•]. In contrast, other investigators have hypothesized that HCV infection may trigger autoimmune hepatitis in susceptible individuals. Postulated mechanisms include molecular mimicry between HCV antigens and autoantigens, formation of complexes between viral and self proteins, processing and presentation of sequestered intracellular self-antigens and antigen presentation by hepatocytes aberrantly expressing HLA class II molecules [2••]. The hypothesis is supported by the study of a young male patient with typical features of chronic hepatitis C and a negative test for anti-LKM1 antibodies who developed anti-LKM1 during treatment with interferon-δ [72•]. The development of anti-LKM1 antibodies was associated with a rise in transaminases and hypergammaglobulinemia. The patient's HLA DR3 haplotype indicated an autoimmune susceptibility. Whether the HCV infection or the immunostimulatory effects of interferon-α triggered an autoimmune pathogenesis of hepatocellular necrosis remains conjectural. However, a previous report clearly indicated that hepatitis A infection can trigger the development of type 1 autoimmune hepatitis in immunogenetically susceptible relatives of index cases [73•].

A new autoantibody, designated anti-liver cytosol antigen type 1, was reported to help differentiate between classic type 2 autoimmune hepatitis and HCV infection associated with anti-LKM1 [74]. This autoantibody, which reacts with a 62 kD peptide antigen from human liver cytosol, was detected in 12 of 37 young patients with autoimmune hepatitis associated with anti-LKM1 antibodies or a second autoimmune disease. In contrast, it was absent in all older patients with both anti-LKM1 and markers of HCV infection.

Type 3

Type 3 autoimmune hepatitis is characterized by the presence of antisoluble liver antigen antibodies that react against epitopes on cytokeratins 8 and 18 [2••]. A newly identified autoantibody that reacts against liver-pancreas antigens was recently reported as an independent marker of autoimmune hepatitis, and frequently coexists with antisoluble liver antigen [75]. Immunoreactive epitopes of 48 and 52 kD were identified, but the specific antigens were not characterized. In a cohort of 660 patients with autoimmune hepatitis, 175 (27%) had complement-fixing anti–liver-pancreas antibodies of the immunoglobulin G1 subclass. Of these patients, 67% also had antisoluble liver antigens indicative of type 3 autoimmune hepatitis. The remaining 33% of the patients had no other autoantibodies except anti–liver-pancreas. Features consistent with a diagnosis of autoimmune hepatitis in these patients included elevated immunoglobulin G levels in 87%, chronic active hepatitis on liver biopsy in 63%, and response to immunosuppressive therapy with decreasing titers of anti–liver-pancreas in 100%. Anti-HCV was detected in 11% of these patients. In contrast, anti–liver-pancreas was found in only 2.9% of patients with chronic viral hepatitis. Validation and extension of these observations is required to assess the utility of anti–liver-pancreas as an independent autoantibody for autoimmune hepatitis.

Other studies

Despite the fact that autoantibodies frequently cannot be identified in patients with cryptogenic cirrhosis [76,77•], the majority of these patients share clinical features, immunogenetic phenotypes, and responsiveness to immunosuppression with autoimmune hepatitis patients. These findings suggest that patients with cryptogenic cirrhosis may indeed have occult autoimmune hepatitis.

Autoantibodies that react against asialoglycoprotein receptor have been of particular interest since the target epitopes are exclusively expressed on the surface membrane of hepatocytes and are accessible to circulating antibodies. In contrast, the antigens reactive with other autoantibodies (with the possible exception of cytochrome P450 IID6) are sequestered intracellularly and are often neither species nor organ specific. Previous studies demonstrated anti-asialoglycoprotein receptor in patients with autoimmune hepatitis as well as other inflammatory liver diseases, indicating a lack of disease specificity. A recent study demonstrated that B-cell secretion of anti-asialoglycoprotein receptor requires T-cell help [78•].

Soluble asialoglycoprotein receptor stimulated in vitro reactions of peripheral T cells obtained from patients with either autoimmune hepatitis or PBC (II). Hepatic T cell clones reacted to asialoglycoprotein receptor presented by autologous (but not allogeneic B cells), indicating self-HLA restriction [79].

Sixty-seven percent of patients with cirrhosis due to various etiologies exhibited redistribution of asialoglycoprotein receptor from the basolateral membrane domains to the canalicular (sinusoidal) domain of hepatocytes [80]. Redistribution may reflect loss of polarity in regenerating hepatocytes and could contribute to the elevated levels of circulating asialoglycoproteins observed in those with cirrhosis.

Primary sclerosing cholangitis

Primary sclerosing cholangitis is considered an autoimmune disease on the basis of HLA haplotype associations, high frequency of autoantibodies and its association with inflammatory bowel disease, particularly chronic ulcerative colitis. An increased frequency of the B8 and DR3 antigens, and a secondary association with DR2 antigens, has been identified in British patients [81].

Following an initial report of an 100% association with HLA DRw52a and PSC, other studies confirmed an association, but at a lower frequency [82]. A recent report in Swedish patients, however, found an insignificant increase in HLA DRw52a in patients with PSC compared with controls using direct DNA hybridization [83•]. The authors contended that the discrepancy with previous findings was due to the increased specificity of their hybridization method. None of the established HLA haplotypes were increased among Israeli patients with PSC [84]. As with PBC and autoimmune hepatitis, the immunogenetics exhibit geographic differences.

Several reports addressed the association between PSC and the perinuclear binding of antineutrophilic cytoplasmic antibodies (ANCAs) [85•]. Perinuclear ANCAs were detected by immunofluorescence in 88% of patients with PSC associated with inflammatory bowel disease and 40% of patients with PSC unassociated with inflammatory bowel disease [86•]. The titers of perinuclear ANCAs ranged widely and were correlated with disease activity only in patients with both PSC and inflammatory bowel disease. Immunoblots performed with sonicated neutrophil antigens demonstrated up to 5 antigenic reactivities in 82% of patients with PSC. In contrast, only 12% of patients with inflammatory bowel disease alone reacted to any of these antigens. Precise identification of the perinuclear ANCA antigens will be required to determine if the spectrum differs between patients with PSC and those with inflammatory bowel disease alone. ANCAs that produce granular cytoplasmic staining were also reported in 77% of patients with PSC and 33% of patients with inflammatory bowel disease alone [87]. The cytoplasmic staining pattern observed with this one-step amino alkaline phosphatase method contrasted with the results of immunofluorescence that demonstrated a perinuclear ANCA pattern in 90% of the patients with PSC and 60% of the patients with inflammatory bowel disease. This cytoplasmic staining pattern of ANCAs was also observed in pediatric patients and aided the diagnosis of PSC in this age group [88]. Further studies are required to validate the observation that a granular cytoplasmic staining pattern is more specific for PSC than conventional patterns of ANCAs observed with immunofluorescence.

Previous studies indicated that ANCAs are not specific for PSC and occur in patients with other chronic liver diseases. In a recent study, ANCAs were observed in 79% of patients with PSC, 88% with autoimmune hepatitis, and 28% with PBC [89•]. In all three patient groups, the presence of ANCAs correlated with the presence of cirrhosis.

Aberrant expression of A and B carbohydrate blood group antigens on both biliary and colonic epithelial cells was recently described in patients with PSC [90•]. The authors speculated that expression of these or other oncofetal antigens may be involved in disease pathogenesis. In addition, blood group antigens may also serve as markers for dysplasia of the biliary epithelia (a possible antecedent of cholangiocarcinoma) in a manner analogous to their association with dysplasia of colonic epithelia. Further studies are necessary to determine whether aberrant expression of blood group antigens is related to the recently reported association between PSC and colonic dysplasia, aneuploidy, and carcinoma in patients with ulcerative colitis [91].

References and recommended reading

Papers of particular interest, published within the annual period of review, have been highlighted as:
• Of special interest
•• Of outstanding interest

1. •• Hu K-Q, Vierling JM: **Immunologic Mechanisms of Hepatobiliary Injury.** In *Liver and Biliary Diseases*. Edited by Kaplowitz N. Baltimore:Williams and Wilkins; 1992:48–69.

A comprehensive review of the immunology of hepatobiliary diseases that emphasizes concepts and mechanisms.

2. •• Meyer zum Bueschenfelde K-H, Poralla T: **Immunology and Autoimmune Liver Diseases.** *Curr Opin Gastroenterol* 1992, **8**:380–387.

A detailed review of the 1991 literature on the immunology of autoimmune liver diseases.

3. • Brubaker DB: **Immunopathogenic Mechanisms of Post-Transfusion Graft-Versus-Host Disease.** *Proc Soc Exp Biol Med* 1993, **202**:122–147.

A review of the allogeneic mechanisms involved in the immunopathogenesis of graft versus host disease.

4. • Vierling JM: **Immunologic Mechanisms of Hepatic Allograft Rejection.** *Semin Liver Dis* 1992, **12**:16–27.

A review of the immunopathogenetic mechanisms of hepatic allograft rejection in human beings and experimental models.

5. • Cohen J: **New Protein Steals the Show as 'Costimulator' of T Cells.** *Science* 1993, **262**:844–845.

An editorial providing a concise overview of the subject of costimulatory signals required for a complete immune response.

6. •• Schwartz RH: **Costimulation of T Lymphocytes: The Role of CD28, CTLA-4, and B7/BB1 in Interleukin-2 Production and Immunotherapy.** *Cell* 1992, **71**:1065–1068.

Landmark study describing the interaction of TCRs CD_{28}/CTLA-4 with the APC ligands B7-1, B7-2 and their role in modulating costimulation.

7. •• Hathcock KS, Laszio G, Dickler HB, Bradshaw J, Linsley P, Hodes RJ: **Identification of an Alternative CTLA-4 Ligand Costimulatory for T Cell Activation.** *Science* 1993, **262**:905–909.

Landmark study describing the interaction of TCRs CD_{28}/CTLA-4 with the APC ligands B7-1, B7-2 and their role in modulating costimulation.

8. •• Freeman GJ, Gribben JG, Boussiotis VA, Ng JW, Restivo VA, Lombard LA, Gray GS, Nadler LM: **Cloning of B7-2: A CTLA-4 Counter-Receptor That Costimulates Human T Cell Proliferation.** *Science* 1993, **262**:909–911.

Landmark study describing the interaction of TCRs CD_{28}/CTLA-4 with the APC ligands B7-1, B7-2 and their role in modulating costimulation.

9. Underhill J, Donaldson P, Bray G, Doherty D, Portmann B, Williams R: **Susceptibility to Primary Biliary Cirrhosis is Associated With the HLA-DR8-DQB10402 Haplotype.** *Hepatology* 1992, **16**:1404–1408.

10. Gregory WL, Mehal W, Dunn AN, Cavanagh G, Chapman R, Fleming KA, Daly AK, Idle JR, James OFW, Bassendine MF: **Primary Biliary Cirrhosis: Contribution of HLA Class II Allele DR8.** *Q J Med* 1993, **86**:393–399.

11. Miyamori H, Kato Y, Kobayashi K, Hattori N: **Antigens in Japanese Patients With Primary Biliary Cirrhosis and Autoimmune Hepatitis.** *Digestion* 1983, **26**:213–217.

12. Seki T, Kiyosawa K, Ota M, Furuta S, Fukushima H, Tanaka E, Yoshizawa K, Kumagai T, Mizuki N, Ando A, Inoko H: **Association of Primary Biliary Cirrhosis With Human Leukocyte Antigen DPB1 0501 in Japanese Patients.** *Hepatology* 1993, **18**:73–78.

13. Morling N, Dalhoff K', Fugger L, Georgsen J, Jakobsen B, Ranek L, Odum N, Svejgaard A: **Polymorphism of HLA Class II Genes in Primary Biliary Cirrhosis.** *Immunogenetics* 1992, **35**:112–116.

14. Leung PS, Watanabe y, Munoz S, Teuber SS, Patel MS, Korenberg JR, Hara P, Coppel R, Gershwin ME: **Chromosome Localization and RFLP Analysis of PDC-E2: The Major Autoantigen of Primary Biliary Cirrhosis.** *Autoimmunity* 1993, **14**:335–340.

15. •• Tuaillon N, Andre C, Briand JP, Penner E, Muller S: **A Lipoyl Synthetic Octapeptide of Dihydrolipoamide Acetyltransferase Specifically Recognized by Anti-M2 Autoantibodies in Primary Biliary Cirrhosis.** *J Immunol* 1992, **148**:445–450.

Evidence that a highly conserved lipoate site in association with lipoic acid is a major conformational epitope of E2.

16. •• Briand JP, Andre C, Tuaillon N, Herve L, Neimark J, Muller S: **Multiple Autoepitope Presentation for Specific Detection of Antibodies in Primary Biliary Cirrhosis.** *Hepatology* 1992, **16**:1395–1403.

Evidence that the major E2 epitope is a conformational epitope requiring lipoic acid binding.

17. • Provenzano G, Diquattro O, Craxi A, Almasio P, Pinzello G, Marino L, Fioentino, Rinaldi F, Pagliaro L: **Immunoblotting as a Confirmatory Test for Antimitochondrial Antibodies in Primary Biliary Cirrhosis.** *Gut* 1993, **34**:544–548.

Evidence that immunoblotting for oxo-acid dehydrogenases is highly specific for PBC.

18. • Fusconi M, Baum H, Caselli A, Cassani F, Ballardini G, Lenzi M, Volta U, Zauli D, Bianchi FB: **Demonstration of Peptide-Specific and Cross-Reactive Epitopes in Proteins Reacting With Antimitochondrial Antibodies of Primary Biliary Cirrhosis.** *J Hepatol* 1992, **15**:162–169.

The authors report that the 2 oxoacid dehydrogenase proteins that react with antimitochondrial antibodies have cross reactive epitopes.

19. Elkhalifa MY, Kiechle FL, Gordon SC, Chen J, Poulik MD: **A Flow Cytometric Method to Detect Anti-Pyruvate Dehy-**

drogenase Antibody in Primary Biliary Cirrhosis. *Am J Clin Pathol* 1992, 97:202–208.

20. • Iwayama T, Leung PS, Rowley M, Munoz S, Nishioka M, Nakagawa T, Dickson ER, Coppel RL, Mackay IR, Gershwin ME: **Comparative Immunoreactive Profiles of Japanese and American Patients With Primary Biliary Cirrhosis Against Mitochondrial Autoantigens.** *Int Arch Allergy Immunol* 1992, 99:28–33.

Only 65% of Japanese patients react by enzyme-linked immunosprbent assay to PDC-E2 compared with 95% of North American PBC patients.

21. •• Van der Water J, Turchany J, Leung PSC, Lake J, Munoz S, Surh CD, Coppel R, Ansari A, Nakanuma Y, Gershwin ME: **Molecular Mimicry in Primary Biliary Cirrhosis.** *J Clin Invest* 1993, 91:2653–2664.

Using confocal microscopy, presents data suggesting the AMA is cross reactive with PDC-E2 and some other biliary antigen on the canalicular surface of biliary epithelial cells.

22. • Joplin R, Lindsay JG, Johnson GD, Strain A, Neuberger J: **Membrane Dihydrolipoamide Acetyltransferase (E2) on Human Biliary Epithelial Cells in PBC.** *Lancet* 1992, 339:93–94.

Suggests that E2 antigens are located in the plasma membranes of rat liver and human biliary epithelial cells, and are reactive to sera of patients with PBC.

23. Sundin U, Sundqvist KG: **Plasma Membrane Association of Primary Biliary Cirrhosis Mitochondrial Marker Antigen M2.** *Clin Exp Immunol* 1991, 83:407–412.

24. Lohse AW, Reckmann A, Kyriatsoulis A, Gerken G, Meyer zum Büschenfelde K-H, Manns M: **In Vitro Secretion of Specific Antimitochoindrial Antibodies in Primary Biliary Cirrhosis.** *J Immunol* 1992, 16:165–170.

25. Nakanuma Y: **Distribution of B Lymphocytes in Nonsuppurative Cholangitis in Primary Biliary Cirrhosis.** *Hepatology* 1993, 18:570–575.

26. • Butler P, Valle F, Hamilton-Miller JMT, Brumfitt W, Baum H, Burroughs AK: **M2 Mitochondrial Antibodies and Urinary Rough Mutant Bacteria in Patients With Primary Biliary Cirrhosis and in Patients With Recurrent Bacteriuria.** *J Hepatol* 1993, 17:408–414.

Recognition of the highly conserved M-2 component of oxoacid dehydrogenases in lower plant forms and bacteria and further supports the possible role of molecular mimicry in the pathogenesis of PBC. PBC specific antibodies are found in patients with M. Tuberculosis infection and react to the plasma membranes of mycobacteria.

27. • Klein R, Wiebel M, Engelhart S, Berg PA: **Sera From Patient With Tuberculosis Recognize the m2a-Epitope (e2-Subunit of Pyruvate Dehydrogenase) Specific for Primary Biliary Cirrhosis.** *Clin Exp Immunol* 1993, 92:308–316.

Recognition of the highly conserved M-2 component of oxoacid dehydrogenases in lower plant forms and bacteria and further supports the possible role of molecular mimicry in the pathogenesis of PBC. PBC specific antibodies are found in patients with M. Tuberculosis infection and react to the plasma membranes of mycobacteria.

28. • Lang P, Klein R, Becker EW, Berg PA: **Distribution of the PBC-Specific-(M2) and the Naturally-Occurring Mitochondrial Antigen-(Nomag) Systems in Plants.** *Clin Exp Immunol* 1992, 90:509–516.

Recognition of the highly conserved M-2 component of oxoacid dehydrogenases in lower plant forms and bacteria and further supports the possible role of molecular mimicry in the pathogenesis of PBC. PBC specific antibodies are found in patients with M. Tuberculosis infection and react to the plasma membranes of mycobacteria.

29. • Caldwell SH, Leung PSC, Spivey JR, Prindiville T, De Medina M, Saicheur T, Rowley M, Reddy KR, Coppel, Jeffers LJ, Mackay IR, Schiff ER, Gershwin ME: **Antimitochondrial Antibodies in Kindreds of Patients With Primary Biliary Cirrhosis: Antimitochondrial Antibodies are Unique to Clinical Disease and Are Absent in Asymptomatic Family Members.** *Hepatology* 1992, 16:899–905.

Confirmation of a hereditary component of PBC but disproves the notion of an increased prevalence of antimitochondrial antibodies in asymptomatic family members.

30. Prieto J, Qian C, García N, Díez J, Medina JF: **Abnormal Expression of Anion Exchanger Genes in Primary Biliary Cirrhosis.** *Gastroenterology* 1993, 105:572–578.

31. Maeda T, Loveland BE, Rowley MJ, IR Mackay: **Autoantibody Against Dihydrolipoamide Dehydrogenase, the e3 Submit of the 2-Oxoacid Dehydrogenase Complexes: Significance for Primary Biliary Cirrhosis.** *Hepatology* 1991, 14:994–999.

32. • Davis PA, Leung P, Manns M, Kaplan M, Munoz SJ, Gorin FA, Dickson ER, Krawitt E, Coppel R, Gershwin ME: **M4 and M9 Antibodies in the Overlap Syndrome of Primary Biliary Cirrhosis and Chronic Active Hepatitis: Epitopes or Epiphenomena?** *Hepatology* 1992, 16:1128–1136.

Evidence that the M4-M9 antigens are not specific for PBC and are of prognostic value.

33. • Palmer JM, Yeaman SJ, Bassendine MF, James OFW: **M4 and M9 Autoantigens in Primary Biliary Cirrhosis- a Negative Study.** *J Hepatol* 1993, 18:251–254.

Evidence that the M4-M9 antigens are not specific for PBC and are of prognostic value.

34. Pawlotsky J-M, Andre C, Metreau J-M, Beaugrand M, Zafrani E-S, Dhumeaux D: **Multiple Nuclear Dots Antinuclear Antibodies are Not Specific for Primary Biliary Cirrhosis.** *Hepatology* 1992, 16:129–131.

35. Onishi S, Saibara T, Nakata S, Maeda T, Iwasaki S, Iwamura S, Miyazaki M, Yamamoto Y, Enzan H: **Cytotoxic Activity of Spleen-Derived T Lymphocytes Against Autologous Biliary Epithelial Cells in Autopsy Patients With Primary Biliary Cirrhosis.** *Liver* 1993, 13:188–192.

36. •• Lohr H, Fleischer G, Gerken G, Yeaman SJ, Meyer zum Buschenfelde KH: **Autoreactive Liver Infiltrating T Cells in Primary Biliary Cirrhosis Recognize Inner Mitochondrial Epitopes and the Pyruvate Dehydrogenase Complex.** *J Hepatol* 1993, 18:322–327.

Contributes evidence that inner mitochondrial epitopes (including PDH-E2 or BCKD-E2) are antigenic for autoreactive T cells.

37. Van de Water J, Ansari AA, Surh CD, Coppel R, Roche T, Bonkovsky H, Kaplan M, Gershwin ME: **Evidence for the Targeting by 2-Oxo-Dehydrogenase Enzymes in the t Cell Response of Primary Biliary Cirrhosis.** *J Immunol* 1991, 146:89–94.

38. Onishi S, Maeda T, Iwasaki S, Saibara T, Miyamoto T: **A Biliary Protein Identified by Immunoblotting Stimulates Proliferation of Peripheral Blood T Lymphocytes in Primary Biliary Cirrhosis.** *Liver* 1991, 11:321–328.

39. Tsuji H, Murai K, Akagi K, Fujishima M: **Familial Primary Biliary Cirrhosis Associated With Impaired Coccanvlin A-Induced Lymphocyte Transformation in Relatives.** *Dig Dis Sci* 1992, 37:353–360.

40. Nouri Aria KT, Lombard M, Williams R: **High Serum Levels of CD8 Antigen in Primary Biliary Cirrhosis: A Possible Cause of Suppressor Cell Dysfunction?** *Clin Exp Immunol* 1991, 86:140–144.

41. Broome U, Eriksson LS, Sundin U, Sundqvist: **Decreased In Vitro Production of Tumor Necrosis Factor in Primary Biliary Cirrhosis Patients.** *Scand J Gastroenterol* 1992, 27:124–128.

42. Spengler U, Moller A, Jung M, Messer G, Zachoval R, Hoffman RM, Eisenburg J, Paumgartner G, Riethmuller G, Weiss EH: **T Lymphocytes From Patients With Primary Biliary Cirrhosis Produce Reduced Amounts of Lymphotoxin, Tumor Necrosis Factor and Interferon-γUpon Mitogen Stimulation.** *J Hepatol* 1992, 15:129–135.

43. Menéndez JL, Girón JA, Manzano L, Garrido A, Abreau L, Albillos A, Durántez A, Alvarez-Mon M: **Deficient Interleukin-2 Responsiveness of T Lymphocytes From Patients With Primary Biliary Cirrhosis.** *Hepatology* 1992, 16:931–936.

44. Kanda K, Onji M, Ohta Y: **Spontaneous Occurrence of Autoimmune Cholangitis in Senescent Mice.** *J Gastroenterol Hepatol* 1993, **8**:7–14.

45. • Bertolini E, Battezzati PM, Zermiani P, Bruno S, Moroni GA, Marelli F, Villa E, Manenti F, Zuin M, Crosgneni A: **Hepatitis C Virus Testing in Primary Biliary Cirrhosis.** *J Hepatol* 1992, **15**:207–210.
The detection of HCV antibodies in PBC patients is rare and of no significant prognostic importance. When present, they often are false-positive reactions secondary to increased globulin levels.

46. • Bertolini E, Marelli F, Zermiani P, Battezzati PM, Zuin M, Moroni GA, Podda M: **Antibodies to Hepatitis C Virus in Primary Biliary Cirrhosis.** *Arch Virol-Suppl* 1992, **4**:205–209.
The detection of HCV antibodies in PBC patients is rare and of no significant prognostic importance. When present, they often are false-positive reactions secondary to increased globulin levels.

47. Ben-Ari Z, Dhillon AP, Sherlock S: **Autoimmune Cholangiopathy: Part of the Spectrum of Autoimmune Chronic Active Hepatitis.** *Hepatology* 1993, **18**:10–15.

48. Terasaki S, Nakanuma Y, Yamazaki M, Unoura M: **Eosinophilic Infiltration of the Liver in Primary Biliary Cirrhosis: A Morphological Study.** *Hepatology* 1993, **17**:206–212.

49. Martinez OM, Asscher NL, Ferrell L, Villanueva J, Lake J, Roberts JP, Krams SM: **Evidence for a Nonclassical Pathway of Graft Rejection Involving Interleukin 5 and Eosinophils.** *Transplantation* 1993, **55**:909–918.

50. •• Wong PYN, Portmann B, O'Grady JG, Devlin JJ, Hegarty JE, Tan K-C, Williams R: **Recurrence of Primary Biliary Cirrhosis After Liver Transplantation Following fk506-Based Immunosuppression.** *J Hepatol* 1993, **17**:284–287.
Description of recurrent PBC post–liver transplantation characterized by the presence of portal granulomas bile duct proliferation, and increased titers of antimitochondrial antibodies.

51. Balan V, Batts KP, Porayko MK, Krom RAF, Ludwig J, Wiesner RH: **Histological Evidence for Recurrence of Primary Biliary Cirrhosis After Liver Transplantation.** *Hepatology* 1993, **18**:1392–1398.

52. Seki T, Kiyosawa K, Inoko H, Ota M: **Association of Autoimmune Hepatitis With hla-bw44 and dr4 in Japanese Patients.** *Hepatology* 1990, **12**:1300–1304.

53. Seki T, Ota M, Furuta S, Fukushima HH, Kondo T, Hino K, Mizuki N, Ando A, Tsuji K, Inkoko H: **HLA Class II Molecules and Autoimmune Hepatitis Susceptibility in Japanese Patients.** *Gastroenterology* 1992, **103**:1041–1047.

54. • Czaja AJ, Carpenter HA, Santrach PJ, Moore SB, Taswell HF, Homburger HA: **Evidence Against Hepatitis Viruses as Important Causes of Severe Autoimmune Hepatitis in the United States.** *J Hepatol* 1993, **18**:342–352.
Evidence against an association between autoimmune hepatitis and viral infection in the United States.

55. • Pawlotsky J-M, Deforges L, Bretagne S, André C, Métreau J-M, Thiers V, Zafrani E-S, Goossens M, Duval J, Mavier J-P, Dhumeaux D: **Hepatitis C Virus Infection Can Mimic Type 1 (Antinuclear Antibody Positive) Autoimmune Chronic Active Hepatitis.** *Gut* 1993, S66–S68.
Describes five patients with the presentation of type 1 autoimmune hepatitis who were HCV-positive and responded to interferon and not to immunosuppressive therapy.

56. Guegen M, Boniface O, Bernard O, Clerc F, Cartwright T, Alvarez F: **Identification of the Main Epitope on Human Cytochrome P450IID6 Recognized by Anti-Liver Microsomal Antibody.** *Autoimmunity* 1991, **4**:607–615.

57. Lunel F, Abuaf N, Frangeul L, Grippon P, Perrin M, Le Coz Y, Valla D, Borotto E, Yamamoto A-M, Huraux J-M, Opolon P, Homberg J-C: **Liver/Kidney Microsome Antibody Type 1 and Hepatitis C Virus Infection.** *Hepatology* 1992, **16**:630–636.

58. • Seelig R, Renz M, Bünger, Schröter, Seelig HP: **Anti-LKM-1 Antibodies Determined by Use of Recombinant P450 2D6 in ELISA and Western Blot and Their Association With Anti-HCV and HCV-RNA.** *Clin Exp Immunol* 1993, **92**:373–380.
Supports the subdivision of Type II autoiommune hepatitis patients into HCV-positive and HCV-negative groups.

59. • Fried MW, Draguesku JO, Shindo M, Simpson LH, Banks SM, Hoofnagle JH, DiBisceglie AM: **Clinical and Serological Differentiation of Autoimmune and Hepatitis C Virus-Related Chronic Hepatitis.** *Dig Dis Sci* 1993, **38**:631–636.
Evidence that autoantibodies are frequently found in chronic hepatitis C, especially in older subjects and in the Mediterranean Basin, but appear to be clinically insignificant. Anti-HCV is frequently present in autoimmune hepatitis but is rarely confirmed by tests of higher specificity.

60. Esteban JI, Esteban R, Viladomiu L, Lopez-Talauera JC, Gonzalez A, Hernandez JM, Roget M, Vargas V, Genesca J, Buti M: **Hepatitis C Virus Antibodies Among Risk Groups in Spain.** *Lancet* 1989, **11**:294–297.

61. • Mitchel LS, Jeffers LJ, Reddy KR, Cheinquer H, Coelho-Little E, Moreda R, Parker T, Silva M, Li XM, de Medina M, Coelho-Morges S, Hill M, Altman R, Manns MP, Schiff ER: **Detection of Hepatitis C Virus Antibody by First- and Second-Generation Assays and Polymerase Chain Reaction in Patients With Autoimmune Chronic Active Hepatitis Types I, II and III.** *Am J Gastroenterol* 1993, **88**:1027–1034.
Further evidence against an association between autoimmune hepatitis and HCV infection in the United States and supports the notion that hepatitis B and C infections are not associated with the production of LKM autoantibodies in US patients.

62. • Czaja AJ, Manns MP, Homburger HA: **Frequency and Significance of Antibodies to Liver/Kidney Microsome Type 1 in Adults With Chronic Active Hepatitis.** *Gastroenterology* 1992, **103**:1290–1295.
Further evidence against an association between autoimmune hepatitis and HCV infection in the United States and supports the notion that hepatitis B and C infections are not associated with the production of LKM autoantibodies in US patients.

63. Lenzi M, Johnson PJ, McFarlane IG, Ballardini G, Smith HM, McFarlane BM, Bridger C, Vergani D, Bianchi FB, Williams R: **Antibodies to Hepatitis C Virus in Autoimmune Liver Disease: Evidence for Geographical Heterogeneity.** *Lancet* 1991, **338**:277–280.

64. Magrin S, Craxi A, Fiorentino G, Fabiano C, Provenzano G, Pinzello GB, Palazzo U, Almasio P, Pagliaro L: **Is Autoimmune Chronic Active Hepatitis a HCV-Related Disease?** *J Hepatol* 1991, **13**:56–60.

65. Manns MP, Griffin KJ, Sullivan KF, Johnson EF: **LKM-1 Autoantibodies Recognize a Short Linear Sequence in P450IId6, a Cytochrome P-450 Monooxygenase.** *J Clin Invest* 1991, **88**:1370–1378.

66. • Loeper J, Descatoire V, Maurice M, Beaune P, Belghiti J, Houssin D, Ballet F, Feldmann G, Guengerich FP, Pessayre D: **Cytochromes P-450 in Human Hepatocytes Plasma Membrane: Recognition by Several Autoantibodies.** *Gastroenterology* 1993, **104**:203–216.
Evidence for and against the role of LKM Ab to cytochrome p450IID6 in the immunopathogenesis of autoimmune hepatitis.

67. • Yamamoto AM, Mura C, De Lemos-Chiarandini C, Krishnamoorthy R, Alvarez Inserm F: **Cytochrome P450IID6 Recognized by LKM 1 Antibody is Not Exposed on the Surface of Hepatocytes.** *Clin Exp Immunol* 1993, **92**:381–390.
Evidence for and against the role of LKM Ab to cytochrome p450IID6 in the immunopathogenesis of autoimmune hepatitis.

68. Yamamoto AM, Cresteil D, Homberg JC, Alvarez F: **Characterization of Anti-Liver-Kidney Microsome Antibody (Anti-LKM1) From Hepatitis C Virus-Positive and Negative Sera.** *Gastroenterology* 1993, **104**:1762–1767.

69. Lohr H, Manns M, Kyriatsoulis A, Lohse AW, Trauwein C, Meyer zum Buschenfelde KH, Fleischer B: **Clonal Analysis of Liver-Infiltrating T Cells in Patients With LKM-1 Antibody-Positive Autoimmune Chronic Active Hepatitis.** *Clin Exp Immunol* 1991, **84**:297–302.

70. Michel G, Ritter A, Gerken G, Meyer zum Buschenfelde KH,
• Decker R, Manns MP: **Anti-GOR and Hepatitis C Virus in Autoimmune Liver Diseases.** *Lancet* 1992, **339**:267–269.

Description of the production of the auto antibody GOR in association with hepatitis C infection and evidence of its insignificance in relationship to clinical, histologic, or therapeutic aspects of hepatitis C infection.

71. Lau JY, Davis GL, Orito E, Qian KP, Mizokami M: **Signifi-**
• **cance of Antibody to the Host Cellular Gene Derived Epitope GOR in Chronic Hepatitis C Virus Infection.** *J Hepatol* 1993, **17**:253–257.

Description of the production of the autoantibody GOR in association with hepatitis C infection and evidence of its insignificance in relationship to clinical, histologic, or therapeutic aspects of hepatitis C infection.

72. Muratori L, Zauli D, Giostra F, Ballardini G, Lenzi M, Cas-
• sani F, Bianchi FB: **LKM-$_1$ Appearance in a HLA-DR3+ Patient With Chronic Hepatitis C During Interferon Treatment [Letter].** *J Hepatol* 1993, **19**:259–260.

Descriptions of viral infections possibly inducing autoimmune hepatitis.

73. Vento S, Garofano T, Di Perri G, Dolci L, Concia E, Bassetti
• D: **Identification of Hepatitis A Virus as a Trigger for Autoimmune Chronic Hepatitis Type I in Susceptible Individuals.** *Lancet* 1991, **337**:1183–1187.

Descriptions of viral infections possibly inducing autoimmune hepatitis.

74. Abuaf N, Johanet C, Chretien P, Martini E, Soulier E, Laperche S, Homberg JC: **Characterization of the Liver Cytosol Antigen Type 1 Reacting With Autoantibodies in Chronic Active Hepatitis.** *Hepatology* 1992, **16**:892–898.

75. Stechemesser E, Klein R, Berg PA: **Characterization and Clinical Relevance of Liver-Pancreas Antibodies in Autoimmune Hepatitis.** *Hepatology* 1993, **18**:1–9.

76. Provenzano G, Marino L, Craxi A: **Features of Autoimmunity in Cryptogenic Chronic Hepatitis.** *Allergol Immunopathol* 1991, **19**:119–122.

77. Czaja AJ, Carpenter HA, Santrach PJ, Moore SB, Hom-
• burger HA: **The Nature and Prognosis of Severe Cryptogenic Chronic Active Hepatitis.** *Gastroenterology* 1993, **104**:1755–1761.

Evidence that patients with cryptogenic cirrhosis infrequently have autoantibodies, but frequently share clinical and therapeutic similarities to patients with autoimmune hepatitis.

78. Lohr H, Treichel U, Poralla M, Manns M, Meyer Zum
• Buschenfelde, Fleischer B: **Liver Infiltrating T Helper Cells in Autoimmune Chronic Active Hepatitis Stimulate the Production of Autoantibodies Against the Human Asialoglycoprotein Receptor In Vitro.** *Clin Exp Immunol* 1992, **88**:45–49.

Adds further evidence for the possible role of the Asialoglycoprotein receptor in the pathogenesis of autoimmune hepatitis.

79. Lohr H, Teichel U, Poralla T, Manns M, Meyer Zum Buschenfelde KH, Fleischer B: **The Human Asialoglycoprotein Receptor is a Target Antigen for Liver Infiltrating T Cells in Autoimmune Chronic Active Hepatitis and Primary Biliary Cirrhosis.** *Hepatology* 1990, **12**:1314–1320.

80. Burgess J, Baenziger JU, Brown W: **Abnormal Surface Distribution of the Human Asialoglycoprotein Receptor in Cirrhosis.** *Hepatology* 1992, **15**:702–706.

81. Donaldson PT, Farrant JM, Wilkinson ML, Hayllar K, Portmann BC, Williams R: **Dual Association of HLA DR2 and DR3 With Primary Sclerosing Cholangitis.** *Hepatology* 1991, **13**:129–133.

82. Prochazka EJ, Terasaki PI, Sik Park M, Goldstein LI, Busuttil RW: **Association of Primary Sclerosing Cholangitis With HLA-DRw52a.** *N Engl J Med* 1990, **322**:1842–1844.

83. Zetterquist H, Broome U, Einarsson K, Olerup O: **HLA Class**
• **II Genes in Primary Sclerosing Cholangitis and Chronic Inflammatory Bowel Disease: No HLA-DRw52a Association in Swedish Patients With Sclerosing Cholangitis.** *Gut* 1992, **33**:942–946.

Evidence for and against an association between PSC and the presence of the HLA haplotype DRw-52a.

84. Amar A, Brautbar C, Goldin E, Sherman L, Barmeir S, Shouval D, Hansen JA, Smith AG: **Serological and Molecular Analysis of HLA in Israeli Primary Sclerosing Cholangitis Patients.** *J Immunogen* 1992, **19**:295–302.

85. Duerr RH, Targan SR, Landers CJ, LaRusso NF, Lindsay KL,
• Wiesner RH, Shanahan F: **Neutrophil Cytoplasmic Antibodies: A Link Between Primary Sclerosing Cholangitis and Ulcerative Colitis.** *Gastroenterology* 1991, **100**:1385–1391.

Evidence that pANCAs are found in both inflammatory bowel disease and PSC.

86. Seibold F, Weber P, Klein R, Berg Pa, Wiedman KH: **Clinical**
• **Significance of Antibodies Against Neutrophils in Patients With Inflammatory Bowel Disease and Primary Sclerosing Cholangitis.** *Gut* 1992, **33**:657–662.

Evidence that different antigens may be involved in the pANCA reaction in the two diseases.

87. Lo SK, Fleming KA, Chapman RW: **Prevalence of Anti-Neutrophil Antibody in Primary Sclerosing Cholangitis and Ulcerative Colitis Using an Alkaline Phosphatase Technique.** *Gut* 1992, **33**:1370–1375.

88. Lo SK, Chapman RWG, Cheeseman P, Charlton CPJ, Walker-Smith JA, Mieli-Vergani G, Fleming KA: **Antineutrophil Antibody: A Test for Autoimmune Primary Sclerosing Cholangitis in Childhood?** *Gut* 1993, **34**:199–202.

89. Leotine Mulder AH, Horst G, Haagsma EB, Limburg PC,
• Kleibeuker JH, Kallenberg CGM: **Prevalence and Characterization of Neutrophil Cytoplasmic Antibodies in Autoimmune Liver Diseases.** *Hepatology* 1993, **17**:411–417.

Evidence that pANCA is nonspecific for PSC and is common in PBC and autoimmune hepatitis as well.

90. Bloom S, Heryet A, Fleming K, Chapman RW: **Inappropri-**
• **ate Expression of Blood Group Antigens on Biliary and Colonic Epithelia in Primary Sclerosing Cholangitis.** *Gut* 1993, **34**:977–983.

Evidence of aberrant blood group antigens on biliary epithelia and the presentation of their possible involvement in the immunopathogenesis of PSC.

91. Broomé U, Linberg G, Löfberg R: **Primary Sclerosing Cholangitis in Ulcerative Colitis-a Risk Factor for the Development of Dysplasia and DNA Aneuploidy.** *Gastroenterology* 1992, **102**:1877–1880.

John M. Vierling, MD, Hepatology Program, Suite 7511 Cedars-Sinai Medical Center, 8700 Beverly Boulevard, Los Angeles, CA 90048, USA.

Role of the immune response in viral hepatitis, hepatocellular carcinoma, and alcoholic hepatitis

Bradley L. Freilich, MD, Ke-Qin Hu, MD, and John M. Vierling, MD

Cedars-Sinai Medical Center, University of California at Los Angeles, Los Angeles, California, USA

Viral infections, malignant transformation, and xenobiotics may elicit immune responses capable of mediating tissue injury. Accumulating evidence indicates that immune responses against viral antigens expressed by infected hepatocytes may mediate hepatocellular necrosis during hepatitis B or C viral infections. Recent studies have clarified the role of T cells, cytokines, and both major histocompatibility complex and adhesion molecules during hepatitis B and C infections. Additional studies have assessed the impact of hepatitis B virus mutants on the immune response and the ability of the hepatitis B virus to alter the phenotype of infected hepatocytes. Emerging data also indicate that hepatitis C infection may play a role in autoimmune reactions. New observations have further defined a relationship between the development of hepatocellular carcinoma and the immune response. In addition, continuing investigations have emphasized the importance of the immune response in the pathogenesis of alcoholic hepatitis. Further understanding of these immune mechanisms may lead to innovative therapeutic strategies.

Current Opinion in Gastroenterology 1994, **10**:269–276

Viral infections, malignant transformation, and xenobiotics can induce both cellular and humoral immune responses. Indeed, immune mechanisms appear to play an important role in the elimination of viral infections, the prevention and retardation of malignant neoplasms, and the prevention of tissue injury associated with a variety of xenobiotics. Whereas the previous paper describes advances in our understanding of the human immune response and putative autoimmune hepatobiliary disease, this article summarizes recent progress with respect to the role of the immune response in hepatitis B and C viral infection, the development of hepatocellular carcinoma, and the pathogenesis of alcoholic hepatitis.

Immunopathogenesis of viral hepatitis

Hepatitis B virus

Although the mechanisms responsible for viral clearance and hepatocellular necrosis during hepatitis B virus (HBV) infection remain poorly defined, a body of evidence indicates that the host-immune response to HBV antigens play a central role. Studies of both hepatic and peripheral blood mononuclear inflammatory cells indicated that T-cell responses to HBV-encoded antigens, including envelope hepatitis B surface antigen and nucleocapsid (hepatitis B core antigen [HBcAg]) proteins, may participate in hepatocellular necrosis. An HLA A2-restricted cytotoxic T lymphocyte (CTL) response was demonstrated against the amino acid sequence 18-27 of HBcAg in patients with the HLA haplotype A2 and acute HBV infection [1••]. This HLA class I-restricted response, however, was not detected in HLA A2-positive patients with chronic hepatitis B. Amino acids 18-27 of HBcAg contain the predicted binding motif for the HLA A2 peptide-binding groove [2•]. HLA A2-restricted CTLs were also identified with antigen specificity for hepatitis B surface antigen in acute hepatitis B infection [3••]. In addition, CTL recognition of the viral epitopes was observed with different HLA class I restrictions. For example, a CTL response to the amino acid sequence 141-151 of HBcAg was restricted to both HLA A31 and HLA Aw68 [1••]. Indeed, circulating CTL responses appeared to be polyclonal and directed against multiple HBV antigens in acute hepatitis [3••]. During acute hepatitis B, peripheral blood mononuclear cells exhibited a significant increase in the proportion of CD8 CTLs that ex-

Abbreviations

CTL—cytotoxic T lymphocyte; **HBcAg**—hepatitis B core antigen; **HBV**—hepatitis B virus; **HCV**—hepatitis C virus; **ICAM**—intercellular adhesion molecule; **MHC**—major histocompatibility complex; **TCR**—T-cell receptor; **TGF**—transforming growth factor; **TNF**—tumor necrosis factor.

 ISBN 1-85922-608-6 ISSN 0267–1379

press CD45R0, a marker of a memory subset [4•]. The above data suggest that accumulation of functional, polyclonal HBV peptide-specific effector T cells may dictate whether acute infection resolves or becomes chronic.

The importance of HBV-specific CTLs in the pathogenesis of hepatocellular necrosis was further confirmed *in vivo* using a transgenic mouse model expressing hepatitis B surface antigen [5••]. Injection of the transgenic mice with exogenous, syngeneic CD8 CTL clones specific for hepatitis B surface antigen resulted in necrosis of hepatocytes expressing hepatitis B surface antigen *in vivo*. The response was major histocompatibility complex (MHC) class I-restricted and *in vitro* studies showed that the CD8 CTL clone secreted interferon-γ when stimulated with hepatitis B surface antigen *in vitro*. Disease severity was correlated with the number of CTLs injected.

Following injection of these interferon-γ-secreting CD8 CTL, severe lethal hepatitis occurred in association with inflammatory infiltrates containing macrophages. Inhibition of macrophage function before administration of the CD8 CTL significantly reduced the severity of liver disease, indicating that macrophages participated in the hepatocellular necrosis. Thus, HBV-specific, MHC class I-restricted CD8 CTL initiate antigen-specific hepatocellular necrosis and elicit (presumably by cytokine secretion) additional macrophage-mediated mechanisms of injury.

Another study documented an association between an HLA class I haplotype and a pre-S2 antigen in patients with high alanine aminotransferase levels. This association was absent in patients with normal alanine aminotransferase levels [6•]. These emerging data strongly indicate that HLA class I-restricted CTL initiate hepatocellular necrosis of HBV-infected cells and contribute to viral clearance during acute infection. However, acute hepatitis B may also occur in the absence of an HLA class I-restricted CTL response. Indeed, HBcAg-specific T-cell responses have been demonstrated in a patient with recurrent hepatitis B in a liver-allograft completely mismatched for HLA class I [7•]. Allogeneic T cell activation and secretion of cytokines presumably leads to recruitment of other effector cells (*eg*, monocyte/macrophages), and may also play an important role in immunopathogenesis.

Recently, lymphoblastoid cells were successfully transformed with the HBV core open reading frame using electroporation [8•]. The constitutive expression of HBcAg should facilitate further study of endogenous antigen processing and the specificity of immune responses against HBcAg.

Hepatitis B virus–infected hepatocytes have been regarded traditionally as passive target cells. Recent studies, however, indicate that HBV infection may substantially alter the hepatocyte phenotype and, thus, modulate the immune response [9••,10••]. For example, the HBV X protein transactivates cellular genes resulting in increased expression of HLA class I molecules and the aberrant expression of HLA class II DR molecules. The former could increase the recognition of infected hepatocytes by HLA class I-restricted CTL. The latter could promote antigen presentation to HLA class II-restricted CD4 T cells or serve as a target for HLA class II-restricted CD4 CTL.

Both effective antigen presentation and cytolysis of target cells require interaction between adhesion molecules in the antigen-presenting cell or target cell and their counter-receptors on the T-cell surface membrane. The most well-studied interaction is that of intercellular adhesion molecule (ICAM)-1 and its T-cell counter receptor lymphocyte activation factor 1. Increased intrahepatic expression of ICAM-1 has been observed during HBV infection and parallels the aberrant expression of HLA class II and infiltration of lymphocyte activation factor 1 positive inflammatory cells [9••,10••]. Intrahepatic expression of ICAM-1 during chronic HBV infection correlated with the magnitude of alanine aminotransferase elevation, the presence of infiltrating CTL, and focal necrosis. However, it did not correlate with viral replication [11•]. Successful treatment with interferon-α2b decreased intrahepatic expression of ICAM-1 [12•].

Although these data suggested that ICAM-1 expression might be the secondary consequence of cytokine (*eg*, interferon-γ) release by infiltrating T cells, a recent study demonstrated increased ICAM-1 expression *in vitro* induced by transactivation of the ICAM-1 gene by HBV X protein in the absence of exogenous inflammatory cytokines [13•]. Lymphocyte activation factor-3, another member of the immunoglobulin supergene family involved in signal transduction between T cells and antigen-presenting cells, is also aberrantly expressed by hepatocytes during hepatitis B infection [9••]. Normal hepatocytes do not express lymphocyte activation factor-3.

The observation that hepatocytes aberrantly express HLA class II and adhesion molecules for antigen-presenting functions led to the speculation that hepatocytes might also express costimulatory molecules (B7-1 and B7-2) required to generate an effective immune response [10••,13•). Alternatively, if infected hepatocytes failed to express costimulatory molecules, activated T-cell subsets would exhibit anergy. Because clearance of HBV infection appears to require a polyclonal T response against multiple HBV antigens, clonal energy of a subset of HBV-specific T cells could promote chronicity. If all T cells were functionally inactivated by clonal anergy, a chronic carrier state without hepatocellular necrosis would ensue.

Patients with chronic hepatitis B are at risk for acute exacerbations of hepatocellular necrosis. Exacerbations are associated with increased markers of viral replication (*eg*, HBV DNA and hepatitis B e antigen). A recent study indicated that exacerbations correlated significantly with the presence of hepatitis B e antigen–specific immune complexes [14•]. These data suggested that increased viral replication and expression of viral proteins might increase susceptibility of infected hepatocytes to antibody-mediated mechanisms of necrosis. T-cell–dependent antibody production may also be directly modified by HBV infection. In the transgenic mouse model antibody, production to T-cell–dependent antigens was reduced due to a defect of the antigen-presenting cell activity of splenic dendritic cells [15•]. There was no functional abnormality of either T or B cells. Another HBV transgenic mouse strain produced modest amounts of anti-HBc after immunization with recombinant HBcAg as a result of tolerance of HBcAg-specific CD4 helper T cells [16•].

Multiple studies addressed the possible role of cytokines and their receptors in the immunopathogenic mechanisms of HBV infection. The expression of both interferon-γ and tumor necrosis factor (TNF) receptors is increased on hepatocytes in both acute and chronic hepatitis B [9••]. In patients with hepatitis B e antigen–positive chronic hepatitis, both spontaneous and interleukin-2–induced production of interleukin-6 was increased [17•]. Treatment of duck HBV-transfected cells with interferon-γ inhibited viral replication [18•]. Interleukin-2 also was observed to down-regulate HBV gene-expression in a transgenic mouse strain [19•]. Interleukin-2–induced down-regulation appeared to be mediated by TNF-α. Human transforming growth factor (TGF)-β1 inhibited the production of interferon-γ and anti-HBc by altering the functions of circulating monocytes, B cells and T cells in patients with chronic hepatitis B [20•]. Thus, TGF-β1, known to be produced in the inflamed livers of patients with hepatitis, may modulate the immunologic response to HBV infection.

As noted above, injection of a CD8 CTL clone that secretes interferon-γ in response to hepatitis B surface antigen resulted in hepatocellular necrosis *in vivo* in a transgenic mouse expressing hepatitis B surface antigen [5••,21•]. Administration of interferon-γ to this transgenic strain caused a transient, severe hepatitis. However, hepatitis was absent following interferon-γ injection into nontransgenic mice and was not cytotoxic for hepatocytes positive for hepatitis B surface antigen *in vitro*. Thus, interferon-γ appeared to be involved in an *in vivo* cascade of immunologic events resulting in hepatocyte necrosis. Indeed, pretreatment of the transgenic mice with a monoclonal antibody specific for interferon-γ before injection of the hepatitis B surface antigen–specific CD8 CTL provided protection against hepatocellular necrosis. Overall, studies in this transgenic model indicated that hepatocellular necrosis can be initiated by HBV-specific CTL and that the magnitude of the resulting hepatitis involves cytokine secretion and recruitment of macrophage effector cell functions.

Variation in the HBV genome may also influence the host immune response and promote chronicity. During HBV infection, a spectrum of variants with mutations in the preC/C and preS/S regions can be identified [22•]. One mutation that has been identified with increasing frequency in the preC/C region is a G to A substitution at position nucleotide 1896 (A_{1896}). This produces a stop codon that prematurely terminates translation of protein from the preC region. Because preC is required for synthesis and secretion of hepatitis B e antigen, the A_{1896} mutant strains are hepatitis B e antigen negative. The consequences of hepatitis B e antigen negativity remain controversial. Because hepatitis B e antigen has been hypothesized to suppress and regulate the immune response to hepatitis B c antigen, the absence of hepatitis B e antigen could result in a more exuberant immune response and increased hepatocellular necrosis. Indeed, this has been proposed as an explanation for fulminant hepatic failure in patients with the A_{1896} mutant. However, most infections with hepatitis B e antigen–negative mutants do not result in clinically severe hepatitis. It was also proposed that absence of hepatitis B e antigen production might facilitate chronicity by blunting host immune surveillance.

PreS/S mutations most often involve a glycine substitution at amino acid position 145 of the "a" determinant of hepatitis B surface antigen [22•]. This mutation inhibits the binding of most anti-HBs antibodies. This raises serious concerns about the ability of current vaccines to elicit anti-hepatitis B surface antigen antibodies that are protective against this mutant strain.

Because the CTL response to HBV appears to be polyclonal and specific for multiple HBV antigens [3••], the presence of HBV mutants could significantly alter the effectiveness of the host-immune-response. Alteration of T-cell peptide epitopes could modulate the CTL response against HBV-infected hepatocytes.

Hepatitis C virus

Identification of hepatitis C virus (HCV) genomic sequences and studies of recombinant HCV polypeptides have advanced our understanding of possible immunologic mechanisms of hepatocellular necrosis in hepatitis C. Cytoplasmic expression of HCV proteins has been demonstrated in the livers of infected patients using serum from HCV-infected humans or chimpanzees as sources of antibodies [23•]. A pool of monoclonal antibodies specific for HCV c100 (derived from the NS3/NS4 region of the HCV genome) demonstrated c100 localization in the cytoplasm, but not the surface membrane of hepatocytes [24•]. Intrahepatic expression of c100 was greater during acute HCV infection than during chronic infection. Expression of c100 was associated with viral replication but was not correlated with the degree of hepatic inflammation or necrosis. It remains unclear whether or not other HCV proteins expressed in the membrane of infected hepatocytes may serve as targets for the host humoral response.

During HCV infection, HLA class I molecules are expressed on hepatocytes and the magnitude of expression is associated with the presence of the T-cell inflammatory infiltrates [25•,26•]. A β2 microglobulin epitope recognized by monoclonal antibody HP-1H8 was expressed by hepatocytes during HCV infection but was absent in normal control livers [26•]. During interferon-α treatment, expression of the β2 microglobulin epitope either decreased or disappeared. As in HBV infection, ICAM-1 was also expressed on the surface membranes of hepatocytes [11•]. The magnitude of expression correlated with the presence of inflammatory infiltrates containing CTL and with disease activity.

Hepatic CD8 T cells from infected patients demonstrated HCV-specific CTL activity *in vitro*. Two HLA class I–restricted viral epitopes were identified in the amino terminal portion of the HCV core protein, indicating that this highly conserved region may be a target for HCV-specific CTL responses [27•]. CD8 T cells from the peripheral blood of the same patients revealed no HCV-specific CTL activity. Hepatic CD4 T cell clones, specific for HCV NS4 proteins, were also identified during chronic HCV infection [28••]. These hepatic T cells provided help for polyclonal immunoglobulin A secretion by B cells, indicating that NS4 is immunogenic for intrahepatic CD4 T cells *in vivo*. CD4 T-cell clones derived from the circulation of the same patients provided less helper function for antibody production. Moreover, they possessed a different T-cell receptor (TCR) repertoire than the hepatic clones. Thus, HCV-specific T-cell reactivity appears to be sequestered in the liver.

In a murine model, CD8 CTL activity was demonstrated against 28 amino acids synthetic peptide from the NS5 region [29•]. The immune response was cross reactive with different HCV strains. CD4 T cells from the peripheral blood of patients with HCV infection were shown to proliferate in response to 6 different recombinant HCV polypeptides: C, E1, E2, NS3/NS4, NS4, and NS5 [30•]. A CD4 T-cell response to the HCV core polypeptide appeared to be associated with a benign clinical course. Repeated stimulation of cells in vitro with synthetic core protein resulted in the generation of CD8 CTL responses [31••]. The CTL reacted with target cells synthesizing HCV core protein endogenously and expressing the HLA class I molecule, B44. Antigenic epitopes recognized by the TCR of the CTL were localized between amino acids 81 and 100 of the core protein. The HLA B44-restricted CTL response was detected in three of five patients with chronic hepatitis C and was absent in two controls. HLA class I–restricted CTLs specific for the E1 and NS2 proteins were also identified in the hepatic inflammatory infiltrates of patients with HCV infection [32•]. In contrast, a population of non-HLA-restricted CTLs (possibly TCRγ/δ CTL) was identified in the circulation of patients with chronic hepatitis C [33•].

The accumulating data strongly suggest that HLA-restricted CTL may mediate necrosis of HCV-infected hepatocytes. Further studies are required to determine whether single or multiple viral proteins serve as targets. The observation that chimpanzees convalescent from HCV infection develop recurrent viremia when rechallenged with the same or a different HCV strain raises questions about both the effectiveness and amnestic quality of the CTL response [34••].

The ability of hepatitis viruses to infect host mononuclear inflammatory cells raises the possibility of a direct viral modulation of monocyte and lymphocyte functions. Replication of HCV in circulating mononuclear cells was confirmed by identification of HCV RNA replicative intermediates and incorporation of radiolabeled nucleotides into nascent viral RNA following mitogen stimulation of the mononuclear cells *in vitro* [35•]. A model of *in vitro* HCV infection was established using a human T-cell line and circulating mononuclear cells from a healthy control [35•,36•]. Successful treatment with interferon-α is associated with disappearance of HCV RNA from both infected hepatocytes and circulating mononuclear cells [37•]. This led to the speculation that relapses of hepatitis following interferon-α treatment are due to a failure to eradicate infected mononuclear cells that serve as a reservoir for HCV.

Several observations indicate that HCV infection is capable of stimulating autoimmune responses. In patients with HCV infection, a novel autoantibody, anti-GOR, has been demonstrated [38•]. Furthermore, approximately 25% of patients with chronic HCV infection have low titer antinuclear antibodies or SMA. In addition, HCV infection is clearly associated with essential mixed cryoglobulinemia [39••,40•–42•]. Among patients with mixed cryoglobulinemia, 55% to 90% have been associated with anti-HCV or HCV RNA positivity. Successful interferon treatment of patients with chronic hepatitis C and cryoglobulinemia results in parallel reduction of serum aminotransferases and cryoglobulins [41•]. Although the specific mechanisms involved in cryoglobulin production during HCV-infection remain undefined, the above data suggests that HCV antigens are present within cryoglobulin immune complexes. Alternatively, both molecular mimicry and HCV-induced alterations of autoantigens have been proposed as sources of antigenicity.

There is a high frequency of genetic variation among HCV strains. Two hypervariable regions (HVR1 and HVR2) have been identified in the *N*-terminal region of the putative envelope glycoprotein (gp70) of HCV [43•]. During HCV infection, variation in HVR1 was shown to range from 0.5 to 1.7 amino acid substitutions per month. Successive mutations in HVR1 were associated with antigenic alterations of the encoded proteins, which might escape recognition by preexisting anti-HVR1 antibodies [44•,45•]. Up to 90% of the mutations observed in HVR sequences result in alterations of amino acid sequences [45•]. By regulating the efficiency of the host-humoral response to HCV, mutations may play a major role in establishing chronicity. This mechanism could also explain fluctuations in disease activity.

Hepatocellular carcinoma

New observations were reported indicating a relationship between the development of hepatocellular carcinoma and the immune response. The frequency of antinuclear antibodies was significantly higher in patients with hepatocellular carcinoma than in patients with either chronic hepatitis or cirrhosis (31% vs 13%, respectively) [46•]. Hepatocellular carcinoma was associated with a variety of antinuclear antibody–staining patterns; however, nucleolar reactivity to three distinct peptides involved in ribosomal synthesis predominated. Some patients with chronic liver disease exhibited increasing titers of antinuclear antibodies specific for these antigens or seroconversion to these antigens at the time hepatocellular carcinoma became clinically detectable. In another report, a change in the specificities of the nuclear antigen reactivity of antinuclear antibodies preceded or occurred concurrently with the development of hepatocellular carcinoma [47•]. These findings suggest that malignant transformation is associated with alterations in intranuclear events resulting in immune recognition of nuclear antigens.

Antibodies against the cellular product of the tumor suppressor gene p53 were also found in patients with hepatocellular carcinoma, but were absent in patients with nonmalignant liver diseases [48•]. Of particular note, 23% of a group of patients with α-fetoprotein–negative hepatocellular carcinoma had anti-p53 antibodies.

Phenotypic analysis of tumor-infiltrating lymphocytes in hepatocellular carcinoma revealed a slight predominance of CD4 T cells (CD4:CD8 ratio 1.3:1) and a TCR repertoire that was 95% TCR-α/β and 5% TCR-γ/δ [49]. The proportion of CD45R0 (memory) T cells was significantly greater in tumor-infiltrating lymphocytes than in peripheral blood. Further analysis of the TCR Vβ of the tumor-infiltrating lymphocyte using semiquantitative polymerase chain reaction revealed a restricted repertoire and indicated that the putative antitumor effector cells expressed TCR Vβ3 [50•].

The cytokine TGF–α appears to play an important role in hepatocarcinogenesis [51•]. In a double transgenic mouse model, which coexpressed *c-myc* and TGF–α transgenes, accelerated neoplasia was observed in the liver, suggesting that the two genes acted synergistically [52•]. The addition of TGF–β1 to a mouse hepatoma cell line *in vitro* induced expression messenger RNA of both jun-B and fos-B [53•]. In a rat model of turpentine-induced hepatic inflammation, the development of hepatocellular carcinoma was associated with significantly increased messenger RNA expression of *c-fos*, *c-jun*, and *c-myc* (nuclear protooncogenes) [54•]. It is attractive to speculate that inflammatory cytokines promote the development of hepatocellular carcinoma in this model. In hepatocellular carcinoma occurring in patients with chronic hepatitis B, TGF–α and hepatitis B surface antigen are coexpressed at high levels suggesting viral induction of cytokine production [55•].

Adhesion molecule CD15 was identified on tumor cells in 29% of 56 patients with hepatocellular carcinoma [56]. Intrahepatic metastases occurred more commonly in patients with CD15-positive hepatocellular carcinoma and there was a trend toward increased survival in patients with CD15-negative tumors. It was previously proposed that advanced hepatocellular carcinoma was associated with increased levels of interferon-γ and decreased lymphokine-activated killer cell activity. A recent report of patients with small hepatocellular carcinoma confirmed decreased lymphokine-activated killer cell activity, but there was no correlation with interferon-γ levels [57].

Alcoholic hepatitis

Multiple observations indicate an important role of the immune response in the pathogenesis of alcoholic hepatitis. Two recent studies demonstrated increased serum levels of interleukin-8 in patients with alcoholic hepatitis, which could explain the neutrophilia and infiltration of the hepatic parenchyma with polymorphonuclear leukocytes in this disease [58•,59•].

In alcoholic cirrhotics, T cells secrete significantly increased amounts of cytokines promoting immunoglobulin G and immunoglobulin A secretion [60]. This may explain, in part, the hypergammaglobulinemia in patients with alcoholic cirrhosis.

Biopsies of patients with alcoholic hepatitis contain an increased proportion of CD8 T cells compared with patients with either alcoholic cirrhosis or chronic hepatitis B [61•]. In subsets of patients with alcoholic hepatitis and liver failure, an increased hepatic ratio of CD4:CD8 T cells was observed compared with that in patients with alcoholic hepatitis alone or chronic hepatitis B. CD8 T cells were the only cells observed to have close contact with Mallory's hyaline.

Titers of antibodies reacting to acetaldehyde-albumin adducts were significantly higher in patients with alcoholic hepatitis than in patients with either alcoholic cirrhosis or steatosis [62•]. This observation suggests a pathogenetic role of the humoral immune response in alcoholic liver disease.

Patients with alcoholic hepatitis exhibited increased expression of ICAM-1 on hepatocytes compared with either normal controls or patients with steatosis. ICAM-1 expression was significantly correlated with the degree of hepatocellular injury and the expression of lymphocyte activation factor-1 by infiltrating leukocytes [63•].

References and recommended reading

Papers of particular interest, published within the annual period of review, have been highlighted as:
- • Of special interest
- •• Of outstanding interest

1. •• Missale G, Redeker A, Person J, Fowler P, Guilhot S, Schlicht HJ, Ferrari C, Chisari FV: **HLA-A31 and HLA-Aw68- Restricted Cytotoxic T Cell Response to a Single Hepatitis B Virus Nucleocapsid Epitope During Acute Viral Hepatitis.** *J Exp Med* 1993, 177:751–762.

Cytotoxic T lymphocyte response to epitope 141-151 of HBcAg is polyclonal and restricted by both the HLA-A31 and HLA-Aw68 alleles during acute viral hepatitis.

2. • Bertoletti A, Chisari FV, Penna A, Guilhot S, Galati L, Missale G, Fowler P, Schlight H-J, Vitiello A, Chesnut RC, Fiaccadori F, Ferrari C: **Definition of a Minimal Optimal Cytotoxic T-Cell Epitope Within the Hepatitis B Virus Nucleocapsid Protein.** *J Virol* 1993, 67:2376–2380.

Residues 18-27 of HBcAg contain a peptide-binding motif for HLA-A2, which stimulates CTL responses to endogenously synthesized HBcAg in patients with acute HBV infection.

3. •• Nayersina R, Fowler P, Guilhot S, Missale G, Gerny A, Schlicht H-J, Vitiello A, Chesnut R, Person JL, Redeker AG, Chisari FV: **HLA A2 Restricted Cytotoxic T Lympho-**

cyte Response to Multiple Hepatitis B Surface Antigen Epitopes During Hepatitis B Virus Infection. *J Immunol* 1993, **150**:4659–4671.

The HLA A-2-restricted CTL response to HBsAg is polyclonal and multispecific in most patients with acute hepatitis, but not in patients with chronic hepatitis.

4. • Jung M-C, Schraut W, Santantonio T, Spengler U, Eichenlaub D, Eisenburg J, Zachoval R, Hoffmann R, Paumgartner G, Postore G, Will H, Riethmuller G, Ziegler Heitbrock H-W L, Pape G-R: **Increased Frequency of CD8+ CD45R0+ Memory T Lymphocytes in Acute Hepatitis B Virus Infection.** *J Hepatol* 1993, **18**:295–300.

Increased CD8+ and CD45R0+ memory cell subsets are present during acute hepatitis B infection.

5. •• Chisari F: **The Role of Cytotoxic T Lymphocytes and Inflammatory Cytokines in the Pathogenesis of Acute Viral Hepatitis.** *Gastroenterol Jpn* 1993, **28(Suppl 4)**:2–6.

Presents evidence linking the role of CTL activity and cytokines during HBV infection.

6. • Yamauchi K, Nakamura T, Yonemitsu H, Sekiya H, Katoh J, Obata H: **Possible Role of PreS2 Peptides Presented by MHC Class I Antigen in the Pathgenesis of Chronic Hepatitis B.** *J Hepatology* 1993, **17 (Suppl 3)**:S6–S9.

In HBV infection, HLA class I presentation of certain PreS2 peptides is associated with high serum ALT levels.

7. • Missale G, Brems JJ, Takiff H, Pockros P, Chisari F: **Human Leukocyte Antigen Class I-Independent Pathways May Contribute to Hepatitis B Virus-Induced Liver Disease After Liver Transplantation.** *Hepatology* 1993, **18**:491–496.

Reports the presence of a HLA class I-independent T-cell immune response in a patient who received a HLA class I mismatched liver.

8. • Shu P-Y, Chang C, Hwang L-H, Hu C-P: **Proliferative and Cytotoxic T-Cell Clones Recognize Endogenously Synthesized HBcAg in an Asymptomatic HBsAg Carrier.** *Hepatology* 1993, **18**:275–283.

Describes successful transformation of lymphoblastoid cells with HBV core gene, and the cloning HBcAg-specific CD4+ and CD8+ cells, indicating that both a HLA class I and II-restricted immune response may play role in HBV clearance.

9. •• Volpes R, van den Oord JJ, Desmet VJ: **Can Hepatocytes Serve as "Activated" Immunodulating Cells in the Immune Response?** *J Hepatol* 1992, **16**:228–240.

Discusses the role of hepatocytes as "accessory" cells in both the afferent and efferent limbs of the cell-mediated immune response.

10. •• Barnaba V, Balsano F: **Immunological and Molecular Basis of Viral Persistence. The Hepatitis B Virus Model.** *J Hepatol* 1992, **14**:391–400.

Reviews the possible mechanisms of persistent HBV infection, including clonal anergy, viral escape, and immunosuppression.

11. • Horiike N, Onji M, Kumon I, Kanaoka M, Michitaka K, Ohta Y: **Intercellular Adhesion Molecule-1 Expression of the Hepatocyte Membrane of Patients With Chronic Hepatitis B and C.** *Liver* 1993, **13**:10–14.

Evidence that the degree of intrahepatic ICAM-1 expression is associated with increased ALT level, CTL infiltration, and focal necrosis during hepatitis B and C. Interferon-αtherapy reduces intrahepatic expression of ICAM-1 in some patients with chronic hepatitis B.

12. • Garcia-Monzon C, Garcia-Buey L, Garcia-Sanchez A, Pajares JM, Moreno-Otero R: **Down-Regulation of Intercellular Adhesion Molecule 1 on Hepatocytes in Viral Chronic Hepatitis Treated With Interferon Alfa-2b.** *Gastroenterology* 1993, **105**:462–469.

In patients responsive to interferon α-2b therapy, decreased intrahepatic expression of ICAM-1, but not LFA3, was observed.

13. • Hu K-Q, Yu C-H, Vierling JM: **Up-Regulation of Intercellular Adhesion Molecule 1 Transcription by Hepatitis B Virus X Protein.** *Proc Natl Acad Sci U S A* 1992, **89**:11441–11445.

Hepatitis B virus X protein directly regulates expression of ICAM-1 in HBV subgenomic transformed hepatoma cell lines in the absence of any cytokine. This article also discusses the possible relationship between clonal anergy and chronic HBV infection.

14. • Maruyama T, Iino S, Koike K, Yasuda K, Milich DR: **Serology of Acute Exacerbation in Chronic Hepatitis B Virus Infection.** *Gastroenterology* 1993, **105**:1141–1151.

Studies the correlation between increasing level of serum HBV DNA, hepatitis B e antigen, hepatitis B e antigen-specific immune complexes and Liver Injury.

15. • Akbar SMF, Onji M, Inaba K, Yamamura K-I, Ohta Y: **Los Responsiveness of Hepatitis B Virus-Transgenic Mice in Antibody Response to T-Cell Dependent Antigen: Defect in Antigen-Presenting Activity of Dendritic Cells.** *Immunology* 1993, **78**:468–475.

Description of an HBV transgenic mouse model showing that a defect in APC cells, rather than T or B cells, results in a lower antigen-specific antibody response.

16. • Takashima H, Araki K, Miyazaki J, Yamamura K, Kimoto M: **Characterization of T- Cell Tolerance to Hepatitis B Virus (HBV) Antigen in Transgenic Mice.** *Immunology* 1992, **75**:398–405.

Hepatitis B virus transgenic mouse model showing that a low anti-HBc response is due to helper T-cell tolerance specific for HBcAg.

17. • Kakumu S, Shinagawa T, Ishikawa T, Yoshioka K, Wakita T, Ida N: **Interleukin 6 Production by Peripheral Blood Mononuclear Cells in Patients With Chronic Hepatitis B Virus Infection and Primary Biliary Cirrhosis.** *Gastroenterol Jpn* 1993, **28**:18–24.

Evidence of spontaneous and interleukin-2 induced production of interleukin-6 increases significantly in patients with hepatitis B e antigen–positive chronic hepatitis.

18. • Lavine JE, Ganem D: **Inhibition of Duck Hepatitis B Virus Replication by Interferon-γ.** *J Med Virol* 1993, **40**:59–64.

Treatment of a DHBV transfected human hepatocellular carcinoma cell line with interferon-γ results in inhibition of DHBV replication.

19. • Guilhot S, Guidotti LG, Chisari FV: **Interleukin-2-Down Regulates Hepatitis B Virus Gene Expression in Transgenic Mice by a Post-Transcriptional Mechanism.** *J Virol* 1993, **67**:7444–7449.

In an HBV transgenic mouse model, TNF-α mediates interleukin-2 down-regulation of the HBV messenger RNA.

20. • Kakumu S, Ito Y, Takayanagi M, Yoshioka K, Wakita T, Ishikawa T, Higashi Y, Yang Z-Q: **Effect of Recombinant Human Transforming Growth Factor β1 on Immune Responses in Patients With Chronic Hepatitis B** *Liver* 1993, **13**:62–68.

Treatment of PMBC with human TGF-β1 inhibits both antigen-dependent and independent immune responses in patients with chronic hepatitis B.

21. • Gilles PN, Guerrette DL, Ulevitch RJ, Schreiber RD, Chisari F: **HBsAg Retention Sensitizes the Hepatocytes to Injury by Physiological Concentrations of Interferon-γ.** *Hepatology* 1992, **16**:655–663.

Report that recombinant interferon-γ cytotoxic for the HBsAg-positive hepatocytes in HBV envelope gene transgenic mice.

22. • Garman W, Thomas H, Domingo E: **Viral Genetic Variation: Hepatitis B Virus as a Clinical Example.** *Lancet* 1993, **341**:349–353.

Reviews current advances in HBV genetic variation and its clinical significance.

23. • Krawczynski K, Beach M, Bradley DW, Kuo G, DiBisceglie AM, Houghton M, Reyes GR, Kim JP, Choo Q-L, Alter MJ: **Hepatitis C Virus Antigen in Hepatocytes: Immunomorphological Detection and Identification.** *Gastroenterology* 1992, **103**:622–629.

Hepatitis C virus antigen can be localized in the cytoplasm of hepatocytes during acute and chronic HCV infection.

24. • Sansonno D, Dammacco F: **Hepatitis C Virus c1070 Antigen in Liver Tissue From Patients With Acute and Chronic Infection.** *Hepatology* 1993, **18**:240–245.

Hepatitis C virus c100-related antigens were localized in the cytoplasm, but not the membrane of hepatocytes, and their expression was related to viral replication.

25. Onji M, Kikuchi T, Kumon I, Masumoto T, Nadano S, Kajino
• K, Horilike N, Ohata Y: **Identification of Intrahepatic Lymphocyte Subpopulations and HLA Class I Expression of Hepatocytes in Patients With Chronic Hepatitis Type C.** *Hepato-Gastroenterology* 1992, **39**:340–343.

Demonstrates a HLA class I expression on hepatocytes and intrahepatic infiltration predominantly of CD8 T cells in patients with chronic hepatitis C.

26. Garcia-Buey L, Lopez-Botet M, Garcia-Sanchez A, Balboa M,
• Aramburu J, Garcia-Monzon C, Acevedo A, Moreno-Otero R: **Variability in the Expression of a β2-Microglobulin Epitope on Hepatocytes in Chronic Type C Hepatitis on Treatment With Interferon.** *Hepatology* 1993, **17**:372–382.

Evidence that a β2-microglobulin epitope is increasingly expressed on hepatocytes of patients with chronic hepatitis C and is down-regulated with an interferon therapy.

27. Koziel MJ, Dudley D, Afahal N, Choo Q-L, Houghton M,
• Palston R, Walker B: **Hepatitis C Virus (HCV)-Specific Cytotoxic T Lymphocytes Recognize Epitopes in the Core and Envelope Proteins of HCV.** *J Virol* 1993, **67**:7522–7532.

Demonstrates that liver-derived, but not PBMC-derived, CD8+ lymphocytes proliferate in response to HCV envelope and core proteins in an HLA class-I restricted manner.

28. Munutello MA, Pileri Piero, Unutmaz D, Censini S, Kuo G,
•• Houghton M, Brunetto MR, Bonino F, Abrignani S: **Compartmentalization of T Lymphocytes to the Site of Disease: Intraheptic CD4 T Cells Specific for the Protein NS4 of Hepatitis C Virus in Patients With Chronic Hepatitis C.** *J Exp Med* 1993, **178**:17–25.

Stimulation of T cells isolated from liver biopsies, but not PBMC, with HCV proteins results in the proliferation of NS4-specific CD4+ T cells, indicating a preferential intrahepatic localization of these T cells.

29. Shirai M, Akatsuka T, Pendleton CD, Houghten R,
• Wychowski C, Mihalik K, Feinstone S, Berzofsky JA: **Induction of Cytotoxic T Cells to a Cross-Reactive Epitope in the Hepatitis C Virus Nonstructural RNA Polymerase-Like Protein.** *J Virol* 1992, **66**:4098–4106.

Evidence that CD8+ CTL recognize an epitope from an RNA polymerase-like protein of HCV in association with a MHC class I molecule.

30. Botarelli P, Brunetto MR, Minutello MA, Calvo P, Unutmaz
• D, Weiner AJ, Choo Q-L, Shuster JR, Kuo G, Bonino F, Houghton M, Abrignani S: **T-Lymphocyte Response to Hepatitis C Virus in Different Clinical Courses of Infection.** *Gastroenterology* 1993, **104**:580–587.

Report that 65% of HCV-positive individuals have T-cell responses to different HCV viral proteins.

31. Kita H, Moriyama T, Kaneko T, Harase I, Nomura M,
•• Miura H, Nakamura I, Yazaki Y, Imawari M: **HLA B44-Restricted Cytotoxic T Lymphocytes Recognizing an Epitope on Hepatitis C Virus Nucleocapsid Protein.** *Hepatology* 1993, **18**:1039–1044.

Cytotoxic T lymphocyte specific for HCV nucleocapsid proteins, restricted by the HLA class I molecule B44, could be generated from PBMC in patients with chronic HCV infection.

32. Koziel MJ, Dudley D, Wong JT, Dienstag J, Houghton M,
• Ralston R, Walker BD: **Intrahepatic Cytotoxic T Lymphocytes Specific for Hepatitis C Virus in Persons With Chronic Hepatitis.** *J Immunol* 1992, **149**:3339–3344.

Hepatitis C virus–specific, HLA class I-restricted CTL react specifically to the epitopes of variable regions of either envelope or nonstructural proteins.

33. Schupper H, Hayashi P, Scheffel J, Aceituno S, Paglieroni
• T, Holland PV, Zeldis JB: **Peripheral-Blood Mononuclear Cell Responses to Recombinant Hepatitis C Virus Antigens in Patients With Chronic Hepatitis C.** *Hepatology* 1993, **18**:1055–1060.

The number of non-HLA–restricted CTL are increased in PBMC in patients with chronic HCV infection.

34. Farci P, Alter HJ, Govindarajan S, Wong DC, Engle R,
•• Lesniewski RR, Mushahwar IK, Desai SM, Miller RH, Ogata N, Purcell RH: **Lack of Protective Immunity Against Reinfection With Hepatitis C Virus.** *Science* 1992, **258**:135–140.

Report that the rechallenge of convalescent chimpanzee with the same or different HCV strain results in the reappearance of viremia, indicating that HCV infection does not elicit protective immunity.

35. Müller HM, Pfaff E, Goeser T, Kallinowski B, Solbach C,
• Theilmann L: **Peripheral Blood Leukocytes Serve as a Possible Extrahepatic Site for Hepatitis C Virus Replication.** *J Gen Virol* 1993, **74**:669–676.

Replicative intermediates of HCV RNA are present in liver and PBML, but not serum. Furthermore, PBML isolates could be infected in vitro by HCV-containing serum.

36. Shimizu YK, Iwamoto A, Hijikata M, Purcell RH, Yoshikura
• H: **Evidence for In Vitro Replication of Hepatitis C Virus Genome in a Human T-Cell Line.** *Proc Natl Acad Sci U S A* 1992, **89**:5477–5481.

Inoculation of a human T-cell line with HCV-containing serum results in infection and replication of the virus.

37. Gil B, Qian C, Riezu-Boj JI, Civeira MP, Prieto J: **Hepatic**
• **and Extrahepatic HCV RNA Strands in Chronic Hepatitis C: Different Patterns of Response to Interferon Treatment.** *Hepatology* 1993, **18**:1050–1054.

Report that replicative intermediates of HCV RNA are present not only in serum and liver, but also in lymphoid cells in patients with chronic HCV infection and that disappearance of the HCV RNA genome from liver and mononuclear cells may predict complete response without post-therapy relapse.

38. Michel G, Ritter A, Gerken G, Meyer zum Buschenfelde KH,
• Decker R, Manns MP: **Anti-GOR and Hepatitis C Virus in Autoimmune Liver Diseases.** *Lancet* 1992, **339**:267–269.

Description of the production of the anti-GOR in association with hepatitis C infection and evidence of its insignificance in relationship to clinical, histologic, or therapeutic aspects of hepatitis C infection.

39. Ferri C, Civita LA, Longombardo G, Greco F, Bombardieri S:
•• **Hepatitis C Virus and Mixed Cryoglobulinemia.** *Eur J Clin Invest* 1993, **23**:399–405.

Review of knowledge of the association of HCV infection and mixed cryoglobulinemia.

40. Misiani R, Bellavita P, Fenili D, Borelli B, Marchesi D, Mas-
• sazza M, Vendramin G, Comotti B, Tanzi E, Schudeller G, Zanetti A: **Hepatitis C Virus Infection in Patients With Essential Mixed Cryoglobulinemia.** *Ann Intern Med* 1992, **117**:573–577.

Describes the high prevalence of anti-HCV antibodies in patients with essential mixed cryoglobulinemia.

41. Marcellin P, Descamps V, Martinot-Peignoux M, Larzul D,
• Xu L, Boyer N, Pham B-N, Crick B, Guillevin L, Belaich S, Erlinger S, Benhamou J-P: **Cryoglobulinemia With Vasculitis Associated With Hepatitis C Virus Infection.** *Gastroenterology* 1993, **104**:272–277.

Describes a direct relationship between cryocrit levels and serum aminotransferases in patients with mixed cryoglobulinemia and hepatitis C who were treated with α-interferon.

42. Agnello V, Chung RT, Kaplan LM: **A Role for Hepatitis C**
• **Virus Infection in Type II Cryoglobulinemia.** *N Engl J Med* 1992, **19**:1490–1495.

Type II cryoglobulinemia is strongly associated with concomitant HCV infection as evidenced by the high prevalence of anti-HCV and HCV RNA in these patients.

43. Kato N, Sekiya H, Ootsuyama Y, Nakazawa T, Hijikata
• M, Ohkoshi S, Shimotohno K: **Humoral Immune Response to Hypervariable Region 1 of the Putative Envelope Glycoprotein (gp70) of Hepatitis C Virus.** *J Virology* 1993, **67**:3923–3930.

Evidence that HVR1 of HCV contains a sequence-specific epitope that induces a strain-specific antibody response. Mutation in this region may result in immune escape and persistent viral infection.

44. Taniguchi S, Okamoto H, Sakamoto M, Kojima M, Tsuda F,
• Tanaka T, Munekata E, Muchmore EE, Peterson DA, Mishiro S: **A Structurally Flexible and Antigenically Variable N-Terminal Domain of the Hepatitis C Virus E2/NS1 Protein:**

Implication for an Escape From Antibody. *Virology* 1993, **195**:297–301.

The hypervariable region of the HCV envelope region appears to be structurally flexible and antigenically variable, providing a potential mechanism for the virus to escape host immunity.

45. • Kurosaki M, Enomoto N, Marumo F, Sato C: **Rapid Sequence Variation of the Hypervariable Region of Hepatitis C Virus During the Course of Chronic Infection.** *Hepatology* 1993, **18**:1293–1299.

Report that rapid sequence variation in hypervariable region of the predominant virus population takes place during chronic HCV infection.

46. • Imai H, Ochs R, Kiyosawa K, Furata S, Nakamura R, Tan E: **Nucleolar Antigens and Autoantibodies in Hepatocellular Carcinoma and Other Malignancies.** *Am J Pathol* 1992, **140**:859–870.

Evidence linking the presence of a nucleolar pattern of antinuclear antibodies and a change in antinuclear antibodies titers and specificities to the development of hepatocellular carcinoma in cirrhotic patients.

47. • Imai H, Nakano Y, Kiyosawa K, Tan EM: **Increasing Titers and Changing Specificities of Antinuclear Antibodies in Patients With Chronic Liver Disease Who Develop Hepatocellular Carcinoma.** *Cancer* 1993, **71**:26–35.

Evidence linking the presence of a nucleolar pattern of antinuclear antibodies and a change in antinuclear antibodies titers and specificities to the development of hepatocellular in cirrhotic patients.

48. • Volkmann M, Muller M, Hofmann WJ, Meyer M, Hagelstein J, Rath U, Kommerell B, Zentgraf H, Galle PR: **The Humoral Immune Response to p53 in Patients With Hepatocellular Carcinoma is Specific for Malignancy and Independent of the Alpha-Fetoprotein Status.** *Hepatology* 1993, **18**:559–565.

Characterizes a subgroup of small α-fetaprotein–negative hepatocellular carcinoma in whom antibodies to the cellular product of the oncogene p53 are found.

49. Shimizu Y, Watanabe A, Whiteside TL: **Memory T-Lymphocytes are the Main Population of Tumor-Infiltrating Lymphocytes Obtained From Human Primary Liver Tumors.** *J Hepatol* 1992, **16**:197–202.

50. • Weidmann E, Whiteside TL, Giorda R, Herberman RB, Trucco M: **The T-Cell Receptor VB Gene Usage in Tumor-Infiltrating Lymphocytes and Blood of Patients With Hepatocellular Carcinoma.** *Cancer Res* 1992, **52**:5913–5920.

Evidence that T lymphocytes in patients with hepatocellular carcinoma may have restricted immunologic reactivity.

51. • Bernuau D, Moreau A, Tournier I, Legres L, Feldmann G: **Activation of Nuclear Protooncogenes and Alpha-Fetoprotein Gene in Rat Liver During the Acute Inflammatory Reaction.** *Liver* 1993, **13**:102–109.

Evidence that serum cytokines in the inflammatory response may be important triggers for oncogene expression and the development of hepatocellular carcinoma.

53. • Collier JD, Guo K, Gullick WJ, Bassendine MF, Burt AD: **Expression of Transforming Growth Factor Alpha in Human Hepatocellular Carcinoma.** *Liver* 1993, **13**:151–155.

Evidence that serum cytokines in the inflammatory response may be important triggers for oncogene expression and the development of hepatocellular carcinoma.

53. • Murukami H, Sanderson ND, Nagy P, Marino PA, Merlino G, Thorgeirsson SS: **Transgenic Mouse Model for Synergistic Effects of Nuclear Oncogenes and Growth Factors in Tumorigenesis: Interaction of C-myc and Transforming Growth Factor a in Hepatic Oncogenesis.** *Cancer Res* 1993, **53**:1719–1723.

Evidence that serum cytokines in the inflammatory response may be important triggers for oncogene expression and the development of hepatocellular carcinoma.

54. • Beauchamp RD, Sheng H-M, Ishizuka J, Townsend CM, Thompson JC: **Transforming Growth Factor (TGF)-b Stimulates Hepatic jun-B Protooncogenes and Decreases Albumin mRNA.** *Ann Surg* 1992, **216**:300–308.

Evidence that serum cytokines in the inflammatory response may be important triggers for oncogene expression and the development of hepatocellular carcinoma.

55. • Hsia CC, Axiotis CA, DiBisceglie AM, Tabor E: **Transforming Growth Factor-Alpha in Human Hepatocellular Carcinoma and Coexpression With Hepatitis B Surface Antigen in Adjacent Liver.** *Cancer* 1992, **70**:1049–1056.

Evidence that serum cytokines in the inflammatory response may be important triggers for oncogene expression and the development of hepatocellular carcinoma.

56. Torii A, Nakayama A, Harada A, Nakao A, Nonami T, Sakamoto J, Watanabe T, Ito M, Takagi H: **Expression of the CD15 Antigen in Hepatocellular Carcinoma.** *Cancer* 1993, **71**:3864–3867.

57. Saibara T, Maeda T, Miyazaki M, Onishi S, Yamamoto Y: **Assessment of Lymphokine-Activated Killer Activity and Gamma-Interferon Production in Patients With Small Hepatocellular Carcinomas.** *Hepatology* 1993, **17**:781–787.

58. • Sheron N, Bird G, Koskinas J, Portmann B, Ceska M, Lindley I, Williams R: **Circulating and Tissue Levels of the Neutrophil Chemotaxin Interleukin-8 are Elevated in Severe Acute Alcoholic Hepatitis and Tissue Levels Correlate With Neutrophil Infiltration.** *Hepatology* 1993, **18**:41–46.

Links elevated interleukin-8 levels with alcoholic hepatitis.

59. • Hill DB, Marsano LS, McClai CJ: **Increased Plasma Interleukin 8 Concentrations in Alcoholic Hepatitis.** *Hepatology* 1993, **18**:576–580.

Links elevated interleukin-8 levels with alcoholic hepatitis.

60. Giron JA, Alvarez-Mon M, Menendez-Caro JL, Abreu L, Albillos A, Manzano L, Durantez A: **Increased Spontaneous and Lymphokine-Conditioned IgA and IgG Synthesis by B Cells From Alcoholic Cirrhotic Patients.** *Hepatology* 1992, **16**:664–670.

61. • Sakai Y, Izumi N, Marumo F, Sato C: **Quantitative Immunohistochemical Analysis of Lymphocyte Subsets in Alcoholic Liver Disease.** *J Gastroenterol Hepatol* 1993, **8**:39–43.

Advances in understanding of a link between the immune response and alcoholic hepatitis.

62. • Teare JP, Carmichael AJ, Burnett FR, Rake MO: **Detection of Antibodies to Acetaldehyde-Albumin Conjugates in Alcoholic Liver Disease.** *Alcohol Alcohol* 1993, **28**:11–16.

Advances in understanding of a link between the immune response and alcoholic hepatitis.

63. • Burra P, Hubscher SG, Shaw J, Elias E, Adams DH: **Is the Intercellular Adhesion Molecule-1/Leukocyte Function Associated Antigen 1 Pathway of Leukocyte Adhesion Involved in the Tissue Damage of Alcoholic Hepatitis?** *Gut* 1992, **33**:268–271.

Advances in understanding of a link between the immune response and alcoholic hepatitis.

John M. Vierling, MD, Hepatology Program, Suite 7511, Cedars-Sinai Medical Center, 8700 Beverly Boulevard, Los Angeles, CA 90048, USA.

Cytokine involvement in the liver

Minhhuyen T. Nguyen, MD, Steven K. Herrine, MD, and Mark A. Zern, MD

Thomas Jefferson University Hospital, Philadelphia, Pennsylvania, USA

An ever-enlarging portion of hepatology research falls under the rubric of molecular biology. Thus, an attempt to summarize all molecular biology studies of liver disease in the past year is less than satisfying. One topic of particular significance relevant to molecular biology during the past year is the study of cytokines. Examples of these studies include: 1) the use of transgenic mouse models and other methodologies to study the effects of growth factors, especially transforming growth factor-α in liver regeneration and oncogenesis, 2) progress in studying the interactions between nonparenchymal cells and growth factors in liver processes, and 3) elucidation of the roles transforming growth factor-β and platelet-derived growth factor play in hepatic fibrogenesis.

Current Opinion in Gastroenterology 1994, **10**:277–284

Over the past decade, a wealth of evidence has accumulated regarding the roles played by various cytokines in hepatic regeneration, carcinogenesis, and fibrogenesis. Cytokines are a group of proteins with autocrine, paracrine, and endocrine activities, which function to provide communication among hepatic cells. Active in minute quantities, cytokines activate and regulate homeostasis and cellular repair through effects on cell growth, differentiation, and receptor expression. In this article, we have chosen for review the most recent advances on a few cytokines that are crucial in the abovementioned liver processes.

Hepatic regeneration

Liver regeneration is a precisely regulated sequence of events that begins at the time of injury or volume loss and ends when the original volume is restored. Hepatocyte growth factor (HGF) as well as transforming growth factor (TGF)-α and TGF-β are the three major cytokines involved in this process.

Hepatocyte growth factor

Hepatocyte growth factor is a pleiotropic mesenchyme-derived growth factor [1••], that was originally isolated and purified from the serum of partially hepatectomized rats and rat platelets. Its mature form is a heterodimer that is composed of a heavy 69-kD α-subunit and a light 34-kD β-subunit. The α-subunit contains four kringle domains and shares structural similarities with plasminogen and other coagulation-related proteins. The β-subunit shares consensus sequence with serine proteases; however, it has no known proteolytic activity. The mature form of HGF is synthesized from a single-chain, 728-amino acid precursor. Another precursor with a few amino acid deletions has been found to be functional [2••]. Both human and rat complementary DNAs of HGF have been cloned and sequenced. The amino acid sequences of human and rat HGFs are more than 90% identical; hence, HGF has no species specificity with regard to biologic activity. The human HGF gene has been localized to chromosome 7 and found to consist of 18 exons interrupted with 17 introns [1••].

Hepatocyte growth factor is the most potent mitogen for cultured hepatocytes, being 100-fold more active than TGF-α or epidermal growth factor (EGF) [1••]. Over the past several years, an increasing body of evidence suggests that HGF may be one of the elusive initiators that trigger hepatic regeneration in the event of liver volume loss or injury with or without inflammation.

Hepatocyte growth factor messenger RNA levels were found to increase rapidly in plasma prior to hepatocyte DNA synthesis in rat models of partial hepatectomy and liver injury caused by carbon tetrachloride administration [3•,4]. In liver ischemia or crush injury, the amount of HGF increase is proportional to the degree of the injury [3•]. HGF expression appears to occur solely in nonparenchymal cells and thus, the peptide appears to stimulate hepatic regeneration, proliferation

Abbreviations

EGF—epidermal growth factor; **HGF**—hepatocyte growth factor; **PDGF**—platelet-derived growth factor; **TGF**—transforming growth factor.

 ISBN 1-85922-608-6 ISSN 0267–1379

and differentiation via a paracrine mechanism [3•,5•]. In her experiments, Maher [2••] showed that in normal liver, HGF and its transcripts can be found in abundance in lipocytes (or Ito cells), with smaller amounts also present in endothelial and Kupffer cells. In the regenerating liver, however, HGF expression is found almost exclusively in the endothelial cells. No change was observed in Ito cells, Kupffer cells, or hepatocytes [2••]. HGF exerts its mitogenic and morphogenic effects mainly on hepatocytes, biliary epithelial cells and certain other epithelial cells, of varying differentiation potentials [6••,7••], but has no effects on Ito cells or endothelial cells [2••].

Hepatocyte growth factor is not only produced locally in the liver, but also in other organs such as lungs and kidneys, especially in the event of liver injury. Therefore, its mechanisms of action may not only be paracrine but also endocrine. Matsumoto *et al.* [8] recently showed evidence for the existence of a humoral factor, so-called injurin, that stimulates HGF expression in rat intact lung following either partial hepatectomy or unilateral nephrectomy. Injurin was purified from CCl_4-treated rat sera and found to be a heat- and acid-stable protein with a molecular weight of 10 to 20 kD. The mechanism by which this protein induces the expression of HGF remains unclear. Ishiki *et al.* [9••] showed that exogenous recombinant human HGF stimulates growth of mouse hepatocytes in several different models of liver injury (CCl_4 and α-naphthylisothiocyanate) and during partial hepatectomy. HGF also prevents marked rises in serum levels of liver enzymes and bilirubin. Because of this *in vivo* protective effect against hepatotoxins, it is suggested that HGF may become clinically useful in the future [9••].

In another experiment to illustrate the complex nature of the role HGF plays in liver regeneration, Tomiya *et al.* [10•] showed that serum levels of HGF in both hepatectomized and nonhepatectomized surgical patients appear to correlate more with liver cirrhosis, serum bilirubin, and peripheral white blood cell counts, than with the liver regeneration process. They concluded that the damaged liver fails to clear HGF or HGF is released from inflammatory cells, resulting in high circulating serum levels. In other words, they suggested that HGF has no direct role in liver regeneration at all. Lindroos *et al.* [4] and Michalopoulous and Zarnegar [11], on the other hand, indicated that the same rapid accumulation of serum HGF as a result of impaired hepatic clearance may actually be the mechanism by which this peptide triggers liver regeneration. In addition, an increase in norepinephrine level, which occurs with the stress of surgery, appears to decrease HGF clearance *in vivo*, and this hormone is known to augment HGF effects on cultured hepatocytes [1••,4,11].

Recent research has further elucidated the nature of the HGF receptor. The receptor is the product of the *c-met* protooncogene, which when transfected into NIH 3T3 fibroblasts, confers to the cells motogenic and invasive responses to HGF [12•]. The HGF receptor belongs to the protein tyrosine kinase receptor family, and in the liver is found mainly in hepatocytes. The receptor is a 190-kD heterodimer (hence the name *p190met*) of a heavily glycosylated and extracellular α-subunit and a membrane-spanning β-subunit. Intracellular transducers include phosphatidylinositol-3 kinase, GTPase-activating protein, phospholipase *C*-gamma, and cytoplasmic *src*-like kinases [13]. Higuchi *et al.* [14] showed that rapid down-regulation of the HGF receptors after liver injury and preceding DNA synthesis suggests that HGF is rapidly supplied to the injured liver, and is quickly internalized after its binding to the receptor. The mechanism of the interaction of HGF and its receptor may be further understood now that a competitive antagonist of HGF has been characterized [15•].

Transforming growth factor-α

Transforming growth factor-α is a secreted 50–amino acid polypeptide with potent mitogenic activity. It is a member of the EGF superfamily of proteins, sharing 30% to 40% sequence homology with EGF. TGF-α is produced by many normal and transformed cell types. In a normal human liver, TGF-α is produced mainly by bile duct epithelial cells [16•] and perivenular hepatocytes [17•]. Mature TGF-α is cleaved from a larger precursor that consists of 160 amino acids and is anchored in the cell membrane. This pro-TGF-α can bind to receptors of neighboring cells and participate in cellular adhesion and proliferation. The TGF-α/EGF receptor is a 170-kD cell-surface protein that, like the HGF receptor, activates tyrosine kinase. It also is the cellular homologue of an oncogene, in this case, *v-erb*B [18••].

In the process of hepatic regeneration, TGF-α is thought to be effective in the G1 phase of the cell replication cycle [19•]. In an experiment done by Burr *et al.* [17•], a new immunohistochemical technique using two antibodies, a polyclonal antibody (26T) against a portion of the C-terminal of the mature rat protein, and a monoclonal (Ab-2) antibody against the recombinant human protein, demonstrated a significant increase in the amount of TGF-α produced by regenerating hepatocytes and in the number of cells making it. These changes immediately precede the wave of DNA synthesis. Therefore, TGF-α seems to stimulate hepatocyte proliferation via an autocrine mechanism [17•]. Tomiya and Fujwara [20•] found that unlike HGF, serum levels of TGF-α appear to correlate closely with the resected volumes and with the regenerated volumes of the liver in patients undergoing partial hepatectomy. In patients with nonhepatic surgery, TGF-α levels do not increase at all [20•]. Thus, HGF may initiate the regeneration process, but TGF-α appears to directly promote further proliferation and differentiation.

In cirrhotic rats, damaged hepatocytes are unable to produce sufficient amount of TGF-α for liver regeneration after partial hepatectomy. Exogenous TGF-α given in these animals results in an increase in hepatic DNA synthesis [21]. In culture, TGF-α is more effective than EGF in stimulating hepatocyte proliferation. There is also an increase in TGF-α/EGF receptors coinciding with increased TGF-α transcripts, and a decrease in the number of these receptors shortly afterward [22]. This down-regulation of the EGF receptor is thought to be a protective mechanism in regenerating cells.

Transforming growth factor-β

The term *TGF-β* represents a growing group of closely related molecules (*eg*, β_1, β_2, and β_3) that constitute the TGF-β superfamily. Only TGF-β_1, β_2, and β_3 have been found in liver tissue. This group of growth factors spans a broad range of biologic activity, including fibrogenesis, angiogenesis, hematopoiesis, morphogenesis, and cell proliferation [23]. Almost all studies in the liver are restricted to the effects of TGF-β_1. In the liver, TGF-β_1 is found mainly in nonparenchymal cells. In the event of liver injury, Ito cells produce high levels of TGF-β_1 transcripts [24••]. Most cells produce the latent form of TGF-β_1, which is then presumed to be activated extracellularly or at the surface of the targeted cells [23]. Hepatocytes express the TGF-β receptors but other cells appear to be the primary source of the cytokine, suggesting a paracrine mechanism of interaction [23,25]. Beauchamp *et al.* [26•] suggest that in hepatocytes, TGF-β may exert its influence by activating other genes. In their experiments, they demonstrated that TGF-β induces oncogenes *jun*-B and *fos*-B, which in turn, decrease albumin synthesis. Earlier studies have not shown this decrease, however [27].

Unlike HGF and TGF-α, TGF-β_1 serves to inhibit unrestrained hepatocyte proliferation and is thought to be involved in the down-regulation of liver regeneration. In the CCl_4 rat model of liver injury, Armendariz-Borunda *et al.* [24••] showed that DNA synthesis, which peaks at 36 hours following the insult, precedes the enhanced accumulation of TGF-β_1 transcript and protein, which peaks at 48 hours. In addition, they found that exogenously added TGF-β_1 inhibits hepatic DNA synthesis and that in the presence of TGF-β_1 antibodies, hepatic proliferation continues at its normal pace. DeJuan *et al.* [28•] have shown that TGF-β_1 inhibits EGF-dependent DNA synthesis in both fetal and regenerating hepatocytes in culture. TGF-β_1 action is partially suppressed by norepinephrine only in regenerating hepatocytes, and TGF-β_1 and dexamethasone exert synergistic inhibitory effects only on fetal liver cells. Hence, there are differences between fetal and regenerating hepatocytes in their response to various growth factors and hormones [28•].

In experiments that examine the interplay among the growth factors discussed thus far, Masuhara *et al.* [29•] discovered that different models of hepatic injury may involve differential expression of these growth factors. For instance, the choline-deficient diet in the rat model resulting in liver necrosis showed gradual increase in the serum levels of all three growth factors, HGF, TGF-α, and TGF-β. On the other hand, a nonnecrosis model with hypolipidemic peroxisome proliferator showed an increase in TGF-α levels but a decrease in HGF and TGF-β levels. TGF-β blocks TGF-α stimulation of cultured hepatocytes when added simultaneously, or a day later [24••].

Hepatic carcinogenesis

The development of a cancer is a multistep event that results in the loss of normal inhibitions upon cellular growth and mobility. These steps may involve activation of protooncogenes, loss of tumor suppression genes, and increased production of certain growth factors.

Hepatic growth factor

Because of the mitogenic and motogenic effects that HGF has on regenerating hepatocytes, one would expect to find that this growth factor would be more likely than not to promote unrestrained hepatocyte proliferation, *ie*, tumorigenesis. Cooper [13] demonstrated in his experiments that transfecting *met* oncogene (HGF receptor) into the NIH 3T3 fibroblasts, which produce HGF, leads to cellular proliferation and transformation via a possible autocrine loop. Thus, it is surprising that HGF is identical to a tumor cytotoxic factor isolated from human fibroblast, IMR-90 cells [30]. Further evidence has established that HGF is a negative growth regulator for hepatocellular carcinoma cells, although it is a growth stimulator in normal hepatocytes as shown in transgenic AlbHGF mice [31]. Furthermore, only six of 35 tumor cell lines are found to express HGF, and no hepatocellular carcinoma cell line does.

Transforming growth factor-α

With the advent of transgenic mouse technology, the role of TGF-α as an initiator and a promoter of liver oncogenesis has been studied in some detail. Lee *et al.* [32] found an increase in TGF-α expression in most α-fetoprotein–positive tumors. TGF-α overexpressing transgenic mice developed well-differentiated hepatocellular carcinoma tumors by 10 to 12 months of age. TGF-α is shown to promote and propagate tumor development via an autocrine mechanism. Double transgenic mice bearing the fusion genes consisting of mouse albumin promoter/mouse *c-myc* complementary DNA and mouse metallothionein 1 promoter/human TGF-α complementary DNA have explosive acceleration of tumor growth compared with those bearing either gene alone [33••].

Two distinct cellular reactions are seen before the development of frank carcinoma: dysplasia and apoptosis followed by hyperplasia in multiple foci. High levels of TGF-α transcripts are found in areas of dysplasia. Therefore, the interaction between TGF-α and nuclear oncogenes such as *c-myc* results in a shortened latency period of tumor formation and high tumor incidence. Sandgren *et al.* [34••] had similar findings in double transgenic mice bearing TGF-α complementary DNA and simian virus 40 T antigen complementary DNA. Moreover, less differentiated or more malignant tumors were observed. Other factors may be synergistic in TGF-α–induced hepatic carcinogenesis, such as sex hormones (male susceptibility), insulin-like growth factor II, and the genetic background of the individuals [35].

Takagi *et al.* [35] studied the effects of diverse chemical carcinogens in TGF-α–overexpressing transgenic mice. Diethylnitrosamine and dimethylnitrosamine are known initiators and phenobarbital is a known promoter of oncogenesis. When these transgenic mice were exposed to each type of chemical, 80% to 100% developed hepatocellular carcinoma in a highly accelerated fashion (24 to 32 weeks instead of 10 to 12 months), as well as larger tumors [18••]. Thus, TGF-α can act as either an initiator or a promoter in tumor development. The postulated mechanisms of tumorigenesis of TGF-α are 1) rapid fixation of genetic mutations, 2) selective enhancement of initiated hepatocytes expressing the largest amount of TGF-α, and 3) down-regulation of EGF receptors, the increased presence of which can be deleterious in cells overexpressing TGF-α.

Other lines of evidence examined the effects of TGF-α in hepatitis B virus–associated hepatocarcinoma. TGF-α is expressed at high levels in 82% of human hepatocellular carcinoma. Localization of hepatitis B surface antigen in the same cells indicates a possible interaction in oncogenesis [36]. Elevated levels of TGF-α are found in both cancerous cells and adjacent nontumorous cirrhotic tissue in patients with hepatitis B virus–related hepatocellular carcinoma; however, it is rarely detected in nontumorous tissue surrounding hepatocellular carcinoma in the absence of hepatitis B virus infection [16•,36]. In *in vitro* studies, TGF-α is found to be increased in HepG2 cells after hepatitis B virus transfection [16•]. Therefore, hepatitis B virus is hypothesized to up-regulate TGF-α expression, which may then initiate and expand malignant transformation.

Transforming growth factor-β

Among the three growth factors reviewed here, the role of TGF-β in hepatic carcinogenesis is the least clearly delineated. Ito *et al.* [37] showed that *in vivo*, hepatocellular carcinoma tissues contain much higher levels of TGF-β than normal human liver does. This suggests an association between the growth factor and oncogenesis, the nature of which is unclear. Other experiments revealed that TGF-β transcripts and the latent protein are seen in desmin-positive perisinusoidal cells surrounding and within preneoplastic nodules or carcinomas. The mature protein is only detected in nonparenchymal cells and connective tissues associated with carcinomas. Thus, the activation of the latent TGF-β may require the proximity of carcinomatous and nonparenchymal cells and TGF-β may exert its effects in a paracrine manner [25]. Recently, Inagaki *et al.* [38•] demonstrated that *in vitro*, TGF-β_1 strongly inhibits the growth of human hepatoma Hep3B cells. In a mutant cell line that lacks the type II TGF-β receptor gene and is thus resistant to this inhibitory effect, transfection of the type II TGF-β receptor complementary DNA restores this inhibition. In addition, types I and II TGF-β receptors coprecipitate in the presence of ligand. This suggests that the TGF-β receptors may act in concert by means of a heteromeric surface complex [38•].

Hepatic fibrogenesis

Hepatic fibrosis can be seen as a final common pathway of a wide variety of chronic liver insults, and it is characterized by a dramatic increase and alteration of hepatic extracellular matrix proteins. The exuberant formation of abnormal extracellular matrix, made up of collagens, proteoglycans, fibronectin, hyaluronic acid, as well as other glycoproteins, seems to be initiated by events in the subendothelial space of Disse, which is bordered by the nonluminal sinusoidal endothelium and the hepatocyte cell membrane. Within this space, normally composed of low-density basement-membrane constituents and quiescent lipocytes, accumulation of a high-density matrix composed of fibril-forming collagens, especially type I, and activated lipocytes is seen in response to chronic injury. Several hepatic cell types have been implicated in these molecular changes, but recently, the hepatic lipocyte (synonymous with Ito, perisinusoidal, stellate, or fat-storing cell) has been shown to be the primary source of extracellular matrix synthesis in chronic liver injury [39].

Increased production of extracellular matrix by lipocytes is preceded by activation of these cells into myofibroblast-like cells, a complex series of events characterized by cell enlargement, local proliferation, enhanced fibrogenesis, and expression of smooth-muscle α-actin [40]. Initiation of lipocyte activation appears to involve soluble factors released by Kupffer cells, hepatocytes, lymphocytes, and platelets resulting in lipocyte expression of cytokines and growth factor receptors. Initiation is followed by perpetuation of lipocyte activation, characterized by the expression of both autocrine and paracrine mediators that perpetuate formation of extracellular matrix [41••]. These mediators include a wide variety of soluble substances, including several of the cytokines.

Cytokines that have been implicated in the pathogenesis of liver fibrosis include TGF-β_1, platelet-derived growth factor (PDGF), TNF-α, γ-interferon, interleukin-1, and various colony-stimulating factors, particularly colony-stimulation factor-1 (also known as macrophage colony-stimulating factor) [42]. Several excellent review articles on the molecular basis of hepatic fibrogenesis have recently been published [41••,43–45]. Recent investigation elucidating the role of the cytokines most implicated in the process of hepatic fibrogenesis, TGF-β_1, and PDGF, will be discussed later.

Transforming growth factor-β_1

Transforming growth factor-β_1 is a homodimer with a molecular weight of 25 kD that has been shown to stimulate fibroblasts to proliferate and produce collagen at sites of tissue injury as well as inhibit collagen degradation [46]. Synthesis of TGF-β_1 has been demonstrated in a variety of hepatic cells including Kupffer cells, hepatocytes, and hepatic lipocytes, while virtually all cells studied have receptors for TGF-β_1 [47]. There are several lines of evidence that place TGF-β_1 at the forefront of the cytokines implicated in the pathogenesis of hepatic fibrogenesis.

Both *in vitro* and *in vivo* models have been used to demonstrate the ability of TGF-β_1 to stimulate the synthesis of extracellular matrix. Animal models of murine schistosomiasis and carbon tetrachloride-induced hepatic fibrosis in rats revealed significant elevation of TGF-β_1 messenger RNA levels and type I procollagen messenger RNA levels in association with fibrosis. Immunohistochemical studies of fibrotic livers from a murine schistosomiasis and streptococcal cell wall–induced models showed increased concentration of TGF-β_1 protein [27,48]. Elevated levels of type I procollagen messenger RNA correlated with increased TGF-β_1 messenger RNA levels were seen by several investigators in human patients with active fibrosis [49]. In a recent brief communication, analysis of liver biopsy specimens from chronic hepatitis C patients showed decreased tissue TGF-β_1 levels after therapy with interferon α-2b [50•]. Further evidence of the role of TGF-β_1 as mediator or marker of hepatic fibrogenesis in humans is provided by a study in autologous bone marrow transplant recipients demonstrating an increased risk for the development of hepatic venoocclusive disease in those patients with higher pretransplant TGF-β_1 levels [51].

In vitro evidence of the role of TGF-β_1 in the pathogenesis of hepatic fibrosis includes studies on cultured hepatic lipocytes isolated from normal human liver exposed to TGF-β_1. These cells displayed a dose-dependent increase in types I and III collagen, and fibronectin protein and messenger RNA production, but no significant increase in collagen IV or laminin production. Furthermore, TGF-β_1 has an autocrine effect [52], inducing its own messenger RNA expression in cultured human hepatic lipocytes [53•]. Recent developments also include the observation that TGF-β_1 gene expression as assayed by *in situ* hybridization is considerably increased in nonparenchymal hepatic cells in a thioacetamide rat model of hepatic fibrosis [54]. Bachem *et al.* [55] demonstrated that TGF-β_1 inhibits the proliferation of cultured rat hepatic lipocytes prior to but not following their activation to myofibroblast-like cells. Further work by this group identified a synergistic effect between TGF-β_1 and TNF-α in the stimulation of fibronectin synthesis while not altering total protein synthesis in cultured rat hepatic lipocytes. The addition of TNF-α to TGF-β_1 in this model also stimulated cell proliferation, an effect opposite to that seen with TGF-β_1 alone [56]. Cultured rat hepatic lipocytes are stimulated by TGF-β_1 to increase production of cellular fibronectin, as assayed by indirect immunofluorescence, in a dose-dependent fashion [57].

Platelet-derived growth factor

Platelet-derived growth factor, a known mitogen of hepatic lipocytes, appears to play a role in hepatic fibrogenesis through its mediation of the Ito cell. Friedman and Arthur [58] have demonstrated that activation of cultured lipocytes is accompanied by a rise in PDGF receptor expression. Increased expression of PDGF receptors has also been observed in *in vivo* models of lipocyte activation [41••]. Stimulation of rat lipocytes with PDGF has been found to be correlated with increased growth and DNA synthesis, an action enhanced by TGF-β_1 [59]. At this time it is not clear if the induction of lipocytes and the induction of PDGF receptors are reliant on the presence of Kupffer cells or other co-factors, but this appears likely. Analysis of ascites and liver tissue of human patients with alcoholic liver disease has revealed a PDGF-like peptide not found in the liver of normal controls [60].

In the past year, it has been shown that PDGF stimulated the growth of myofibroblast-like cells, but not of pretransdifferentiated cultured rat hepatic lipocytes, an effect opposite that of TGF-β_1. Furthermore, unlike TGF-β_1, PDGF does not stimulate glycosaminoglycan synthesis in either lipocytes or myofibroblast-like cells [55]. PDGF is shown by Win *et al.* [61•] to play a central role, with TGF-β_1, in the mitogenesis of human hepatic lipocytes *in vitro* using two lines of evidence: 1) blockage of TGF-β_1–induced mitogenesis by anti-PDGF antibodies and 2) increased PDGF messenger RNA in TGF-β_1–stimulated lipocytes [61•]. Human hepatic lipocytes in culture demonstrated increased [^{3}H]thymidine uptake when exposed to PDGF, an effect counteracted in dose-dependent form by pretreatment with retinoic acid. However, PDGF receptor abundance or activation was not affected by pretreatment with retinoic acid [62]. Possible therapeutic applications of the inhibition of PDGF are implied by Peterson [63•], who demonstrated that pretreatment with pentoxifylline prevents increased hepatic collagen in a pig yellow phosphorus–induced model of hepatic fibrosis.

Conclusions

With increasing availability of more sensitive and advanced molecular biological techniques, a fuller and more complex picture of cytokine involvement in various liver processes begins to emerge. Their modes of action and interaction, if further clarified, will provide invaluable insights into these processes and influence the future direction of therapy for liver diseases.

References and recommended reading

Papers of particular interest, published within the annual period of review, have been highlighted as:

- • Of special interest
- •• Of outstanding interest

1. •• LaBrecque DR: **Hepatocyte Growth Factor-How Do I Know Thee? Let Me Count the Ways.** *Gastroenterology* 1992, **103**:1686–1691.
In-depth review of various functions of HGF.

2. •• Maher JJ: **Cell-Specific Expression of Hepatocyte Growth Factor in Liver. Upregulation in Sinusoidal Endothelial Cells After Carbon Tetrachloride.** *J Clin Invest* 1993, **91**:2244–2252.
A closer look at the types of cell populations that express HGF during liver regeneration: endothelial cells, Kupffer cells, and lipocytes.

3. • Hamanoue M, Kawaida K, Takao S, Shimazu H, Noji S, Matsumoto K, Nakamura T: **Rapid and Marked Induction of Hepatocyte Growth Factor During Liver Regeneration After Ischemic or Crush Injury.** *Hepatology* 1992, **16**:1485–1492.
Hepatocyte growth factor acts as a hepatotropic factor for liver regeneration in the event of liver ischemia or crush injury.

4. Lindroos PM, Zarnegar R, Michalopoulous GK: **Hepatic Growth Factor (Hepatopoietin A) Rapidly Increases in Plasma Before DNA Synthesis and Liver Regeneration Stimulated by Partial Hepatectomy and Carbon Tetrachloride Administration.** *Hepatology* 1991, **13**:743–750.

5. • Hu Z, Evarts RP, Fujio K, Marsden ER, Thorgeirsson SS: **Expression of Hepatocyte Growth Factor and c-met Genes During Hepatic Differentiation and Liver Development in the Rat.** *Am J Pathol* 1993, **142**:1823–1830.
The roles of HGF and *c-met* genes are examined in rat hepatic differentiation and development.

6. •• Joplin R, Hishida T, Tsubouchi H, Daikuhara Y, Ayres R, Neuberger JM, Strain AJ: **Human Intrahepatic Biliary Epithelial Cells Proliferate In Vitro in Response to Human Hepatocyte Growth Factor.** *J Clin Invest* 1992, **90**:1284–1289.
Hepatocyte growth factor stimulates the growth of human biliary epithelial cells *in vitro*. This experiment affords a better look at other cell types involved in hepatic regeneration.

7. •• Johnson M, Koukoulis G, Matsumoto K, Nakamura T, Lyer A: **Hepatocyte Growth Factor Induces Proliferation and Morphogenesis in Nonparenchymal Epithelial Liver Cells.** *Hepatology* 1993, **17**:1052–1061.
Another study that examines the stimulatory effects of HGF on nonparenchymal epithelial liver cells.

8. Matsumoto K, Tajima H, Hamanoue M, Kohno S, Kinoshita T, Nakamura T: **Identification and Characterization of "Injurin," an Inducer of Expression of the Gene for Hepatocyte Growth Factor.** *Proc Natl Acad Sci U S A* 1992, **89**:3800–3804.

9. •• Ishiki Y, Ohnishi H, Muto Y, Matsumoto K, Nakamura T: **Direct Evidence That Hepatocyte Growth Factor is a Hepatotropic Factor for Liver Regeneration and Has a Potent Antihepatitis Effect In Vivo.** *Hepatology* 1992, **16**:1227–1235.
Intravenously injected recombinant human HGF stimulates the growth of hepatocytes in mouse liver and protects the liver against injurious effects of hepatotoxins.

10. • Tomiya T, Tani M, Yamada S, Hayashi S, Umeda N, Fujiwara K: **Serum Hepatocyte Growth Factor Levels in Hepatectomized and Nonhepatectomized Surgical Patients.** *Gastroenterology* 1992, **103**:1621–1624.
The rise in HGF levels is not related to the hepatic regeneration process, but to the presence of cirrhosis, necrosis, and systemic inflammation.

11. Michalopoulous GK, Zarnegar R: **Hepatocyte Growth Factor [Editorial].** *Hepatology* 1992, **15**:149–155.

12. • Giordana S, Zhen Z, Medico E, Gaudino G, Galimi F, Comoglio PM: **Transfer of M Otogenic and Invasive Response to Scatter Factor/Hepatocyte Growth Factor by Transfection of Human MET Protooncogene.** *Proc Natl Acad Sci U S A* 1993, **90**:649–653.
Possessing the *met* oncogene product and its ligand HGF allows NIH3T3 fibroblasts to pursue a motogenic-invasive course.

13. Cooper CS: **The Met Oncogene: From Detection by Transfection to Transmembrane Receptor for Hepatocyte Growth Factor.** *Oncogene* 1992, **7**:3–7.

14. Higuchi O, Nakamura T: **Identification and Change in the Receptor for Hepatocyte Growth Factor in Rat Liver After Partial Hepatectomy or Induced Hepatitis.** *Biochem Biophys Res Commun* 1991, **176**:599–607.

15. • Lokker NA, Godowski PJ: **Generation and Characterization of a Competitive Antagonist of Human Hepatocyte Growth Factor, HGF/NK1.** *J Biol Chem* 1993, **268**:17145–17150.
A competitive antagonist of HGF is characterized. This may enable future studies looking at HGF receptor-ligand binding.

16. • Collier JD, Guo K, Gullick WJ, Bassendine MF, Burt AD: **Expression of Transforming Growth Factor α in Human Hepatocellular Carcinoma.** *Liver* 1993, **13**:151–155.
Transforming growth factor-α is found in high levels in some cases of hepatocellular carcinoma.

17. • Burr AW, Carpenter MR, Hines JE, Gullick WJ, Burt AD: **Intrahepatic Distribution of Transforming Growth Factor-α (TGF-α) During Liver Regeneration Following Carbon Tetrachloride-Induced Necrosis.** *J Pathol* 1993, **170**:95–100.
This study establishes the spatial and temporal relationships between TGF-α expression and cell proliferation, suggesting a stimulatory response and an autocrine mechanism.

18. •• Takagi H, Sharp R, Takayama H, Anver MR, Ward JM, Merlino G: **Collaboration Between Growth Factors and Diverse Chemical Carcinogens in Hepatocarcinogenesis of Transforming Growth Factor α Transgenic Mice.** *Cancer Res* 1993, **53**:4329–4336.
A close examination of the synergistic effects of various types of chemical carcinogens and TGF-α expression in transgenic mice.

19. • Hashimoto M, Kothary PC, Raper SE: **The Effects of Transforming Growth Factor-α and Somatostatin on Regenerating Hepatocytes in the Rat.** *Regul Pept* 1993, **44**:49–59.
Exogenous peptide influence is limited to the early phase of hepatic regeneration. Subsequent steps of the process appear to be unresponsive to external stimuli.

20. • Tomiya T, Fujiwara K: **Serum Levels of Transforming Growth Factor-α in Patients After Partial Hepatectomy As Determined With an Enzyme-Linked Immunosorbent Assay.** *Hepatology* 1993, **18**:304–308.
Unlike HGF, TGF-α expression is closely related to the kinetics of hepatic regeneration.

21. Kokudo N, Kothary PC, Eckhauser FE, Raper SE: **Transforming Growth Factor-α (TGF-α) Improves Hepatic DNA Synthesis After Hepatectomy in Cirrhotic Rats.** *J Surg Res* 1992, **52**:648–655.

22. Mead JE, Fausto N: **Transforming Growth Factor-α May Be a Physiological Regulator of Liver Regeneration by Means of an Autocrine Mechanism.** *Proc Natl Acad Sci U S A* 1989, **86**:1558–1562.

23. Fausto N: **Multifunctional Roles for Transforming Growth Factor-β_1.** *Lab Invest* 1991, **65**:497–499.

24. Armendariz-Borunda J, Katai H, Jones M, Seyer JM, Kang
•• AH, Raghow R: **Transforming Growth Factor β Gene Expression is Transiently Enhanced at a Critical Stage During Liver Regeneration After CCl_4 Treatment.** *Lab Invest* 1993, **69**:283–294.

Conclusive evidence demonstrates the inhibitory effects of TGF-β in liver regeneration.

25. Nakatsukasa H, Evarts RP, Hsia CC, Marsden E, Thorgeirsson SS: **Expression of Transforming Growth Factor-β_1 During Chemical Hepatocarcinogenesis in the Rat.** *Lab Invest* 1991, **65**:511–517.

26. Beauchamp RD, Sheng HM, Ishizuka J, Townsend CM,
• Thompson JC: **Transforming Growth Factor (TGF)-β Stimulates Hepatic jun-B and fos-B Proto-Oncogenes and Decreases Albumin mRNA.** *Ann Surg* 1992, **216**:300–308.

TGF-β exerts its effects via the induction of another gene.

27. Czaja MJ, Weiner FR, Flanders KC, Giambrone MA, Wind R, Biempica L, Zern MA: **In Vitro and In Vivo Association of Transforming Growth Factor-beta With Hepatic Fibrosis.** *J Cell Biol* 1989, **108**:2477–2482.

28. De Juan C, Benito M, Alvarez A, Fabregat I: **Differential**
• **Proliferative Response of Cultured Fetal and Regenerating Hepatocytes to Growth Factors and Hormones.** *Exp Cell Res* 1992, **202**:495–500.

A study looking at differential proliferative response of fetal and regenerating hepatocytes to various hormones and growth factors such as EGF, TGF-β, glucagon, norepinephrine, and dexamethasone.

29. Mashuhara M, Katyal SL, Nakamura T, Shinozuka H: **Differ-**
• **ential Expression of Hepatocyte Growth Factor, Transforming Growth Factor-alpha and Transforming Growth Factor-β_1 Messenger RNAs in Two Experimental Models of Liver Cell Proliferation.** *Hepatology* 1992, **16**:1241–1249.

Different models of liver injury causes differential expression of various growth factors.

30. Higashio K, Shima N, Goto M, Itagaki Y, Nagao M, Yasuda H, Morinaga T: **Identity of a Tumor Cytotoxic Factor From Human Fibroblasts and Hepatocyte Growth Factor.** *Biochem Biophys Res Commun* 1990, **170**:397–404.

31. Shiota G, Rhoads DB, Wang T, Nakamura T, Schmidt EV: **Hepatocyte Growth Factor Inhibits Growth of Hepatocellular Carcinoma Cells.** *Proc Natl Acad Sci U S A* 1992, **89**:373–377.

32. Lee GH, Merlino G, Fausto N: **Development of Liver Tumors in Transforming Growth Factor α Transgenic Mice.** *Cancer Res* 1992, **52**:5162–5170.

33. Murakami H, Sanderson ND, Nagy P, Marino PA, Merlino G,
•• Thorgeirsson: **Transgenic Mice Model for Synergistic Effects of Nuclear Oncogenes and Growth Factors in Tumorigenesis: Interaction of c-myc and Transforming Growth Factor-α in Hepatic Oncogenesis.** *Cancer Res* 1993, **53**:1719–1723.

Transgenic mouse model looking at the synergistic effects of nuclear oncogene c-myc and TGF-α in hepatic oncogenesis.

34. Sandgren EP, Luetteke NC, Qiu TH, Palmiter RD, Brinster
•• RL, Lee DC: **Transforming Growth Factor α Dramatically Enhances Oncogene-Induced Carcinogenesis in Transgenic Mouse Pancreas and Liver.** *Mol Cell Biol* 1993, **13**:320–330.

Transgenic mouse model looking at the carcinogenic effects of constitutive expression of TGF-α in the liver and pancreas.

35. Takagi H, Sharp R, Hammermeister C, Goodrow T, Bradley MO, Fausto N, Merlino G: **Molecular and Genetic Analysis of Liver Oncogenesis in Transforming Growth Factor-α Transgenic Mice.** *Cancer Res* 1992, **52**:5171–5177.

36. Hsia CC, Axiotis CA, Di Bisceglie AM, Tabor E: **Transforming Growth Factor-α in Human Hepatocellular Carcinoma and Coexpression With Hepatitis B Surface Antigen in Adjacent Liver.** *Cancer* 1992, **70**:1049–1056.

37. Ito N, Kawata S, Tamura S, Takaishi K, Shirai Y, Kiso S, Yabuuchi I, Matsuda Y, Nishioka M, Tarui S: **Elevated Levels of Transforming Growth Factor β Messenger RNA and Its Polypeptide in Human Hepatocellular Carcinoma.** *Cancer Res* 1991, **51**:4080–4083.

38. Inagaki M, Moustakas A, Lin HY, Lodish HF, Carr BI: **Growth**
• **Inhibition by Transforming Growth Factor β (TGF-β) Type I is Restored in TGF-β-Resistant Hepatoma Cells After Expression of TGF-β Receptor Type II cDNA.** *Proc Natl Acad Sci U S A* 1993, **90**:5359–5363.

Types I and II TGF-β receptors appear to form a heteromeric surface complex in the receptor-ligand binding process.

39. Arenson DM, Friedman SL, Bissell DM: **Formation of Extracellular Matrix in Normal Rat Liver: Lipocytes As a Major Source of Proteoglycan.** *Gastroenterology* 1988, **95**:441–447.

40. Geerts A, Vrijsen R, Rauteeberg J, Burt A, Schelink P, Wisse E: **In Vitro Differentiation of Fat-Storing Cells Parallels Marked Increase of Collagen Synthesis and Secretion.** *J Hepatol* 1989, **9**:59–68.

41. Friedman S: **The Cellular Basis of Hepatic Fibrosis: Mech-**
•• **anisms and Treatment Strategies.** *N Engl J Med* 1993, **328**:1828–1835.

A review of the cellular events within the subendothelial space, and a summary of current and future therapies for hepatic fibrosis.

42. Weiner FR, Degli Esposti S, Zern MA: **A Role of Cytokines As Regulators of Hepatic Fibrogenesis.** *Gastroenterol Jpn* 1993, **28**:97–101.

43. Clement B, Loreal O, Levavasseur, Guillouzo A: **New Challenges in Hepatic Fibrosis.** *J Hepatol* 1993, **18**:1–4.

44. Lissoos TW, Beno DWA, Davis BH: **Hepatic Fibrogenesis and Its Modulation by Growth Factors.** *J Pediatr Gastroenterol* 1992, **15**:225–231.

45. Burt AD: **C. L. Oakley Lecture (1993): Cellular and Molecular Aspects of Hepatic Fibrosis.** *J Pathol* 1993, **170**:105–114.

46. Amento EP, Beck LS: **TGF-β and Wound Healing.** In *Clinical Applications of TGFβ*. Edited by Bock GR, Marsh J. West Sussex, England: John Wiley; 1991:115–129.

47. Sporn MB, Roberts AB, Wakefield LML, Assoian RK: **Transforming Growth Factor-beta: Biological Function and Chemical Structure.** *Science* 1986, **233**:532–534.

48. Manthey CL, Allen JB, Ellingsworth LR, Wahl SM: **In Situ Expression of Transforming Growth Factor-beta in Streptococcal Cell Wall-Induced Granulomatous Inflammation and Hepatic Fibrosis.** *Growth Factors* 1990, **4**:17–26.

49. Annoni G, Weiner FR, Zern MA: **Increased Transforming Growth Factor-beta (TGF-β) Gene Expression in Human Liver Disease.** *J Hepatol* 1992, **14**:259–264.

50. Bedossa P, Poynard T, Mathurin P, Lemaigre G, Chaput JC:
• **Transforming Growth Factor β_1: In Situ Expression in the Liver of Patients With Chronic Hepatitis C Treated With Alpha Interferon.** *Gut* 1993, **34**:S146–S147.

A brief report noting reduction in TGF-β_1 expression in liver biopsy specimens in six of seven chronic hepatitis C patients treated with interferon-α-2b.

51. Anscher MS, Peters WP, Reisenbichler H, Petros WP, Jirtle RL: **Transforming Growth Factor β As a Predictor of Liver and Lung Fibrosis After Autologous Bone Marrow Transplantation for Advanced Breast Cancer.** *N Engl J Med* 1993, **328**:1592–1598.

52. Weiner FR, Giambrone MA, Czaja MJ, Shah A, Annoni G, Takahashi S, Eghbali M, Zern MA: **Ito Cell Gene Expression and Collagen Regulation.** *Hepatology* 1990, **11**:111–117.

53. Casini A, Pinzani M, Milani S, Grappone C, Galli G, Jeze-
• quel AM, Schuppan D, Rotella CM, Surrenti C: **Regulation of Extracellular Matrix Synthesis by Transforming Growth Factor-β_1 in Human Fat-Storing Cells.** *Gastroenterology* 1993, **105**:245–253.

Transforming growth factor-β_1 was shown to induce a dose-dependent increase in procollagen I, III and fibronectin in human hepatic lipocytes in culture. Increased expression of procollagen, fibronectin and TGF-β_1 was also shown in TGF-β_1–stimulated Ito cells *in vitro.*

54. Krull NB, Zimmerman T, Gressner AM: **Spatial and Temporal Patterns of Gene Expression for the Proteoglycans Biglycan and Decorin and for Transforming Growth Factor-β_1 Revealed In Situ Hybridization During Experimentally Induced Liver Fibrosis in the Rat.** *Hepatology* 1993, **18**:581–589.

55. Bachem MG, Meyer D, Schafer W, Riess U, Melchior R, Sell K, Gressner AM: **The Response of Rat Liver Perisinusoidal Lipocytes to Polypeptide Growth Regulator Changes With Their Transdifferentiation Into Myofibroblast-Like Cells in Culture.** *J Hepatol* 1993, **18**:40–52.

56. Bachem MG, Sell K, Melchior R, Kropf J, Eller T, Gressner AM: **Tumor Necrosis Factor Alpha (TNF-α) and Transforming Growth Factor Beta (TGF-β_1) Stimulate Fibronectin Synthesis and the Transdifferentiation of Fat-Storing Cells in the Rat Liver Into Myofibroblasts.** *Virchows Archiv B Cell Pathol* 1993, **63**:123–130.

57. Ramadori G, Knittel ZT, Odenthal M, Schwogler S, Neubauer K, Zum Buschenfelde KM: **Synthesis of Cellular Fibronectin by Rat Liver Fat-Storing (Ito) Cells: Regulation by Cytokines.** *Gastroenterology* 1992, **103**:1313–1321.

58. Friedman SL, Arthur MJP: **Activation of Cultured Rat Hepatic Lipocytes by Kupffer Cell Conditioned Medium.** *J Clin Invest* 1989, **84**:1780–1785.

59. Pinzani M, Gesualdo L, Sabbath GM, Abboud HE: **Effects of Platelet-Derived Growth Factor and Other Polypeptide Mitogens on DNA Synthesis and Growth of Cultured Rat Liver Fat-Storing Cells.** *J Clin Invest* 1989, **84**:1786–1789.

60. Penchev D, Lee WM, Kowalyk KK, Grotendorst GR: **Increased Levels of a PDGF-Like Factor in Ascites in Fibrotic Liver From Individuals With Alcoholic Liver Disease [Abstract].** *Hepatology* 1988, **8**:1228A.

61. • Win KM, Charlotte F, Mallat A, Cherqui D, Martin N, Mavier P, Preaux A, Dhumeaux D, Rosenbaum J: **Mitogenic Effect of Transforming Growth Factor-β_1 on Human Ito Cells in Culture: Evidence for Mediation by Endogenous Platelet-Derived Growth Factor.** *Hepatology* 1993, **18**:137–145.

Using human hepatic lipocytes in culture, the authors demonstrate that TGF-β_1 is mitogenic for these cells, an effect apparently mediated through induction of autocrine PDGF secretion.

62. Davis BH, Coll D, Beno DW: **Retinoic Acid Suppresses the Response to Platelet-Derived Growth Factor in Human Hepatic Ito-Cell-Like Myofibroblasts: A Post Receptor Mechanism Independent of raf/fos/jun/egr Activation.** *Biochem J* 1993, **294**:785–791.

63. • Peterson TC: **Pentoxifylline Prevents Fibrosis in an Animal Model and Inhibits Platelet-Derived Growth Factor-Driven Proliferation of Fibroblasts.** *Hepatology* 1993, **17**:486–493.

Based on the observation that pentoxyifylline reduces interleukin-1–driven fibroproliferation, the authors demonstrate decreased collagen concentration in livers of a pig hepatic fibrosis model in animals pretreated with pentoxifylline.

Minhhuyen T. Nguyen, MD, and Steven K. Herrine, MD, Thomas Jefferson University Hospital, Division of Gastroenterology and Hepatology, 132 South 10th Street, Philadelphia, PA 19107, USA.

Mark A. Zern, MD, Thomas Jefferson University Hospital, Division of Gastroenterology and Hepatology, 1025 Walnut Street, 901 College Building, Philadelphia, PA 19107, USA.

Radiologic procedures and imaging in hepatology

William E. Torres, MD

Emory Clinic, Atlanta, Georgia, USA

In the past few years, there have been dramatic advances in the field of radiology—in technology, in contrast agents, and in therapeutic procedures. The new computed tomography and magnetic resonance technology will permit new imaging protocols to be used, thus revolutionizing how the radiologist images the liver. Likewise, advances in both computed tomography and magnetic resonance contrast agents will aid in lesion localization and increase diagnostic confidence. In patients with known or suspected hepatocellular carcinoma, techniques such as ultrasound-guided percutaneous biopsy of portal vein thrombi and percutaneous ethanol ablation therapy are changing how physicians deal with this group of patients. Transjugular intrahepatic portosystemic shunt, a new therapeutic nonoperative procedure for management of variceal bleeding, is effective in lowering portal pressure and in controlling variceal bleeding both in patients unresponsive to sclerotherapy and in patients with chronic variceal bleeding before liver transplantation.

Current Opinion in Gastroenterology 1994, **10**:285–288

Imaging

Spiral computed tomography

Computed tomography has undergone significant changes since its clinical introduction in the 1970s. Spiral or helical computed tomography is a new rapid scanning technique that allows the volumetric acquisition of data [1•] as the patient advances through a computed tomography unit at a constant rate. The total scan time is greatly reduced, *ie*, one image per second and the study usually can be obtained in one breath hold. Because the images are obtained volumetrically, the images can be reconstructed, not only in the usual axial fashion, but in two-dimensional (*eg*, coronal or sagittal) or three-dimensional formats and as maximum intensity projection images [2•,3,4]. Computed tomographic angiography images can be created using two-dimensional, three-dimensional, and maximum intensity projection reconstruction techniques; in some cases, the need for routine angiography is eliminated. Additionally, the ability to reconstruct images in different planes can aid in lesion localization and, at times, increase diagnostic confidence.

With spiral computed tomography, the liver in a patient with known or suspected hepatic lesions can usually be imaged within 24 seconds. Owing to fast scanning now available and because of the rapid injection of contrast, hepatic images can now be obtained in either the arterial or venous phases; some authors advocate acquiring images in both phases to increase diagnostic confidence. With spiral computed tomography, images are now often obtained at 5-mm intervals; this smaller interscan spacing should result in better lesion identification and, thus, better diagnostic confidence in the diagnosis of hepatic lesions. Recent work with spiral computed tomography has demonstrated that smaller interscan intervals (4 mm instead of 8 mm) increases both the confidence in detecting lesions and the rate of detection [5]. Future improvements in imaging technology and in contrast agents most likely will improve lesion detection within the liver.

Imaging strategies

Strategies for imaging of patients with suspected or known hepatic neoplasms have undergone major changes in the past few years with the development of new computed tomographic imaging techniques and with the advent of magnetic resonance and new magnetic resonance contrast agents [6••,7]. Currently, no single imaging method is optimal in the detection of hepatic lesions. Hepatic imaging, therefore, requires a combination of examinations to be performed. This is especially true in the patient who is a candidate for hepatic metastasectomy. In order to optimize lesion detection, the following sequence of examinations are performed: dynamic sequential bolus iodine computed tomography, computed tomography with arterial portography, delayed computed tomography with iod-

Abbreviations

PEAT—percutaneous ethanol ablation therapy; **TIPS**—transjugular intrahepatic portosystemic shunt.

 ISBN 1-85922-608-6 ISSN 0267–1379

inated contrast material, and magnetic resonance imaging. Using the listed techniques, the patient with multiple lesions would be excluded early in the process. A prior study [8] suggested that when using the more advanced techniques of magnetic resonance and computed tomography with arterial portography, a combined sensitivity of 97% is possible for the detection of liver lesions. A recent study [9] evaluated 404 patients from three institutions who had computed tomography during arterial portography for potential hepatic metastasectomy. The study found that 64% of patients were spared unnecessary surgery. Thirteen percent of patients who were considered resectable based on the computed tomography during arterial portography findings were found at surgery to have unresectable tumors; in this group of patients the local extension of the tumor was greater than predicted or additional lesions were seen.

The small hepatic lesion

The advances in computed tomography technology have led to the detection of an increasing number of small hepatic lesions. Detecting these small lesions often creates a problem for both the referring clinician as well as the radiologist. Are the lesions 15 mm or smaller within the liver benign or malignant? In a recent study [10••], the computed tomography scans on 1454 outpatients were reviewed. In 254 (17%) of the original 1454 patients, hepatic lesions less than or equal to 15 mm were detected. The study demonstrated that there is a high probability that hepatic lesions 15 mm and under are benign, even in patients with a known extrahepatic malignancy.

Hepatocellular carcinoma

Asian versus non-Asian type

Much has been written in Western medical literature regarding the radiologic findings of hepatocellular carcinoma; however, most of the work reflects data from Asian populations, especially from Korea and Japan. Recent studies [11••,12••] have demonstrated that computed tomography features thought to be specific for hepatocellular carcinoma (tumor encapsulation, fatty metamorphosis, portal or hepatic venous involvement, and arterioportal shunting) occur at a lower frequency in the non-Asian population as follows: tumor encapsulation, 12%; fatty metamorphoses, 0%; and arterioportal shunting, 4%. Of the four features thought to be specific for hepatocellular carcinoma, only venous invasion was seen at high percentages both in the Asian and non-Asian groups (48%).

Portal vein thrombosis

The detection of small hepatocellular carcinomas has increased in asymptomatic patients because of screening of high-risk patients. Portal vein thrombosis, a complication of hepatic cirrhosis, can be caused by either benign or malignant processes. Neoplastic invasion of the portal vein is a contraindication to either transplantation or hepatic resection. Imaging studies often cannot differentiate malignant from benign portal vein thrombi. Several authors [13•,14,15] have evaluated the safety and efficacy of sonographically guided percutaneous biopsy of portal vein thrombi and have found it to be safe and sensitive in establishing the benign or malignant nature of portal vein thrombosis.

Percutaneous ethanol ablation therapy

Therapy

In addition to surgery and chemoembolization, a recent study [16••] has demonstrated good long-term results in the treatment of small hepatocellular carcinomas with percutaneous ethanol ablation therapy (PEAT). This treatment technique has shown better long-term survival over surgery in patients who are poor surgical candidates with single lesions smaller than 3 cm. In general, ethanol is usually administered over several sessions.

Recently, the use of high-dose PEAT in patients with small hepatocellular carcinoma, *ie*, greater than 10 mL of ethanol per session, was examined [17••]. The authors found that no serious complication occurred. Pain and fever were the most common complications; a higher frequency of these complications occurred at the higher doses, but this was felt to be related to the greater degree of tumor necrosis occurring from the larger volumes. Investigators have also looked at the feasibility and effectiveness of PEAT performed with general anesthesia in a single session [18]. Thirty patients with hepatocellular carcinoma and metastasis were included in the study; the authors felt that PEAT performed with general anesthesia decreased the treatment time and allowed larger and more numerous lesions to be treated. It should be noted, however, that in only 10 of the original 30 patients were the authors able to achieve complete necrosis of the tumor in one session; presumably, the remaining patients will need additional sessions.

Imaging

Imaging in patients with known or suspected hepatocellular carcinoma can be performed with ultrasound, computed tomography, or magnetic resonance imaging. The typical sonographic findings of treated hepatocellular carcinoma lesions have been described previously. The computed tomography, magnetic resonance, and color-Doppler sonographic findings have recently been reported [19•,20•,21,22]. In a study in patients with biopsy-proven hepatocellular carcinoma [19•], the authors found that computed tomographic evidence of necrosis and lack of nodularity after PEAT was suggestive of absence of disease. Two reports [20•,21] examined the role of magnetic resonance in the follow-up of patients treated with PEAT. One report [20•] suggested that magnetic resonance imaging alone is insufficient in the evaluation and follow-up of hepatocellular carcinoma treated with PEAT because of its lack of specificity. The other study [21] looked at contrast-enhanced computed tomography and T_2-weighted magnetic resonance images and felt that magnetic resonance imaging was an alternative to computed tomography in the follow-up of patients treated with PEAT. This subject should be further studied to determine the role of magnetic resonance in this group of patients. The function of color Doppler sonography was examined in a group of 31 patients with hepatocellular carcinoma before and after transcatheter arterial embolization [22]. The authors felt that color Doppler sonography is highly reliable in determining vascularity and in looking for recurrence of hepatocellular carcinoma; if tumoral blood flow is noted after therapy, further treatment should be considered.

Transjugular intrahepatic portosystemic shunts

Esophageal variceal hemorrhage is a major life-threatening complication of portal hypertension. In the United States alone, there are over 15,000 hospital admissions annually. Transjugular intrahepatic portosystemic shunt (TIPS) is a new therapeutic nonoperative procedure for management of variceal bleeding [23••]. In the TIPS procedure, the portal venous system is decompressed partially by using a stent creating a channel between a hepatic and portal vein. In a recent study with 100 patients, TIPS was reliable and effective in lowering portal pressure and in controlling variceal bleeding both in patients unresponsive to sclerotherapy and in patients with chronic variceal bleeding before liver transplantation. In one study [23••], the portal vein pressure was reduced from 34.5±7.6 mm Hg (SD) to 24.5±6.2 mm Hg. Acute variceal bleeding was controlled in 29 of 30 patients. The feasibility of using TIPS in patients with preexisting portal vein occlusion was evaluated in a group of 10 patients [24]. In six of 10 patients, using a transjugular approach, the portal veins were successfully recanalized and TIPS was established in three of six patients. In the remaining four patients, a transhepatic approach was used for portal vein recanalization prior to the TIPS procedure; in all four patients, TIPS was successful.

Angiography, until recently, has been the standard technique to evaluate the post-TIPS patient. Investigators examined the role of color Doppler ultrasound in the evaluation of patents that have had the TIPS procedure [25]. Color Doppler ultrasound easily identified the prosthesis, determined shunt patency, and defined the direction of flow in 23 patients both immediately following the TIPS procedure and after 2 to 3 months.

Hepatic transplantation

In patients with end-stage liver disease, hepatic transplantation has become the treatment of choice. A variety of radiologic techniques are being used to evaluate these patients postoperatively. Usually, color flow duplex ultrasound is the method of choice to evaluate the transplanted liver. Hepatic arterial thrombosis, most common in the first 6 weeks posttransplant, is a serious complication. Patients have not yet formed collateral and thrombosis often results in the loss of the transplanted liver. In a recent study [26•], 160 hepatic transplant recipients were evaluated over a 3-year period. Thirty patients demonstrated aberrant diastolic flow in the hepatic artery following transplantation; 20 patients had reversed flow and 10 had no flow during diastole. In the 30 patients with abnormal flow, complications occurred in six patients, although only two were vascular in nature. The authors felt that reversed or absent diastolic flow in the hepatic artery of recently transplanted patients has little correlation with subsequent hepatic artery thrombosis.

Computed tomography examinations performed on patients post–hepatic transplant, have demonstrated periportal halos seen as circumferential zones of decrease attenuation around the peripheral or subsegmental post venous branches on contrast-enhanced computed tomography [27•]. Although the finding is nonspecific, it should alert the physician to evaluate the liver for the underlying etiology. In the patient who is post-hepatic transplant, the periportal halo is felt to be secondary to disruption and engorgement of lymphatic vessels.

References and recommended reading

Papers of particular interest, published within the annual period of review, have been highlighted as:
- • Of special interest
- •• Of outstanding interest

1. • Zeman RK, Fox SH, Silverman PM, Davros WJ, Carter LM, Griego D, Weltman DI, Ascher SM, Cooper CJ: **Helical (Spiral) CT of the Abdomen**. *AJR Am J Roentgenol* 1993, **160**:719–725.

Reviews the technical features of spiral computed tomography and looks at its advantages and disadvantages.

2. • Bluemke DA, Fishman EK: **Spiral CT of the Liver**. *AJR Am J Roentgenol* 1993, **160**:787–792.

This paper looks at spiral computed tomography of the liver in the preoperative evaluation of patients with neoplastic liver disease.

3. Dillon EH, van Leeuwen MS, Fernandez MA, Mali WPTM: **Spiral CT Angiography**. *AJR Am J Roentgenol* 1993, **160**:1273–1278.

4. Rubiln GD, Dake MO, Napel SA, McDonnell CH, Jeffrey RB Jr: **Three-Dimensional Spiral CT Angiography of the Abdomen: Initial Clinical Experience**. *Radiology* 1993, **186**:147–152.

5. Urban BA, Fishman EK, Kuhlman JE, Kawashima A, Hennessey JG, Siegleman SS: **Detection of Focal Hepatic Lesions With Spiral CT: Comparison of 4- and 8-Mm Interscan Spacing**. *AJR Am J Roentgenol* 1993, **160**:783–785.

6. Harned RK II, Chezmar JL, Nelson RC: **Imaging of Patients**
•• **With Potentially Resectable Hepatic Neoplasms**. *AJR Am J Roentgenol* 1993, **159**:1191–1194.

Describes an imaging approach to patients with potentially resectable liver disease.

7. Saini S: **Contrast-Enhanced MR Imaging of the Liver**. *Radiology* 1992, **182**:12–14.

8. Nelson RC, Chezmar JL, Bernardino ME: **Comparison of Angiography CTA-Portography, Delayed CT and MRI for the Preoperative Evaluation of Hepatic Tumors**. *Radiology* 1989, 172:27–34.

9. Small WC, Mehard WB, Langmo LS, Dagher AP, Fishman EK, Heiken JP, Bernardino ME: **Preoperative Determination of the Resectability of Hepatic Tumors: Efficacy of CT During Arterial Portography**. *AJR Am J Roentgenol* 1993, 161:319–322.

10. Jones EC, Chezmar JL, Nelson RC, Bernardino ME: **The Fre-**
•• **quency and Significance of Small (<15mm) Hepatic Lesions Detected by CT**. *AJR Am J Roentgenol* 1992, **158**:535–539.

This excellent article looks at the small hepatic lesion found on computed tomography and concludes that there is a high probability that lesions smaller than 15 mm are benign, even in patients with known extrahepatic malignant tumor.

11. Freeny PC, Baron RL, Teefey SA: **Hepatocellular Carci-**
•• **noma: Reduced Frequency of Typical Findings With Dynamic Contrast-Enhanced CT in a Non-Asian Population**. *Radiology* 1992, **182**:143–148.

Four computed tomography findings thought to be typical of hepatocellular carcinoma were evaluated; the authors found that the computed tomography findings are more often seen in Asian as opposed to non-Asian patients with hepatocellular carcinoma.

12. Nelson PC, Chezmar JL: **Pathology and Imaging of Hepa-**
•• **tocellular Neoplasms: Are Findings From Asian Populations Applicable to Non-Asian Groups?** *AJR Am J Roentgenol* 1993, 1188–1190.

The authors looked at the key differences and similarities between Asian and non-Asian patients with primary liver tumors.

13. Dodd GD III, Carr BI: **Percutaneous Biopsy of Portal Vein**
• **Thrombus: a New Staging Technique for Hepatocellular Carcinoma**. *AJR Am J Roentgenol* 1993, **161**:229–233.

Ultrasound guided percutaneous biopsy of portal vein thrombi is accurate, safe, and well-tolerated.

14. Joly JP, Delamarre J, Razafimahaleo A, Sevestre H, Tossou H, Capron JP: **Occult Hepatocellular Carcinoma in Cirrhosis: Value of Ultrasound-Guided Biopsy of Portal Vein System Thrombus**. *Abdom Imag* 1993, **18**:344–346.

15. Vilana R, Bru C, Bruix J, Castells A, Sole M, Rodes J: **Fine-Needle Aspiration Biopsy of Portal Vein Thrombus: Value in Detecting Malignant Thrombosis**. *AJR Am J Roentgenol* 1992, **160**:1285–1287.

16. Shinna S, Tagawa K, Niwa Y, Unuma T, Komatsu Y,
•• Yoshiura K, Hamada E, Takahashi M, Shiratori Y, Terano A, *et al.*: **Percutaneous Ethanol Injection Therapy for Hepatocellular Carcinoma: Results in 146 Patients**. *AJR Am J Roentgenol* 1993, **160**:1023–1028.

The experience in treating a large group of patients with hepatocellular carcinoma was reviewed and showed that PEAT is a valuable treatment.

17. Redvanly RD, Chezmar JL, Strauss RM, Galloway JR, Boyer
•• TD, Bernardino ME: **Malignant Hepatic Tumors: Safety of High-Dose Percutaneous Ethanol Ablation Therapy**. *Radiology* 1993, **188**:283–285.

The safety of high-dose PEAT was evaluated and found to be both safe and effective.

18. Livraghi T, Lassaroni S, Pellicano S, Ravasi S, Torzilli, Vettori C: **Percutaneous Ethanol Injection of Hepatic Tumors: Single-Session Therapy With General Anesthesia**. *AJR Am J Roentgenol* 1993, **161**:1065–1069.

19. Joseph FB, Baumgarten DA, Bernardino ME: **Hepatocellu-**
• **lar Carcinoma: CT Appearance After Percutaneous Ethanol Ablation Therapy**. *Radiology* 1993, **186**:553–556.

The computed tomography appearance of patients treated with PEAT was discussed. Necrosis and lack of nodularity immediately after PEAT is suggestive of absence of disease.

20. Nagel HS, Bernardino ME: **Contrast-Enhanced MR Imaging**
• **of Hepatic Lesions Treated With Percutaneous Ethanol Ablation Therapy**. *Radiology* 1993, **189**:265–270.

The authors found that the magnetic resonance appearance of PEAT-treated hepatic lesions is not indicative of residual or recurrent tumor.

21. Sironi S, Livraghi T, Angeli E, Vanzulli A, Villa G, Colombo E, Taccagni G, Del Maschio A: **Small Hepatocellular Carcinoma: MR Follow-up of Treatment with Percutaneous Ethanol Injection**. *Radiology* 1993, **187**:119–123.

22. Tanaka K, Inoue S, Numata K, Takamura Y, Takebayashi S, Ohaki Y, Misugi K: **Color Doppler Sonography of Hepatocellular Carcinoma Before and After Treatment by Transcatheter Arterial Embolization**. *AJR Am J Roentgenol* 1992, **158**:541–546.

23. LaBerge HJM, Ring EJ, Gordon RL, Lake JR, Doherty MM,
•• Somberg KA, Roberts JP, Ascher NL: **Creation of Transjugular Intrahepatic Portosystemic Shunts With Wallstent Endoprosthesis: Results in 100 Patents**. *Radiology* 1993, **187**:413–420.

Transjugular intrahepatic portosystemic shunt is an effective method to lower portal pressure and control variceal bleeding in patients with chronic variceal bleeding before liver transplantation.

24. Radosevich PM, Ring EJ, LaBerge JM, Peltzer MY, Haskal ZJ, Doherty MM, Gordon RL: **Transjugular Intrahepatic Portosystemic Shunts in Patients With Portal Vein Occlusion**. *Radiology* 1993, **186**:523–527.

25. Longo JM, Bilbao JI, Rousseau HP, Garcia-Villareal L, Vinel JP, Zozaya JM, Joffre FG, Prieto J: **Transjugular Intrahepatic Portosystemic Shunt: Evaluation With Doppler Sonography**. *Radiology* 1993, **186**:529–534.

26. Propeck PA, Scanlan KA: **Reversed Or Absent Hepatic Ar-**
• **terial Diastolic Flow in Liver Transplants Shown by Duplex Sonography: a Poor Predictor of Subsequent Hepatic Artery Thrombosis**. *AJR Am J Roentgenol* 1993, **159**:1199–1201.

Absent or reversed hepatic artery diastolic flow in the patient with a recently transplanted liver has no correlation with subsequent hepatic artery thrombosis.

27. Lawson TL, Thorsen MK, Erickson SJ, Perret RS, Quiroz FA:
• **Periportal Halo: a CT Sign of Liver Disease**. *Abdom Imag* 1992, **18**:42–46.

The computed tomography sign of periportal halo was discussed. Although the pathophysiology has not been proven, it appears to represent an important sign of occult liver disease.

William E. Torres, MD, Department of Radiology, Outpatient Section, Emory Clinic, 1365 Clifton Road, NE, Atlanta, GA, 30322, USA.

Complications of cirrhosis

David Bernstein, MD, and Eugene R. Schiff, MD

University of Miami School of Medicine and
Veteran Affairs Medical Center, Miami, Florida, USA

The pathogenesis of ascites formation, hepatic encephalopathy, and the hepatorenal syndrome are still uncertain. Recent studies have furthered our understanding of these processes. This paper reviews current understanding of these processes and discusses current developments that may have therapeutic implications in these areas. Recent studies regarding spontaneous bacterial peritonitis and the malnutrition of cirrhosis are also reviewed.

Current Opinion in Gastroenterology 1994, **10**:289–294

Ascites

Pathophysiology

The precise mechanism of ascites formation in cirrhosis remains unclear. The contradictory features of the two traditional theories have not been resolved [1]. The *underfilling hypothesis* proposes that the primary event in ascites formation is spillover of fluid into the peritoneal cavity, which results in intravascular hypovolemia. The kidney then responds to this hypovolemia with sodium and water retention. The *overfilling hypothesis* proposes that sodium retention by the kidney is the primary event, and spillover into the peritoneal cavity is a result of intravascular hypervolemia. The vasodilation hypothesis unifies many aspects of the underfilling and overfilling hypotheses [2]. This hypothesis proposes that peripheral arterial vasodilation is the initiating event that leads to a decreased effective arterial blood volume. Decreased effective arterial blood volume leads to an increase in circulating levels of renin, aldosterone, noradrenaline, and vasopressin, which leads to renal vasoconstriction with sodium and water retention. These factors, together with a decrease in plasma oncotic pressure due to hypoalbuminemia and an increase in hydrostatic pressure in the splanchnic vessels, result in extravasation of fluid. Once the resorptive capabilities of the lymphatic vessels are exceeded, ascites develops. As liver disease progresses, these hormonal, renal, and hemodynamic changes are amplified, leading to further ascites formation [3•,4•]. (Table 1). Nevertheless, studies correlating hemodynamic parameters with sodium retention do not support the hypothesis that arterial underfilling is the stimulus for sodium retention in alcoholic cirrhosis [5•].

Table 1. The sequence of events in vasodilation hypothesis of ascites formation*

1. Cirrhosis
2. Peripheral arterial vasodilation
3. Decrease in effective blood volume
4. Activation of volume-retaining hormones
5. Renal sodium retention
6. Increase in blood volume
7. Ascites

*From Gerbes [3•]; with permission.

The pathogenesis of sodium and water retention in cirrhosis remains undefined. Activation of the renin-angiotensin-aldosterone neuroendocrine system in cirrhotic patients is believed to stimulate sodium resorption in the distal nephron [1]. Hayes *et al.* [6] expanded on this theory and found that altered relationships between intrarenal hormone systems, such as the renin-angiotensin and kallikrein-kinin systems, may be important in salt and water retention. However, in this small study not all ascitic cirrhotic patients showed activation of the renin-angiotensin-aldosterone system, which makes one wonder what other neuroendocrine factors may be involved in sodium retention.

Ascitic cirrhotic patients have been shown to have higher than normal plasma levels of atrial natriuretic peptide, a vasodilatory substance. Angeli *et al.* [7•] showed variable levels of circulating atrial natriuretic peptide that may reflect different pathophysiological features among ascitic cirrhotic patients. Among such patients requiring increased diuretic therapy, atrial natriuretic peptide levels and the ratio of atrial natriuretic

Abbreviations

BCAA—branched-chain amino acids; **CNNA**—culture-negative neutrocytic ascites; **GABA**—γ-aminobutyric acid; **SBP**—spontaneous bacterial peritonitis.

 ISBN 1-85922-608-6 ISSN 0267–1379

peptide to plasma renin activity levels fall progressively, suggesting that patients become progressively underfilled and that antinatriuretic factors predominate. These antinatriuretic factors were reversed by Tobe *et al.* [8•], who showed improvement in sodium homeostasis and atrial natriuretic peptide response in six cirrhotic patients with refractory ascites after peritoneovenous shunting.

Ascites fluid production in cirrhosis represents a steady state between the formation and the reabsorption of fluid across peritoneal membranes. Dilution techniques have been used to indirectly estimate the free-water peritoneal turnover in cirrhosis. Recently, the methylene blue dilution test was shown to safely estimate free-water transperitoneal dynamics in a direct fashion [9]. This simple test may lead to a greater understanding of ascites dynamics.

Treatment

Survival of patients with ascitic cirrhosis is considerably shorter than survival of patients with nonascitic cirrhosis. The presence of refractory ascites, a serum albumin less than 3 g/dL, and a Pugh score greater than 10 have all been shown to be independent risk factors for early demise in patients with ascitic cirrhosis [10]. Dietary sodium restriction, diuretic therapy, and paracentesis have been the mainstay of treatment for ascites. The reported incidence of bleeding or bowel perforation from paracentesis is less than 1% [11]. Large volume paracentesis, peritoneovenous shunting, transjugular intrahepatic portosystemic shunt, or liver transplantation may be required for patients who fail to respond to the mainstays of treatment. Hillaire *et al.* [12] inserted a LeVeen shunt into 56 patients with intractable ascites, with a cumulative rate of recurrent ascites of 22% at 3 years. This low rate of recurrent ascites was believed to be due to the addition of a titanium tip to the venous catheter. Survival of patients without a history of variceal bleeding or episodes of spontaneous bacterial peritonitis prior to shunt placement was 71% at 2 years. LeVeen shunts have a high incidence of serious complications, with the most common being bacterial infection, intravascular coagulation, and gastrointestinal hemorrhage. Planas *et al.* [13] recently reported the development of a right pulmonary artery embolus following rupture of the venous segment of a LeVeen shunt. Transjugular intraheptic portosystemic shunting shows promise in treating refractory ascites, with a recent study showing ascites resolution in 80% to 90% of patients [14].

Intravenous ascitic fluid reinfusion following ultrafiltration is another option that has been reassessed in the treatment of ascites [15] (Fig. 1). This technique has the theoretical advantage of conserving the patient's opsonins and therefore protecting against the development of spontaneous bacterial peritonitis. In addition, reinfusion of ultrafiltered ascites is significantly less expensive than albumin infusion. One study has shown this technique to be as effective as large volume paracentesis in the treatment of refractory ascites [16•].

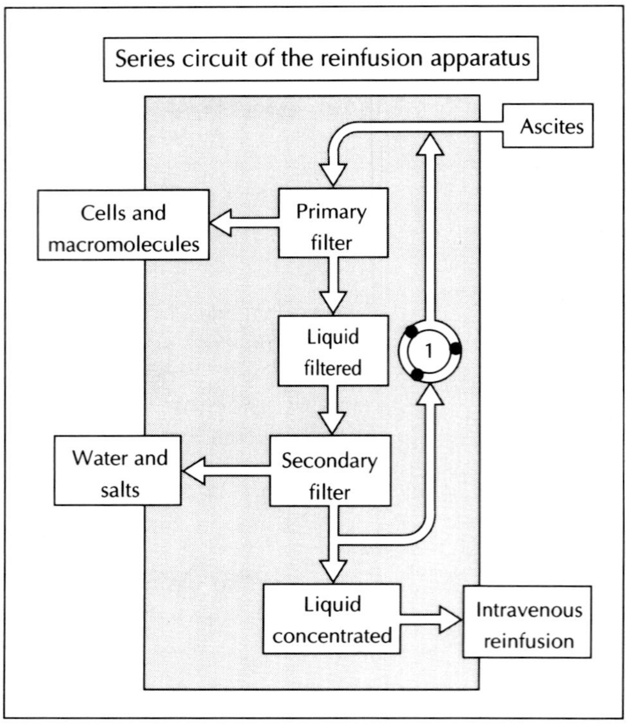

Fig. 1. Left, the ascitic fluid constituents are either trapped in the primary filter (cells and macromolecules) or discarded by the secondary filter or concentrator (water and salts). The end result (5% to 10% of its initial volume) is a protein-enriched fluid that is intravenously reinfused in the patient (*right side*). 1—peristaltic pump. (*From* Rossaro *et al.* [15]; with permission.)

Complications

Spontaneous infection

Spontaneous ascitic fluid infection can be divided into three categories. Spontaneous bacterial peritonitis (SBP) is defined as an ascitic fluid polymorphonuclear leukocyte count of greater than 250 cells/μL with a positive ascitic fluid culture for a single organism. Bacterascites is defined as an ascitic fluid polymorphonuclear leukocyte count of less than 250 cells/μL with a positive ascitic fluid culture for a single organism. Culture-negative neutrocytic ascites (CNNA) is defined as an ascitic fluid count of greater than 250 cells/μL with a negative ascites fluid culture. A recent study by Terg *et al.* [17•] comparing the clinical course of patients with SBP and those with CNNA showed the same mortality and prognosis in both groups. This study, along with previous studies by Runyon and Hoefs [18] and by Pelletier *et al.* [19], question whether SBP and CNNA are different forms of the same disease. Belghitti *et al.* [20] have shown that the ascitic fluid polymorphonuclear leukocyte count of greater than 250 cells/μL is diagnostic for SBP in patients with cirrhosis who have had surgical laparotomy.

Two recent studies have shown the incidence of SBP in patients with ascitic cirrhosis to be 9% [21] and 7% [22•]. Conte *et al.* [21] found the 3-month recurrence and mortality rates of SBP to be 36% and 42%, respectively. Multiple studies have shown the most common organisms to be *Escherichia coli, Klebsiella* spp, and *Streptococcus* species [21,23]. Because of the high incidence and mortality associated with SBP, several investigators have evaluated possible risk factors for the development of this infection. Llach *et al.* [24••], in a prospecitve study of 127 patients with ascitic cirrhosis, found that an ascitic fluid protein concentration of less than 1 g/dL was the best predictor for development of SBP. Several similar studies performed in the past year have reached similar conclusions [21,23]. Andreu *et al.* [23] found a serum bilirubin concentration of greater than 2.5 mg/dL and an ascitic fluid protein concentration of less than 1 g/dL to be the most relevant independent predictors of an initial episode of SBP. The recognition of patients at risk for SBP may be important in selecting patients for antibiotic prophylaxis with norfloxacin, which selectively inhibits aerobic enteric gram-negative flora while preserving anaerobic flora in the gut. Norfloxacin has been shown to be effective in the prophylaxis of SBP in hospitalized patients with cirrhosis who have low ascitic fluid total protein [25•].

Cefotaxime has been shown to be adequate initial therapy for SBP. Infection resolution and patient survival can be predicted on the basis of laboratory and clinical variables including blood urea nitrogen level and whether the SBP was community or hospital acquired [26].

Hernia

Hurst *et al.* [27] reported the surgical repair of femoral and symptomatic inguinal hernias in 11 patients with ascitic cirrhosis without increased morbidity or mortality. The presence of poorly controlled ascites did not contraindicate the repair of symptomatic hernias. However, control of ascites is recommended, if possible, prior to herniorrhaphy.

Malnutrition

Malnutrition is often forgotten when clinical strategies in cirrhotic patients are planned [28•]. However, the prevalence of protein-calorie malnutrition in cirrhotic patients is high. In a comparison of a North American and an Italian population, one study found that 5% to 45% of male patients with cirrhosis and 10% to 30% of female patients with cirrhosis had signs of malnutrition [29]. Multiple factors contribute to the development of malnutrition in cirrhotic patients. Impaired dietary intake secondary to anorexia, nausea, or iatrogenic protein restriction as a result of treatment of hepatic encephalopathy are the principal causes of nutritional deficiencies in cirrhotic patients. Fat and muscle wasting occur as a result of impaired nutrient absorption, despite energy intake well above estimated requirements. Changes in energy metabolism contribute to the development of malnutrition. Carbohydrate metabolism is abnormal due to the development of carbohydrate intolerance, peripheral insulin resistance, hyperinsulinemia, and reduced hepatic glycogen stores. Fat stores are depleted due to an increased rate of fat oxidation. Severely malnourished patients exhibit deficiencies of essential and long-chain polyunsaturated fatty acids [30]. Fat-soluble vitamin deficiencies frequently develop. Zinc and magnesium levels are frequently reduced, which contributes to the impaired wound healing, depressed cellular immunity, and generalized weakness seen in these patients.

Cirrhosis is typically associated with low levels of the branched-chain amino acids (BCAA) valine, leucine, and isoleucine. The pathogenesis of this association is unclear, although it is felt by many to be a result of enhanced skeletal muscle uptake secondary to hyperinsulinemia. Several studies, however, have failed to show any correlation between insulin levels and BCAA levels. Eriksson and Soderman [31] reported an increase in BCAA levels after β-blocker administration in cirrhotic patients. Their results suggest that catecholamines, especially norepinephrine, might contribute to the low levels of BCAA seen in cirrhotic patients.

The assessment of malnutrition in cirrhosis is difficult because routine techniques to assess nutrition are not reliable in liver disease. Weight is an unreliable measurement because it reflects fluid retention caused by ascites and edema as well as body mass. Albumin levels are unreliable because impaired hepatic synthetic function will also decrease serum levels. Unfortunately, the best tests for nutritional assessment in cirrhotic patients, *ie*, dual energy absorptiometry, neutron activation, and measurement of total body potassium, are not routinely available and are quite expensive [28•].

Portal systemic encephalopathy

Pathophysiology

A prospective study using noninstrumental psychomotor tests estimated the prevalence of latent portosystemic encephalopathy to be 71% in patients with cirrhosis [32•]. Despite the frequency of portosystemic encephalopathy, its mechanisms are poorly understood. This condition usually occurs in cirrhotic patients with portal hypertension or in patients with surgical portosystemic anastomoses. Exogenous factors such as bacterial infection, upper gastrointestinal bleeding, and electrolyte imbalance may lead to acute worsening of hepatic encephalopathy. These changes are usually reversible with treatment of the precipitating factor [33]. Sekido *et al.* [34] described hepatic encephalopathy secondary to an acquired large-caliber portohepatic venous shunt that was reversed with surgery. Several theories have been proposed to explain the pathophysiology of latent or chronic portosystemic encephalopathy, although none have been experimentally proven. Alterations in the blood-brain barrier allowing neurotoxins from the splanchnic circulation to reach the brain are a common feature of these theories. Knudsen *et al.* [35••] found no evidence of general or selective blood-brain barrier disturbances in portosystemic encephalopathy. These results question the most basic principle of our current understanding of the pathophysiology of portosystemic enceophalopathy.

The ammonia hypothesis that links elevated levels of ammonia to hepatic encephalopathy has been proposed for almost 60 years. Ammonia interferes with brain function at several sites. It may induce 1) changes of blood-to-brain transport of amino acids, 2) metabolic changes resulting in a decreased cerebral concentration of the excitatory amino acid neurotransmitter glutamate, 3) alterations of brain energy metabolism, and 4) alterations in neuronal electric activity by inhibiting the generation of excitatory and inhibitory potentials [36•]. Despite these activities, it seems highly unlikely that ammonia is the sole neurotoxin precipitating portosystemic encephalopathy because several studies have noted normal ammonia levels in the presence of portosystemic encephalopathy.

Over the past several years, increased tone in the γ-aminobutyric acid (GABA) neurotransmitter system has been implicated in the pathogenesis of portosystemic encephalopathy. The GABA-benzodiazepine receptor is a complex of functionally coupled receptors for GABA, benzodiazepines, and picrotoxine linked to a chloride channel. Binding of GABA to its receptor leads to an influx of chloride, which generates an inhibitory postsynaptic potential. Chloride fluxes are augmented by benzodiazepine agonists and barbiturates and thus increase GABA–mediated neural inhibition [37]. Cirrhotic patients have an increased sensitivity to benzodiazepine agonists, which may explain the ease with which benzodiazepines precipitate portosystemic encephalopathy. Patients with portosystemic encephalopathy have been shown to have elevated levels of endogenous benzodiazepine-like substances [38]. Elevated levels of benzodiazepine receptor agonits in the brains of rats have been shown to contribute to the severity of hepatic encephalopathy [36•]. In contrast, a recent study reported that endogenous benzodiazepines do not precipitate hepatic encephalopathy in rats with thioacetamide-induced liver failure [39•]. Several anecdotal reports have described either transient improvement or no effect in portosystemic encephalopathy with administration of the benzodiazepine antagonist flumazenil. In a recent animal study, Puspok *et al.* [37] reported no improvement in hepatic encephalopathy with administration of the pure benzodiazepine antagonist Ro 14-7437. In contrast, the administration of an antagonist with partial inverse agonistic activity, Ro 14-4513, resulted in an immediate improvement of the hepatic encephalopathy. This study is one of several that show improvement of portosystemic encephalopathy with the administration of a benzodiazepine antagonist with partial inverse agonistic activity, and it emphasizes the therapeutic importance that these substances may have. The therapeutic potential of these substances must be further evaluated.

Treatment

The mainstays of therapy of portosystemic encephalopathy are 1) the correction of any precipitant factors, 2) the reduction of protein in the diet, and 3) the amelioration of ammonia production and absorption in the intestine. Low levels of BCAA are found in portosystemic encephalopathy. Plauth *et al.* [40•] showed improvement of latent portosystemic encephalopathy with long-term BCAA therapy. Bianchi *et al.* [41], in a study of 25 cirrhotic patients with chronic portosystemic encephalopathy, showed that the favorable effects of BCAA on mental state are not mediated by changes in cerebral neurotransmission but are due mainly to maintained liver function, probably as a result of improved nutrition. The use of BCAA in portosystemic encephalopathy remains controversial.

Nonabsorbable carbohydrates, especially lactulose, are routinely used in portosystemic encephalopathy to decrease ammonia absorption by modifying the metabolic activity of intestinal flora. A recent study showed that lactulose improved psychometric test results in 88% of patients with latent portosystemic encephalopathy [32•]. Lactitol, a more palatable nonabsorbable disaccharide, has been shown by meta-analysis to be equally as effective as lactulose in treating portosystemic encephalopathy, with fewer side effects and a quicker onset of action [42•].

Antibiotics are used to reduce the load of aerobic, urease-splitting bacterial flora in the gut in chronic portosystemic encephalopathy. Strauss *et al.* [33] treated cirrhotic patients who had exogenously precipitated hepatic encephalopathy using neomycin alone without any improvement in the encephalopathy. Hepatic encephalopathy improved with treatment of the precipitating event. Bucci and Palmieri [43•] compared a 15-day course of the antibiotic rifaximin (1200 mg/d) with lactulose (30 g/d for 15 days) in 58 cirrhotic patients with portosystemic encephalopathy. They found equal improvement in signs and symptoms of portosystemic encephalopathy in both groups. The rifaximin group had a greater rapidity of action with significantly greater tolerability. Further studies need to be performed to evaluate the potential therapeutic benefit of this new antibiotic.

Hepatorenal syndrome

The hepatorenal syndrome may be defined as renal failure that occurs in patients with liver disease in the absence of clinical, laboratory, or anatomical evidence of other known causes. It is characterized by functional renal failure with preserved renal architecture. This syndrome usually occurs in patients with cirrhosis, although cirrhosis is not necessary for its development. The pathogenesis of the hepatorenal syndrome remains uncertain. It involves mechanisms that lead to renal vasoconstriction and cortical hypoperfusion resulting in the development of renal failure. Multiple factors including the renin-angiotensin system, the sympathetic nervous system, eicosanoids, renal kallikrein, endotoxemia, and nitric oxide have been postulated to play a role in the development of this syndrome [44•]. Moore *et al.* [45••] measured the plasma concentrations of endothelin-1 and endothelin-3 (potent long-acting vasoconstrictors that also stimulate contraction of glomerular mesangial cells and thereby decrease the glomerular filtration rate, in patients with liver disease with and without the hepatorenal syndrome. This study found increased plasma endothelin concentrations in patients with the hepatorenal syndrome, suggesting that endothelins may play a role in the pathogenesis of the hepatorenal syndrome.

Treatment of the hepatorenal syndrome has remained difficult, with the only effective therapy being liver transplantation. Oral misoprostol and intravenous prostaglandin E_2 have recently been shown not to improve renal function in cirrhosis with ascites [46••]. Nitric oxide, a vasodilator, has received attention as a mediator of both hyperdynamic circulation and renal failure. McCormick *et al.* [47] used the nitric oxide synthase inhibitor N^g-monomethyl-L-arginine to treat a patient with the hepatorenal syndrome and noted an increase in the mean arterial pressure without any beneficial or deleterious effects on renal function. The authors postulated that their dose may have been inappropriately low. Further investigation with this agent may be warranted. Liver size, plasma renin activity, and serum sodium concentration are all prognostic parameters for the hepatorenal syndrome and may be applicable to the timing of patient selection for liver transplantation [48].

References and recommended reading

Papers of particular interest, published within the annual period of review, have been highlighted as:
• Of special interest
•• Of outstanding interest

1. Arroyo V, Gines P: **Mechanism of Sodium Retention and Ascites Formation in Cirrhosis.** *J Hepatol* 1993, **17(Suppl 2)**:S24–S28.

2. Schrier RW, Arroyo V, Bernardi M, Epstein M, Henriksen JH, Rodes J: **Peripheral Arterial Vasodilation Hypothesis: A Proposal for the Initiation of Renal Sodium and Water Retention in Cirrhosis.** *Hepatology* 1988, **8**: 1151–1157.

3. • Gerbes AL: **Medical Treatment of Ascites in Cirrhosis.** *J Hepatol* 1993, **17(Suppl 2)**:S4–S9.
A concise updated review of the medical treatment of ascites.

4. • Longmire-Cook SJ: **Pathophysiologic Factors and Management of Ascites.** *Surg Gynecol Oncol* 1993, **176**:191–202.
This review provides an excellent list of references on the pathophysiology of ascites.

5. • Rector WG, Robertson AD, Lewis FW: **Arterial Underfilling Does Not Cause Sodium Retention in Cirrhosis.** *Am J Med* 1993, **95**:286–295.
The data presented in this study refute the peripheral vasodilatation theory for the pathogenesis of ascites.

6. Hayes PC, Cumming AD, Craig KJ, Watson M, Bouchier IAD: **Portal and Systemic Hemodynamics and Humoral Factors in Cirrhosis With and Without Ascites.** *Am J Gastroenterol* 1992, **87**:1433–1438.

7. • Angeli P, Caregaro L, Menon F, Sacerdoti, De Toni R, Merkel C, Gatta A: **Variability of Atrial Natriuretic Peptide Plasma Levels in Ascitic Cirrhotics: Pathophysiological and Clinical Implications.** *Hepatology* 1992, **16**:1389–1394.
Patients requiring higher doses of diuretics developed a compensatory decrease in atrial natriuretic peptide plasma levels.

8. • Tobe SW, Morali GA, Greig PD, Logan A, Blendis LM: **Peritoneovenous Shunting Restores Atrial Natriuretic Factor Responsiveness in Refractory Hepatic Ascites.** *Gastroenterology* 1993, **105**:202–207.
Successful peritoneovenous shunting was associated with improved atrial natriuretic factor–induced natriuresis.

9. Milani A, Ciammella AM, Degen C, Siciliano M, Rossi L: **Ascites Dynamics in Cirrhosis.** *J Hepatol* 1992, **16**:369–375.

10. Salerno F, Borroni G, Moser P, Badalamenti S, Cassara L, Maggi A, Fusini M, Cesana B: **Survival and Prognostic Factors of Cirrhotic Patients With Ascites: A Study of 134 Outpatients.** *Am J Gastroenterol* 1993, **88**:514–519.

11. Qureshi WA, Harshfield D, Shah H, Netchvolodoff C, Banerjee B: **An Unusual Complication of Paracentesis.** *Am J Gastroenterol* 1992, **87**:1209–1211.

12. Hillaire S, Labianca M, Borgonovo G, Smadja C, Grange D, Franco D: **Peritoneovenous Shunting of Intractable Ascites in Patients With Cirrhosis: Improving Results and Predictive Factors of Failure.** *Surgery* 1993, **113**:373–379.

13. Planas R, Domenech E, Montana X, Rodriguez MP, Rodriguez N, Cabre E, Gassull MA: **Rupture and Migration of the Venous Segment of LeVeen Shunt: An Unreported Complication.** *Am J Gastroenterol* 1993, **88**:1101–1103.

14. Adams L, Soulen MC: **TIPS: A New Alternative for the Variceal Bleeder.** *Am J Crit Care* 1993, **2**:196–201.

15. Rossaro L, Graziotto A, Bonato S, Plebani M, VanThiel DH, Burlina A, Naccarato R, Salvagnini M: **Concentrated Ascitic Fluid Reinfusion After Cascade Filtration in Tense Ascites.** *Dig Dis Sci* 1993, **38**:903–908.

16. • Bruno S, Borzio M, Romagnoni M, Battezatti PM, Rossi S, Chiesa A: **Extracorporeal Ultrafiltration and Intravenous Reinfusion of Ascitic Fluid vs. Large Volume Paracentesis: A Randomized Controlled Trial.** *BMJ* 1992, **304**:1655–1658.
Reinfusion of ascitic fluid has the advantage of the conservation of protein, in contrast to large-volume paracentesis, which may require replacement albumin infusions.

17. • Terg R, Levi D, Lopez P, Rafaelli C, Rojter S, Abecasis R, Villamil F, Aziz H, Podesta A: **Analysis of Clinical Course and Prognosis of Culture-Positive Spontaneous Bacterial Peritonitis and Neutrocytic Ascites.** *Dig Dis Sci* 1992, **37**:1499–1504.
Culture-negative neutrocytic ascites was as likely to recur following treatment as culture-positive SBP was.

18. Runyon BA, Hoefs JC: **Culture-Negative Neutrocytic Ascites: A Variant of Spontaneous Bacterial Peritonitis.** *Hepatology* 1984, 4:1209–1211.

19. Pelletier G, Salmon D, Ink O, Hannoun S, Attali P, Buffet C, Ettiene JP: **Culture-Negative Neutrocytic Ascites: A Less Severe Variant of Spontaneous Bacterial Peritonitis.** *J Hepatol* 1990, **10**:327–331.

20. • Belghiti J, Panis Y, Chiche R, Faivre E, Fekete F: **Polymorphonuclear Count in Ascitic Fluid After Laparotomy in Cirrhotic Patients.** *Hepatogastroenterology* 1992, **39**:584–585.
Polymorphonuclear counts above 250/mm^3 were indicative of SBP in postlaparotomy patients with cirrhosis.

21. Conte D, Bolzoni P, Bodini P, Mandelli C, Ranzi ML, Cesarini L, Fraquelli M, Penagini R, Bianchi PA: **Frequency of Spontaneous Bacterial Peritonitis in 265 Cirrhotics With Ascites.** *Eur J Gastroenterol Hepatol* 1993, **5**:41–45.

22. • Hurwich DB, Lindor KD, Hay JE, Gross JB, Kaese D, Rakela J: **Prevalence of Peritonitis and the Ascitic Fluid Protein Concentration Among Chronic Liver Disease Patients.** *Am J Gastroenterol* 1993, **88**:1254–1257.
In contrast to the findings of Llach *et al.* (*Hepatology* 1992, 16:724–727), these authors could not demonstrate a correlation of ascitic fluid protein content with predisposition to the development of SBP.

23. Andreu M, Sola R, Sitges-Serra A, Alia C, Gallen M, Vila MC, Coll S, Oliver MI: **Risk Factors for Spontaneous Bacterial Peritonitis in Cirrhotic Patients With Ascites.** *Gastroenterology* 1993, **104**:1133–1138.

24. Llach J, Rimola A, Navasa M, Gines P, Salmeron JM, Gines
•• A, Arroyo V, Rodes J: **Incidence and Predictive Factors of First Episode of Spontaneous Bacterial Peritonitis in Cirrhosis With Ascites: Relevance of Ascitic Fluid Protein Concentration.** *Hepatology* 1992, **16**:724–727.

The most important predictor of SBP is ascitic fluid protein concentration. The probability for development of SBP was sixfold greater in those patients with ascitic fluid protein concentrations of less than 1 g/dL.

25. Soriano G, Guarner C, Tomas A, Villanueva C, Torras X,
• Gonzalez D, Sainz S, Anguera, Cusso X, Balanzo J, Vilardell F: **Norfloxacin Prevents Bacterial Infection in Cirrhotics With Gastrointestinal Hemorrhage.** *Gastroenterology* 1992, 1267–1272.

Norfloxicin proved to be effective as prophylaxis against bacterial infections following gastrointestinal bleeding in cirrhotic patients.

26. Toledo C, Salmeron JM, Rimola A, Navasa M, Arroyo V, Llach J, Gines A, Gines P, Rodes J: **Spontaneous Bacterial Peritonitis in Cirrhosis: Predictive Factors of Infection Resolution and Survival in Patients Treated With Cefotaxime.** *Hepatology* 1993, **17**:251–257.

27. Hurst RD, Butler BN, Soybel DI, Wright HK: **Management of Groin Hernias in Patients With Ascites.** *Ann Surg* 1992, **216**:696–700.

28. Crawford DHG, Cuneo RC, Shepherd RW: **Pathogenesis and**
• **Assessment of Malnutrition in Liver Disease.** *J Gastroenterol Hepatol* 1993, **8**:89–94.

Dual-energy absorptiometry and neutron activation are reliable techniques for nutritional assessment, but unfortunately they are expensive and have a limited availability.

29. Lolli R, Marchesini G, Bianchi G, Fabbri G, Bugianesi E, Zoli M, Pisi E: **Anthropometric Assessment of the Nutritional Status of Patients With Liver Cirrhosis in an Italian Population.** *Ital J Gastroenterol* 1992, **24**:429–435.

30. Gonzalez J, Periago JL, Cabre E, Abad-Lacruz, Gassull MA, deMedina FS: **Malnutrition Related Polyunsaturated Fatty Acid Changes in Plasma Lipid Fractions of Cirrhotic Patients.** *Metabolism* 1992, **9**:954–960.

31. Eriksson LS, Soderman C: **Influence of Beta Blockade on Branched Chain Amino Acid Concentrations in Cirrhosis.** *Hepatogastroenterology* 1992, **39**:451–454.

32. Schomerus H, Schreiegg J: **Prevalence of Latent Porto-Sys-**
• **temic Encephalopathy in an Unselected Population of Patients With Liver Cirrhosis in General Practice.** *Z Gastroenterol* 1993, **31**:231–234.

An underutilized noninvasive simple technique for outpatient screening of subclinical encephalopathy was found to be quite practical.

33. Strauss E, Tramote R, Silva EPS, Caly WR, Honain NZ, Maffei RA, Sa MFG: **Double-Blind Randomized Clinical Trial Comparing Neomycin and Placebo in the Treatment of Exogenous Hepatic Encephalopathy.** *Hepatogastroenterology* 1992, **39**:542–545.

34. Sekido H, Nakano A, Takahashi T, Matsuo K, Mochizuki Y, Tsuchiya S, Shimada H: **Hepatic Encephalopathy Secondary to a Large-Caliber Porto-Hepatic Venous Shunt: Case Report.** *Hepatogastroenterology* 1992, **39**:316–318.

35. Knudsen GM, Schmidt J, Almdal T, Paulson OB, Vilstrup H:
•• **Passage of Amino Acids and Glucose Across the Blood-Brain Barrier in Patients With Hepatic Encephalopathy.** *Hepatology* 1993, **17**:987–992.

These authors failed to find evidence of a blood-brain barrier disturbance in hepatic encephalopathy.

36. Ferenci P, Puspok A, Steindl P: **Current Concepts in the**
• **Pathophysiology of Hepatic Encephalopathy.** *Eur J Clin Invest* 1992, **22**:573–581.

The salient features of the pathogenesis of hepatic encephalopathy are reviewed.

37. Puspok, Herneth A, Steindl P, Ferenci P: **Hepatic Encephalopathy in Rats With Thioacetamide-Induced Acute Liver Failure is Not Mediated by Endogenous Benzodiazepines.** *Gastroenterology* 1993, **105**:851–857.

38. Basile AS, Hughes RD, Harrison PM, Murata Y, Pannell L, Jones EA, Williams R, Skolnick P: **Elevated Brain Concentrations of 1,4-Benzodiazepines in Fulminant Hepatic Failure.** *N Engl J Med* 1991, **325**:473–478.

39. Yurdaydin C, Gu ZQ, Nowak G, Fromm C, Holt AG, Basile
• AS: **Benzodiazepine Receptor Ligands are Elevated in an Animal Model of Hepatic Encephalopathy.** *J Pharmacol Exp Ther* 1993, **265**:565–571.

The findings support the previous observations on the role of benzodiazepine-like substances in the pathogenesis of hepatic encephalopathy.

40. Plauth M, Egberts EH, Hamster W, Torok M, Muller PH,
• Brand O, Furst P, Dolle W: **Long-Term Treatment of Latent Porto-Systemic Encephalopathy With Branched Chain Amino Acids.** *J Hepatol* 1993, **17**:308–314.

Branched-chain amino acid supplementation was given for 8 weeks and was found to be effective in improving automobile driving performance among cirrhotic patients with subclinical encephalopathy.

41. Bianchi GP, Marchesini G, Abbiati, Ferrario E, Fabbri A, Pisi E: **Oral BCAA Supplementation in Cirrhosis With Chronic Encephalopathy: Effect on Prolactin and Estradiol Levels.** *Hepatogastroenterology* 1992, **39**:443–446.

42. Camma C, Fiorello F, Tine F, Marchesini G, Fabbri A,
• Pagliaro L: **Lactitol in Treatment of Chronic Hepatic Encephalopathy: A Meta-Analysis.** *Dig Dis Sci* 1993, **5**:916–922.

Lacititol was found to be as effective as lactulose in the treatment of hepatic encephalopathy and was more palatable.

43. Bucci L, Palmieri GC: **Double-Blind, Double-Dummy Compar-**
• **ison Between Treatment With Rifaximin and Lactulose in Patients With Medium to Severe Degree Hepatic Encephalopathy.** *Curr Med Res Opin* 1993, **13**:109–118.

Rifaximin was as effective as lactulose, with fewer side effects.

44. Epstein M: **The Hepatorenal Syndromes-Newer Prospectives.**
• *N Engl J Med* 1992, **327**:1810–1811.

This editorial accompanied the study by Moore *et al.* (*N Engl J Med* 1992, 327:1774–1778) and provides an excellent update of the hepatorenal syndrome. Vasoconstrictor mediators are foremost in the pathogenesis.

45. Moore K, Wendon J, Frazer M, Karani J, Williams R,
•• Badr K: **Plasma Endothelin Immunoreactivity in Liver Disease and the Hepatorenal Syndrome.** *N Engl J Med* 1992, **327**:1774–1778.

Plasma levels of endothelin-1 and -3, potent long-acting vasoconstrictors, were observed to be elevated in the hepatorenal syndrome.

46. Gines A, Salmeron JM, Gines P, Arroyo V, Jimenez W, Rivera
•• F, Rodes J: **Oral Misoprostol or Intravenous Prostaglandin E_2 Do Not Improve Renal Function in Patients With Cirrhosis and Ascites With Hyponatremia or Renal Failure.** *J Hepatol* 1993, **17**:220–226.

Although prostaglandin supplementation would be anticipated to improve the renal dysfunction associated with cirrhosis, these studies failed to show any benefit from such therapy.

47. McCormick PA, Chin JKT, Nair DR, Sweny P, Karatapanis S, Varghese Z, Jacobs M, McIntyre N, Burroughs AK: **Nitric Oxide Synthase Inhibitors in the Hepatorenal Syndrome.** *Eur J Gastroenterol Hepatol* 1993, **5**:59–60.

48. Gines A, Escorsell A, Gines P, Salo J, Jimenez W, Inglada L, Navasa M, Claria J, Rimola A, Arroyo V, Rodes J: **Incidence, Predictive Factors, and Prognosis of the Hepatorenal Syndrome in Cirrhosis With Ascites.** *Gastroenterology* 1993, **105**:229–236.

David Bernstein, MD, and Eugene R. Schiff, MD, University of Miami School of Medicine and Veteran's Affairs Medical Center, Division of Hepatology (R-10), P.O. Box 016960, Miami, FL 33101, USA.

Portal hypertension

Andres T. Blei, MD

Lakeside VA Medical Center, Chicago, Illinois, USA

Portal hypertension arises from an elevated resistance to portal flow combined, in many cases, with an increased portal venous inflow. The pathogenesis of the hyperdynamic circulation in portal hypertensive states, with its subsequent increase in splanchnic blood flow, continues to be a central focus of research in this area. Further evidence continues to accumulate in experimental models that nitric oxide may be a key mediator in the peripheral vasodilation seen in portal hypertension; however, the pathogenesis of the increase in nitric oxide remains obscure. Contradictory human studies have been reported on whether the gastric mucosa in portal hypertensive gastropathy participates in this hyperemic response. A wide array of noninvasive technology is being examined in order to detect the presence of esophageal varices. With regard to therapy, several trials have shown benefit with the administration of octreotide in the management of acute variceal bleeding. Three randomized controlled trials have shown the advantages of esophageal variceal band ligation over sclerotherapy in the management of variceal hemorrhage. Increasing experience with transjugular intrahepatic portal-systemic stent has highlighted the risks and benefits associated with its use: its precise role in the management of variceal hemorrhage is still under examination.

Current Opinion in Gastroenterology 1994, **10**:295–302

Pathophysiology

Portal hypertension arises from a combination of increased portal vascular resistance and a variable rise in venous inflow. The latter is part of the hyperdynamic state, seen in all forms of portal hypertension. Arteriolar vasodilation may be the initial event leading to sodium retention and plasma volume expansion; the end result is a decrease in peripheral resistance with a high cardiac output, features of the hyperdynamic state. In support of this hypothesis, octreotide, an arterial vasoconstrictor agent, corrected the vasodilation and sodium retention seen in rats after partial portal vein ligation at doses that did not affect arterial pressure or the extracellular sodium space in normal rats [1]. An alternative view emphasizes the expansion of plasma volume (owing to sodium retention) as the primary event that leads to arteriolar vasodilation [2•].

Nitric oxide, derived from L-arginine by the action of nitric oxide synthase, may be the endogenous mediator of the peripheral arteriolar vasodilation. Released by vascular endothelium, it diffuses into vascular smooth muscle and results in relaxation via the activation of cyclic GMP [3••]. Specific inhibitors of nitric oxide synthesis correct the peripheral vasodilation seen in a portal hypertensive rat model [4]. Furthermore, such an antagonist can reduce the extent of portal-systemic shunting in the absence of changes in portal pressure, suggesting that nitric oxide may be involved in the genesis of the collateral circulation [5]. The unstable nature of nitric oxide precludes its easy measurement; it is rapidly converted to serum nitrite and nitrate, whose levels are increased in cirrhotic patients [6•]. By administering colistin (a nonabsorbable antibiotic with antiendotoxin activity) to 15 patients, both endotoxin, nitrite, and nitrate levels were reduced. The authors propose that endotoxin may be the trigger that increases nitric oxide synthesis in portal hypertensive subjects (Fig. 1).

Abbreviation

TIPS—transjugular intrahepatic portal systemic stent.

 ISBN 1-85922-608-6 ISSN 0267–1379

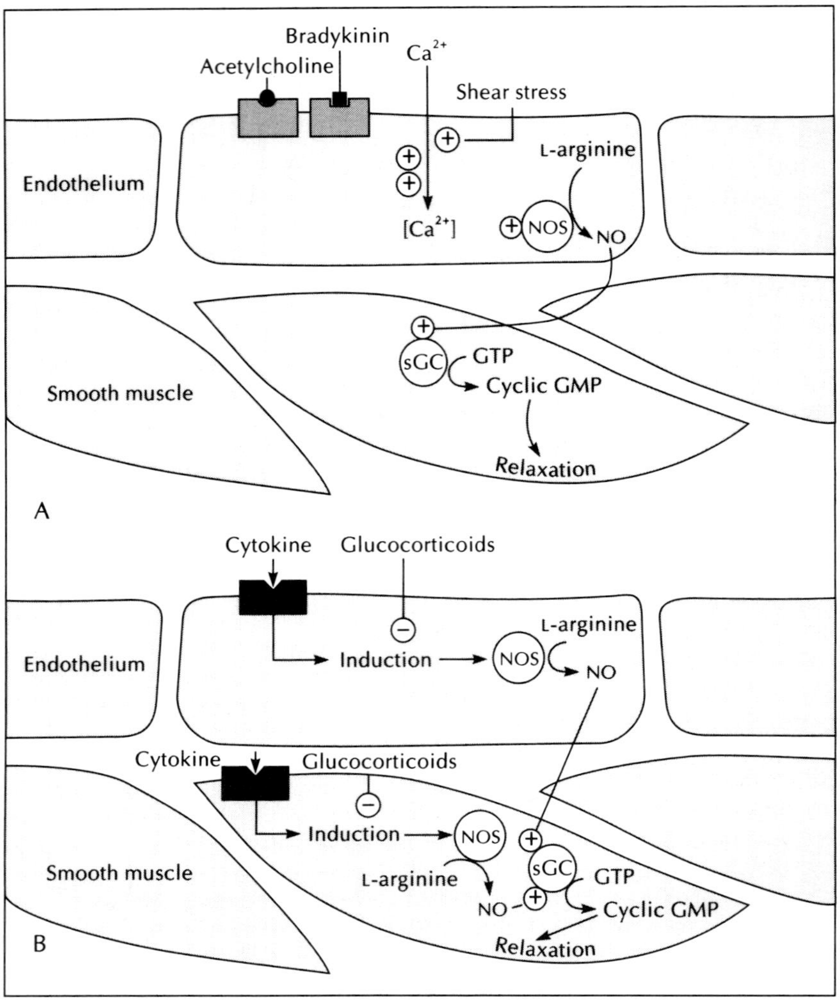

Fig. 1. A, Binding of vasodilators to endothelial receptors or shear stress activate nitric oxide synthase (NOS) via a calcium-mediated pathway. Nitric oxide (NO) is generated from L-arginine, and diffuses into vascular smooth muscle to cause relaxation after activation of soluble guanylate cyclase (sGC) and generation of cyclic GMP. **B**, In portal hypertension, endotoxin [6•] or tumor necrosis factor [82] may be the initial trigger that results in NO production. The role of glucocorticoids is uncertain. (*Adapted from* Moncada and Higgs [3••]; with permission.)

Other mediators continue to be sought. Prostaglandins, acting via independent mechanisms from nitric oxide, may play a pathogenic role in gastric [7] and splanchnic [8] hyperemia; prostacyclin may be one of such compounds [9] whose levels are increased in humans with portal-systemic shunting [10]. Bile salts can induce splanchnic vasodilation at the high levels seen in cirrhotic rats [11]. Even more puzzling, the administration during the neonatal period of capsaicin, an agent that induces afferent nerve denervation, prevents development of the hyperdynamic circulation when portal hypertension is induced during adulthood [12•]. If confirmed, the source of the afferent signals would have to be sought. In rats, the cerebral circulation does not participate in this hyperdynamic state [13].

Regardless of its cause, peripheral arterial vasodilation is associated with a decreased response to vasoconstrictive agents. This was confirmed in the intestinal circulation of portal hypertensive rats [14] and observed in the isolated forearm circulation *in vivo* in stable alcoholic cirrhotics [15]. This hyporesponsiveness to pressor agents was more pronounced in aged portal hypertensive animals [16•], raising the question as to whether older cirrhotics are less responsive to pharmacologic agents.

Clinical aspects

Portal hypertension can arise from multiple causes and can be classified according to the site of resistance to portal flow. A common cause of prehepatic portal hypertension in certain geographic areas is the so-called "idiopathic portal hypertension" [17]. A careful histologic study of 25 biopsy specimens of Japanese patients revealed changes in both the portal triads and the parenchyma [18•]. Phlebosclerosis and fibro-elastosis of the stroma was seen in the portal areas; curiously, capillary and necroinflammatory bridging disturbed the lobular architecture, including evidence of early nodular regeneration in 25% of the cases. Incomplete septal cirrhosis may be a late manifestation of idiopathic portal hypertension.

Portal hypertension in lymphoproliferative disorders arise from the combined effects of a high splenic (and hence portal) flow, together with an increased presinusoidasl resistance site [19]. In another study, 20 patients with portal vein thrombosis, no evidence of liver disease and portal-systemic shunts had evidence of a compensated, mild disseminated intravascular coagulation with activation of fibrinolysis [20]. A high prevalence of rectal varices, with 15% of them bleeding, was seen in 116 patients with extrahepatic portal hypertension [21]. Otherwise, many signs of portal hypertension can be absent, and ultrasound can aid in the diagnosis of extrahepatic portal hypertension [22].

A case report highlights the association of portal and pulmonary hypertension in a patient with multiple focal nodular hyperplasia of the liver [23].

Investigation

A diverse array of technology is increasingly used to examine the portal hypertensive state. At a time when understanding the natural history of varices in cirrhosis has led to measures to prevent the first hemorrhage [24••], less invasive but accurate methods to detect the presence of varices are being sought. Endoscopic ultrasonography is superior to conventional endoscopy in the diagnosis of gastric varices [25]; at this time, this expensive technology is not as useful for the diagnosis of esophageal varices. For the latter, a transnasal thin endoluminal ultrasound appears more sensitive than conventional endoscopy [26] and may prove extremely useful to screen cirrhotic individuals. Another version of an endoscopic capsule has been tested with a satisfactory ability to measure variceal pressure [27]. For the iconoclast, a study reevaluated the utility of the barium swallow [28]; in 47 patients, the length and the width of the folds representing varices on barium swallow correlated well with the degree of varices on endoscopy.

The ability to predict the presence of esophageal varices has been examined in different diseases. In hepatosplenic schistosomiasis, an ultrasound score that incorporates periportal vein changes and diameter, spleen size, and the echographic detection of collaterals had good specificity in predicting the presence of esophageal varices [29]; it was not used in cirrhotic individuals. In the latter subjects, a higher splenic than portal venous flow, as measured by Doppler ultrasound [30], indicated the presence of portal-systemic collaterals; however, limitations in the accuracy of flow measurements with Doppler have not been fully resolved. In Japan, where a thin body habitus makes ultrasound insonation easier, reversal of flow in the left gastric vein was a good predictor of the presence of esophageal varices [31]. Transvaginal sonography was used to detect the presence of rectal and pararectal varices in female patients with different portal hypertensive etiologies [32]. Application of all these techniques to primary prophylaxis of variceal bleeding is still in its infancy.

Phase-contrast cine magnetic resonance angiography can provide anatomic detail [33] and estimation of flow [34]. The use of contrast agents for computed tomography can be problematic in cirrhotic patients with ascites, and magnetic resonance angiography can be useful in this setting.

Portal hypertensive gastropathy

Although iron-deficiency anemia from chronic bleeding is the usual presentation of portal hypertensive gastropathy, a small number of patients have an acute presentation [35•]. This is likely to recur and may evolve into a chronic picture. Pharmacologic therapy with propranolol may improve the picture by reducing portal hypertension. Splenic arterial embolization has been shown to reduce gastric hemoglobin content, a reflection of gastric blood flow [36]. The safety of splenic embolization to treat hypersplenism [37] needs to be confirmed in other centers; this question is of importance in view of the use of interferon in cirrhotic patients with chronic viral hepatitis.

An area of striking controversy is the nature of gastric mucosal perfusion in portal hypertensive gastropathy. Using similar techniques, laser Doppler flowmetry and reflectance spectrophotometry, two groups have reached diametrically opposite conclusions [38,39•]. It is difficult to reconcile the notion of a reduced mucosal flow [38] when splanchnic inflow is actually increased; the increased perfusion, related to some of the humoral mediators previously discussed, has been reported to decrease with propranolol administration [39•].

Changes in jejunal biopsies in cirrhotic patients, with increase in size and number of vessels, has been termed congestive jejunopathy [40].

Pharmacologic therapy

Pharmacologic agents are now widely used in the treatment of acute bleeding, in the prophylaxis of the first hemorrhage and in the prevention of rebleeding [41,42]. Investigations continue on the mechanisms by which these drugs may be effective in portal hypertension. Many of the agents used were shown to reduce intravariceal pressure. In a double-blind investigation, propranolol reduced intravariceal pressure from a mean of 13.1 to 10.2 mm Hg [43]. In eight of 37 subjects, there was no decrease in hepatic venous pressure gradient with propranolol; however, four of these subjects had a reduction (>10%) in intravariceal pressure. Thus, some individuals will have reductions in intravariceal pressure that are not detected by hepatic venous pressure measurements. Both vasopressin [44] and nitroglycerin [45] were shown to significantly reduce intravariceal pressure; this was not the case with metoclopramide [45], an agent thought to reduce variceal pressure by increasing the pressure of the lower esophageal sphincter.

For the treatment of acute variceal hemorrhage, somatostatin and its long-acting analogue, octreotide, have received increasing attention [46]. In a detailed hemodynamic study in patients with hepatitis B–related cirrhosis, somatostatin (250-mg bolus with a 250 mg/h infusion) was associated with a reduction in portal pressure [47]. Vasoconstrictive effects were seen, also confirmed with octreotide by a reduction in superior arterial mesenteric blood flow using intra-arterial Doppler catheters [48]. When compared with sclerotherapy in a randomized controlled trial of 84 patients in Hong Kong, octreotide (in infusion followed by subcutaneous injections) was a efficacious as the endoscopic therapy in controlling hemorrhage (67% vs 72%) as well as in transfusion needs [49••]. Also, octreotide was slightly more effective in controlling acute hemorrhage than the combination of a vasopressin analogue (terlipressin) and nitroglycerin in a multicenter randomized trial in France [50••]. Vasopressin could be effective in variceal hemorrhage via binding to both V_1 (in vascular smooth muscle) and V_2 (procoagulant effects) receptors; the addition of desmopressin, a V_2 receptor analogue, did not result in additional control of variceal hemorrhage as seen with terlipressin alone [51].

For the chronic treatment of portal hypertension, efficacy of therapy is greater when portal pressure is reduced by 20% or more [52]. New approaches include the development of combination therapy. A new agent that combines the effects of β-blockers with those of nitrates, nipradilol, was tested in portal hypertensive rats [53]. The addition of isosorbide dinitrate to propranolol, although potentiating the reduction of portal pressure seen with the latter, resulted in greater problems with management of ascites [54]. Indeed, the acute administration of isosorbide-5-mononitrate was associated with a 20% reduction of glomerular filtration rate [55]. Most of the drugs used in the treatment of portal hypertension have renal effects [56••]; those that reduce arterial pressure (such as nitrates) may be especially prone to worsening of renal status.

A reduction of plasma volume may be a new therapeutic approach. In 15 subjects, a 4-week course of 100 mg/d of spironolactone reduced the portal pressure gradient from a mean of 16.5 to 12.9 mm Hg, with an approximate 10% reduction in plasma volume [57•]; furosemide, at 40 mg/d, had no effects. Ritanserin, a serotonin S_2 receptor antagonist, was further evaluated in rats with secondary biliary cirrhosis showing a clear portal hypotensive effect [58].

Prevention of rebleeding

Sclerotherapy

Endoscopic treatment is the mainstay of therapy in many centers [59]. When compared with propranolol, sclerotherapy was significantly more efficacious, with rebleeding occurring in 37 of 58 patients of the propranolol group as compared with 26 of 58 in the sclerotherapy patients [60•]. However, complications of sclerotherapy were more frequent and severe, some of which were documented in a consecutive series of patients with alcoholic cirrhosis [61]. Three studies examined the potential benefits of adding propranolol to chronic sclerotherapy. In one study from Athens [62], the combination group was not only more efficacious in preventing bleeding from esophageal varices, but patients were also less likely to bleed from congestive gastropathy and gastric varices compared with

Table 1. Comparison of sclerotherapy with variceal band ligation in acute bleeding and prevention of rebleeding

Site of study and therapy used*	Patients, *n*	Alcoholic, %	Child's C class, %	Active bleeding, %	Bleeding controlled, %	Recurrent bleeding, %	Mean sessions to obliteration, *n*	Complications, %	Complications due to bleeding, %
Denver [68]									
SCT	65	80	20	20	77	48	5	22	12
VBL	64	82	17	22	86	36	4	2†	4
London [67••]									
SCT	54	45	28	39	81	53	4.9	69	63‡
VBL	49	52	24	47	82	30†	3.5†	57	48‡
Los Angeles [66]									
SCT	39	77	13	23	89	31	6.2	56	8
VBL	38	82	34†	24	89	24	4.1†	24†	8

*Numbers in brackets represent reference numbers.
†Significant from sclerotherapy
‡Either dead or withdrawn from transplantation.
SCT—sclerotherapy; VBL—variceal band ligation.

the patients on sclerotherapy alone (total 22 bleeding episodes in 45 patients vs 35 episodes in 40 patients, $P<0.012$). However, in two studies, from Taiwan and New Delhi, propranolol did not confer additional benefits [63,64]. Omeprazole was useful in the healing of postsclerotherapy esophageal ulcerations [65•].

Variceal band ligation

The past year saw the publication of two randomized controlled trials of variceal band ligation versus sclerotherapy in the prevention of rebleeding [66,67••], which can be compared with the initial study from Colorado [68] (Table 1). The three reports do not coincide in the statistically favorable effects of banding: a reduced incidence of rebleeding [67••], a decrease in the number of complications [66], or an increased survival (Fig. 2) [68] in the banding group. All three studies note a reduced number of sessions required to obliterate varices with banding. Prophylactic banding (Fig. 3) has also been reported [69], though not rigorously compared with pharmacologic therapy. A postmortem analysis has confirmed the mechanism by which banding is effective: strangulation of the tissue with subsequent thrombosis of the submucosal varix [70]. Ulcerations may be present; though they are seldom deep as with sclerotherapy, they may be associated with hemorrhage [71].

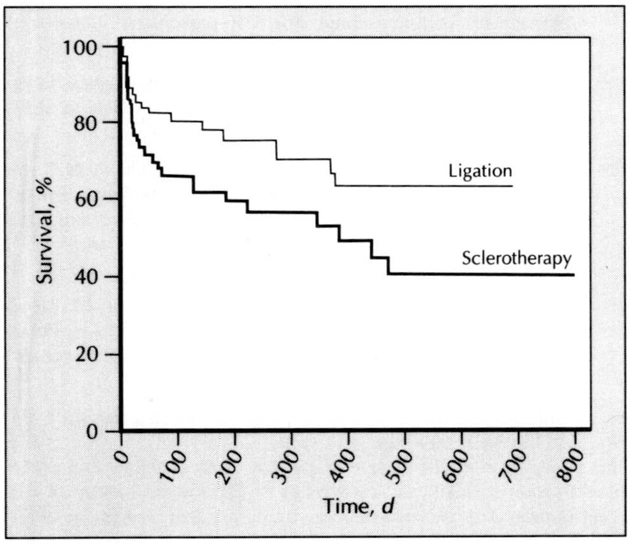

Fig. 2. Survival was significantly better with band ligation compared with sclerotherapy. Two other trials [66,67••] did not show such benefit. (*From* Stiegmann *et al.* [68]; with permission.)

Transjugular intrahepatic portal-systemic stent

Enthusiasm with transjugular intrahepatic portal-systemic stent (TIPS), a nonsurgical approach to the treatment of variceal bleeding [72••], has been tempered by the observation of complications (especially at the initial stage), stenosis of the effluent hepatic vein in 8% to 10% of the cases, as well as occlusion of the shunt in a similar number [72••,73–75]. In one series, 25 patients were actively bleeding at the time of TIPS; in a quarter bleeding could not be controlled [74]. Hepatic encephalopathy, as expected in a side-to-side portacaval shunt, occurred in up to 20% of individuals. Controlled trials comparing TIPS with other therapeutic modalities are eagerly awaited. In the meantime, technical refinements continue to be developed [76].

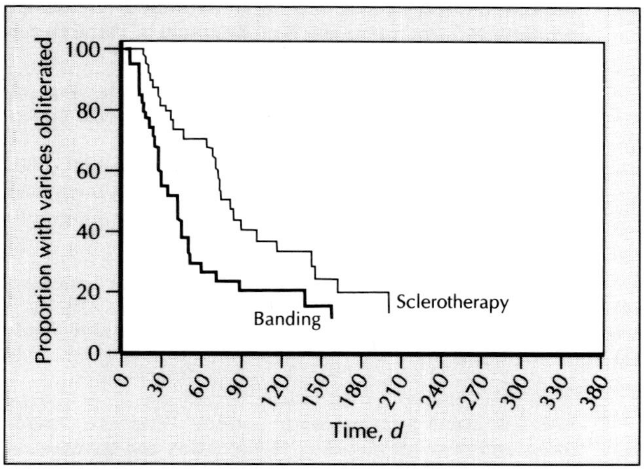

Fig. 3. Time to obliteration of varices was reduced with banding as compared with sclerotherapy. (*From* Gimson *et al.* [67••]; with permission.)

Surgery

Shunt surgery, especially the distal splenorenal shunt and the small diameter interposition portacaval graft, is still a viable option for patients with compensated cirrhosis [77]. A final report of a controlled trial in a nonurban area showed an increased benefit of surgery over sclerotherapy [78•]; long geographic distances conspire against an endoscopic treatment that requires multiple sessions. Patients over 60 years of age with compensated liver function tolerate this surgery well [79].

Portal hypertension and liver transplantation

In a large series, a prior variceal hemorrhage did not impact adversely on the survival after liver transplantation [80]. Variceal hemorrhage is not an indication per se for replacement of the cirrhotic liver; however, its occurrence may precipitate additional acute problems (infection, liver decompensation) that may worsen the outcome in individual subjects. This view has led to a comparison of prophylactic versus therapeutic endoscopy in patients awaiting liver transplantation [81]. Fewer complications of sclerotherapy were seen in the prophylactic setting; the optimal prophylactic treatment in this setting has not been defined.

References and recommended reading

Papers of particular interest, published within the annual period of review, have been highlighted as:
- • Of special interest
- •• Of outstanding interest

1. Albillos A, Colombato LA, Lee FY, Groszmann RJ: **Octreotide Ameliorates Vasodilation and NA+ Retention in Portal Hypertensive Rats**. *Gastroenterology* 1993, **104**:575–579.

2. • Wong F, Massio D, Colman J, Dudley F: **Glomerular Hyperfiltration in Patients With Well-Compensated Alcoholic Cirrhosis**. *Gastroenterology* 1993, **104**:884–889.

Although the study by Albillos *et al.* (*Gastroenterology* 1993, 104:575–579) was is in rats and this study was in humans, the papers reflect two sides of a key controversy that encompasses pathogenesis of both ascites and portal hypertension.

3. •• Moncada S, Higgs A: **Mechanisms of Disease: The l-Arginine-Nitric Oxide Pathway**. *N Engl J Med* 1993, **329**:2002–2012.

A review that encompasses many areas in biology where nitric oxide has been implicated.

4. Lee FY, Colombato LA, Albillos A, Groszmann RJ: **N Omega-Nitro-L-Arginine Administration Corrects Peripheral Vasodilation and Systemic Capillary Hypotension and Ameliorates Plasma Volume Expansion and Sodium Retention in Portal Hypertensive Rats**. *Hepatology* 1993, **17**:84–90.

5. Lee, F-Y, Colombato A, Albillos A, Groszmann R: **Administration of N^{w}-Nitro-L-Arginine Ameliorates Portal-Systemic Shunting in Portal-Hypertensive Rats**. *Gastroenterology* 1993, **105**:1464–1470.

6. • Guarner C, Soriano G, Tomas A, Bulbena O, Novella MT, Balanzo J, Villardell F, Mourelle M, Moncada S: **Increased Serum Nitrite and Nitrate Levels in Patients With Cirrhosis: Relationship to Endotoxemia**. *Hepatology* 1993, **18**:1139–1143.

Indirect evidence to support increased nitric oxide synthesis in cirrhotic patients as a result of endotoxinemia. Colistin, an antiendotoxin antibody, reduced nitrate and nitrite levels, though hemodynamic studies were not performed to assess a potential reversal of the hyperdynamic state.

7. Casadevall M, Panes J, Pique JM, Marroni N, Bosch J, Whittle BJ: **Involvement of Nitric Oxide and Prostaglandins in Gastric Mucosal Hyperemia of Portal-Hypertensive Anesthetized Rats**. *Hepatology* 1993, **18**:628–634.

8. Wu Y, Bums RC, Sitzmann JV: **Effects of Nitric Oxide and Cyclooxygenase Inhibitation on Splanchnic Hemodynamics in Portal Hypertension**. *Hepatology* 1993, **18**:1416–1421.

9. Oberti F, Sogni P, Cailmail S, Moreau R, Pipy B, Lebrec D: **Role of Prostacyclin in Hemodynamic Alterations in Conscious Rats With Extrahepatic Or Intrahepatic Portal Hypertension**. *Hepatology* 1993, **18**:621–627.

10. Sitzmann JV, Campbell KA, Wu Y, Cameron JL: **Effect of Portosystemic Shunting on PG12 and Glucagon Levels in Humans**. *Ann Surg* 1993, **217**:248–252.

11. Pak JM, Lee SS: **Vasoactive Effects of Bile Salts in Cirrhotic Rats: *In Vivo* and *In Vitro* Studies**. *Hepatology* 1993, **18**:1175–1181.

12. • Lee SS, Sharkey KA: **Capsaicin Treatment Blocks Development of Hyperkinetic Circulation in Portal Hypertensive and Cirrhotic Rats**. *Am J Physiol* 1993, **264**:G868–873.

A provocative, well-designed study that implicates afferent nerve signals probably emanating from the portal hypertensive liver in the pathogenesis of the hyperdynamic circulation.

13. Srivastava A, Gottstein J, Blei AT: **Cerebral Blood Flow and the Hyperdynamic Circulation of Rats After Portacaval Anastomosis**. *J Hepatol* 1993, **17**:15–19.

14. John T, Granger DN, Benoit JN: **Endogenous Vasoconstrictor Tone in Intestine of Normal and Portal Hypertensive Rats**. *Am J Physiol* 1993, **264**:H171–177.

15. Ryan J, Sudhir K, Jennings G, Esler M, Dudley F: **Impaired Reactivity of the Peripheral Vasculature to Pressor Agents in Alcoholic Cirrhosis**. *Gastroenterology* 1993, **105**:1167–1172.

16. • Polio J, Sieber CC, Lerner E, Groszmann RJ: **Cardiovascular Hyporesponsiveness to Norepinephrine, Propranolol, and Nitroglycerin in Portal-Hypertensive and Aged Rats**. *Hepatology* 1993, **18**:128–136.

Aging has been shown to alter normal cardiovascular responsiveness, especially to adrenergic stimuli. In older portal hypertensive rats, norepinephrine caused less vasoconstriction than in younger counterparts. It is worth examining whether the effects of propranolol are different in an older cirrhotic population.

17. Ludwig J, Hashimoto E, Obata H, Baldus WP: **Idiopathic Portal Hypertension**. *Hepatology* 1993, **17**:1157–1162.

18. • Ludwig J, Hashimoto E, Obata H, Baldus WP: **Idiopathic Portal Hypertension; a Histopathological Study of 26 Japanese Cases**. *Histopathology* 1993, **22**:227–234.

A distinct histologic entity is described in patients from Japan, suggesting more than a vascular insult in its pathogenesis. It Is unclear whether idiopathic portal hypertension in other areas of the world exhibits the same histologic changes.

19. Dubois A, Dauzat M, Pignodel C, Pomier-Layrargues G, Marty-Double C, Lopez FM, Janbon C: **Portal Hypertension in Lymphoproliferative and Myeloproliferative Disorders: Hemodynamic and Histological Correlations**. *Hepatology* 1993, **17**:246–250.

20. Robson SC, Kahn D, Kruskal J, Bird AR, Kirsch E: **Disordered Hemostasis in Extrahepatic Portal Hypertension**. *Hepatology* 1993, **18**:853–857.

21. Pai CG, Thomas V, Hariharan M, Nair KV: **Rectal Varices in Extrahepatic Portal Hypertension**. *J Gastroenterol Hepatol* 1993, **8**:244–246.

22. Sugiura N, Matsutani S, Ohto M, Ebara M, Yoshikawa M, Yamaguchi T, Okuda K, Miki M: **Extrahepatic Portal Vein Obstruction in Adults Detected by Ultrasound With Frequent Lack of Portal Hypertension Signs**. *J Gastroenterol Hepatol* 1993, **8**:161–167.

23. Portmann B, Stewart S, Higenbottam TW, Clayton PT, Lloyd JK, Williams R: **Nodular Transformation of the Liver Associated With Portal and Pulmonary Arterial Hypertension**. *Gastroenterology* 1993, **104**:616–621.

24. •• Burroughs AK: **The Natural History of Varices**. *J Hepatol* 1993, **17(Suppl 2)**:510–513.

The ability to alter the course of patients with cirrhosis and portal hypertension is based on knowledge of the natural history of this complication. This review article encompasses several decades of important clinical observations.

25. Boustiere C, Dumas O, Jouffre C, Letard JC, Patouillard B, Etaix JP, Barthelemy C, Audigier JC: **Endoscopic Ultrasonography Classification of Gastric Varices in Patients With Cirrhosis. Comparison With Endoscopic Findings**. *J Hepatol* 1993, **19**:268–272.

26. Liu JB, Miller LS, Feld RI, Barbarevech CA, Noodleman L, Goldberg BB: **Gastric and Esophageal Varices: 20-MHz Transnasal Endoluminal US**. *Radiology* 1993, **187**:363–366.

27. Gertsch P, Fischer G, Kleber G, Wheatley AM, Geigenberger G, Sauerbruch T: **Manometry of Esophageal Varices: Comparison of an Endoscopic Balloon Technique With Needle Puncture**. *Gastroenterology* 1993, **105**:1159–1166.

28. Ginai AZ, van Buuren HR, Hop WC, Schlolm SW: **Oesophageal Varices: How Reliable Is a Barium Swallow?** *Br J Radiol* 1993, **56**:322–326.

29. Abdel-Wahab MF, Esmat G, Farrag A, al-Boracy Y, Strickland GT: **Ultrasonographic Prediction of Esophageal Varices in Schistosomiasis Manoni.** *Am J Gastroenterol* 1993, **88**:560–563.

30. Nelson RC, Sharbourne GM, Spencer HB, Chazmar JL: **Splenic Venous Flow Exceeding Portal Venous Flow at Doppler Sonography: Relationship to Portosystemic Varices.** *AJR Am J Roentgenol* 1993, **161**:563–567.

31. Matsutani S, Furuse J, Ishii H, Mizumoto H, Kimura K, Ohto M: **Hemodynamics of the Left Gastric Vein in Portal Hypertension.** *Gastroenterology* 1993, **105**:513–518.

32. Malde H, Nagral A, Shah P, Joshi MS, Bhatia SJ, Abraham P: **Detection of Rectal and Pararectal Varices in Patients With Portal Hypertension: Efficacy of Transvaginal Sonography.** *AJR Am J Roentgenol* 1993, **161**:335–337.

33. Burkart DJ, Johnson CD, Morton MJ, Ehman RL: **Phase-Contrast Cine MR Angiography in Chronic Liver Disease.** *Radiology* 1993, **187**:407–412.

34. Burkart DJ, Johnson CD, Ehman RL, Weaver AL, Ilstrup DM: **Evaluation of Portal Venous Hypertension With Cine Phase-Contrast MR Flow Measurements: High Association of Hyperdynamic Portal Flow With Variceal Hemorrhage.** *Radiology* 1993, **188**:643–648.

35. • Gostout CJ, Viggiano TR, Balm RK: **Acute Gastrointestinal Bleeding From Portal-Hypertensive Gastropathy: Prevalence and Clinical Features.** *Am J Gastroenterol* 1993, **88**:2030–2034.

A rare presentation of portal hypertensive gastropathy is well described.

36. Ohmagari K, Toyonaga A, Tanikawa K: **Effects of Transcatheter Splenic Arterial Embolization on Portal Hypertensive Gastric Mucosa.** *Am J Gastroenterol* 1993, **88**:1837–1841.

37. Sangro B, Bilbao I, Herraro I, Corolla C, Longo J, Beloqui O, Ruiz J, Zozaya JM: **Partial Splenic Embolization for the Treatment of Hypersplenism in Cirrhosis.** *Hepatology* 1993, 19:309–314.

38. Iwao T, Toyonaga A, Ikegami M, Oho K, Sumino M, Harada H, Sakaki M, Shigemori H, Aoki T, Tanikawa K: **Reduced Gastric Mucosal Blood Flow in Patients With Portal-Hypertensive Gastropathy.** *Hepatology* 1993, **18**:36–40.

39. • Panes J, Bordas JM, Pique JM, Garcia-Pagan JC, Feu F, Teres J, Bosch, Rodes J: **Effects of Propranolol on Gastric Mucosal Perfusion in Cirrhotic Patients With Portal Hypertensive Gastropathy.** *Hepatology* 1993, **17**:213–218.

How could two groups using the same technology arrive at diametrically opposite conclusions as to the nature of gastric mucosal perfusion in cirrhosis? Hemoglobin values affect readings with laser Doppler velocimetry, but this may not be the full explanation.

40. Nagral AS, Joshi AS, Bhatia SJ, Abraham P, Mistry FP, Vora IM: **Congestive Jejunopathy in Portal Hypertension.** *Gut* 1993, 34:694–697.

41. Blei AT: **Pharmacological Therapy for Portal Hypertension.** *Probl Gen Surg* 1992, 9:415–430.

42. Lebrec D: **Pharmacologic Prevention of Variceal Bleeding and Rebleeding.** *J Hepatol* 1993, **17**:S29–S33.

43. Feu F, Bordas JM, Luca A, Garcia-Pagan JC, Escorsell A, Bosch J, Rodes J: **Reduction of Variceal Pressure by Propranolol: Comparison of the Effects on Portal Pressure and Azygos Blood Flow in Patients With Cirrhosis.** *Hepatology* 1993, **18**:1082–1089.

44. Chao Y, Wang SS, Loo FY, Lin HC, Lo GH, Tsai YT, Lee SD: **Measurement of Intravariceal Pressure by Fine Needle Direct Puncture in Hepatitis B Surface Antigen-Positive Cirrhotic Patients: The Effect of Vasopressin.** *J Gastroenterol Hepatol* 1993, **8**:157–160.

45. Saraya A, Sarin SK: **Effects of Intravenous Nitroglycerin and Metoclopramide on Intravariceal Pressure: a Double-Blind, Randomized Study.** *Am J Gastroenterol* 1993, **88**:1850–1854.

46. Cello JP, Chan MF: **Octreotide Therapy for Variceal Hemorrhage.** *Digestion* 1993, **54(Suppl 1)**:20–25.

47. Hsia HC, Lin HC, Lee FY, Tsai YT, Lee SD, Meng HC, Chao Y, Wang SS, Lo KJ: **Changes of Hepatic and Systemic Haemodynamics Following Somatostatin Administration in Patients With Hepatitis B-Related Cirrhosis.** *J Gastroenterol Hepatol* 1993, 9:15–20.

48. McCormick PA, Seifalian AM, Stansby G, McGann G, Collins P, Chin J, McIntyre N, Dick R, Burroughs AK: **Superior Mesenteric Artery Blood Flow in Man Measured With Intra-Arterial Doppler Catheters: Effect of Octreotide.** *J Hepatol* 1993, 17:20–27.

49. •• Sung JJ, Chung SC, Lai CW, Chan FK, Leung JW, Yung MY, Kastianides O, Li AK: **Octreotide Infusion or Emergency Sclerotherapy for Variceal Haemorrhage.** *Lancet* 1993, 342:637–641.

In subsequent correspondence, the statistical analysis of this study was severely criticized. However, a Spanish cooperative trial (*Hepatology* 1993, 18:383A) showed similar effectiveness of somatostatin to sclerotherapy in the control of acute bleeding.

50. •• Silvain C, Carpantier S, Sautoreau D, Ozornichow B, Motreau JM, Fort E, Ingrand P, Boyer J, Pillegand B, Doffel M, *et al.*: **Terlipressin Plus Transdermal Nitroglycerin Vs Octreotide in the Control of Acute Bleeding From Esophageal Varices: a Multicenter Randomized Trial.** *Hepatology* 1993, **18**:61–65.

Terlipressin is simpler to administer (single injection) than its parent compound, vasopressin; no other differences are obvious. Combination with nitroglycerin is standard therapy in many centers; again, octreotide was as effective, if not better.

51. DeFranchis R, Arcidiacono PG, Carpinelli L, Andreoni B, Cestari L, Brunati S, Zambelli A, Battaglia G, Mannucci PM, and The New Italian Endoscopic Club: **Randomized Controlled Trial of Desmopressin Plus Terlipressin Vs Terlipressin Alone for the Treatment of Acute Variceal Hemorrhage in Cirrhotic Patients: a Multicenter, Double-Blind Study.** *Hepatology* 1993, 18:1102–1107.

52. Bosch J, Garcia-Pagan JC, Feu F, Luca A, Fernandez M, Pizcueta P, Rodes J: **New Approaches in the Pharmacologic Treatment of Portal Hypertension.** *J Hepatol* 1993, **17**:S41–S45.

53. Ohsuga M, Cailmail S, Lebrec D: **Hemodynamic Effects of Nipradilol, a New Beta-Adrenergic Antagonist Combined With a Nitroxy Base, in Rats With Intra- Or Extra-Hepatic Portal Hypertension.** *J Hepatol* 1993, 17:236–240.

54. Vorobioff J, Picabea E, Gamen M, Villavicencio R, Bordato J, Bessone F, Tanno H, Palazzi J, Sarano H, Pozzoli L, *et al.*: **Propranolol Compared With Propranolol Plus Isosorbide Dinitrate in Portal-Hypertensive Patients: Long-Term Hemodynamic and Renal Effects.** *Hepatology* 1993, **18**:477–484.

55. Salmeron JM, Ruiz del Arbol L, Gines A, Garcia-Pagan JC, Gines P, Feu F, Claria J, Rivera F, Bosch J, Arroyo V, *et al.*: **Renal Effects of Acute Isosorbide-5-Mononitrate Administration in Cirrhosis.** *Hepatology* 1993, 17:800–806.

56. •• Henriksen JH, Ring-Larsen H: **Renal Effects of Drugs Used in the Treatment of Portal Hypertension [Editorial].** *Hepatology* 1993, **18**:688–695.

A review of pharmacologic therapy that emphasizes the impact of pharmacologic agents in the relation between the hemodynamic derangement that leads to variceal hemorrhage and that of ascites.

57. • Katsuta Y, Aramaki T, Sekiyama T, Satomura K, Okumura K: **Plasma Volume Contraction in Portal Hypertension.** *J Hepatol* 1993, 17:S19–S23.

A new approach to the treatment of portal hypertension may be the combination of propranolol with spironolactone.

58. Fernandez M, Pizcueta P, Garcia-Pagan JC, Feu F, Cirera I, Bosch J, Rodes J: **Effects of Ritanserin, a Selective and Specific S2-Serotonergic Antagonist, on Portal Pressure and Splanchnic Hemodynamics in Rats With Long-Term Bile Duct Ligation.** *Hepatology* 1993, **18**:389–393.

59. Westaby D: **The Management of Active Variceal Bleeding.** *J Hepatol* 1993, **17**:S34–S37.

60. Teres J, Bosch J, Bordas JM, Garcia-Pagan JC, Feu F, Cirera I, Rodes J: **Propranolol Versus Sclerotherapy in Preventing Variceal Rebleeding: a Randomized Controlled Trial.** *Gastroenterology* 1993, **105**:1508–1514.
•
The choice of propranolol vs. sclerotherapy to prevent variceal rebleeding may need to be reexamined with the widespread acceptance of the practicing community of variceal band ligation.

61. Pugh S, Lewis S, Ross Smith P: **Bleeding Esophageal Varices in Alcoholic Cirrhosis: Long-Term Follow-Up of Endoscopic Sclerotherapy.** *Q J Med* 1993, **86**:241–245.

62. Avgerinos A, Rekoumis G, Klonis C, Papadimitriou N, Gouma P, Pournaras S, Raptis S: **Propranolol in the Prevention of Recurrent Upper Gastrointestinal Bleeding in Patients With Cirrhosis Undergoing Endoscopic Sclerotherapy. A Randomized Controlled Trial.** *J Hepatol* 1993, **19**:301–311.

63. Acharya SK, Dasarathy S, Saksena S, Pande JN: **A Prospective Randomized Study to Evaluate Propranolol in Patients Undergoing Long-Term Endoscopic Sclerotherapy.** *J Hepatol* 1993, **19**:291–300.

64. Lo GH, Loi KH, Loo SD, Tsai YT, Lo KJ: **Does Propranolol Maintain Post-Sclerotherapy Variceal Obliteration? A Prospective Randomized Study.** *J Gastroenterol Hepatol* 1993, **8**:359–362.

65. Shepherd H, Barkin JS: **Omeprazole Heals Mucosal Ulcers Associated With Endoscopic Injection Sclerotherapy.** *Gastrointest Endosc* 1993, **39**:474–475.
•
Confirmation that complete acid suppression may be useful to prevent bleeding from esophageal ulcers induced by sclerotherapy.

66. Laine L, al-Nowihi HM, Migikovsky B, Sloane R, Garcia F: **Endoscopic Ligation Compared With Sclerotherapy for the Treatment of Bleeding Esophageal Varices.** *Ann Intern Med* 1993, **119**:11–17.

67. Gimson AE, Ramage JK, Panos MZ, Hayllar K, Harrison PM, Williams R, Westaby D: **Randomized Trial of Variceal Banding Ligation Versus Injection Sclerotherapy for Bleeding Esophageal Varices.** *Lancet* 1993, **342**:391–394.
••

68. Sticgmann GV, Goff JS, Michaletz-Onody PA, Korula J, Lieberman D, Saeed ZA, Reveille RM, Sun J, Lowenstein SR: **Endoscopic Sclerotherapy As Compared With Endoscopic Ligation for Bleeding Esophageal Varices.** *N Engl J Med* 1992, **32S**:1527–1532.

69. Hashizumo M, Ohta M, Uono K, Tanouc K, Kitano S, Sugimachi K: **Endoscopic Ligation of Esophageal Varices Compared With Injection Sclerotherapy; a Prospective Randomized Trial.** *Gastrointest Endosc* 1993, **39**:123–125.

70. Marks RD, Arnold MD, Baron TH: **Gross and Microscopic Findings in the Human Esophagus After Esophageal Variceal Band Ligation: a Postmortem Analysis.** *Am J Gastroenterol* 1993, **88**:272–274.

71. Young MF, Sanowski RA, Rasche R: **Comparison and Characterization of Ulcerations Induced by Endoscopic Ligation of Esophageal Varices Versus Endoscopic Sclerotherapy.** *Gastrointest Endosc* 1993, **39**:119–122.

72. Conn HO: **Transjugular Intrahepatic Portal-Systemic Shunts: the State of the Art.** *Hepatology* 1993, **17**:148–158.
••
A review that encompasses technical aspects, clinical results, and complications of this procedure.

73. LaBorge JM, Ring EJ, Gordon RL, Lake JR, Doherty MM, Somberg KA, Roberts JP, Ascher NL: **Creation of Transjugular Intrahepatic Portosystemic Shunts With the Wall Stent Endoprosthesis: Results in 100 Patients.** *Radiology* 1993, **197**:413–420.

74. Helton WS, Belshaw A, Althaus S, Park S, Coldwell D, Johansen K: **Critical Appraisal of the Angiographic Portacaval Shunt (TIPS).** *Am J Surg* 1993, **165**:566–571.

75. Simpson KJ, Chalmers N, Redhead DN, Finalyson ND, Bouchier IA, Hayes PC: **Transjugular Intrahepatic Portosystemic Stent Shunting for Control of Acute and Recurrent Upper Gastrointestinal Haemorrhage Related to Portal Hypertension.** *Gut* 1993, **34**:968–973.

76. Maynar M, Cabrera J, Pulido-Duque JM, Reyes R, Gorriz E, Rostagno R, Ferral H, Castaneda-Zuniga WR: **Transjugular Intrahepatic Portosystemic Shunt: Early Experience With a Flexible Trocar/Catheter System.** *AJR Am J Roentgenol* 1993, **161**:301–306.

77. Henderson JM: **Portal Hypertension and Shunt Surgery.** *Adv Surg* 1993, **26**:233–257.

78. Rikkers LF, Jin G, Burnett DA, Buchi KN, Cormier RA: **Shunt Surgery Versus Endoscopic Sclerotherapy for Variceal Hemorrhage: Late Results of a Randomized Trial.** *Am J Surg* 1993, **165**:27–32.
•
The choice of endoscopic therapy or shunt surgery to prevent variceal rebleeding is influenced by local factors, such as technical expertise and geographic location.

79. Gusberg RJ: **Selective Shunts in Selected Older Cirrhotic Patients With Variceal Hemorrhage.** *Am J Surg* 1993, **166**:274–278.

80. Ho KS, Lashner BA, Emond JC, Baker AL: **Prior Esophageal Variceal Bleeding Does Not Adversely Affect Survival After Orthotopic Liver Transplantation.** *Hepatology* 1993, **19**:66–72.

81. Van Thiel DH, Dindzana VJ, Schade RR, Rabinovitz M, Gavaler JS: **Prophylactic Versus Emergency Sclerotherapy of Large Esophageal Varices Prior to Liver Transplantation.** *Dig Dis Sci* 1993, **39**:1505–1510.

82. Lopez-Talavera JC, Merril W, Groszmann RJ: **Treatment With Anti-Tumor Necrosis Factor-α Polyclonal Antibodies Prevents the Development of the Hyperdynamic Circulation and Reduces Portal Pressure in Portal Hypertensive Rats.** *Hepatology* 1993, **18**:140A.

Andres T. Blei, MD, Section of Gastroenterology, Northwestern Medical Faculty Foundation, 680 North Lake Shore Drive #822, Chicago, IL 60611, USA.

Cholestatic diseases and mechanisms of cholestasis

Leslie B. Lilly, MD, and John L. Gollan, MD, PhD

Brigham and Women's Hospital, Boston, Massachusetts, USA

Primary biliary cirrhosis and primary sclerosing cholangitis are distinct hepatobiliary disorders that are both characterized by bile duct injury, the development of cirrhosis, and, in many cases, liver failure, often necessitating transplantation. Research continues to focus on the pathogenesis of these disorders and on the efficacy and mechanism of action of ursodeoxycholic acid, which currently is the therapy of choice. The association of primary biliary cirrhosis with HLA-DR8 was confirmed, the involvement of both activated B- as well as T-cell populations has been documented, and the T-cell response to the pyruvate dehydrogenase complex has been shown to be blocked by antibodies to HLA class II antigens. B cells were found in significant numbers within the portal tracts of affected livers, and were shown to be maximally stimulated to produce specific antimitochondrial antibodies. It was proposed that antigen recognition may be triggered through a process involving immunoglobulin A secretion into bile, whereas another report confirmed significant cross-reactivity with bacterial antigens. Research into the mechanism of action of ursodeoxycholic acid demonstrated a direct cytoprotective effect against toxic bile acids, as well as effects on interleukin-2 production and on bile acid pools. In primary sclerosing cholangitis, the role of neutrophil cytoplasmic antibodies was further evaluated, and the benefits and timing of liver transplantation were analyzed. Other cholestatic disorders investigated include drug-induced jaundice, cholestasis of pregnancy, cystic fibrosis, and Caroli's disease, as well as the role of ursodeoxycholic acid and other therapeutic modalities.

Current Opinion in Gastroenterology 1994, **10**:303–312

Primary biliary cirrhosis

Laboratory abnormalities

Serum cholesterol concentrations are often elevated in primary biliary cirrhosis (PBC), although the true incidence of atherosclerosis in this disorder has not been determined. Propst *et al.* [1], following comprehensive noninvasive cardiac evaluation of 19 PBC patients, suggested that the elevated high-density lipoprotein-2 cholesterol noted in patients is protective against atherogenesis and questioned the need for treatment with cholesterol-lowering drugs. Similarly, Hiraoka *et al.* [2] concluded that the hyper-alphalipoproteinemia commonly seen in PBC patients is entirely different from the familial variety attributed to cholesteryl ester transfer protein deficiency, because the activity of this protein appears to be increased in PBC.

Briand *et al.* [3] reported the development of a potential new diagnostic test for antimitochondrial antibodies (AMAs). The test uses a cross-linked synthetic peptide with sequence homology with residues 40-52 of the pyruvate dehydrogenase complex (PDC), a region essentially identical to residues 167-79, which is the lipoic acid–binding moiety of the PDC. The assay demonstrated 100% specificity for M2-positive PBC patients, with a sensitivity of 74%.

Serologic markers other than AMAs also have been examined. Mulder *et al.* [4•] measured the prevalence of antineutrophil cytoplasmic antibodies (ANCAs) in patients with autoimmune liver diseases, and detected them in 28% of patients with PBC. ANCA positivity was found to correlate significantly with the presence of cirrhosis; it appears likely, however, that these antibodies are markers of chronic inflammatory states.

Genetics and immunopathogenesis

There is incomplete evidence of an HLA association in PBC. Previous studies support an association between PBC and HLA-DR8; other associations also have been

Abbreviations

AMA—antimitochondrial antibody; **ANCA**—antineutrophil cytoplasmic antibody; **PBC**—primary biliary cirrhosis; **PDC**—pyruvate dehydrogenase complex; **PSC**—primary sclerosing cholangitis.

 ISBN 1-85922-608-6 ISSN 0267–1379

described. Several reports describing further efforts to clarify the role of HLA phenotype in PBC emerged. The King's College group [5] employed Taq1 restriction-fragment-length polymorphism analysis in 159 PBC patients from southern England. The only DR antigen to show a significant increase when compared with a local control population was DR8 (11% vs 4%; $P<0.01$). Only one DQB allele (DQB1•0402) was found to substantially differ in frequency from controls (10% vs 3%), although this association failed to stand up under more rigorous statistical analysis.

Investigators from Newcastle-upon-Tyne [6] analyzed 130 PBC patients from northern England using the same technique and again confirmed the association with HLA-DR8 (18.5% vs 9.2% in local controls; $P<0.005$). They further noted that the DR8-positive patients tended to have a higher serum bilirubin level, and suggested that this haplotype might identify a subgroup of patients with more severe disease. It should be noted that both these reported rates of DR8 association are significantly less than the literature values, a discrepancy attributed to the different racial groups studied and to the fact that previous determinations were carried out using serological, rather than molecular, methods.

Finally, Seki *et al.* [7] applied similar techniques to assess HLA associations in a series of 47 Japanese patients with PBC, and observed an increase in the DPB1•0501 allele compared with controls (85.1% vs 55.3%; $P<0.01$) and a decrease in the DPB1•0402 allele (2.2% vs 23.3%; $P<0.05$). They proposed that a specific amino acid substitution (Leu at position 35 of the DPB1 chain) might play a role in the susceptibility of Japanese patients to develop PBC.

Since their first description in 1965, AMAs have been intensively investigated to determine their role in the pathogenesis of PBC. Efforts have been concentrated on the M2 subset, although M4, M8, and M9 also have been implicated in PBC patients. The E2 subunit of the pyruvate dehydrogenase complex (PDC), which has been identified as dihydrolipoamide acetyltransferase, is the principal target of the M2 AMAs (recognized by about 85% of all PBC sera).

It is unclear why PBC patients are stimulated to make antibodies to an enzyme complex located on the inner mitochondrial membrane and why these antibodies should specifically target intrahepatic biliary duct cells (cholangiocytes) and not other cells expressing this particular antigen. These two questions were addressed in some detail by Van de Water *et al.* [8•], using a panel of monoclonal antibodies raised against various regions of PDC-E2, as well as an antibody derived from a PBC lymph node combinatorial library, described separately [9]. The authors concluded that the PDC epitopes expressed at the cell surface differ from those within the mitochondria, suggesting either modification of the antigen as it is targeted to the cell surface, or the existence of distinct molecules with an epitope shared with PDC-E2. Additional studies revealed high levels of immunoglobulin A staining in the lumenal region of bile duct epithelial cells of PBC patients, along with PDC-E2–specific immunoglobulin A in bile, suggesting a possible role of immunoglobulin A in antigen processing as it is transported through the hepatocytes into bile [8•].

It has been proposed that the target antigen of the AMA is actually a bacterial membrane component, as cross-reactivity of PBC sera with M2 antigen components and bacterial antigens has been demonstrated. Rough bacterial mutants, which have an abnormal cell wall, can induce AMA production in immunized animals, and are present in high frequency in the stool of PBC patients. In a study by Butler *et al.* [10], the relationship between bacteriuria and M2 antibodies in PBC patients, and in women with recurrent urinary tract infections, was examined. M2 antibodies were detected in 69% of women with recurrent urinary tract infections and, conversely, a higher than predicted incidence of recurrent infections, often involving bacterial R-forms, was noted in PBC patients when compared with women having other forms of chronic liver disease.

Several other issues involving AMAs have recently been addressed. Chen *et al.* [11] presented evidence for the conformational nature of the PDC-E2 epitope in studies using a recombinant form of the lipoyl binding site along with a variety of antibody-binding substrates. Anti-idiotype antibodies to AMAs in the serum of PBC patients were detected by Zhang *et al.* [12], and their potential role in the regulation of AMAs was discussed. Two studies examined the role of M4 and M9 antibodies in PBC, and the so-called overlap syndrome of PBC and chronic active autoimmune hepatitis. Davis *et al.* [13] performed detailed analysis of sera from patients with PBC, chronic active autoimmune hepatitis, primary sclerosing cholangitis (PSC), the overlap syndrome, and other chronic liver and autoimmune disorders. These investigators were unable either to demonstrate the presence of M4 and M9 antigens or to confirm their proposed identities as sulfite oxidase and glycogen phosphorylase, respectively [13]. In a study of 149 patients with PBC and 85 patients with other forms of chronic liver disease, Palmer *et al.* [14] also were unable to confirm the identities of the M4 and M9 autoantigens, supporting the notion that the nature of the antigens in M4- and M9-positive patients is still unclear, as is the clinical significance of the presence of these AMA subtypes.

On the basis of earlier studies demonstrating AMA secretion by B lymphocytes isolated from PBC patients, Lohse *et al.* [15] showed that these cells have been maximally stimulated to synthesize antibodies of PBC subspecificities, suggesting a high level of stimulation of B lymphocytes *in vivo*. Immunohistochemical studies on biopsies from PBC patients confirmed the presence of varying densities of B cells within the portal tracts, always in conjunction with activated T cells [16];

these data support a sequence of events that is initiated by T-cell activation, followed by B-cell recruitment and the subsequent production of antibodies responsible for the destruction of biliary epithelial cells.

The presence of autoreactive T-cell clones in PBC has previously been documented; the proliferative response of cells derived from these clones to crude mitochondrial extracts and to PDC and PDC-E2 was examined and compared with cells from other forms of chronic liver disease [17]. Upon exposure to PDC, T cells obtained from PBC patients exhibited a maximal proliferative response, whereas cells from other patient groups exhibited no response, although they were able to proliferate when exposed to the crude mitochondrial preparation. The T-cell response to PDC in PBC patients was blocked by antibodies to HLA class II antigens, providing a possible etiologic link to the HLA-association noted above.

The search for clues to the pathogenesis of PBC has not been confined to analysis of the antigens recognized by the AMA. Guldner *et al.* [18] studied the expression of Sp100, an intranuclear protein to which approximately 30% of PBC patients produce autoantibodies. The expression of this protein was dramatically increased by type I and II interferon, and the authors propose that, in PBC, elevated interferon levels result in up-regulation of this protein with enhanced immune recognition and autoantibody production. However, the etiology of the initial interferon elevation is unclear, although viruses or other microbes are possible candidates. Increased expression of heat-shock protein in the biliary epithelium of patients with PBC (and PSC) was reported, and it was suggested that this may serve as an immune target [19]. Suou *et al.* [20] looked at cellular sensitivity to native human type IV collagen using an *in vitro* assay of leukocytes from PBC patients, and reported an increased sensitivity, possibly reflecting accelerated basement membrane metabolism. It appears unlikely, however, that this sensitivity to collagen would serve as a primary trigger for the development of bile duct injury.

Pathology

Detailed histologic analysis of portal tracts in the liver biopsies of 162 PBC patients revealed a 29% incidence of focal eosinophilic infiltrates, a finding reported in the biopsies of only 4% of patients with chronic active viral hepatitis [21]. The eosinophils appeared particularly abundant around the damaged bile ducts, and it was proposed that these cells may have a role in the ductular epithelial injury in PBC.

Hiley *et al.* [22], using glutathione-*S*-transferase isoform analysis, provided data suggesting that the proliferating bile duct cells observed in PBC and other cholestatic diseases are a form of transdifferentiating hepatocyte. However, as noted in response by Matthew and Burt [23], this does not exclude a role of primary proliferation of bile duct cells in more acute injury, nor does it disprove the notion of stem cells present within the portal tract.

Primary biliary cirrhosis–associated disorders

Although PSC is the hepatobiliary disease most frequently associated with ulcerative colitis, there are now a total of six reported cases of PBC diagnosed in association with ulcerative colitis, the most recent provided by Lever *et al.* [24]. A case of pulmonary hemorrhage and focal proliferative glomerulonephritis complicating PBC has been reported [25]; separate associations with pulmonary dysfunction and with glomerulonephritis have previously been documented.

The association of PBC with polyglandular exocrine failure is well-documented; Prieto *et al.* [26] proposed that these disorders are linked by abnormal expression of anion exchanger genes. The authors demonstrated reduced messenger RNA expression of anlon exchanger-2 gene in the liver and lymphoid tissues of PBC patients when compared with healthy controls and with patients having other cholestatic diseases. The consequences of this altered message at the protein level remain to be fully elucidated.

Therapy

Ursodeoxycholic acid

With few new treatment strategies on the immediate horizon [27], ursodeoxycholic acid remains the drug of choice for PBC. The final analyses of several large multicenter clinical trials are pending; interim reports have appeared in the literature in abstract form only. Hwang *et al.* [28] reported the results of a small, randomized, double-blind trial of ursodeoxycholic acid in 12 Chinese patients with PBC, and noted improvements in pruritus in seven of seven patients treated on a long-term basis and improvement in the biochemical indices of all patients. Unfortunately, only one patient was biopsied both before and 2 years after treatment; some histologic decrease in inflammation was observed, with no change in fibrosis.

Battezzati *et al.* [29] reported the preliminary results of a double-blind multicenter trial of ursodeoxycholic acid in a series of Italian PBC patients. Only patients with pruritus or a serum bilirubin in excess of 2 mg/dL were randomly assigned to receive ursodeoxycholic acid or placebo. Forty-four patients were enrolled in each group, and only clinical and biochemical parameters were assessed, with no histologic follow-up. After 6 months, all ursodeoxycholic acid–treated patients exhibited a significant reduction in pruritus, serum bilirubin, immunoglobulin G, immunoglobulin M, high-density lipoprotein cholesterol, serum cholic acid, and chenodeoxycholic acid levels. No data on the effect of ursodeoxycholic acid treatment on survival or likelihood of transplantation were available and, at the end of the 6-month interval, all patients were switched to receive either ursodeoxycholic acid alone or ursodeoxycholic acid plus colchicine.

Poupon *et al.* [30] evaluated the impact of ursodeoxycholic acid treatment on serum cholesterol in PBC patients, as their prior studies had indicated a drop in cholesterol levels. The decline was attributed largely to a decline in low-density lipoprotein cholesterol, coupled with a decrease in very low density lipoprotein cholesterol. Total high-density lipoprotein cholesterol levels remained stable, although the high-density lipoprotein-2 to high-density lipoprotein-3 ratio decreased. The authors concluded that the reduction in low-density lipoprotein cholesterol could be explained by both an improvement in cholestasis as well as modification of cholesterol metabolism.

Ursodeoxycholic acid has been postulated to improve hepatocyte function in PBC via various mechanisms (Table 1). Reports have appeared that address each of these hypotheses. Ursodeoxycholic acid appears to consistently modify bile acid pools, and several recent studies have evaluated the effects of ursodeoxycholic acid on bile acid metabolism.

Table 1. Proposed mechanisms of action of ursodeoxycholic acid in primary biliary cirrhosis

Mechanism	Study
Modification of bile acid pools	Battezzati *et al.* [29], Batta *et al.* [31], Poupon *et al.* [32], Mazzella *et al.* [33]
Immunomodulation	Lacaille and Paradis [35•], Kurtschiev *et al.* [36]
Choleresis	Nakai *et al.* [37]
Cytoprotection	Ohiwa *et al.* [34••], Guldutuna *et al.* [38]

In a small, double-blind study, Batta *et al.* [31] reported the results of ursodeoxycholic acid treatment in 14 PBC patients for periods up to 2 years. Improvement in pruritus and fatigue were noted, as well as a significant decline in alkaline phosphatase (44%), alanine aminotransferase (34%), and aspartate aminotransferase (41%) levels, consistent with earlier findings. Only four patients underwent serial liver biopsies; three of them were reported to show some histologic improvement over the 2-year treatment period. Analysis of serum and urinary bile acids following therapy revealed a decrease in total serum endogenous bile acid concentration, that could not be fully explained by a rise in urinary bile acid excretion, suggesting improved hepatic clearance of endogenous bile acids by ursodeoxycholic acid. Biliary bile acid analysis demonstrated that cholic acid predominated pretreatment; this declined during ursodeoxycholic acid administration, and was accompanied by a small decrease in biliary chenodeoxycholic acid, as ursodeoxycholic acid came to represent 30% of total biliary bile acids. These authors also identified abnormal patterns of bile acid conjugation in patients with PBC [31].

Poupon *et al.* [32] measured alterations in serum bile acids in 73 ursodeoxycholic acid–treated and 73 control patients. A significant increase in total serum bile acid concentrations in the ursodeoxycholic acid–treated group was observed after 6 months of therapy; the proportion of ursodeoxycholic acid also increased progressively throughout the study, representing 60% of total serum bile acids after 2 years. Both cholic acid and chenodeoxycholic acid exhibited a sustained substantial decrease throughout ursodeoxycholic acid therapy, whereas deoxycholic acid concentrations were unchanged, and the levels of lithocholic acid increased significantly. The authors speculated that the sustained reduction in the concentration of endogenous bile acids, along with the presence of ursodeoxycholic acid, accounted for the associated improvement in hepatocyte function. In a study of nine PBC patients, Mazzella *et al.* [33] obtained similar findings.

The effect of tauro-ursodeoxycholic acid on hepatic bile acid concentrations was examined by Ohiwa *et al.* [34••], using rat liver hepatocytes isolated by collagenase perfusion. Changes in intracellular taurochenodoxycholate concentrations and in cell viability were measured in response to treatment with tauro-ursodeoxycholic acid or tauro-β-muricholate plus taurochenodoxycholate. Tauro-ursodeoxycholic acid appeared to exert a cytoprotective effect, which correlated with a decrease in intrahepatocyte taurochenodoxycholate content. The authors concluded that bile acid hydrophilicity is reflected in the protective actions of tauro-ursodeoxycholic acid and tauro-β-muricholate.

The immunomodulatory effects of ursodeoxycholic acid also have received close attention during this period. The proliferative responses of peripheral blood mononuclear cells from healthy volunteers were used to assess the immunosuppressive effects of ursodeoxycholic acid, its glycine and taurine conjugates, and chenodeoxycholic acid [35•]. All of the compounds tested inhibited mitogen-stimulated peripheral blood mononuclear cells proliferation and mixed lymphocyte cultures; chenodeoxycholic acid was the most potent, and ursodeoxycholic acid the least effective, with the ursodeoxycholic acid conjugates having intermediate effects. All of these bile acids also inhibited proliferation of a rat helper T-cell clone, and ursodeoxycholic acid markedly decreased interleukin-2 production. Thus, the authors proposed that, in patients with PBC, replacement of more toxic bile acids with ursodeoxycholic acid would facilitate inhibition of autoactivation and produce a decrease in cytokine production, possibly through a diminution of abnormal HLA expression. In contrast to these findings, Kurtschiev *et al.* [36] demonstrated that ursodeoxycholic acid restored interleukin-2 production to normal levels in patients with PBC.

The choleresis produced by ursodeoxycholic acid administration was investigated in isolated perfused livers from rats treated with colchicine (which inhibits microtubule polymerization) and in isolated perfused livers from normal control rats [37]. Tauro-ursodeoxycholic acid increased bile flow, bile acid output, and phospholipid output in both groups, whereas taurocholic acid administration after colchicine pretreatment induced marked cholestasis. Tauro-ursodeoxycholic acid (and, to a lesser extent, ursodeoxycholic acid) resulted in a reduction in the cholestatic effect of taurocholic acid when coadministered, supporting the concept of a direct action of tauro-ursodeoxycholic acid on the hepatocyte rather than on the bile acid pool.

The effect of ursodeoxycholic acid and chenodeoxycholic acid on cell membranes was examined using electron paramagnetic resonance spectroscopy [38], and it was concluded that chenodeoxycholic acid solubilizes membrane lipids, enabling water molecules to permeate into plasma membranes, whereas ursodeoxycholic acid is bound to the apolar domain (and it conjugates to the membrane interface), resulting in stabilization of membrane structure. These data support the proposal that cytoprotection is a mechanism of ursodeoxycholic acid action in PBC and in other cholestatic disorders.

Other drug therapies

A number of investigators have reported a beneficial effect of methotrexate on the serum biochemistry and clinical symptoms in small groups of patients with PBC. Buscher *et al.* [39] added methotrexate (2.5 mg 6d/wk) to the treatment regimen of eight patients who had an unsatisfactory response to ursodeoxycholic acid (10 to 15 mg/kg/d for a mean of 11 months). Pruritus and fatigue disappeared in those patients affected and, following initial deterioration, transaminases improved, as did alkaline phosphatase levels. Unfortunately, no histologic analysis was performed. Larger and longer trials are still awaited to validate this form of combination therapy.

A multicenter trial of cyclosporin A in PBC was conducted by Lombard *et al.* [40••], involving 349 patients randomly assigned to either cyclosporin A or placebo; the group randomly assigned to cyclosporin A had more advanced disease. There was no benefit achieved in terms of fatigue or liver histology, and improvements in pruritus were minimal. Time to death or liver transplantation was prolonged by cyclosporin A treatment, but this difference failed to achieve statistical significance and cyclosporin A was associated with significant side effects (*eg*, renal toxicity and hypertension). Thus, although confirming that immunosuppressive therapy may have a role in the treatment of PBC, this study failed to justify the use of cyclosporin A in this disease [41].

A randomized, double-blind trial of malotilate (di-isopropyl 1,3-dithiol-2-ylidene malonate) in PBC demonstrated no benefit [42], and a proposal that thalidomide might be a useful therapy [43] has thus far yielded no tangible results.

Liver transplantation

Orthotopic liver transplantation is a proven effective therapy for advanced PBC. Two recent reports [44,45•] appear to confirm earlier findings of disease recurrence in the transplanted liver. Wong *et al.* [44] reported histologic recurrence in two patients (at 11 months and 1 year post-transplant) maintained on FK-506 immunosuppression, and Hubscher *et al.* [45•] provided a detailed review of the literature, and of 353 liver biopsies performed at more than 12 months posttransplant. Evidence consistent with or diagnostic of recurrence in 16 biopsies from 13 patients was detected. All of these patients had undergone liver transplantation for PBC. These data reflected a recurrence rate of 16% after 1 year. However, the findings unfortunately did not address the natural history or prognosis of these patients, or the effect, if any, of concurrent liver injury on the course of the recurrent disease.

Primary sclerosing cholangitis

Laboratory abnormalities and immunopathogenesis

Primary sclerosing cholangitis is a chronic inflammatory hepatobiliary disorder that may progress to biliary cirrhosis, and is generally presumed to be of autoimmune etiology. The identity of the autoantigen in PSC remains unknown. Most of the studies reported to date focus on ANCAs, which may represent a useful marker of PSC in the setting of ulcerative colitis, with which it coexists in up to two thirds of cases. This topic has been addressed directly by several groups.

Mulder *et al.* [4•] detected ANCAs in 79% of patients with PSC, consistent with earlier findings by other investigators. Three putative antigens were detected; lactoferrin, a 67/66-kD protein combination or a 40-kD polypeptide. Although the presence of ANCAs did correspond with the presence of cirrhosis, there was no other apparent relationship to disease severity. Lo *et al.* [46] had previously described an ANCA that was highly specific for adult PSC detecting using immunoalkaline phosphatase. In a later study [47], they went on to assess the diagnostic potential of this method in children, where eight of 10 PSC patients in a total patient group of 72 were correctly identified, and the particular pattern of staining was not observed in any other patient group apart from chronic active hepatitis. In a letter to the editor, Lo *et al.* [48] describe a modification of previous methods using Western blotting and immunoprecipitation, in which the presence of a specific autoantigen was not confirmed. Berg and Klein [49] dispute these conclusions, however, and it is apparent that the role of ANCAs as a diagnostic test in PSC is yet to be established.

The expression of blood group antigens on colonic and biliary epithelium, previously noted to be abnormal in ulcerative colitis, was examined in patients with PSC [50]. Inappropriate expression of A and B antigens on both epithelia was noted, and it was suggested that the PSC autoantigen may share an epitope with one or more blood group antigens. Unfortunately, liver biopsy specimens from patients with ulcerative colitis but without evidence of PSC were not examined.

A number of other lymphocyte-mediated inflammatory process exhibit epithelial coexpression of intracellular adhesion molecule-1 and HLA-DR alleles, although there is no evidence that this was the case in PSC [51].

Therapy

A limited number of trials reported to date suggest that ursodeoxycholic acid may improve both the liver biochemical parameters and histology in patients with PSC [52]. However, definitive data from large, placebo-controlled, randomized trials are not yet available. The effect of ursodeoxycholic acid on bile acid kinetics in PSC patients was analyzed in six patients treated for 3 months, in whom significant improvements in biochemical markers of cholestasis were noted [53]. Endogenous bile acid levels declined, due mainly to a decrease in cholic acid. Compared with normal subjects, the pretreatment pool sizes of cholic acid and chenodeoxycholic acid were small, and they were unaffected by ursodeoxycholic acid therapy, although fractional turnover of both bile acids was increased.

Total proctocolectomy for refractory ulcerative colitis or for severe dysplasia-carcinoma can be complicated by the presence of coexistent PSC, particularly if end-stage liver disease is present. It was demonstrated that the development of peristomal varices in an ileostomy could be prevented completely if an ileal pouch–anal anastomosis was performed, and that this procedure could be performed safely in this difficult subgroup of patients, without interfering with subsequent liver transplantation [54].

Strasser *et al.* [55•] compared liver transplantation for PBC and PSC. An increased incidence of postoperative sepsis in PSC patients was noted, particularly in those with recurrent septic cholangitis before transplantation. In addition, they reported several cases of incidental cholangiocarcinoma in the PSC patients, and outline measures to increase diagnostic efficiency prior to liver transplant surgery.

Drug-induced cholestasis

In order to attribute cholestatic hepatitis to a specific drug, three criteria generally should be met: 1) commencement of the illness within 5 days of the start of drug administration, 2) normalization of laboratory abnormalities within 6 months of cessation of drug therapy, and 3) exclusion of other causes of hepatitis and cholestasis. Several compounds that fulfilled these criteria were reported or evaluated in the literature during the review period (Table 2). These include macrolide antibiotics (erythromycin, troleandomycin, and spiramycin [56–58], flucloxacillin [59,60], propafenone [61], danazol [62,63], flutamide [64], lovastatin [65], and bupivacaine [66].

Derby *et al.* [60] estimated the frequency of cholestatic hepatitis due to flucloxacillin as 7.6 per 100,000 users in a population-based study that included more than 4 million patients and over 130,000 prescriptions.

Table 2. Drug-induced cholestasis reported in the review period

Drug	Study	ALP	TBili	ALT	AST
Macrolide antiobiotics					
Erythromycin	Derby *et al.* [56]*	—	—	—	—
Spiramycin	Denie *et al.* [58]	2×N	2.4 mg/dL	5–10×N	NR
Troleandomycin	Uzzan *et al.* [57]	1.6×N	234 µmol/L	NR	2×N
Flucloxacillin	Fairley *et al.* [59]*	—	—	—	—
	Derby *et al.* [60]*	—	—	—	—
Danazol	Qaseem *et al.* [62]	316 IU	284 µmol/L	35 IU	NR
	Bray *et al.* [63]†	336 IU	936 µmol/L	NR	120 IU
Flutamide	Rosman *et al.* [64]	3054 IU	26.1 mg/dL	443-IU	305 IU
Lovastatin	Yoshida and Levin [65]‡	190 IU	23 µmol/L	NR	184 IU
Propafenone	Mondardini *et al.* [61]	553 IU	8.8 mg/dL	127 IU	64 IU
Bupivacaine	Billstrom *et al.* [66]	330 IU	10 µmol/L	70 IU	NR
		1080 IU	69 µmol/L	335 IU	NR
		1122 IU	43 µmol/L	498 IU	NR

*Large series. Details provided in text.
†Responded to treatment with *S*-adenosylmethionine.
‡Total of 15 reported cases.
ALP—alkaline phosphatase; ALT—alanine aminotransferase; AST—aspartate aminotransferase; N—normal; NR—not reported; TBili—total bilirubin.

Women appeared to be at higher risk than men, but no correlation of risk with age, dose, or duration of use was identified. In contrast, Fairley *et al.* [59], in a review of 51 patients, determined that increasing age and a prolonged duration of treatment constitute risk factors for the development of jaundice.

Erythromycin, particularly the estolate form, has frequently been linked to cholestasis. An incidence of 3.6 per 100,000 users was determined after analysis of over 360,000 patients who received all forms of the drug [56], although the frequency with the estolate salt was not specifically increased. The risk of cholestatic hepatitis appeared to be increased in patients over 39 years of age.

Two reports of jaundice due to danazol appeared. In one case, clinical and laboratory abnormalities resolved spontaneously upon discontinuation of the drug [62]. The other patient, in whom jaundice was complicated by renal failure [63], responded to treatment with *S*-adenosylmethionine, which has previously been shown to partially alleviate estrogen-induced cholestasis in animal models.

There was one case reported of toxic epidermal necrolysis with severe cholestasis after treatment with fenfluramine chloride, although the authors felt that a direct association was unproven [67•]. Serial biopsies documented the disappearance of bile ducts; however, 1 year after onset of the cholestasis, biopsy revealed reappearance of bile ducts, accompanied by normalization of serum bilirubin levels.

Other cholestatic disorders

Autoimmune cholangitis (or immunocholangitis) is a term that has been coined to describe patients who have clinical, biochemical, and histologic findings indistinguishable from PBC, but are AMA negative and antinuclear antibody positive. These cases also have been referred to an "overlap syndrome" of PBC with autoimmune chronic hepatitis. Ben-Ari *et al.* [68••] described in detail four such patients, three of whom had an excellent response to corticosteroids, supporting the authors' contention that this syndrome represents a subgroup of autoimmune hepatitis type I, rather than a separate disease process. The term *autoimmune cholangiopathy* is proposed to describe these unusual patients.

A lengthy review of the epidemiology, clinical manifestations, and management of *intrahepatic cholestasis of pregnancy* was published by Reyes [69], commenting on earlier reports of the efficacy of ursodeoxycholic acid in this enigmatic disorder. Although the drug has an excellent safety profile in pregnancy, no convincing data are yet available to justify its routine use in intrahepatic cholestasis of pregnancy [70]. Two cases were reported of an unusually prolonged postpartum course of intrahepatic cholestasis of pregnancy [71]; both had no apparent response to ursodeoxycholic acid, but each demonstrated clinical and biochemical improvement upon treatment with corticosteroids.

Caroli's syndrome, a congenital disorder characterized by cystic dilatations of the intrahepatic bile duct system, has traditionally been resistant to medical management. Ros *et al.* [72] described 12 patients with primary hepatolithiasis treated with ursodeoxycholic acid. All displayed clinical improvement and evidence of at least partial stone dissolution, supporting the use of ursodeoxycholic acid in this rare cholestatic disease.

In a dose-response study involving nine patients, the efficacy of ursodeoxycholic acid in *cystic fibrosis*—associated liver disease was evaluated by Colombo *et al.* [73•]. The authors recommended doses of at least 20 mg/kg/d in order to achieve desired modifications in biliary bile acid composition; they also acknowledge that no long-term clinical benefit of ursodeoxycholic acid treatment in cystic fibrosis has been documented.

An exhaustive review of the hepatobiliary complication of *total parenteral nutrition* was published [74], as well as data on bilirubin metabolism in a rat model of total parenteral nutrition–induced cholestasis [75]. In another interesting report, reversal of intractable total parental nutrition–induced cholestasis in premature infants was achieved by biliary irrigation [76], supporting the potential role of ductal obstruction by viscous bile in this disorder.

Several *animal models of cholestasis* and biliary cirrhosis have been studied. A variety of procedures that produce obstructive jaundice are available, including a novel new technique [77]. Studies of hepatic macrophage function have been conducted in these animals [78,79]. Ursodeoxycholic acid therapy has generally failed to show any beneficial effects in such models [80], although Frezza *et al.* [81•] did show reduced bile duct proliferation in animals treated with ursodeoxycholic acid after bile duct ligation. In cholestasis induced by estrogen and its derivatives, multiple alterations in canalicular membrane transport have been described [82], and some beneficial effects of ursodeoxycholic acid and tauro-ursodeoxycholic acid [83] and ursodeoxycholic acid-3-O-glucuronide [84,85] have been reported.

Pruritus

Pruritus is one of the potentially disabling symptoms of cholestasis, and efforts to both understand its pathogenesis and provide more effective treatment modalities continue. A comprehensive summary of current knowledge in this area has been presented by Gillespie and Vickers [86•]. In addition, the role of the opioid system and the potential therapeutic applications of opioid antagonists were reviewed [87]. The results of a retrospective analysis of the use of rifampicin in childhood cholestasis suggested that it represents a safe and effective treatment option [88]. Finally, in a case report, ondansetron, a serotonin receptor antagonist, was reported to offer effective short-term relief of pruritic symptoms in a patient with PBC [89].

References and recommended reading

Papers of particular interest, published within the annual period of review, have been highlighted as:
- • Of special interest
- •• Of outstanding interest

1. Propst A, Propst T, Lechleitner M, Hoppichler F, Kathrein H, Vogel W, Judmaier G, Knapp E, Braunsteiner H: **Hypercholesterolemia in Primary Cirrhosis Is No Risk Factor for Atherosclerosis.** *Dig Dis Sci* 1993, **38**:379–380.

2. Hiraoka H, Yamashita S, Matsuzawa Y, Kubo M, Nozaki S, Sakai N, Hirano K, Kawata S, Tarui S: **Decrease of Hepatic Triglyceride Lipase Levels and Increase of Cholesteryl Ester Transfer Protein Levels in Patients With Primary Biliary Cirrhosis: Relationship to Abnormalities in High-Density Lipoprotein.** *Hepatology* 1993, **18**:103–110.

3. Briand JP, Andre C, Tuaillon N, Herve L, Neimark J, Muller S: **Multiple Autoepitope Presentation for Specific Detection of Antibodies in Primary Biliary Cirrhosis.** *Hepatology* 1992, **16**:1395–1403.

4. • Mulder AHL, Horst G, Haagsma EB, Limburg PC, Kleibeuker JH, Kallenbert CG: **Prevalence and Characterization of Neutrophil Cytoplasmic Antibodies in Autoimmune Liver Diseases.** *Hepatology* 1993, **17**:411–417.

A total of 28% of PBC patients and 79% of PSC patients were positive for ANCA. The presence of the antibodies correlated with the presence of cirrhosis.

5. Underhill J, Donaldson P, Bray G, Doherty D, Portmann B, Williams R: **Susceptibility to Primary Biliary Cirrhosis Is Associated With the HLA-DR8-DQB1•0402 Haplotype.** *Hepatology* 1992, **16**:1404–1408.

6. Gregory WL, Mehal W, Dunn AN, Cavanagh G, Chapman R, Fleming KA, Daly AK, Idle JR, James OFW, Bassendine MF: **Primary Biliary Cirrhosis - Contribution of HLA Class-II Allele DR8.** *Q J Med* 1993, **86**:393–399.

7. Seki T, Kiyosawa K, Ota M, Furuta S, Fukushima H, Tanaka E, Yoshizawa K, Kumagai T, Muziku M, Ando A, Inoko H: **Association of Primary Biliary Cirrhosis With Human Leukocyte Antigen DPB1•0501 in Japanese Patients.** *Hepatology* 1993, **18**:73–78.

8. • Van de Water J, Turchany J, Leung PSC, Lake J, Munoz S, Surh CD, Coppel R, Ansari A, Nakanuma Y, Gershwin ME: **Molecular Mimicry in Primary Biliary Cirrhosis - Evidence for Biliary Epithelial Expression of a Molecule Cross-Reactive With Pyruvate Dehydrogenase Complex-E2.** *J Clin Invest* 1993, **91**:2653–2664.

Expression of an antigen that shares epitopes with, but is not identical to, pyruvate dehydrogenase complex-E2 near the surface of biliary epithelial cells was demonstrated in PBC patients but not in patients with other forms of chronic liver disease. Elevated biliary concentrations of immunoglobulin A support its role in altered antigen presentation.

9. Cha S, Leung PSC, Gershwin ME, Fletcher MP, Ansari AA, Coppel RL: **Combinatorial Autoantibodies to Dihydrolipoamide Acetyltransferase, the Major Autoantigen of Primary Biliary Cirrhosis.** *Proc Natl Acad Sci U S A* 1993, 90:2527–2531.

10. Butler P, Valle F, Hamiltonmiller JMT, Brunfitt W, Baum H, Burroughs AK: **M2 Mitochondrial Antibodies and Urinary Rough Mutant Bacteria in Patients With Primary Biliary Cirrhosis and in Patients With Recurrent Bacteriuria.** *J Hepatol* 1993, **17**:408–414.

11. Chen QY, Rowley MJ, Mackay IR: **Antibody to Two Forms of Dihydrolipoamide Acetyltransferase (PDC-E2) in Primary Biliary Cirrhosis.** *Liver* 1993, **13**:130–135.

12. Zhang L, Jayne DRW, Oliveira DBG: **Anti-Idiotype Antibodies to Anti-Mitochondrial Antibodies in the Sera of Patients With Primary Biliary Cirrhosis.** *J Autoimmun* 1993, **1**:93–105.

13. Davis PA, Leung P, Manns M, Kaplan M, Munoz SJ, Gorin FA, Dickson ER, Krawitt E, Coppel R, Gershwin ME: **M4 and M9 Antibodies in the Overlap Syndrome of Primary Biliary Cirrhosis and Chronic Active Hepatitis: Epitopes or Epiphenomena?** *Hepatology* 1992, **16**:1128–1136.

14. Palmer JM, Yeaman SJ, Bassendine MF, James OFW: **M4 and M9 Autoantigens in Primary Biliary Cirrhosis - A Negative Study.** *J Hepatol* 1993, **18**:251–254.

15. Lohse AW, Reckmann A, Kytiatsoulis A, Gerken G, zum Buschenfelde KHM, Manns M: **In Vitro Secretion of Specific Antimitochondrial Antibodies in Primary Biliary Cirrhosis.** *J Hepatol* 1992, **16**:165–170.

16. Nakanuma Y: **Distribution of B-Lymphocytes in Nonsuppurative Cholangitis in Primary Biliary Cirrhosis.** *Hepatology* 1993, **18**:570–575.

17. Lahr H, Fleishcher B, Gerken G, Yeaman SJ, zum Buschenfelde KHN, Manns M: **Autoreactive Liver-Infiltrating T-Cells in Primary Biliary Cirrhosis Recognize Inner Mitochondrial Epitopes and the Pyruvate Dehydrogenase Complex.** *J Hepatol* 1993, **18**:322–327.

18. Guldner HH, Szostecki C, Grotzinger T, Will H: **IFN Enhance Expression of Sp100, an Autoantigen in Primary Biliary Cirrhosis.** *J Immunol* 1992, **149**:4067–4073.

19. Broome U, Scheynius A, Hultcrantz R: **Induced Expression of Heat-Shock Protein on Biliary Epithelium in Patients With Primary Sclerosing Cholangitis and Primary Biliary Cirrhosis.** *Hepatology* 1993, **18**:298–303.

20. Suou T, Ago H, Sawada H, Hirayama C: **Cellular Sensitivity to Native Type IV Collagen in Primary Biliary Cirrhosis.** *Res Commun Chem Pathol Pharmacol* 1993, **79**:275–291.

21. Terasaki S, Nakanuma Y, Yamazaki M, Unoura M: **Eosinophilic Infiltration of the Liver in Primary Biliary Cirrhosis: A Morphological Study.** *Hepatology* 1993, **17**:206–212.

22. Hiley CG, Strange RC, Davies MH, Elias E, Hubscher SG: **Glutathione S-Transferase Expression in Primary Biliary Cirrhosis Supports Concept of Ductular Metaplasia of Hepatocytes.** *J Clin Pathol* 1993, **46**:381.

23. Matthew, Burt: **Glutathione S-Transferase Expression in Primary Biliary Cirrhosis Supports Concept of Ductular Metaplasia of Hepatocytes - Comment.** *J Clin Pathol* 1993, **46**:381.

24. Lever E, Balasubramarian K, Condon S, Wat BY: **Primary Biliary Cirrhosis Associated With Ulcerative Colitis.** *Am J Gastroenterol* 1993, **6**:945–947.

25. Bissuel F, Bizollon T, Dijoud F, Bouletreau P, Cordier JF, Chazot C, Gouillat C, Trepo C: **Pulmonary Hemorrhage and Glomerulonephritis in Primary Biliary Cirrhosis.** *Hepatology* 1992, **16**:1357–1361.

26. Prieto J, Qian C, Garcia N, Diez J, Medina JF: **Abnormal Expression of Anion Exchanger Genes in Primary Biliary Cirrhosis.** *Gastroenterology* 1993, **105**:572–578.

27. **Bile Acid Therapy in the 1990s [Editorial].** *Lancet* 1992, 340:1260–1261.

28. Hwang SJ, Chan CY, Lee SD, Wu JC, Tsay SH, Lo KJ: **Ursodeoxycholic Acid in the Treatment of Primary Biliary Cirrhosis - A Short-Term, Randomized, Double-Blind Controlled, Cross-Over Study With Long-Term Follow-Up.** *J Gastroenterol Hepatol* 1993, **18**:217–233.

29. Battezzati PM, Podda M, Bianchi FB, Naccarato R, Orlandi F, Surrenti C, Pagliaro L, Manenti F, Bertolini E, Camisasca M, Crosignani A, Zuin M, Fusconi M, Ballardini G, Cassani F, Orlandi F, Macarri GP, Benedetti A, Chiaramonte M, Floreani AR, Pozzi M, Biagini MR, Almasio P, Provenzano G, Scalisi L, Bellentani S, Tabarroni G, Roda A, Annoni G, Bisiani G: **Ursodeoxycholic Acid for Symptomatic Primary Biliary Cirrhosis - Preliminary Analysis of a Double-Blind Multicenter Trial.** *J Hepatol* 1993, **17**:332–338.

30. Poupon RE, Chretien Y, Poupon R, Paumgartner G: **Serum Bile Acids in Primary Biliary Cirrhosis - Effect of Ursodeoxycholic Acid Therapy.** *Hepatology* 1993, **17**:599–604.

31. Batta AK, Salen G, Mirchandani R, Tint GS, Shefer S, Batta M, Abroon J, O'Brien CB, Senior JR: **Effect of Long-Term Treatment With Ursodiol on Clinical and Biochemical Features and Biliary Bile Acid Metabolism in Patients With Primary Biliary Cirrhosis.** *Am J Gastroenterol* 1993, **88**:691–700.

32. Poupon RE, Ouguerram K, Chretien Y, Bemeau C, Eschwege E, Magot T, Poupon R: **Cholesterol-Lowering Effect of Ursodeoxycholic Acid in Patients With Primary Biliary Cirrhosis.** *Hepatology* 1993, **17**:577–582.

33. Mazzella G, Parini P, Bazzoli F, Villanova N, Fest D, Aldini R, Roda A, Cipolla A, Polimeni C, Tonelli D, Roda E: **Ursodeoxycholic Acid Administration on Bile Acid Metabolism in Patients With Early Stages of Primary Biliary Cirrhosis.** *Dig Dis Sci* 1993, **38**:896–902.

34. •• Ohiwa T, Katagiri K, Hoshino M, Hayakawa R, Nakai T: **Tauroursodeoxycholate and Tauro-β-Muricholate Exert Cytoprotection by Reducing Intrahepatocyte Taurochenodeoxycholate Content.** *Hepatology* 1993, **17**:470–476.

Studies using hepatocytes isolated by collagenase perfusion demonstrated the cytoprotective effect of certain bile salts, with decreased intracellular concentrations of taurochenodeoxycholate and improved cell viability. Bile salt hydrophilicity is correlated with protective capacity.

35. • Lacaille F, Paradis K: **The Immunosuppressive Effect of Ursodeoxycholic Acid - A Comparative In Vitro Study on Human Peripheral Blood Mononuclear Cells.** *Hepatology* 1993, **18**:165–172.

Bile salts inhibited mitogen-stimulated peripheral monocyte proliferation, as well as T-cell clone proliferation, and ursodeoxycholic acid inhibited interleukin-2 production.

36. Kurtschiev D, Subat S, Adler D, Schentke KU: **Immunomodulating Effect of Ursodeoxycholic Acid Therapy in Patients With Primary Biliary Cirrhosis.** *J Hepatol* 1993, **18**:373–377.

37. Nakai T, Katagiri K, Hoshino M, Hayakawa T, Ohiwa T: **Microtubule-Independent Choleresis and Anti-Cholestatic Action of Tauroursodeoxycholate in Colchicine-Treated Rat Liver.** *Biochem J* 1992, **288**:613–617.

38. Guldutuna S, Zimmer G, Irnhof M, Bhati S, You T, Leuschner U: **Molecular Aspects of Membrane Stabilization by Ursodeoxycholate.** *Gastroenterology* 1993, **104**:1736–1744.

39. Buscher HP, Zitzschmann Y, Gerok W: **Positive Responses to Methotrexate and Ursodeoxycholic Acid in Patients With Primary Biliary Cirrhosis Responding Insufficiently to Ursodeoxycholic Acid Alone.** *J Hepatol* 1993, **18**:9–14.

40. •• Lombard M, Portmann B, Neuberger J, Williams R, Tystrup N, Ranek L, Ring-Larsen H, Rodes J, Navasa M, Trepo C, Pape G, Schou G, Badsberg JH, Andersen PK: **Cyclosporin: A Treatment in Primary Biliary Cirrhosis: Results of a Long-Term Placebo Controlled Trial.** *Gastroenterology* 1993, **104**:519–526.

A large multicenter trial of Cyclosporin A in 349 patients demonstrated no significant improvement in biochemical or clinical parameters. Interval to death or liver transplantation was prolonged (not statistically significant). Marked renal toxicity was observed.

41. Kaplan MN: **New Strategies Needed for Treatment of Primary Biliary Cirrhosis?** *Gastroenterology* 1993, **104**:651–653.

42. Mitchison HC, Mutimer DJ, James OFW, Triger DR, Moller B, Hopf U, Hahn EG, Raedsch R, Gmelin K, Kommerell B, Liehr H, Schalm SW, van Buuren HR, Brandt KH, Henegouwen GPV, Trepo C, Adler M, Geubel AP, Fevery J, Tenkate FJW, Hop WCJ: **The Results of a Randomized Double Blind Controlled Trial Evaluating Malotilate in Primary Biliary Cirrhosis.** *J Hepatol* 1993, **17**:227–235.

43. Rhoton AJ: **Role for Thalidomide in Primary Biliary Cirrhosis Treatment? [Letter].** *Gastroenterology* 1993, **105**:956.

44. Wong PYN, Portmann B, Ogrady JG, Devlin JJ, Hegarty JE, Tan KC, Williams R: **Recurrence of Primary Biliary Cirrhosis After Liver Transplantation Following FK-506-Based Immunosuppression.** *J Hepatol* 1993, **17**:284–287.

45. • Hubscher SG, Elias E, Buckels JAC, Mayer AD, McMaster P, Neuberger JM: **Primary Biliary Cirrhosis: Histological Evidence of Disease Recurrence After Liver Transplantation.** *J Hepatol* 1993, **18**:251–254.

A recurrence rate of 16% after 1 year was documented, with no data on prognosis.

46. Lo SK, Chapman RW, Fleming KA: **Tissue Distribution of Autoantigen Specific for Primary Sclerosing Cholangitis.** *J Clin Pathol* 1993, **46**:246–249.

47. Lo SK, Chapman RWG, Cheeseman P, Charlton CPJ, Walker-Smith JA, Mieli-Vergani G, Fleming KA: **Antineutrophil Antibody: A Test for Autoimmune Primary Sclerosing Cholangitis in Childhood?** *Gut* 1993, **34**:199–202.

48. Lo SK, Chapman RW, Fleming KA: **Investigation of the Specimen Autoantigen of Primary Sclerosing Cholangitis by Western Blot and Immunoprecipitation.** *Hepatology* 1993, **18**:469–471.

49. Berg PA, Klein R: **Reply.** *Hepatology* 1993, **18**:471–474.

50. Bloom S, Heryet A, Fleming K, Chapman RW: **Inappropriate Expression of Blood Group Antigen on Biliary and Colonic Epithelia in Primary Sclerosing Cholangitis.** *Gut* 1993, **34**:977–983.

51. Broome U, Hultcrantz R, Scheynius A: **Lack of Concomitant Expression of ICAM-1 and HLA-DR on Bile Duct Cells From Patients With Primary Sclerosing Cholangitis and Primary Biliary Cirrhosis.** *Scand J Gastroenterol* 1993, **28**:126–130.

52. Gross Jr. JB: **Promises, Promises: Ursodeoxycholic Acid for Primary Sclerosing Cholangitis.** *Gastroenterology* 1993, **104**:941–943.

53. Rudolph G. Endele R, Senn M, Stiehl A: **Effect of Ursodeoxycholic Acid on the Kinetics of Cholic Acid and Chenodeoxycholic Acid in Patients With Primary Sclerosing Cholangitis.** *Hepatology* 1993, **17**:1028–1032.

54. Kartheuser AH, Dozois RR, Wiesner RH, Larusso NF, Ilstrup DM, Schleck CD: **Complications and Risk Factors After Ileal Pouch-Anal Anastomosis for Ulcerative Colitis Associated With Primary Sclerosing Cholangitis.** *Ann Surg* 1993, **217**:314–320.

55. • Strasser S, Sheil AGR, Gallagher ND, Waugh R, Mccaughan GW: **Liver Transplantation for Primary Sclerosing Cholangitis Versus Primary Biliary Cirrhosis - A Comparison of Complications and Outcome.** *J Gastroenterol Hepatol* 1993, **8**:238–243.

Recurrent septic cholangitis pretransplant was associated with an increased incidence of post-operative septic complications. Cholangiocarcinoma was diagnosed post-transplant in several PSC patients, despite rigorous efforts to identify it prior to transplantation.

56. Derby LE, Jick H, Henry DA, Dean AD: **Erythromycin-Associated Cholestatic Hepatitis.** *Med J Aust* 1993, **158**:600–602.

57. Uzzan B, Vassy R, Nicolas P, Chapman A, Perret G: **Troleandomycin Hepatotoxicity: A Case Report of Overt Jaundice and a Placebo-Controlled Trial.** *Therapie* 1993, **48**:59–62.

58. Denie C, Henrion J, Schapira M, Schmitz A, Heller FR: **Spiramycin-Induced Cholestatic Hepatitis.** *J Hepatol* 1992, 16:386.

59. Fairley CK, McNeil JJ, Desmond P, Smallwood R, Young H, Forbes A, Purcell P, Boyd I: **Risk Factors for Development of Flucloxacillin Associated Jaundice.** *BMJ* 1993, **306**:233–235.

60. Derby LE, Jick H, Henry DA, Dean AD: **Cholestatic Hepatitis Associated With Flucloxacillin.** *Med J Aust* 1993, **158**:596–600.

61. Mondardini A, Pasquine P, Bernardi P, Aluffi E, Tartaglino B, Mazzucco G, Bonino F, Verme G, Negro F: **Propafenone-Induced Liver Injury: Report of a Case and Review of the Literature.** *Gastroenterology* 1993, **104**:1524–1526.

62. Qaseem T, Jafri W, Khurshid M, Khan H: **Cholestatic Jaundice Associated With Danazol Therapy.** *Postgrad Med J* 1992, **68**:984–985.

63. Bray GP, Tredger JM, Williams R: **Resolution of Danazol-Induced Cholestasis With S-Adenosylmethionine.** *Postgrad Med J* 1993, **69**:237–239.

64. Rosman AS, Frissorarodeo C, Marshall AT, Reiter BP, Paronetto F: **Cholestatic Hepatitis Following Flutamide.** *Dig Dis Sci* 1993, **38**:1756–1759.

65. Yoshida E, Levin A: **Lovastatin and Cholestasis.** *Can Med Assoc J* 1993, **148**:374.

66. Billstrom R, Blomberg HMS: **Cholestasis After Interpleural Bupivacaine for Chronic Upper Limb Pain.** *Anesth Analg* 1993, **76**:1158–1159.

67. • Chamuleau RAFM, Dickman MJM, Bos PJM, Smitt JHS, Bosma A, Schellekens PTA: **Reappearance of Vanished Bile Ducts.** *Hepatogastroenterology* 1992, **39**:523–524.

Bile duct disappearance following probable drug-induced hepatotoxicity was documented on serial biopsies. One year after onset of jaundice, bile ducts reappeared on biopsy and bilirubin levels had normalized with no specific therapy.

68. •• Ben-Ari Z, Dhillon AP, Sherlock S: **Autoimmune Cholangiopathy - Part of the Spectrum of Autoimmune Chronic Active Hepatitis.** *Hepatology* 1993, **18**:10–15.

The authors propose that autoimmune cholangitis represents a subset of chronic autoimmune hepatitis, rather than a distinct disease entity or a variant of PBC, and document response of several patients to corticosteroid therapy.

69. Reyes H: **The Spectrum of Liver and Gastrointestinal Disease Seen in Cholestasis of Pregnancy.** *Gastroenterol Clin North Am* 1992, **21**:905–921.

70. Dubner H, Fromm H: **Ursodeoxycholic Acid Treatment of Intrahepatic Cholestasis of Pregnancy: Observations of Safety and Efficacy.** *Gastroenterology* 1993, **104**:660–661.

71. Olsson R, Tysk C, Aldenborg F, Holm B: **Prolonged Postpartum Course of Intrahepatic Cholestasis of Pregnancy.** *Gastroenterology* 1993, **105**:267–271.

72. Ros E, Navarro S, Bru C, Gilabert R, Bianchi L, Bruguera M: **Ursodeoxycholic Acid Treatment of Primary Hepatolithiasis in Caroli's Syndrome.** *Lancet* 1993, **342**:404–406.

73. • Colombo C, Crosignani A, Assaisso M, Battezzati PM, Podda M, Giunta Z, Zimmermechemias L, Setchell KDR: **Ursodeoxycholic Acid Therapy in Cystic Fibrosis Associated Liver Disease - A Dose Response Study.** *Hepatology* 1992, 16:924–930.

Because of impaired gastrointestinal absorption, higher than expected doses of ursodeoxycholic acid are required in cystic fibrosis to modify biliary bile acid concentrations.

74. Quigley EMM, Marsh MN, Shaffer JL, Markin RS: **Hepatobiliary Complications of Total Parenteral Nutrition.** *Gastroenterology* 1993, **104**:286–301.

75. Culebras JM, Garcia-Vielba J, Garcia-Diez F, Delahoz MD, Collado PS, Gonzalez-Gallego F: **The Effects of Total Parenteral Nutrition on the Hepatic Handling of Bilirubin in the Rat.** *JPEN J Parenter Enterol Nutr* 1993, **17**:125–129.

76. Rintala R, Lindahl H, Pohjavuori M, Saxen H, Sariola H: **Surgical Treatment of Intractable Cholestasis Associated With Total Parenteral Nutrition in Premature Infants.** *J Pediatr Surg* 1993, **5**:716–719.

77. Aller MA, Lorente L, Alonso S, Arias J: **A Model of Cholestasis in the Rat, Using a Microsurgical Technique.** *Scand J Gastroenterol* 1993, **28**:10–14.

78. Hines JE, Johnson SJ, Burt AD: **In Vivo Responses of Macrophages and Perisinusoidal Cells to Cholestatic Liver Injury.** *Am J Pathol* 1992, **142**:511–518.

79. Adachi Y, Arii S, Sasaoki T, Funaki N, Higashitsuji H, Fujita S, Furutani M, Mise M, Shang WH, Tobe T: **Hepatic Macrophage Malfunction in Rats With Obstructive Jaundice and Its Biological Significance.** *J Hepatol* 1992, 16:171–176.

80. Zimmerman H, Reichen J: **Ursodeoxycholate Has no Beneficial Effect on Liver Function or Histology in Biliary Cirrhosis in the Rat.** *J Hepatol* 1992, **16**:355–359.

81. • Frezza EE, Gerunda GE, Plebani M, Galligioni A, Giacomini A, Neri D, Faccioli AM, Tiribelli C: **Effect of Ursodeoxycholic Acid Administration on Bile Duct Proliferation and Cholestasis in Bile Duct Ligated Rat.** *Dig Dis Sci* 1993, **38**:1291–1296.

Administration of ursodeoxycholic acid in bile duct ligand rats inhibited bile duct proliferation.

82. Bossard R, Stieger B, O'Neill B, Fricker G, Meier PJ: **Ethinylestradiol Treatment Induces Multiple Canalicular Membrane Transport Alterations in Rat Liver.** *J Clin Invest* 1993, **91**:2714–2720.

83. Bouchard G, Yousef IM, Tuchweber B: **Influence of Oral Treatment With Ursodeoxycholic and Tauroursodeoxycholic Acids on Estrogen-Induced Cholestasis in Rats - Effects on Bile Formation and Liver Plasma Membranes.** *Liver* 1993, 13:193–202.

84. Takikawa H, Minagawa K, Sano N, Yamanaka M: **Lithocholate-3-O-Glucuronide-Induced Cholestasis: A Study With Congenital Hyperbilirubinemic Rats and Effects of Ursodeoxycholate Conjugates.** *Dig Dis Sci* 1993, **38**:1543–1548.

85. Sano N, Takikawa H, Yamanaka M: **Estradiol-17 β-Glucuronide-Induced Cholestasis - Effects of Ursodeoxycholate-3-O-Glucuronide and 3,7-Disulfate.** *J Hepatol* 1993, **17**: 241–246.

86. • Gillespie DA, Vickers CR: **Pruritus and Cholestasis - Therapeutic Options.** *J Gastroenterol Hepatol* 1993, **8**:168–173.

A concise review of the current available therapies for pruritus.

87. Jones EA, Bergasa NV: **The Pruritus of Cholestasis and the Opoid System.** *JAMA* 1992, **268**:3359–3362.

88. Gregorio GV, Ball CS, Mowat AP, Mielivergani G: **Effect of Rifampicin in the Treatment of Pruritus in Hepatic Cholestasis.** *Arch Dis Child* 1993, **69**:141–143.

89. Schworer H, Ramadori G: **Improvement of Cholestatic Pruritus by Ondansetron.** *Lancet* 1993, **341**:1277.

John L. Gollan, MD, PhD, Department of Medicine, Gastroenterology Division, Brigham and Women's Hospital, Harvard Medical School, 75 Francis Street, Boston, MA 02115, USA.

New developments in drug hepatotoxicity

Carolyn Holeski, MD, PhD, and Neil Kaplowitz, MD

University of Southern California School of Medicine, Los Angeles, California, USA

Drug hepatotoxicity continues to be a major concern in health care today. Many commonly used drugs are known to have possible hepatotoxic side effects. There are drug-drug interactions that are known to potentiate the hepatotoxicity of some drugs. In this review, we discuss the current developments in the field of hepatotoxicity and review recent literature on several known hepatotoxic agents. Of the many drugs and toxins known to produce liver injury, only those that have received the most attention in the recent literature are discussed. Nonsteroidal anti-inflammatory drugs are a class of drugs that is widely used, but the potential hepatotoxic side effects are not always appreciated. Total parenteral nutrition has become increasingly used in medicine today. Recent studies have discussed possible mechanisms by which total parenteral nutrition may produce liver injury. Other commonly used drugs with possible hepatotoxic side effects are also discussed.

Current Opinion in Gastroenterology 1994, **10**:313–318

Diagnosing drug hepatotoxicity relies on a clinical index of suspicion and recognition of drug or toxin exposure. However, understanding the mechanisms involved may provide the information for possible treatment or prevention of hepatotoxicity. Until recently, the study of hepatotoxicity was limited by the available animal models. Since the early 1980s, investigators have been attempting to isolate and culture human hepatocytes. Recent major advances have provided new tools with which to study the effects of drugs and toxins on the human liver. One example is the refined methods available for maintaining functional drug-metabolizing enzyme activities in culture. Moshage and Yap [1•] have written a useful review on the use of cultured human hepatocytes in the study of disease mechanisms.

Nonsteroidal anti-inflammatory drugs

Nonsteroidal anti-inflammatory drugs (NSAIDs) are commonly used today. The gastrointestinal side effects are widely recognized; however, many health care professionals are less aware of the potential hepatotoxic side effects. The hepatotoxic side effects of these drugs are rare, but the liver injury may be severe or even fatal when it occurs. Many case reports continue to appear in the literature documenting the hepatotoxicity of these drugs; a recent review by Rabinovitz and Van Thiel [2••], published within the past year, discusses the hepatotoxicity of the many drugs within the category of NSAIDs. Although the mechanism by which aspirin results in hepatotoxicity appears to be an intrinsic one, most of the other NSAIDs appear to cause toxicity through an idiosyncratic or hypersensitivity reaction.

Hepatotoxicity of aspirin appears to be dependent on dosage, plasma levels, duration of exposure, and age. Plasma levels over 15 mg/mL have been associated with hepatic injury, and duration of exposure varies between 1 and several weeks. Children appear to be at greater risk of aspirin hepatotoxicity. Preexisting liver disease is also a risk factor for developing aspirin-induced hepatotoxicity. It has been suggested that hypoalbuminemia associated with preexisting liver disease may result in decreased protein binding of aspirin. Thus, higher serum levels of aspirin, which may result in hepatotoxic side effects, occur [3].

Phenylbutazone is known to have potentially serious hepatic side effects, with an incidence of hepatotoxicity ranging from 1% to 5% [4]. In their series of 23 cases of phenylbutazone hepatotoxicity, Benjamin *et al.* [5] found a fatality rate of nearly 25%.

The incidence of indomethacin-induced hepatotoxicity is rare, estimated to be less than 5% of reported side effects. However, because indomethacin was attributed to several early cases of fatal hepatotoxicity, it has been suggested that indomethacin should not be prescribed to patients with underlying liver disease [4].

Abbreviations

NSAID—nonsteroidal anti-inflammatory drug; **TPN**—total parenteral nutrition.

 ISBN 1-85922-608-6 ISSN 0267–1379

Sulindac is also associated with hepatotoxicity. Although asymptomatic elevations in liver enzymes occur in approximately 15% of patients, serious hepatotoxicity can also occur, but infrequently. Sulindac-induced hepatotoxicity may be diagnosed within 1 to 4 weeks of initiating therapy, with general symptoms of fatigue, nausea, vomiting, and abdominal discomfort. Histologically, a cholestatic or mixed hepatocellular injury can occur. Symptoms resolve after discontinuation of the drug. Rechallenge of the drug is not recommended because it may result in serious side effects.

Piroxicam (Feldene; Charles Pfizer & Co., New York, NY) is an oxicam that is chemically unrelated to the other NSAIDs. It has a long half-life and therefore has a more convenient daily dosing schedule. It is generally believed that hepatotoxicity with this agent is less common than with the other NSAIDs. However, new cases of serious hepatotoxicity continue to be reported. Within the past year, Paterson *et al.* [6•] reported two additional cases of fulminant hepatic failure believed to be due to piroxicam. Piroxicam is believed to act as an idiosyncratic hepatotoxin, producing hepatocellular injury from 1.5 to 15 months after initiation of therapy.

Although transient, asymptomatic elevations of liver enzymes occur with diclofenac (Voltaren; Ciba-Geigy, Basel, Switzerland) therapy, severe toxicity was previously thought to be rare. However, increasing numbers of cases of diclofenac hepatotoxicity have been published within the past 10 years. Scully *et al.* [7•] described three cases of diclofenac-induced hepatitis diagnosed by one hepatology practice during a single year. They suggest that cases of diclofenac hepatotoxicity may be more common than previously recognized because their cases were initially misdiagnosed as autoimmune hepatitis and were treated using corticosteroid therapy before being referred to their practice. All three patients developed positive antinuclear antibody titers, which resolved after discontinuation of diclofenac. However, each patient developed recurrent liver injury with elevated antinuclear antibodies when rechallenged with diclofenac or a related drug. All were later able to tolerate naproxen without significant side effects.

Ibuprofen and naproxen appear to be better tolerated than most NSAIDs. Although transient liver enzyme abnormalities have been reported with these drugs, the incidence appears to be less than with other NSAIDs. Few cases of hepatotoxicity have been reported with these drugs.

In a retrospective case-control study using Medicaid billing data from Michigan and Florida to identify patients who were hospitalized with acute idiopathic hepatitis between 1980 and 1987, Carson *et al.* [8•] calculated an incidence rate of 2.2 per 100,000 people per year. Nine cases had been exposed to NSAIDs, yielding an odds ratio of 1.4 (0.6 to 3.1), which after adjusting for potential confounding variables, was 1.2 (0.5 to 2.8). The authors concluded that there was no association between NSAIDs and acute hepatitis in their study. However, there were several problems with this study that may have affected the results and conclusions. The first was that data on NSAID use were determined by computed pharmacy records for an NSAID prescription filled within the 30 days prior to hospitalization. No attempt was made to document whether NSAIDs were taken as prescribed, whether over-the-counter NSAIDs were taken, or what was the duration of NSAID exposure. Only 52% of the medical records requested were obtained. No hepatitis C testing was available at the time of the study, and other hepatitis serologies were not performed in 17% of the cases for which the authors had medical records. Although the validity of the study is questionable due to the many methodologic problems, it does illustrate the difficulty involved in performing a study of this nature.

Total parenteral nutrition

Hepatobiliary complications of total parenteral nutrition (TPN) has been a major topic in the recent literature (Table 1). A review by Quigley *et al.* [9•] discusses the recent literature involving the effects of TPN in adults and children. These authors have divided the TPN-related complications into three clinical syndromes (Table 2): cholestasis (which is most frequently observed in children), steatosis and steatohepatitis (seen predominantly in adults), and biliary sludge formation and cholelithiasis (seen in both children and adults).

Table 1. Hepatobiliary disorders reported in patients undergoing total parenteral nutrition*

Adults
Steatosis†
Steatohepatitis†
Cholestasis
Fibrosis
Micronodular cirrhosis
Phospholipidosis
Biliary sludge†
Cholelithiasis and its complications†
Acalculous cholecystitis
Infants
Cholestasis†
Fibrosis
Cirrhosis
Hepatocellular carcinoma
Biliary sludge
Abdominal pseudotumor (distended gallbladder)†
Cholelithiasis and its complications

*From Quigley *et al.* [9•]; with permission.
†More common disorders.

It has been difficult to determine the incidence of TPN-induced hepatic injury because the many studies evalu-

Table 2. Patient factors and total parenteral nutrition–related effects proposed to contribute to the pathophysiology of hepatobiliary dysfunction during total parenteral nutrition*

		TPN-related effects	
Complication	Patient factors	Major	Minor or controversial
Steatosis	Starvation Protein-calorie malnutrition Glucose intolerance	Calorie excess Carbohydrate excess Carbohydrate-nitrogen imbalance	Essential fatty-acid deficiency Carnitine deficiency Impaired drug oxidation Absence of dietary "protective factor" L-glutamine deficiency Lipid excess
Cholestasis			
Children	Immaturity of biliary secretory system Absence of oral intake (loss of enteric stimulation) Sepsis Major surgery (especially gastrointestinal) Disturbed enterohepatic circulation Small intestinal bacterial overgrowth Hypoxia	Amino acid excess Prolonged duration of TPN	Serine deficiency Methionine deficiency Taurine deficiency Selenium, vitamin E deficiency TPN contaminants (sodium bisulphite, aluminum) Bacterial translocation L-glutamine deficiency Lithocholate toxicity
Adults	Absence of oral intake (loss of enteric stimulation) Sepsis Ileal disease or resection Short bowel syndrome Inflammatory bowel disease Malignant disease Bacterial overgrowth Lithocholate toxicity	Duration of TPN	Low energy-to-nitrogen ratio Continuous administration Bacterial translocation L-glutamine deficiency Copper in TPN solution Lipid content Lithocholate toxicity
Gallbladder disease and gallstones	Fasting, loss of enteric stimuli gallbladder stasis, and impaired bile flow	Decreased bile flow	Altered bile composition

*From Quigley *et al.* [9•]; with permission.
TPN—total parenteral nutrition.

ating this injury involve varied patient populations and TPN compositions, and their results are not consistent with one another. Most studies agree that TPN-induced liver injury in adults is evident between 1 and 4 weeks of initiating therapy. Enzyme elevations are often mild and enzyme levels may return to normal with continuance of TPN. Patients are usually asymptomatic, but may complain of right upper quadrant tenderness. Histologic evidence of periportal fat accumulation is often seen, with progression to panlobular distribution in more advanced cases. Many studies have investigated the mechanism underlying the TPN-induced steatosis. It is generally believed that excess calories delivered as dextrose or glucose stimulate insulin release that results in hepatic fat deposition and lipogenesis, inhibits fatty acid oxidation and lipoprotein synthesis, and impairs triglyceride secretion. The mechanism by which TPN results in cholestasis in children is poorly understood.

Halothane

Halothane is an anesthetic agent well known for its potential hepatotoxicity. Two types of hepatotoxicity may result from halothane exposure: a mild form and a more severe, fulminant form. Patients with halothane hepatotoxicity have been shown to have specific serum antibodies to liver microsomal proteins bound with halothane metabolites. Martin *et al.* [10••] attempted to isolate and characterize these specific target proteins, and they report that one of these antigens is the enzyme protein disulfide isomerase, bound to a trifluoroacetyl metabolite of halothane. These researchers had earlier identified three other antigenic proteins, carboxylesterase, calreticulin, and a protein with unknown function, termed *ERp72* [10••,11,12]. Future work is needed to further identify the liver antigens involved in this specific antibody response and to further identify the nature of the immune reaction and whether it is T-cell or antibody mediated. Hopefully, this research will bring us closer to a treatment or prevention of halothane hepatotoxicity.

Amiodarone

Amiodarone is an anti-arrhythmic drug associated with a range of hepatic side effects, from asymptomatic liver enzyme elevation to cirrhosis. The use of amiodarone has greatly increased over the past several years. Recently, a case of acute hepatitis due to intravenous administration of amiodarone was reported by Rhodes *et al.* [13•]. There are three other case reports in the literature documenting an amiodarone-induced acute hepatitis [14–16]. However, in the case reported by Rhodes *et al.* [13•], amiodarone was re-administered orally with no adverse sequelae noted. The authors speculate that amiodarone itself may not have caused the initial acute hepatitis, but that the intravenous vehicle, polysorbate 80, may have been responsible. This explanation is very intriguing, but there is little information provided to support it.

Propafenone

Another antiarrhythmic agent, propafenone, used to treat supraventricular and ventricular arrhythmias, is also potentially hepatotoxic. Mondardini *et al.* [17•] reported a case of propafenone hepatotoxicity and reviewed the limited literature on this subject. Propafenone toxicity appears to be rare; however, health care workers should be aware of the potential for hepatotoxicity with increased use of this agent. Propafenone produces an acute cholestatic syndrome, with onset of symptoms occurring 2 to 4 weeks after initiation of therapy. Histology showed cholestasis with inflammatory infiltrates in the portal tracts. The patient described by Mondardini *et al.* recovered initially, but he developed a similar syndrome when rechallenged with propafenone. He recovered fully after discontinuation of the drug.

Propylthiouracil

Propylthiouracil is a thiourea commonly used in the treatment of hyperthyroidism. There have been a small number of cases of presumed propylthiouracil-induced liver injury reported in the literature since 1953. Because most of these cases had been reported before the introduction of serologic testing for hepatitis C, Liaw *et al.* [18••] designed a study to estimate the incidence of propylthiouracil-induced liver injury using state of the art technologies to rule out other possible causes of liver injury (namely, second-generation tests for hepatitis C virus). The study found that 30% of 54 patients (15 patients) treated with propylthiouracil developed asymptomatic liver test abnormalities. None of the enzyme abnormalities were due to viral hepatitis infection. In 13 of the 15 patients, these enzyme abnormalities returned to baseline within 3 months, even though the drug was continued at a lower dose (Fig. 1). Liver biopsies done in three patients showed pericentral necrosis and granuloma-like lesions. No clinical hepatitis was diagnosed in this series of patients. The authors suggest that subclinical liver injury is relatively common in patients treated with propylthiouracil for hyperthyroidism. In addition, they suggest that propylthiouracil may be cautiously continued in patients who develop mild liver test abnormalities, but at a reduced dose. However, because this was a small study, further data need to be collected to determine the true incidence of propylthiouracil-induced liver disease.

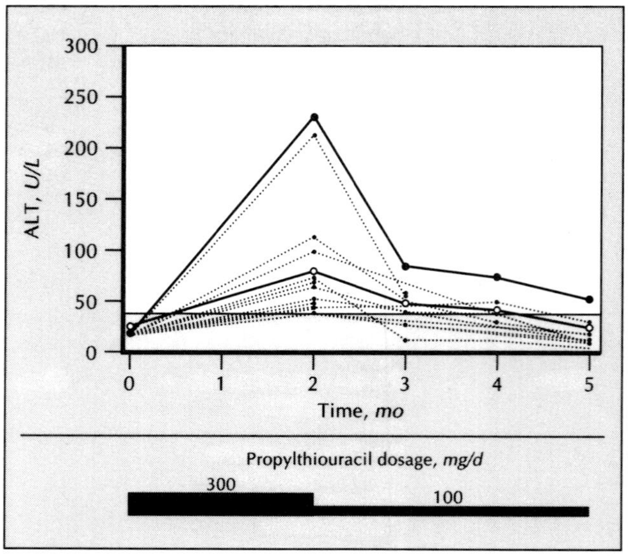

Fig. 1. Changes of alanine aminotransferase (ALT) levels over time for each of the 15 patients with ALT elevation during propylthiouracil therapy (*dotted lines*). The *solid line with open circles* represents the mean level of ALT over time. The *solid line with closed circles* represents the ALT changes over time in the patient with the highest ALT elevations (231 U/L [3.85 μkat/L]), who received a liver biopsy 5 months after starting therapy. (*From* Liaw *et al.* [18••]; with permission.)

Other hepatotoxic drugs

A study by Tavani *et al.* [19•] confirms the risk of hepatocellular carcinoma in patients using oral contraceptive hormones, and shows that this risk persists for more than 10 years after discontinuing the therapy. The investigators also found a correlation with duration of use of oral contraceptives, but found no increased risk associated with the use of estrogen replacement therapy.

The antiestrogen, tamoxifen, used in the treatment of breast cancer, is now being used as a prophylactic therapy in healthy women with a family history of breast cancer. A recent report by Williams *et al.* [20••] has shown that tamoxifen is a potent hepatocarcinogen in female rats, producing tumors after 1 year in 75% of rats receiving high doses. The authors raise serious concerns about the use of this drug for long-term prophylaxis against breast cancer in healthy women.

Acetaminophen toxicity is known to be potentiated by alcohol. Recent reports have been published showing possible potentiation of acetaminophen toxicity by "starvation" diets [21•] and by isoniazid therapy [22•].

The unfortunate story that received headline news in major cities in the United States involved an investigational drug used to treat hepatitis B, Fialuridine. This drug was used to treat a small group of patients with hepatitis B at the National Institutes of Health, as part of a study protocol. Early reports were encouraging, suggesting that this drug was effective in treating the hepatitis B virus. However, after several weeks of therapy, many of the patients developed lactic acidosis and liver failure [23•]. In some cases, toxicity developed months after the drug had been discontinued. Liver biopsy specimens showed steatosis and mitochondrial abnormalities. Several of the patients died before liver transplantation could be arranged. This unfortunate experience further emphasizes the serious nature of hepatotoxic side effects of drugs, especially the possible risks associated with newer drugs for which years of clinical experience are not yet available.

References and recommended reading

Papers of particular interest, published within the annual period of review, have been highlighted as:
- • Of special interest
- •• Of outstanding interest

1. • Moshage H, Yap SH: **Primary Cultures of Human Hepatocytes: A Unique System for Studies in Toxicology, Virology, Parasitology, and Liver Pathophysiology in Man.** *J Hepatol* 1992, **15**:404–413.
A useful review on the applications of cultured human hepatocytes in the study of toxicology and in other fields.

2. •• Rabinovitz M, Van Thiel DH: **Hepatotoxicity of Nonsteroidal Anti-Inflammatory Drugs.** *Am J Gastroenterol* 1992, **87**:1696–1704.
A thorough review on the hepatotoxicity of NSAIDs.

3. Gitlin N: **Salicylate Hepatotoxicity: The Potential Role of Hypoalbuminemia.** *J Clin Gastroenterol* 1980, **2**:281–285.

4. Lewis JH: **Hepatic Toxicity of Nonsteroidal Anti-Inflammatory Drugs.** *Clin Pharm* 1984, **3**:128–138.

5. Benjamin SB, Ishak KG, Zimmerman JH: **Phenylbutazone Liver Injury: A Clinical Pathologic Survey of 23 Cases and Review of the Literature.** *Hepatology* 1981, **1**:255–263.

6. • Paterson D, Kerlin P, Walker N, Lynch S, Strong R: **Piroxicam Induced Submassive Necrosis of the Liver.** *Gut* 1992, **33**:1436–1438.
Three additional cases of piroxicam-induced hepatitis are described, and the possible mechanisms of toxicity are discussed.

7. • Scully LJ, Clarke D, Barr RJ: **Diclofenac Induced Hepatitis: 3 Cases With Features of Autoimmune Chronic Active Hepatitis.** *Dig Dis Sci* 1993, **38**:744–751.
Reports three cases of diclofenac-induced hepatitis and provides an excellent discussion of the current literature available. This study also suggests that diclofenac-induced hepatotoxicity may be more common than was previously appreciated and emphasizes the need to recognize possible hepatotoxicity when it occurs.

8. • Carson JL, Strom, BL, Dugg, A, Gupta A, Das K: **Safety of Nonsteroidal Anti-Inflammatory Drugs With Respect to Acute Liver Disease.** *Arch Intern Med* 1993, **153**:1331–1336.
Although hampered by methodologic difficulties, this study provides an assessment of the incidence and risks of hepatotoxicity due to NSAIDs.

9. • Quigley EM, Marsh MN, Shaffer JL, Markin RS: **Hepatobiliary Complications of Total Parenteral Nutrition.** *Gastroenterology* 1993, **104**:286–301.
A thorough review of TPN-induced liver toxicity, including a discussion of the possible mechanisms involved.

10. •• Martin JL, Kenna JG, Martin BM, Thomassen D, Reed GF, Pohl LR: **Halothane Hepatitis Patients Have Serum Antibodies That React With Protein Disulfide Isomerase.** *Hepatology* 1993, **18**:858–863.
Reports the purification and characterization of the fourth liver microsomal protein antigen that reacts with antibodies in sera from patients with halothane hepatitis.

11. Satoh H, Martin BM, Schulick AH, Christ DD, Kenna JG, Pohl LR: **Human Anti-Endoplasmic Reticulum Antibodies in Sera of Patients With Halothane-Induced Hepatitis are Directed Against a Trifluoroacetylated Carboxylesterase.** *Proc Natl Acad Sci U S A* 1989, **86**:322–326.

12. Butler LE, Thomassen D, Martin JL, Martin BM, Kenna JG, Pohl LR: **The Calcium-Binding Protein Calreticulin is Covalently Modified in Rat Liver by a Reactive Metabolite of the Inhalation Anesthetic Halothane.** *Chem Res Toxicol* 1992, **5**:406–410.

13. • Rhodes A, Eastwood JB, Smith SA: **Early Acute Hepatitis With Parenteral Amiodarone: A Toxic Effect of the Vehicle?** *Gut* 1993, **34**:565–566.
Describes a recent case of acute hepatotoxicity from parenteral amiodarone, in which oral amiodarone was later reintroduced with no toxic side effects. This paper is of special interest because it suggests that the acute hepatotoxicity observed may not be due to amiodarone itself, but to the vehicle in which is was administered.

14. Stevenson RNS, Nayam TH, Davies JR: **Acute Hepatic Dysfunction Following Parenteral Amiodarone Administration.** *Postgrad Med J* 1989, **65**:707–708.

15. Lupon-Roses J, Simo-Canonge R, Lu-Cortez L, Permanyer-Miralda G, Allende-Mondus J: **Probable Early Acute Hepatitis With Parenteral Amiodarone.** *Clin Cardiol* 1986, **9**:225–229.

16. Pye M, Northcote RJ, Cobbe SM: **Acute Hepatitis After Parenteral Amiodarone Administration.** *Br Heart J* 1988, **59**:690–691.

17. • Mondardini A, Pasquino P, Bernardi P, Aluffi E, Tartaglino B, Mazzucco G, Bonino F, Verme G, Negro F: **Propafenone-Induced Liver Injury: Report of a Case and Review of the Literature.** *Gastroeneterology* 1993, **104**:1524–1526.
Describes a case of acute cholestasis induced by the antiarrhythmic agent propafenone and discusses the currently available (although limited) literature.

18. •• Liaw YF, Huang MJ, Fan KD, Li KL, Wu SS, Chen TJ: **Hepatic Injury During Propylthiouracil Therapy in Patients With Hyperthyroidism: A Cohort Study.** *Ann Intern Med* 1993, **118**:424–428.
A useful paper evaluating the incidence of propylthiouracil-induced hepatotoxicity in a cohort study. Results indicated that mild liver enzyme elevation induced by propylthiouracil is common; however, more severe hepatotoxicity is rare.

19. • Tavani A, Negri E, Parazzini F, Franceschi S, La Vecchia C: **Female Hormone Utilisation and Risk of Hepatocellular Carcinoma.** *Br J Cancer* 1993, **67**:635–637.
Reports a case-control study to assess the risk of oral contraceptive–induced hepatocellular carcinoma.

20. •• Williams GM, Iatropoulos MJ, Djordjevic MV, Kaltenberg OP: **The Triphenylethylene Drug Tamoxifen is a Strong Liver Carcinogen in the Rat.** *Carcinogenesis* 1993, **14**:315–317.

Discusses a 1-year animal study done to assess possible risks of hepatotoxicity associated with the antiestrogenic drug, tamoxifen. This report raises concerns about the current use of tamoxifen (under study protocol) in healthy women as a prophylactic treatment for breast cancer.

21. • Eriksson LS, Broome U, Kalin M, Lindholm M: **Hepatotoxicity Due to Repeated Intake of Low Doses of Paracetamol.** *J Intern Med* 1992, **231**:567–570.

Discusses two cases of patients with acetaminophen toxicity who were evaluated for liver transplantation. It is suggested that acetaminophen toxicity was potentiated by low food intake that resulted in relative starvation.

22. • Crippin JS: **Acetaminophen Hepatotoxicity: Potentiation by Isoniazid.** *Am J Gastroenterol* 1993, **88**:590–592.

Discusses a case of acetaminophen toxicity potentiated by isoniazid.

23. • MacIlwain C: **NIH, FDA Seek Lessons From Hepatitis B Drug Trial Deaths.** *Nature* 1993, **364**:275.

An interesting report discussing the unfortunate incidents of hepatotoxicity due to a newer drug under study for the treatment of hepatitis B.

Carolyn Holeski, MD, PhD, and Neil Kaplowitz, MD, University of Southern California School of Medicine, GI/Liver Division, Department of Medicine, 2025 Zonal Avenue, Los Angeles, CA 90033, USA.

Alcoholic liver disease

Charles S. Lieber, MD

Bronx Veterans Affairs Medical Center, and Mount Sinai School of Medicine, New York, New York, USA

During the past year, abundant new information was gained on the metabolism and hepatotoxicity of ethanol. The molecular biology of hepatic alcohol dehydrogenase and the contribution of gastric alcohol dehydrogenase to the first-pass metabolism of ethanol and to alcohol-drug interactions were further described. The mechanism of the induction of the hepatic cytochrome P4502E1 (2E1) by chronic ethanol consumption was elucidated, and its contribution to hepatotoxicity via free radical formation and xenobiotic activation has been delineated. New roles for factors such as hepatitis C, cytokines, gender, genetics, and age have emerged. A better understanding of the pathology induced by ethanol (including enhanced fibrogenesis) has generated improved prospects for therapy.

Current Opinion in Gastroenterology 1994, **10**:319–330

Microsomal ethanol metabolism

Chronic ethanol consumption results in the induction of a specific hepatic microsomal cytochrome P450 enzyme (namely 2E1) that oxidizes ethanol. In contrast to other 2E1 inducers (such as acetone), chronic ethanol consumption had no effect on rates of 2E1 degradation but it increased the synthesis of the protein [1•]. Hepatic 2E1 messenger RNA, detected by *in situ* hybridization, was also increased with a selective perivenular response [1•]. This was confirmed in humans [2•]. In rats, the induction was shown to be dose dependent, with largely posttranslational mechanisms at low ethanol concentrations and an additional transcriptional or messenger RNA stabilization mechanism at high ethanol levels [3•]. The induction was caused primarily by ethanol rather than undernutrition or a combination of ethanol and undernutrition [4•]. Another substrate of 2E1, namely isoniazid, was also shown to be an inducer when given chronically, whereas acutely, it inhibited the metabolism of other 2E1 substrates such as acetaminophen and chlorozoxazone [5•].

As illustrated in figure 1, the medical significance of the microsomal ethanol metabolism (MEOS), and its ethanol-inducible 2E1, results not only from the oxidation of ethanol, but also from the unusual and unique capacity of 2E1 to generate reactive oxygen intermediates, such as superoxide radicals [6•], and to activate many xenobiotic compounds to toxic metabolites. These include various industrial solvents [7••,8•], such as *m*–xylene [9•]. Activation of hepatotoxins also pertains to analgesics. Studies in isolated periportal and perivenous hepatocytes illustrated the zonal distribution of acetaminophen metabolism and cytochrome P450 2E1-mediated toxicity [10]. Increased hepatotoxicity also pertains to anesthetics. 2E1 was found to be the predominant, if not singular, enzyme catalyzing defluorination (in human liver) of enflurane [11•], sevoflurane, isoflurane, and methoxyflurane [12]. Hepatotoxicity of xenobiotics may also be promoted by the decrease, after long-term ethanol treatment, in the activities of glutathione *S*-transferase and epoxide hydrolase [13].

Levels of 2E1 in humans were found to be extremely variable, and these variations were not simply related to liver disease nor to alcohol drinking or smoking habits and are as yet unexplained [14•].

When the existence of the MEOS was first proposed, it was argued that this activity may represent contaminating catalase. Reconstitution of MEOS with purified enzymes (including 2E1) laid this objection to rest, but catalase continues to be proposed as a participant in alcohol metabolism under special circumstances, *eg*, methanol metabolism in alcohol dehydrogenase–negative deermice, using H_2O_2 generated from fatty-acid oxidation. These data obtained with methanol were extrapolated to the metabolism of ethanol [15,16], which is questionable because ethanol metabolism via alcohol dehydrogenase is known to inhibit oxidation of fatty acids [17] and because H_2O_2 generation from fatty acids is small or virtually absent in the intact liver [18].

Abbreviations

CDT—carbohydrate-deficient transferrin; **MEOS**—microsomal ethanol metabolism; **TNF**—tumor necrosis factor.

ISBN 1-85922-608-6 ISSN 0267–1379

Long-term alcohol consumption pleiotropically increases microsomal activities other than that of the P–450 2E1 [7••]. One recent example of this effect was the observation that long-term ethanol administration to rats increases hepatic microsomal ω-hydroxylation of fatty acids and that this effect is greater in male than in female rats. These changes were associated with parallel alterations in the content of cytochrome P-450 4A1 (previously known as P-452) [19•].

Enhanced product formation from ω-oxidation may explain the increase in liver cytosolic fatty-acid binding protein [20], an effect recently confirmed [21]. 2E1, when induced, could contribute significantly to the formation of the ω-1 and ω-2 hydroxylated metabolites of arachidonic acid [22•]. In addition to gender, species differences in the induction properties of ethanol have been described, especially in extrahepatic tissues, and not only with regard to 2E1, but also in terms of 1A [23].

One alcohol-drug interaction of particular practical impact is that with cocaine. Ethanol potentiates cocaine-induced liver injury by mechanisms that are still not fully elucidated. Of interest are the observations that cocaine ethyl ester is formed in the presence of ethanol, may reach concentrations similar to those of cocaine, and was found to be equally injurious [24•]. Cocaine ethyl ester was also detected in plasma of volunteers given 100 mg of intranasal cocaine in acute alcohol intoxication [25].

In addition to the activation of hepatoxic agents, 2E1 was also confirmed in its role of promoter of lipid peroxidation [6•, 26].

Cytochrome P4502E1 genetic polymorphism with racial variation was described but it could not be related to genetic susceptibilities to disease [27•].

Alcohol metabolism mediated via alcohol dehydrogenase

Although the MEOS is of great interest because of its inducibility after chronic ethanol consumption and its interaction with various other xenobiotics (Fig. 1), the bulk of ethanol metabolism proceeds via alcohol dehydrogenase, the activity of which is determined by various genetic factors as reviewed by Bosron *et al.* [28••]. Progress was made in our understanding of factors that modulate alcohol dehydrogenase activity in the liver. For instance, a novel negative element in the promoter of the mouse alcohol dehydrogenase gene *ADH*-1 [29] was defined. Growth hormone, known to increase the transcription of the rat class I alcohol dehydrogenase gene, was found to probably act by enhancing alcohol dehydrogenase promoter activity, mediated by liver activator protein binding to the enhancer binding-protein site [30].

It was also suggested that alcohol dehydrogenase dimerization may play a role in activity [31]. However, some factors that are known to accelerate ethanol metabolism, such as carbohydrates, were found not to act via an alteration in hepatic alcohol dehydrogenase activity [32]. Furthermore, although it has been postulated before that the presence of an "atypical" alcohol dehydrogenase may play a role in the development of alcoholism or alcoholic liver disease, this was not found to be the case in a Spanish population [33•].

The liver represents the main site of ethanol metabolism, but extrahepatic oxidation of ethanol also occurs, primarily because of the existence of various forms of extrahepatic alcohol dehydrogenase, as described by Engeland and Maret [34]. Purification and determination of the partial amino acid sequence of a high-activity human stomach alcohol dehydrogenase (σADH) was accomplished by Stone *et al.* [35•]. The affinity of this form for ethanol is lower than that of the alcohol dehydrogenase classes that prevail in the liver but, because of the extraordinarily high concentration of ethanol in the stomach after alcohol consumption, even gastric alcohol dehydrogenase forms with a high K_m for ethanol participate; significant gastric ethanol oxidation ensues, as recently confirmed *in vivo* [36] and *in vitro* in cultured gastric cells [37].

Experimental studies showed that this gastric oxidation of ethanol can explain the decreased bioavailability of alcohol when taken orally, as compared with the same dose given intravenously (the so-called "first-pass metabolism of ethanol"). The role of the stomach was further illustrated by the disappearance of this first-pass metabolism when the stomach was bypassed (by intraduodenal or intraportal infusion), whereas bypassing the liver (via portal ligation and portocaval shunts) had no appreciable effect [38•]. Thus, the stomach can be viewed as a "protective" barrier against the penetration of alcohol into the body, and the lesser gastric alcohol dehydrogenase activity in women than in men [39] may contribute to their greater vulnerability to alcohol. This gender difference in alcohol dehydrogenase has now been confirmed [40•], at least in subjects less than 50 years old. In older individuals, this gender difference disappeared.

Because of the importance of concentration for the activity of gastric alcohol dehydrogenase, alcoholic beverages of relatively low concentration (such as beer), when taken with a meal, undergo less gastric metabolism and result in higher blood alcohol levels than equal amounts of ethanol taken as more concentrated distilled beverages [41•]. Several studies had shown before that H_2 blockers, which inhibit gastric alcohol dehydrogenase activity *in vitro*, also reduce ethanol first-pass metabolism and increase blood alcohol levels *in vivo* (Fig. 1*E*). A consensus has been reached for these effects, at least at low doses of alcohol. For higher doses the effect is still debated, as shown by a recent negative report [42]. However, the latter investigation did not specify whether first-pass

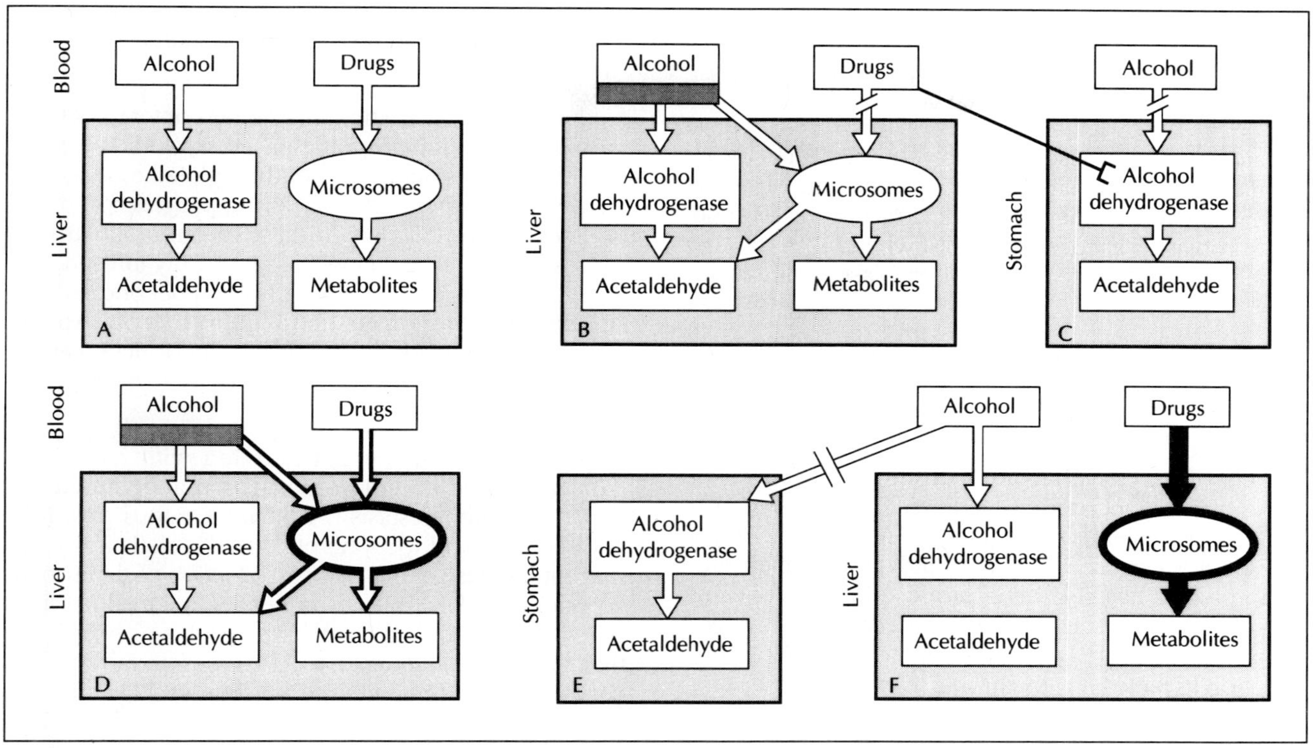

Fig. 1. Hepatic ethanol-drug interactions involving the alcohol dehydrogenase pathway and liver microsomes. **A**, Hepatic metabolism of alcohol by alcohol dehydrogenase and drugs by microsomes. **B**, Inhibition of hepatic microsomal drug metabolism in the presence of high concentrations of ethanol, in part through competition for a common microsomal detoxification process. **C**, Inhibition, by other drugs, of ethanol metabolism mediated by gastric alcohol dehydrogenase. **D**, Induction of microsomal enzymes, including cytochrome P450 2E1 (2E1), after chronic alcohol consumption and its contribution to accelerated hepatic metabolism of ethanol at high blood levels. **E**, Decreased gastric alcohol dehydrogenase activity and gastric ethanol metabolism after chronic alcohol abuse. **F**, Increased hepatic drug metabolism and xenobiotic activation to hepatotoxic agents and carcinogens because of the persisting microsomal induction after withdrawal from chronic alcohol consumption.

metabolism was present to begin with in the subjects studied; furthermore, dilute concentrations of alcohol were used, shown to minimize gastric ethanol metabolism. The existence of various confounding factors and the need for proper controls in studies of acute effects of alcohol and alcoholic beverages on the stomach was emphasized [43].

The respective roles of gastric alcohol dehydrogenase and the hepatic MEOS were studied in a strain of deermice lacking the hepatic low-K_m enzyme (ADH$^-$). It was concluded that in such deermice, when ethanol is given parenterally, the MEOS rather than gastric alcohol dehydrogenase is a major pathway of ethanol oxidation [44•], whereas both pathways contribute significantly to the metabolism of orally administered ethanol.

Because of the presence of high activity (and high-K_m) alcohol dehydrogenase as well as low-activity aldehyde dehydrogenase in human esophageal mucosa, it was postulated that there may be local accumulation of intracellular acetaldehyde during alcohol ingestion, which may be involved in the pathogenesis of alcohol-induced esophageal disorders [45•].

Acetaldehyde and markers of alcohol consumption

Acetaldehyde is the first oxidation product of ethanol by all pathways discussed above. Because of its high reactivity, it continues to be explored as the intermediate responsible for many aspects of alcoholic liver injury. Acetaldehyde measurements, however, still present difficulties, both in blood [46•] and in breath [47•].

Protein adduct formation is a key mode of acetaldehyde hepatotoxicity [48•]. Acetaldehyde binds covalently to various circulating proteins and lipoproteins [49•], as well as to liver proteins [50], one of which was identified as collagen-like [51•]. Koskinas *et al.* [52•] showed that circulating antibodies from patients with alcoholic liver disease recognize a 200-kD acetaldehyde–liver protein adducts, again most likely a collagen-acetaldehyde adduct [53]. That the immune response to acetaldehyde adducts may be involved, at least partly, in the pathogenesis of inflammation observed in alcoholic liver disease was suggested by the production of hepatitis in guinea pigs by immunization with acetaldehyde adducts and ethanol treatment [54•]. The zonal distribution of protein-acetaldehyde adducts in the liver of rats [55] or pigs [56] fed alcohol for long periods is consistent with the preferential damage of perivenous hepatocytes induced by long-term alcohol consumption.

Acetaldehyde may also be involved more directly in hepatic collagen metabolism via stimulation of collagen production by hepatic lipocytes, fibroblasts, and myofibroblasts, as described elsewhere [7••,8•]. Acetaldehyde may also stimulate fibroblast proliferation [57].

Hemoglobin-acetaldehyde adduct [58•] and measurement of hemoglobin- or whole blood-associated acetaldehyde levels by high-performance liquid chromatography [59•] have been proposed as biologic markers of excessive alcohol consumption. However, whole blood-associated acetaldehyde levels were also found in teetotalers, with significant age and sex differences [60]. Decreased activity of aldehyde dehydrogenase in blood has also been proposed as an adjuvant marker [61]. The usefulness of serum carbohydrate-deficient transferrin (CDT) as a marker of alcohol consumption in patients with chronic liver diseases was reassessed [62,63]: the observation that, when measured with a commercial radio immunoassay, CDT is a specific marker for chronic alcohol abuse, except in some patients with other chronic liver diseases [64], was confirmed [62]. Possible effects of gender [65], sensitivity, and specificity of various CDT methods [66] and usefulness of these and some of the other markers were addressed [67].

Ethanol toxicity, oxidative stress, and lipid peroxidation

Lipid peroxidation (and associated membrane damage) is a key feature of alcoholic liver injury. It results in increased excretion of malondialdehyde in the urine of rats following short-and long-term administration of relatively small doses of ethanol [68]. Lipid peroxidation results not only from the increased oxygen radical production by the induced 2E1 [6•, 26], but also from the enhanced generation of acetaldehyde, shown to be capable of causing lipid peroxidation [7••], and from the hepatic depletion of natural antioxidants such as carotenoids and tocopherol [69•]. In humans, increased ethane exhalation (as an *in vivo* index of lipid peroxidation) correlated with the Pugh's score in alcoholic patients with cirrhosis [70•]. However, the weakness of this correlation suggests that other factors contribute to the development of severe liver disease in such patients.

Polyunsaturated phospholipids may be especially vulnerable to peroxidation, and a significant correlation was obtained between the level of 2E1 and the decrease in arachidonic acid from baseline levels. The latter also correlated with the increase in conjugated dienes [71•], suggesting that these processes may be interlinked and caused by the 2E1 induction [22•].

Previously, it had been shown that long-term ethanol feeding reduces hepatic glutathione content [7••]. Hirano *et al.* [72•] now report a progressive and selective depletion of hepatic mitochondrial glutathione associated with lipid peroxidation during progression of experimental alcoholic liver disease to centrilobular liver necrosis and fibrosis in rats intragastrically infused with a high-fat diet plus ethanol. The mitochondrial glutathione depletion may contribute to the well-known changes in mitochondrial structure and functions [7••], now documented by breath analysis in alcoholics [73].

Rat fetal hepatocytes also provide evidence that ethanol-induced injury is associated with membrane damage caused by lipid peroxidation and altered cell glutathione homeostasis [74•]. Simultaneous treatment with ethanol and tocopherol caused a statistically significant increase of the *in vitro* reduction of *p*-nitrobenzoic acid and reversal of the hepatic microsomal lipid peroxidation induced by ethanol [75]. It was postulated that the tocopheral acts by obviating free-radical processes that interfere with the function of P450 after the treatment with ethanol. However, when electron paramagnetic resonance spectroscopy was used to study free-radical signals in freeze-clamped frozen liver tissue from rats after dietary supplementation with alcohol, there was no increase in the stable free-radical signal, even in the presence of considerable hepatic damage; this does not support the hypothesis of free-radical–mediated alcoholic liver disease in this animal model [76]. This was the case even with large dietary iron supplementation, although iron increases ethanol toxicity in rat liver [77]. In any event, hepatocytes isolated from alcohol-fed rats exhibit an increased ability to take up ferritin-bound iron. However, this process did not appear to contribute to iron deposition in these hepatocytes, but may reflect increased general iron uptake in response to lowered liver iron status, following a decrease in transferrin-bound iron uptake [78].

Role of immunologic factors, associated viral infections, and cytokines

As reviewed by Paronetto [79••], various derangements of immune systems are present in alcoholic liver disease. A quantitative immunohistochemical analysis of lymphocyte subsets suggested that in alcoholic hepatitis, hepatocyte necrosis may be partly mediated by immunologic mechanisms involving cytotoxic T cells infiltrating the hepatic lobule [80]. There is still some debate, however, as to whether immunologic changes represent a consequence or a cause of the liver injury. A significant interaction of some immunologic factors with gender was found in rats: ethanol increased the percentage population of CD4 (T-helper cells) in males, but not in females, and it raised both immunoglobulin M and immunoglobulin G secretions in spleen lymphocytes from females but not males [81]. Also, female cells secreted significantly more immunoglobulins than did male cells [81].

In many subjects with alcoholic cirrhosis there is no evidence for antecedent viral hepatitis, but alcoholism and viral hepatitis B or hepatitis C are commonly associated, and the latter may play an important role. Depending on the groups, but regardless of the severity of liver injury, hepatitis C virus replication by polymerase chain reaction was observed either in a minority [82] or in a majority [83] of subjects. Portal or lobular inflammation was strongly associated with hepatitis C virus antibody, even in the absence of hepatitis C virus risk factors [84•]. In another study [85], however, only 2 of 32 patients without risk factors had anti–hepatitis C virus detected by recombinant immunoblot assay. Parenteral drug use and multiple heterosexual contacts were significantly associated with anti–hepatitis C virus [85].

Despite the increasing evidence for the involvement of viruses in the pathogenesis of chronic liver disease in alcoholics, Takase *et al.* [86] concluded that hepatitis C virus markers were not related to development of cirrhosis. However, hepatocellular carcinoma developed more frequently in the hepatitis C virus marker–positive patients, as already shown for hepatitis B virus carriers [87]. Ikeda *et al.* [88] also found that positive hepatitis C virus antibodies as well as total alcohol intake were independently associated with the appearance rate of hepatocellular carcinoma.

Increased interleukin-8 concentrations in patients with alcoholic hepatitis suggests its role in the neutrophilia and hepatic polymorphonuclear leukocyte infiltration of alcoholic hepatitis [89,90]. Bacterial infections are also common in patients with cirrhosis [91]. The most frequent type was spontaneous bacterial peritonitis, a probable source of endotoxins. Furthermore, experimentally, after chronic alcohol administration, there was a strong positive correlation between plasma endotoxin levels and severity of liver injury [92•].

In infected cirrhotics, initial levels of both tumor necrosis factor (TNF–α) and interleukin-6 were significantly higher than in noninfected cirrhotic patients [93]. Ruiz *et al.* [94] also reported that serum concentrations of TNF-α, interleukin-1β and interleukin-6 were significantly raised in patients with alcoholic cirrhosis. It has been proposed that TNF, a mediator of endotoxic shock and sepsis, also plays a role in alcoholic hepatitis [95••]. Thus, on the one hand, TNF appears to be elevated in multiple types of experimental injury and in alcoholic liver disease, as are the levels of some other cytokines, and anticytokines therapies, including specific antibodies, are being developed [95••]. On the other hand, low physiologic amounts of cytokines appear to be important for liver regeneration (and perhaps are beneficial to the organism as a whole). It is noteworthy that the general response to ethanol of the Kupffer cells (which play a major role in cytokine secretion) is also bimodal; whereas exposure to high levels of ethanol depresses Kupffer cell function, lower levels may be stimulatory [96].

A role for cytokines in liver fibrosis has been observed in *in vitro* systems or in animal models and it has been speculated that a balance between profibrogenic and antifibrogenic cytokines normally exists but that, in the presence of hepatic insults, a relative superabundance of the fibrogenic factors may promote the development of liver fibrosis [97]. Thus, the task at hand is to acquire further knowledge on how cytokines and ethanol interact, and to find ways to attenuate the cytotoxic effects of cytokines while conserving their positive growth-enhancing effects. Liver regeneration and its impairment remains an elusive process, however, with ethanol-induced disturbances in expression and inhibition of cyclic AMP–dependent signaling [98•], responsiveness to TNF during liver regeneration [99], and insulin-like growth factor 1 [100], all now being recognized as playing a role.

Alcohol-induced disorders of collagen metabolism and cirrhosis

Alcoholics have high morbidity and mortality rates owing to cirrhosis. Parish *et al.* [101] showed in an American population that three drinks per day was associated with a significantly higher percentage of cirrhosis deaths compared with lifetime abstainers, confirming prior similar European results. Death rates from cirrhosis declined a decade ago, partly due to the impact of alcohol abuse treatment and Alcoholics Anonymous [102]; they have now stabilized [103•]. Improved diagnostic modalities include ultrasonographic diagnosis of acute alcoholic hepatitis by a "pseudoparallel channel sign" of intrahepatic artery dilatation [104], characteristic appearance at computed tomography of confluent hepatic fibrosis in advanced cirrhosis [105], and magnetic resonance images that are statistically significantly associated with periportal and lobular necrosis and portal inflammation [106]. By contrast, the measurement of serum P-III-P (procollagen III peptide) was reported to be of little use in the evaluation of cirrhotic patients [107], but a significant correlation was found between serum and liver type IV collagen content, and the increase was more prominent in alcoholic than in nonalcoholic liver disease [108].

Current concepts of pathogenesis and therapy were reviewed [7••,109••,110••]. Oxandrolone is now shown to be effective in patients with moderate malnutrition [111•]. Prevention of cirrhosis by polyenephosphatidylcholine was demonstrated in nonhuman primates [112] and is now being tested in humans. One possible mechanism of the effect is the stimulation of collagenase activity by hepatic lipocytes. Another, not mutually exclusive, mechanism is the attenuation by polyenephosphatidylcholine of the ethanol-induced activation of lipocytes, now considered to play a major role in hepatic fibrogenesis, especially when stimulated by acetaldehyde [7••], injured hepatocytes, or secretions of activated Kupffer cells [113].

S-adenosyl-L-methionine was shown to prevent and reverse erythrocyte membrane alterations in experimental cirrhosis [114]. Prior studies also demonstrate the therapeutic effectiveness of *S*-adenosyl-L-methionine in experimental liver injury induced by alcohol and other agents; beneficial effects have now been shown in pilot studies in humans [115•]. Betaine administration was reported to have the capacity to elevate hepatic *S*-adenosyl-L-methionine and to prevent the ethanol-induced fatty liver in rats [116]. Lack of methionine may also result from a deficit in methylation of homocysteine to methionine, mainly by the folate and vitamin B_{12}-dependent enzyme methionine synthase. Because a disturbed folate metabolism is present in most alcoholics (attributable to multiple mechanisms, including an inadequate diet), elevated plasma homocysteine levels in alcoholics could have been anticipated and have now indeed been noted in a group of alcoholics [117•]. These observations illustrate again the need to correct underlying malnutrition in the alcoholic, which may exist irrespective of the social and medical situation of the patient and is mostly related to caloric undernutrition [118]. Nutrition support was successful in decreasing nutrition-associated complications in patients with alcoholic liver disease [119]. The rationale for the various modalities of nutritional intervention was also reviewed [120•].

Another emerging treatment modality is liver transplantation. Originally not applied to alcoholic liver disease, it is now increasingly being considered for individuals who have stopped drinking [121•] with no absolute period of abstinence from alcohol being required [122]. One-year survival rates of 80% or higher were reported, even in patients with alcoholic hepatitis [123•].

Finally, early intervention was shown to be effective in reducing alcohol consumption among at-risk patients [124]. It was also emphasized that alcoholic liver disease is a public health issue that could greatly benefit from a public health approach, based on early diagnosis of vulnerable individuals and early onset of treatment, prior to the medical or social disintegration of the patients [67•, 125].

References and recommended reading

Papers of particular interest, published within the annual period of review, have been highlighted as:

- • Of special interest
- •• Of outstanding interest

1. • Tsutsumi M, Lasker JM, Takahashi T, Lieber CS: **In Vivo Induction of Hepatic P4502E1 by Ethanol: Role of Increased Enzyme Synthesis.** *Arch Biochem Biophys* 1993, **304**:209–218.

Experiments with rats fed ethanol in adequate liquid diets revealed that the 2E1 content of liver microsomes increases rapidly and reaches a new steady-state level after 10 days, with an associated enhanced incorporation of radio-labeled methionine and δ-aminolevulinic acid in 2E1 apoprotein and heme, respectively, indicating increased synthesis of the protein, thereby settling a controversy in the field.

2. • Takahashi T, Lasker JM, Rosman AS, Lieber CS: **Induction of P4502E1 in Human Liver by Ethanol Is Due to a Corresponding Increase in Encoding mRNA.** *Hepatology* 1993, 17:236–245.

To assess the mechanism of hepatic 2E1 induction in humans and its zonal localization, liver sections derived from needle biopsy specimens were obtained from recently drinking alcoholics and control subjects. *In situ* hybridization of these liver sections with a human 2E1 complementary DNA probe was used to localize 2E1 messenger RNA transcripts. Quantitative image analysis of hybridized sections from control subjects revealed that 2E1 transcript content in perivenular (zone 3) hepatocytes was significantly higher than in midzonal (zone 2) and periportal (zone 1) cells. These results indicate that the induction, by ethanol, of 2E1 protein in human liver stems, at least in part, from a corresponding increase of 2E1 messenger RNA.

3. • Ronis MJ, Haung J, Crouch J, Mercado C, Irby D, Valentine C, Lumpkin C, Ingelman-Sundberg M, Badger T: **Cytochrome P450 CYP 2E1 Induction During Chronic Alcohol Exposure Occurs by a Two-Step Mechanism Associated With Blood Alcohol Concentrations in Rats.** *J Pharmacol Exp Ther* 1993, **264**:944–950.

The results of this study suggest that ethanol induces CYP 2E1 by two separate mechanisms: a largely posttranslational mechanism at low ethanol concentrations and an additional transcriptional or messenger RNA stabilization mechanism at high ethanol levels.

4. • Badger T, Ronis MJ, Lumpkin C, Valentine C, Shahare M, Irby D, Haung J, Mercado C, Thomas P, Ingelman-Sundberg M, Crouch J: **Effects of Chronic Ethanol on Growth Hormone Secretion and Hepatic Cytochrome P450 Isozymes of the Rat.** *J Pharmacol Exp Ther* 1993, **246**:438–447.

The results of this study suggest that the reduced CYP 2C11 activities, apoprotein levels and steady-state messenger RNA concentrations during chronic alcohol exposure are causally related to the alterations in growth hormone secretion. By contrast, chronic alcohol exposure elevated CYP 2E1 activities, apoprotein levels and steady-state messenger RNA levels, and these changes occur primarily as the result of ethanol rather than undernutrition or as the combination of ethanol and undernutrition.

5. • Zand R, Nelson S, Slattery J, Thummel K, Kalhorn T, Adams S, Wright J: **Inhibition and Induction of Cytochrome P4502E1-Catalyzed Oxidation by Isoniazid in Humans.** *Clin Pharmacol Ther* 1993, **54**:142–149.

The effect of isoniazid administration on the cytochrome P4502E1-catalyzed elimination of chlorzoxazone and acetaminophen was studied in 10 volunteer slow acetylators. Isoniazid inhibited the clearance of chlorzoxazone by 58% and reduced the formation of acetaminophen thioether metabolites. By contrast, 2 days after the discontinuations of isoniazid, the clearance of chlorzoxazone was increased over the value before isoniazid by 56%, and acetaminophen thioether by 56%. The mechanism of this biphasic effect is probably induction by protein stabilization, with inhibition of catalytic activity while isoniazid is present.

6. • Dai Y, Rashba-Step J, Cederbaum AI: **Stable Expression of Human Cytochrome P4502E1 in HepG2 Cells: Characterization of Catalytic Activities and Production of Reactive Oxygen Intermediates.** *Biochemistry* 1993, 32:6928–6937.

Liver microsomes are the site of an inducible ethanol metabolizing system comprising a specific cytochrome, namely P4502E1 [Lieber, *Medical and Nutritional Complications of Alcoholism: Mechanisms and Management 1992*.]. However, when cultured under standard conditions, hepatocytes (whether human or from experimental animals) do not express this cytochrome in a stable manner. This difficulty was overcome recently by Dai *et al.* who succeeded in stabilizing and constitutively expressing the coding sequence of the human cytochrome P4502E1 in HepG2 cells (a human hepatoma–derived cell line), by recombinant retroviral expression. Southern blot analysis showed a successful integration of a single copy of unaltered viral DNA into the genome of each transduced clone tested. Northern blot analysis revealed that the transduced clones produced an RNA species that hybridized to the CYP2E1 complementary DNA probe. Western blot analysis using anti–human P4502E1 immunoglobulin G indicated that the transduced clones produced a protein band with molecular weight of 54,000. Microsomes from transduced clones were catalytically active with *p*-nitrophenol, dimethylnitrosamine, aniline, and ethanol as substrates. Rates of superoxide and H_2O_2 production and of lipid peroxidation were 7- to 20-fold higher on a per nanomole of P450 basis compared with human liver microsomes, indicating that the P4502E1 is especially reactive in production of active oxygen intermediates and in catalysis of lipid peroxidation. Thus, these cells may serve as an appropriate model to develop antioxidants and to test their effectiveness.

7. Lieber CS: *Medical and Nutritional Complications of Alcoholism: Mechanisms and Management.* New York: Plenum Medical Book Company; 1992.
•• This book provides an in-depth review of the pathogenesis and treatment of medical disorders associated with alcoholism, including an abundant bibliography of about 5000 references.

8. Lieber CS: **Biochemical Factors in Alcoholic Liver Disease.** *Semin Liver Dis* 1993, **13**:136–153.
• Comprehensive up-to-date review of the topic.

9. Kaneko T, Wang P-Y, Sato A: **Enzyme Induction by Ethanol Consumption Affects the Pharmacokinetics of Inhaled m-Xylene Only at High Levels of Exposure.** *Arch Toxicol* 1993, **67**:473–477.
• It was observed that induction of microsomal enzymes (presumably 2E1) affects the pharmacokinetics of inhaled *m*-xylene but only at high levels of exposure. If the results of this rat study can be extrapolated to humans, they may be reassuring with regard to the toxicity of low levels of industrial exposure to *m*-xylene.

10. Anundi I, Lahteenmaki T, Rundgren M, Moldeus P, Lindros K: **Zonation of Acetaminophen Metabolism and Cytochrome P450 2E1-Mediated Toxicity Studied in Isolated Periportal and Perivenous Hepatocytes.** *Biochem Pharmacol* 1993, **45**:1250–1259.

11. Thummel KE, Kharasch ED, Podoll T, Kune K: **Human Liver Microsomal Enflurane Deflurination Catalyzed by Cytochrome P-450 2E1.** *Drug Metab Dispos* 1993, **21**:350–357.
• In view of the potentiation of enflurane toxicity by chronic ethanol consumption and 2E1 induction demonstrated in rats, this observation in humans is of obvious clinical relevance when surgery has to be performed in alcohol abusers.

12. Kharasch ED, Thummel KE: **Identification of Cytochrome P4502E1 as the Predominant Enzyme Catalayzing Human Liver Microsomal Defluorination of Sevoflurane, Isoflurane, and Methoxyflurane.** *Anesthesiology* 1993, **79**:795–807.

13. Van De Wiel JAG, Fijneman PHS, Teeuw KB, Van Ommen B, Noordhoek J, Bos RP: **Influence of Long-Term Ethanol Treatment on Rat Liver Biotransformation Enzymes.** *Alcohol* 1993, **10**:397–402.

14. Lucas D, Berthou F, Dreano Y, Lozac'h P, Volant A, Menez J-F: **Comparison of Levels of Cytochromes P-450, CYP1A2, CYP2E1, and Their Related Monooxygenase Activities in Human Surgical Liver Samples.** *Alcohol Clin Exp Res* 1993, **17**:900–905.
• Much emphasis has been placed on CYP1A2 and CYP2E1 induction by smoking and drinking, respectively. Surprisingly, this study revealed that other environmental factors, diet habits, or genetic factors are responsible for even much larger interindividual variations.

15. Bradford B, Forman D, Thurman R: **4-Methylpyrazole Inhibits Fatty Acyl Coenzyme Synthetase and Diminishes Catalase-Dependent Alcohol Metabolism: Has the Contribution of Alcohol Dehydrogenase to Alcohol Metabolism Been Previously Overestimated?** *Mol Pharmacol* 1992, **43**:115–119.

16. Bradford B, Seed C, Handler J, Forman D, Thurman R: **Evidence That Catalase Is a Major Pathway of Ethanol Oxidation in vivo: Dose-Response Studies in Deer Mice Using Methanol as a Selective Substrate.** *Arch Biochem Biophys* 1993, **303**:172–176.

17. Williamson JR, Scholz R, Browning ET, Thurman RG, Fukami MH: **Metabolic Effects of Ethanol in Perfused Rat Liver.** *J Biol Chem* 1969, **244**:5044–5054.

18. Foerster EC, Fahrenkemper T, Rabe U, Graf P, Sies H: **Peroxisomal Fatty Acid Oxidation as Detected by H_2O_2 Production in Intact Perfused Rat Liver.** *Biochem J* 1981, **196**:705–712.

19. Ma X-L, Baraona E, Lieber CS: **Alcohol Consumption Enhances Fatty Acid ω-Oxidation, With a Greater Increase in Male Than in Female Rats.** *Hepatology* 1993, **18**:1247–1253.
• Fatty acid ω-oxidation is an accessory pathway that accounts for less than 5% of the fatty acids oxidized by the liver of normal rats. However an increase in ω-oxidation may pertain to conditions in which the activity in the main mitochondrial oxidation pathway is decreased. Thus the induction of the cytochrome P450 4A1-catalyzed ω-hydroxylation can provide an alternate pathway for disposition of fatty acids that accumulate as a result of the impairment of mitochondrial oxidation caused by ethanol. Quantitatively, more important may be the fact that products of ω-oxidation have been shown to enhance the peroxisomal oxidation, another alternate pathway for fatty-acid oxidation, and to increase liver cytosolic fatty acid–binding protein (L-FABPc), which in turn is known to stimulate fatty acid-esterifying activities of microsomes. Thus, the enhancement of ω–oxidation after long-term alcohol consumption might play a compensatory role in the prevention of potentially deleterious accumulation of fatty acids both by providing alternate pathways for their oxidation and by promoting L-FABPc–mediated esterification.

20. Pignon JP, Bailey NC, Baraona E, Lieber CS: **Fatty-Acid–Binding Protein: A Major Contributor to the Ethanol-Induced Increase in Liver Cytosolic Proteins in the Rat.** *Hepatology* 1987, 7:865–871.

21. Watanabe S, Wakatsuki Y, Yoshioka H, Inada M, Ono T, Kita T: **Biochemical and Histochemical Studies of Liver Fatty Acid Binding Protein in Alcohol-Treated Rats.** *J Clin Biochem Nutr* 1993, **14**:171–181.

22. Laethem RM, Balazy M, Falck JR, Laethem CL, Koop DR: **Formation of 19(S)-, 19(R)-, and 18(R)-Hydroxyeicosatetraenoic Acids by Alcohol-Inducible Cytochrome P4502E1.** *J Biol Chem* 1993, **268**:12912–12918.
• It was shown that, when reconstituted with cytochrome b_5 and NADPH cytochrome P450 oxidoreductase, cytochrome P4502E1 metabolized lauric, stearic, oleic, linoleic, linolenic, and arachiodonic acids to multiple metabolites. The oxidation of fatty acids by P4502E1 may have two potentially important consequences: 1) the formation of pharmacologically active metabolites of arachiodonic acid, and 2) because of the ethanol-induced increase in lipids, fatty acids as potential substrates for P4502E1 may become important in terms of uncoupled NADPH oxidation, formation of oxygen-derived radicals, and increased lipid peroxidation.

23. Ueng TH, Ueng YF, Tsai JN, Chao IC, Chen TL, Park SS, Iwasaki M, Guengerich FP: **Induction and Inhibition of Cytochrome P450-Dependent Monooxgyenase in Hamster Tissues by Ethanol.** *Toxicology* 1993, **81**:145–154.

24. Boelsterli UA, Wolf A, Goldlin C: **Oxygen Free Radical Production Mediated by Cocaine and Its Ethanol-Derived Metabolite, Cocaethylene, in Rat Hepatocytes.** *Hepatology* 1993, **18**:1154–1161.
• Biotransformation of cocaine to cocaine ethyl ester (cocaethylene) has been demonstrated in rat hepatocytes. This study shows that cocaine and its ethanol-derived metabolite, cocaethylene, are equally injurious. Furthermore, both cocaine and cocaethylene induced massive NADPH-dependent reactive oxygen species production in hepatic microsomal suspensions and in homogenates of cultured hepatocytes. Thus, prooxidants may be responsible for the cocaine-induced hepatocyte injury and for the exacerbation of cocaine hepatotoxicity by ethanol.

25. Farre M, De La Torre R, LLorente M, Lamas X, Ugena B, Segura J, Cami J: **Alcohol and Cocaine Interactions in Humans.** *J Pharmacol Exp Ther* 1993, **266**:1364–1373.

26. Castillo T, Koop D, Kamimura S, Triadafilopoulos G, Tsukamoto H: **Role of Cytochrome P450 2E1 in Ethanol-, Carbon Tetrachloride- and Iron-Dependent Microsomal Lipid Peroxidation.** *Hepatology* 1992, **16**:992–996.

27. • Kato S, Shields PG, Caporaso NE, Hoover RN, Trump BF, Sugimura H, Weston A, Harris CC: **Cytochrome P450IIE1 Genetic Polymorphisms, Racial Variation, and Lung Cancer Risk.** *Cancer Res* 1992, **52**:6712–6715.

Restriction fragment length polymorphisms have been identified in the cytochrome P4502E1 transcription regulatory region that may affect expression. It was postulated that the ethnic differences of these restriction fragment-length polymorphisms might be related to genetic susceptibilities for lung cancer among Caucasians and for gastric or esophageal cancer among Japanese but the data indicated no evidence for an association of cytochrome P4502E1 PstI of RsaI restriction fragment-length polymorphism with lung cancer in this US population.

28. •• Bosron WF, Ehrig T, Li T–K: **Genetic Factors in Alcohol Metabolism and Alcoholism.** *Semin Liver Dis* 1993, **13**:126–135.

Comprehensive and up-to-date review.

29. Lin RC, Edenberg HJ, Carr LG: **A Novel Negative Element in the Promotor of the Mouse Alcohol Dehydrogenase Gene Adh-1.** *J Biol Chem* 1993, **268**:10260–10267.

30. Potter JJ, Yang VW, Mezey E: **Regulation of the Rat Class Alcohol Dehydrogenase Gene by Growth Hormone.** *Biochem Biophys Res Commun* 1993, **191**:1040–1045.

31. Ehrig T, Muhoberac B, Brems D, Bosron W: **Monomers of Human $B_1\beta_1$ Alcohol Dehydrogenase Exhibit Activity that Differs From the Dimer.** *J Biol Chem* 1993, **268**:11721–11726.

32. Keegan A, Batey R: **Dietary Carbohydrate Accelerates Ethanol Elimination, but Does Not Alter Hepatic Alcohol Dehydrogenase.** *Alcohol Clin Exp Res* 1993, **17**:431–433.

33. • Vidal F, Perez J, Panisello J, Toda R, Gutierrez C, Richart C: **Atypical Liver Alcohol Dehydrogenase in the Spanish Population: Its Relation With the Development of Alcoholic Liver Disease.** *Alcohol Clin Exp Res* 1993, **17**:782–785.

Atypical alcohol dehydrogenase was present in 14.9% of alcoholics and in 17.4% of nonalcoholics, a nonsignificant difference, inconsistent with the role of the atypical enzyme in the pathogenesis of the disease.

34. Engeland K, Maret W: **Extrahepatic, Differential Expression of Four Classes of Human Alcohol Dehydrogenase.** *Biochem Biophys Res Commun* 1993, **193**:47–53.

35. • Stone CL, Thomasson HR, Bosron WF, Li T-K: **Purification and Partial Amino Acid Sequence of a High-Activity Human Stomach Alcohol Dehydrogenase.** *Alcohol Clin Exp Res* 1993, **17**:911–918.

A stomach-specific alcohol dehydrogenase (σ-alcohol dehydrogenase) was purified to homogeneity from human transplant donor and surgical tissues, and its activity for ethanol oxidation was found to be much higher than that of other hepatic or gastric isoenzymes.

36. Huang MT, Huang CC, Chen MY: **In Vivo Uptake of Ethanol and Release of Acetate in Rat Liver and GI.** *Life Sci* 1993, **53**:165–170.

37. Mirmiran-Yazdy SA, Haber PS, Mak KM, Gentry RT, Batra S, Korsten MA, Lieber CS: **Ethanol Metabolism by Gastric Cells in Culture and Its Inhibition by Cimetidine [Abstract].** *Hepatology* 1993, **18**:106A.

38. • Lim Jr RT, Gentry RT, Ito D, Yokoyama H, Baraona E, Lieber CS: **First Pass Metabolism of Ethanol in Rats is Predominantly Gastric.** *Alcohol Clin Exp Res* 1993, **17**:1337–1344.

Consumption of alcohol results in much lower blood alcohol concentrations than does the same dose administered intravenously, suggesting significant first-pass metabolism. Questions remain, however, such as 1) whether this difference truly represents first-pass metabolism or simply results from slower absorption of alcohol, and 2) if there is first-pass metabolism, is it mainly of gastric or hepatic origin. To study this, rats were given the same dose alcohol (1 g/kg) by either intragastric intubation or by intravenous, intraportal and intraduodenal infusions at a rate which mimicked the loss of alcohol from the stomach. Higher blood alcohol concentration levels after intravenous than intragastric alcohol indicated true first-pass metabolism. Higher levels after intraportal or intraduodenal infusions (in fact, comparable to those obtained with the intravenous route) demonstrated negligible first-pass metabolism when the route of delivery bypassed the stomach, yet included the liver. Furthermore, rats that had developed portosystemic shunts after ligation of the portal vein exhibited blood alcohol curves and first-pass metabolism equivalent to those of sham-operated controls, indicating that first-pass metabolism is not dependent on first-pass flow through the liver, but reflects gastric metabolism. Finally, the *in vivo* gastric metabolism of alcohol in pylorus-ligated rats was demonstrated by significantly lower blood alcohol concentration when alcohol was administered intragastrically than when an amount identical to that lost from the ligated stomach was given intraportally.

39. Frezza M, Di Padova C, Pozzato G, Terpin M, Baraona E, Lieber CS: **High Blood Alcohol Levels in Women: Role of Decreased Gastric Alcohol Dehydrogenase Activity and First Pass Metabolism.** *N Engl J Med* 1990, **322**:95–99.

40. • Seitz HK, Egerer UA, Waldherr R, Eckey R, Agarwal DP, Goedde HW, von Wartburg JP: **Human Gastric Alcohol Dehydrogenase Activity: Effect of Age, Sex and Alcoholism.** *Gut* 1993, **34**:1433–1437.

Consistent with prior observations, the activity of gastric alcohol dehydrogenase was found to be decreased in young women, in elderly men, and in subjects with alcoholism. It was concluded that this decrease in alcohol dehydrogenase activity may contribute to the reduced first-pass metabolism of ethanol and associated raised ethanol blood concentrations.

41. • Roine RP, Gentry RT, Lim Jr RT, Heikkonen E, Salaspuro M, Lieber CS: **Comparison of Blood Alcohol Concentrations After Beer and Whiskey.** *Alcohol Clin Exp Res* 1993, **17**:709–711.

Peak blood alcohol levels were higher with beer than with whiskey in the postprandial and prandial conditions, whereas the opposite was true in the preprandial state. Similarly, the area under the blood alcohol curve was higher with beer in the prandial state, and higher with whiskey in the preprandial condition. Wine and sherry yielded peak concentrations intermediate between those of beer and whiskey in the postprandial state. The results indicate that a dilute alcoholic drink can yield either higher or lower blood alcohol levels than a concentrated beverage, depending on the prandial state.

42. Raufman JP, Notar-Francesco V, Raffaniello RD, Straus EW: **Histamine-2 Receptor Antagonists Do Not Alter Serum Ethanol Levels in Fed, Nonalcoholic Men.** *Ann Intern Med* 1993, **118**:488–494.

43. Chari ST, Teyssen S, Singer MV: **What Controls Should Be Used in Studies of Acute Effects of Alcohol and Alcoholic Beverages on the Stomach and the Pancreas?** *Scand J Gastroenterol* 1993, **28**:289–295.

44. • Ito D, Lieber CS: **Ethanol Metabolism in Deermice: Role of Extrahepatic Alcohol Dehydrogenase.** *Alcohol Clin Exp Res* 1993, **17**:919–925.

The relative contributions to ethanol metabolism of extrahepatic alcohol dehydrogenase and of liver microsomes were assessed in deermice that lack hepatic low-K_m alcohol dehydrogenase. With deuterated ethanol, a poor correlation between the rate of exchange and the rate of metabolism was found. Furthermore, gastrectomized low-km alcohol dehydrogenase deermice still showed an exchange of reducing equivalents, thereby dissociating exchange from gastric alcohol dehydrogenase activity. It was concluded that when ethanol is given parenterally, the microsomal ethanol oxidizing system rather than gastric alcohol dehydrogenase is a major pathway of ethanol oxidation in low-km alcohol dehydrogenase deermice, whereas both pathways contribute significantly to the metabolism of orally administered ethanol.

45. • Yin SJ, Chou FJ, Chao SF, Tsai SF, Liao CS, Wang SL, Wu CW, Lee SC: **Alcohol and Aldehyde Dehydrogenase in Human Esophagus: Comparison With the Stomach Enzyme Activity.** *Alcohol Clin Exp Res* 1993, **17**:376–381.

Alcohol dehydrogenase and aldehyde dehydrogenase isoenzymes from surgical esophageal and gastric mucosa were compared by agarose isoelectric focusing. The esophageal alcohol dehydrogenase activity was approximately fourfold and the aldehyde dehydrogenase activity 20% that of the stomach enzyme. A resulting acetaldehyde accumulation and associated adverse consequences are postulated.

46. • Eriksson CJP, Fukunaga T: **Human Blood Acetaldehyde (Update 1992).** *Alcohol Alcohol Suppl* 1993, **28**:9–25.

Highly critical review of available methods of acetaldehyde measurements.

47. • Jones AW: **Breath Acetaldehyde Concentration.** *Alcohol* 1993, **10**:325–326.

This review provides a critique of breath acetaldehyde measurements and their significance.

48. • Tuma DJ, Klassen LW: **Immune Responses to Acetaldehyde-Protein Adducts: Role in Alcoholic Liver Disease.** *Gastroenterology* 1992, **103**:1969–1973.

This editorial reviews the evidence of the role of immune responses to acetaldehyde-protein adducts in the pathogenesis of alcoholic liver disease.

49. • Wehr H, Rodo M, Lieber CS, Baraona E: **Acetaldehyde Adducts and Autoantibodies Against VLDL and LDL in Alcoholics.** *J Lipid Res* 1993, **34**:1237–1244.

Alcoholics develop acetaldehyde adducts in apolipoprotein B–containing lipoproteins, particularly very low density lipoprotein. The immune response to these neoantigens could result in accelerated clearance of very low density lipoprotein and low-density lipoprotein and decreased conversion of very low density lipoprotein to low-density lipoprotein, thereby explaining, at least in part, why alcohol consumption, while markedly increasing the hepatic output of very low density lipoprotein, nevertheless decreases the resulting low-density lipoprotein levels.

50. Nomura F, Lieber CS: **Binding of Acetaldehyde to Rat Liver Microsomes: Enhancement After Chronic Alcohol Consumption.** *Biochem Biophys Res Commun* 1981, **100**:131–137.

51. • Baraona E, Liu W, Ma XL, Svegliati-Baroni G, Lieber CS: **Acetaldehyde-Collagen Adducts in N-Nitrosodimethylamine-Induced Liver Cirrhosis in Rats.** *Life Sci* 1993, **52**:1249–1255.

In cytosol and microsomes of rats with cirrhosis produced by *N*-nitrosodimethylamine, an acetaldehyde-protein adduct of approximately 200 kD was recognized by rabbit immunoglobin G raised against either an *in vitro*–produced hemocyanin-acetaldehyde adduct or an *in vivo*–occurring P4502E1-acetaldehyde adduct isolated from alcohol-fed rats, as well as by anti-rat collagen (I) immunoglobulin G. Its immune complexes contained three proteins that reacted with the anticollagen immunoglobulin G and were digested by collagenase: two proteins with molecular weights similar to procollagens $\alpha1$ and $\alpha2$, and a $\beta1$, 2(I)-like protein that was readily produced by *in vitro* modification of cytosol with acetaldehyde. This liver acetaldehyde-protein adduct may correspond to the findings of Svegliati-Baroni *et al.* (*Alcohol Clin Exp Res* 1993, 17:447A) in patients with alcoholic liver disease and may be responsible for the circulating antibody described in alcoholics by Koskinas *et al.* (*Gastroenterology* 1992, 103:1860–1867).

52. • Koskinas J, Kenna JG, Bird GL, Alexander GJM, Williams R: **Immunoglobulin A Antibody to a 200-Kilodalton Cytosolic Acetaldehyde Adduct in Alcoholic Hepatitis.** *Gastroenterology* 1992, **103**:1860–1867.

Immunoglobulin A antibodies to a 200-kD acetaldehyde-protein adduct were found to be present in a large proportion of patients with alcoholic liver disease.

53. Svegliati-Baroni G, Baraona E, Rosman A, Lieber CS: **Liver Collagen-Acetaldehyde Adducts in Alcoholic and Non-Alcoholic Liver Disease [Abstract].** *Alcohol Clin Exp Res* 1993, 17:447A.

54. • Yokoyama H, Ishii H, Nagata S, Kato S, Kamegaya K, Tsuchiya M: **Experimental Hepatitis Induced by Ethanol After Immunization With Acetaldehyde Adducts.** *Hepatology* 1993, 17:14–19.

Guinea pigs were immunized with human hemoglobin-acetaldehyde adducts and were simultaneously given ethanol for 40 days. These treatments induced hepatic necrosis with infiltration of mononuclear cells in the hepatic lobules. Peripheral blood lymphocytes obtained from the animals with hepatitis were shown to be stimulated by acetaldehyde adducts. This study reveals that acetaldehyde-protein adducts may play a pathogenic role in alcohol-induced liver injury.

55. Lin RC, Zhou FC, Fillenwarth MJ, Lumeng L: **The Zonal Distribution of Protein-Acetaldehyde Adducts in the Liver of Rats Fed Alcohol for Long Periods.** *Hepatology* 1993, **18**:864–869.

56. Halstead CH, Villanueva J, Chandler CJ, Ruebner B, Munn RJ, Parkkila S, Niemela O: **Centrilobular Distribution of Acetaldehyde and Collagen in the Ethanol-Fed Micropig.** *Hepatology* 1993, **18**:954–960.

57. Matias A, da-Silva PS, Azevedo I: **Neurotoxicity and Induction of Fibroblast Proliferation by Acetaldehyde in the Rabbit Liver.** *J Auton Pharmacol* 1993, **13**:275–280.

58. • Lin RC, Shahidi S, Kelly TJ, Lumeng C, Lumeng L: **Measurement of Hemoglobin-Acetaldehyde Adduct in Alcoholic Patients.** *Alcohol Clin Exp Res* 1993, **17**:669–674.

This study reports the measurement of hemoglobin-acetaldehyde adducts in alcoholic patients by a sandwich enzyme-liked immunosorbent assay and concluded that hemoglobin-acetaldehyde adduct has the potential of being a good marker for alcohol abuse.

59. • Peterson CM: **Review: Development of a Fluid Phase Measure of Acetaldehyde for Biological Samples.** *Alcohol* 1993, **10**:327–332.

This paper reviews earlier studies of acetaldehyde adducts with hemoglobin and of a new assay based on the reaction of free or liberated bound acetaldehyde. As stated by the author, "Whether the fluid phase assay will be advantageous for the study of acetaldehyde in breath or tissue samples remains to be determined."

60. Halvorson MR, Noffsinger JK, Peterson CM: **Studies of Whole Blood-Associated Acetaldehyde Levels in Teetotalers.** *Alcohol* 1993, **10**:409–413.

61. Helander A: **Aldehyde Dehydrogenase in Blood: Distribution Characteristics and Possible Use as Marker of Alcohol Misuse.** *Alcohol Alcohol* 1993, **28**:135–145.

62. Bell H, Tallaksen C, Sjaheim T, Weberg R, Raknerud N, Orjasaeter H, Try K, Haug E: **Serum Carbohydrate-Deficient Transferrin as a Marker of Alcohol Consumption in Patients With Chronic Liver Diseases.** *Alcohol Clin Exp Res* 1993, 17:246–252.

63. Sillanaukee P, Seppa K, Lof K, Koivula T: **CDT by Anion-Exchange Chromatography Followed by RIA as a Marker of Heavy Drinking Among Men.** *Alcohol Clin Exp Res* 1993, 17:230–233.

64. Xin Y, Rosman AS, Lasker JM, Lieber CS: **Measurement of Carbohydrate-Deficient Transferrin by Isoelectric Focusing/Western Blotting and by Micro Anion-Exchange Chromatography/Radioimmunoassay: Comparison of Diagnostic Accuracy.** *Alcohol Alcohol* 1992, 27:425–433.

65. Halvorson MR, Campbell JL, Sprague G, Slater K, Noffsinger JK, Peterson CM: **Comparative Evaluation of the Clinical Utility of Three Markers of Ethanol Intake: The Effect of Gender.** *Alcohol Clin Exp Res* 1993, 17:225–229.

66. Lieber CS, Xin Y, Lasker JM, Rosman AS: **Comparison of New Methods for Measuring Carbohydrate-Deficient Transferrin (CDT): Application to a Public Health Approach for the Prevention of Alcoholic Cirrhosis.** *Alcohol Alcohol Suppl* 1993, **28**:111–116.

67. Rosman AS, Lieber CS: **Biological Markers of Alcoholism.** In *Medical and Nutritional Complications of Alcoholism: Mechanisms and Management.* Edited by Lieber CS. New York: Plenum Medical Book Company; 1992:531–563.

68. Moser J, Bagci D, Akubue PI, Stohs SJ: **Excretion of Malondialdehyde, Formaldehyde, Acetaldehyde and Acetone in the Urine of Rats Following Acute and Chronic Administration of Ethanol.** *Alcohol Alcohol* 1993, **28**:287–295.

69. Leo MA, Rosman AS, Lieber CS: **Differential Depletion of Carotenoids and Tocopherol in Liver Disease.** *Hepatology* 1993, **17**:977–986.
•
Compared with controls (transplant donors), levels of carotenoids and retinoids were extremely low at all stages of liver disease. Patients with alcoholic cirrhosis had 20- and 25-fold decreases of lycopene and α + β carotene, respectively. Even in subjects with less severe alcoholic liver disease (steatosis, perivenular fibrosis, and portal fibrosis), the levels were four to six times lower than those of normal subjects. By contrast, levels of α-tocopherol were decreased significantly only in the patients with cirrhosis, with a threefold reduction. In the serum of most patients, lycopene and tocopherol concentrations were not depressed, whereas one third of the α + β carotene levels were low, probably reflecting poor dietary intake.

70. Letteron P, Duchatelle V, Berson A, Fromenty B, Degott C, Benhamou JP, Pessayre D: **Increased Ethane Exhalation, an In Vivo Index of Lipid Peroxidation, in Alcohol-Abusers.** *Gut* 1993, **34**:409–414.
•
Peroxidation may be assessed noninvasively by determining the exhalation of volatile hydrocarbons (pentane and ethane) in breath. In this study, ethane exhalation was similar in control subjects and in patients with nonalcoholic liver diseases, but was five times higher in alcohol abusers, and showed slow improvement during abstinence, suggesting that it ws not related, at that time, to the production of free radicals during the metabolism of ethanol. One of the possible mechanisms may be the presence of increased amounts of oxidizable fat in the liver.

71. Nanji AA, Zhao S, Lamb RG, Sadradeh SMH, Dannenberg AJ, Waxman DJ: **Changes in Microsomal Phospholipase and Arachidonic Acid in Experimental Alcoholic Liver Injury: Relationship to Cytochrome P4502E1 Induction and Conjugated Diene Formation.** *Alcohol Clin Exp Res* 1993, **17**:598–603.
•
These data demonstrate a correlation between the decline in microsomal arachidonic acid, induction of CYP2E1, and the formation of conjugated dienes, thus supporting the hypothesis that induction of 2E1 is associated with formation of free-radical intermediates and active oxygen species that may play a role in liver injury. The results also showed increased phospholipase C and phospholipase A activities in microsomes, suggesting that phospholipids are the likely source of arachidonic acid in that model.

72. Hirano T, Kaplowitz N, Tsukamoto H, Kamimura S, Fernandez-Checa JC: **Hepatic Mitochondrial Glutathione Depletion and Progression of Experimental Alcoholic Liver Disease in Rats.** *Hepatology* 1992, **16**:1423–1427.
•
This study confirmed that mitochondrial glutathione is selectively depleted in livers of ethanol-fed rats and shows that the depletion becomes progressively more profound as histologic liver disease progresses with increased lipid peroxidation in the mitochondria.

73. Lauterburg BH, Liang D, Schwarzenbach FA, Breen KJ: **Mitochondrial Dysfunction in Alcoholic Patients as Assessed by Breath Analysis.** *Hepatology* 1993, **17**:418–422.

74. Devi BG, Henderson GI, Frosto TA, Schenker S: **Effect of Ethanol on Rat Fetal Hepatocytes: Studies on Cell Replication, Lipid Peroxidation and Glutathione.** *Hepatology* 1993, **18**:648–659.
•
Pretreatment of fetal rat hepatocytes with 0.1 mmol/L *N*-acetylcysteine or *S*-adenosylmethionine for 24 hours prevented the ethanol-induced reduction of ATP and glutathione levels, essentially restoring cell replication. Pretreatment with 0.1 mmol/L of vitamin E fully normalized malonaldehyde and diene conjugated levels and ^{51}Cr leakage but failed to improve ATP levels or to increase significantly cell replication and glutathione levels. Concomitant administration of glutathione precursors with ethanol, rather than pretreatment, did not alter the impaired cell replication. These data underscore the importance of cellular glutathione and ATP in preventing ethanol-induced decreases in fetal cell replication and suggest that alleviation of cellular lipid peroxidation alone is not sufficient to prevent this abnormality in fetal rat hepatocyte function.

75. Tani E, Kourounakis PN: **Effect of Ethanol and of its Interaction With Ascorbic Acid or Tocopherol-Acetate on p-Nitrobenzoic Acid Reduction and on Lipid Peroxidation.** *Res Commun Subst Abuse* 1993, **14**:7–15.

76. Butcher GP, Deighton N, Batt RM, Ding B, Haywood S, Hoffman J, Jackson MJ, Symons MCR, Rhodes JM: **Electron Paramagnetic Resonance Spectroscopy of Stable Free Radicals in the Liver Compared With Ultrastructural and Functional Damage in Rat Model of Alcohol- and Iron-Overload.** *Clin Sci* 1993, **84**:339–348.

77. Stal P, Hunltcrantz R: **Iron Increases Ethanol Toxicity in Rat Liver.** *J Hepatol* 1993, **17**:108–115.

78. Zhang H, Loney LA, Potter BJ: **Effect of Chronic Alcohol Feeding on Hepatic Iron Status and Ferritin Uptake by Rat Hepatocytes.** *Alcohol Clin Exp Res* 1993, **17**:394–400.

79. Paronetto F: **Immunologic Reactions in Alcoholic Liver Disease.** *Semin Liver Dis* 1993, **13**:183–195.
••
Comprehensive review of a complex topic.

80. Sakai Y, Izumi N, Marumo F, Sato C: **Quantitative Immunohistochemical Analysis of Lymphocyte Subsets in Alcoholic Liver Disease.** *J Gastroenterol Hepatol* 1993, **8**:39–43.

81. Grossman CJ, Nienaber M, Mendenhall CL, Hurtubise P, Roselle GA, Rouster S, Weber N, Schmitt G, Gartside PS: **Sex Differences and the Effect of Alcohol on Immune Response in Male and Female Rats.** *Alcohol Clin Exp Res* 1993, **17**:832–840.

82. Zarski JP, Thelu MA, Moulin C, Rachail M, Seignerurin JM: **Interest of the Detection of Hepatitis C Virus RNA in Patients With Alcoholic Liver Disease.** *J Hepatol* 1993, **17**:10–14.

83. Caldwell SH, Li X, Rourk RM, Millar A, Sosnowski KM, Sue M, Barritt AS, McCallum RW, Schiff ER: **Hepatitis C Infection by Polymerase Chain Reaction in Alcoholics: False-Positive ELISA Results and the Influence of Infection on a Clinical Prognostic Score.** *Am J Gastroenterol* 1993, **88**:1016–1021.

84. Rosman AS, Paronetto F, Galvin K, Williams RJ, Lieber CS: **Hepatitis C Virus Antibody in Alcoholic Patients.** *Arch Intern Med* 1993, **153**:965–969.
•
Even in the absence of known risk factors, antibody to hepatitis C virus (as confirmed by the recombinant immunoblot assay) was strongly associated with the presence of portal or lobular inflammation (91% seropositivity) but was only present in 16% of patients without such histologic findings (P<0.001). This association indicates that hepatitis C virus is responsible, at least in part, for the portal or lobular hepatitis associated with alcoholic liver disease.

85. McHutchison JG, Leal R, Govindarajan S, Redeker AG: **Hepatitis C Antibodies in Patients With Alcoholic Liver Disease Commonly Have an Identifiable Risk Factor.** *J Clin Gastroenterol* 1992, **15**:233–235.

86. Takase S, Tsutsumi M, Kawahara H, Takada N, Takada A: **The Alcohol-Altered Liver Membrane Antibody and Hepatitis C Virus Infection in the Progression of Alcoholic Liver Disease.** *Hepatology* 1993, **17**:9–13.

87. Chen D-S: **From Hepatitis to Hepatoma: Lessons From Type B Viral Hepatitis.** *Science* 1993, **262**:369–370.

88. Ikeda K, Saitoh S, Koida I, Arese Y, Tsubota A, Chayama K, Kumada H, Kawanishi M: **A Multivariate Analysis of Risk Factors for Hepatocellular Carcinogenesis: A Prospective Observation of 795 Patients With Viral and Alcoholic Cirrhosis.** *Hepatology* 1993, **18**:47–53.

89. Hill DB, Marsano LS, McClain CJ: **Increased Plasma Interleukin-8 Concentrations in Alcoholic Hepatitis.** *Hepatology* 1993, **18**:576–580.

90. Sheron N, Bird G, Koskinas J, Portmann B, Ceska M, Lindley I, Williams R: **Circulating and Tissue Levels of the Neutrophil Chemotaxin Interleukin-8 are Elevated in Severe Acute Alcoholic Hepatitis, and Tissue Levels Correlate With Neutrophil Infiltration.** *Hepatology* 1993, **18**:41–46.

91. Caly WR, Strauss E: **A Prospective Study of Bacterial Infections in Patients With Cirrhosis.** *J Hepatol* 1993, **18**:353–358.

92. • Nanji AA, Khettry U, Sadrzadeh SMH, Yamanaka T: **Severity of Liver Injury in Experimental Alcoholic Liver Disease Correlation With Plasma Endotoxin, Prostaglandin E_2, Leukotriene B_4 and Thromboxane B_2.** *Am J Pathol* 1993, **142**:367–373.

This study shows the importance of endotoxin in the pathogenesis of experimental alcoholic liver disease and suggests that endotoxin modulates production of eicosanoids that contribute to the severity of liver injury.

93. Byl B, Roucloux I, Crusiaux A, Dupont E, Deviere J: **Tumor Necrosis Factor α and Interleukin 6 Plasma Levels in Infected Cirrhotic Patients.** *Gastroenterology* 1993, **104**:1492–1497.

94. Ruiz AD, Perez JLS, Martinez GL, Calvin JG, Extremera BG, Gea FG: **Tumor Necrosis Factor, Interleukin-1 and Interleukin-6 in Alcoholic Cirrhosis.** *Alcohol Alcohol* 1993, **28**:319–323.

95. •• McClain C, Hill D, Schmidt J, Diehl AM: **Cytokines and Alcoholic Liver Disease.** *Semin Liver Dis* 1993, **13**:170–182.

Excellent review of a complex topic.

96. Basista MH, Gavaler J, Stieffenhofer A, Love K, Rosenblum E, Dindzans V: **Effect of Ethanol on Kupffer Cell Function.** *Alcohol Clin Exp Res* 1993, **17**:556–560.

97. Weiner FR, Esposti SD, Zern MA: **A Role for Cytokines as Regulators of Hepatic Fibrogenesis.** *Gastroenterol Jpn* 1993, **28**:97–101.

98. • Diehl AM, Yang SQ, Cote P, Wand GS: **Chronic Ethanol Consumption Disturbs G-Protein Expression and Inhibits Cyclic AMP-Dependent Signaling in Regenerating Rat Liver.** *Hepatology* 1992, **16**:1212–1219.

Ethanol treatment significantly reduced hepatic accumulation of cyclic AMP after partial hepatectomy. Activation of adenyl cyclase by agents acting through receptors (*eg*, glucagon or isoproterenol), GTP–binding proteins and directly on adenylyl cyclase (*eg*, forskolin) was significantly inhibited. Ethanol also significantly depressed post–partial hepatectomy induction of the stimulatory G protein and phosphoenolpyruvate carboxykinase expression. It was concluded that ethanol-induced desensitization of signaling by way of cyclic AMP–dependent paths may constitute a major obstacle to the orderly process of liver regeneration.

99. Akerman PA, Cote PM, Yang SQ, McClain C, Nelson S, Bagby G, Diehl AM: **Long-Term Ethanol Consumption Alters the Hepatic Response to the Regenerative Effects of Tumor Necrosis Factor-α.** *Hepatology* 1993, **17**:1066–1073.

100. Resnicoff M, Sell C, Ambrose D, Baserga R, Rubin R: **Ethanol Inhibits the Autophosphorylation of the Insulin-Like Growth Factor 1 (IGF-1) Receptor and the IGF-1-Mediated Proliferation of 3T3 Cells.** *J Biol Chem* 1993, **268**:21777–21782.

101. Parrish KM, Dufour MC, Stinson FS, Harford TC: **Average Daily Alcohol Consumption During Adult Life Among Decedents With and Without Cirrhosis: The 1986 National Mortality Followback Survey.** *J Stud Alcohol* 1993, **54**:450–456.

102. Smart RG, Mann RE: **Recent Liver Cirrhosis Declines: Estimates of the Impact of Alcohol Abuse Treatment and Alcoholics Anonymous.** *Addiction* 1993, **88**:193–198.

103. • Dufour MC, Stinson FS, Fe Caces M: **Trends in Cirrhosis Morbidity and Mortality: United States, 1979-1988.** *Semin Liver Dis* 1993, **13**:109–125.

Recent trends are put in perspective.

104. Sumino Y, Kravetz D, Kanel GC, McHutchison JG, Reynolds TB: **Ultrasonographic Diagnosis of Acute Alcoholic Hepatitis 'Pseudoparallel Channel Sign' of Intrahepatic Artery Dilation.** *Gastroenterology* 1993, **105**:1477–1488.

105. Ohtomo K, Baron RL, Dodd III GD, Federle MP, Miller WJ, Campbell WL, Cofner SR, Weber KM: **Confluent Hepatic Fibrosis in Advanced Cirrhosis: Appearance at CT.** *Radiology* 1993, **188**:31–35.

106. Marti-Bonmati L, Talens A, del Olmo J, del Val A, Serra MA, Rodrigo JM, Ferrandez A, Torres V, Rayon M, Vilar JS: **Chronic Hepatitis and Cirrhosis: Evaluation by Means of MR Imaging With Histologic Correlation.** *Radiology* 1993, **188**:37–43.

107. Diaz F, Collazos J, Genolla J: **Study of Serum Procollagen Type III Peptide in Patients With Hepatic Cirrhosis From a Clinical Point of View.** *Clin Invest Med* 1993, **71**:416–418.

108. Tsutsumi M, Urashima S, Matsuda Y, Takase S, Takada A: **Changes in Type IV Collagen Content in Livers of Patients With Alcoholic Liver Disease.** *Hepatology* 1993, **17**:820–827.

109. •• Schenker S, Halff GA: **Nutritional Therapy in Alcoholic Liver Disease.** *Semin Liver Dis* 1993, **13**:196–209.

New insights are provided by this review.

110. •• Mezey E: **Treatment of Alcoholic Liver Disease.** *Semin Liver Dis* 1993, **13**:210–216.

Broad review of an evolving field.

111. • Mendenhall CL, Moritz TE, Roselle GA, Morgan TR, Nemchausky BA, Tamburro CH, Schiff ER, McClain CJ, Marsano LS, Allen JI, Samanta A, Weesner RE, Henderson W, Gartside P, Chen TS, French SW, Chedid A, Veterans Affairs Cooperative Study Group 275: **A Study of Oral Nutritional Support With Oxandrolone in Malnourished Patients With Alcoholic Hepatitis: Results of a Department of Veterans Affairs Cooperative Study.** *Hepatology* 1993, **17**:564–576.

This study involving 273 male subjects concluded that, in patients with moderate malnutrition, oxandrolone should be added to the regimen.

112. Lieber CS, Li J, Robins SJ, DeCarli LM, Mak KM, Leo MA: **Dietary Dielinoleoylphosphatidylcholine (DLPC) is Incorporated into Liver Phospholipids, Protects Against Alcoholic Cirrhosis, Enhances Collagenase Activity and Prevents Acetaldehyde-Induced Collagen Accumulation in Cultured Lipocytes [Abstract].** *Hepatology* 1992, **16**:87A.

113. Gressner AM, Lofti S, Gressner G, Haltner E, Kroph J: **Synergism Between Hepatocytes and Kupffer Cells in the Activation of Fat Storing Cells (Perisinusoidal Lipocytes).** *J Hepatol* 1993, **19**:117–132.

114. Muriel P: **S-Adenosyl-L-Methionine Prevents and Reverses Erythrocyte Membrane Alterations in Cirrhosis.** *J Appl Toxicol* 1993, **13**:179–182.

115. • Osman E, Owens JS, Burroughs AK: **Review Article: S-Adenosyl-L-Methionine – A New Therapeutic Agent in Liver Disease?** *Aliment Pharmacol Ther* 1993, **7**:21–28.

This paper reviews the established biochemical effects of exogenous *S*-adenosyl-L-methionine. The deficiency of *S*-adenosyl-L-methionine synthetase in cirrhosis can be bypassed by exogenous *S*-adenosyl-L-methionine, leading to increased levels of sulphur–containing amino acids and glutathione which are protective against oxidant stress and drug-induced hepatotoxicity. Moreover, *S*-adenosyl-L-methionine appears to act by improving membrane fluidity as well as symptoms and biochemical parameters of cholestasis.

116. Barak A, Beckenhauer HC, Junnila M, Tuma DJ: **Dietary Betaine Promotes Generation of Hepatic S-Adenosylmethione and Protects the Liver From Ethanol-Induced Fatty Infiltration.** *Alcohol Clin Exp Res* 1993, **17**:552–555.

117. • Hultberg B, Berglund M, Andersson A, Frank A: **Elevated Plasma Homocysteine in Alcoholics.** *Alcohol Clin Exp Res* 1993, **17**:687–689.

A significantly higher concentration of plasma homocysteine (compared with controls) was noted in a group of alcoholics. Because hyperhomocysteinemia has been associated with premature vascular disease, the increased plasma homocysteine in alcoholics might cause the increased incidence of stroke found in these patients.

118. Koehn V, Burnand B, Niguille M, Paccaud F, Magnenat P, Yersin B: **Prevalence of Malnutrition in Alcoholics and Non Alcoholic Medical Inpatients: A Comparative Anthropometric Study.** *JPEN J Parenter Enteral Nutr* 1993, **17**:35–40.

119. Hirsch S, Bunout D, de la Maza P, Iturriaga H, Petermann M, Icazar G, Gattas V, Ugarte G: **Controlled Trial on Nutrition Supplementation in Outpatients With Symptomatic Alcohol Cirrhosis.** *JPEN J Parenter Enteral Nutr* 1993, **17**:119–124.

120. Lieber CS: **Herman Award Lecture, 1993: A Personal Perspective on Alcohol, Nutrition, and the Liver.** *Am J Clin Nutr* 1993, **58**:430–442.
•
Review of the interactions of nutrition and direct hepatoxicity of alcohol.

121. Lucey MR: **Liver Transplantation for the Alcoholic Patient.** *Adv Liver Transplant* 1993, **22**:243–256.
•
This review of the data from the University of Michigan and other transplant centers suggests that the outcome of liver transplantation, when considered as either mortality or psychological morbidity, is similar for alcoholics and nonalcoholics alike.

122. Gish RG, Lee AH, Keeffe EB, Rome H, Concepcion W, Esquivel CO: **Liver Transplantation for Patients With Alcoholism and End-Stage Liver Disease.** *Am J Gastroenterol* 1993, **88**:1337–1342.

123. Bonet H, Manez R, Kramer D, Wright HI, Gavaler JS, Baddour N, Van Thiel DH: **Liver Transplantation for Alcoholic Liver Disease: Survival of Patients Transplanted With Alcoholic Hepatitis Plus Cirrhosis as Compared With Those With Cirrhosis Alone.** *Alcohol Clin Exp Res* 1993, **17**:1102–1106.
•
Of 147 patients with alcoholic liver disease who had received liver transplantation, 30% had alcoholic hepatitis plus cirrhosis, whereas 70% had cirrhosis alone. One-year survival was 80% for patients with alcoholic hepatitis and 84% for those with cirrhosis. Thus, liver transplantation could be accomplished as successfully with alcoholic hepatitis as with cirrhosis, although, the diagnosis of alcoholic hepatitis implies a briefer period of alcohol abstention.

124. Anderson P: **Management of Alcohol Problems: The Role of the General Practitioner.** *Alcohol Alcohol* 1993, **28**:263–272.

125. Lieber CS: **Alcoholic Liver Disease: A Public Health Issue In Need of a Public Heatlh Approach.** *Semin Liver Dis* 1993, **13**:108A–108C.

Charles S. Lieber, MD, VAMC #151-G, 130 West Kingsbridge Road, Bronx, NY 10468, USA.

Progress in pediatric hepatology

James V. Higgins, MD, and William F. Balistreri, MD

Children's Hospital Medical Center, Cincinnati, Ohio, USA

Hepatitis B virus, one of the most common worldwide causes of acute and chronic liver disease, remains of concern to pediatricians. Efforts at universal immunization have been only marginally successful, despite recommendations by the American Academy of Pediatrics and the Centers for Disease Control and despite several studies conducted during the past year that have confirmed the efficacy of hepatitis B immunization. These reports place continued emphasis on physician understanding and acceptance of infant vaccination. Liver transplantation is being considered more often in patients less than 1 year of age with end-stage liver disease. New surgical techniques, which provide alternatives to the diminishing cadaver donor pool, have included living-related donors and split segment grafts. Nonsurgical options for the treatment of pediatric liver disease are mentioned briefly.

Current Opinion in Gastroenterology 1994, **10**:331–336

Pediatric hepatology is a rapidly maturing field. The past year has brought advances in several areas of diagnosis, treatment, and prevention of childhood liver disease. We have limited our review to two areas of major importance in which there has been significant activity during the past year: hepatitis B vaccination and pediatric liver transplantation. Extrahepatic biliary atresia remains the most common disease leading to liver transplantation in pediatric patients, and this subject has been extensively reviewed in a recent article by Strauss *et al.* [1••]. There are two reports of interest that continue to support the safety and efficacy of hepatitis A vaccine [2•,3•].

Hepatitis B immunization

One of the important developments within the past year has been the increased emphasis on implementation of a universal vaccination program for the prevention of hepatitis B infection. Hepatitis B virus (HBV) has been the subject of several reviews detailing the effects of acute and chronic infection [4••,5•]. The reported incidence of acute hepatitis B increased by 37% from 1979 to 1989, with an estimated 200,000 to 300,000 new infections occurring annually from 1980 to 1991. This increase has given rise to an estimated 1.25 million persons with chronic HBV infection in the United States. Each is at long-term risk for significant sequelae such as chronic liver disease and hepatocellular carcinoma [6]. The benefit of HBV vaccine in children has been reviewed [7••,8••]; however, there is still a general reluctance of health care providers to incorporate the vaccine into their practices.

Strategy

Based on the continued increase in new hepatitis B infections, the Centers for Disease Control have developed a strategy for universal immunization of children through a comprehensive HBV vaccination program [9]. The need for such a program is underscored by the high incidence of new HBV infections in health care workers with high blood exposure (1.5% per year) compared with those with low exposure (0.2% per year) [10], the increased risk of children with early hepatitis B surface antigen (HBsAg) positivity to develop hepatocellular carcinoma [11], and the detection of HBV DNA in the colostrum of hepatitis B e antigen–positive mothers [12].

The recommendations were followed by an educational effort of the Centers for Disease Control to encourage pediatricians and family practitioners to incorporate HBV immunization into their practices. In order to evaluate the effectiveness of these efforts, Freed *et al.* [13••] studied the response of North Carolina pediatricians and the effect of the recommendations on clinical practice. Although a majority of pediatricians (82%) stated that they were aware of the new recommendations, only 32% agreed that immunizations were warranted in their practices. The study revealed that noneconomic barriers (concern regarding multiple injections at a single visit, anticipation of severe reactions, and unknown long-term immunogenicity) were

Abbreviations

HBsAg—hepatitis B surface antigen; **HBV**—hepatitis B virus; **LRLT**—living-related liver transplantation; **OLT**—orthotopic liver transplantation.

 ISBN 1-85922-608-6 ISSN 0267–1379

often cited by practitioners as obstacles in the immunization program. Similar results were also found in a survey of family practitioners [14]. Further discouraging results were reported by the American Academy of Pediatrics [15]. Twenty-four percent of the members surveyed opposed universal early HBV immunization, and 23% said that they were unsure. These reports confirm the need for further education of the medical community, in order to successfully implement that we view as a sound and cost-effective universal HBV immunization program.

Immune response

The use of the vaccine in preterm infants has been evaluated in China [16••]. Over a 2-year period, 132 infants weighing less than 1750 g were immunized with HBV vaccine. In the group of patients weighing between 1000 and 2000 g at the time of the immunization, there was a 79% seropositivity rate (anti-HBs titer > 10 mIU/mL) after the third dose of vaccine. In the group weighing greater than 2000 g there was a 91% seropositivity rate to the HBV vaccine. In full-term infants there was 100% seropositivity rate following the third dose of vaccine. The maternal HBsAg status bore no correlation to the final response of the three groups of infants. This study suggests that routine immunization of preterm infants should begin after they reach 2000 g (*ie*, prior to discharge from the hospital). The study also showed that delaying the immunization of infants of HBsAg-positive mothers for up to 59 days did not affect the seroconversion rate or the HBV carrier status of the infants as long as 0.5 mL of HBV immune globulin was given at birth.

Cost effectiveness

A Canadian study evaluated the immune response of 145 full-term infants, born to HBsAg-positive mothers, from birth to 5 years of age [17••]. Doses were given at 1,2, and either 6,7, or 8 months of age after the vaccine series. One-hundred thirty-four children (93%) developed anti-HBs titers greater than 10 mIU/mL, five (3%) became HBsAg positive, and six (4%) failed to seroconvert but did not become infected. Fifteen children (11%) lost detectable anti-HBs levels during follow-up, but none became HBsAg positive, suggesting that the protection may last longer than the detectable antibody titers. The probability of maintaining a protective concentration of antibody in the vaccine responders was 86% at 5 years of age.

Seroconversion rates of over 90% have also been demonstrated in areas in which HBV is endemic, such as Italy [18•] and Gambia [19••]. A study of the effect of a comprehensive aggressive hepatitis B vaccination program on the prevalence of HBV infection in children was carried out in an area of American Samoa in which HBV infection is endemic [20••]. The vaccination strategy was to target the entire population through the immunization of newborns, children less than 6 years of age, and persons at high risk greater than 6 years of age. The chronic infection rate was 7% prior to the institution of the program. Five years after beginning this program, the overall prevalence of HBV infection declined by 50%, and the carrier rate declined by 80%. There were no children with acute HBV infection and the prevalence rate of chronic HBV infection in children was less than 1.5%. There were no carriers among 3- to 4-year-old children, indicating that perinatal transmission was prevented.

The question of type and dose of HBV vaccine was addressed in a randomized trial comparing HBV recombinant-DNA yeast vaccine with plasma-derived vaccine in 305 children having a mean age of 5.5 years [21••]. Both of the vaccines were shown to be highly immunogenic, with a 93% to 99% seropositivity rate (anti-HBs response) at 8 months. There was no difference between a two-dose and three-dose regimen of the plasma-derived vaccine. The only side effects reported were fever of less than 39.5°C (9%) and tenderness at the injection site (5%). All groups of patients were found to have a slow decrease in mean titers of anti-HBs over a 5-year follow-up period. Although all of the patients were close relatives of HBV carriers, and therefore at high risk of repeated exposure to HBV, there were no breakthrough HBV infections reported. Anamnestic responses (a significant increase in anti-HBs titers after 12 months) were also found in 42 patients (13%) (mean age, 8.7 years) during the 5-year follow-up period. Although the majority of the subjects were not infants, the anamnestic response in patients with titers less than 10 mIU/mL suggests that long-term protective immunogenicity may be better than previously thought. Other promising long-term immunogenicity results have been reported. Tabor *et al.* [22] noted a 74% seropositivity rate at 9 years after vaccination in both adult and pediatric patients in a rural African setting. Lo *et al.* [23] reported a 100% seropositivity rate at 10 years after vaccination in neonates born to HBsAg-carrier mothers in a plasma-derived HBV vaccine trial in China.

The cost-effectiveness of a universal HBV immunization program has been studied. Bloom *et al.* [24••] performed a cost-effectiveness analysis of several potential immunization strategies including no vaccination, universal vaccination, and screening and vaccination. It was estimated that the optimal cost-effectiveness would result from a strategy in which 1) all pregnant women are screened for active HBV infection, 2) HBV vaccine and hepatitis B immune globulin are administered to babies born to hepatitis B–positive mothers, and 3) HBV vaccine is administered to all children at 10 years of age and then again 10 years later. If this strategy is followed, the projected cost per year of life saved would be $375 compared with $3332 using the strategy of universal newborn immunization alone. Programs targeted at adolescents ($13,938) or the general adult population ($54,524) were less cost-effective. Although vaccine cost is clearly a concern, other impediments to implementation have now emerged. Pediatricians have been reluctant to endorse HBV immunizations of infants because few of them have seen a case of HBV infection in their practice, and they tend to view their patients as being at low risk for exposure to the virus [13••,25]. They are also reluctant to give another injection to an infant to prevent what is perceived to be an adult disease. As educational efforts continue, and further studies are carried out to clarify the most effective immunization schedule and cost-effectiveness, practitioners should become more willing to vaccinate their patients.

Liver transplantation

Liver transplantation has become a commonly accepted therapy for children with end-stage liver disease. Advances in surgical techniques and improved immunosuppression and postoperative care have allowed broader application of transplantation in many pediatric liver diseases.

Fulminant hepatic failure is defined as acute liver failure and the development of encephalopathy within 8 weeks of the onset of symptoms in patients with no evidence of previous liver disease [26]. Mortality is near 90% when supportive measures alone are used. Therefore, orthotopic liver transplantation (OLT) is a viable option to improve the outcome. Tan *et al.* [27] reported a 66% survival rate in a group of 12 children who received transplants for fulminant hepatic failure or late-onset hepatic failure. Another report of 35 children (aged 3 months to 15 years) who underwent OLT for fulminant hepatic failure resulted in a nearly identical (68%) survival rate [28••]. Of the 35 patients, 22 met established criteria for OLT (hepatic encephalopathy and factor V level <25% of control). Nineteen (86%) subsequently received transplants and 13 (68%) are alive without sequelae. Ten patients in the original group died, either before or after transplantation, as a result of severe irreversible brain damage. This study shows that the degree of encephalopathy at the time of transplantation is, as in adults, an important indicator of patient survival. Whereas no patient with grade 1 or 2 encephalopathy died, 54.1% of patients with grade 3 or 4 encephalopathy died. This study also reported that patients who died or progressed to transplantation had significantly reduced levels of factor V compared with those who recovered spontaneously. Because of the rapid neurologic deterioration in pediatric fulminant hepatic failure patients and the high mortality associated with higher grades of encephalopathy, the authors stress the importance of early referral of patients to a liver transplant facility.

According to the American United Network for Organ Sharing, children less than 1 year of age have the highest mortality of any age group awaiting transplantation [29••]. Therefore, these children have been the subject of closer evaluation. In a study comparing the survival of 46 children who underwent OLT (15 of whom were less than 1 year of age), 2-year survival was 80% for those less than 1 year of age and 91% for those greater than 1 year of age [29••]. The postoperative course was similar for the two groups, except that the younger group required more reoperations (87%) than the older group (48%). The authors concluded that although children less than 1 year of age present technical challenges, they are not a high-risk group for OLT and should be listed for transplantation when medically indicated, regardless of age. Another study evaluating OLT in infants and children with extrahepatic biliary atresia found similar results [30]. The authors reported a 79% survival for patients less than 1 year of age compared with 65% for patients greater than 1 year of age. There was no increase in operative complications.

Donor options

As the indications for and capabilities of pediatric liver transplant continue to expand, the pool of available size-matched donor organs diminishes. This has led to the development of alternative surgical procedures to supplement cadaveric organs, including living-related liver transplantation (LRLT) and split segment grafts. There is currently a great deal of excitement concerning LRLT as a way to secure more organs for both emergent and elective OLT [31••]. Survival rates have been reported to be between 85% and 94% in series from Japan [32•,33] and from the United States [34••]. However, a small series from Turkey reported a survival rate of only 33% [35]. The major emphasis has been on minimizing the degree of risk and the operative stress on the donor, while providing grafts with a high degree of viability and immunohistocompatibility. The risk to the donor was analyzed by Shimahara *et al.* [36••] in a series of 28 patients who received parent/donor livers. The authors showed that the risk to the donor is minimal when the left lobe or left lateral segment of the liver is used as a graft. In their series, one right lobe donor developed transient icterus, but this was the only postoperative complication encountered in the entire series. Edmond *et al.* [34••] reported on 45 consecutive patients treated with either living-related, whole-cadaver, or reduced-size liver transplantation. The survival rate for LRLT was 94% (16 of 17 patients) compared with 86% (12 of 14) for whole-cadaver transplants and 90% (nine of 10) for reduced-size liver transplantation. Graft survival was slightly higher in LRLT (84%) than in whole-cadaver (73%) and reduced-size liver transplantation (75%). One teenager in their series was also successfully treated, raising the possibility that LRLT may also be used for adult patients awaiting organs.

Another option to increase the number of donor livers is controlled splitting of a single organ for transplantation into two recipients. Houssin *et al.* [37•] reported on a series of 16 patients who received transplants from eight livers using split grafts. The postoperative survival rate was 75%, with an immediate graft survival rate of 69%. They reported an increased incidence of bleeding from the right graft following revascularization and an overall increased incidence of hepatic artery thrombosis (25% vs 3% to 10% in other series). The authors point out that although this concept is promising, new ethical and technical issues are being raised. For example, if there is a risk related to controlled splitting, should it be shared between two recipients? If the two grafts are to be used at different transplant centers, then decisions on splitting technique need to be shared and coordinated.

New indications

There are a number of reports on the use of OLT in specific liver diseases that may not have previously been treated with transplantation. Tzakis *et al.* [38•] studied a series of 23 children with Alagille's syndrome and end-stage liver disease who underwent liver transplantation. They reported a 57% survival rate, with an increase in mortality noted in patients who had associated cardiopulmonary disease or in those with a previous hepatoportoenterostomy procedure. This finding underscores the importance of confirming the diagnosis before performing an unnecessary surgical procedure. We would also caution that the decision to perform transplantation on patients with Alagille's syndrome should be made carefully and only with clear indications.

Sokal *et al.* [39] reported on a series of five patients who received transplants for hereditary tyrosinemia. Four patients survived and one patient died from hyperacute rejection following retransplantation. Because this study shows good outcome for early transplantation, the authors suggest that liver transplantation should be considered in these patients even at a young age (*ie*, < 1 year), before the onset of long-term complications. Other reports describe successful OLT in patients with cystic fibrosis [40], type I glycogenosis unresponsive to medical therapy [41], and familial hypercholesterolemia before the onset of cardiovascular complications [42].

Nontransplant options

Along with continued advances in surgical techniques, nonsurgical alternatives to liver transplantation are also being reported with increasing frequency (Table 1). For example, development of a bioartificial liver [43••] may offer hope to patients by providing a bridge to transplantation or by allowing time for the injured liver to recover spontaneously. Somatic gene transfer has been used to treat the hepatobiliary disease of cystic fibrosis [44]. And bile acid therapy for an inborn error of bile acid metabolism has led to the resolution of liver biopsy alterations [45]. Further research should provide other advances in biomedical treatment of several metabolic liver diseases.

Table 1. Strategies for the management of metabolic disease*

Replacement of deficient end-product or substrate
Oral administration of primary bile acids in inborn errors of bile acid metabolism
Oral administration of corn starch in glycogen storage disease type 1 (glucose-6-phosphatase deficiency)
Oral administration of cholesterol in Smith-Lemli-Opitz syndrome
Enzyme inhibition
Treatment of tyrosinemia type 1 by inhibition of 4-hydroxyphenylpyruvate dioxygenase with 2-(2–nitro-4-trifluro methyl benzoyl)-1,3-cyclohexanedione
Treatment of acute hepatic porphyria by inhibition of Δ-amino levelonic acid synthase with heme
Enzyme induction
Phenobarbital therapy in Crigler-Najjar syndrome type II (partial deficiency of glucuronyltransferase)
Removal of toxic product
Iron chelation and antioxidant therapy for neonatal iron storage disease
Copper chelation in Wilson's disease
Stimulation of alternative pathways of waste nitrogen excretion with benzoate and phenylacetate in urea cycle defects
Use of cysteamine to reduce cystine storage in cystinosis
Dietary restriction of the substrate
Galactose in galactose-1-phosphate uridyl transferase deficiency
Fructose in fructose-1-phosphate aldolase deficiency
Molecular manipulation
Inhibition of polymerization of α_1 antitrypsin (PiZZ)
Receptor-based, targeted enzyme replacement therapy
Targeting of purified glucocerebroside to Kupffer cells via macrophage-specific cell-surface mannose receptors in Gaucher's disease
Gene therapy (animal models)
Hepatocyte-directed gene transfer for hyperchlolesterolemia in low-density lipoprotein receptor–deficient rabbits
Receptor-mediated gene delivery for partial correction of genetic analbuminemia in Nagase rats
Somatic gene transfer in cystic fibrosis–associated hepatobiliary disease
Organ transplantation

*From Balistreri [46]; with permission.

Conclusions

Advances in immunization strategies for hepatitis B virus hold the potential for the eradication of one of the world's most common causes of chronic liver disease. Further education of medical personnel and continued studies into the long-term immunogenicity and cost-effectiveness of HBV vaccine should eventually result in a successful universal immunization program. The advances in liver transplantation continue to provide alternative approaches to meet the shortage of size-matched donor organs for pediatric patients. Early referral to transplant centers is imperative for good outcome in fulminant hepatic failure. As further research continues in the area of metabolic liver disease, genetics, and molecular biology nonsurgical therapies are expected to take a primary role in the treatment of chronic liver disease in children.

References and recommended reading

Papers of particular interest, published within the annual period of review, have been highlighted as:

- • Of special interest
- •• Of outstanding interest

1. •• Strauss RS, Weisselberg B, Grand RJ: **Pediatric Biliary Disease.** *Curr Opin Gastroenterol* 1993, 9:841–846.

A comprehensive review of pediatric hepatobiliary disease including biliary atresia, cholelithiasis, and cystic fibrosis.

2. • Horng Y, Chang M, Lee C, Safary A, Andre FE, Chen D: **Safety and Immunogenicity of Hepatitis A Vaccine in Healthy Adult Volunteers.** *J Gastroenterol Hepatol* 1993, **8**:338–341.

An immunogenicity study of a three-dose hepatitis A virus vaccine regimen. A seropositivity rate of 100% is reported at 7 months after injections at 0, 1, and 6 months.

3. • Hilleman MR, Calacdra GB, Hesley TM, Nalin DR, Ryan JL, West DJ: **Vaccines Against Hepatitis A and B.** *J Gastroenterol Hepatol* 1993, **8**:S21–S26.

A brief review article that discusses the recent advances in the areas of hepatitis A and B immunizations. Both adult and pediatric patient data are presented.

4. •• Margolis HS: **Prevention of Acute and Chronic Liver Disease Through Immunization: Hepatitis B and Beyond.** *J Infect Dis* 1993, **168**:9–14.

A review article examining current trends in hepatitis A and B infection. Emphasis is placed on hepatitis B immunization programs, with a comparison of the effectiveness of various strategies.

5. • Ruiz-Moreno M: **Chronic Hepatitis B in Children: Natural History and Treatment.** *J Hepatol* 1993, 17:S64–S66.

A brief review of the experience of treating chronic hepatitis B infection in Spanish children. The authors suggest that interferon-alpha treatment (10 mU/m^2 three times weekly x 6 months) of chronic HBV is associated with a 50% response rate compared with untreated control subjects.

6. Center for Disease Control.: **Protection Against Viral Hepatitis: Recommendations of the Immunization Practices Advisory Committee (ACIP).** *MMWR Morb Mortal Wkly Rep* 1990, 39:5–22.

7. •• Greenberg DP: **Pediatric Experience With Recombinant Hepatitis B Vaccines and Relevant Safety and Immunogenicity Studies.** *Pediatr Infect Dis J* 1993, 12:438–445.

A review of the development of the currently available HBV vaccines with emphasis on safety, immunogenicity, and protective efficacy as reported in studies of infants and children.

8. •• West DJ, Calandra GB, Hesley TM, Ioli V, Miller WJ: **Control of Hepatitis B Through Routine Immunization of Infants: The Need for Flexible Schedules and New Combination Vaccine Formulations.** *Vaccine* 1993, **11**:S21–S27.

An evaluation of the rationale for the universal immunization of infants, including the importance of screening pregnant women for HBsAg, the use of HBV immunoglobulin immunoprophylaxis, age, and the schedule of immunization. Prospects for combined vaccines are also reviewed. Several alternative vaccine schedules are presented, based on the future availability of combined vaccines.

9. Center for Disease Control: **Hepatitis B Virus: A Comprehensive Strategy for Eliminating Transmission in the United States Through Universal Childhood Vaccination. Recommendations of the Immunization Practices Advisory Committee (ACIP).** *MMWR Morb Mortal Wkly Rpt* 1991, 40:1–19.

10. Gibas A, Blewett DR, Schoenfeld DA, Dienstag JL: **Prevalence and Incidence of Viral Hepatitis in Health Workers in the Prehepatitis B Vaccination Era.** *Am J Epidemiol* 1992, 136:603–610.

11. Hsieh CC, Tzonou A, Zavitsanos X, Kaklamani E, Lan SJ, Trichopoulos D: **Age at First Establishment of Chronic Hepatitis B Virus Infection and Hepatocellular Carcinoma Risk.** *Am J Epidemiol* 1992, **136**:1115–1121.

12. Lin H, Hsu H, Chang M, Chen P, Chen D: **Hepatitis B Virus in the Colostra of HBeAg-Positive Carrier Mothers.** *J Pediatr Gastroenerol Nutr* 1993, **17**:207–210.

13. •• Freed GL, Bordley WC, Clark SJ, Konrad TR: **Reactions of Pediatricians to a New Centers for Disease Control Recommendation for Universal Immunization of Infants With Hepatitis B Vaccine.** *Pediatrics* 1993, **91**:699–702.

An appraisal of the efforts of the Centers for Disease Control to disseminate HBV universal immunization information. The study identifies practical concerns of pediatricians who consider compliance with the recommendations.

14. Freed GL, Bordley WC, Clark SJ, Konrad TR: **Family Physician Acceptance of Universal Hepatitis B Immunization of Infants.** *J Fam Pract* 1993, **36**:153–157.

15. **Survey Reveals Views on HBV Recommendations.** *Am Acad Pediatr News* 1993, October p. 2.

16. •• Lau Y, Tam AYC, Ng KW, Tsoi NS, Lam B, Lam P, Yeung CY: **Response of Preterm Infants to Hepatitis B Vaccine.** *J Pediatr* 1992, **121**:962–965.

A study comparing various HBV vaccine dose schedules in preterm neonates, which suggests that routine immunization should begin after infants reach 2000 g. Delay in administration of the vaccine to infants weighing less than 2000 g (and with HBsAg-positive mothers) did not increase the risk for HBV infection.

17. •• Delage G, Remy-Prince S, Montplaisir S: **Combined Active-Passive Immunization Against the Hepatitis B Virus: Five-Year Follow-Up of Children Born to Hepatitis B Surface Antigen-Positive Mothers.** *Pediatr Infect Dis J* 1993, **12**:126–130.

A study of the long-term protective response to HBV vaccine in children born to HBsAg-positive mothers suggesting that protection may be provided long after antibody titers fall. This study addresses concerns about the need for and timing of booster doses of vaccine.

18. • Zanetti AR, Tanzi E, Romano L, Grappasonni I: **Vaccination Against Hepatitis B: The Italian Strategy.** *Vaccine* 1993, **11**:521–524.

A report of the Italian strategy for HBV immunization of neonates, 12-year-old children, and high-risk older individuals, in an effort to completely immunize the population that is less than 24 years of age within 12 years time.

19. •• Chotard J, Inskip HM, Hall AJ, Loik F, Mendy M, Whittle H, George MO, Lowe Y: **The Gambia Hepatitis Intervention Study: Follow-Up of a Cohort of Children Vaccinated Against Hepatitis B.** *J Infect Dis* 1992, **166**:764–768.

A 3-year follow-up report of the Gambian Hepatitis Intervention Study that started in 1986, showing a 95% response rate in patients receiving vaccines. The study reports promising data for the prevention of chronic HBV carrier status, and ultimately a reduced incidence of hepatocellular carcinoma.

20. •• Mahoney FJ, Woodruff BA, Erben JJ, Coleman PJ, Reid EC, Schatz GC, Kane MA: **Effect of a Hepatitis B Vaccination Program on the Prevalence of Hepatitis B Virus Infection.** *J Infect Dis* 1993, **167**:203–207.

This study showed the impact of HBV universal immunization in an area in which HBV is endemic (American Somoa). Strong support for infant immunization is provided, because none of the vaccinated newborns were later found to be HBV carriers.

21. •• Lai C, Wong BC, Yeoh E, Lim W, Chang W, Lin H: **Five-Year Follow-Up of a Prospective Randomized Trial of Hepatitis B Recombinant DNA Yeast Vaccine vs. Plasma-Derived Vaccine in Children: Immunogenicity and Anamnestic Responses.** *Hepatology* 1993, **18**:763–767.

This study showed comparable immunogenicity between yeast-derived and plasma-derived vaccines. The study also documented a similar antibody response to a two-dose and a three-dose schedule of plasma-derived vaccine.

22. Tabor E, Cairns J, Gerety RJ, Bayley AC: **Nine-Year Follow-Up of a Plasma-Derived Hepatitis B Vaccine in a Rural African Setting.** *J Med Virol* 1993, **40**:204–209.

23. Lo KJ, Lee SD, Tsai YT, Wu TC, Yu MY, Wang YJ, Chan CY: **Hepatitis B Vaccine Trial in Neonates.** *J Gastroenterol Hepatol* 1993, **8**:S99–S102.

24. Bloom BS, Hillman AL, Fendrick AM, Schwartz JS: **A Reappraisal of Hepatitis B Virus Vaccination Strategies Using Cost-Effectiveness Analysis.** *Ann Intern Med* 1993, **118**:298–306.
•• A decision analysis showing that a strategy of screening and vaccinating newborns, combined with routine vaccination of 10-year-old children, is the most cost-effective approach to HBV immunization.

25. Dickinson CJ, Olson A: **Hepatitis B Vaccine: Should We Give it a Shot?** *Hepatology* 1993, **18**:458–460.

26. Bernuau J, Rueff B, Benhamou JP: **Fulminant and Subfulminant Liver Failure: Definitions and Causes.** *Semin Liver Dis* 1986, 6:97–106.

27. Tan KC, Mondragon RS, Vougas V, Mieli-Vergani G, Heaton ND, Mowat AP, Chiyende J, Baker A, Koukoulis G, Portmann B, *et al.*: **Liver Transplantation for Fulminant Hepatic Failure and Late-Onset Hepatic Failure in Children.** *Br J Surg* 1992, 79:1192–1194.

28. Devictor D, Desplanques L, Debray D, Ozier Y, Dubousset A, Valayer J, Houssin D, Bernard O, Huault G: **Emergency Liver Transplantation for Fulminant Liver Failure in Infants and Children.** *Hepatology* 1992, **16**:1156–1162.
•• A report of liver transplantation as an effective treatment for children with fulminant hepatic failure. The results suggest that the outcome is improved when patients are transferred to transplant centers before the onset of hepatic encephalopathy.

29. Dunn SP, Weintraub W, Vinocur CD, Billmire DF, Falkenstein K: **Is Age Less Than 1 Year a High-Risk Category for Orthotopic Liver Transplantation?** *J Pediatr Surg* 1993, **28**:1048–1050.
•• A study challenging the common belief that children less than 1 year of age are high-risk patients for OLT. The results show survival rates to be similar to those attained in older children, suggesting that liver transplantation should not be delayed based solely on the age of the patient.

30. Beath S, Pearmain G, Kelly D, McMaster P, Mayer A, Buckels J: **Liver Transplantation in Babies and Children With Extrahepatic Biliary Atresia.** *J Pediatr Surg* 1993, **28**:1044–1047.

31. Tanaka K, Uemoto S, Tokunaga Y, Fujita S, Sano K, Nishizawa T, Sawada H, Shirahase I, Kim HJ, Yamaoka Y, *et al.*: **Surgical Techniques and Innovations in Living Related Liver Transplantation.** *Ann Surg* 1993, **217**:82–91.
•• A report of LRLT as an option for increasing the number of available organs for OLT. Techniques are described that broaden the donor/recipient body weight ratio, allowing for wider application of LRLT.

32. Ozawa K, Uemoto S, Tanaka K, Kumada K, Yamaoka Y, Kobayashi N, Inamoto T, Shimahara Y, Mori K, Honda K, *et al.*: **An Appraisal of Pediatric Liver Transplantation From Living Relatives.** *Ann Surg* 1992, **216**:547–553.
• A study of 20 pediatric patients who were treated with LRLT. An 85% survival rate is reported, with no complication in donors.

33. Tanaka K, Uemoto S, Tokunaga Y, Fujita S, Sano K, Mori K, Yamaoka Y, Ozawa K: **Liver Transplantation in Children From Living-Related Donors.** *Transplant Proc* 1993, **25**:1084–1086.

34. Edmond JC, Heffron TG, Kortz EO, Gonzalez-Vallina R, Contis JC, Black DD, Whitington PF: **Improved Results of Living-Related Liver Transplantation With Routine Application in a Pediatric Program.** *Transplantation* 1993, **55**:835–840.
•• A comparison study of LRLT, whole-organ (cadaver), and reduced-size liver transplantation in 45 children, which indicated that LRLT is an important option in the management of pediatric transplantation candidates.

35. Haberal M, Abbasoglu O, Büyükpamukçu N, Bilgin N, Telatar H, Besim A: **Segmental Living Related Donor Liver Transplantation in Childhood.** *Transplant Proc* 1993, **25**:2200–2202.

36. Shimahara Y, Awane M, Yamaoka Y, Tanaka A, Morimoto T, Mori K, Higashiyama H, Yamaguchi T, Kumada K, Takada Y, *et al.*: **Analyses of the Risk and Operative Stress for Donors in Living-Related Partial Liver Transplantation.** *Transplantation* 1992, **54**:983–988.
•• This study addresses donor safety in LRLT. The study population includes one right lobe donor (a procedure that is usually not performed), which raises issues concerning the higher risk procedure of right lobectomy for larger graft recipients as a future extension of LRLT into adult patients.

37. Houssin D, Boillot O, Soubrane O, Couinaud C, Pitre J, Ozier Y, Devictor D, Bernard O, Chapuis Y: **Controlled Liver Splitting for Transplantation in Two Recipients: Technique, Results and Perspectives.** *Br J Surg* 1993, **80**:75–80.
• This study evaluated liver splitting as another option for increasing available donor organs in pediatric liver transplantation patients. The favorable patient survival rate (75%) suggests that this technique warrants further investigation.

38. Tzakis AG, Reyes J, Tepetes K, Tzoracoleftherakis V, Todo S, Starzl TE: **Liver Transplantation for Alagille's Syndrome.** *Liver Transplant* 1993, **128**:337–339.
• A retrospective analysis of 23 children with Alagille's syndrome and end-stage liver disease suggesting that OLT is a therapeutic option in these patients. A high risk is assigned to those patients with cardiopulmonary disease.

39. Sokal EM, Bustos R, Van Hoof F, Otte JB: **Liver Transplantation for Hereditary Tyrosinemia-Early Transplantation Following the Patient's Stabilization.** *Transplantation* 1992, **54**:937–939.

40. Revell SP, Noble-Jamieson G, Roberton NRC, Barnes ND: **Liver Transplantation in Cystic Fibrosis.** *J R Soc Med* 1993, **86**:111–112.

41. Sokal EM, Lopez-Silvarrey A, Buts JP, Otte JB: **Orthotopic Liver Transplantation for Type I Glycogenosis Unresponsive to Medical Therapy.** *J Pediatr Gastroenterol Nutr* 1993, **16**:465–467.

42. Sokal EM, Ulla L, Harvengt C, Otte JB: **Liver Transplantation for Familial Hypercholesterolemia Before the Onset of Cardiovascular Complications.** *Transplantation* 1993, **55**:432–433.

43. Rozga J, Williams F, Ro M, Neuzil DF, Giorgio TD, Backfisch G, Moscioni AD, Hakim R, Demetriou AA: **Development of a Bioartificial Liver: Properties and Function of a Hollow-Fiber Module Inoculated With Liver Cells.** *Hepatology* 1993, **17**:258–265.
•• A report of the use of a bioartificial liver in the treatment of acute ischemic liver failure in dogs, resulting in improvement in metabolic derangements. The results provide hope for future clinical trials.

44. Yang Y, Raper SE, Cohn JA, Engelhardt JF, Wilson JM: **An Approach for Treating the Hepatobiliary Diseases of Cystic Fibrosis by Somatic Gene Transfer.** *Proc Natl Acad Sci U S A* 1993, **90**:4601–4605.

45. Daugherty CC, Setchell KDR, Heubi JE, Balistreri WF: **Resolution of Liver Biopsy Alterations in Three Siblings With Bile Acid Treatment of an Inborn Error of Bile Acid Metabolism.** *Hepatology* 1993, **18**:1096–1101.

46. Balistreri WF: **Non-Transplant Options for the Treatment of Metabolic Liver Disease - Saving Livers While Saving Lives.** *Hepatology* 1994, **19**:782–787.

James V. Higgins, MD, and William F. Balistreri, MD, Division of Pediatric Gastroenterology and Nutrition, Children's Hospital Medical Center, 3333 Burnet Avenue, Cincinnati, OH 45229-4415, USA.

Primary and secondary liver tumors

Dominique Franco, MD, and Corinne Vons, MD

Hôpital Antoine Béclère, Université Paris, Clamart, France

The year 1993 has been rather quiet in the field of liver tumors. Some of the excitement raised by the discovery of site-specific mutations of the p53 gene in hepatocellular carcinoma is decreasing; it may just be another gene alteration occurring at a late stage of cancer development. Hepatitis C virus is becoming the most frequent etiologic factor of hepatocellular carcinoma, even in countries with high hepatitis B virus endemicity. Cirrhosis is a key step in the development of hepatocellular carcinoma in patients with viral hepatitis. Frequently, macroegenerative nodules in cirrhotic livers may be preneoplastic lesions. There were no major advances in the diagnosis and treatment of hepatocellular carcinoma. Molecular variants of α-fetoprotein may be the next most promising biological markers of hepatocellular carcinoma. The indications for liver transplant in the treatment of hepatocellular carcinoma have become very limited. At last, gene therapy seems to be effective for treating liver metastases (from human colon carcinoma cell lines) in mice.

Current Opinion in Gastroenterology 1994, **10**:337–343

Although 1993 was not a great year in the field of liver tumors, there were some advances in the knowledge of epidemiology, tumorigenesis, and diagnostic and therapeutic procedures of hepatocellular carcinoma and liver metastases.

The p53 gene

Genetic alterations seem to play an important role in the carcinogenetic process, including integration of viral genoma, activation of protooncogenes, and inactivation of tumor suppressor genes. Attention has recently focused on the p53 gene. Mutations of the p53 gene, a tumor suppressor gene located on chromosome 17*p*, are present in about 20% of hepatocellular carcinoma cases [1•]. A large spectrum of p53 DNA changes are observed in hepatocellular carcinoma cases. In hepatocellular carcinoma cases from geographic areas with high dietary exposure to the liver carcinogen aflatoxin B1 p53 mutations are particularly frequent (more than 50% of tumors) and might specifically cluster at the third base of codon 249 [2,3,4•,5]. Because geographic areas with high aflatoxin B1 exposure are also areas with high hepatitis B virus (HBV) endemicity, the role of chronic HBV infection in p53 gene alterations may be suggested. However, the rate of mutations at codon 249 is low in geographic areas with high HBV endemicity and low aflatoxin B1 exposure [2,6–8]. There is no correlation between the state of HBV DNA and p53 mutations [4•]. In addition, p53 mutations were not detected in hepatocellular carcinoma cell lines that were positive for genomic integration of HBV X-gene and surface antigen gene, whereas cell lines with p53 mutations did not contain HBV sequences [9••]. Mutations of p53 are more frequent in advanced hepatocellular carcinomas (*eg*, large diameter, invasiveness, presence of cancerous portal thrombi) than in early stage hepatocellular carcinomas [6,7,10–13]. Whether p53 mutation precedes the development of cancer or appears at a later stage of development is not yet known. In the rat fed an aflatoxin B1–rich diet, hepatic hyperplastic nodules did not exhibit a site-specific mutation within the p53 gene [14•].

Many other chromosomal alterations have been recently found in human hepatocellular carcinomas [15,16]. Their role in carcinogenesis remains to be determined.

Association with hepatitis C virus

Although many case-control studies strongly support an association between chronic hepatitis C virus (HCV) infection and hepatocellular carcinoma, the prevalence of this infection in patients with hepatocellular carcinoma is disputed. In a previous cohort study from Italy

Abbreviations

HBsAg—hepatitis B surface antigen; **HBV**—hepatitis B virus; **HCV**—hepatitis C virus; **ELISA**—enzyme-linked immunosorbent assay; **PEI**—percutaneous ethanol injection.

 ISBN 1-85922-608-6 ISSN 0267–1379

[17], there was no clear relationship between the viral status and the risk of cancer in patients with cirrhosis. In two cohort studies of Japanese patients with cirrhosis from Osaka (917 patients) [18••] and Tokyo (795 patients) [19••], the cumulative appearance rates of hepatocellular carcinoma at 3, 5, 10, and 15 years were respectively 12.5%, 19.4%, 44.3%, and 58.2%. The positivity of HCV antibodies by enzyme-linked immunosorbent assay (ELISA) at enrollment increases fourfold the risk of developing hepatocellular carcinoma during follow-up [18••]. Hepatocellular carcinoma occurred more frequently (75.2% at 15 years) in patients with only HCV antibodies at enrollment than in those with only hepatitis B surface antigen (HBsAg) (27.2%) [19••] (Fig. 1).

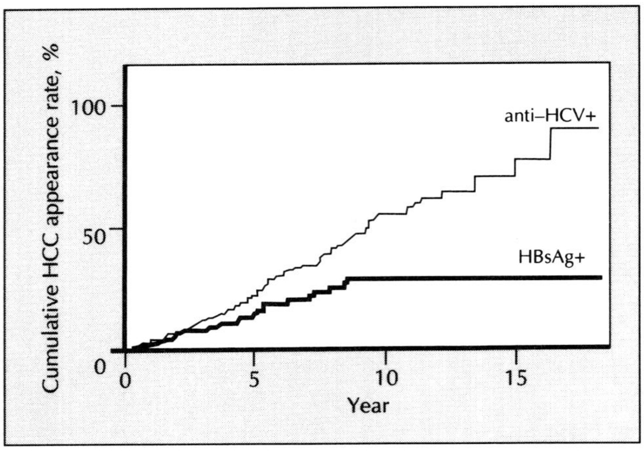

Fig. 1. Cumulative hepatocellular carcinoma (HCC) appearance rates in patients with cirrhosis positive for hepatitis B surface antigen (HBsAg+) or for hepatitis C virus antibody (anti-HCV+). (*Adapted from* Ikeda *et al.* [19••]; with permission.)

It has been suggested that the high prevalence of chronic HCV infection found in many series of patients with hepatocellular carcinoma resulted from the low specificity of the first generation enzyme immunoassays. In Greek patients tested for chronic HCV infection by second-generation ELISA or by recombinant immunoblot assay-2, its prevalence in patients with hepatocellular carcinoma was lower than expected (13.3% and 12.5%, respectively) [20•]. However, in one Spanish study [21] where HCV infection was evaluated by second-generation ELISA and by the presence of HCV RNA, HCV RNA was found in 62% of patients with hepatocellular carcinoma. There was a high (95%) correlation between the presence of HCV antibodies and of HCV RNA in the serum of these patients. Virus markers (B or C) were present in 89% of patients with hepatocellular carcinoma. There were no simultaneous positivities of HBsAg and anti-HCV–antibodies or HCV RNA found in this study [21] nor in another series of South African blacks [22••]. In a series of 22 French patients with hepatocellular carcinoma negative for HBsAg, HCV RNA was detected in the serum of about half the patients and HBV DNA in roughly another half [23•]. Coinfection by both viruses was not frequent (18%).

The heterogeneity of the HCV genome is now well admitted [24] and at least 12 genotypes have been identified with uneven distribution around the world [25••]. The severity of chronic liver disease and the response to interferon therapy seem to be associated with the genotype of HCV [26,27]. In countries with predominantly less severe genotypes resulting in a more chronic evolution towards cirrhosis, patients might be more exposed to the risk of hepatocellular carcinoma. Finally, HCV seems to become predominant as compared with HBV in the etiology of hepatocellular carcinoma, even in geographic areas with high HBV endemicity [28•].

Precursor lesions

Macroregenerative nodules

It has been suggested by Japanese investigators that large regenerative nodules (>0.5 or 1 cm in diameter) were frequently present in cirrhotic livers. These macroregenerative nodules are benign but are difficult to distinguish from small malignant nodules. In addition, foci of well-differentiated hepatocellular carcinomas have been found within macroregenerative nodules, suggesting that macroregenerative nodules might be preneoplastic lesions. In two studies from the United States, macroregenerative nodules and hepatocellular carcinomas were systematically searched for in all livers explanted from patients with cirrhosis during orthotopic liver transplantation [29••,30••]. The incidence of macroregenerative nodules (25% and 17.3%) was similar to that of previous Japanese reports. Some nodules contained both hepatocellular carcinoma and a residual rim of tissue with architectural and cytologic features of macroregenerative nodules (Fig. 2). Patients with macroregenerative nodules (one or more) had a significantly higher rate of hepatocellular carcinoma than those without macroregenerative nodules (26.3% vs 4.2%) [30••]. These results further support the hypothesis that macroregenerative nodules might be premalignant lesions. The recent first report of macroregenerative nodules containing multiple foci of hepatocellular carcinoma in a patient with chronic hepatitis C but without cirrhosis suggests that cirrhosis is not a prerequisite for these nodules [31]. The finding of infracentimetric nodules on morphologic examination in cirrhotic livers should lead to histologic analysis. Decreased reticulin, infiltrating border or multilobular areas of atypia, intranodular fibrosis, and thickening of cellular plates (more than two cells thick) are good indicators of malignancy in patients with macroregenerative nodules [31]. Whether liver cell dysplasia (large-cell or small-cell) is associated with hepatocellular carcinoma is still debated [29••].

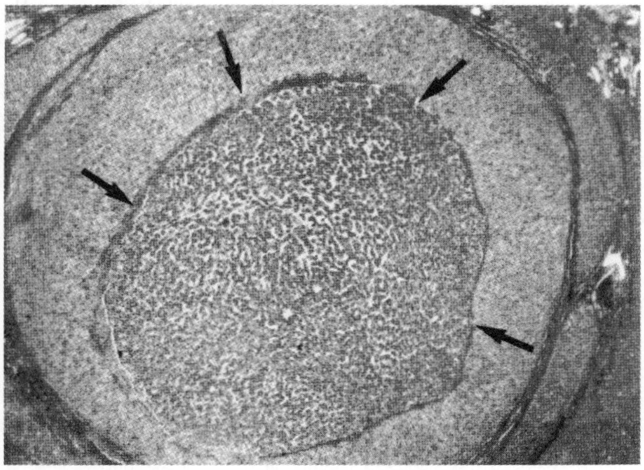

Fig. 2. Surgical specimen of a cirrhotic liver; macroregenerative nodule with hepatocellular carcinoma arising within it (*arrows*) (original magnification x 22). (*Courtesy of* G. Lemaigre and F. Capron, Clamart, France.)

Oval cells

Proliferation of oval cells occurs during chemical hepatocarcinogenesis in the rat and also in the woodchuck virus-related hepatitis. The simultaneous expression by oval cells of hepatocytes specific proteins such as α-fetoprotein and albumin and of biliary specific cytokeratins suggests that oval cells might be stem cells directly involved in the histogenesis of hepatocellular carcinoma. However some authors believe that oval cells are only bile duct epithelial cells occurring during liver regeneration with no essential role in the emergence of hepatocellular carcinoma. Small epithelial "oval-like cells" were found in the tumor adjacent liver parenchyma of patients with HBV-related hepatocellular carcinoma [32]. They were present in all 14 patients studied. These cells reacted with an antibody directed against murine oval cells. They were positive for a wide spectrum of cytokeratins. Subpopulations of these "oval-like cells" were positive for α-fetoprotein, albumin, or both or negative for both. These results strengthen the hypothesis of a role of oval cells in hepatocarcinogenesis in humans.

Detection and diagnosis

Early recognition of hepatocellular carcinoma is a prerequisite to successful treatment. However, surveillance of populations at risk by serial ultrasonographies and measurements of serum concentration of α-fetoprotein often fails to detect hepatocellular carcinomas at an early stage. Human α-fetoprotein has several molecular variants with different affinities for lectines. The serum α-fetoprotein of patients with hepatocellular carcinoma is characterized by an increased proportion of some of these variants. The appearance of these variants in the serum of cirrhotic patients preceded the occurrence of visible cancerous nodules by several months or years [33,34••]. Routine measurement of α-fetoprotein variants might therefore be a good mean of surveying patients with cirrhosis. Mutations of the p53 gene result in increased p53 protein levels in tumor cells and in the appearance of circulating p53 antibodies. Serologic testing for p53 antibodies using immunoblotting with a recombinant purified p53 was positive in 25% of European patients with hepatocellular carcinoma [35]. There was no complete overlap between patients positive for α-fetoprotein and those positive for p53 antibodies. None of the patients with chronic liver disease without hepatocellular carcinoma were positive for p53 antibodies. p53 Antibodies may be another specific marker of hepatocellular carcinoma.

The future may lie in artificial neural network in order to compute clinical, biological, and morphologic results obtained in patients with hepatic tumors in order to identify those with hepatocellular carcinoma [36].

The malignant nature of portal thrombi was ascertained in patients with a 93% sensitivity and a 100% specificity by percutaneous transhepatic fine-needle aspiration biopsy of the thrombus. Great care must be taken during puncture under ultrasonographic guidance to avoid hepatocellular carcinoma nodules in the parenchyma [37•]. This procedure is very helpful for diagnosing malignant thrombi in patients with visible or nonvisible cancerous nodules.

Treatment

Liver resection

Large series of liver resections have been now published confirming previous results with less than one third of patients surviving 5 years after surgery. Approximately 75% of patients have intrahepatic recurrence 3 to 5 years after potentially curative resection [38,39•]. The strongest predictors of recurrence are tumor multiplicity [38,39•], local invasiveness [39•], and the proliferative capacity of the adjacent parenchyma [40]. The high recurrence rate might be partly related to the presence of occult cancerous foci in the non-resected part of the liver. Hepatic artery injection of iodized oil and of ^{131}I-labeled iodized oil could be valuable in order to detect multiple minute nodules in patients with apparent solitary tumors [41].

There is some good news:

1. Neoplastic portal thrombus is generally considered as an absolute contraindication to resection of hepatocellular carcinoma. However, tumor thrombi in main portal branches or in the portal trunk can be removed together with the resected liver [42•]. This does not increase the operative mortality rate. Removal of the portal thrombus allows subsequent chemoembolization.

2. The small size of the left liver when a right hepatectomy is considered is another contraindication to resection. Preoperative percutaneous right portal branch embolization did result in atrophy of the right liver and hypertrophy of the left liver by about 30%, even in cirrhosis [43•,44]. This may allow resection of an atrophic right liver to be performed safely, leaving a large hypertrophic left liver.

3. Repeated (2 to 9 sessions) preoperative chemoembolization with cisplatin, mitomycin C, 5-fluorouracil, and ethiodized oil resulted in a mean decrease of tumor size by 31% of its volume, a return to normal of serum α-fetoprotein concentration in 23% of the patients, and complete tumor necrosis in 17% [45]. The 3-year survival rate after resection was 77%, a figure somehow higher than in most other series of resection. The possible advantage of preoperative chemoembolization was not confirmed however by other authors [39•].

Is liver transplantation any better than liver resection in the treatment of hepatocellular carcinoma? Increasingly, it seems that the results of both therapies are not very different. A retrospective comparison between the two types of treatment showed that the overall survival rate was the same [46•]. Although disease-free-survival rate was higher in the group of patients with a solitary tumor less than 3 cm in diameter than in other groups, the crude survival rate was similar. Given the shortage of donors, there is much less incentive to perform liver transplantation for treating hepatocellular carcinomas.

Transarterial chemoembolization

There is increasing evidence that transarterial chemoembolization does not improve much the life-expectancy of nonselected patients with inoperable hepatocellular carcinomas. However, in a selected group of patients with a high retention of the drug into the tumor, there was a high rate of partial or complete tumoral response and a high survival rate reaching 79% at 1 year and 61% at 2 years [47]. Superselective segmental transarterial chemoembolization might increase the tumor response and the survival rates [48•]. Complete necrosis of the tumor was observed in seven of 11 patients with subsequent resection. Segmental transarterial chemoembolization is well tolerated by patients.

All types of arterial treatments of hepatocellular carcinoma (transcatheter arterial chemoembolization or infusion of anticancer agents) are responsible for biliary complications. The incidence of biliary complications has been clearly analyzed in a series of 56 consecutive autopsies of patients with hepatocellular carcinoma and intra-arterial therapy [49••]. Seven (12.5%) had bile duct necrosis resulting in biloma in four. Necrosis occurred in large (> 200 μm) intrahepatic ducts and may result from destruction of the peribiliary capillary plexus. Because biliary complications occur after infusion of cytotoxic drugs with or without embolization, drug toxicity rather than arterial obstruction might be the prominent factor in inducing such lesions.

Percutaneous ethanol injection

Although percutaneous ethanol injection (PEI) is widely used as a treatment of hepatocellular carcinoma because of its easiness and the absence of major side effects, very few scientific publications report its results. Recent studies suggest that PEI can be applied to lesions larger than previously recommended, above 3 cm in diameter [50]. Ethanol should be injected in and around the nodules to improve efficacy [51]. More than one nodule can be treated during the same treatment session. The recurrence (60%) and survival (52% at 5 years) rates were not very different from those reported in the series of patients with resection [51]. Randomized studies should definitely be undergone in order to compare liver resection and PEI in patients with potentially resectable hepatocellular carcinomas.

Liver metastases

The lack of good animal models is still a difficulty in working on pathogenesis, growth, and treatment of liver metastases, particularly from primary colorectal adenocarcinomas. The severe combined immunodeficiency mice, with congenital lack of functional T and B lymphocytes, seem a better model than nude mice for the implantation of human colon cancer cell lines [52].

There have been very few advances in the treatment of liver metastases from colorectal cancers. There is no convincing evidence that adjuvant chemotherapy decreases the recurrence rate or increases the survival rate following surgery. The results of a pilot study suggest that a combined therapy including hepatic arterial infusion of floxuridine (0.25 mg/kg/d during 14 days), followed by systemic administration of 5-fluorouracil (280 mg/m^2) and leucovorin (200 mg/m^2) for 5 days, repeatedly, decreases the risk of recurrence [53]. The eight patients treated with this regimen were alive and disease-free after a median postoperative follow-up of 25 months.

Gene therapy may offer new ways of treating liver metastases by modifying the host environment or the tumor aggressiveness. The herpes virus simplex type 1 thymidine kinase converts nontoxic nucleoside analogues such as ganciclovir into phosphorylated compounds that specifically kill dividing cells. This property has already been successfully used for the treatment of gliomas in rats and has been recently tested in rats for the treatment of rapidly growing liver metastases from colon carcinoma [54••]. The herpes virus simplex type 1 thymidine kinase gene was inserted into metastases by direct injection of fibroblastic cells transfected with a recombinant retrovirus. Rats were then treated with ganciclovir. This resulted in a marked and significant decrease of tumor size and in a 60-fold decrease of cancerous cell mass. One third of treated rats had no residual tumor. There were no toxic lesions nor viral contamination of the adjacent liver tissue. Recombinant retroviruses may also be transfected to the tumors cells by selective perfusion of the liver *in situ*. This procedure could be applied to human with multiple liver metastases.

Intraoperative cryotherapy [55] and percutaneous interstitial laser photocoagulation [56] are still being tested.

References and recommended reading

Papers of particular interest, published within the annual period of review, have been highlighted as:
• Of special interest
•• Of outstanding interest

1. • Buetow KH, Sheffield VC, Zhu M, Zhou T, Shen FM, Hino O, Smith M, McMahon BJ, Lanier AP, London WT, Redeker AG, Govindarajan S: **Low Frequency of p53 Mutations Observed in a Diverse Collection of Primary Hepatocellular Carcinomas.** *Proc Natl Acad Sci U S A* 1992, **89**:9622–9626.

A study of p53 mutations in hepatocellular carcinomas from several countries. The mutation rate is lower in this study than in those previously published.

2. Hsu IC, Metcalf RA, Sun T, Welsh JR, Wang NJ, Harris CC: **Mutational Hotspot in the p53 Gene in Human Hepatocellular Carcinoma.** *Nature* 1991, **350**:427–428.

3. Bressac B, Kew M, Wands J, Ozturk M: **Selective G to T Mutations of p53 Gene in Hepatocellular Carcinoma From South Africa.** *Nature* 1991, **350**:429–431.

4. • Li D, Cao Y, He L, Wang NJ, Gu JR: **Aberrations of p53 Gene in Human Hepatocellular Carcinoma From China.** *Carcinogenesis* 1993, **14**:169–173.

In Chinese patients with hepatocellular carcinoma, the rate of p53 mutations is much higher in geographical areas with high exposure to dietary AFB1. In hepatocellular carcinoma patients from Shangaï, a low AFB1 exposure area with a high HBV endemicity, the p53 mutation rate was low.

5. Coursaget P, Depril N, Chabaud M, Nandi R, Mayelo V, Lecann P, Yvonnet B: **High Prevalence of Mutations At Codon 249 of the p53 Gene in Hepatocellular Carcinomas From Senegal.** *Br J Cancer* 1993, **67**:1395–1397.

6. Oda T, Tsuda H, Scarpa A, Sakamoto M, Hirohashi S: **p53 Gene Mutation Spectrum in Hepatocellular Carcinoma.** *Cancer Res* 1992, **52**:6358–6364.

7. Nose H, Imazeki F, Ohto M, Omata M: **p53 Gene Mutations and 17p Allelic Deletions in Hepatocellular Carcinoma From Japan.** *Cancer* 1993, **72**:355–360.

8. Sheu JC, Huang GT, Lee PH, Chung JC, Chou HC, Lai MY, Wang JT, Lee HS, Shih LN, Yang PM, Wang TH, Chen DS: **Mutation of p53 Gene in Hepatocellular Carcinoma in Taiwan.** *Cancer Res* 1992, **52**:6098–6100.

9. •• Hsu IC, Tokiwa T, Bennett W, Metcalf RA, Welsh JA, Sun T, Harris CC: **p53 Gene Mutation and Integrated Hepatitis B Viral DNA Sequences in Human Liver Cancer Cell Lines.** *Carcinogenesis* 1993, **14**:987–992.

Human hepatocellular carcinoma cell lines with integrated HBV DNA sequences do not have p53 mutations. A very strong argument against a correlation between HBV infection and p53 mutations.

10. Nishida N, Fukuda Y, Kokuryu H, Toguchida J, Yandell DW, Ikenega M, Imura H, Ishikazi K: **Role and Mutational Heterogeneity of the p53 Gene in Hepatocellular Carcinoma.** *Cancer Res* 1993, **53**:368–372.

11. Laurent-Puig P, Flejou JF, Fabre M, Bedossa P, Belghiti J, Gayral F, Franco D: **Overexpression of p53 : A Rare Event in a Large Series of White Patients With Hepatocellular Carcinoma.** *Hepatology* 1992, **16**:1171–1175.

12. Tanaka S, Toh Y, Adachi E, Matsumata T, Mori R, Sugimachi K: **Tumor Progression in Hepatocellular Carcinoma May Be Mediated by p53 Mutation.** *Cancer Res* 1993, **53**:2884–2887.

13. Lai MY, Chang HC, Li HP, Ku CK, Chen PJ, Sheu JC, Huang GT, Lee PH, Chen DS: **Splicing Mutations of the p53 Gene in Human Hepatocellular Carcinoma.** *Cancer Res* 1993, **53**:1653–1656.

14. • Hulla JE, Chen ZY, Eaton DL: **Aflatoxin B_1-Induced Rat Hepatic Hyperplastic Nodules Do Not Exhibit a Site-Specific Mutation Within the p53 Gene.** *Cancer Res* 1993, **53**:9–11.

No p53 mutations were detected in preneoplastic nodules induced by AFB1 in rats. This is against a major role of p53 mutation at the early stage of liver carcinogenesis. p53 Mutation may occur only at a late stage of tumor development as suggested by clinical observations.

15. Lasserre C, Christa L, Simon MT, Vernier P, Brechot C: **A Novel Gene (HIP) Activated in Human Primary Liver Cancer.** *Cancer Res* 1992, **52**:5089–5095.

16. Takahasi K, Kudo J, Ishibashi H, Hirata Y, Niho Y: **Frequent Loss of Heterozygosity on Chromosome 22 in Hepatocellular Carcinoma.** *Hepatology* 1993, **17**:794–799.

17. Colombo M, De Franchis R, Del Ninno E, Sangiovanni A, De Fazio C, Tommasini M, Donato MF, Piva A, Di Carlo V, Dioguardi N: **Hepatocellular Carcinoma in Italian Patients With Cirrhosis.** *N Engl J Med* 1991, **325**:675–680.

18. •• Tsukuma H, Hiyama T, Tanaka S, Nakao M, Yabuuchi T, Kitamura T, Nakanishi K, Fujimoto I, Inoue A, Yamazaki H, Kawashima T: **Risk Factors for Hepatocellular Carcinoma Among Patients With Chronic Liver Disease.** *N Engl J Med* 1993, **328**:1797–1801.

A very good study of a cohort of 917 patients with chronic liver disease followed-up for 6 to 51 months. The 3-year cumulative risk of cancer was 12.5%. The risk of hepatocellular carcinoma was increased sevenfold in patients positive for hepatitis B surface antigen at enrollment and it was increased fourfold in patients with HCV antibodies. A strong argument in favor of the role of HCV in the pathogenesis of hepatocellular carcinoma.

19. •• Ikeda K, Saitoh S, Koida I, Arase Y, Tsubota A, Chayama K, Kumada H, Kawanishi M: **A Multivariate Analysis of Risk Factors for Hepatocellular Carcinogenesis: A Prospective Observation of 795 Patients With Viral and Alcoholic Cirrhosis.** *Hepatology* 1993, **18**:47–53.

A study of a cohort of 795 patients with viral or alcoholic cirrhosis followed-up for a median period of 5.8 years. The cumulative risk of hepatocellular carcinoma was 58.2% at 15 years. In patients with HCV antibodies, it was 75.2%.

20. • Zavitsanos X, Hatzakis A, Kaklamani F, Tzonou A, Toupadaki N, Broeksma C, Chrispeels J, Troonen H, Hadziyannis S, Hsieh CC, Alter H, Trichopoulos D: **Association Between Hepatitis C Virus and Hepatocellular Carcinoma Using Assays Based on Structural and Non Structural Hepatitis C Virus Peptides.** *Cancer Res* 1992, **52**:3564–3567.

The prevalence of HCV markers in patients with hepatocellular carcinoma depends on the type of assay used.

21. Ruiz J, Sangro B, Cuende JI, Beloqui O, Riezu-Boj JI, Herrero JI, Prieto J: **Hepatitis B and C Viral Infections in Patients With Hepatocellular Carcinoma.** *Hepatology* 1992, **16**:637–641.

22. •• Bukh J, Miller RH, Kew MC, Purcell RH: **Hepatitis C Virus RNA in Southern African Blacks With Hepatocellular Carcinoma.** *Proc Natl Acad Sci U S A* 1993, **90**:1848–1851.

This work suggests that there is a clear association between HCV infection and hepatocellular carcinoma in southern African Blacks. HCV infection was more frequently involved in the etiology of hepatocellular carcinoma in urban areas and HBV infection was more frequently involved in rural residents. Coinfection was not frequent.

23. • Paterlini P, Driss F, Nalpas B, Pisi E, Franco D, Berthelot P, Brechot C: **Persistence of Hepatitis B and Hepatitis C Viral Genomes in Primary Liver Cancers From HBsAg-Negative Patients : A Study of a Low-Endemic Area.** *Hepatology* 1993, 17:20–29.

Eighty-two percent of patients with hepatocellular carcinoma who were hepatitis B surface antigen negative had signs of virus infection when evaluated by HBV DNA or HCV RNA. Only four patients were negative for both viruses. Coinfection by viruses B and C is not frequent in patients with hepatocellular carcinoma.

24. Hayashi N, Higashi H, Kaminaka K, Sugimoto H, Esumi M, Komatsu K, Hayashi K, Sugitani M, Suzuki K, Tadao O, Nozaki C, Mizuno K, Shikata T: **Molecular Cloning and Heterogeneity of the Human Hepatitis C Virus (HCV) Genome.** *J Hepatol* 1993, **17**:94–107.

25. •• Bukh J, Purcell RH, Miller RH: **At Least 12 Genotypes of Hepatitis C Virus Predicted by Sequence Analysis of the Putative E1 Gene of Isolates Collected Worldwide.** *Proc Natl Acad Sci U S A* 1993, **90**:8234–8238.

Some genotypes of HCV are widely distributed around the world whereas other genotypes are found in specific geographic regions. This may be an explanation for discrepancies between different countries in the role of HCV in the development of hepatocellular carcinoma.

26. Pozzato G, Moretti M, Franzin F, Croce LS, Tiribelli C, Masayu T, Kaneko S, Unoura M, Kobayashi K: **Severity of Liver Disease With Different Hepatitis C Viral Clones.** *Lancet* 1991, **338**:509.

27. Yoshioka K, Kakumu S, Wakita T, Ishikawa T, Itoh Y, Takayanagi M, Higashi Y, Shibata M, Morishima T: **Detection of Hepatitis C Virus by Polymerase Chain Reaction and Response to Interferon-α Therapy: Relationship to Genotypes of Hepatitis C Virus.** *Hepatology* 1992, **16**:293–299.

28. • Hamasaki K, Nakata K, Tsutsumi T, Tsuruta S, Nakao K, Kato Y, Shima M, Koji T, Nagataki S: **Changes in the Prevalence of Hepatitis B and C Infection in Patients With Hepatocellular Carcinoma in the Nagasaki Prefecture, Japan.** *J Med Virol* 1993, **40**:146–149.

Presently HCV infection plays a more important role than HBV infection in the development of hepatocellular carcinoma, even in regions with a high rate of HBV infection.

29. •• Theise ND, Schwartz M, Miller C, Thung SN: **Macroregenerative Nodules and Hepatocellular Carcinoma in Forty-Four Sequential Adult Liver Explants With Cirrhosis.** *Hepatology* 1992, **16**:949–955.

Macroregenerative nodules are common in chronic liver disease in non-Japanese patients. They may represent precancerous lesions. Results obtained from 44 explanted livers.

30. •• Ferrell L, Wright T, Lake J, Roberts J, Ascher N: **Incidence and Diagnostic Features of Macroregenerative Nodule Vs. Small Hepatocellular Carcinoma in Cirrhotic Livers.** *Hepatology* 1992, **16**:1372–1381.

Macroregenerative nodules seem to be precancerous lesions. Histological differentiation between benign macroregenerative nodules and hepatocellular carcinoma may be difficult. Architectural features such as the thickening of cell plates and the loss of reticulin are argument for hepatocellular carcinoma. Results obtained from examination of 110 explanted livers.

31. Theise ND, Lapook JD, Thung SN: **A Macroregenerative Nodule Containing Multiple Foci of Hepatocellular Carcinoma in a Non Cirrhotic Liver.** *Hepatology* 1993, 17:993–996.

32. Hsia CC, Evarts RP, Nakatsukasa H, Marsden ER, Thorgeirsson SS: **Occurrence of Oval-Type Cells in Hepatitis B Virus-Associated Human Hepatocarcinogenesis.** *Hepatology* 1992, 16:1327–1333.

33. Aoyagi Y, Saitoh A, Suzuki Y, Igarashi K, Oguro M, Yokota T, Mori S, Suda T, Isemura M, Asakura H: **Fucosylation Index of α-Fetoprotein, a Possible Aid in the Early Recognition of Hepatocellular Carcinoma in Patients With Cirrhosis.** *Hepatology* 1993, **17**:50–52.

34. •• Sato Y, Nakata K, Kato Y, Shima M, Ishii N, Koji T, Taketa K, Endo Y, Nagataki S: **Early Recognition of Hepatocellular Carcinoma Based on Altered Profiles of Alpha-Fetoprotein.** *N Engl J Med* 1993, **328**:1802–1806.

The proportion of some variants of α-fetoprotein increases early in patients with chronic liver disease and small increase of α-fetoprotein on repeated measurements who will lately develop hepatocellular carcinoma. Is this a better way to detect hepatocellular carcinoma at an early stage?

35. Volkmann M, Müller M, Hofmann WJ, Meyer M, Hagelstein J, Rath U, Kommerell B, Zentgraf H, Galle PR: **The Humoral Immune Response to p53 in Patients With Hepatocellular Carcinoma Is Specific for Malignancy and Independent of the α-Fetoprotein Status.** *Hepatology* 1993, **18**:559–565.

36. Maclin PS, Dempsey J: **Using an Artificial Neural Network to Diagnose Hepatic Masses.** *J Med Systems* 1992, **16**:215–225.

37. • Vilana R, Bru C, Bruix J, Castells A, Sole M, Rodes J: **Fine-Needle Aspiration Biopsy of Portal Vein Thrombus: Value in Detecting Malignant Thrombosis.** *Am J Roentgenol* 1993, **160**:1285–1287.

A smart technique in order to differentiate noncancerous from cancerous portal thrombi.

38. Ikeda K, Saitoh S, Tsubota A, Arase Y, Chayama K, Kumada H, Watanabe G, Tsurumaru M: **Risk Factors for Tumor Recurrence and Prognosis After Curative Resection of Hepatocellular Carcinoma.** *Cancer* 1993, **71**:19–25.

39. • Nagasue N, Uchida M, Makino Y, Takemoto Y, Yamanoi A, Hayashi T, Chang YC, Kohno H, Nakamura T, Yukaya H: **Incidence and Factors Associated With Intrahepatic Recurrence Following Resection of Hepatocellular Carcinoma.** *Gastroenterology* 1993, **105**:488–494.

These results confirm, in a large number of patients, that satellite nodules, distal portal thrombi, the absence of a capsule, and a positive surgical margin are predictors of hepatic recurrence after resection of hepatocellular carcinoma.

40. Chiu JH, Wu LH, Kao HL, Chang HM, Tsay SH, Loong CC, Chau GY, Lui WY: **Can Determination of the Proliferative Capacity of the Nontumor Portion Predict the Risk of Tumor Recurrence in the Liver Remnant After Resection of Human Hepatocellular Carcinoma?** *Hepatology* 1993, **18**:96–102.

41. Raoul JL, Duvauferrier R, Bretagne JF, Bourguet P, Heresbach D, Siproudhis L, Gosselin M: **Usefulness of Hepatic Artery Injection of Iodized Oil and ^{131} I-Labeled Iodized Oil Before the Therapeutic Decision in Hepatocellular Carcinoma.** *Scand J Gastroenterol* 1993, **28**:217–223.

42. • Yamaoka Y, Kumada K, Ino K, Takayasu T, Shimahara Y, Mori K, Tanaka A, Morimoto T, Taki Y, Washida M, Manaka D, Hayashi M, Fujita T, Ozawa K: **Liver Resection for Hepatocellular Carcinoma (HCC) With Direct Removal of Tumor Thrombi in the Main Portal Vein.** *World J Surg* 1992, 16:1172–1177.

Large cancerous portal thrombi are no longer a contraindication to liver resection and may be safely removed. This is an important surgical step.

43. • De Baere T, Roche A, Vavasseur D, Therasse E, Indushekar S, Elias D, Bognel C: **Portal Vein Embolization: Utility for Inducing Left Hepatic Lobe Hypertrophy Before Surgery.** *Radiology* 1993, **188**:73–77.

Smart. This paper demonstrated how to induce atrophy of the lobe to be resected and how to maintain hypertrophy of the lobe after resection.

44. Lee KC, Kinoshita H, Hirohashi K, Kubo S, Iwasa R: **Extension of Surgical Indications for Hepatocellular Carcinoma by Portal Vein Embolization.** *World J Surg* 1993, 17:109–115.

45. Yu YQ, Xu DB, Zhou XD, Lu JZ, Tang ZY, Mack P: **Experience With Liver Resection After Hepatic Arterial Chemoembolization for Hepatocellular Carcinoma.** *Cancer* 1993, 71:62–65.

46. • Bismuth H, Chiche L, Adam R, Castaing D, Diamond T, Dennison A: **Liver Resection Versus Transplantation for Hepatocellular Carcinoma in Cirrhotic Patients.** *Ann Surg* 1993, **218**:145–151.

Is there any indication of transplantation for hepatocellular carcinoma in cirrhotic patients? Crude survival is no better than following resection even in patients with a small tumor. A randomized study is awaited.

47. Ngan H, Lai CL, Fan ST, Lai ECS, Yuen WK, Tso WK: **Treatment of Inoperable Hepatocellular Carcinoma by Transcatheter Arterial Chemoembolization Using an Emulsion of Cisplatin in Iodized Oil and Gelfoam.** *Clin Radiol* 1993, 47:315–320.

48. • Matsui O, Kadoya M, Yoshikawa J, Gabata T, Arai K, Demachi H, Miyayama S, Takashima T, Unoura M, Kogayashi K: **Small Hepatocellular Carcinoma : Treatment With Subsegmental Transcatheter Arterial Embolization.** *Radiology* 1993, **188**:79–83.

If performing a transcatheter arterial embolization, do it segmentally. There is better efficacy and less risk of complications.

49. •• Kobayashi S, Nakanuma Y, Terada T, Matsui O: **Postmortem Survey of Bile Duct Necrosis and Biloma in Hepatocellular Carcinoma After Transcatheter Arterial Chemoembolization Therapy : Relevance to Microvascular Damages of Peribiliary Capillary Plexus.** *Am J Gastroenterol* 1993, **88**:1410–1415.

A nice assessment of local complications of intra-arterial therapy, which are frequent and often related to large intrahepatic bile duct necrosis.

50. Redvanly RD, Chezmar JL, Strauss RM, Galloway JR, Boyer TD, Bernardino ME: **Malignant Hepatic Tumors : Safety of High-Dose Percutaneous Ethanol Ablation Therapy.** *Radiology* 1993, **188**:283–285.

51. Shiina S, Tagawa K, Niwa Y, Unuma T, Komatsu Y, Yoshiura K, Hamada E, Takahashi M, Shiratori Y, Terano A, Omata M, Kawauchi N, Inoue H: **Percutaneous Ethanol Injection Therapy for Hepatocellular Carcinoma : Results in 146 Patients.** *AJR Am J Roentgenol* 1993, **160**:1023–1028.

52. Furukawa T, Kubota T, Watanabe M, Nishibori H, Kuo TH, Saikawa Y, Kase S, Tanino H, Teramoto T, Ishibiki K, Kitajima M: **A Suitable Model for Experimental Liver Metastasis of Human Colon Cancer Xenografts Using Mice With Severe Combined Immunodeficiency.** *J Surg Oncol* 1993, **52**:64–67.

53. Kemeny N, Conti JA, Sigurdson E, Cohen A, Seiter K, Lincer R, Niedzwiecki D, Botet J, Chapman D, Costa P, Budd A: **A Pilot Study of Hepatic Artery Floxuridine Combined With Systemic 5-Fluorouracil and Leucovorin. A Potential Adjuvant Program After Resection of Colorectal Hepatic Metastases.** *Cancer* 1993, 71:1964–1971.

54. •• Caruso M, Panis Y, Gagandeep S, Houssin D, Salzmann JL, Klatzmann D: **Regression of Established Macroscopic Liver Metastases After In Situ Transduction of a Suicide Gene.** *Proc Natl Acad Sci U S A* 1993, **90**:7024–7028.

Gene therapy is coming. Using a killer gene it was possible to destroy most implanted liver metastases in rats. A clinical trial is awaited.

55. Morris DL, Horton MDAC, Dilley AV, Warlters A, Clingan PR: **Treatment of Hepatic Metastases by Cryotherapy and Regional Cytotoxic Perfusion.** *Gut* 1993, **34**:1156–1157.

56. Amin Z, Donald JJ, Masters A, Kant R, Steger AC, Bown SG, Lees WR: **Hepatic Metastases : Interstitial Laser Photocoagulation With Real-Time US Monitoring and Dynamic CT Evaluation of Treatment.** *Radiology* 1993, **187**:339–347.

Dominique Franco, and Corinne Vons, Hôpital Antoine Béclère, Service de Chirurgie, 92141 Clamart Cedex, France.

Liver transplantation

Rowen K. Zetterman, MD

University of Nebraska Medical Center, Omaha, Nebraska, USA

The increased use of liver transplantation for the management of endstage liver disease has resulted in the need for more donors, for more careful selection of recipients, and for reduction or control of postoperative complications if they occur. In this review, selected issues are highlighted, including the use of nonhuman primate donors, the management of biliary complications, and the selection and outcome of patients undergoing liver transplantation as therapy for controversial indications such as chronic hepatitis B and hepatocellular carcinoma.

Current Opinion in Gastroenterology 1994, **10**:344–348

There has been a continuing proliferation of reports regarding liver transplantation. Because of the volume of these reports, I will review only articles from 1993. This article is not meant to be an exhaustive review of these topics but rather a compilation of selected areas of research including studies of donor organs, biliary complications, recipient selection, and outcome of transplantation in diseases such as chronic hepatitis and hepatocellular carcinoma.

Donor issues

Donor gender

It has not been thought that gender plays a significant role in matching donors and recipients, except for the obvious differences in body and liver size. However, in a study of 798 liver transplant recipients at the University of Pittsburgh, the early (60 day) outcome of male and female recipients of human livers from male and female donors was determined concerning retransplantation rate and early death [1•]. Female recipients of male or female donor livers and male recipients of male donor livers had similar outcomes (28% to 36% retransplantation or death rates). However, in 50 male recipients of livers from female donors, a significantly poorer outcome was observed. Sixty percent required retransplantation (11 of 50) or died (19 of 50). In this analysis, male recipients of female livers were 3.7 times more likely to develop graft failure than recipients of male livers. Graft failure in these men was not affected by the age of the recipient or by the type of preexisting liver disease. Does this mean that we should change the policy of donor allocation based on gender? I think not. This is a small series that requires evaluation by other centers. Furthermore, the cause of the difference in outcome is not readily apparent. Whereas there are differences in estrogen and androgen receptors on the hepatocytes of men and women, the mechanism by which such receptors might influence graft outcome is unclear. Furthermore, we need additional information about the clinical urgency of liver transplantation in these recipients. Women tend to wait longer for a donor liver than men do because of a smaller body habitus. Perhaps this was true of the men receiving these (smaller) organs from female donors. In addition, men receiving organs from female donors may have had a worse preoperative status than male recipients of livers from male donors.

Baboon to human xenotransplantation

As the number of patients awaiting liver transplantation increases and the number of donors remains constant, other sources of donor livers must be explored. A 35-year-old hepatitis B surface antigen (HBsAg)–positive and HIV-positive man with endstage hepatitis B virus (HBV) cirrhosis received a baboon liver using standard immunosuppression, with additional cyclophosphamide to control B-cell proliferative response [2]. During the first 24 days, the liver appeared to regenerate as it increased in volume from 600 to 1555 g. Ultimately, the patient's course was complicated by bacterial, viral, and fungal infection, with death due to a subarachnoid hemorrhage as a consequence of aspergillus infection of the brain. Significant cholestasis and biliary sepsis began the cascade of infectious complications. This case does demonstrate, however, the potential utility of nonhuman donors as a temporary measure when human donor organs are not available. There is no question that there are numerous ethical, medical, and animal rights questions to be raised about such use. Even if these issues are resolved, we will also need to determine just how many baboon donors would be available.

Abbreviations

FCH—fibrosing cholestatic hepatitis; **HBeAg**—hepatitis B e antigen; **HBIG**—anti–hepatitis B surface immune globulin; **HBsAg**—hepatitis B surface antigen; **HBV**—hepatitis B virus; **HCV**—hepatitis C virus; **HDV**—hepatitis D virus.

 ISBN 1-85922-608-6 ISSN 0267–1379

In an attempt to answer this question, 30 baboons at a French primate center were evaluated for factors that would exclude them from human use [3]. Only eight were suitable donors, with 10 lost because of a history of disease or prior experimental use, another seven dropped for anatomic reasons, three for renal failure or sepsis, and two because of abnormal liver test results. The blood types of the baboons are also of interest, as 18 were blood type AB, 10 were type B, two were type A, and none were type O. Thus, even if there were plenty of baboons for use as a source of xenografts, they would not significantly improve the donor supply for our greatest need because of their blood type. These data suggest that the use of baboon xenografts will be limited.

Chimerism

Cells of donor origin have been identified in liver transplantation recipients either by identification of cells containing the Y chromosome in female recipients, or by expression of mixed histocompatibility products and DNA sequences specific to the donor in the recipient tissues. This raises several questions about the potential for development of chimerism and its attendant effects on the recipient. For example, chimerism could influence the host immune system with development of tolerance to donor tissues. In fact, Starzl *et al.* [4], reported that some liver recipients have been successfully weaned from immunosuppressive agents without developing allograft rejection. Furthermore, the transfer of donor cells to the recipient could alleviate metabolic deficiencies, as has been described for patients with type IV glycogen storage disease and type 1 Gaucher's disease [5•]. In these cases, a decrease in tissue storage of amylopectin and glucocerebroside, respectively, has been observed. Transfer of donor stem cells with graft-versus-host disease and hematopoiesis by donor cells has also been noted [6]. Although it seems clear that stem cells and leukocytes can be transferred via the donor liver, the question remains whether dendritic cells are necessary for development of tolerance.

Complications

Bile duct complications can develop following liver transplantation due to surgical complications, ischemic injury, premature dislodgement of t-tubes and biliary stents, anastomotic dehiscence, biliary sludge, and biliary infections. In addition, ABO blood group incompatibility of the donor and recipient can also result in biliary injury. When 18 patients who received an ABO-incompatible allograft were compared with 18 recipients of an ABO-compatible graft, biliary complications were observed in 82% of patients receiving the incompatible grafts compared with only 6% of patients receiving the compatible grafts [7•]. Biliary complications included attenuation of the bile ducts, strictures, and bile duct leaks. Hepatic artery thrombosis and rejection were also more frequent and overall survival was less (44% vs 78%) in patients receiving incompatible grafts, although the severity of the underlying liver disease that mandated choosing an incompatible graft may also have influenced the outcome. This finding suggests that biliary injury might be a consequence of immune injury of either the biliary epithelium or the vascular supply to the bile duct. Patients who receive ABO-incompatible grafts should be prospectively evaluated for hepatic artery patency and observed for signs of biliary complications.

Ischemic biliary strictures also develop following liver transplantation [8•]. Of 128 liver transplantation patients, ischemic biliary strictures developed in 25 patients and involved the bifurcation in 17 (68%) and the right or left main ducts or the segmental ducts in four (16%). Ischemic strictures occurred early in the postoperative interval, with most being diagnosed within 4 months of transplantation. If the diagnosis was established in the first month, the outcome was poor; five of six patients required repeat transplantation. Of the 18 surviving patients, duct dilation and stent placement led to satisfactory resolution in 16, with stents left in place for a mean time of 310 days (range 52 days to 530 days). Cholangitis following duct manipulation was common (occurring in 11 of 18 patients) despite use of preprocedure antibiotics. There was a reduction of 1 year graft survival with ischemic strictures (69% vs 88%) although patient survival was unaffected (91% vs 89%). This evaluation suggests that early ischemic biliary strictures develop in the setting of more severe ischemic injury and will often require retransplantation, whereas late strictures should be managed medically.

Two additional studies also confirm that medical therapy is satisfactory for most biliary complications [9,10]. In 18 patients with biliary fistulae, the placement of a nasobiliary catheter (13 patients) or stent (five patients) led to relief of pain within 12 hours in 17 patients [9]. Of the 13 patients with nasobiliary tubes, closure of the fistula occurred at a mean time of 6.3 days. Stents were left in place for an average of 45 days, with one of five developing cholangitis. Not surprisingly, patients with biliary leaks from Roux-en-Y choledochojejunostomies usually required surgery for control of the leaks (six of nine patients) whereas those with leaks following choledochocholedochostomy did not (four of 65 patients) [10].

Indications for and outcome of liver transplantation

Hepatitis B virus–related cirrhosis

The long-term result of liver transplantation in patients with cirrhosis due to HBV has been poor. At present, we are unable to identify all of the patients who will do well following liver transplantation. However, although the choice of candidates remains difficult, there is some hope that recurrence rates can be partially controlled by long-term infusion of antibody to HBsAg.

In 15 patients with cirrhosis due to HBV, six of 14 transplant survivors developed serologic evidence of recurrent HBsAg after liver transplantation [11]. Although only two of 11 patients tested preoperatively were HBV DNA–positive by dot blot hybridization, five of 13 became positive following transplantation. Similarly, only four were hepatitis B e antigen (HBeAg)-positive preoperatively, with six of 14 becoming positive postoperatively. Three deaths due to recurrent hepatitis B occurred. In another eight patients, six developed recurrent HBV infection following transplantation [12]. Of three HBeAg-negative patients, two became reinfected with HBV (one of whom was HBeAg positive) and in one patient the virus cleared . Evidence of HBV in the liver allograft was identified as early as 22 days postoperatively. One additional study of 14 patients who received transplants for HBV disease (11 for cirrhosis and three for fulminant hepatitis) revealed that of the 11 with cirrhosis, two died early, two were lost to follow-up, and seven developed recurrent HBV infection. Among these seven patients, five developed cirrhosis and six had histologic evidence of hepatocyte HBV [13]. Theses studies all indicate that liver transplant recipients with cirrhosis due to HBV are likely to develop recurrent infection. Unfortunately, the lack of circulating HBeAg and HBV DNA (assayed by dot blot hybridization) does not identify a group at less risk of recurrent infection.

Fibrosing cholestatic hepatitis (FCH) is an unusual syndrome that can occur with HBV allograft infection. The syndrome is characterized by progressive hepatic failure and a histologic picture of severe cholestasis, minimal inflammation, and periportal fibrosis. It accounts for many of the deaths of patients with chronic hepatitis B who undergo liver transplantation [12,13]. However, the mechanism of liver injury in this syndrome is unknown. Marked HBV viral expression is observed, as indicated by *in situ* hybridization studies of liver tissue from 14 patients with recurrent HBV liver infection [14•]. When compared with biopsy results from 18 patients with chronic hepatitis B who did not receive transplants, high-intensity HBV DNA signals (53% in recurrent HBV vs 0% in chronic hepatitis) and HBV RNA signals (42% vs 17%) were noted. The highest grades of HBV RNA signals were seen in those with FCH (92% had grades 2 or 3) when compared with those with posttransplantation HBV infection without FCH (17%). These data suggest that FCH is associated with marked viral transcription of HBV and also suggest that the virus might be cytopathic in such circumstances. FCH has also been described in posttransplantation infection with an HBV precore mutant [15]. Is it possible that excessive expression of precore mutant forms accounts for some cases of FCH after liver transplantation?

If the results of transplantation for chronic hepatitis B are poor and the ability to predict those with successful outcome is difficult, is there any other manipulation that can improve success? In a multicenter trial of 334 patients who received transplants as therapy for acute and chronic HBV disease, long-term postoperative administration of high-titer anti–hepatitis B surface immune globulin (HBIG) appeared to decrease the recurrence of HBV disease [16••]. Patients who were studied included those with HBV cirrhosis, cirrhosis due to coexisting HBV and hepatitis D virus (HDV), fulminant HBV, and fulminant HBV and HDV. Recurrence of HBV was highest in those with HBV cirrhosis (67% ± 4%) and lowest in those with fulminant HBV (17% ± 7%). When only those with HBV cirrhosis were considered, the recurrence of HBV was 83% ± 6% in those who were seropositive for HBV DNA (assayed by dot blot hybridization) at transplantation compared with 58% ±7% in those who were HBV DNA– and HBeAg-negative. If patients with HBV cirrhosis received HBIG prophylaxis for 6 months or more, the recurrence rate decreased to 36%±4%. By multivariate analysis of the entire study group, predictors of reduced HBV recurrence included long-term administration of HBIG, coexisting HDV infection, and acute HBV liver disease.

Although this study [16••] confirmed that the risk of HBV recurrence cannot be determined by pretransplantation serologic criteria such as HBeAg or HBV DNA (by molecular hybridization), it does suggest that long-term administration of antibody to HBsAg can reduce early reinfection. Whether this effect is a consequence of delayed evidence of recurrence from excess circulating antibody to HBsAg is unclear, although a significant reduction in early mortality is seen which suggests that recurrent disease is ameliorated. We will need additional information regarding the pretransplantation status of HBV DNA by polymerase chain reaction to see if we can predict risk of reinfection. The quantity and duration of administration of hepatitis B immune globulin used in this study will add significantly to the postoperative costs of these patients. Any information that permits reduction in the use of HBIG is needed.

One other brief report [17] of recurrent HBV infection is of potential interest. In a single case of recurrent severe HBV liver disease that occurred after transplantation, a more significant clinical improvement followed continuous administration of foscarnet and ganciclovir than followed ganciclovir given alone for 12 months [17]. Although this is a preliminary report, the associated reduction of serum HBV DNA, improved liver test results, and the decrease in number of infected hepatocytes detected histologically after treatment suggests that these agents had a positive effect. If HBV recurrence develops despite administration of HBIG, this might be another (although again very expensive) alternative.

Hepatitis D virus–related cirrhosis

There are additional studies indicating that coexisting infection with HDV reduces the risk of recurrent HBV infection following liver transplantation [17,18]. In 49 patients who received transplants because of HBV and HDV cirrhosis and who also received HBIG postoperatively, the 2-year actuarial recurrence of HBV infection was only 13% [18]. Such data suggest that the reduction of HBV replication by coexisting infection with HDV may be in part responsible for this effect, perhaps by reducing the HBV burden or by decreasing replication in nonhepatic sites.

Hepatitis C virus–related cirrhosis

Using the serum bank at the liver transplantation unit at the University of Pittsburgh, 516 patients with stored preoperative sera and corresponding donor sera were assessed for pretransplantation presence of antibody to hepatitis C virus (HCV) by second-generation enzyme-linked immunosorbent assay, and subsequent post-operative histologic evidence of hepatitis or cirrhosis was correlated with the preoperative anti-HCV results [19•]. Of the 516 patients, 473 underwent postoperative liver biopsies (mean, 3.7 ± 2.0 biopsies per patient) that were available for review. When patients were grouped by pretransplantation donor and recipient anti-HCV status, 375 were negative and negative (group 1), 111 negative and positive (group 2), 25 positive and negative (group 3), and five positive and positive (group 4). Histologic evidence of hepatitis after transplantation occurred in 11.2% of group 1, 25.2% of group 2, 24% of group 3, and in none of the group 4 patients. Cirrhosis was observed in only two group 1 patients during follow-up of up to 5 years. These data suggest that the risk of recurrent HCV infection (as identified by the presence anti-HCV) is approximately 25%, with infrequent progression to cirrhosis during the first 5 years after liver transplantation.

Hepatocellular carcinoma

It would seem that liver transplantation should be the ideal treatment for the patient with hepatocellular carcinoma because of its multicentric nature and the likelihood of coexisting cirrhosis. Unfortunately, the promise of liver transplantation has not been fulfilled, and was again confirmed by studies reported in 1993. However, one study [20••] raises a hope that adjuvant chemotherapy might improve the outcome, in these cases.

Most clinicians have considered the resection of hepatocellular carcinoma to be inappropriate for patients with cirrhosis. However, in a comparison study of 60 cirrhotic patients who received liver resection versus 60 patients with hepatocellular carcinoma who underwent liver transplantation, the overall survival at 3 years was similar (52% resection vs 49% transplantation) [21•]. However, the tumor-free survival rate was quite different (27% vs 46%, respectively). Surprisingly resection was better for large (>3 cm) solitary tumors, suggesting that the development of a single large nodule indicates that no additional lesions are likely to be present. When small (<3 cm) single or double tumors were compared, disease-free survival at 2 years was 18% for resection and 83% for transplantation, again indicating that additional tumors were likely to be present. Hepatic resection resulted in six early deaths (three from hepatic failure) compared with three early cardiac deaths in patients who received transplants.

That tumor size and number of tumors influence the outcome of liver transplantation for hepatocellular carcinoma is apparent from the results of 56 surviving patients with nonfibrolamellar hepatocellular carcinoma [22•]. Thirty-nine patients had single tumors (four of them incidental) and 23 had multifocal tumors varying from 0.8 to 21 cm in maximum diameter. Tumor recurrence was 0% if the solitary tumor was less than 4 cm, 40% if the single tumor was 4 to 8 cm, and 78% if the single tumor was more than 8 cm in diameter or if tumors were multifocal. Unfortunately, normalization of a preoperatively elevated α-fetoprotein level after liver transplantation did not predict lack of recurrence. Five patients received transplants because of multifocal fibrolamellar variant hepatocellular carcinoma, with recurrence of the tumor in four of five surviving patients. Additional studies also confirm that tumor size [23] and vascular invasion by the tumor [24] are predictors of poor outcome.

There is one bit of hope for the management of hepatocellular carcinoma by liver transplantation, however. In a study of 20 patients receiving preoperative (one to three doses of 10 mg/m^2), intraoperative, and post-operative chemotherapy to a total dose of 200 mg/m^2, enhanced tumor-free survival seems apparent [20••]. All patients received doxorubicin, with 17 of 20 patients completing therapy. There were eight patients with tumor recurrence (three other patients died of HBV reinfection). Disease-free actuarial survival was 54% at 3 years, and for those 17 patients with tumors greater than 5 cm in diameter at transplantation, tumor-free survival at 3 years was 49%. This significantly improved result deserves additional study in a randomized multicenter trial.

References and recommended reading

Papers of particular interest, published within the annual period of review, have been highlighted as:

- • Of special interest
- •• Of outstanding interest

1. • Kahn D, Gavaler JS, Makowka L, van Thiel DH: **Gender of Donor Influences Outcome After Orthotopic Liver Transplantation in Adults**. *Dig Dis Sci* 1993, **38**:1485–1488.

The failure rate of liver grafts in male recipients of livers from female donors was 60% within 60 days of orthotopic liver transplantation compared with 28% to 36% failure rates in other donor-recipient gender combinations.

2. Starzl TE, Fung J, Tzakis A, Todo S, Demetris AJ, Marino IR, Doyle H, Zeevi A, Warty V, Michaels M, *et al.*: **Baboon-to-Human Liver Transplantation**. *Lancet* 1993, **341**:65–71.

3. Chiche L, Adam R, Caillat-Zucman S, Castaing D, Bach JF, Bismuth H: **Xenotransplantation: Baboons as Potential Liver Donors? Scientific and Ethical Issues**. *Transplantation* 1993, **55**:1418–1421.

4. Starzl TE, Demetris AJ, Trucco M, Murase N, Ricordi C, Ildstad S, Ramos H, Todo S, Tzakis A, Fung JJ, *et al.*: **Cell Migration and Chimerism After Whole-Organ Transplantation: The Basis of Graft Acceptance**. *Hepatology* 1993, **17**:1127–1152.

5. • Starzl TE, Demetris AJ, Trucco M, Ricordi C, Ildstad S, Terasaki PI, Murase N, Kendall RS, Kocova M, Rudert WA, *et al.*: **Chimerism After Liver Transplantation for Type IV Glycogen Storage Disease and Type 1 Gaucher's Disease**. *N Engl J Med* 1993, **328**:745–749.

A report of two patients with type IV glycogen storage disease and a third with lysosomal glucocerebrosidase deficiency (type 1 Gaucher's disease) who had improvement of amylopectin and glucocerebroside deposition following orthotopic liver transplantation. Examination of tissue and blood samples identified donor-specific cells, indicating that systemic microchimerism may be able to ameliorate enzymatic deficiencies after liver transplantation.

6. Collins RH, Anastasi J, Terstappen LW, Nikaein A, Feng J, Fay JW, Klintmalm G, Stone MJ: **Donor-Derived Long-Term**

Multilineage Hematopoesis in a Liver Transplant Recipient. *N Engl J Med* 1993, **328**:762–765.

7. • Sanchez-Urdazpal L, Batts KP, Gores GJ, *et al.*: **Increased Bile Duct Complications in Liver Transplantation Across the ABO Barrier.** *Ann Surg* 1993, **218**:152–158.

In 18 recipients of ABO-incompatible orthotopic liver grafts, an increase in bile duct complications and a corresponding decrease in 1-year survival were observed. An increased frequency of hepatic artery thrombosis and allograft rejection was also observed.

8. • Sanchez-Urdaspal L, Gores GJ, Ward EM, *et al.*: **Diagnostic Features and Clinical Outcome of Ischemic-Type Biliary Complications After Liver Transplantation.** *Hepatology* 1993, **17**:605–609.

Ischemic-type biliary complications were identified in 25 of 128 orthotopic liver transplant recipients. Of six patients developing such complications during the first month postoperatively, five required repeat transplantation. Patients developing ischemic-type biliary complications 1 month or more after transplantation could be treated medically with bile duct dilation and stent placement. These patients were at increased risk of biliary sepsis from duct manipulation.

9. Sherman S, Shaked A, Cryer HM, Goldstein LI, Busuttil RW: **Endoscopic Management of Biliary Fistulas Complicating Liver Transplantation and Other Hepatobiliary Operations.** *Ann Surg* 1993, **218**:167–175.

10. Osorio RW, Freise CE, Stock PG, Lake JR, Laberge JM, Gordon RL, Ring EJ, Ascher NL, Roberts JP: **Nonoperative Management of Biliary Leaks After Orthotopic Liver Transplantation.** *Transplantation* 1993, **55**:1074–1077.

11. Gonzalez EM, Loinaz C, Garcia I, Lumbreras C, Gomez R, Moraleda G, G-Pinto I, Colina F, Jimenez C, Carreno V, *et al.*: **Liver Transplantation in Chronic Viral B and C Hepatitis.** *J Hepatol* 1993, **17(Suppl 3)**:S116–S122.

12. Walker N, Apel R, Kerlin P, Horn M, Tinniswood R, Lynch S, Strong R: **Hepatitis B Virus Infection of Liver Allografts.** *Am J Surg Pathol* 1993, **17**:666–677.

13. Harrison RF, Davies MH, Goldin RD, Hubscher SG: **Recurrent Hepatitis B in Liver Allografts: A Distinctive Form of Rapidly Developing Cirrhosis.** *Histopathology* 1993, **23**:21–28.

14. • Mason AL, Wick M, White HM, Benner KG, Lee RG, Regenstein F, Riely CA, Bain VG, Campbell C, Perrillo RP: **Increased Hepatocyte Expression of Hepatitis B Virus Transcription in Patients With Features of Fibrosing Cholestatic Hepatitis.** *Gastroenterology* 1993, **105**:237–244.

Liver biopsy specimens from patients with recurrent HBV were evaluated by *in situ* hybridization studies. The intensities of HBV DNA and HBV RNA signals were greatest in those with FCH, suggesting a cytopathic role in these cases.

15. Fang JWS, Tung FYT, Davis GL, Dolson DJ, VanThiel DH, Lau JY: **Fibrosing Cholestatic Hepatitis in a Transplant Recipient With Hepatitis B Virus Precore Mutant.** *Gastroenterology* 1993, **105**:901–904.

16. •• Samuel D, Muller R, Alexander G, *et al.*: **Liver Transplantation in European Patents With the Hepatitis B Surface Antigen.** *N Engl J Med* 1993, **329**:1842–1847.

In a multicenter study of patients who did or did not receive anti-HBIG during and after liver transplantation for acute and chronic HBV disease, a reduced likelihood of HBV reinfection of the allograft was noted with the long-term administration of hepatitis B immune globulin. This reduced likelihood was also seen in transplant patients who had fulminant hepatitis B or coexisting HDV disease.

17. Angus P, Richards M, Bowden S, Ireton J, Sinclair R, Jones R, Locarnini S: **Combination Antiviral Therapy Controls Severe Post-Liver Transplant Recurrence of Hepatitis B Virus Infection.** *J Gastroenterol Hepatol* 1993, **8**:353–357.

18. Samuel D, Bismuth H, Benhamou J-P: **Liver Transplantation in Cirrhosis Due to Hepatitis D Virus Infection.** *J Hepatol* 1993, **17(Suppl 3)**:S154–S156.

19. • Shah G, Demetris AJ, Irish W, Scheffel J, Mimms L, VanThiel DH: **Frequency and Severity of HCV Infection Following Orthotopic Liver Transplantation: Effect of Donor and Recipient Serology for HCV Using a Second Generation ELISA Test.** *J Hepatol* 1993, **18**:279–283.

A retrospective analysis of preoperative patient and donor sera indicates a risk of approximately 25% for infection after liver transplantation in patients who have preexisting HCV infection or receive a allograft from an HCV-positive donor (as indicated by the presence of anti-HCV by a second-generation enzyme-linked immunosorbent assay test).

20. •• Stone MJ, Klintmalm GBG, Polter D, Husberg BS, Mennel RG, Ramsay MA, Flemens ER, Goldstein RM: **Neoadjuvant Chemotherapy and Liver Transplantation for Hepatocellular Carcinoma: A Pilot Study in 20 Patients.** *Gastroenterology* 1993, **104**:196–202.

When 20 patients with hepatocellular carcinoma received preoperative, intraoperative, and postoperative doxorubicin, an improved postoperative outcome was observed.

21. • Bismuth H, Chiche L, Adam R, Castaing D, Diamond T, Dennison A: **Liver Resection Versus Transplantation for Hepatocellular Carcinoma in Cirrhotic Patients.** *Ann Surg* 1993, **218**:145–151.

A comparison of 120 patients with cirrhosis and hepatocellular carcinoma who underwent either resection or liver transplantation (60 patients each). Disease-free outcome is better with liver transplantation than with resection.

22. • McPeake JR, O'Grady JG, Zaman S, Portmann B, Wight DG, Tan KC, Calne RY, Williams R: **Liver Transplantation for Primary Hepatocellular Carcinoma: Tumor Size and Number Determine Outcome.** *J Hepatol* 1993, **18**:226–234.

After liver transplantation, the recurrence of hepatocellular carcinoma is highest in patients with large or multifocal tumors.

23. Gennari L, Mazzaferro V, Regalia E, Colella G, Doci R, Bozzetti F, Ammatuna M, Andreola S, Montalto F, Manzi R, *et al.*: **Reappraisal of the Role of Liver Transplantation in the Treatment of HCC Arising in Cirrhosis.** *J Surg Oncol Suppl* 1993, **3**:83–86.

24. Moreno-Gonzalez E, Loinaz C, Gomez R, Garcia I, Gonzalez-Pinto I, Jimenez C, Maffettone V, Colina F, Palomo JC, Vorwald P, *et al.*: **Orthotopic Liver Transplantation in Primary Liver Tumors.** *J Surg Oncol Suppl* 1993, **3**:74–77.

Rowen K. Zetterman, MD, Professor, Internal Medicine, University of Nebraska Medical Center, 600 South 42nd Street, Omaha, NE, 68198-2000, USA.

Miscellaneous liver disorders

Norman Gitlin, MD, and Johan Fevery, MD, PhD

School of Medicine, Emory University, Atlanta, Georgia, USA, and University Hospital, Gasthuisberg, Leuven, Belgium

Amyloidosis can involve the liver. It should be suspected in patients with amyloid who have an unexplained elevation of alkaline phosphatase. Inflammatory pseudotumor of the liver is a rare condition that should be considered in the differential diagnosis of hepatocellular cancer. Venoocclusive disease of the liver occurs after bone marrow transplantation, especially if the following risk factors are present: pretransplant elevation of aminotransferases, or previous therapy with cyclovir, vancomycin, or abdominal radiation. Hepatobiliary complications of total parenteral nutrition may not be due to the actual nutrients, but may reflect a decrease in enteric enzyme stimulation (less cholecystokinin release). Another possible mechanism may be the colonization of the gut by bacterial flora that produce toxins. Prophylactic antimicrobial therapy in experimental animal models reduced the incidence of hepatobiliary sequelae.

Current Opinion in Gastroenterology 1994, **10**:349–354

Hepatic amyloidosis

Amyloidosis is caused by the extracellular deposit of an insoluble fibrillar protein called amyloid. Amyloid is classified biochemically according to the dominant fibril type. Clinically, amyloid is either focal or systemic (throughout the body). In primary amyloidosis there is no apparent underlying disease, except for plasma cell myeloma in 25% of patients. Secondary amyloid is associated with chronic inflammatory disorders, neoplasia, and connective tissue disorders. Amyloid can also be associated with genetic disorders. Most commonly, amyloid syndromes are associated with kidney, cardiac, and neurologic involvement. It has been stated that a percutaneous liver biopsy carries a higher complication rate than normal in patients with hepatic amyloid [1,2]. However, many hepatologists dispute this association, and a review from the Mayo Clinic of 80 patients with hepatic amyloid described bleeding in two patients [3]. Capsular tears of the liver were not encountered. The Mayo report identified four features that should alert one to the diagnosis of hepatic amyloidosis: proteinuria, abnormal serum protein electrophoresis, hyposplenism (showing Howell-Jolly bodies on the peripheral blood smear), and hepatomegaly with a biochemical profile showing an infiltrative pattern (elevated alkaline phosphatase and γ-glutamyl transpeptidase). Amyloidosis can be confirmed by fat biopsy, rectal biopsy, or bone marrow aspiration. Hepatic involvement occurs in over 50% of all patients with amyloidosis, yet serious hepatic complications are rare [4]. Occasionally hepatic amyloidosis can occur with severe intrahepatic cholestasis [5]. A liver-spleen technetium sulphur colloid scan has been shown to be helpful in the diagnosis of amyloidosis with hepatosplenomegaly that mimics portal hypertension. In hepatic amyloidosis, splenic uptake is less than hepatic uptake, and bone marrow uptake may be normal or decreased [6•].

Inflammatory pseudotumor of the liver

Inflammatory pseudotumor of the liver (also referred to as plasma cell granuloma, histiocytoma, pseudolymphoma, fibroxanthoma or plasmacytoma) is rare. Approximately 47 cases have been reported. It is more common in males, it can occur at any age (10 months to 83 years of age), and the lesion is mostly solitary, spherical, and may vary from 1 to 25 cm in diameter [7••,8••]. The presenting features in these reports were fever, weight loss, malaise, and upper abdominal pain.

Histologic findings in inflammatory psuedotumor of the liver include a tumor composed of spindle cells intermixed with varying numbers of plasma cells, lymphocytes, and histiocytes. The spindle cells are plump and are arranged in interlacing fascicles with moderate amounts of intercellular collagen. Mitotic figures are very rare. The lesions are rarely vascular. On gross examination the tumors have a variegated appearance, with areas of hemorrhage and necrosis resembling a hepatocellular carcinoma. The prompt recognition and differentiation of an inflammatory pseudotumor of the liver from hepatocellular carcinoma is extremely im-

 ISBN 1-85922-608-6 ISSN 0267–1379

portant, in order to avoid unwarranted radical surgery or chemotherapy. Pseudotumors are best managed by local resection, although occasionally steroids or antibiotics are effective alone. The prognosis is good provided that the diagnosis is recognized. Fine-needle biopsy is the best diagnostic modality, because ultrasonography and angiography can be misleading. Focal areas of fatty infiltrate or focal sparing in a diffuse abnormal process have been noted on ultrasonography. Measurement of computed tomography attenuation may reveal fatty infiltration, thus favoring a specific diagnosis of a pseudotumor [9•].

The pathogenesis of inflammatory psuedotumor is uncertain. The α-fetoprotein level is usually normal. There is no proven association with other hepatobiliary diseases, but an isolated association with sclerosing cholangitis has been reported [10•].

Ischemic hepatitis

Ischemic hepatitis as a consequence of systemic hypotension is not uncommon. It is often overlooked or misdiagnosed because it is mostly a self-limiting process, provided that the underlying cause for hypotension (myocardial ischemia or cardiac dysrhythmia) is corrected. The biochemical profile is very characteristic, with a rapid massive rise in alanine aminotransferase, aspartate aminotransferase and lactate dehydrogenase, and a slight rise in bilirubin and a prolongation of the prothrombin time [11]. Approximately 3 to 5 days later there is an equally rapid resolution of these biochemical abnormalities and, provided hepatic perfusion and oxygenation is maintained, a total recovery occurs. In a rat model, arterial and venous ischemia resulted in more severe enzyme and plasma aminogram changes in cirrhotic rats than in healthy rats [12•]. In humans with cirrhosis, ischemic hepatitis appears to be rare even after massive variceal bleeding. However, if sepsis is also present, then ischemic hepatitis occurs [13•]. Focal ischemic necrosis (also known as anoxic pseudolobular necrosis) can occur in patients with cirrhosis or hepatocellular cancer. Ultrasonography and computed tomography scans can help diagnose ischemic hepatitis [14•]. Transitory hepatic ischemia can follow a surgical pancreaticoduodenectomy, and it can result from postsurgical celiac axis compression [15•].

Other liver disorders

Hyperammonemia

Noncirrhotic hyperammonemia has been reported in a number of conditions. These range from congenital metabolic disorders of the urea cycle to urinary sepsis due to *Escherichia coli* or *Pseudomonas mirabilis* (which are both urease-producing bacteria). Intestinal ischemia is also associated with raised ammonia levels, and congenital portosystemic shunts have been associated with symptomatic hyperammonemia and coma [16•]. Severe exercise, heat stroke, and a high-protein meal can cause a rise in ammonia levels even in healthy individuals.

Vitamin A hepatotoxicity

Vitamin A abuse, a daily oral intake in excess of 50,000 IU for 6 months, can damage the liver. An interesting report documented that over a 6-year period, a 35-year-old male patient with vitamin A–induced liver disease progressed from extensive perivenular sclerosis and perisinusoidal fibrosis with Ito cell hyperplasia to cirrhosis, despite having discontinued the excessive vitamin A intake after the hepatic dysfunction was diagnosed [17•]. Clearly, progression was independent of further vitamin A toxicity and indicated that fibroblastic activity, once initiated, appears to progress regardless of the presence of the vitamin.

Systemic lupus erythematosus

The spectrum of hepatic abnormalities associated with systemic lupus erythematosus includes cirrhosis, chronic active hepatitis, and chronic persistent hepatitis in nearly one third of patients with this disease [18]. A Japanese report of 51 autopsies in patients with systemic lupus erythematosus found steatosis in most cases and arteritis in 22% [19•]. Hepatic infarction was not detected.

Oral contraceptive agents

The role (if any) that oral contraceptive agents contribute to the pathogenesis of hepatocellular carcinoma is uncertain. Certainly an association has been established between these agents and hepatic adenomas. Hepatic adenomas are not regarded as premalignant. An important report, albeit a solitary case, of a hepatocellular carcinoma developing in a large multilobulated adenoma in the noncirrhotic liver of a 29-year-old woman demonstrates that malignant transformation can occur on rare occasions [20•]. The patient had a distant limited exposure to oral contraceptives, but she had no other exposure to carcinogenic agents.

Hepatic hematoma

Spontaneous hepatic hematomas are rare even in patients taking anticoagulants on a long-term basis. Hematomas can be associated with trauma, pregnancy, or toxemia of pregnancy. There are a number of reports of spontaneous hepatic hematomas developing in patients without cirrhosis who are receiving long-term oral anticoagulant therapy [21•]. The precipitating role of concurrent antibiotic therapy (especially metronidazole, sulfonamides, or ampicillin) has been noted in most cases. Altered hepatic metabolism of warfarin, prolonging its half-life, may be the mechanism of this association. Reports of hepatic hemotomas associated with antifibrinolytic therapy are appearing. The initial symptom in all patients with hepatic hematomas is right upper quadrant pain. Other features include hepatomegaly, pyrexia, and abnormal biochemistry in some instances. Early diagnosis, discontinuation of the anticoagulation, and drainage and antibiotics (if infection is evident) are the cornerstones of management.

A rare case of hemoperitonium caused by focal hemorrhagic necrosis of the liver was reported [22•]. Although not clearly defined, it was most probably due to early stage of peliosis (because sinusoidal dilatation was recorded) resulting from a 10-year intake of conjugated estrogens (Premarin, Wyeth-Ayerst Laboratories, Philadelphia, PA). Bleeding secondary to preeclampsia is more frequently seen as a cause of hemoperitoneum. The history of a 25-year-old woman, gravida II, para I at 25 weeks of gestation has also been reported [23•]. The patient had a nearly daily recurrence of severe upper abdominal pain, nausea, and vomiting, with a fluctuating transaminase level of approximately 1000 IU/L, which rapidly fell but soon rose again. After 10 days, she developed hypertension and proteinuria. A Cesarean section was performed to deliver a healthy son, this was followed by peritoneoscopical examination of the liver, which showed multiple foci of subcapsular hemorrhages.

Liver biopsy

Procedures to obtain liver tissue safely remain a topic of investigation. One report compared the risks involved in obtaining one (n=834 patients), two (n=983), or three (n=829) specimens with a needle [24•]. No significant difference was present in the incidence of pain, hypotension, or death; however, the overall mortality rate due to intraperitoneal bleeding (0.3%) was unacceptably high. In our opinion, this could be decreased by using ultrasonographic monitoring of the procedure. A comparison between transjugular (n=44) and plugged-percutaneous (n=56) liver biopsies in patients with impaired blood coagulation (platelet count below 80 $\times 10^9$/L or prothrombin time prolonged by 3 seconds) showed that the latter procedure was less time-consuming and provided larger biopsy specimens (12±5 mm vs 6±4 mm, P>0.001), but that it was associated with hemorrhage requiring transfusion in two patients [25•]. The plugged-percutaneous procedure allows one to perform a biopsy on a focal lesion, whereas the transjugular approach is easier when pressure studies are done simultaneously.

Percutaneous needle biopsy was performed to establish the diagnosis of cavernous hemangioma in 38 patients [26•]. A 20-gauge needle was used and an average of 2.7 passes were made. No hemorrhage was reported. One should, however, ensure that enough normal liver tissue is interposed between the liver capsule and the targeted lesion to prevent intraperitoneal leakage.

A comparison between wedge and needle biopsies has also been reported [27•]. Two points raised in this paper are important. First, a parenchymal cell volume ratio was calculated (from 10 randomly selected areas) as the ratio of hepatocytes, sinusoids, and bile canaliculi to the total area. This differs from the classical way to quantitate fibrosis. Note that the liver capsule was not accounted for in this calculation. Second, the parenchymal cell volume ratio in the subcapsular area was 99.3%±6.6% of that in the intralobular area, demonstrating that wedge biopsy samples do not overestimate fibrosis (as thought by several pathologists), provided that the assessment is made from hepatic tissue more than 0.2 cm deep to the capsule [28] (because most individuals have fibrous extensions from the capsule into the portal and even the central venous tracts). This conclusion was reached in both near-normal and in cirrhotic tissue.

Laparoscopic cholecystectomy

The increasing use of laparoscopic cholecystectomy has led to the reconsideration of the diagnostic aspects of laparoscopy. An overview is give by Boyce [29•]. His suggestion that laparoscopy with biopsy be used as a substitute for autopsy in certain circumstances is a very interesting one. Liver biopsy represents the most effective way to finally diagnose diffuse parenchymatous disease. The sensitivity of ultrasonography to disease such as cirrhosis is rather low. At present, ultrasonography and computed tomography are able to detect focal lesions in approximately 90% of cases. Laparoscopy might add to the diagnosis in cases in which all imaging techniques give unsatisfactory answers but malignancy is suspected [30•]. Probably of greater interest is the development of ultrasonolaparoscopy [31•]. Its place in our diagnostic armamentarium needs further evaluation.

Hepatic venoocclusive disease

A major prospective study that determined the incidence and clinical course of hepatic venoocclusive disease after bone marrow transplantation was reported by McDonald *et al.* [32••]. Venoocclusive disease developed in 190 of 355 patients (54%) and it was severe in one quarter of these patients. Pretransplant elevated transaminase levels or acyclovir therapy were independent risk factors. Somewhat less important were vancomycin therapy preceding radiation to the abdomen, a mismatched or unrelated donor, and a high-dose regimen for cytoreduction. Venoocclusive disease is frequently associated with renal and cardiopulmonary failure. The mortality rate before day 100 was 98% in the severe cases of venoocclusive disease, 23% in the moderate cases, and 9% in the mild cases.

Parenteral nutrition and hepatobiliary complications

Hepatobiliary complications of total parenteral nutrition remain of major interest [33••] because an increasing number of patients are being treated with this modality. Increasing evidence is accumulating that it is not a specific detrimental effect of carbohydrate or lipid excess that is the major determinant but rather the loss of enteric stimulation that causes the complications [33••]. In this respect, a significant increase in the number of gram-negative bacteria has been observed in the cecum of rats receiving total parenteral nutrition. These bacteria could lead to enhanced production of endotoxin and tumor necrosis factor, both of which are known to produce cholestasis, cholestatic hepatitis, or steatosis. Metronidazole has previously been demonstrated to decrease the severity of these derangements [34]. Similarly, polymyxin B was shown to reduce liver steatosis in experimental rats [35•]. Although oral administration of polymyxin B induced a significantly greater decrease in the amount of gram-negative bacteria in the cecum than it did when given intravenously, the latter route was more effective in reducing steatosis and production of tumor necrosis factor by peritoneal macrophages. Therefore, it was concluded that polymyxin B protects the liver through an antimicrobial effect that prevents overgrowth and subsequent translocation of endotoxin, and through its specific antilipolysaccharide activity.

Hepatatrophic agents

It has long been noted that portal blood contains hepatatrophic factors partly derived from the pancreas. To study the effect of portal perfusion, a rat model was developed in which the subcutaneously transposed spleen was perfused by portal blood due to portal vein ligation at the hilum of the liver. Isolated hepatocytes were injected into the spleen. Greater numbers of hepatocytes survived the first 6 weeks when perfused with portal blood than when perfused normally [36•]. In another study [37•], 10 patients receiving peripheral intravenous nutritional support were compared with 10 patients receiving a similar infusion into the gastroepiploic vein near the portal vein trunk. The nitrogen balance was significantly more positive during day 5 and day 6 in the portal vein nutrition group than in the standard control. Further studies to evaluate this approach are needed.

Pulmonary hypertension

The interest in pulmonary arterial hypertension present in patients with portal hypertension has increased in the era of liver transplantation, because it greatly complicates transplant surgery. Pulmonary arterial hypertension should be differentiated from the functional hepatopulmonary syndrome [38,39]. A case report from India [40•] of pulmonary hypertension in a patient with noncirrhotic portal fibrosis stresses again that the duration of portal hypertension and not the presence of cirrhosis is the cause of the fibrosis. The exact pathogenesis is unknown but circulating vasoactive agents are probably involved. Sclerotherapy might accelerate the process, and caution is needed in using β-blocking drugs in the treatment of portal hypertension because they have a deleterious effect on pulmonary hypertension.

References and recommended reading

Papers of particular interest, published within the annual period of review, have been highlighted as:
• Of special interest
•• Of outstanding interest

1. Stauffer MH, Gross JB, Faulk WT, Dahlin DC: **Amyloidosis: Diagnosis With Needle Biopsy of the Liver in 18 Patients.** *Gastroenterology* 1961, **41**:92–96.

2. Volwiler W, Jones EM: **The Diagnostic and Therapeutic Value of Liver Biopsies With Particular Reference to Trocar Biopsy.** *N Engl J Med* 1947, **237**:651–656.

3. Gertz MA, Kyle RA: **Hepatic Amyloidosis (Primary [AL], Immunoglobulin Light Chain): The Natural History in 80 Patients.** *Am J Med* 1988, **85**:73–80.

4. O'Doherty DP, Neoptolemos JP, Wood KF: **Place of Surgery in the Management of Amyloid Disease.** *Br J Surg* 1987, **74**:83–88.

5. Hoffman MS, Stein BE, Davidian MM, Rosenthal WS: **Hepatic Amyloidosis Presenting as Severe Intrahepatic Cholestasis: A Case Report and Review of the Literature.** *Am J Gastroenterol* 1988, **83**:783–785.

6. • Straub RF, Boyer TD: **The Liver-Spleen Scan in Systemic Amyloidosis: A Clue to the Diagnosis.** *J Clin Gastroenterol* 1993, **16**:1–4.

A technetium sulphur colloid liver-spleen scan showed splenic uptake less than hepatic uptake in three patients with systemic amyloidosis. This differentiates the condition from cirrhosis with portal hypertension, and this test is easy to perform.

7. •• Shek WH, Ng OL, Chan KW: **Inflammatory Pseudotumor of the Liver: Report of Our Cases and Review of the Literature.** *Am J Surg Pathol* 1993, **17**:231–238.

Four cases of pseudotumor of the liver are reported. This is an excellent review of every published case report (47 in all) and a comprehensive review of their overall findings. This report includes a very thorough bibliography.

8. •• Hata Y, Sasaki F, Matuoka S, Hamada H, Taguchi K, Hasumi T, *et al.*: **Inflammatory Pseudotumor of the Liver in Children: Report of Cases and Review of the Literature.** *J Pediatr Surg* 1992, **27**:1549–1552.

Two pediatric patients with inflammatory pseudotumor of the liver are reported. Fever and vague abdominal symptoms were present. Both patients were suspected to have hepatic malignancies and they both underwent radical surgery. A more conservative approach might have been pursued if a histologic diagnosis had been obtained originally.

9. • Scriven MW, Shandall A, Fitzgerald EJPG, Puntis MCA: **Hepatic 'Pseudotumours': An Important Diagnostic Pitfall.** *Ann R Coll Surg Engl* 1993, **75**:43–45.

Hepatic pseudotumors have the radiological appearance of a neoplasm. However, focal areas of fatty infiltration or focal sparing in a diffuse process have been noted on ultrasonography. Measurement of computed tomography attenuation may permit a confident diagnosis of fatty infiltration with focal sparing, thus avoiding a misdiagnosis of cancer.

10. • Gough J, Chakrabarti S: **Inflammatory Pseudotumor of the Liver in a Patient With Chronic Sclerosing Cholangitis.** *Am J Gastroenterol* 1993, **88**:1452–1453.

A report of inflammatory pseudotumor of the liver in a patient with sclerosing cholangitis and hepatic abscesses.

11. Gitlin N, Serio KM: **Ischemic Hepatitis: Widening Horizons.** *Am J Gastroenterol* 1992, **87**:871–836.

12. • Nishimura T, Nakahara M, Kobayashi S, *et al.*: **Ischemic Injury in Cirrhotic Livers: An Experimental Study of the Temporary Arrest of Hepatic Circulation.** *J Surg Res* 1992, **53**:227–233.

In an experimental cirrhotic rat model, hepatic ischemia (to only the left hepatic lobe) resulted in a higher aspartate aminotransferase level, a reduction in the hepatic adenine nucleotidase level, and alteration in serum aminograms (the ratio of valine, leucine, and isoleucine decreased relative to the ratio of tyrosine to phenylalanine) compared with noncirrhotic control rats.

13. • Henrion J, Colin L, Schmitz A, Schapira M, Heller FR: **Ischemic Hepatitis in Cirrhosis: Rare But Lethal.** *J Clin Gastroenterol* 1993, **16**:35–39.

Two patients with cirrhosis and portal hypertension developed ischemic hepatitis as a consequence of their acute variceal bleeding. They subsequently died. In addition, both patients had sepsis that might have aggravated their ischemia. Ischemic hepatitis in cirrhosis is a rare entity. The role of sepsis superimposed on the pathogenesis of ischemic hepatitis in patients with cirrhosis is raised.

14. • Fukui N, Kitagawa K, Matsui O, Takashima T, Kidani H, Hirano M, Masuda S, Nakanuma Y: **Focal Ischemic Necrosis of the Liver Associated With Cirrhosis: Radiologic Findings.** *AJR Am J Roentgenol* 1992, **159**:1021–1022.

Focal ischemic necrosis of the liver (also known as anoxic pseudolobular necrosis) occurs in patients with cirrhosis or liver cancer. Sonography reveals a hypoechoic nodular lesion and computed tomography showed a subtle low-density area on contrast-enhanced scan.

15. • Bull DA, Hunter GC, Crabtree TG, Berhard VM, Putnam CW: **Hepatic Ischemia, Caused by Celiac Axis Compression, Complicating Pancreaticoduodenectomy.** *Ann Surg* 1993, **217**:244–247.

A report of two patients with operative hepatic ischemia due to celiac axis compression during pancreaticoduodenectomy. The hepatic ischemia was only arterial and of limited duration. Moderate elevation of aminotransferase levels ensued.

16. • Kitagawa S, Gleason WA, Northrup H, Middlebrook MR, Ueberschar E: **Symptomatic Hyperammonemia Caused by a Congenital Portosystemic Shunt.** *J Pediatr* 1992, **121**:917–919.

A case report of hyperammonemia and coma in a 3.5-year-old boy with a congenital portosystemic shunt and normal hepatic function.

17. • Jorens PG, Michielsen PP, Pelckmans PA, Fevery J, Desmet VJ, Geubel AP, Rahier J, Vam Maercke YM: **Vitamin A Abuse: Development of Cirrhosis Despite Cessation of Vitamin A: A Sixty-Year Clinical and Histopathologic Follow-Up.** *Liver* 1992, **12**:381–386.

A case report in which a 35-year-old man was followed beginning in December 1983, when he was found to have extensive perivenular sclerosis, perisinusoidal fibrosis, centrolobular atrophy, and Ito cell hyperplasia, secondary to vitamin A abuse (200,000 IU/d for 12 months). By 1989 his disease had progressed to cirrhosis even though he had not taken any further vitamin A and had not been exposed to any other recognized hepatotoxic agent.

18. Runyon BA, LaBrecque DR, Anuras S: **The Spectrum of Liver Disease in Systemic Lupus Erythematosus.** *Am J Med* 1980, **69**:187–194.

19. • Matsumoto T, Yoshimine T, Shimouchi K, Shiotu H, Kiwabara N, Fukuda Y, Hoshi T: **The Liver in Systemic Lupus Erythematosus: Pathologic Analysis of 52 Cases and Review of Japanese Autopsy Registry Data.** *Hum Pathol* 1992, **23**:1151–1158.

A report of 51 Japanese patients with systemic lupus erythematosus. Their hepatic pathology as determined by autopsy is reviewed. Arteritis was evidence in 20% of the patients but actual infarction was rare. Nodular regenerative hyperplasia was present in 7% of the patients (it also occurs with Felty's syndrome). Approximately 2% of the patients had chronic active hepatitis or cirrhosis.

20. • Ferrell LD: **Hepatocellular Carcinoma Arising in a Focus of Multilobular Adenoma.** *Am J Surg Path* 1993, **17**:525–529.

An important report (albeit a solitary case) of a hepatocellular carcinoma developing in a large multilobulated adenoma in the noncirrhotic liver of a 29-year-old woman. Hepatocyte proliferation that is sufficient to induce malignant transformation in the absence of other known carcinogenic agents is rare and fortunately unusual. The patient had taken oral contraceptives for a period of 6 months, beginning 5 years earlier.

21. • Erichsen C, Sndenna K, Streide JA, Andersen E, Tysvoer A: **Spontaneous Liver Hematomas Induced by Anticoagulation Therapy.** *Hepatogastroenterology* 1993, **40**:402–406.

A case report of a nonfatal spontaneous hepatic hematoma in a patient without liver disease who was on long-term oral anticoagulant therapy. Seven other similar reports are reviewed, as are five reports of hepatic hemotomas associated with antifibrinolytic therapy. The role of concurrent antimicrobial therapy (metronidazole, sulfonamides, and ampicillin) in the pathogenesis of the bleeding is discussed.

22. • Takiff H, Brems JJ, Pockros PJ, Elliott ML: **Focal Hemorrhagic Necrosis of the Liver.** *Dig Dis Sci* 1992, **37**:1910–1914.

Case report.

23. • Gordon SC, Meyer RA, Rosenberg BF: **Laparoscopic Diagnosis of Subcapsular Hepatic Hemorrhage in Pre-Eclamptic Liver Disease.** *Gastrointest Endosc* 1992, **38**:718–720.

Case report.

24. • Maharaj B, Bhoora IG: **Complications Associated With Percutaneous Needle Biopsy of the Liver When One, Two or Three Specimens Are Taken.** *Postgrad Med J* 1992, **68**:964–967.

Comparison of side effects.

25. • Sawyerr AM, McCormick PA, Tennyson GS, Chin J, Dick R, Scheuer PJ, Burroughs AK, McIntyre N: **A Comparison of Transjugular and Plugged-Percutaneous Liver Biopsy in Patients With Impaired Coagulation.** *J Hepatol* 1993, **17**:81–85.

Comparative study.

26. • Tung GA, Cronan JJ: **Percutaneous Needle Biopsy of Hepatic Cavernous Hemangioma.** *J Clin Gastroenterol* 1993, **16**:117–122.

Study advocating needle biopsy in cases suspected of hemangioma.

27. • Imamura H, Kawasaki S, Bandai Y, Sanjo K, Idezuki Y: **Comparison Between Wedge and Needle Biopsies for Evaluating the Degree of Cirrhosis.** *J Hepatol* 1993, **17**:215–219.

Comparative study.

28. Petrelli M, Scheuer PJ: **Variation in Subcapsular Liver Structure and Its Significance in the Interpretation of Wedge Biopsies.** *J Clin Pathol* 1967, **20**:743–748.

29. • Boyce HW: **Diagnostic Laparoscopy in Liver and Biliary Disease.** *Endoscopy* 1992, **24**:676–681.

Review paper.

30. • Leuschner M, Leuschner U: **Diagnostic Laparoscopy in Focal Parenchymal Disease of the Liver.** *Endoscopy* 1992, **24**:689–692.

Review paper.

31. • Fukuda M, Hirata K, Mima S: **Preliminary Evaluation of Sonolaparoscopy in the Diagnosis of Liver Diseases.** *Endoscopy* 1992, **24**:701–708.

Prototype instrument.

32. •• McDonald GB, Hinds MS, Fisher LD, Schoch HG, Wolford JL, Banaji M, Hardin BJ, Shulman HM, Clift RA: **Veno-Occlusive Disease of the Liver and Multiorgan Failure After Bone Marrow Transplantation: A Cohort Study of 355 Patients.** *Ann Intern Med* 1993, **118**:255–267.

Thorough overview of a large series of patients.

33. •• Quigley EM, Marsh MN, Shaffer JL, Markin RS: **Hepatobiliary Complications of Total Parenteral Nutrition.** *Gastroenterology* 1992, **104**:286–301.

Thorough review of total parenteral nutrition.

34. Capron JP, Herve MA, Gineston JL, Braillon A: **Metronidazole in Prevention of Cholestasis Associated With Total Parenteral Nutrition.** *Lancet* 1983, **1**:446.

35. Pappo I, Bercovier H, Berry EM, Haviv Y, Gallily R, Freund
• HR: **Polymyxin B Reduces Total Parenteral Nutrition-Associated Hepatic Steatosis by its Antibacterial Activity and by Blocking Deleterious Effects of Lipopolysaccharide.** *JPEN J Parenter Enteral Nutr* 1992, **16**:529–532.
Well designed experimental study.

36. Jaffé V, Darby H, Hodgson HJ: **The Effect of Portal Perfusion**
• **on Intrasplenic Hepatocytes.** *Scand J Gastroenterol* 1992, **27**:837–841.
Development of a new experimental animal model.

37. Bozzetti F, Regalia E, Barbieri A, Facchetti G, Bombardieri
• E, Montlato F, Cozzaglio L, Gennari L: **Does Portal Nutrition Benefit Liver Protein Synthesis?** *JPEN J Parenter Enteral Nutr* 1993, **17**:20–24.
Experimental study of intraportal nutrition in patients.

38. Hadengue A, Benhayoun MK, Lebrec D, Benhamou J-P: **Pulmonary Hypertension Complicating Portal Hypertension: Prevalence and Relation to Splanchnic Hemodynamics.** *Gastroenterology* 1991, **100**:520–528.

39. Krowka MJ, Cortese DA: **Hepatopulmonary Syndrome: An Evolving Perspective in the Era of Liver Transplantation.** *Hepatology* 1990, **11**:138–141.

40. Goenka MK, Mehta SK, Malik AK, Kumar YR, Kochhar
• R: **Fatal Pulmonary Arterial Hypertension Complicating Noncirrhotic Portal Fibrosis.** *Am J Gastroenterol* 1992, **87**:1203–1205.
Case report.

Norman Gitlin, MD, Division of Digestive Diseases, Emory University School of Medicine, Drawer AL, Atlanta, GA 30322, USA.

Johan Fevery, MD, PhD, University Hospital Gasthuisberg, v.s. Gasthuisberg, Herestraat 49, 3200 Leuven, Belgium.

Inflammatory bowel disease

Commentary

Richard P. MacDermott, MD

Lahey Clinic, Burlington, Massachusetts, USA

Current Opinion in Gastroenterology 1994, **10**:355–357

This has been a landmark year in the development of fundamental advances that will shape the future approaches to research in inflammatory bowel disease (IBD). During the past decade, a unifying hypothesis describing the immunopathologic alterations that lead to IBD has been developed and now provides the starting point for basic investigational studies into the etiopathogenesis of ulcerative colitis and Crohn's disease research. Within the past year, we have seen important new observations obtained in both human and animal studies that allow us to more confidently support this working hypothesis. In the following paragraphs, I will discuss the components as well as the implications of the current working hypothesis and then summarize the reasons for the excitement regarding the recent advances in animal model systems and the implications for future research studies.

The stimulatory molecules present in the intestinal lumen that activate and induce subsequent mucosal immunologic and inflammatory events now appear most likely to be bacterial cell wall products such as peptidoglycans, lipopolysaccharides, and other chemotactic and toxic bacterial products that are produced by the many different types of bacteria within the gastrointestinal tract. These highly stimulatory bacterial cell wall products are capable of activating macrophages and T lymphocytes to release a group of potent proinflammatory cytokines including interleukin-1, interleukin-6, and tumor necrosis factor (TNF)-α. The proinflammatory cytokines normally augment protective immune processes. Interleukin-1, interleukin-6, and TNF-α as well as interferon-γ increase the presence of HLA class II antigen-presenting molecules on the surfaces of epithelial cells, endothelial cells, macrophages, and B cells, thus increasing their ability to present lumenal antigens and bacterial products.

The proinflammatory cytokines interleukin-1 and TNF-α also increase the ability of epithelial cells, endothelial cells, macrophages, and fibroblasts to secrete potent chemotactic cytokines such as interleukin-8 and macrophage chemotactic and activating factor. The chemokines along with other chemotactic molecules, such as leukotriene B_4, complement components, and bacterial products, such as *N*-formyl-methionine-leucine-phenylalanine, all serve to markedly increase the movement of macrophages and granulocytes from the circulation into the inflamed mucosa. The heightened stimulatory and activation events are not confined solely to the mucosal inflammatory network, but also include heightened antibody (immunoglobulin G) synthesis and secretion with resultant complement activation as well as heightened T-cell activation.

Thus, through lumenal exposure to potent, nonspecific stimulatory bacterial products, the state of activation of the intestinal immune system and mucosal inflammatory pathways are markedly up-regulated. This raises the question of whether there is a deficiency in effective down-regulation through the absence of normally suppressive cytokines such as interleukin-10, transforming growth factor-β, interleukin-4, and interleukin-1 receptor antagonist. Normally, the turning off of the active and destructive immunologic and inflammatory events should occur following the resolution of a bacterial or viral infection that has been appropriately defended against and controlled by the mucosal immune system. In IBD, however, the down-regulatory events and processes that should turn off the immunologic and inflammatory protective processes once the pathogenic agent has been cleared, appear to be deficient or only partially effective.

One of the major questions that arises from the above working hypothesis and is the current focus of very active investigation is the question of why up-regulated immunologic and inflammatory intestinal activities are not turned off, thus allowing the destructive processes to continue. Another critical area of investigation is delineation of the genetic factors that predispose certain individuals to having either a heightened immune and inflammatory response, or not being able to down-regulate ongoing chronic immunologic and inflammatory events. An unresolved issue is the precise nature of the bacterial species or substrains of bacteria that produce the bacterial cell wall products, antigens, chemotactic peptides, or bacterial toxins that continuously stimulate the nonspecific activation of immune and inflammatory processes in ulcerative colitis and Crohn's disease patients.

Abbreviations

IBD—inflammatory bowel disease; **TNF**—tumor necrosis factor.

 ISBN 1-85922-609-4 ISSN 0267–1379

A rapidly advancing area has been delineation of the nature of the molecules that mediate the destruction and damage during chronic intestinal inflammation. Excellent progress is being made in characterizing the destructive and inflammatory capabilities of nitrous oxide in addition to oxygen radicals, proteases, leukotrienes, and the other molecules released from activated macrophages and granulocytes in IBD. A critical question is which of the large number of diverse pathways is central to driving the entire chronic inflammatory process and might be, therefore, specifically targeted for the development of new therapeutic strategies. Alternatively, perhaps the numerous backup systems and redundancy involved in the normal protective mechanisms associated with mucosal immunity and intestinal inflammation may indicate that future pharmacologic and therapeutic strategies will need to focus on the development of drugs that have multiple mechanisms of action.

During the past year, several enormously exciting and extremely important developments have occurred which clearly indicate that valuable novel animal models are now in hand and which will allow rapid exploration of the working hypothesis and the questions outlined above. The advances in animal models that have occurred are in the area of genetically engineered animals that develop intestinal inflammation. All of the genetically manipulated models were developed by basic immunologists and geneticists who were carrying out molecular biologic approaches in order to answer questions regarding the effect of these alterations on normal immune function. It is interesting to note that in none of the animal models published to date were the basic immunologists seeking to establish an animal model of colitis, but rather, the colitis occurred for as yet unclear reasons because of the specific genetic alteration.

The first genetic animal model developed was a transgenic model that consisted of human HLA B-27 and β-2 microglobulin genes introduced into rats, which developed small and large bowel inflammation as well as arthritis, iritis, and epididymitis. The next two models were specific gene deletion ("knock-out") models in which interleukin-2 knock-out mice developed inflammation of the colon and interleukin-10 knock-out mice developed inflammation of the entire intestinal tract. The third type of model is that of a mutated T-cell receptor in mice who then developed chronic intestinal inflammation without ulcers. In contrast, there have also been a number of specifically genetically altered animals that have not developed colitis or enteritis and further models are in the process of being described. All of these models are described and discussed in detail by three of our section authors.

This rapidly exploding area of genetically engineered animal models is of extraordinary excitement and importance for many reasons. First of all, after crossbreeding, some of the animal models do or do not develop intestinal inflammation depending on the specific inbred strains of mouse or rat with which the animal is back-crossed. Thus, an exploration of both the background genes in addition to the specifically altered genes that influence the development of intestinal inflammation can now begin to be examined.

Secondly, studies now indicate that when animal strains that are likely to develop intestinal inflammation are raised in a totally germ-free (gnotobiotic) environment, intestinal inflammation does not develop. This demonstrates the central importance of bacterial pathogens or bacterial cell wall products or toxins in these particular animal models. These observations support the concepts of the nonspecific stimulatory role of bacterial cell wall products, antigens, chemotactic molecules, or toxins in ulcerative colitis and Crohn's disease.

The role of cells and cytokines that specifically up-regulate or down-regulate the immune response can be evaluated in these genetically engineered animal models. One overall conclusion from evaluating the animal models that appears likely is that the normal intestinal immune system is under a careful balance in which proinflammatory and anti-inflammatory cells and molecules are usually regulated in order to promote a normal host mucosal defense capability without destruction of intestinal tissue. The genetically engineered animal models indicate that once this carefully regulated balance is disturbed, nonspecific stimulation and activation can lead to marked up-regulatory and destructive immunologic and inflammatory events. An intriguing issue that is raised by these studies of balance and regulation of normal mucosal immune and inflammatory events is how perilously close we all may be to developing intestinal inflammation. That is, it is surprisingly easy with disruption of any one of a number of specific immune defense mechanisms to develop chronic intestinal inflammation. In retrospect, this may not be entirely surprising because we have always recognized that the normal mucosal immune system is constantly stimulated by normal lumenal contents and bacteria, *ie*, the mucosal immune system's "engine" must always be turned on and ready to go into high gear at a moment's notice. It now appears that defects in a wide variety of different regulatory events can quickly switch the mucosal immune system's engine into a high powered (inflamed) racing machine.

Another issue raised by these observations is that different genetic defects can each lead to different types of intestinal inflammatory events. This may suggest that parts of the overall working hypothesis discussed above may need to be amended in the future as we begin to characterize the different clinical subtypes of IBD, ulcerative colitis, and Crohn's disease. We may find that we ultimately are dealing with disease processes that have more than one genetic or cellular basis. That is, the different disease subgroups that we see clinically may be due to different specific genetic alterations.

A final important implication of the advances made in animal models of genetically altered immune animals is that these systems will allow new experimental approaches to the development of therapy. These models can be used to help determine the effects and mechanisms of action of currently used medications that are used to treat IBD. In addition, the genetically engineered animal models will allow exploration of novel immunologic and genetic approaches such as gene replacement therapy, administration of the missing cytokine or altered cell surface antigen, administration of monoclonal antibodies directed against overexpressed cytokines, or development of newer strategies against fundamental cell biologic mechanisms such as adhesion molecules.

Thus, the development of genetically engineered animal models has made this a landmark year with regard to the emergence of exciting new approaches and strategies that will now allow the dissection and understanding of basic mechanisms of IBD pathogenesis. The true importance of these powerful new animal models will be seen in the forthcoming rapid progress and advances that are absolutely certain to occur in the coming few years.

Richard P. MacDermott, MD, Chief, Gastroenterology Section, Lahey Clinic, 41 Mall Road, Burlington, MA 01805, USA.

Genetically engineered models of inflammatory bowel disease

Elaine M. Conner, PhD, Satoshi Aiko, MD, and Matthew Grisham, PhD

Louisiana State University Medical Center, Shreveport, Louisiana, USA

Recent advances in genetic engineering techniques have made possible new and exciting approaches to generating models of inflammatory bowel disease in mice and rats. Several recent studies have demonstrated that targeted deletions of genes encoding for interleukin-2, interleukin-10, or certain T-cell receptor proteins produce mice that spontaneously develop chronic intestinal inflammation similar to human inflammatory bowel disease. In addition, it has been demonstrated that the introduction of HLA-B27 and human β_2-microglobulin genes into rats produces transgenic animals that spontaneously develop chronic gastrointestinal inflammation. Data derived from these studies suggest that T cells play an important role in regulating B-cell activity, such that an unrestrained or unregulated B-cell response to normal luminal antigens or bacterial products promotes chronic gut inflammation. In addition, these studies demonstrate that endogenous luminal bacteria are important in promoting or exacerbating chronic gut inflammation. Indeed, these studies indicate that the production of very different defects in the immune system leads, in many cases, only to gut mucosal inflammation, suggesting that the gut mucosa is subjected to substantially more antigenic "stress" than are other tissues. Thus, these new models offer new and exciting avenues of research for the study of the pathogenesis of inflammatory bowel disease as well as providing new and possibly more appropriate models for the development and testing of new therapeutic agents for the treatment of these diseases.

Current Opinion in Gastroenterology 1994, **10**:358–364

Progress in understanding the pathogenetic mechanisms responsible for the inflammation and injury of the intestine and colon in idiopathic inflammatory bowel disease (IBD) (*eg*, ulcerative colitis, Crohn's disease) has been slowed by the lack of availability of animal models that exhibit the chronic and spontaneously relapsing inflammation characterized by these diseases. A number of animal models have been developed over the past 20 years that possess some but not all of the features of human IBD. The large majority of these models are induced by administration of exogenous agents in the form of noxious chemicals, bacterial products, polysaccharides or immune complexes [1–3] (Table 1). However, recent advances in genetic engineering techniques have made possible new and exciting approaches to generating models of IBD in small animals, without the use of exogenous agents (Table 1).

Several recent reports have demonstrated that targeted deletions of genes encoding for interleukin-2 [4••], interleukin-10 [5••], or certain T-cell receptor (TCR) proteins [6••] result in the spontaneous development of chronic intestinal inflammation similar to human IBD. Another genetically engineered model of chronic gut inflammation has been reported by Hammer *et al.* [7] in which they demonstrated that the introduction of HLA-B27 and human β_2-microglobulin genes into rats produces transgenic animals that develop systemic inflammatory disease. The inflammatory disorders observed in this model include intestinal and colonic lesions, arthritis, alopecia, hyperkeratosis, testicular atrophy, and myocardial lesions. These observations cor-

Abbreviations

IBD—inflammatory bowel disease; **MHC**—major histocompatibility complex; **TCR**—T-cell receptor.

 ISBN 1-85922-609-4 ISSN 0267–1379

relate well with the level of B27 expression and concur with the strong association of IBD with HLA-B27 in ankylosing spondylitis patients [8].

Table 1. Animal models of inflammatory bowel disease

Experimentally induced by exogenous agents
Acetic acid–induced colitis
Ethanol/trinitrobenzene sulfonic acid–induced colitis
Peptidoglycan/polysaccharide–induced enterocolitis
Indomethacin-induced colitis
Freunds adjuvant–induced colitis
Immune complex–induced colitis
Dextran sulfate–induced colitis
Genetically engineered
Interleukin-2–deficient mice
Interleukin-10–deficient mice
T-cell receptor–deficient mice
HLA-B27 Transgenic rate

This discussion will review the salient features of each of these models with special emphasis on incidence, clinical symptoms, severity of intestinal inflammation, and histopathology. In addition, the potential mechanisms by which the deletion or introduction of certain genes all give rise to chronic gut inflammation will also be discussed.

Interleukin-2–deficient mice

Interleukin-2 is produced by activated T cells and is proposed to be a key regulator of the immune and inflammatory responses. This cytokine appears to be intimately involved in the activation of cytotoxic responses in that it promotes T-cell proliferation and B-cell differentiation as well as activation of natural killer cells, lymphokine-activated killer cells, and macrophages [9]. A recent report [10] has demonstrated that targeted disruption of the gene that encodes for interleukin-2 in pluripotent mouse embryonic stem cells produces mice that are deficient for interleukin-2. These interleukin-2 "knockout" mice spontaneously developed an ulcerative colitis–like disease [4••]. Homozygous interleukin-2 deficient mice exhibited a 50% mortality between 4 and 9 weeks of age. Mice surviving beyond 9 weeks of age spontaneously developed IBD with an incidence of 100%. Overt signs of IBD included chronic diarrhea, bleeding, and anorectal prolapse. Death usually occurred within 10 to 25 weeks. Intestinal lesions were found to be confined almost exclusively to the large intestine with inflammation increasing in severity from proximal to distal bowel. The most severe involvement appeared to be localized in the rectum and distal colon with less intense involvement in the more proximal portions of the colon and cecum. Macroscopically, the colon appeared thick, rigid, and inflamed. Enlarged spleens and lymph nodes were also apparent.

Histologically, mucosal ulcerations were prominent, with the presence of occasional crypt abscesses. Bowel wall thickening, goblet cell depletion, inflammatory cell infiltration, disruption of the crypt architecture, and dysplasia were also evident. These interleukin-2–deficient animals also exhibited extraintestinal manifestations in the form of amyloidosis in the liver, spleen, and kidneys. Interleukin-2–deficient mice housed in a germ-free environment did not develop IBD, although at 17 to 20 weeks, histologic signs of mild inflammation were observed.

Both B- and T-cell populations in the inflamed bowel were dramatically increased above control levels at 17 weeks. During the terminal stages of the disease, B-cell populations were reduced to almost negligible levels from 22 weeks onward. T-cell populations were also dramatically reduced at 22 weeks, compared with numbers determined at 17 weeks of age. Analysis of T-cell subsets indicated that there was a relative reduction in $CD8^+$ $\alpha\beta$ TCR^+ cells. The importance of these observations in the development of chronic gut inflammation is not known because the role of $CD8^+$ TCR^+ cells in mucosal immune regulation remains controversial [11,12]. Enhanced expression of epithelial cell class II major histocompatibility complex (MHC) molecules in interleukin-2–deficient mice was also found. The absence of a pathogenic agent along with the failure of interleukin-2–deficient mice to develop IBD in a germ-free environment suggest that an abnormal immune response to the normal nonpathogenic microflora may play an important role in the pathogenesis of chronic gut inflammation in this model.

The role (or lack thereof) of interleukin-2 in human IBD remains controversial. For example, *in vitro* studies demonstrate decreased levels of interleukin-2 activity and messenger RNA expression in isolated lamina propria mononuclear cells [13,14]. The loss of interleukin-2 activity was associated with loss of interleukin-2 production by mucosal $CD4^+$ T cells [14]. In contrast, enhanced interleukin-2 secretion was found in isolated peripheral blood mononuclear cells from ulcerative colitis patients, which correlated well with disease activity [15]. Studies *in vivo* indicate enhanced secretion of interleukin-2 in IBD patients [16], although correlation with clinical activity was not comparable. The time course of interleukin-2 activity in lamina propria mononuclear cells in experimental colitis demonstrated that interleukin-2 levels were enhanced during the chronic but not acute phase [17•]. One proposed mechanism underlying IBD is that interleukin-4–producing T-helper subset 2 cells become predominant because of the loss of interleukin-2–producing $CD4^+$ cells, resulting in unregulated B-cell activity and decreased T-cell suppressor activity [18•]. The high incidence of IBD in interleukin-2–deficient mice supports a strong role for abnormal immune function contributing to the pathogenesis of IBD.

Interleukin-10–deficient mice

Interleukin-10 is produced by T-helper cell subset 2 cells and by activated Ly-1B (B-1) cells, macrophages, thymocytes, and keratinocytes [19]. Interleukin-10 enhances the expression of class II MHC molecules on the surface of murine B cells, whereas it inhibits a variety of functions of macrophages including activation, production of interleukin-1, interleukin-6, and tumor necrosis factor [20]. In addition, interleukin-10 inhibits the interferon-γ induced up-regulation of NO (nitric oxide) synthase [21].

A recent publication by Kuhn *et al.* [5••] has demonstrated that targeted mutation of the gene specific for interleukin-10 produced mice susceptible to chronic enterocolitis. The growth of these interleukin-10–deficient mice was significantly retarded exhibiting approximately a 30% reduction in bodyweight at 7 to 11 weeks of age. At this time about 90% of the mutant mice were anemic. A rapid increase in mortality (reaching 30%) between 4 to 6 weeks was also observed. Mutants surviving beyond this age developed a chronic enterocolitis affecting the entire intestinal tract. Intestinal lesions were more severe in the proximal colon, proximal jejunum, and duodenum. Marked thickening of the intestinal wall and regenerative mucosal hyperplasia was observed in the duodenum and adjoining jejunum. Histologically, branching of crypts and villi, multiple superficial erosions, and subepithelial basement membrane thickening were also observed. Inflammatory cell infiltration (plasma cells, lymphocytes, macrophages, neutrophils, giant cells, and eosinophils) of the lamina propria and submucosa was evident. No major extraintestinal manifestations were observed in these animals. Animals maintained in a defined microbiological environment (*eg*, specific pathogen-free conditions) did not develop small intestinal inflammation but instead suffered from a local colitis.

These studies demonstrated that interleukin-10 is not essential for the generation of $CD4^+$ and $CD8^+$ T or B cells because there was no significant difference in these lymphocyte populations compared with wild-type controls. This was reflected in a normal T-cell response to haptenated γ-globulin by interleukin-10–deficient mice. Because interleukin-10 is known to inhibit cytokine production by macrophages, the absence of interleukin-10 may result in uncontrolled macrophage activation and enhanced cytokine production in response to normal enteric antigens with the subsequent stimulation of T-helper and natural killer cells [5••]. Continuous overproduction of macrophage-activating cytokines such as tumor necrosis factor, interleukin-1, and interferon-γ, coupled to enhanced expression of epithelial cell class II MHC and antigen presentation, may promote epithelial cell injury. Barrier disruption would facilitate the introduction of large amounts of luminal antigens and bacterial products into the mucosal interstitium where their interactions with the mucosal lymphoid tissue would perpetuate the inflammatory response.

T-cell receptor–deficient mice

Recent studies by Mombaerts *et al.* [22,23] have demonstrated that mice with a mutation at either the TCR-α or TCR-β locus are selectively deficient in αβ T cells, whereas a mutation at the TCR-δ locus are selectively deficient in γδ T cells [24]. Furthermore, they found that by crossing TCR-β x TCR-δ, they were able to produce mice deficient in both αβ and γδ T cells [23]. Although the TCR-α and TCR-β animals appeared normal for approximately 3 to 4 months, the authors observed that the αβ T-cell–deficient mice began to gradually develop chronic diarrhea associated with anorectal prolapse and a wasting syndrome. In the terminal stages of the disease, the incidence of mortality was substantial after 6 months and only a few mice survived 1 year [6••].

Intestinal lesions affected mainly the large bowel. Macroscopically, the rectum and colon were markedly dilated and thickened. Histologically, crypt abscesses, elongation and proliferation occurred with crypt distortion observed in severe cases. Mucin-producing goblet cells were also markedly depleted and inflammatory cell infiltration within the lamina propria, and in severe cases, the muscularis mucosa and submucosa was also evident.

The major difference between these αβ T-cell mutant mice and human IBD was the absence of mucosal ulceration and fecal blood in the TCR-deficient animals. Of the 3000 αβ T-cell–deficient mice studied, only 30% of these animals actually developed diarrhea and clinical signs of IBD. Analysis of other major organs ruled out the intestinal disorder as part of a multiorgan disease. In addition to the TCR-α and TCR-β mutant mice, IBD was also found in TCR-β x δ double mutant mice and mice with a mutation in the class II MHC αβ gene [25]. No chronic gut inflammation was observed in wild-type mice nor in TCR-δ mutants, *RAG-1* (recombination-activating gene) mutant mice, or nude mice. The possibility that an infectious pathogen was responsible for the chronic gut inflammation was ruled out since housing mice such as the *RAG-1* mutant mouse (deficient in both T and B cells) in the same environment as αβ TCR-deficient mice did not result in chronic gut inflammation. Furthermore, the immunodeficient mice were found to be free of microorganisms known to be pathogenic for mice.

The mechanisms by which targeted deletions of genes specific for certain TCR genes promote chronic inflammatory bowel disease in mice remain to be elucidated. One feature that appears common to all of these immunodeficient mice that eventually develop IBD is that they possess B cells but no class II MHC-restricted $CD4^+$ αβ T cells. It would appear that the absence of αβ T cells, and not B cells, is a prerequisite for generation of IBD, because *RAG-1* mutant mice that are deficient in T and B cells do not develop IBD.

Mombaerts *et al.* [6••] suggest that the chronic gut inflammation in these mice is caused by the inappropriate control of B cells, which may be due to the lack of the interleukin-2 producing class II MHC-restricted $CD4^+$ αβ T cells. Indeed, as described previously, Sadlack *et al.* [4••] have demonstrated that interleukin-2–deficient mice develop spontaneous IBD. Furthermore, Kusugami *et al.* [14] have demonstrated a loss of interleukin-2–producing $CD4^+$ T cells in gut obtained from human IBD [14]. Thus, the absence of αβ T-cell suppression of B-cell activity by whatever mechanism may lead to subsequent autoimmunity to epithelial cell constituents or cross-reactive bacterial products and promotion of gut inflammation.

Transgenic HLA-B27 rats

Several kinds of human diseases have an association with class 1 or class 2 alleles of the HLA complex. Among them, HLA-B27, a serologically defined class 1 MHC allele, is known to have a striking association with inflammatory human disorders including ankylosing spondylitis, reactive arthritis, juvenile spondyloarthropathy, psoriatic arthropathy, and enteropathic arthropathy [26–28]. Recently, Hammer *et al.* [7] have developed transgenic rats expressing the HLA-B27 and human β_2 microglobulin genes that have been found to spontaneously develop inflammatory disease that includes most of the clinical and pathologic features of B27-associated disorders in humans. These HLA-B27 rats present with inflammation of the gut, male genital tract, nails, skin, heart, and peripheral and axial joints.

Hammer *et al.* [7] report that the most prevalent site of inflammation in the transgenic rats appeared to be localized within the gastrointestinal tract and the most common and persistent finding was diarrhea. They also report that overt gastrointestinal inflammation affects 100% of the transgenic rats that survived beyond 10 weeks. The most common observation was the development of watery diarrhea and loose stools that developed in 100% of animals at 3 months of age and occurred in both males and females. Histologic inspection of the tissue revealed chronic inflammation of the stomach, small intestine, and colon with the severity of inflammation occurring to a much greater extent in the colon than the other organ systems. The inflammatory infiltrate consisted of large and small lymphocytes (commonly aggregated into lymphoid foci), plasma cells, and eosinophils that were confined primarily to the lamina propria but occasionally extended into the submucosa in severe cases of inflammation. Hyperplasia of crypt epithelial cells was also a common finding. Interestingly, neither crypt destruction nor crypt abscesses were observed to significant degree in these animals. As with the other genetically engineered models of gut inflammation, a contagious pathogen did not appear responsible for the chronic inflammation as no pathogen could be cultured from the transgenic animals expressing IBD. Furthermore, other transgenic rats and normal Lewis rats maintained in the same cages and environment as the HLA-B27 rats did not develop the spontaneous IBD.

In addition to chronic gastrointestinal inflammation, HLA-B27 rats developed significant peripheral and axial joint inflammation. Hammer *et al.* [7] found that approximately 70% of the males and only 10% of the females developed this arthritic condition, which was characterized by swelling, erythema, and tenderness of the tarsal joints of one or both hindlimbs. They reported that the arthritis persisted for a few days to several weeks and occasionally exhibited an undulating pattern of remission and exacerbations. A preliminary study suggests that HLA-B27 rats maintained in strict germ-free conditions have a much attenuated IBD and arthritis [29].

We have recently completed a series of experiments using commercially available HLA-B27 transgenic male rats as well as their littermate controls (GenPharm International, Mountain View, CA). Animals were obtained at 8 weeks of age, housed in a conventional rodent facility, and observed for clinical symptoms of colitis and arthritis until the age of 30 weeks (Aiko and Grisham, Unpublished observations.) In contrast to what was originally published by Hammer *et al.* [7], we found that diarrhea occurred in only five of 10 HLA-B27 transgenic males beginning at the age of 17 weeks. In addition, the incidence of peripheral arthritis was also substantially less than originally reported, with only three of 10 transgenic rats developing arthritis. No arthritis was observed in those HLA-B27 rats that did not develop colitis nor in their litter mate controls. The arthritis was manifested in all cases by swelling and erythema of a single hindleg, which persisted for 3 to 4 days and then disappeared.

Macroscopically, the most characteristic finding in the gastrointestinal system in the transgenic rats was colonic dilatation and bowel wall thickening, especially of the proximal colon (Aiko and Grisham, Unpublished observations). Mucosal lesions such as erosions and ulcerations were not present in the stomach, ileum, or colon of any transgenic animal. Blood-to-lumen clearance of ^{51}Cr-EDTA, gastrointestinal myeloperoxidase activity, and plasma nitrate and nitrite levels were measured and used to quantify gastrointestinal mucosal permeability (epithelial integrity), gastrointestinal inflammation, and NO production, respectively. We found that there were no significant increases in mucosal permeability in either the stomach, ileum, or colon when compared with littermate controls. However, myeloperoxidase activity of the stomach and colon was significantly higher in transgenic rats with clinical signs of IBD (diarrhea) than in littermate controls (Fig. 1). Myeloperoxidase activity in the

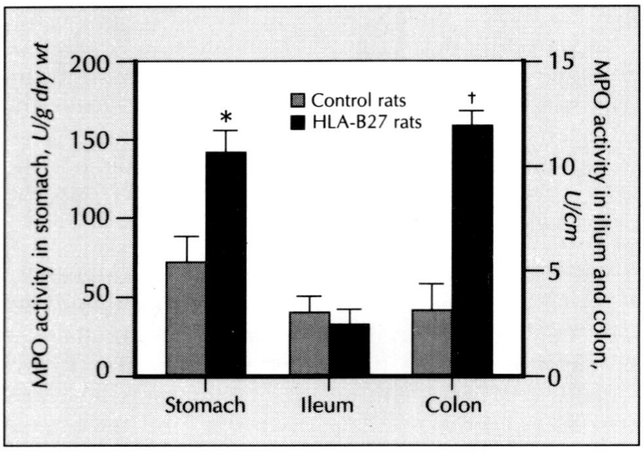

Fig. 1. Myeloperoxidase (MPO) activity in the stomach, ileum and colon in control and HLA-B27 rats. Gastrointestinal tissue was obtained from healthy controls (n=5) and transgenic (n=5) rats that developed chronic diarrhea and assayed for MPO activity. MPO activity correlates well with granulocyte infiltration into the tissues. *Asterisk* indicates $P<0.05$; *dagger* indicates $P<0.01$.

ileum was not significantly different than that found in controls (Fig. 1). Plasma levels of nitrate and nitrite and the stable decomposition products of NO were also significantly higher (fourfold) in those transgenic animals that developed diarrhea than in healthy control rats (Fig. 2). These results suggest that granulocyte (neutrophils, eosinophils, and monocytes) infiltration is prominent in the stomach as well as the colon. Histologic inspection of the tissue appears to confirm this finding. In addition, these inflammatory cells in the gastrointestinal tract may be the major source of NO in the transgenic rats. It is becoming increasingly apparent that the chronic gut inflammation associated with human IBD is accompanied by enhanced NO metabolism [30,31,32•–34•]. Whether or not NO plays an important role in mediating or exacerbating gut inflammation remains to be defined. The reasons for the relatively low incidence of chronic gastrointestinal and joint inflammation in this study are not known.

Although the molecular mechanisms by which addition of the HLA-B27/human$\beta_2$microglobulin genes promote chronic gastrointestinal and joint inflammation have not been delineated, there is some suggestion that HLA-B27 and bacterial products may interact to promote some types of chronic inflammation, such as arthritis. One hypothesis proposes that HLA-B27 is the element that presents bacterial antigen to disease-causing T lymphocytes [35]. Indeed, presentation of antigenic peptides to T lymphocytes is the physiologic function of HLA class I molecules [36]. A second hypothesis proposes that HLA-B27 antigens act as receptors for factors released by organisms that produce arthritis [37]. Finally, it has been proposed that there is molecular mimicry or cross-reactivity between HLA-B27 and some epitope on arthritis-causing bacteria [38,39]. A recent report [40] suggests that B27 need not be expressed in nonmarrow-derived elements in the thymus, or in sites of disease such as intestinal mucosa, synovium, or skin in order for B27-mediated disease in rats to be induced at these sites. These results may provide clues to develop new directions to elucidate the pathogenesis of B27-associated multiorgan disease.

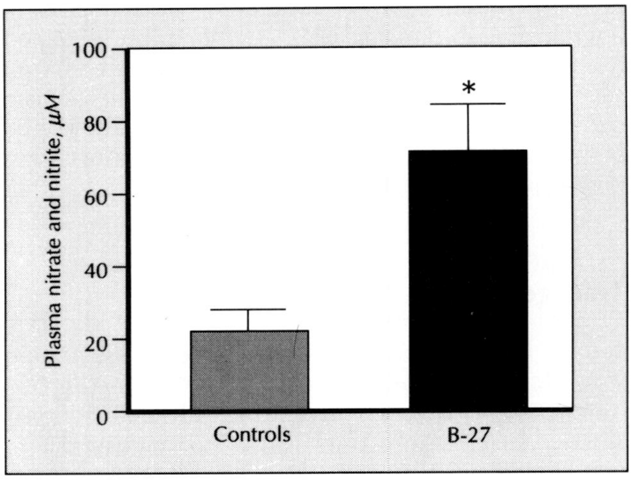

Fig. 2. Plasma nitrate and nitrite levels. Fasted plasma was obtained from healthy controls ($n=5$) and transgenic ($n=5$) rats that developed chronic diarrhea. Nitrate and nitrite are the stable decomposition products of nitric oxide. *Asterisk* indicates $P<0.001$.

The aforementioned model of IBD possesses three major advantages over our presently used model of chronic granulomatous colitis [32•] or the more common chemically induced models of colitis used by our laboratory and others [41]. First, no exogenous bacterial product (or noxious chemical) is required for the induction of gastrointestinal inflammation. Second, the time-consuming and tedious nature of survival surgery is not required. Finally, the inflammation is chronic, thereby allowing for observations over a relatively long period of time without the problem of spontaneous resolution of the inflammation that occurs in virtually all rodent models of colitis. The major disadvantages of this model are the high cost of the animals (approximately $300 per rat), the long time required to house these animals until colitis develops (4 to 5 months), and the relatively low incidence of gastrointestinal inflammation and arthritis, all of which increase substantially the effective cost of each animal well beyond the initial investment of $300 per rat. Nevertheless, HLA-B27 transgenic rats represent an interesting model that may provide new and important information on the pathogenesis of IBD and other multiorgan inflammatory disorders.

Conclusions

The recent development of several different genetically engineered models of IBD in rodents has revealed some important clues to our understanding of how uncontrolled regulation of the immune system may promote chronic gut inflammation. These studies demonstrate that deletions or additions of specific genes that appear, at least superficially, unrelated promote IBD in mice and rats. Strober and Ehrhardt [18••] have described the concept that homeostatic regulation of the mucosal immune system is dependent on a "delicate balance between the ability to react to the presence of potential gut pathogens and the ability not to react with common, ubiquitous gut constituents."

It has been suggested that an uncontrolled (or inappropriate) response to naturally occurring luminal antigens or bacterial products may lead to chronic gut inflammation and may represent an important pathogenetic mechanism in human IBD. Although it is still too early (and probably unrealistic) to propose one hypothesis to account for the chronic gut inflammation observed in these genetically engineered models, two important concepts appear to have emerged from these studies. One concept that has been proposed in the past and strengthened by the recent experiments involving the interleukin-2–, interleukin-10–, and TCR-deficient mice is the important role that T cells play in regulating B-cell responses. These studies demonstrate that unrestrained B-cell responses promote chronic gut inflammation.

A second concept that has emerged from the studies using the interleukin-2– and interleukin-10–deficient mice, as well as the HLA-B27 rats is the importance of endogenous luminal bacteria in promoting or exacerbating chronic gut inflammation. The importance of luminal constituents is supported by the fact that very different defects in the immune system may lead, in many cases, only to gut mucosal inflammation suggesting that the gut mucosa is subjected to substantially more antigenic "stress" by luminal constituents than are other tissues. Taken together, these studies offer new and exciting avenues of research for the study of the pathogenesis of IBD, as well as providing new and possibly more appropriate models for the development and testing of new therapeutic agents for the treatment of IBD.

Acknowledgments

Some of the work reported in this manuscript was supported by grants from the National Institutes of Health (DK43785; Project 6 and DK47663).

References and recommended reading

Papers of particular interest, published within the annual period of review, have been highlighted as:
• Of special interest
•• Of outstanding interest

1. Grisham MB: **Animal Models of Inflammatory Bowel Disease.** *Curr Opin Gastroenterol* 1993, 9:524–533.

2. Sartor RB: **Animal Models of Intestinal Inflammation: Relevance to Inflammatory Bowel Disease.** In *Inflammatory Bowel Disease.* Edited by MacDermott RP, Stenson WF. New York: Elsevier; 1992: 332–353.

3. Stenson WF: **Animal Models of Inflammatory Bowel Disease.** In *Inflammatory Bowel Disease: From Bench to Bedside.* Edited by Targan SR, Shanahan F. Baltimore: Williams and Wilkins; 1994: 180–192.

4. •• Sadlack B, Merz H, Schorle H, Schimpl A, Feller AC, Horak I: **Ulcerative Colitis-Like Disease in Mice With a Disrupted Interleukin-2 Gene.** *Cell* 1993, **75**:253–261.

This study describes an IBD in interleukin-2–deficient mice with striking clinical and histologic similarities to human ulcerative colitis. A primary role for the immune system in the etiology of ulcerative colitis is suggested.

5. •• Kuhn R, Lohler J, Rennick D, Rajewsky K, Muller W: **Interleukin-10-Deficient Mice Develop Chronic Enterocolitis.** *Cell* 1993, **75**:263–274.

The chronic enterocolitis that develops in interleukin-10–deficient mice was attenuated in a specific pathogen-free environment, suggesting that an uncontrolled immune response to enteric antigens may precipitate IBD.

6. •• Mombaerts P, Mizoguchi E, Grusby MJ, Glimcher LH, Bhan AK, Tonegawa S: **Spontaneous Development of Inflammatory Bowel Disease in T Cell Receptor Mutant Mice.** *Cell* 1993, **75**:275–282.

These studies implicate a role for certain T-cell subsets in the pathogenesis of IBD.

7. Hammer RE, Maika SD, Richardson JA, Tang J, Taurog JD: **Spontaneous Inflammatory Disease in Transgenic Rats Expressing HLA-B27 and Human β2m: An Animal Model of HLA-B27-Associated Human Disorders.** *Cell* 1990, **63**:1099–1112.

8. Mielants H, Veys E, Cuvelier C, De Vos M, Botelberghe L: **HLA-B27 Related Arthritis and Bowel Inflammation. Part 2. Ileocolonoscopy and Bowel Histology in Patients With HLA-B27 Related Arthritis.** *J Rheumatol* 1985, **12**:293–298.

9. Smith KA: **Interleukin-2.** *Curr Opin Immunol* 1992, 4:271–276.

10. Schorle H, Holtschke T, Hunig T, Schimpl A, Horak I: **Development and Function of T Cells in Mice Rendered IL-2 Deficient by Gene Targeting.** *Nature* 1991, **352**:621–624.

11. Fujihashi K, Taguchi T, McGhee JR, Eldridge JH, Bruce MG, Green DR, Singh B, Kiyono H: **Regulatory Function for Murine Epithelial Lymphocytes.** *J Immunol* 1990, **145**:2010–2019.

12. Hoang P, Dalton HR, Jewell DP: **Human Colonic Intraepithelial Lymphocytes Are Suppressor Cells.** *Clin Exp Immunol* 1991, **85**:498–503.

13. Fiocchi C, Hilfiker ML, Youngman KR, Deorder NC, Finke JH: **Interleukin-2 Activity of Human Intestinal Mucosal Mononuclear Cells: Decreased Levels of Inflammatory Bowel Disease.** *Gastroenterology* 1984, **86**:734–742.

14. Kusugami K, Matsuura T, West GA, Youngman KR, Rachmilewitz D, Fiocchi C: **Loss of Interleukin-2 Producing Intestinal CD4+ T Cells in Inflammatory Bowel Disease.** *Gastroenterology* 1991, **101**:1594–1605.

15. Mullin GE, Lazenby AJ, Harris ML, Bayless TM, James SP: **Increased Interleukin-2 Messenger RNA in the Intestinal Mucosal Lesions of Crohn's Disease but Not Ulcerative Colitis.** *Gastroenterology* 1992, **102**:1620–1627.

16. Brynskov J, Trede N, Andersen CB, Vilien M: **Increased Concentrations of Interleukin-1B, Interleukin-2, and Soluble Interleukin-2 Receptor in Endoscopical Mucosal Biopsy Specimens With Active Inflammatory Bowel Disease.** *Gut* 1992, **33**:55–58.

17. • Gurbindo C, Russo P, Sabbah S, Lohoues M-J, Seidman E: **Interleukin-2 Activity of Colonic Lamina Propria Mononuclear Cells in a Rat Model of Experimental Colitis.** *Gastroenterology* 1993, **104**:964–972.

This study demonstrates that interleukin-2 levels are significantly increased during the chronic, but not acute, phase of experimental colitis, indicating the variability of interleukin-2 production depending on the seventy and duration of inflammation.

18. • Strober W, Ehrhardt RO: **Chronic Intestinal Inflammation: An Unexpected Outcome in Cytokine or T Cell Receptor Mutant Mice.** *Cell* 1993, **75**:203–205.

Provides an excellent overview of the newer, genetically engineered mouse models of IBD.

19. Moore KW, O'Garra A, de Waal Maelfyt R, Vieira P, Mosmann TR: **Interleukin-10.** *Ann Rev Immunol* 1993, **11**:165–190.

20. Fiorentino DF, Zlotnik A, Vieira P, Mosmann TR, Howard M, Moore KW, O'Garra A: **IL-10 Acts on the Antigen-Presenting Cell to Inhibit Cytokine Production by Th1 Cells.** *J Immunol* 1991, **146**:3444–3451.

21. Gazzinelli RT, Oswald IP, James SL, Sher A: **IL-10 Inhibits Parasite Killing and Nitric Oxide Production by IFN-γ-activated Macrophages.** *J Immunol* 1992, **148**:1792–1796.

22. Mombaerts P, Clarke AR, Hooper ML, Tonegawa S: **Creation of a Large Genomic Deletion at the T-Cell Antigen Receptor β Subunit Locus in Mouse Embryonic Stem Cells by Gene Targeting.** *Proc Natl Acad Sci U S A* 1991, **88**:3084–3087.

23. Mombaerts P, Clarke AR, Rudnicki MA, Iacomini J, Itohara I, Lafaille JJ, Wang L, Ichikawa Y, Jaenisch R, Hooper ML, Tonegawa S: **Mutations in T-Cell Antigen Receptor Genes α and β Block Thymocyte Development at Different Stages.** *Nature* 1992, **360**:225–231.

24. Itohara S, Mombaerts P, Lafaille J, Iacomini J, Nelson A, Clarke AR, Hooper ML, Farr A, Tonegawa S: **T Cell Receptor δ Gene Mutant Mice: Independent Generation of αβ T Cells and Programmed Rearrangements of γδ TCR Genes.** *Cell* 1993, **72**:337–348.

25. Grusby MJ, Johnson RS, Papaionannou VE, Glimcher LH: **Depletion of CD4+ T Cells in Major Histocompatibility Complex Class II-Deficient Mice.** *Science* 1991, **253**:1417–1420.

26. Schlosstein L, Terasaki PI, Bluestone R, Pearson CM: **High Association of an HL-A Antigen, W27, With Ankylosing Spondylitis.** *N Engl J Med* 1973, **5**:704–706.

27. Brewerton DA, Caffrey M, Nicholls A, Walters D, Oates JK, James DCO: **Reiter's Disease and HL-A 27.** *Lancet* 1973, **3**:996–998.

28. Carpenter CB: **The Major Histocompatibility Gene Complex.** In *Harrison's Principles of Internal Medicine.* Edited by Wilson JD, Braunwalt E, Fauci AS, Isselbacher KJ, Martin JB, Petersdorf RG, Root RK. New York: McGraw-Hill; 1990: 86–92.

29. Taurog JD, Hammer RE, Montanez S, Hadavand R, Breban M, Croft JT, Balish E: **Effect of the Germfree State on the Inflammatory Disease of HLA-B27 Transgenic Rats: A Split Result [Abstract].** *Am Coll Rheum 57th Annual Meeting* 1993: S46.

30. Hegesh E, Shiloah J: **Blood Nitrate and Infantile Methemoglobinemia.** *Clin Chim Acta* 1982, **125**:107–115.

31. Roediger WEW, Lawson MJ, Nance SH, Radcliffe BC: **Detectable Colonic Nitrite Levels in Inflammatory Bowel Disease - Mucosal or Bacterial Malfunction?** *Digestion* 1986, **35**:199–204.

32. • Yamada T, Sartor RB, Marshall S, Specian RD, Grisham MB: **Mucosal Injury and Inflammation in a Chronic Granulomatous Colitis in Rats.** *Gastroenterology* 1993, **104**:759–771.

The colitis produced by submucosal injection of bacterial polymers is similar to Crohn's disease and is characterized by enhanced NO production.

33. • Middleton SJ, Shorthouse M, Hunter JO: **Increased Nitric Oxide Synthesis in Ulcerative Colitis.** *Lancet* 1993, **341**:465–466.

Suggests that immune cell–derived NO may have a pathogenic role in ulcerative colitis.

34. • Boughton-Smith NK, Evans SM, Hawkey CJ, Cole AT, Balsitis M, Whittle BJR, Moncada S: **Nitric Oxide Synthase Activity in Ulcerative Colitis and Crohn's Disease.** *Lancet* 1993, **342**:338–340.

Increase in NO synthase activity in ulcerative colitis but not Crohn's disease may be involved in mucosal vasodilation and increased vascular permeability.

35. Yu DT, Choo SY, Schaack T: **Molecular Mimicry in HLA-B27-Related Arthritis.** *Ann Intern Med* 1989, **111**:581–591.

36. Sprent J, Schaefer M: **Antigen Presenting Cells for CD8+ T Cells.** *Immunol Rev* 1990, **117**:213–234.

37. Taurog JD, Maika SD, Simmons WA, Breban M, Hammer RE: **Susceptibility to Inflammatory Disease in HLA-B27 Transgenic Rat Lines Correlates with the Level of B27 Expression.** *J Immunol* 1993, **150**:4168–4178.

38. Raybourne RB, Williams KM: **Monoclonal Antibodies Against an HLA-B27-Derived Peptide React With an Epitope Present on Bacterial Proteins.** *J Immunol* 1990, **145**:2539–2544.

39. Stieglitz H, Fosmire S, Lipsky P: **Identification of a 2-Md Plasmid From Shigella flexneri Associated With Reactive Arthritis.** *Arthritis Rheum* 1989, **32**:937–946.

40. Breban M, Hammer RE, Richardson JA, Taurog JD: **Transfer of the Inflammatory Disease of Bone Marrow Engraftment.** *J Exp Med* 1993, **178**:1607–1616.

41. Yamada T, Marshall S, Specian RD, Grisham MB: **A Comparative Analysis of Two Models of Colitis in Rats.** *Gastroenterology* 1992, **102**:1524–1534.

Matthew Grisham, PhD, Department of Physiology, LSU Medical Center, 1501 Kings Highway, Shreveport, LA 71130, USA.

Cell-mediated immunity and mucosal immunity

George T. Fantry, MD, and Stephen P. James, MD

University of Maryland at Baltimore and Department of Veterans Affairs, Baltimore, Maryland, USA

Studies of intraepithelial lymphocytes have shown that these cells have specialized characteristics and functions. Although their function is uncertain *in vivo,* they appear to have the potential to function as regulatory or cytolytic cells in response to a limited array of antigens. There have been no convincing abnormalities of these cells in inflammatory bowel disease (IBD). The most important advance in basic immunology in IBD has been the observation of spontaneous colitis or enterocolitis in mice having experimentally induced genetic deficiencies of cytokines or T-cell receptors. Further studies in human IBD have shown that there are some differences in the cytokine profile in Crohn's disease and ulcerative colitis, consistent with differences in underlying pathogenesis. Adhesion molecules are important for entry of lymphoid cells into sites of inflammation and may serve as potential targets for immunotherapy in IBD. The relevance of antineutrophil antibodies to the pathogenesis of IBD remains unclear. Further work suggests that IBD may be associated with HLA genes. One potential colon epithelial cell autoantigen has been identified in ulcerative colitis.

Current Opinion in Gastroenterology 1994, **10:**365–373

Intraepithelial and lamina propria lymphocyte function

Intraepithelial lymphocytes

Lymphocytes in the intestinal mucosa appear to be intimately involved in the pathogenesis of inflammatory bowel disease (IBD) and their function in the normal and diseased mucosa continues to be an area of active investigation. T cells located in the epithelium (intraepithelial lymphocytes) are a relatively homogeneous population of cells, suggesting that they have very specialized functions, although at the moment their physiologic role is still uncertain. Intraepithelial lymphocytes in humans are nearly all CD8 positive, have a large granular lymphocyte morphology, (which suggests they are activated), express the CD45RO antigen found on memory cells, have cytolytic potential *in vitro,* and are capable of producing cytokines *in vitro.* Although a significant proportion of intraepithelial lymphocytes in humans express the γ,δ T-cell receptor (of interest because cells with these receptors are found primarily in the intestinal epithelium), the majority of cells have α,β T-cell receptors.

Blumberg *et al.* [1•] investigated the T-cell receptor repertoire of human jejunal intraepithelial lymphocytes from patients without intestinal disease and found evidence that the majority of intraepithelial lymphocytes are derived from a relatively small number of T-cell clones, but that a large number of different V beta genes can be used by these cells. The fact that these cells seem to have undergone oligoclonal expansion suggests that these cells have a relatively limited repertoire for antigens, and therefore their role as a specific primary recognition system for host defense against pathogens remains questionable.

Because of their location in the epithelium, the possible interactions of intraepithelial lymphocytes and epithelial cells have been studied, both with regard to potential effects on both the epithelium and lymphocytes. Previously, it has been shown that intestinal epithelial cells can stimulate proliferation of CD8 T cells in an mixed lymphocyte reaction. In an extension of these studies, Panja *et al.* [2] have now shown that antibodies against CD1d, a nonpolymorphic major histocompatibility complex molecule expressed primarily on intestinal epithelial cells, blocks, and epithelial cell–lymphocyte mixed lymphocyte reaction. These results suggest the possibility that CD1d may play a significant and potentially unique role in activation of intraepithelial lymphocytes. Studies of murine in-

Abbreviations

ADCC—antibody-dependent cellular toxicity; **ANCA**—antineutrophil cytoplasmic antibody; **IBD**—inflammatory bowel disease; **TNF**—tumor necrosis factor.

ISBN 1-85922-609-4 ISSN 0267–1379

traepithelial lymphocytes provide further evidence that these cells may carry out relatively restricted functions. Fujihashi *et al.* [3,4] have demonstrated that α,β-positive intraepithelial lymphocytes produce a Th2 pattern of cytokines, indicating that they may provide help for B-cell antibody production in the underlying lamina propria. Further studies in mice confirm that γ,δ-bearing intraepithelial lymphocytes may be a special lineage that is T-cell independent, having specialized activation requirements and potential for cytolytic function [5–8].

Because of the considerable difficulty in obtaining sufficient quantities of human intraepithelial lymphocytes for study, few studies have investigated their function in IBD. Prior murine studies have suggested that intraepithelial lymphocytes may have a role in regulating the function of lamina propria B cells through production of cytokines [3,4]. Sachdev *et al.* [9] carried out studies of the immunoregulatory potential of isolated human intraepithelial lymphocytes by determining whether they could alter production of immunoglobulins by autologous peripheral blood or lamina propria lymphocytes *in vitro*. Intraepithelial lymphocytes from both control subjects and patients with IBD inhibited the spontaneous production of total immunoglobulin, and in particular immunoglobulin A *in vitro*. The inhibitory activity appeared to be due to a soluble factor, although this was not identified in the study. However, there was no significant difference comparing controls with patients having IBD. These findings suggest that intraepithelial lymphocytes may have the potential to down-regulate immunoglobulin production *in vivo*; however, the significance of these observations requires further study. It is unclear whether the inhibitory activity occurs because of antigen-specific triggering or is a nonspecific effect of these cells. Furthermore, although abnormal regulation of antibody production may be important in ulcerative colitis, at this point it is very unclear whether abnormal production of antibodies is of primary pathologic significance in Crohn's disease.

In another study, the same group of investigators evaluated antigen- and mitogen-induced proliferation of allogeneic peripheral blood lymphocytes and found that intraepithelial lymphocytes from patients with IBD had a diminished ability to inhibit proliferation [10]. This observation suggested that patients with IBD may have a defective ability to inhibit proliferative responses on the underlying lamina propria lymphocytes. Again, the significance of this observation is uncertain: the test system used is artificial in that allogeneic co-cultures were used. Furthermore, relatively few lymphocytes in the lamina propria appear to undergo cell division either in the normal physiologic state or in IBD, so that the significance of diminished inhibition of proliferation to the pathogenesis of IBD is at the moment unclear. As in all studies of this nature, it remains difficult to determine whether the abnormality is a primary one or secondary to the inflammatory process. Nonetheless, these observations, together with previous observations that the epithelial cell–lymphocyte mixed lymphocyte reaction may be abnormal in IBD, suggest that abnormal function of intraepithelial lymphocytes could play a role in IBD.

Lymphocyte cytotoxicity

As indicated above, previous studies have suggested that intraepithelial lymphocytes have cytolytic function. Roberts *et al.* [11] studied the spontaneous cytolytic function of normal human intraepithelial lymphocytes using a panel of target cells and found that although these cells had low cytotoxicity against the conventional natural killer target K562, they did have cytotoxicity against other cell lines such as epithelial tumor cells. Furthermore, specific antibodies against intraepithelial lymphocyte cell surface antigens such as HML-1 blocked cytotoxicity. These studies show that there are important differences in the cytolytic function of intraepithelial lymphocytes compared with that of circulating lymphocytes.

Rüthlein *et al.* [12] examined spontaneous and antibody (anti-CD2 or CD3, so-called *redirected cytotoxicity*) or mitogen-induced cytotoxicity using human intraepithelial lymphocytes and lamina propria lymphocytes. Although lamina propria lymphocytes had both spontaneous and antibody-induced cytotoxicity as previously described, intraepithelial lymphocytes had only antibody-induced cytotoxicity. Furthermore, patients with both inflammatory disease (diverticulitis) and IBD had diminished induced cytotoxicity. These observations indicate that human intraepithelial lymphocytes might not be efficient cytolytic cells; furthermore, it suggests that decreased cytotoxicity may simply reflect a non-selective effect of inflammatory disease. Interestingly, similar conclusions have been reached in the past based on studies of circulating lymphocytes in IBD and nonspecific spontaneous cytotoxicity.

Van Tol *et al.* [13] reached conclusions somewhat at odds with this study. They examined spontaneous cytotoxicity of lamina propria mononuclear cells against K562 and Caco-2 target cells in a relatively large number of subjects. Cytotoxicity was found in all patient groups, including IBD. However, when patients with IBD were stratified according to Crohn's disease or ulcerative colitis, patients with Crohn's disease had higher spontaneous cytotoxicity and patients with ulcerative colitis had lower spontaneous cytotoxicity. These observations suggest that there may be significant, although subtle, differences in cytotoxic function of intestinal lymphocytes in IBD. Unfortunately, in this study there was no attempt to prove the identity of the cytotoxic cells or to determine whether the mechanisms of the differences. As indicated further on, differences in the cytokine environment of the mucosa in Crohn's disease and ulcerative colitis might account for differences in nonspecific cytotoxic function. Finally, whether spontaneous cytotoxicity against tumor target cells *in vitro* is a relevant physiologic immune function is unclear.

Although spontaneous cytotoxicity may or may not be relevant in IBD, another mechanism of cellular cytotoxicity that could be mediated by the same cellular population (natural killer cells) is antibody-dependent cellular cytotoxicity (ADCC). Thus, in the presence of relevant anticellular antibodies, these cells could mediate injury. Hibi *et al.* [14] examined the effect of cytokines on ADCC. The *in vitro* system was potentially IBD relevant in that sera from patients with IBD and anticolon antibodies were used as a source of antibodies, and a colon cancer cell line was used as the target cell. Normal peripheral blood lymphocytes were used as the effector cells. In this system, interleukin-2 enhanced the effector function of cytolytic cells, as would be expected based on prior work. Interestingly, interferon-γ treatment of target cells enhanced their susceptibility to lysis, possibly due to up-regulation of the adhesin intercellular adhesion molecule-1. Finally, prednisolone inhibited this form of cytotoxicity. These interesting studies again reveal the potential that ADCC could be a relevant mechanism in IBD, particularly in ulcerative colitis, as has been suggested for many years. Furthermore, the study illustrates how cytokines and therapeutic agents could modulate the cytotoxicity. Again, the difficult problem has been to find experimental systems that indicate that this form of injury occurs *in vivo* in IBD.

Many studies concerning the role of lymphocyte mediated cytotoxicity in IBD have been flawed by the failure to use relevant potential target cells that are necessary to study the question as to whether there is antigen-specific T-cell–mediated cytotoxic tissue injury in IBD. This is largely due to the considerable difficulty of obtaining and maintaining autologous human epithelial cells. Ten years ago, Shorter *et al.* [15] described cytotoxicity of circulating lymphocytes from patients with IBD against autologous epithelial cells, but it was concluded that this form of cytotoxicity was mediated by natural killer cells, not T cells. The question of T-cell cytotoxicity against autologous epithelial cells has been reexamined by Okazaki *et al.* [16•] using more recently developed methods to examine cytotoxicity. In this study, there is evidence that circulating lymphocytes have higher cytotoxic activity against autologous intestinal epithelial cells than allogeneic epithelial cells, and that this cytotoxicity is mediated predominantly by CD8 T cells. However, there are important limitations of this study. Most importantly, lymphocyte cytotoxic activity against autologous epithelial cells from control subjects was not presented, and it is unclear whether this form of cytotoxicity is specific for IBD. Furthermore, it could not be shown that there was any clear relationship to the activity of disease. Thus, although this represents a better approach to trying to determine whether there is T-cell–mediated cytolytic injury against epithelial cells in IBD, the question remains far from resolved.

Role of cytokines and other mediators

Genetically altered animal models with intestinal inflammation

One of the most important advances in IBD research has been the observation that genetically altered animals spontaneously develop gastrointestinal disease. These observations, which were largely unexpected, provide important new insights into possible mechanisms of inflammation in the gastrointestinal tract in IBD.

The human HLA-B27 allele is strongly associated with the spondyloarthropathy syndrome, and proof that the product of this gene plays a direct role in the disease has been obtained in rats that are transgenic for human HLA-B27. These animals develop multisystem inflammatory disease, resembling the human disease, including inflammatory disease of joints, skin, genital tract, and heart. Interestingly, these animals also develop a severe panenteritis. The most recent advance in this model system was the demonstration by Breban *et al.* [17••] that the disease could be transferred to nontransgenic rats with stem cells, but not with mature spleen or lymph node cells. This finding indicates that the critical element in the disease expression is the presence of the transgene on a stem cell, possibly antigen-presenting cells. It is considered very likely that the presence of this specific gene in the presence of specific environmental antigens, most likely intestinal bacterial flora antigens, is the essential trigger for the disease. Further work in this field will undoubtedly provide more insight into the mechanisms of HLA-B27 disease, and possibly provide clues to the genetic associations in IBD.

Mombaerts *et al.* [18••], in carrying out immunologic studies of T-cell–deficient and major histocompatability complex–deficient mice, observed that many animals failed to thrive and in particular this was associated with the presence of colitis. Many different strains of mice were studied, and the common elements that seemed to correlate with colitis were the presence of B cells and the absence of mature CD4 T cells. Animals with deficiency of γ,δ cells or severe combined immunodeficiency did not develop colitis. This observation is consistent with current theories of pathogenesis of human ulcerative colitis that inadequately down-regulated activity of the immune system, including B cells, may play a role in the disease.

Sadlack *et al.* [19••] also found the unexpected observation of spontaneous colitis in a completely different model. These investigators disrupted the interleukin-2 gene and produced animals completely deficient in this lymphokine (interleukin-2 "knockout" animals). These animals have demonstrable T-cell functional defects, but surprisingly the most important abnormality that they seem to have is a spontaneous, hemorrhagic inflammatory colitis associated with anticolon antibodies. There is no evidence for a specific infectious etiology for colitis in these animals, but germ-free animals have little clinical evidence of intestinal disease. These important observations suggest that deficiency of interleukin-2, particularly in the gastrointestinal mucosa, in the presence of a normal flora, results in uncontrolled inflammation that resembles ulcerative colitis.

Another unexpected and different pattern of intestinal inflammation was observed in interleukin-10–deficient animals in studies of Kühn *et al.* [20••]. These animals had a panenterocolitis that was also much less severe in a specific pathogen-free environment. The immunodeficiency of these animals is distinctly different from interleukin-2–deficient animals, in that the interleukin-10–deficient animals mounted an aberrant TH1-type response, rather than a Th2-type response to the parasite *Nipposteongylus brasiliensis.*

These exciting animal models are distinctly different from human IBD, in which profound deficiency of T cells, interleukin-2, or interleukin-10 does not occur. However, the models indicate that multiple events, presumably a combination of immunologic, environmental, bacterial and genetic, that shift the normal balance of immune regulation in the gut can result in ulcerative colitis–like lesions or a panenteritis-like lesions [21••,22,23]. These models provide potential new clues to examine pathogenic mechanisms in human disease. As discussed in part below, emerging new data on cytokine regulation in human IBD suggests that ulcerative colitis and Crohn's disease are distinctly different.

Interleukin-2 and interleukin-2 receptors

The intestinal lamina propria contains a mixed population of T cells and B cells that are more differentiated compared with circulating lymphocytes and have a variety of functions, including cytokine production, help for B-cell activation, cytolytic function, and antibody synthesis. Previous studies in IBD have shown evidence of activation of all immune cells in the lamina propria in IBD, including T cells, B cells, and macrophages. Matsuura *et al.* [24•] carefully examined the expression of interleukin-2 and the interleukin-2 receptor α- and β-chains using both RNA and protein assays. Using purified lymphocytes isolated from surgical specimens, resting lymphocytes had very low expression of interleukin-2; following *in vitro* activation, lamina propria cells from normal individuals had very high interleukin-2 production compared with peripheral blood lymphocytes, and consistent with previous studies from the same laboratory, levels of interleukin-2 produced by stimulated intestinal lymphocytes were lower using cells from both Crohn's disease and ulcerative colitis patients. In contrast, IBD mucosal lymphocytes had high expression of interleukin-2 receptors, suggesting that they could be responsive to local interleukin-2 produced by T cells. Furthermore, this observation suggests that the previously observed serum interleukin-2 receptors found in patients with active disease is produced by activated mucosal lymphoid cells.

Gurbindo *et al.* [25•] also studied interleukin-2 production by lymphocytes isolated from peripheral blood and the mucosa of IBD patients. Unlike the study by Matsuura, stimulated lamina propria lymphocytes from patients with Crohn's disease produced higher levels of interleukin-2 than controls and values from patients with ulcerative colitis were not significantly different from controls. This data is consistent with other recent studies also demonstrating differences comparing Crohn's disease and ulcerative colitis patients: patients with Crohn's disease generally have been found to have higher levels of interleukin-2 messenger RNA and protein compared with controls and patients with ulcerative colitis in the mucosa. These observations support the concept that the pathogenesis of the two diseases, while overlapping in some respects, also have distinct immunologic differences.

Interestingly, in one of the commonly used experimental models of induced colitis, trinitrobenzene sulfonic acid–induced colitis in rats, up-regulation of interleukin-2 production in the chronic phase of colitis was observed [26]. This experiment indicates that increased interleukin-2 production can be a secondary effect of severe inflammatory injury. This study should also raise a note of caution concerning this animal model of ulcerative colitis, in that most of the human data show low levels of interleukin-2 in the mucosa. Thus this particular model, although a useful one for studying acute inflammation mechanisms in the gut, may not replicate some of the other important immunological characteristics of ulcerative colitis.

Interleukin-1

Numerous previous studies have suggested that the proinflammatory cytokine interleukin-1 has increased expression in the mucosa in IBD. In order to determine more directly the effects of interleukin-1 on the mucosa, Mowat *et al.* [27] studied the role of interleukin-1 in a murine model of enteropathy, graft-versus-host disease, and the direct effect of interleukin-1 administration on the gut. Anti-interleukin-1 treatment ameliorated crypt hyperplasia in graft-versus-host disease without altering the increase in intraepithelial lymphocytes in the mucosa. Administration of recombinant interleukin-1 to mice induced crypt hyperplasia, villous atrophy, and increase in the numbers of intraepithelial lymphocytes. These results indicate that the observed increase in interleukin-1 expression in IBD could have pathologic effects and further suggest that therapy directed at reducing interleukin-1 production could be beneficial.

Interleukin-8

Interleukin-8 is a cytokine expressed at high levels in monocytes and at lower levels on many other cell types following activation. There is *in vitro* evidence of production of interleukin-8 in epithelial cells that are activated, such as by invasion with pathogenic bacteria [28•], however, it is presently still unclear whether intestinal epithelial cells produce interleukin-8 *in vivo*. Interleukin-8 has as a primary function chemotaxis and also activation of granulocytes, and there is evidence of production of this cytokine in inflammatory diseases characterized by neutrophil infiltration. Izzo *et al.* [29] found that colonic tissue levels of immunoreactive interleukin-8 were 10-fold higher in patients with Crohn's disease compared with controls. Interestingly, myeloperoxidase, a marker of neutrophils, was not increased, and interleukin-8 was higher regardless of the histologic or endoscopic degree of activity. These interesting findings suggest that interleukin-8 may be a sensitive marker of the presence of Crohn's disease, presumably owing to monocyte activation. This would be consistent with previous observations of elevations of other inflammatory cytokines in IBD, such as interleukin-1 and interleukin-6. Furthermore, the presence of interleukin-8 but apparent lack of a neutrophilic infiltrate in Crohn's disease was suggested by the authors to indicate that some other mechanism might interfere with neutrophil migration into the intestine in Crohn's disease, as has been suggested in other studies.

Raab *et al.* [30•] used a different method to assess local production of interleukin-8 in patients with ulcerative colitis, by obtaining colonic fluid samples using a perfusion system. Concentrations of interleukin-8, tumor necrosis factor (TNF)-α and myeloperoxidase were increased in perfusates from ulcerative colitis patients compared with normal controls. As would be expected in a study of this design, neither the mechanism of induction of interleukin-8 or its cellular source could be determined, but the data do indicate that this proinflammatory cytokine might be important in ulcerative colitis.

Nicholls *et al.* [31] took a more direct approach to studying cytokine in IBD by assaying for cytokines in stool samples from children with IBD and controls. Low levels of TNF-α and occasionally interleukin-6 could be detected in stools of normal children. Higher levels of TNF-α were detected in active IBD, with levels similar to normal in active disease. Very high levels of both cytokines were found in children with acute shigellosis. Variability in interleukin-6 levels were shown to be possibly confounded by the presence of stool factors that rapidly destroy interleukin-6. These findings confirm that the gut is a site of cytokine production under normal physiologic circumstances, and that there may be a marked, nonselective increased in these cytokines in inflammatory diseases.

Novel cytokines

Abnormalities of mucin are present in IBD, particularly ulcerative colitis, including the typical appearance of mucin depletion from goblet cells and biochemical abnormalities of mucin. Sperber *et al.* [32] have studied a novel macrophage-derived protein, termed *MMS-68*, that has previously been shown to be a mucin secretagogue. It was demonstrated that MMS-68 enhances mucin secretion from normal and IBD-afflicted tissues, and that it is present in intestinal macrophages in normal individuals and patients with IBD. Paradoxically, in the small number of ulcerative colitis tissues examined there was lower staining for MMS-68 in some samples. Thus, this novel protein could potentially be involved in mucin secretion in IBD.

Other peptide mediators

In addition to cytokines, there has been a growing interest in other peptides and proteins that may potentially play a role in inflammation and tissue repair in IBD. Wright *et al.* [33,34] have studied the expression of trefoil peptides in intestinal tissue in Crohn's disease. The trefoil peptides are a group of homologous molecules whose function remains to be more completely defined. The prototype peptide pS2 has homology with the gastrointestinal peptide pancreatic spasmolytic polypeptide. In rodents, this molecule inhibits intestinal muscular contraction and gastric acid secretion. Wright *et al.* [33,34] found that pS2 and human spasmolytic peptide messenger RNA localized to areas of injury in goblet cells and neuroendocrine cells. Unfortunately, the study was flawed by lack of any description of the clinical materials, data analysis, or control studies so that it is difficult to draw other than the most limited conclusions. It appears that trefoil peptide expression in intestinal lesions may be associated with tissue injury or repair in IBD and is worthy of further investigation.

Adhesion molecules

An important characteristic of lymphoid and myeloid cells is their ability to disseminate throughout the body via blood and lymphatics. However, in order for these cells to exert their functions, they must gain access to particular sites, such as organized lymphoid tissue and the gut, both in normal physiologic conditions and during inflammation. Once cells have reached an appropriate site, they also must communicate with other cells. These processes require adhesion of cells of the immune system to vascular endothelium, to each other, and to other cell types. Thus, there is great interest in the subject of adhesion molecules in immunology. Adhesion molecules belong to three distinct families: the immunoglobulin supergene family, the integrins, and the selectins. The first two groups contain a large number of molecules, while the third consists of only three. A detailed understanding of these molecules and their functions is not only necessary for a fundamental understanding of immune function, but, more practically, these molecules have become potential targets for interrupting immune and inflammatory responses with selective therapeutic agents. This area of research has considerable practical potential in IBD.

Mishra *et al.* [35] made the surprisingly simple but intriguing observation that peripheral blood lymphocytes from patients with Crohn's disease, when incubated with glass beads, form small "granulomas" around the beads consisting primarily of CD4 T cells and non-T cells. The formation of granulomas is considerably greater than in control subjects and correlates with activity of disease. Furthermore, as would be predicted, antibodies against certain cell surface molecules that are involved in adhesion and cell-cell interactions (LFA-2, LFA-3, MAC-1) blocked the formation of granulomas. The abnormal behavior of *in vitro* cells from patients with Crohn's disease suggests that they had undergone prior activation and up-regulation of adhesion molecules, and this interesting model system could be of use in further understanding of the granuloma process in Crohn's disease.

In a study exploring the potential for therapy with antiadhesins, Podolsky *et al.* [36•] treated cotton-top tamarins that developed spontaneous colitis with antibodies against the E-selectin and α4 integrins in a placebo-controlled trial. Whereas anti-E selectins bound to endothelial cells, they had little effect on colitis. In contrast, antibodies against the α4 integrin (found in very late activation-4 integrin on lymphocytes and the α4, β7 integrin that is thought to be important for mucosal homing) significantly decreased colitis. These observations suggest that it might be possible to interrupt the immune and inflammatory events in human IBD by therapy directed at blocking lymphocyte adhesion and homing. Greenfield *et al.* [37] showed that sulfasalazine inhibits up-regulation of the critical CD11b/CD18 adhesin on granulocytes that was stimulated by activating agents such as TNF-α. Thus, drugs known to have efficacy in IBD may work in part by interfering with adhesion of inflammatory cells.

Specific antibodies and autoantibodies

Antineutrophil cytoplasmic antibodies

The role of antibodies and autoantibodies continues to be of considerable interest in IBD. Numerous studies have examined their potential role in disease pathogenesis and their usefulness as clinical tests for diagnosis and management. Antineutrophil cytoplasmic antibodies (ANCAs) [38] can be found in the majority of patients with ulcerative colitis. However, there is wide variation in frequency in reported studies. ANCAs are found with a much higher frequency in ulcerative colitis than in Crohn's disease.

The relationship between the presence of ANCAs and disease activity has been variable. Several studies have confirmed these findings. Oudkerk *et al.* [39] showed that 79% of patients with ulcerative colitis had ANCAs, compared with only 13% of patients with Crohn's disease. In this study, there was a wide variation in the frequency of ANCAs that correlated with the method of detection used. The indirect immunofluorescence assay had a sensitivity of 75% with a high degree of correlation between laboratories compared with a sensitivity of 39% for the enzyme-linked immunosorbent assay. There was no relationship between the frequency of ANCA positivity and clinical variables such as disease activity, duration, or location. Using the immunofluorescence method, Hardarson *et al.* [40] also found ANCAs in 72% of patients with ulcerative colitis or primary sclerosing cholangitis. Dalekos *et al.* [41] demonstrated the presence of a number of autoantibodies including rheumatoid factor, antinuclear antibody, anticardiolipin antibody, and anti–double-stranded DNA antibodies in patients with ulcerative colitis. In this study, using the immunofluorescence method, ANCAs were found in only 30% of patients with ulcerative colitis, which again shows the wide variability in the frequency of ANCAs in ulcerative colitis. The variability in ANCA positivity in ulcerative colitis may be related to the method of detection used and differences in technique. The clinical significance and precise role of ANCAs in pathogenesis of IBD remains unclear.

Many disorders associated with cellular activation including IBD have been shown to have increased serum concentrations of soluble interleukin-2 receptors that correlate with disease activity. Dalekos *et al.* [41] found that 32.5% of patients with ulcerative colitis had elevated concentrations of soluble interleukin-2 receptors that correlated with disease activity and ANCA positivity. This suggests that in ulcerative colitis, where clinical markers of disease activity are not well defined, these concentrations are potentially useful as markers of disease activity.

Major histocompatibility complex class II genes have been studied in an attempt to define their potential role as factors in the pathogenesis of IBD. Toyoda *et al.* [42•] demonstrated an association of the HLA DR2 allele with ulcerative colitis and an association of the combination of HLA DR1 and DQ5 alleles with Crohn's disease. In both ulcerative colitis and Crohn's disease, these findings suggest genetic heterogeneity of susceptibility.

A familial distribution of ANCAs in families with ulcerative colitis suggests heterogeneity within the disease. Yang *et al.* [43] demonstrated that this heterogeneity of ANCA seropositivity in ulcerative colitis may have a genetic basis that resides within the HLA region. They found that ANCA-positive ulcerative colitis patients had a significantly increased frequency of DR2. In addition, ANCA-negative ulcerative colitis patients had an increase in the DR4 allele.

Recently, there has been a focus on the specific autoantigens recognized by ANCAs. The target antigen appears to be different from the serine protease 3 in patients with Wegener's granulomatosus. Myeloperoxidase and elastase do not seem to be target antigens of ANCAs. Candidate antigens suggested by previous studies include myeloid proteinase cathepsin G and β-glucuronidase. Peen *et al.* [44] found antilactoferrin antibodies in 50% of patients with ulcerative colitis and 50% of those with primary sclerosing cholangitis, respectively. Only 8% of patients with Crohn's disease had antilactoferrin antibodies. This data suggests that lactoferrin may be a target antigen and that antibodies directed against it may be of pathogenic significance. In a small study [45], none of the ANCA-positive serum samples from patients with ulcerative colitis reacted with β-glucuronidase, which raises some question about β-glucuronidase as a target antigen.

M_r 40-kD autoantigen

Serum autoantibodies to colonic goblet cells and surface epithelial cells have been identified in patients with ulcerative colitis. Das *et al.* [46••] have suggested that the one autoantigen is a M_r 40-kD colonic protein that belongs to the tropomyosin family. Halstensen *et al.* [47] examined the distribution of M_r 40-kD using two- and three-color immunofluorescence staining including the murine monoclonal antibody $7E_{12}H_{12}$. The authors found that the M_r 40-kD antigen is found in goblet cells in the terminal ileum and proximal colon and is expressed on biliary epithelium and the apical surface of colonic enterocytes where it colocalized with apical immune complexes (immunoglobulin G1 and activated complement) in active ulcerative colitis. These findings support the hypothesis that an autoimmune reaction to this antigen is a potential pathogenic mechanism in ulcerative colitis. The M_r 40-kD colonic protein has also been shown to be expressed by the colon tumor cell line DLD-1. Biancone *et al.* [48] showed that serum from ulcerative colitis patients induced significantly more cytotoxicity than did normal serum against DLD-1 colon cancer cells. In addition, anti-M_r 40-kD monoclonal antibodies significantly inhibited the ulcerative colitis serum-induced cytotoxicity. These findings suggest that the M_r 40-kD protein may be a target of cytotoxic antibodies in ulcerative colitis.

Other autoantibodies

Rheumatoid factor

Increased levels of rheumatoid factor have been found in patients with Crohn's disease but not ulcerative colitis. MacDermott *et al.* [49] studied the spontaneous *in vitro* secretion of rheumatoid factor by intestinal lamina propria mononuclear cells in IBD. They found increased rheumatoid factor secretion from Crohn's disease intestinal mononuclear cells compared with controls, which correlated with the activity of the disease from which the intestinal mononuclear cells were isolated. There was decreased rheumatoid factor secretion in ulcerative colitis mononuclear cells compared with controls. These findings suggest that serum rheumatoid factor in Crohn's disease may be produced in the small intestine and supports the concept that Crohn's disease and ulcerative colitis have a different pathogenesis. These data are also interesting because they sharply contrast with our current knowledge about specific antibodies and autoantibodies that are predominantly present in ulcerative colitis as opposed to Crohn's disease.

Antiendothelial antibodies

Intestinal vascular injury has been implicated as a possible early event in the pathogenesis of IBD. Circulating levels of von Willebrand factor, an endothelial cell product released into the circulation following vascular injury, are elevated in patients with IBD. Antiendothelial antibodies have been found in some vasculitic disorders. Stevens *et al.* [50] investigated the potential role of antiendothelial antibodies in the pathogenesis of IBD. The authors found that antiendothelial antibodies were significantly elevated in IBD patients compared with healthy controls. In ulcerative colitis, antibody levels were related to disease activity and correlated with circulating levels of von Willebrand factor. These antiendothelial antibodies, however, were not cytotoxic to endothelial cells *in vitro*.

Antilipocortin-I antibodies

Corticosteroids are commonly used to treat IBD. Their activity is thought to be in part related to the induction of specific anti-inflammatory proteins such as lipocortin-1. Lipocortin-1 is autoantigenic and raised levels of autoantibodies have been implicated as a possible cause of steroid resistance in rheumatoid arthritis. Stevens *et al.* [51] investigated whether antibody to lipocortin-1 could be responsible for the variable clinical response to corticosteroids in IBD. The authors found high levels of immunoglobulin M lipocortin-1 antibodies in IBD patients not taking steroids and low levels of immunoglobulin M lipocortin-1 antibodies in patients on long-term corticosteroid therapy. These results are in sharp contrast with those previously described in rheumatoid arthritis patients. In addition, high levels of antibodies were associated with good clinical outcome, which suggests a pathogenic role in IBD is unlikely.

Antimycobacterial antibodies

The role of mycobacterial antigens in IBD continues to get some attention, however, their potential role remains unclear. In one study, antibodies to three mycobacterial antigens were found in some patients with Crohn's disease, but only a small percentage were positive for all three [52].

References and recommended reading

Papers of particular interest, published within the annual period of review, have been highlighted as:
- • Of special interest
- •• Of outstanding interest

1. • Blumberg RS, Yockey CE, Gross GG, Ebert EC, Balk SP: **Human Intestinal Intraepithelial Lymphocytes are Derived From a Limited Number of T Cell Clones That Utilize Multiple V Beta T Cell Receptor Genes.** *J Immunol* 1993, 150:5144–5153.

This paper presents evidence that intraepithelial lymphocytes are derived from a limited number of precursors, suggesting that the antigenic repertoire of this cell population is limited. This suggests that this cell subpopulation may play only a limited role in antigen-specific immune responses in the epithelium.

2. Panja A, Blumberg RS, Balk SP, Mayer L: **CD1d is Involved in T Cell Intestinal Epithelial Cell Interactions**. *J Exp Med* 1993, **178**:1115–1119.

3. Fujihashi K, Yamamoto M, McGhee JR, Beagley KW, Kiyono H: **Function of Alpha Beta TCR+Intestinal Intraepithelial Lymphocytes: Th1- and Th2-Type Cytokine Production by CD4+CD8- and CD4+CD8+ T Cells for Helper Activity**. *Int Immunol* 1993, **5**:1473–1481.

4. Fujihashi K, Yamamoto M, McGhee JR, Kiyono H: **Alpha Beta T Cell Receptor-Positive Intraepithelial With CD4+CD8- and CD4+CD8+ Phenotypes From Orally Immunized Mice Provide Th2-Like Function for B Cell Responses**. *J Immunol* 1993, **151**:6681–6691.

5. Sydora BC, Mixter PF, Houlden B, Hershberg R, Levy R, Comay M, Bluestone J, Kronenberg M: **T Cell Receptor Gamma Delta Diversity and Specificity of Intestinal Intraepithelial Lymphocyts: Analysis of IEL Derived Hybridomas**. *Cell Immunol* 1993, **152**:305–322.

6. Poussier P, Teh HS, Julius M: **Thymus Independent Positive and Negative Selection of T Cells Expressing a Major Histocompatibility Complex Class I Restricted Transgenic T Cell Receptor Alpha/Beta in the Intestinal Epithelium**. *J Exp Med* 1993, **178**:1947–1957.

7. Stickney D, Mosley RL, Whetsell M, Whetsell L, Schaefer FV, Miller KS, Klein JR: **T Cell Receptor Delta Gene Repertoire and Diversity of Intestinal Intraepithelial Lymphocytes in Athymic Mice**. *Mol Immunol* 1993, **30**:813–819.

8. Sydora BC, Mixter PF, Holcombe HR, Eghtesady P, Williams K, Amaral MC, Nel A, Kronenberg M: **Intestinal Intraepithelial Lymphocytes are Activated and Cytolytic but do not Proliferate as Well as Other T Cells in Response to Mitogenic Signals**. *J Immunol* 1993, **150**:2179–2191.

9. Sachdev GK, Dalton HR, Hoang P, DiPaolo MC, Crotty B, Jewell DP: **Human Colonic Intraepithelial Lymphocytes Suppress In Vitro Immunoglobulin Synthesis by Autologous Peripheral Blood Lymphocytes and Lamina Propria Lymphocytes**. *Gut* 1993, **34**:257–263.

10. Dalton HR, DiPaolo MC, Sachdev GK, Crotty B, Hoang P, Jewell DP: **Human Colonic Intraepithelial Lymphocytes From Patients With Inflammatory Bowel Disease Fail to Down-Regulate Proliferative Responses of Primed Allogeneic Peripheral Blood Mononuclear Cells After Rechallenge With Antigens**. *Clin Exp Immunol* 1993, **93**:97–102.

11. Roberts AI, O'Connell SM, Biancone L, Brolin RE, Ebert EC: **Spontaneous Cytotoxicity of Intestinal Intraepithelial Lymphocytes: Clues to the Mechanism**. *Clin Exp Immunol* 1993, **94**: 527–532.

12. Rüthlein J, Heinze G, Auer IO: **Anti-CD2 and Anti-CD3 Induced T Cell Cytotoxicity of Human Intraepithelial and Lamina Propria Lymphocytes**. *Gut* 1993, **33**:1626–1632.

13. Van Tol EAF, Verspaget HW, Pena AS, Lamers CBHW: **Normal Inflammatory Bowel Disease Mucosa Conceals Alterations in Natural Killer Cell Activity**. *Scand J Gastroenterol* 1992, **27**:999–1005.

14. Hibi T, Ohara M, Watanabe M, Kanai T, Takaishi H, Hayashi A, Hosoda Y, Ogata H, Iwao Y, Aiso S, Watanabe N, Toda K, Tsuchiya M: **Interleukin 2 and Interferon G Augment Anticolon Antibody Dependent Cellular Cytotoxicity in Ulcerative Colitis**. *Gut* 1993, **34**:788–793.

15. Shorter RG, McGill DB, Bahn RC: **Cytotoxicity of Mononuclear Cells for Autologous Colonic Epithelial Cells in Colonic Disease**. *Gastroenterology* 1984, **86**:13–22.

16. • Okazaki K, Morita M, Nishimori I, Sano S, Toyonaga M, Nakazawa Y, Yamamoto Y, Yamamoto Y: **Major Histocompatibility Antigen-Restricted Cytotoxicity in Inflammatory Bowel Disease**. *Gastroenterology* 1993, **104**:384–391.

This paper provides evidence that intestinal mononuclear cells may mediate cytotoxicity against autologous intestinal epithelial cells; however, control studies are not presented to determine the specificity for IBD.

17. •• Breban M, Hammer RE, Richardson JA, Taurog JD: **Transfer of the Inflammatory Disease of HLA-B27 Transgenic Rats by Bone Marrow Engraftment**. *J Exp Med* 1993, **178**:1607–1616.

This paper demonstrates that the disease of HLA-B27 transgenic rats can be transferred to naive rats by hematopoietic stem cells, indicating that the transgene does not need to be expressed on any other cell types for disease to occur.

18. •• Mombaerts P, Mizoguchi E, Grusby MJ, Glimcher LH, Bhan AK, Tonegawa S: **Spontaneous Development of Inflammatory Bowel Disease in T Cell Receptor Mutant Mice**. *Cell* 1993, **75**:275–282.

This is a second genetic knockout model, in which animals were manipulated to have different forms of T-cell deficiency, in which an ulcerative colitis–like disease occurs. The absence of CD4 T cells and presence of B cells may create immune imbalance leading to colitis.

19. •• Sadlack B, Merz H, Schorle H, Schimpl A, Feller AC, Horak I: **Ulcerative Colitis-Like Disease in Mice With a Disrupted Interleukin-2 Gene**. *Cell* 1993, **75**:253–261.

A very important paper demonstrating that interleukin-2 "knockout" animals may have a severe, ulcerative colitis like disease that may be immunologically mediated and may depend on the presence of antigens in the intestinal flora.

20. •• Kühn R, Löhler J, Rennick D, Rajewsky K, Müller W: **Interleukin 10 Deficient Mice Develop Chronic Enterocolitis**. *Cell* 1993, **75**:263–274.

This paper presents a second example of cytokine knockout mice (interleukin-10) that has a different form of intestinal inflammation, a panenteritis. This animal model has enhanced TH1 types of immune responses, and the immune imbalance causes intestinal disease that may depend on antigens in the intestinal flora.

21. •• Strober W, Ehrhardt RO: **Chronic Intestinal Inflammation: An Unexpected Outcome in Cytokine or T Cell Receptor Mutant Mice**. *Cell* 1993, **75**:203–205.

An editorial accompanying the three papers on knockout animals that suggests possible mechanisms whereby immune imbalance in the gastrointestinal mucosa results in inflammatory disease.

22. Shanahan F: **Pathogenesis of Ulcerative Colitis**. *Lancet* 1993, **342**:407–411.

23. Fiocchi C: **Cytokines and Animal Models: A Combined Path to Inflammatory Bowel Disease Pathogenesis**. *Gastroenterology* 1993, **104**:1202–1219.

24. • Matsuura T, West GA, Youngman KR, Klein JS, Fiocchi C: **Immune Activation Genes in Inflammatory Bowel Disease**. *Gastroenterology* 1993, **104**:448–458.

This paper provides evidence that increased serum interleukin-2 receptor in active IBD is due to local production by activated lymphocytes.

25. • Gurbindo C, Sabbah S, Menzes J, Justinich C, Marchand R, Seidman EG: **Interleukin-2 Production in Pediatric Inflammatory Bowel Disease: Evidence for Dissimilar Mononuclear Cell Function in Crohn's Disease and Ulcerative Colitis**. *J Pediatr Gastroenterol Nutr* 1993, **17**:247–254.

This paper demonstrates higher interleukin-2 production by intestinal mononuclear cells from Crohn's disease patients compared with controls and those with ulcerative colitis, providing further evidence for differences in immunopathogenesis. This is particularly interesting in light of the cytokine knockout animal studies showing panenteritis in animals predisposed to a TH1 type of immune response.

26. Gurbindo C, Russo P, Sabbah S, Lohoues M-J, Seidman E: **Interleukin-2 Activity of Colonic Lamina Propria Mononu-**

clear Cells in a Rat Model of Experimental Colitis. *Gastroenterology* 1993, **104**:964–972.

27. Mowat AM, Hutton AK, Garside P, Steel M: **A Role for Interleukin-1a in Immunologically Mediated Intestinal Pathology.** *Immunology* 1993, **80**:110–115.

28. • Eckmann L, Kagnoff MF, Fierer J: **Epithelial Cells Secrete the Chemokine Interleukin-8 in Response to Bacterial Entry.** *Infect and Immun* 1993, **61**:4569–4574.

This paper suggests a mechanism whereby intestinal epithelial cells injured by invasive bacteria could produce IL-8 that plays a role in recruiting inflammatory cells to the site of injury.

29. Izzo RS, Witkon K, Chen AI, Hadjiyane C, Weinstein MI, Pellecchia C: **Neutrophil-Activating Peptide (Interluekin-8) in Colonic Mucosa from Patients With Crohn's Disease.** *Scand J Gastroenterol* 1993, **28**:296–300.

30. • Raab Y, Gerdin B, Ahlstedt S, Hällgren R: **Neutrophil Involvement is Accompanied by Enhanced Local Production of Interleukin-8 in Ulcerative Colitis.** *Gut* 1993, **34**:1203–1206.

Interleukin-8 is produced locally in the colon in patients with ulcerative colitis and may play a role in neutrophil recruitment to the mucosa.

31. Nicholls S, Stephens S, Braegger CP, Walker-Smith JA, MacDonald TT: **Cytokines in Stools of Children With Inflammatory Bowel Disease or Infective Diarrhoea.** *J Clin Pathol* 1993, **46**:757–760.

32. Sperber K, Ogata S, Sylvester C Aisenberg J, Chen A, Mayer L, Itzkowitz S: **A Novel Human Macrophage-Derived Intestinal Mucin Secretagogue: Implications for the Pathogenesis of Inflammatory Bowel Disease.** *Gastroenterology* 1993, **104**:1302–1309.

33. Wright NA, Poulsom R, Stamp G, Van Norden S, Sarraf C, Elia G, Ahnen D, Jeffery R, Longcroft J, Pike C, Rio M-C, Chambon P: **Trefoil Peptide Gene Expression in Gastrointestinal Epithelial Cells in Inflammatory Bowel Disease.** *Scand J Gastroenterol* 1992, **27(Suppl 193)**:76–82.

34. Wright NA, Poulsom R, Stamp G, Van Norden S, Sarraf C, Elia G, Ahnen D, Jeffery R, Longcroft J, Pike C, Rio M-C, Chambon P: **Trefoil Peptide Gene Expression in Gastrointestinal Epithelial Cells in Inflammatory Bowel Disease.** *Gastroenterology* 1994, **104**:12–20.

35. Mishra L, Mishra BB, Harris M, Bayless TM, Muchmore AV; **In Vitro Cell Aggregation and Cell Adhesion Molecules in Crohn's Disease.** *Gastroenterology* 1993, **104**:772–779.

36. • Podolsky DK, Lobb R, King N, Benjamin CD, Pepinsky B, Sehgal P, deBeaumont M: **Attenuation of Colitis in the Cotton-Top Tamarin by Anti-a4 Integrin Monoclonal Antibody.** *J Clin Invest* 1993, **92**:372–380.

This paper suggests that antibodies that interfere with lymphocyte adhesion and homing may improve inflammation in this model of ulcerative colitis.

37. Greenfield SM, Hamblin AS, Shakoor ZS, Teare JP, Punchard NA, RPH Thompson: **Inhibition of Leucocyte Adhesion Molecule Upregulation by Tumor Necrosis Factor A: A Novel Mechanism of Action of Sulphasalazine.** *Gut* 1993, **34**:252–256.

38. Kallenberg CG, Mulder AH, Tervaert JW: **Antineutrophil Cytoplasmic Autoantibodies: A Still-Growing Class of Autoantibodies in Inflammatory Disorders.** *Am J Med* 1992, **93**:675–682.

39. Oudkerk Pool M, Ellerbroek PM, Ridwan BU, Goldschmeding R, von Blomberg BM, Pena AS, Dolman KM, Bril H, Dekker W, Nauta JJ, Gans RO, Breed H, Meuwissen SG: **Serum Antineutrophil Cytoplasmic Autoantibodies in Inflammatory Bowel Disease are Mainly Associated With Ulcerative Colitis. A Correlation Study Between Perinuclear Antineutrophil Cytoplasmic Autoantibodies and Clinical Parameters, Medical, and Surgical Treatment.** *Gut* 1993, **34**:46–50.

40. Hardarson S, LaBrecque DR, Mitros FA, Neil GA, Goeken JA: **Antineutrophil Cytoplasmic Autoantibody in Inflammatory Bowel and Hepatobiliary Diseases. High Prevalence in Ulcerative Colitis, Primary Sclerosing Cholangitis, and Autoimmune Hepatitis.** *Am J Clin Pathol* 1993, **99**:277–281.

41. Dalekos GN, Manoussakis MN, Goussia AC, Tsianos EV, Moutsopolous HM: **Soluble Interleukin-2 Receptors, Antineutrophil Cytoplasmic Autoantibodies, and Other Autoantibodies in Patients With Ulcerative Colitis.** *Gut* 1993, **34**:658–664.

42. • Toyoda H, Wang S-J, Yang H-Y, Redford A, Magalong D, Tyan D, McElree C, Pressman SR, Shanahan F, Targan SR, Rotter JI: **Distinct Associations of HLA Class II Genes With Inflammatory Bowel Disease.** *Gastroenterology* 1993, **104**:741–748.

This paper describes a separation of ulcerative colitis and Crohn"s disease on a genetic basis with distinct HLA class II gene associations.

43. Yang H, Rotter JI, Toyoda H, Landers C, Tyan D, McElree CK, Targan SR: **Ulcerative Colitis: A Genetically Heterogeneous Disorder Defined by Genetic (HLA Class II) and Subclinical (Antineutrophil Cytoplasmic Autoantibodies) Markers.** *J Clin Invest* 1993, **92**:1080–1084.

44. Peen E, Almer S, Bodemar G, Ryden BO, Sjolin C, Tejle K, Skogh T: **Anti-Lactoferrin Antibodies and Other Types of ANCA in Ulcerative Colitis, Primary Sclerosing Cholangitis, and Crohn's Disease.** *Gut* 1993, **34**:56–62.

45. Kanecko K, Suzuki Y, Yamashiro Y, Yabuta K: **Is p-ANCA in Ulcerative Colitis Directed Against B-Glucuronidase.** *Lancet* 1993, **341**:320.

46. •• Das KM, Dasgupta A, Mandal A, Geng X: **Autoimmunity to Cytoskeletal Protein Tropomyosin. A Clue to the Pathogenic Mechanism for Ulcerative Colitis.** *J Immunol* 1993, **150**:2487–2493.

This paper demonstrates that one of the autoantigens that may be involved in the pathogenesis of ulcerative colitis belongs to the tropomyosin family.

47. Halstensen TS, Das KM, Brandtzaeg P: **Epithelial Deposits of ImmunoglobulinG1 and Activated Complement Colocalise With the Mr 40 kD Putative Autoantigen in Ulcerative Colitis.** *Gut* 1993, **34**:650–657.

48. Biancone L, Das KM, Roberts AI, Ebert EC: **Ulcerative Colitis Serum Recognizes the Mr 40K Protein on Colonic Adenocarcinoma Cells for Antibody- Dependent Cellular Cytotoxicity.** *Digestion* 1993, **54**:237–242.

49. MacDermott RP, Schreiber S, Nash GS, Koopman WJ: **Increased Spontaneous Secretion of Rheumatoid Factor by Intestinal Lamina Propria Mononuclear Cells From Crohn's Disease but not Ulcerative Colitis Patients.** *Clin Exp Immunol* 1993, **92**:152–157.

50. Stevens TR, Harley SL, Groom JS, Cambridge G, Leaker B, Blake DR, Rampton DS: **Anti-Endothelial Cell Antibodies in Inflammatory Bowel Disease.** *Dig Dis Sci* 1993, **38**:426–432.

51. Stevens TR, Smith SF, Rampton DS: **Antibodies to Human Recombinant Lipocortin-I in Inflammatory Bowel Disease.** *Clin Sci* 1993, **84**:381–386.

52. Elsagheir A, Prantera C, Moreno C, Ivanyi J: **Antibodies to *Mycobacterium paraatuberculosis*-Specific Protein Antigens in Crohn's Disease.** *Clin Exp Immunol* 1992, **90**:503–508.

George T. Fantry, MD, and Stephen P. James, MD, Room N3W62, Division of Gastroenterology, University of Maryland at Baltimore, 22 South Greene Street, Baltimore, MD 21201, USA.

Clinical epidemiology of inflammatory bowel disease

Bret A. Lashner, MD, MPH, and Aaron Brzezinski, MD

Cleveland Clinic Foundation, Cleveland, Ohio, USA

Publications involving the clinical epidemiology of inflammatory bowel disease were plentiful in 1993. Greater understanding was made in the diagnosis, etiology, and natural history of disease. Specifically, a newer diagnostic technique of technetium-labeled leukocyte scanning appeared to be as accurate with lower radiation exposure than other nuclear medicine alternatives. Etiologically, work continued on two fronts. Genetic studies demonstrated homogenous groups within these heterogenous diseases, groups that may share etiologic, prognostic, and therapeutic advantages. Also, promising work continued the search for the infectious agents responsible for inflammatory bowel disease. Prognosis in patients with ulcerative colitis appears to be directly related to extent of disease at diagnosis. Inroads were made in finding some of the genetic mutations responsible for neoplastic transformation and cancer-related motility reduction through either risk factor intervention or surveillance of high-risk patients remained an area of considerable interest. Despite these insights, this year's literature seemed to uncover more questions than were answered.

Current Opinion in Gastroenterology 1994, **10**:374–383

Advances in the understanding of the clinical epidemiology of inflammatory bowel disease (IBD) were made in 1993. Conveniently, the literature could be divided into diagnostic, etiologic, and prognostic hypotheses. The literature on cancer in IBD is presented in the section on natural history of disease.

Diagnosis

Incidence rates

Two European studies exemplified the disparity of information reported for incidence rates. Such differences may have been due to genetic and environmental differences between populations or differences in reporting rates. Over a 10-year period, the incidence of ulcerative colitis in Granada, Spain was two per 100,000 and the incidence of Crohn's disease was 0.9 per 100,000 [1•]. Both incidence figures were markedly below rates reported elsewhere in Europe. In Bologna, Italy, the incidence rate for either ulcerative colitis or Crohn's disease was 7.7 per 100,000 with former smokers more likely to develop ulcerative colitis and current smokers more likely to develop Crohn's disease [2•].

Familial ties

Relatives of IBD patients were much more likely to develop IBD themselves, usually concordant disease, than others in the community. Fully 5.2% of ulcerative patients and 1.6% of Crohn's disease patients had first-degree relatives affected with IBD at the time of diagnosis of the proband [3••]. Higher rates were reported in relatives of Jewish patients. In ulcerative colitis patients, the relative risk for a family member to develop ulcerative colitis was 15 and was not elevated for a family member to develop Crohn's disease [4••]. Likewise, in Crohn's disease patients, family members had a relative risk of 15 for developing Crohn's disease and 3 for developing ulcerative colitis.

Identification of family members at risk was a subject of active investigation. Increased intestinal permeability to environmental toxins has been an attractive theory for identifying a population at risk. Newer diagnostic techniques have been developed to identify the "highly permeable small bowel" population, a population who may be at high risk for developing Crohn's disease by allowing passage to toxic substances that initiate disease [5•]. Fractional excretion of lactulose, a measure of intestinal permeability, was elevated in approximately 16% of asymptomatic first-degree relatives of Crohn's disease patients [6••]. Of note, approximately 10% of relatives of Crohn's disease patients in this population are expected to develop Crohn's disease in the future. Only time will tell whether "permeable" populations will actually develop the disease.

Abbreviations

ANCA—antineutrophil cytoplasmic antibody; **IBD**—inflammatory bowel disease.

 ISBN 1-85922-609-4 ISSN 0267-1379

Unusual presentations

The diagnosis of IBD can humble even the most experienced clinician. Unusual presentations are being reported with greater frequency and with a wider array of signs and symptoms. Seemingly commonplace diseases are at times diagnosed as the relatively rare IBD, especially Crohn's disease. Moonka *et al.* [7•] reported on a case of recurrent chronic gastric ulcers that were due to unsuspected upper gastrointestinal Crohn's disease. Scapa *et al.* [8•] described a child with a "miliary" appearance in a large portion of small bowel that was neither lymphoma nor tuberculosis, but Crohn's disease. Calder *et al.* [9•] reported on a child who developed pulmonary Crohn's disease when granulomas were found in the lungs and microscopic skip lesions were found in the colon. It is known that Crohn's disease can affect any part of the gastrointestinal tract, and now Crohn's disease isolated to the appendix has been reported [10•]. Alternatively, disease that appears to be Crohn's disease may not be, as in the case of an enterocutaneous fistula that was caused by a ruptured appendiceal diverticulum [11•].

Alcantara *et al.* [12•] reported that Crohn's disease can be diagnosed in patients with "indeterminate" colitis if aphthoid ulcers or granulomas can be identified in an asymptomatic upper gastrointestinal tract. Indeed, aphthoid ulcers in the stomach were found in 35% of patients and granulomas were found in 20% of patients with Crohn's disease elsewhere in the gastrointestinal tract, most of whom had no symptoms referable to the upper gastrointestinal tract.

Diagnostic testing

Much work has been done to evaluate newer diagnostic tools in comparison with established techniques. Endoscopic ultrasound is an excellent tool and may be the best method for carefully mapping perianal fistulas and abscesses in Crohn's disease [13•]. The use of a rectal probe can be limited, though, by pain and strictures, features present in most patients with perianal disease.

When compared with conventional methods of assessing Crohn's disease activity, technetium-99m hexamethyl propylene amine oxime granulocyte scintigraphy had a sensitivity of 95% and a specificity of 100% for detecting active inflammation, abscess, and fistula [14•]. Furthermore, scintigraphy also could assess any therapeutic response of inflammation, especially in the large bowel. When compared with the now established indium-111-granulocyte scanning, technetium scanning was less time consuming, offered less radiation exposure, and was equally effective in detecting more active from less active IBD [15•]. Such scanning, be it with technetium- or indium-labeled granulocytes, correlated well with endoscopically severe lesions but was not able to detect subtle lesions or smaller changes in clinical activity [16•].

Other attempts at finding objective measures of disease activity have included the determination of cytokine levels in the stool of IBD patients [17•]. As expected, stool concentrations of tumor necrosis factor-α were elevated in active ulcerative colitis. Surprisingly, low levels of interleukin-6 were detected, a phenomenon attributed to local destruction by an as yet unidentified heat labile factor. Biopsies of rectal mucosa in ulcerative colitis patients, and not Crohn's disease patients, exhibit the neurotransmitter substance P [18•]. Levels of substance P correlate with both the severity of inflammation and the quantity of neutrophils and eosinophils. Kokoszka *et al.* [19•] reported that breath pentane, generated by peroxidation of cellular fatty acids, correlated well with activity of disease as determined by indium-111–labeled leukocyte scanning in both ulcerative colitis and Crohn's disease patients.

Etiology

Genetic predisposition

There is a clear genetic predisposition for the development of IBD. The disease occurs much more commonly than expected in relatives and disease developing in spouses, persons who share many environmental exposures, is rare. Recently, patterns of genetic homogeneity within these heterogenous disorders have been reported. Should these homogenous populations exist, there may be etiologic factors, prognostic outcomes, and therapeutic options uniquely suited to these populations. Particularly interesting has been the work on antineutrophil cytoplasmic antibodies (ANCAs) and HLA classification. Of note, patients with IBD share some of the same genetic markers as patients with other autoimmune diseases such as multiple sclerosis (HLA DR2), insulin-dependent diabetes mellitus, and rheumatoid arthritis (HLA DR4) [20•,21••].

Perinuclear ANCA is a distinct feature of ulcerative colitis. Hardarson *et al.* [21••] reported that 72% of ulcerative colitis patients and only 10% of other patients including Crohn's disease patients, were positive for perinuclear ANCA. The highest rates were in patients with both ulcerative colitis and primary sclerosing cholangitis. Sung *et al.* [22•] found 73% of Chinese ulcerative colitis patients to be ANCA positive. Even in children, 66% of ulcerative colitis patients were ANCA positive and only 19% of Crohn's disease patients were ANCA positive [23•]. Interestingly, ANCA positivity did not correlate with disease activity.

Yang *et al.* [24••] also found a large proportion (79%) of ulcerative colitis patients to be positive for perinuclear ANCA. Forty-four percent of ANCA-positive patients expressed HLA DR2, a figure much higher than expected (Fig. 1). Only 21% of ANCA-negative patients expressed DR2, a figure similar to the 50 ethnically matched controls. Also, 42% of ANCA-negative ulcerative colitis patients expressed the DR4 allele, more than ANCA-positive patients (13%) or controls (20%) (Fig. 2). In another study by the same group [25••], Crohn's disease patients, who usually are ANCA negative, often exhibited HLA DR1 and DQw5, a pattern distinctly different from ulcerative colitis patients. Therefore, genetically distinct IBD populations exist.

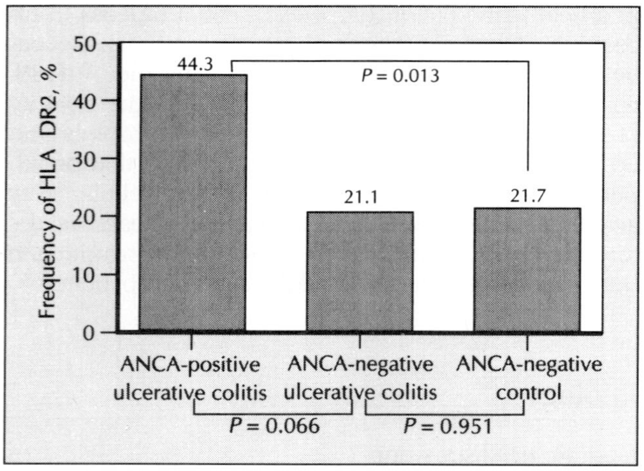

Fig. 1. HLA-DR2 allele frequency in antineutrophil cytoplasmic antibody (ANCA)-positive and -negative ulcerative colitis patients, compared with ANCA-negative controls. (*From* Yang *et al.* [3••]; with permission.)

The clinical utility of defining ANCA and HLA status in IBD patients has not been determined. Treem *et al.* [26•] reported on a mother and son who both had ulcerative colitis and total alopecia. Both were ANCA positive and not HLA identical. Treatment of the son with 6-mercaptopurine led to ulcerative colitis remission and nascent hair growth. It is hoped that this line of research will lead to the characterization of homogeneous populations of IBD who will exhibit unique disease features, course, prognosis, and response to therapy.

Infectious agents

Whereas genetic predisposition appears to be an important determinant of disease, promising work has demonstrated that environmental, and hence preventable, agents play an important role. Van Kruiningen *et al.* [27••] reported on an epidemic of Crohn's disease when multiple siblings in two French families developed the disease within a short period of time. No infectious agent or common HLA haplotype could be discerned. Aisenberg and Janowitz [28•] theorized an environmental etiology for three close college friends who developed IBD (two with Crohn's disease, one with ulcerative colitis) within a decade of graduation. Rutgeerts and Geboes [29•] provided support for a theory of the pathogenesis of Crohn's disease whereby a toxic substance, possibly an infectious organism, causes a microvascular lesion (pre-aphthoid ulceration) that triggers an unchecked immune response and fibrinogenesis.

From cluster studies, enough evidence exists to study *Mycobacteria paratuberculosis* as a cause of Crohn's disease in greater depth [30•]. Wall *et al.* [31••] described a non–acid-fast, cell wall–deficient, spheroplast-like form of mycobacteria isolated from Crohn's disease patients and identified by polymerase chain reaction to have DNA from either *M. paratuberculosis* or mycobacteria of unknown specific origin. Although certain mycobacteria may be important etiologic factors for Crohn's disease, mycobacterial antibodies do not correlate with disease activity [32•]. In general, the evidence supporting the etiologic role of *M. paratuberculosis* and other mycobacteria is weak. However, because mycobacteria are potentially treatable, Ciclitira [33•] suggested that certain Crohn's disease patients should be treated with a trial of quadruple antimycobacterial therapy (rifampin, ethambutol, isoniazid, and pyrazinamide or clofazimine).

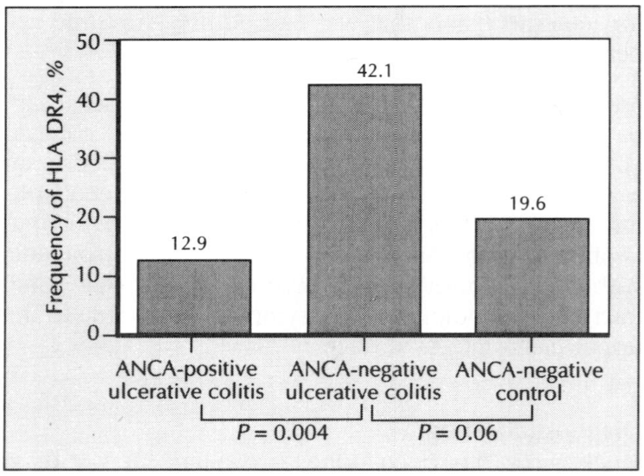

Fig. 2. HLA-DR4 allele frequency in antineutrophil cytoplasmic antibody (ANCA)-positive and -negative ulcerative colitis patients, compared with ANCA-negative controls. (*From* Yang *et al.* [3••]; with permission.)

Other organism have potential etiologic associations. Viral studies on tissue demonstrated paramyxovirus-like particles, nuclear inclusions, and measles virus *N*-protein genomic RNA in Crohn's disease patients localized in the lymphocytes of granulomas [34••]. The authors conclude that a persistent measles virus may cause a chronic intestinal granulomatous inflammation that is, or is indistinguishable from, Crohn's disease. Two South American children were described with enterocolitis from the filiform nematode *Angiostrongylus costaricensis* whose inflammatory disease in the distal and terminal ileum is indistinguishable from Crohn's disease [35•]. Patients with active ulcerative colitis were colonized less frequently with *Escherichia coli* than patients with inactive or no disease [36•]. Furthermore, in contrast to previous work, the adhesive properties of the bacteria in the groups did not differ. *E. coli* is not likely to be etiologic.

Other environmental agents

Cigarette smoking continues to be the single most important environmental agent associated with the development of IBD. Smokers are more likely than control subjects to develop Crohn's disease and less likely than controls to develop ulcerative colitis. Former smokers have an increased risk of developing ulcerative colitis and smoking history does not correlate with extent of disease or frequency of colectomy [37•]. Smoking in the household (passive smoking) increases a child's risk of developing IBD, either Crohn's disease or ulcerative colitis [38••]. Katschinski *et al.* [39••] theorized that this phenomenon may be confounded by a higher sugar intake in beverages among nonsmokers. After adjusting for cigarette smoking, the risk of developing ulcerative colitis in populations consuming added sugar in beverages was not significantly elevated (odds ratio 1.4, 95% confidence interval 0.70 to 2.9).

Oral contraceptive use is not felt to be an important risk factor for the development of Crohn's disease or ulcerative colitis. Katschinski *et al.* [40••] reported that oral contraceptive use was associated with a threefold increased risk of developing Crohn's disease in nonsmokers only. There was no such association in smokers.

Natural history

Disease exacerbation and mortality

From a large referral population, Farmer *et al.* [41••] theorized that the major determinant of the natural history of ulcerative colitis is extent of disease at diagnosis. At diagnosis, patients most commonly presented with proctosigmoiditis (46%) and pancolitis (37%), whereas left-sided disease (17%) was less common. Patients with pancolitis had the worst prognosis; 24% developed toxic, fulminant, or severe colitis and 61% required colectomy (Table 1). A total of 13% of left-sided colitis patients developed toxic colitis and 52% required surgery. Only 4% of patients with proctosigmoiditis developed toxic symptoms and 14% eventually required colectomy. Of note, colectomy rates for cancer or dysplasia were similar (approximately 9%) among groups. During the course of the evaluation period, fully 70% of left-sided patients and 34% of proctosigmoiditis patients extended disease and developed pancolitis. Disease progression was significantly associated with either toxic symptoms or joint symptoms.

Jayanthi *et al.* [42•] underscored the importance of correct extent of ulcerative colitis at diagnosis in epidemiologic surveys or therapeutic trials. As compared with patients having proctosigmoiditis, patients with proctitis more often achieved a long-term remission or had their diagnosis changed to non-IBD. Tysk and Jarnerot [43••] reported that although the month of diagnosis of ulcerative colitis is distributed evenly throughout the year, exacerbations of ulcerative colitis occur more frequently in the spring and the fall. Gryboski [44•] and Ahsgren *et al.* [45•] concur that children who present with ulcerative colitis usually have only mildly active disease, infrequent relapses, a lower colectomy rate, and lower incidence of colorectal cancer than patients who present as adults. Probert *et al.* [46••] calculated a standardized mortality ratio for European ulcerative patients of just 93, an innocuous figure that did not appreciably vary with extent of disease, age at diagnosis, year of diagnosis, or surgical treatment.

The course of Crohn's disease is less well defined. Tan and Allan [47••] reported on 34 patients with diffuse

Table 1. Frequency of primary indications for surgery by clinical pattern*

	Extent of disease at diagnosis, *n (%)*			
Indication	Pancolitis (*n* = 243)	Left-sided colitis (*n* = 98)	Proctitis (*n* = 72)	Overall (*n* = 413)†
Intractability/chronicity	87 (35.8)	42 (42.9)	37 (51.4)	166 (40.2)
Acute medical failure	42 (17.3)	19 (19.4)	9 (12.5)	70 (16.9)
Colonic dilation	59 (24.3)	9 (9.2)	8 (11.1)	76 (18.4)
Cacer prophylaxis or dysplasia	12 (4.9)	8 (8.2)	5 (6.9)	25 (6.1)
Cancer	9 (3.7)	3 (3.1)	1 (1.4)	13 (3.1)
Bleeding	10 (4.1)	3 (3.1)	2 (2.8)	15 (3.6)
Growth retardation	2 (0.8)	1 (1.0)	0	3 (0.7)
Extraintestional manifestations	3 (1.2)	0	0	3 (0.7)
Free perforation	7 (2.9)	1 (1.0)	0	8 (1.9)
Perianal disease	1 (0.4)	3 (3.1)	7 (9.7)	11 (2.7)
Strong patient pressure	4 (2.4)	2 (2.0)	1 (1.4)	7 (1.7)
Other‡	7 (2.4)	7 (7.1)	2 (2.8)	16 (3.9)

**From* Farmer *et al.* [41••]; with permission.

†Data were not available for six pancolitis patients and one proctitis patient.

‡Consists of small percentages of peritonitis, obstruction, mass/abscess, and internal fistula.

jejunoileitis of Crohn's disease. These patients usually present with colicky abdominal pain, weight loss, and diarrhea and most receive prolonged steroid administration. Surgery is common, but with the advent of strictureplasty, short bowel syndrome is rare and prolonged remissions can be attained. Heimann *et al.* [48•] demonstrated that microscopic inflammation at the resection margin and primary anastomosis are the two principal determinants of early recurrence after surgery for Crohn's disease.

Inflammatory complications

Thrombotic and thromboembolic diseases are important inflammatory complications of IBD. Once mechanisms are better understood, these severe complications might be prevented. Webberley *et al.* [49••] suspected that a hypercoagulable state exists because of abnormal platelet function. Spontaneous platelet aggregation, hypersensitive platelet aggregation, and high thromboxane B2 were found in IBD patients in the face of normal platelet count and normal platelet life span. These findings are not related to disease activity and may contribute to the hypercoagulable state.

The suppurative process in Crohn's disease patients can extend to a variety of regions. Sung *et al.* [50•] reported the first two cases of mesenteric abscesses extending to the rectus sheath. Attanoos *et al.* [51•] presented intriguing evidence that patients with Crohn's disease and hidradenitis suppurativa may have cutaneous Crohn's disease, because granulomas of the dermis are found away from the site of active inflammation. Church *et al.* [52••] reported on 24 patients with Crohn's disease, mostly Crohn's colitis (79%) and hidradenitis suppurativa of the perineum. The treatment difficulties are reflected in the fact that only 46% became asymptomatic following surgery.

Hughes' pathogenic classification of perianal Crohn's disease correlates with outcome [53•]. Primary lesions (*eg*, fissures, cavitating ulcers, or condylomas with Crohn's disease) had a worse prognosis (32% continence after treatment) than patients with secondary lesions (*eg*, abscess and fistulas, 63% continence). The inflammatory process in IBD may have remote effects and include remote organs. Motil *et al.* [54••] determined that the degree of inflammation, not steroid use or surgery, correlated best with growth failure in children with Crohn's disease. Chugh *et al.* [55•] described a 78-year-old woman who had ulcerative colitis for 15 years who was diagnosed with concomitant polymyositis. Corticosteroids and 5-acetylsalicylic acid therapy successfully treated both disease.

Hepatobiliary complications

Hepatobiliary complications of IBD are numerous and plentiful. Hashimoto *et al.* [56••] reported that among 163 consecutive Japanese ulcerative colitis patients studied, seven patients (4.3%) had chronic liver disease, five had primary sclerosing cholangitis, and two had chronic viral hepatitis. Primary sclerosing cholangitis was present in all patients who developed cholestasis. Interestingly, primary sclerosing cholangitis need not be symptomatic. Bornman *et al.* [57•] described nine cases of asymptomatic primary sclerosing cholangitis with diffuse ductal involvement. All had a benign course and only two ever exhibited mild hyperbilirubinemia. Two reports surfaced reported the coincidence between ulcerative colitis and primary biliary cirrhosis [58•,59•]. One of these unlucky patients also had chronic pancreatitis. Crohn's disease also can affect the gallbladder, as reported by Post *et al.* [60•] in a patient who had upper gastrointestinal disease.

Unusual complications

Several unusual complications of IBD have been reported this year. Lindgren *et al.* [61•] report that approximately one third of ulcerative colitis patients will suffer from autonomic vagal neuropathy, a figure independent of activity of disease or colectomy. In contrast, the autonomic neuropathy of Crohn's disease usually is sympathetic dysfunction. Norton *et al.* [62•] described three cases of Crohn's disease with rheumatoid arthritis and negative antinuclear antibody, rheumatoid factor, and HLA-B27. Gower-Rousseau *et al.* [63•] reported remission of myasthenia gravis after proctocolectomy in a patient with ulcerative colitis, implying a colonic source for an autoantibody of myasthenia gravis. Eisner *et al.* [64•] asserted that acute pancreatitis may occur in patients with Crohn's disease from duodenal disease and ductal obstruction or as an extraintestinal manifestation from remote disease.

Cancer in ulcerative colitis patients

Both oncogenes and tumor-suppresser genes are believed to be necessary components of the dysplasia-carcinoma sequence in both sporadic colorectal cancer and ulcerative colitis–associated cancer. The two oncogenes that are most studied in sporadic colorectal cancer are from *ras* gene family and the C-*myc* gene. Mutations in these oncogenes induce cellular proliferation. The tumor-suppressor genes include the retinoblastoma (*RB*) gene, the adenomatous polyposis coli (*APC*) gene, the mutated in colon cancer (*MCC*) gene, the deleted in colon cancer (*DCC*) gene, and the *p53* gene.

Yin *et al.* [65••] studied 45 ulcerative colitis patients with dysplasia or cancer, 20 of whom (44%) exhibited *p53* point mutations that resulted in inactivation and loss of heterozygosity. These mutations were present in both dysplastic lesions and malignancies. The findings suggest that neoplastic transformation in ulcerative colitis involved point mutations in the *p53* gene that may occur in dysplastic epithelium long before malignancy develops.

These findings were corroborated by Taylor *et al.* [66•] who used an immunohistochemical method with a monoclonal antibody specific to the human p53 protein on archival samples from patients with colorectal carcinoma complicating ulcerative colitis. Six of 20 samples with dysplasia and 11 of 21 samples with cancer exhibited mutations in the p53 protein. Ten of 21 samples of sporadic colorectal cancer also exhibited such mutations. These studies support the hypothesis that tumor-suppressor gene mutations are associated with colorectal cancer in ulcerative colitis patients.

Epidemiologic studies are underway to identify etiologic associations. In a case-control study, Lashner [67••] studied 67 consecutive patients enrolled in a cancer surveillance program for ulcerative colitis. The risk of developing dysplasia or cancer increased by 18% for each 10 ng/mL decrease in red blood cell folic acid. Folic acid deficiency may be caused by a number of factors, such as intestinal losses, poor intake, or competitive inhibition from sulfasalazine, that require more complete elucidation. Still, folic acid supplementation is safe and inexpensive, and may decrease cancer risk.

D'Haens *et al.* [68••], in a matched case-control study, found that patients with cholestatic liver disease, either primary sclerosing cholangitis or pericholangitis, and ulcerative colitis were nine times as likely to develop cancer or dysplasia as patients without cholestasis. It is theorized that patients with cholestatic liver disease have increased levels of the carcinogenic secondary bile acids in the enterohepatic circulation and consequently have an increased risk for neoplastic transformation.

Sugita *et al.* [69•] demonstrated that survival of 102 patients with colorectal cancer in ulcerative colitis was critically dependent on histologic stage and was not appreciably different from noncolitic cancer. Choi *et al.* [70•] demonstrated that asymptomatic cancers found during the course of surveillance were detected at an earlier histologic stage and consequently had a better survival than symptomatic cancers detected outside of a surveillance program. Still, surveillance programs have yet to demonstrate dramatically improved cancer-related survival among the total group of screened patients.

Lynch *et al.* [71••] reported cancer detection rates from a surveillance program. In a program of 160 patients, one Dukes' A lesion was detected. Eight other colorectal malignancies were detected at their institution outside of the screening program, implying either a failure to enroll all high-risk patients or a tremendously successful program that prevents cancer by performing colectomy on all high-risk patients. The latter scenario did not appear to be the case.

Cancer in Crohn's disease patients

The risk of a Crohn's disease patient developing adenocarcinoma is much lower than the risk in ulcerative colitis patients. Quantifying these risks are important in determining the maximal effectiveness of cancer surveillance. Munkholm *et al.* [72••] determined that 373 Crohn's disease patients in a Danish regional inception cohort had a relative risk for intestinal cancer of 1.7 (not significant), 50 for small bowel cancer, and 1.1 for colorectal cancer. Michelassi *et al.* [73••] reported on 14 cases of adenocarcinoma, seven in the large bowel and seven in the small bowel, in Crohn's disease patients evaluated at a single large referral center. The diagnosis was made preoperatively in only four cases of large bowel cancer and only two patients developed carcinoma within 10 years of diagnosis of Crohn's disease. Mean survival was only 6 months for small bowel cancer, reflecting the advanced stage of disease at diagnosis. The cumulative incidence for small bowel cancer was 0.6% and for large bowel cancer was 1.4%.

Even though there is an increased risk of colorectal and small intestinal cancer in patients with Crohn's disease, the risk is still small and routine surveillance in this population cannot be cost effective. Perhaps chemoprevention through vitamin supplementation could provide a benefit. Kuroki *et al.* [74•] demonstrated that patients with Crohn's disease had diminished vitamins A, E, B1, B2, B6, and folic acid, some of which may be protective for the development of cancer.

Definite advances were made in the clinical epidemiology of IBD in 1993, opening many challenging areas of clinical research. A few questions were answered, but many more remain and new questions have been posed.

References and recommended reading

Papers of particular interest, published within the annual period of review, have been highlighted as:
- • Of special interest
- •• Of outstanding interest

1. • Martinez-Salmeron JF, Rodrigo M, de Teresa J, Nogueras F, Garcia-Montero M, de Sola C, Salmeron J, Caballero C: **Epidemiology of Inflammatory Bowel Disease in the Province of Granada, Spain: A Retrospective Study From 1979 to 1988.** *Gut* 1993, 34:1207–1209.

Over a 10-year period, the incidence of ulcerative colitis in Spain was two per 100,000 and the incidence of Crohn's disease was 0.9 per 100,000.

2. • Tragnone A, Hanau C, Bazzocchi G, Lanfranchi GA: **Epidemiological Characteristics of Inflammatory Bowel Disease in Bologna, Italy - Incidence and Risk Factors**. *Digestion* 1993, 54:183–188.

This study of descriptive epidemiology calculated an incidence rate for IBD of 7.7 per 100,000 population with former smokers likely to develop ulcerative colitis and smokers likely to develop Crohn's disease.

3. •• Yang H, McElree C, Roth M-P, Shanahan F, Targan SR, Rotter JI: **Familial Empirical Risks for Inflammatory Bowel Disease: Differences Between Jews and Non-Jews.** *Gut* 1993, 34:517–524.

Seven point eight percent of Jewish ulcerative colitis patients, 5.2% of non-Jewish ulcerative colitis patients, 4.5% of Jewish Crohn's disease patients, and 1.6% of non-Jewish Crohn's disease patients have first-degree relatives affected with IBD, differences that are statistically significant.

4. Probert CSJ, Jayanthi V, Hughes AO, Thompson JR, Wicks
•• ACB, Mayberry JF: **Prevalence and Family Risk of Ulcerative Colitis and Crohn's Disease: An Epidemiologic Study Among Europeans and South Asians in Leicestershire.** *Gut* 1993, **34**:1547–1551.

In ulcerative colitis patients, the relative risk of a family member developing ulcerative colitis was 15 (not elevated for a family member developing Crohn's disease). Likewise, in Crohn's disease patients, relatives had a relative risk of 15 for developing Crohn's disease and 3 for developing ulcerative colitis.

5. Hollander D: **Permeability in Crohn's Disease: Altered Bar-**
• **rier Functions in Healthy Relatives?** *Gastroenterology* 1993, **104**:1848–1873.

The history and importance of intestinal permeability studies are reviewed. Newer diagnostic techniques may be useful in identifying "highly permeable small bowel" populations who may be at high risk for developing Crohn's disease.

6. May GR, Sutherland LR, Meddings JB: **Is Small Intestinal**
•• **Permeability Really Increased in Relatives of Patients With Crohn's Disease?** *Gastroenterology* 1993, **104**:1627–1632.

Lactulose permeabily was elevated in small proportion (10%) of asymptomatic relatives of Crohn's disease patients. Of note, approximately 10% of relatives of Crohn's disease patients are expected to develop Crohn's disease.

7. Moonka D, Lichtenstein GR, Levine MS, Rombeau JL, Furth
• EE, MacDermott RP: **Giant Gastric Ulcers: An Unusual Manifestation of Crohn's Disease.** *Am J Gastroenterol* 1993, **88**:297–299.

This patient with recurrent giant gastric ulcers, outlet obstruction perforation, achlorhydria, and granulomatous had unsuspected Crohn's disease.

8. Scapa E, Marcus EL, Kaufman S, Vinograd I, Reif R, Es-
• hchar J: **Miliary Crohn's Disease: Early or Different?** *J Clin Gastroenterol* 1993, **16**:222–226.

A 14-year-old boy is described with suspected lymphoma who is found to have granulomatous inflammation of the serosal surface of 110 cm of small bowel with a "miliary" appearance.

9. Calder CJ, Lacy D, Raafat F, Weller PH, Booth IW: **Crohn's**
• **Disease With Pulmonary Involvement in a 3 Year Old Boy.** *Gut* 1993, **34**:1636–1638.

This 3-year-old boy had granulomas in the lung and microscopic colitis with findings concentrated in the transverse colon.

10. Haddad M, Azim F, Koran A, Stelman E, Mor C, Ze-
• likovski: **Crohn's Disease of the Appendix.** *Eur J Surg* 1993, **159**:191–192.

A rare case of Crohn's disease isolated to the appendix is reported.

11. Dunstan SP, Balfour TW: **Fistulas are not Always due to**
• **Crohn's Disease: An Unusual Groin Abscess.** *Am J Gastroenterol* 1993, **88**:120–121.

A chronic enterocutaneous fistula in a 38-year-old was due to a ruptured appendiceal diverticulum.

12. Alcantara M, Rodriguez R, Potenciano JLM, Carrobles JL,
• Munoz C, Gomez R: **Endoscopic and Bioptic Findings in the Upper Gastrointestinal Tract in Patients With Crohn's Disease.** *Endoscopy* 1993, **25**:282–286.

Aphthoid ulcers in the stomach were found in 35% and granulomas were found in 20% of patients with Crohn's disease elsewhere in the gastrointestinal tract, most of whom had no upper gastrointestinal symptoms. The authors suggest that upper endoscopy with biopsy may be useful in the diagnosis of indeterminate colitis.

13. Schratter-Sehn AU, Lochs H, Handl-Zeller L, Tschalakoff
• D, Schratter M: **Endosonographic Features of Lower Pelvic Region in Crohn's Disease.** *Am J Gastroenterol* 1993, **88**:1054–1057.

Endoscopic ultrasound can map fistulas and abscesses in perirectal Crohn's disease. The technique is limited, though, by pain and strictures.

14. Sciarretta G, Furno A, Mazzoni M, Basile C, Malaguti P:
• **Technetium-99m Hexamethyl Propylene Amine Oxime Granulocyte Scintigraphy in Crohn's Disease: Diagnostic and Clinical Relevance.** *Gut* 1993, **34**:1364–1369.

In 103 patients with Crohn's disease, scintigraphy had a sensitivity of 95% and a specificity of 100% for detecting active inflammation, abscess, and fistula. Scintigraphy also could assess response of inflammation, especially in the large bowel, to treatment.

15. Arndt J-W, van der Sluys Veer A, Blok D, Griffoen F,
• Werspaget HW, Lamers CBHW, Pauwels EKJ: **Prospective Comparative Study of Technetium-99m-WBCs and Indium-111-Granulocytes for the Examiniation of Patients With Inflammatory Bowel Disease.** *J Nucl Med* 1993, **34**:1052–1057.

Technetium-labeled leukocyte scintigraphy is less time consuming, offers less radiation exposure, and as useful as indium-labeled leukocyte scintigraphy is assessing activity in IBD.

16. Heresbach D, Bretagne J-F, Raoul J-L, Moisan A, Siproudhis
• L, Devillers A, Gosselin M: **Indium Scanning in Assessment of Acute Crohn's Disease: A Prospective Study of Sensitivity and Correlation With Severity of Mucosal Damage.** *Dig Dis Sci* 1993, **38**:1601–1607.

Scanning correlates well with endoscopically severe lesions, but poorly with subtle lesions.

17. Nicholls S, Stephens S, Braegger CP, Walker-Smith JA, Mac-
• Donald TT: **Cytokines in Stools of Children With Inflammatory Bowel Disease or Infective Diarrhea.** *J Clin Pathol* 1993, **46**:757–760.

Children with active ulcerative colitis had elevated stool concentrations of tumor necrosis factor-α but low levels of interleukin-6 whose immunoreactivity was destroyed by a heat-labile factor.

18. Bernstein CN, Robert ME, Eysselein VE: **Rectal Substance P**
• **Concentrations are Increased in Ulcerative Colitis but not Crohn's Disease.** *Am J Gastroenterol* 1993, **88**:908–913.

The neurotransmitter substance P is found in the rectal mucosa of ulcerative colitis patients, not Crohn's disease patients, and correlates with the degree of inflammation and the presence of neutrophils and eosinophils.

19. Kokoszka J, Nelson RL, Swedler WI, Skosey J, Abicarian
• H: **Determination of Inflammatory Bowel Disease Activity by Breath Pentane Analysis.** *Dis Colon Rectum* 1993, **36**:597–601.

Breath pentane, generated by peroxidation of cellular fatty acids, correlated well with indium-111–labeled leukocyte scanning in IBD patients.

20. Sofaer J: **Crohn's Disease: The Genetic Contribution.** *Gut*
• 1993, **34**:869–871.

Autoimmunity, associated chromosomal and monogenetic disorders, frequencies among relatives, and associated genetic markers point directly to one or more defective gene products as a "genetic liability" for developing Crohn's disease.

21. Hardarson S, LaBrecque DR, Mitros FA, Neil GA, Goeken
•• JA: **Antineutrophil Cytoplasmic Antibody in Inflammatory Bowel and Hepatobiliary Diseases: High Prevalence in Ulcerative Colitis, Primary Sclerosing Cholangitis, and Autoimmune Hepatitis.** *Am J Clin Pathol* 1993, **99**:277–281.

Perinuclear ANCA was positive in 72% of patients with ulcerative colitis or sclerosing cholangitis. The specificity of the test was 90%. Such information may be useful for diagnosing indeterminate colitis and cholestatic liver disease.

22. Sung JY, Chan KL, Hsu R, Liew CT, Lawton JWM: **Ulcerative**
• **Colitis and Antineutrophil Cytoplasmic Antibodies in Hong Kong Chinese.** *Am J Gastroenterol* 1993, **88**:864–869.

Of 19 ulcerative colitis patients, 73% were ANCA positive. Surprisingly, cytoplasmic staining was more common than perinuclear staining.

23. Proujansky R, Fawcett PT, Gibney KM, Treem WR, Hyams
• JS: **Examination of Anti-Neutrophil Cytoplasmic Antibodies**

in Childhood Inflammatory Bowel Disease. *J Pediatr Gastroenterol Nutr* 1993, **17**:193–197.
ANCA was positive in 66% of children with ulcerative colitis and 19% of children with Crohn's disease and did not correlate with disease activity.

24. •• Yang H, Rotter JI, Toyoda H, Landers C, Tyan D, McElree CK, Targan SR: **Ulcerative Colitis: A Genetically Heterogeneous Disorder Defined by Genetic (HLA Class II) and Subclinical (Antineutrophil Cytoplasmic Antibodies) Markers.** *J Clin Invest* 1993, **92**:1080–1084.
Among ulcerative colitis patients, two distinct genetic patterns have been described: ANCA-positive/DR2 patients and ANCA-negative/DR4 patients.

25. •• Toyoda H, Wang S-J, Yang H-Y, Redford A, Magalong D, Tyan D, McElree CK, Pressman SR, Shanahan F, Targan SR, Rotter JI: **Distinct Associations of HLA Class II Genes With Inflammatory Bowel Disease.** *Gastroenterology* 1993, **105**:741–748.
In ulcerative colitis patients, there were positive associations with HLA DR2 and negative associations with DR4 and DRw6. In Crohn's disease patients, there were positive associations with the combination of HLA DR1 and DQw5. There are genetic distinctions between Crohn's disease and ulcerative colitis.

26. • Treem WR, Veligati LM, Rotter JI, Targan SR, Hyams JS: **Ulcerative Colitis and Total Alopecia in a Mother and Her Son.** *Gastroenterology* 1993, **104**:1187–1191.
These patients with ulcerative colitis and alopecia areata were both ANCA positive, but not HLA identical. Treatment of the son wtih 6-mercaptopurine led to ulcerative colitis remission and hair growth.

27. •• Van Kruningen HJ, Colombel JF, Cartun RW, Whitlock RH, Koopmans M, Hangro HO, Hoogkamp-Korstanje AA, Lecomte-Houcke M, Devred M, Paris JC, Cortot A: **An In-Depth Study of Crohn's Disease in Two French Families.** *Gastroenterology* 1993, **104**:351–360.
Epidemic Crohn's disease was postulated when multiple siblings developed disease within a short period of time. No infectious agent or common HLA haplotype could be discerned.

28. • Aisenberg J, Janowitz HD: **Cluster of Inflammatory Bowel Disease in Three Close College Friends?** *J Clin Gastroenterol* 1993, **17**:18–20.
Within a decade of graduation, three close college friends developed IBD (two Crohn's disease, one ulcerative colitis).

29. • Rutgeerts P, Geboes K: **Crohn's Disease and Pre-Aphthoid Lesions.** *Lancet* 1993, **341**:1443–1444.
A theory of the pathogenesis of Crohn's disease is outlined beginning with a microvascular lesion that triggers an unchecked immune response and fibrinogenesis.

30. • Hermon-Taylor J: **Causation of Crohn's Disease: The Impact of Clusters.** *Gastroenterology* 1993, **104**:643–646.
Enough evidence exists to study *M. paratuberculosis* as a cause of Crohn's disease in much greater depth.

31. •• Wall S, Kunze AZM, Saboor S, Soufleri I, Seechurn P, Chiodini R, McFadden JJ: **Identification of Spheroplast-Like Agents Isolated From Tissues of Patients With Crohn's Disease and Control Tissues by Polymerase Chain Reaction.** *J Clin Microbiol* 1993, **31**:1342–1345.
Non–acid-fast, cell wall–deficient, spheroplast-like forms of mycobacteria were isolated from Crohn's disease patients and identified to have DNA from either *M. paratuberculosis* or mycobacteria of unknown specific origin.

32. • Stansby KJ, Lowes JR, Allen RN, Ibbotson JP: **Antibodies to *Mycobacterium paratuberculosis* and Species of Environmental Mycobacteria in Crohn's Disease and Control Subjects.** *Gut* 1993, **34**:371–374.
There were no important or significant differences in antibodies to a variety of mycobacteria among active and inactive Crohn's disease populations, as well as controls.

33. • Ciclitira PJ: **Does Crohn's Disease Have a Mycobacterial Basis? The Case is Unproved.** *BMJ* 1993, **306**:733–734.
Evidence supporting the etiologic role of *M. paratuberculosis* and other mycobacteria is weak. However, treatment of Crohn's disease patients with quadruple therapy (rifampin, ethambutol, isoniazid, and pyrazinamide or clofazimine) may be of value in select patients.

34. •• Wakefield AJ, Pittilo RM, Sim R, Cosby SL, Stephenson JR, Dhillon AP, Pounder RE: **Evidence for Persistent Measles Virus Infection in Crohn's Disease.** *J Med Virol* 1993, 39:345–353.
Viral studies on tissue from Crohn's disease and control patients demonstrated *Paramyxovirus*-like particles, nuclear inclusions, and measles virus N-protein genomic RNA in Crohn's disease patients localized in the lymphocytes of granulomas. The authors conclude that measles virus may cause a chronic intestinal granulomatous inflammation, namely Crohn's disease.

35. • Liacouras CA, Bell LM, Aljabi MC, Piccoli DA: ***Angiostrongylus costaricensis* Enterocolitis Mimics Crohn's Disease.** *J Pediatr Gastroenterol Nutr* 1993, **16**:203–207.
Two children are described who were infected with this filiform nematode in South America and developed an inflammatory disease in the distal and terminal ileum.

36. • Hartley MG, Hudson MJ, Swarbrick ET, Gent AE, Hellier MD, Grace RH: **Adhesive and Hydrophobic Properties of *Escherichia coli* From the Rectal Mucosa of Patients With Ulcerative Colitis.** *Gut* 1993, **34**:63–67.
Patients with active ulcerative colitis were colonized less frequently with *E. coli* than patients with inactive or no disease. Furthermore, in contrast to previous work, the adhesive properties of the bacteria in the groups did not differ. *E. coli* is not likely to be etiologic.

37. • Srivasta ED, Newcombe RG, Rhodes J, Avaramidis P, Mayberry JF: **Smoking and Ulcerative Colitis: A Community Study.** *Int J Colorectal Dis* 1993, **8**:71–74.
Ulcerative colitis patients are more likely than controls to never have smoked or be former smokers. Smoking history did not correlate with extent of disease or frequency of colectomy.

38. •• Lashner BA, Shaheen NJ, Hanauer SB, Kirschner BS: **Passive Smoking is Associated With an Increased Risk of Developing Inflammatory Bowel Disease in Children.** *Am J Gastroenterol* 1993, **88**:336–359.
Cigarette smoking in the household increases the risk of children developing IBD, either Crohn's disease or ulcerative colitis.

39. •• Katschinski BD, Fisel W, Schmialek J-P, Bract J, Goebell H: **Smoking and Sugar Intake in Ulcerative Colitis: A Case-Control Study.** *Eur J Gastroenterol Hepatol* 1993, **5**:91–95.
Smokers, protected from developing ulcerative colitis, may consume less added sugar to beverages than former smokers, a group not so protected. However, after adjusting for the effects of cigarette smoking, added sugar intake is not associated with the development of ulcerative colitis (odds ratio 1.4, 95% confidence interval 0.70 to 2.9). After adjusting for added sugar intake, cigarette smoking protects against the development of ulcerative colitis (odds ratio 0.18, 95% confidence interval 0.07 to 0.50).

40. •• Katschinski B, Fingerle D, Scherbaum B, Goebell H: **Oral Contraceptive Use and Cigarette Smoking in Crohn's Disease.** *Dig Dis Sci* 1993, **38**:1596–1600.
Oral contraceptive use increased the risk of developing Crohn's disease by threefold in nonsmokers only. There was no such association in smokers.

41. •• Farmer RG, Easley KA, Rankin GB: **Clinical Patterns, Natural History, and Progression of Ulcerative Colitis: A Long-Term Follow-Up of 1116 Patients.** *Dig Dis Sci* 1993, **38**:1137–1146.
In this large Cleveland Clinic series, extent of disease at diagnosis was the major determinant of prognosis. In patients with pancolitis, 61% required surgery and 11.5% developed arthritis. Interestingly, 70% of patients initially diagnosed as having left-sided colitis eventually developed pancolitis.

42. • Jayanthi V, Chuah SY, Probert CSJ, Mayberry M, Mayberry JF: **Proctitis and Proctosigmoiditis - A Need to Identify the Extent of Disease in Epidemiological Surveys.** *Digestion* 1993, **54**:61–64.
As compared with patients with proctosigmoiditis, patients with proctitis more often achieved a long-term remission or had their diag-

nosis changed to non-IBD. Caution may be necessary when entering proctitis patients into epidemiologic studies or therapeutic trials.

43. Tysk C, Jarnerot G: **Seasonal Variation in Exacerbations of Ulcerative Colitis.** *Scand J Gastroenterol* 1993, **28**:95–96.
••
While month of diagnosis of ulcerative colitis is distributed evenly throughout the year, exacerbations of ulcerative colitis occur more frequently in the spring (observed/expected 1.097) and the fall (observed/expected 1.144) as compared with the summer (observed/expected 0.787) and the winter (observed/expected 0.973).

44. Gryboski JD: **Ulcerative Colitis in Children 10 Years Old or Younger.** *J Pediatr Gastroenterol Nutr* 1993, **17**:24–31.
•
Of the 38 children with ulcerative colitis reviewed, most had mildly active disease with infrequent relapses.

45. Ahsgren L, Jonsson B, Stenling R, Rutegard J: **Prognosis After Early Onset of Ulcerative Colitis: A Study From an Unselected Patient Population.** *Hepatogastroenterology* 1993, **40**:467–470.
•
Among 32 patients with disease onset before age 20, 75% had pancolitis, 22% required colectomy within 15 years of disease, and 22% developed low-grade dysplasia. No patient had developed cancer within a mean follow-up of 18 years.

46. Probert CSJ, Jayanthi V, Wicks ACB, Mayberry JF: **Mortality in Patients With Ulcerative Colitis in Leicestershire, 1972-1989: An Epidemiologic Study.** *Dig Dis Sci* 1993, **38**:538–541.
••
The standardized mortality ratio for Europeans with ulcerative colitis was 93 (95% confidence interval 75 to 114). The standardized mortality ratios did not appreciably vary with extent of disease, age at diagnosis, year of diagnosis, or surgical treatment.

47. Tan WC, Allan RN: **Diffuse Jejunoileitis of Crohn's Disease.** *Gut* 1993, **34**:1374–1378.
••
The 34 patients described with diffuse jejunoileitis usually present with colicky abdominal pain, weight loss, and diarrhea. Most require prolonged steroid administration and repeated surgical resections are common. With the advent of strictureplasty, short-bowel syndrome is rare and prolonged remissions can be attained.

48. Heimann TM, Greenstein AJ, Lewis B, Kaufman D, Heimann DM, Aufsus AH: **Prediction of Early Symptomatic Recurrence After Intestinal Resection in Crohn's Disease.** *Ann Surg* 1993, **218**:294–299.
•
Microscopic inflammation at the resection margin and primary anastomosis are the two principal determinants of early recurrence following surgery for Crohn's disease.

49. Webberley MJ, Hart MT, Melikian V: **Thromboembolism in Inflammatory Bowel Disease: Role of Platelets.** *Gut* 1993, **34**:247–251.
••
Some patients with either ulcerative colitis or Crohn's disease have spontaneous platelet aggregation, hypersensitive platelet aggregation, and high thromboxane B2, as well as normal platelet life span. Such findings were not related to disease activity may contribute to the high risk of thromboembolic disease and microvascular disease in these patients.

50. Sung W-C, McKinley MJ, Harvey LP: **Rectus Sheath Abscess in Crohn's Disease.** *Am J Gastroenterol* 1993, **88**:793–794.
•
These are the first two cases reported of mesenteric abscesses extending to the rectus sheath.

51. Attanoos RL, Aooleton MAC, Hughes LE, Ansell ID, Douglas-Jones AG, Williams GT: **Granulomatous Hidradenitis Suppurativa and Cutaneous Crohn's Disease.** *Histopathology* 1993, **23**:111–115.
•
Both Crohn's disease and sarcoidosis patients who have hidradenitis suppurativa may have granulomas of the dermis away from the site of active inflammation.

52. Church JM, Fazio VW, Lavery IC, Oakley JR, Milsom JW: **The Differential Diagnosis and Comorbidity of Hidradenitis Suppurativa and Perianal Crohn's Disease.** *Int J Colorectal Dis* 1993, **8**:117–119.
••
Of 24 patients with Crohn's disease and hidradenitis suppurativa of the perineum, 19 had disease of the large bowel alone and only 11 became asymptomatic following surgery.

53. Frabcois Y, Vignal J, Descos L: **Outcome of Perianal Fistulae in Crohn's Disease - Value of Hughes' Pathogenic Classification.** *Int J Colorectal Dis* 1993, **8**:39–41.
•
Primary lesions (fissures, cavitating ulcers, condylomas with Crohn's disease) had a worse prognosis (32% continence after treatment) than patients with secondary lesions (abscess and fistulas, 63% continence).

54. Motil KJ, Grand RJ, Davis-Kraft L, Ferlic LL, Smith EO: **Growth Failure in Children With Inflammatory Bowel Disease: A Prospective Study.** *Gastroenterology* 1993, **105**:681–691.
••
The degree of inflammation, not steroid use or surgery, correlated with growth failure in children with Crohn's disease.

55. Chugh S, Dilawari JB, Sawhney IMS, Dang N, Radotra BD, Chawla YK: **Polymyositis Associated With Ulcerative Colitis.** *Gut* 1993, **34**:567–569.
•
This report from India describes a 78-year-old woman who had 15 years of symptoms suggestive of ulcerative colitis who presented with polymyositis. Corticosteroids and 5-acetylsalicylic acid therapy successfully treated both diseases.

56. Hashimoto E, Ideta M, Taniai M, Watanabe U, Okuda H, Nagasako K, Hisamitsu T, Obata H: **Prevalence of Primary Sclerosing Cholangitis and Other Liver Diseases in Japanese Patients With Chronic Ulcerative Colitis.** *J Gastroenterol Hepatol* 1993, **8**:146–149.
••
Among 163 consecutive ulcerative colitis patients, 4.3% (seven patients) had chronic liver disease; 5 patients had PSC and two had chronic viral hepatitis. Primary sclerosing cholangitis was present in all patients with alkaline phosphatase at least twice the upper limit of normal with mild transaminase elevations.

57. Bornman PC, Lemmer ER, Robson SC, Wright JP, Girdwood AH: **Asymptomatic Primary Sclerosing Cholangitis in Association With Inflammatory Bowel Disease.** *J Clin Gastroenterol* 1993, **16**:263–264.
•
Nine cases of asymptomatic primary sclerosing cholangitis are described with alkaline phosphatase elevations and diffuse ductal involvement. All had a benign course and only two ever exhibited mild hyperbilirubinemia.

58. Lever E, Balasubramanian K, Condon S, Wat BY: **Primary Biliary Cirrhosis Associated With Ulcerative Colitis.** *Am J Gastroenterol* 1993; **88**:945–947.
•
This is the sixth reported association between ulcerative colitis and primary biliary cirrhosis.

59. Tavarela Veloso F, Dias LM, Carvalho J, Fraga J, Saleiro J: **Ulcerative Colitis, Primary Biliary Cirrhosis, and Chronic Pancreatitis: Coincident or Coexistent?** *J Clin Gastroenterol* 1993, **16**:55–57.
•
This is the sixth case of ulcerative colitis and primary biliary cirrhosis and the first to include chronic pancreatitis.

60. Post AB, van Stolk R, Broughan TA, Tuthill RJ: **Crohn's Disease of the Gallbladder.** *J Clin Gastroenterol* 1993, **16**:139–142.
•
The 57-year-old woman developed Crohn's disease of the duodenum and gallbladder with biliary obstruction relieved surgically and with corticosteroids.

61. Lindgren S, Stewenius J, Sjolund K, Lilja B, Sundkvist G: **Autonomic Vagal Nerve Dysfunction in Patients With Ulcerative Colitis.** *Scand J Gastroenterol* 1993, **28**:638–642.
•
Approximately one-third of patients with ulcerative colitis suffer from autonomic vagal neuropathy, a figure independent of activity of disease or colectomy. In contrast, the autonomic neuropathy of Crohn's disease tends to be sympathetic dysfunction.

62. Norton KI, Eichenfield AH, Rosh JR, Stern MT, Hermann G: **Atypical Arthropathy Associated With Crohn's Disease.** *Am J Gastroenterol* 1993, **88**:948–952.
•
Three cases are described of Crohn's disease patients with rheumatoid arthritis and negative antinuclear antibody, rheumatoid factor, and HLA-B27.

63. Gower-Rousseau C, Reumauz D, Bellard M, Delecourt L, Ribet M, Colombel JF: **Remission of Myasthenia Gravis After**
•

Proctocolectomy in a Patient With Ulcerative Colitis. *Am J Gastroenterol* 1993, **88**:1136–1138.

Known autoimmune disorders in ulcerative colitis are primary sclerosing cholangitis, thyroid disorders, vitiligo, insulin dependent diabetes mellitus, rheumatoid arthritis, and myasthenia gravis, the last of which is reported to remit following proctocolectomy.

64. Eisner TD, Goldman IS, McKinley MJ: **Crohn's Disease and**
• **Pancreatitis.** *Am J Gastroenterol* 1993, **88**:583–586.

Acute pancreatitis may occur in patients with Crohn's disease from duodenal disease and ductal obstruction or as an extraintestinal manifestations from remote disease.

65. Yin J, Harpaz N, Tong Y, Huang Y, Laurin J, Greenwald
•• BD, Hontanosas M, Newkirk C, Meltzer SJ: **p53 Point Mutations in Dysplastic and Cancerous Ulcerative Colitis Lesions.** *Gastroenterology* 1993, **104**:1633–1639.

Of 45 ulcerative colitis patients with dysplasia or cancer, 20 exhibited *p53* point mutations that resulted in decreased expression and loss of heterozygosity. These mutations are associated with loss of tumor suppression and malignant transformation.

66. Taylor HW, Boyle M, Smith SC, Bustin S, Williams NS: **Ex-**
• **pression of p53 in Colorectal Cancer and Dysplasia Complicating Ulcerative Colitis.** *Br J Surg* 1993, **80**:442–444.

In archival samples of ulcerative colitis patients, six of 20 samples with dysplasia and 11 of 21 samples with cancer exhibited the p53 protein, a product of tumor suppresser genes. Ten of 21 samples of sporadic colorectal cancer exhibited such a protein.

67. Lashner BA: **Red Blood Cell Folate is Associated With the**
•• **Development of Dysplasia and Cancer in Ulcerative Colitis.** *J Cancer Res Clin Oncol* 1993, **119**:549–554.

In this case-control study, the risk of developing dysplasia or cancer increased by 18% for each 10 ng/mL decrease in erythrocyte folic acid.

68. D'Haens GR, Lashner BA, Hanauer SB: **Pericholangitis and**
•• **Sclerosing Cholangitis are Risk Factors for Dysplasia and Cancer in Ulcerative Colitis.** *Am J Gastroenterol* 1993, **88**:1174–1178.

This matched case-control study found that patients with cholestatic liver disease and ulcerative colitis were nine times as likely to develop cancer or dysplasia as patients without cholestasis.

69. Sugita A, Greenstein AJ, Ribeiro MB, Sachar DB, Bodian C,
• Panday AKN, Szporn A, Pozner J, Heimann T, Palmer M, Aufses AH: **Survival With Colorectal Cancer in Ulcerative Colitis: A Study of 102 Cases.** *Ann Surg* 1993, **218**:189–195.

Survival with colorectal cancer in ulcerative colitis is critically dependent on histologic stage and is not appreciably different from noncolitic cancer.

70. Choi PM, Nugent FW, Schoetz DJ, Silverman ML, Haggitt
• RC: **Colonoscopic Surveillance Reduces Mortality From Colorectal Cancer in Ulcerative Colitis.** *Gastroenterology* 1993, **105**:418–424.

Asymptomatic cancers detected during the course of surveillance were detected at an earlier histologic stage and consequently had a better survival than symptomatic cancers detected outside of a surveillance program.

71. Lynch DAF, Lobo AJ, Sobala GM, Dixon MF, Axon ATR:
•• **Failure of Colonoscopic Surveillance in Ulcerative Colitis.** *Gut* 1993, **34**:1075–1080.

In a surveillance program of 160 patients, 1 Dukes' A lesion was detected. Eight other malignancies were detected outside the screening program implying either a failure to enroll all high-risk patients or a tremendously successful program the prevents cancer by performing colectomy on all high-risk patients.

72. Munkholm P, Langholz E, Davidsen M, Binder V: **Intestinal**
•• **Cancer Risk and Mortality in Patients With Crohn's Disease.** *Gastroenterology* 1993, **105**:1716–1723.

A total of 373 Crohn's disease patients in a Danish regional inception cohort had a relative risk of 1.7 (not significant) for intestinal cancer, 50 for small bowel cancer, and 1.1 for colorectal cancer.

73. Michelassi F, Testa G, Pomidor WJ, Lashner BA, Block GE:
•• **Adenocarcinoma Complicating Crohn's Disease.** *Dis Colon Rectum* 1993, **36**:654–661.

Fourteen cases of adenocarcinoma, seven in the large bowel and seven in the small bowel, in Crohn's disease are reported. The diagnosis was made preoperatively in only four cases of large bowel cancer. Mean survival was only 6 months for small bowel cancer, reflecting the advanced stage of disease at diagnosis.

74. Kuroki F, Iida M, Tominaga M, Matsumoto T, Hirakawa K,
• Sugiyama S, Fujishima M: **Multiple Vitamin Status in Crohn's Disease: Correlation With Disease Activity.** *Dig Dis Sci* 1993, **38**:1614–1618.

Patients with Crohn's disease had diminished vitamins A, E, B1, B2, B6, and folic acid.

Bret A. Lashner, MD, MPH, Director, Center for Inflammatory Bowel Disease, Department of Gastroenterology, Cleveland Clinic Foundation, Desk S-40, 9500 Euclid Avenue, Cleveland, OH 44195, USA.

Aaron Brzezinski, MD, Department of Gastroenterology, Cleveland Clinic Foundation, Desk S-40, 9500 Euclid Avenue, Cleveland, OH 44195, USA.

Inflammatory mediators in inflammatory bowel disease

William F. Stenson, MD

Washington University School of Medicine, St. Louis, Missouri, USA

The most important development in the study of the pathogenesis of inflammation in inflammatory bowel disease was the publication of three papers demonstrating that genetically manipulated mice developed chronic intestinal inflammation similar to human inflammatory bowel disease. Two of these genetic models comprised cytokine knockouts (interleukin-2 and interleukin-10), the third model included a series of genetic defects in the T-cell receptor (α and β chains) or the class II major histocompatibility complex. One striking characteristic of these models was the limitation of pathology to the gastrointestinal tract, even though these were all defects in systemic immunity that might have been expected either to cause widespread pathology or to be incompatible with life. The second striking characteristic of these models was the influence of colonic bacteria on the development of pathology.

Current Opinion in Gastroenterology 1994, **10**:384–389

Inflammatory bowel disease in genetically determined animal models

The October 22, 1993 issue of *Cell* contained three papers describing inflammatory bowel disease (IBD) in genetically manipulated mice [1••–3••]. Two of these genetic models contained cytokine knockouts, interleukin-2 and interleukin-10, the third model contained defects in several T-cell receptor genes.

The interleukin-2 knockout mice developed normally during the first 3 to 4 weeks of life, but then became severely compromised; approximately 50% of the animals died between the 4th and 9th week of age [1••]. These animals developed splenomegaly, lymphadenopathy, and severe anemia. Of the surviving animals, 100% developed IBD. The first signs were observed between 6 and 15 weeks of age and involved the mucosa and submucosa of the colon with sparing of the small bowel. Analysis of colonic lymphocytes revealed increased numbers of both B and T cells. The B-cell responses were marked by increased production of immunoglobulin G1 and immunoglobulin E, which are supported by Th2 T cells. These animals also had anticolon antibodies, although the identity of the antigen was not explored. Immunohistochemistry demonstrated a large number of epithelial cells in the inflamed colon that expressed class II major histocompatibility complex (MHC) molecules. In the healthy gut, class II antigen expression is limited to the small intestine and is not seen in the colon. To determine the role of microorganisms in the induction of IBD in the interleukin-2 knockout, mice were transferred and bred in a germ-free facility and in a facility with a restricted and defined microbial environment. Germ-free mice followed for 5 months did not develop clinical symptoms or histologic signs of IBD. Mice grown in an environment with restricted and defined microbial agents did not develop clinical signs of IBD; however, histologic and immunologic analysis of colons from 17- to 20-week-old animals showed the beginnings of an inflammatory process.

The clinical picture of the interleukin-10 knockout mice was somewhat different from that of the interleukin-2 knockouts. The interleukin-10 knockout mice developed gastrointestinal inflammation that involved the entire small bowel and colon rather than just the colon as in the interleukin-2 knockouts [2••]. The histology was marked by desquamation of apical epithelial cells, multiple small superficial erosions, and thickening of the subepithelial basement membranes. There was also extensive lymphoplasmocytic and histiocytic infiltration of the lamina propria. The interleukin-10 knockout mice had abnormalities of the Th1 T cells with production of increased amounts of interferon-γ. They were not tested in a germ-free environment; however, when grown in a restricted and defined microbial environment, the interleukin-10 knockout mice developed lesions in the proximal colon but not in the small intestine or distal colon, as were seen in animals grown under conventional conditions.

Abbreviations

IBD—inflammatory bowel disease; **MHC**—major histocompatability complex; **PAF**—platelet-activating factor; **TNF**—tumor necrosis factor.

 ISBN 1-85922-609-4 ISSN 0267–1379

The third paper describes the spontaneous development of IBD in several immunodeficient mouse strains created by targeting genes for the T-cell receptor and the MHC [3••]. Chronic colitis was observed in mutants of the T-cell receptor α chain, the T-cell receptor β chain, double mutants of the T-cell receptor β and γ chains, and mutants of the class II MHC. The authors interpreted this pattern to suggest that IBD requires the presence of B cells and the absence of class II MHC-restricted $CD4^+$ αβ T cells. The authors postulate that these mice suffered from a loss of tolerance to dietary or microbial antigens due to the lack of the αβ T-cell mediated suppression of B cells. This lack of suppression eventually produced an autoimmune attack on the colonic epithelium resulting from autoantibodies. The only pathology frequently observed in the αβ T-cell–deficient mice was inflammation of the colon with loss of goblet cells, elongation of crypts, microabcesses, and inflammatory cell infiltration of the lamina propria. The role of intestinal dietary and microbial antigens in the development of colitis in these mutants was not fully addressed. These animals were raised in a pathogen-free facility, but their intestinal lymphocytes were still exposed to normal microbial and dietary antigens.

The previous three articles were accompanied by an editorial by Strober and Ehrhardt [4••] that analyzed the implications of the three models for the pathogenesis of IBD and put them in the context of earlier work on immune mechanisms in IBD. This editorial took three implications from this group of studies. The first was that chronic intestinal inflammation can occur as a result of a variety of immunologic defects. The second was that these models bring out the role of the T cells as regulators of B-cell responses, *ie*, that uncontrolled inflammation can result from the failure of the T-cell system to shut down B-cell responses. The third implication of these studies is that intestinal mucosal tissue can be the sole site of pathology in animals with profound systemic immune abnormalities. Presumably, the localization of pathology to the gastrointestinal tract is a result of the large number of dietary and microbial antigens to which the intestinal mucosa is exposed. This suggestion is supported by the absence of intestinal pathology in interleukin-2 knockout mice grown in a germ-free environment and the diminished inflammatory response seen in the intestines of interleukin-10 knockout mice grown in a controlled microbial environment.

The presence of IBD-like lesions in mice with genetic T-cell defects grown in a conventional environment, along with lessened lesions in similar animals grown in a germ-free environment, supports the widely held opinion that the pathogenesis of human IBD involves both a genetically determined immune defect and exposure to intestinal antigens. One surprising aspect of these models is that systemic immune defects can result in pathology that is confined to the gastrointestinal tract. Equally surprising was the finding that genetic defects in central elements of the immune system, especially the interleukin-2 knockout and the T-cell receptor mutations, were compatible with life.

Patients with IBD, to the best of our knowledge, have normal T-cell receptors and are capable of producing interleukin-2 and interleukin-10; thus, the direct relevance of genetically determined immune defects to human IBD has to be interpreted carefully. The fact that a specific, genetically determined immune defect produces a clinical picture similar to IBD does not necessarily imply that patients with IBD share a similar immune defect.

Interleukin-2

The high degree of immune activation in IBD suggests that interleukin-2 levels should be high. Moreover, the efficacy of cyclosporine, which affects T-cell function, in IBD also suggests that interleukin-2 levels might be elevated. However, studies that have measured interleukin-2 production and interleukin-2 messenger RNA levels in IBD have had conflicting findings. In one set of studies, interleukin-2 production by both peripheral and intestinal lymphocytes in IBD was lower than in normal subjects [5,6]. In another study, interleukin-2 production by isolated lymphocytes was undetectable under unstimulated conditions, whereas phytohemagglutinin-induced interleukin-2 levels were similar in lymphocytes of patients with IBD and controls. Studies using quantitative polymerase chain reaction showed that levels of interleukin-2 messenger RNA transcripts were significantly increased in inflamed mucosa of Crohn's disease compared with those of ulcerative colitis and controls [7]. In a recent study, interleukin-2 production was assessed in pediatric IBD patients. Lamina propria mononuclear cells isolated from colonic resections of IBD patients had significantly lower spontaneous proliferation and interleukin-2 production *in vitro* than did lamina propria mononuclear cells of control patients [8]. In contrast, significantly greater interleukin-2 production was detected when lamina propria mononuclear cells of Crohn's disease patients were cultured with phytohemagglutinin in comparison with those of ulcerative colitis or control patients. In another study [9•], the expression of interleukin-2 messenger RNA and interleukin-2 receptor messenger RNA was measured in mucosal and peripheral blood lymphocytes. In all cases, intestinal lymphocytes produced more interleukin-2 than peripheral blood cells. IBD cells produced slightly greater amounts of interleukin-2 receptor messenger RNA than controls, but significantly lower interleukin-2 messenger RNA [9•]. Viewed together, these studies suggest that the relative rates of interleukin-2 production by control and IBD patients may be influenced by the lymphocyte population under study, the method of isolation, and the presence or absence of stimulation.

The trinitrobenzene sulfonic acid model of colitis in the rat goes through a phase of acute inflammation followed by a phase of chronic inflammation followed by healing. Spontaneous lamina propria mononuclear cell interleukin-2 activity is significantly increased in the chronic but not in the acute or resolving colitis groups. Concanavalin A–stimulated interleukin-2 activity was the highest in the groups of resolved and chronic colitis and lowest in the group with acute colitis [10].

High-dose interleukin-2 has been used to treat advanced renal cell carcinoma. In a group of 300 patients who received interleukin-2 as part of their therapy for renal cell carcinoma, two patients had a past history of Crohn's disease and both developed apparent exacerbations of their Crohn's disease during treatment with interleukin-2 [11•]. Thus, excess interleukin-2 exacerbates Crohn's disease; whereas, in apparent contradiction, the inability to make interleukin-2 in mice induces a picture very much like IBD [1••]. There appears to be an important role for T-cell activation in IBD but the exact role of interleukin-2 is still uncertain.

Proinflammatory cytokines

In contrast to the somewhat conflicting data on the production of interleukin-2 in IBD, the data on the production of most proinflammatory cytokines (interleukin-1, interleukin-6, and interleukin-8) consistently demonstrate enhanced production. Tumor necrosis factor (TNF)-α production in IBD has varied from study to study. Lamina propria mononuclear cells isolated from involved IBD mucosa spontaneously produced increased amounts of interleukin-1β, interleukin-6, and TNF-α compared with normal subjects [12]. TNF-α secretion from IBD lamina propria mononuclear cells could be further enhanced by stimulation with pokeweed mitogen. The secretion pattern of TNF-α and interleukin-1β by lamina propria mononuclear cells from patients with either ulcerative colitis or Crohn's disease demonstrated a close correlation with the degree of tissue involvement and mucosal inflammation. The enhanced production of interleukin-1 is not specific to IBD and is likely to occur in any intestinal disorder marked by chronic inflammation; for example, enhanced production of interleukin-1 has been demonstrated in graft versus host reaction [13], where it appears to play an important part in pathogenesis. Treatment of animals undergoing graft versus host reaction with rabbit anti-interleukin-1 antibodies abolished the jejunal crypt hyperplasia and significantly reduced the parallel decrease in crypt length.

Although several studies have convincingly demonstrated that interleukin-1 is increased in the involved areas from IBD, assessment of TNF production has given less consistent results. At least three groups have been unable to demonstrate increased TNF messenger RNA and protein in biopsies or resected tissues from patients with IBD, even though the same patients expressed high tissue levels of interleukin-1 and interleukin-6 [14–16]. More recently there have been two reports of increased TNF in IBD tissue. One study used immunohistochemical staining in tissue sections from pediatric patients who had received no therapy [17]. The other demonstrated increased TNF-α in stools from children with active IBD [18]. It is not clear whether the finding of increased TNF in IBD is peculiar to children or if it relates to the stage of the disease, the time from onset, or therapy.

Of particular interest was an anecdotal report of a teenaged girl with Crohn's disease who was successfully treated with anti-TNF monoclonal antibodies [19•]. In this girl, who had been resistant to conventional Crohn's disease therapy, there was an immediate improvement in clinical symptoms after the first dose of anti-TNF. If these results can be confirmed in other patients, there would be firm evidence for an important role of TNF in the pathogenesis of IBD and a potential new area for therapeutic intervention.

Interleukin-8 has received increasing attention as a mediator of neutrophil activation and chemotaxis. Increased interleukin-8 levels were found throughout the colonic mucosa in patients with Crohn's disease compared with a control group [20]. The relative contribution of interleukin-8 versus leukotriene B4 and other chemotactic factors towards neutrophil infiltration in IBD remains to be determined.

Inflammatory mediators

Increased production of prostaglandins and leukotrienes in active IBD is well established. Uninflamed areas from colons of patients with IBD produce levels of eicosanoids similar to those seen in normal tissue. However, coculture of quiescent plus inflamed tissue generates a marked increase in eicosanoid (prostaglandin E2 and leukotriene C4) production [21]. These findings suggest that in some patients with limited IBD, quiescent mucosa is sensitized. A small but significant increase in the macrophage population may be partly responsible, but it is likely that these and other cells are primed to release eicosanoids and may be induced to do so by soluble mediators produced by actively inflamed tissue.

The influence of eicosanoids from inflamed areas of IBD tissue on mucosal transport function was assessed by coculture with rat distal colonic mucosa *in vitro* [22]. Colonic tissue from patients with colitis and control subjects was cultured. Media from inflamed tissue contained more prostaglandin E2 and leukotriene D4 and evoked a greater secretory response in rat colonic mucosa than did control tissue media. Incubation of inflamed tissue with cyclooxygenase inhibitors or lipoxygenase inhibitors used individually had little effect on the secretory response; however, incubation of inflamed IBD tissue with a combination of cyclooxygenase and a lipoxygenase inhibitor profoundly decreased ion secretion.

The lack of specificity of enhanced eicosanoid production for IBD was demonstrated by the measurement of eicosanoids by rectal dialysis in patients undergoing pelvic radiotherapy [23]. Patients undergoing radiotherapy had increased levels of leukotriene B4, prostaglandin E2, and thromboxane B2 compared with normal subjects.

Lipoxygenase products are primarily produced by inflammatory cells. Immunohistochemical studies of human colon demonstrated 12-lipoxygenase in epithelial cells from involved but not uninvolved areas of ulcerative colitis and Crohn's colitis surgical resections [24]. Colonic epithelial cells from normal colon did not demonstrate 12-lipoxygenase. Inflamed tissue from ulcerative colitis also produced 12-hydroxyeicosatatraenoic acid, the metabolic of arachidonic acid produced by 12-lipoxygenase. This study raises the possibility that inflammatory cytokines may induce lipoxygenases in epithelial cells.

The conventional wisdom has been that platelet-activating factor (PAF) is primarily the product of neutrophils, macrophages, and other inflammatory cells rather than epithelial cells. Epithelial cells and lamina propria mononuclear cells were isolated from surgical resections from control, Crohn's disease, and ulcerative colitis patients and assayed for production of PAF when stimulated with the calcium ionophore A23187 [25]. Epithelial cells and lamina propria mononuclear cells produced PAF in approximately equivalent quantities. Basal and stimulated PAF activity of epithelial and lamina propria cells from ulcerative colitis, but not Crohn's disease patients, was appreciably higher than that of controls.

Mucosal and submucosal mast cell hyperplasia is a feature of ulcerative colitis and Crohn's disease. Degranulated mast cells are often seen in areas of active disease, suggesting that inflammatory mediators released from these cells contribute to the pathophysiology of IBD. Human intestinal mucosal mast cells suspensions were obtained from surgical resections of colon and small intestine and were incubated with colon or small bowel derived mouse epithelial-cell–associated components [26]. Histamine release from IBD mast cells incubated with epithelial-cell–associated components was significantly greater than that from control mast cells. These data raise the possibility that epithelial-cell protein–induced release of intestinal mast cell mediators may contribute to the inflammation in IBD.

Substance P is a neuromodulator that is released from gastrointestinal intrinsic substance P neurons as well as extrinsic nerve fibers whose cell bodies are in the dorsal root ganglia. In the colon, substance P can affect smooth muscle contractility, vascular permeability, inflammatory cell traffic, and cytokine production. Mucosal substance P levels were measured by radioimmunoassay in extracts of endoscopically obtained rectal mucosal biopsies [27]. There were significantly increased concentrations of substance P in biopsies from patients with ulcerative colitis compared with controls and compared with patients having Crohn's disease. Mucosal levels of substance P in Crohn's disease patients were significantly lower than in controls.

Reactive oxygen species

The epithelial cell damage seen in IBD is thought to be the product of activated neutrophils and macrophages. One of the primary effector mechanisms for activated neutrophils and macrophages is the production of reactive oxygen species. Resting neutrophils and macrophages have only a limited ability to produce reactive oxygen species; their ability to generate reactive oxygen species is greatly enhanced when they undergo priming. Priming does not in itself cause the production of reactive oxygen species, but rather increases the quantity of reactive oxygen species produced when these cells are activated. One of the agents known to prime neutrophils and macrophages is bacterial lipopolysaccharide. The generation of superoxide was assessed in freshly isolated monocytes from patients with active untreated Crohn's disease and controls [28]. Monocytes from patients with active Crohn's disease showed enhanced stimulated release of superoxide when compared with normal monocytes. To address the hypothesis that the monocyte priming factor in Crohn's disease serum may be lipopolysaccharide, the priming ability of Crohn's disease serum was assayed before and after the removal of lipopolysaccharide. Removal of lipopolysaccharide eliminated the ability of Crohn's disease serum to prime normal monocytes. These studies indicate that bacterial cell wall products which cross the intestinal epithelial barrier in active Crohn's disease may be important proinflammatory molecules involved in the initiation or perpetuation of inflammation in Crohn's disease.

Cells capable of generating superoxide were identified in inflamed human gastrointestinal mucosa by the use of nitroblue tetrazolium as a probe [29]. Biopsy specimens from control subjects and patients with ulcerative colitis were studied. Superoxide production was noted in epithelial cells, vascular endothelium, and infiltrating mononuclear cells of the mucosa. Superoxide production by vascular epithelial and infiltrating mononuclear cells was greater in inflamed mucosa.

Nitric oxide

Nitric oxide is produced in tissues by nitric oxide synthase with liberation of equimolar amounts of citrulline. Citrulline concentrations are significantly higher in rectal biopsy specimens from patients with active ulcerative colitis than in those from patients with quiescent disease or with normal histology [30]. Citrulline production was inhibited in ulcerative colitis specimens by incubation with an inhibitor of nitric oxide synthase. These findings suggest that the mucosal production of nitric oxide by nitric oxide synthase is increased in ulcerative colitis. Increased mucosal nitric oxide may be an important pathogenic factor in ulcerative colitis, underlying some of the pathologic features of this disease including relaxation of colonic circular smooth muscle as seen in toxic megacolon and epithelial damage.

References and recommended reading

Papers of particular interest, published within the annual period of review, have been highlighted as:
• Of special interest
•• Of outstanding interest

1. •• Sadlack B, Merz H, Schorle H, Schimpl A, Feller AC, Horak I: **Ulcerative Colitis-Like Disease in Mice With a Disrupted Interleukin-2 Gene.** *Cell* 1993, **75**:253–261.

All surviving interleukin-2 knockout mice develop IBD confined to the colon. Similar mice raised in a germ-free environment did not develop IBD.

2. •• Kuhn R, Lohler J, Rennick D, Rajewsky K, Muller W: **Interleukin-10-Deficient Mice Develop Chronic Enterocolitis.** *Cell* 1993, **75**:263–274.

Interleukin-10 knockout mice developed gastrointestinal inflammation that involved the entire small bowel and colon.

3. •• Mombaerts P, Mizoguchi E, Grusby MJ, Glimcher LH, Bhan AK, Tonegawa S: **Spontaneous Development of Inflammatory Bowel Disease in T Cell Receptor Mutant Mice.** *Cell* 1993, **75**:275–282.

Chronic colitis developed in mice with mutations in the T-cell receptor (α or β chain) or the class II major histocompatibility complex.

4. •• Strober W, Ehrhardt RO: **Chronic Intestinal Inflammation: An Unexpected Outcome in Cytokine or T Cell Receptor Mutant Mice.** *Cell* 1993, **75**:203–205.

An excellent review of the articles listed above.

5. Fiocchi C, Hilfiker ML, Youngman KR, Doerder NC, Finke JH: **Interleukin-2 Activity of Human Intestinal Mucosa Mononuclear Cells. Decreased Levels in Inflammatory Bowel Disease.** *Gastroenterology* 1984, **86**:734–742.

6. Gurbindo C, Russo P, Sabbah S, Lohoues MJ, Seidman E: **Interleukin-2 Activity of Colonic Lamina Propria Mononuclear Cells in a Rat Model of Experimental Colitis.** *Gastroenterology* 1993, **104**:964–972.

7. • Pullman WE, Doe WF: **IL-2 Production by Intestinal Lamina Propria Cells in Normal, Inflamed and Cancer-Bearing Colons.** *Clin Exp Immunol* 1992, **88**:132–137.

8. Gurbindo C, Sabbah S, Menezes J, Justinich C, Marchand R, Seidman EG: **Interleukin-2 Production in Pediatric Inflammatory Bowel Disease: Evidence for Dissimilar Mononuclear Cell Function in Crohn's Disease and Ulcerative Colitis.** *J Pediatr Gastrointerol Nutr* 1993, **17**:247–254.

Lamina propria mononuclear cells isolated from colonic resections of inflammatory bowel disease patients had significantly lower spontaneous proliferation and interleukin-2 production *in vitro* than did lamina propria mononuclear cells of control patients. In contrast, significantly greater interleukin-2 production was detected when lamina propria mononuclear cells of Crohn's disease patients were cultured with phytohemagglutinin in comparison with those of ulcerative colitis or control patients.

9. • Matsuura T, West GA, Youngman KR, Klein JS, Fiocchi C: **Immune Activation Genes in Inflammatory Bowel Disease.** *Gastroenterology* 1993, **104**:448–458.

Expression of interleukin-2 messenger RNA and interleukin-2 receptor messenger RNA were measured in mucosal and peripheral blood lymphocytes. Intestinal lymphocytes produced more interleukin-2 than peripheral blood cells. IBD cells produced slightly greater amounts of interleukin-2 receptor messenger RNA than controls, but significantly lower interleukin-2 messenger RNA.

10. Gurbindo C, Russo P, Sabbah S, Lohoues MJ, Seidman E: **Interleukin-2 Activity of Colonic Lamina Propria Mononuclear Cells in a Rat Model of Experimental Colitis.** *Gastroenterology* 1993, **104**:964–972.

11. • Sparano JA, Brandt LJ, Dutcher JP, Dubois JS, Atkins MB: **Symptomatic Exacerbation of Crohn's Disease After Treatment With High-Dose Interleukin-2.** *Ann Intern Med* 1993, **118**:617–618.

Patients with Crohn's disease who were treated for renal cell carcinoma with interleukin-2 developed exacerbations of their Crohn's disease.

12. Reinecker HC, Steffen M, Witthoeft T, Pfleuger I, Schreiber S, MacDermott RP, Raedler A: **Enhanced Secretion of Tumour Necrosis Factor-α, IL-6, and IL1β by Isolated Lamina Propria Mononuclear Cells From Patients With Ulcerative Colitis and Crohn's Disease.** *Clin Exp Immunol* 1993, **94**:174–181.

13. Mowat AM, Hutton AK, Garside P, Steel M: **A Role for Interleukin-1α in Immunologically Mediated Intestinal Pathology.** *Immunology* 1993, **80**:110–115.

14. Isaacs KL, Sartor RB, Haskill S: **Cytokine mRNA Profiles in Inflammatory Bowel Disease Mucosa Detected by PCR Amplification.** *Gastroenterology* 1992, **103**:1587–1595.

15. Mahida YR, Wu K, Lamming CED, Jewell DP, Hawkey CJ: **Human Colonic Tumor Necrosis Factor Production.** *Gastroenterology* 1989, **96**:A313.

16. Stevens C, Walz G, Zanker B, Singaran C, Lipman M, Strom T: **Interleukin 6, IL-1 and Tumor Necrosis Factor Expression in Inflammatory Bowel Disease [Abstract].** *Gastroenterology* 1990, **98**:A475.

17. Olson AD, Ayass M, Chensue S: **Tumor Necrosis Factor and Interleukin-1β Expression in Pediatric Patients With Inflammatory Bowel Disease.** *J Pediatr Gastroenterol Nutr* 1993, **16**:241–246.

18. Nicholls S, Stephens S, Braegger CP, Walker-Smith JA, MacDonald TT: **Cytokines in Stools of Children With Inflammatory Bowel Disease or Infective Diarrhoea.** *J Clin Pathol* 1993, **46**:757–760.

19. • Derkx B, Taminiau J, Radema S, Stronkhorst A, Wortel C, Tytgat G, Van Deventer S: **Tumour-Necrosis-Factor Antibody Treatment in Crohn's Disease.** *Lancet* 1993, **342**:173–174.

A patient whose Crohn's disease was treated with a single infusion of TNF antibody developed a prompt and dramatic improvement in Crohn's disease activity.

20. Izzo RS, Witkon K, Chen AI, Hadjiyane C, Weinstein MI, Pellechia C: **Neutrophil-Activating Peptide (Interleukin-8) in Colonic Mucosa From Patients With Crohn's Disease.** *Scand J Gastroenterol* 1993, **28**:296–300.

21. Wardle TD, Hall L, Turnberg LA: **Use of Coculture of Colonic Mucosal Biopsies to Investigate the Release of Eicosanoids by Inflamed and Uninflamed Mucosa From Patients With Inflammatory Bowel Disease.** *Gut* 1992, **33**:1644–1651.

22. Wardle TD, Hall L, Turnberg LA: **Inter-Relationships Between Inflammatory Mediators Released From Colonic Mucosa in Ulcerative Colitis and Their Effects on Colonic Secretion.** *Gut* 1993, **34**:503–508.

23. Cole AT, Slater K, Sokal M, Hawkey CJ: **In Vivo Rectal Inflammatory Mediator Changes With Radiotherapy to the Pelvis.** *Gut* 1993, **34**:1210–1214.

24. • Shannon VR, Stenson WF, Holtzman MJ: **Induction of Epithelial Arachidonate 12-Lipoxygenase at Active Sites of Inflammatory Bowel Disease.** *Am J Physiol (Gastrointest Liver Physiol 27)* 1993, **264**:G104–G111.

Immunohistochemical studies of human colonic surgical resections demonstrate the presence of arachidonate 12-lipoxygenase in epithelial cells from areas of active inflammation with ulcerative colitis and Crohn's disease. Epithelial cells from normal colons or from uninvolved areas of IBD colons did not express 12-lipoxygenase.

25. Ferraris L, Karmeli F, Eliakim R, Klein J, Fiocchi C, Rachmilewitz D: **Intestinal Epithelial Cells Contribute to the Enhanced Generation of Platelet Activating Factor in Ulcerative Colitis.** *Gut* 1993, **34**:665–668.

26. Fox CC, Lichtenstein LM, Roche JK: **Intestinal Mast Cell Responses in Idiopathic Inflammatory Bowel Disease. Histamine Release From Human Intestinal Mast Cells in Response to Gut Epithelial Proteins.** *Dig Dis Sci* 1993, **38**:1105–1112.

27. Bernstein CN, Robert ME, Eysselein VE: **Rectal Substance P Concentrations are Increased in Ulcerative Colitis but not in Crohn's Disease.** *Am J Gastroenterol* 1993, **88**:908–913.

28. Baldassano RN, Schreiber S, Johnston RB Jr, Fu RD, Muraki T, MacDermott RP: **Crohn's Disease Monocytes are Primed for Accentuated Release of Toxic Oxygen Metabolites.** *Gastroenterology* 1993, **105**:60–66.

29. Oshitani N, Kitano A, Okabe H, Nakamura S, Matsumoto T, Kobayashi K: **Location of Superoxide Anion Generation in Human Colonic Mucosa Obtained by Biopsy.** *Gut* 1993, **34**: 936–938.

30. Middleton SJ, Shorthouse M, Hunter JO: **Increased Nitric Oxide Synthesis in Ulcerative Colitis.** *Lancet* 1993, **341**:465–466.

William F. Stenson, MD, Professor of Medicine, Washington University School of Medicine, Gastroenterology Division, 660 South Euclid Avenue, Box 8124, St. Louis, MO 63110, USA.

Medical therapies for inflammatory bowel disease

Gary R. Lichtenstein, MD

Hospital of the University of Pennsylvania, and University of Pennsylvania School of Medicine, Philadelphia, Pennsylvania, USA

Inflammatory bowel disease comprises a group of chronic idiopathic inflammatory disorders of the intestine, ulcerative colitis and Crohn's disease. These disorders currently afflict over 1 million Americans and have an annual incidence of 70,000 to 100,000 cases in the United States alone. Despite an inability to identify the etiologic agents of ulcerative colitis and Crohn's disease, we are still able to diagnose and treat these disorders effectively. Although Crohn's disease currently has no medical or surgical cure, we are able to effectively alter its natural course and achieve and maintain symptomatic remission pharmacologically. Total proctocolectomy with ileoanal pouch construction is not the panacea it was initially thought to be, because it can be associated with a small perioperative morbidity and subsequent development of pouchitis, a clinical syndrome that has symptoms often indistinguishable from those of ulcerative colitis. Thus, medical therapy remains the mainstay of treatment for ulcerative colitis. Effective treatment of ulcerative colitis and Crohn's disease is dependent on establishing a precise diagnosis and determining the extent and severity of disease. In this paper, the current standard medical therapies available for treatment of patients with inflammatory bowel disease will be reviewed along with their efficacy and side effects, as well as the status of other investigative drugs.

Current Opinion in Gastroenterology 1994, **10**:390–403

Despite intense investigative efforts, the etiologies of ulcerative colitis and Crohn's disease remain elusive. Thus, at present, the mainstay of medical therapy focuses on inhibition of the effects of the inflammatory mediators operant in inflammatory bowel disease (IBD). Over recent years, the physician's armamentarium for medical treatment of IBD has increased substantially.

Aims of medical therapy

The primary goals of medical therapy for treatment of IBD are severalfold and include the following: 1) providing symptomatic relief, *ie*, induction of disease remission, 2) maintaining adequate nutritional status, 3) abatement of inflammation in the intestine, and 4) reducing the incidence of recurrent flares, *ie*, maintenance of disease remission. The ideal medication should be safe (have a low side-effect profile), simple to administer, and affordable.

Aminosalicylates

Oral compounds

The first aminosalicylate used to treat patients with IBD, sulfasalazine, was initially used to treat rheumatoid arthritis in the 1930s by Nana Svartz, a Scandinavian rheumatologist [1]. It is currently the most commonly used medication to treat IBD. Sulfasalazine is formed by a sulfa moiety (a sulfonamide), sulfapyridine, which is covalently bonded by an azo bond to an aspirin analogue, 5-aminosalicylate. The sulfasalazine molecule is cleaved by the enzyme azo-reductase found in enteric bacteria to yield its constituent moieties, 5-aminosalicylate and sulfapyridine. The 5-aminosalicylate portion confers its anti-inflammatory activity as was initially demonstrated by Azad Khan *et al.* [2] in 1977. The sulfapyridine serves as the "carrier" portion for the delivery of the 5-aminosalicylate. The sulfapyridine moiety of sulfasalazine is the portion of the compound that is responsible for most of the side effects of and the intolerance to sulfasalazine. Side effects are commonly seen in patients taking sul-

Abbreviations

EPA—eicosapentanoic acid; **IBD**—inflammatory bowel disease; **ROM**—reactive oxygen metabolite; **SCFA**—short-chain fatty acid.

 ISBN 1-85922-609-4 ISSN 0267–1379

fasalazine, occurring in approximately 15% of patients. With use of sulfasalazine, side effects are seen in a dose-dependent fashion occurring in 13% to 60% of patients [3]. In light of the frequency of side effects, other 5-aminosalicylate (termed mesalamine in the United States and mesalazine in Europe) compounds have been developed (Table 1). Approximately 80% to 90% of people who are intolerant of sulfasalazine are tolerant of other mesalamine derivatives.

In individuals with mild to moderately active ulcerative colitis, oral sulfasalazine will induce remission in 35% to 80% of patients when taken in doses of 4 to 6 g for a period of up to 1 month and it is more effective than placebo for maintenance of remission [3–7], regardless of disease distribution. This observed rate of induction of remission is approximately twice the spontaneous remission rate seen in patients treated with placebo [4–6]. The use of sulfasalazine is also effective for the treatment of mild to moderately active Crohn's colitis and ileocolitis. The efficacy is most proven in Crohn's colitis with less utility in Crohn's ileitis. Its use in severely active ulcerative colitis and severely active Crohn's disease has not been well established.

It is generally accepted that the oral aminosalicylates are therapeutically equivalent to sulfasalazine for treatment of active ulcerative colitis. Olsalazine, Asacol (Tillots Labs, Henlow, Bedfordshire, UK; Proctor & Gamble Pharmaceuticals, Norwich, NY) and Pentasa (Ferring AB, Malmö, Sweden; Marion Merrell Dow, Kansas City, MO) are equally efficacious in treating mildly and moderately severe active ulcerative colitis when compared with sulfasalazine. A recent meta-analysis concluded that there is insufficient evidence to suggest that any of the newer 5-aminosalicylate compounds are superior to sulfasalazine [8]. Similarly, oral aminosalicylates are as effective as sulfasalazine when used in equivalent dosage for the maintenance of patients with ulcerative colitis in remission [9]. The goal in formulating the multiple 5-aminosalicylate delivery systems that are in use is to deliver an adequate amount of active drug to the area of inflammation, the intestinal mucosa, whether it is in the colon or small bowel.

Patients with active Crohn's colitis and ileocolitis have been shown to benefit from use of Dipentum (Pharmacia Labs, Piscataway, NJ), Asacol, and Pentasa. There is limited data available for evaluating the effect of sulfasalazine or mesalamine on maintenance of remission.

Table 1. Oral 5-aminosalicylate derivatives

Drug and trade name	Constituents	Release area	Formulation
Sulfasalazine			
Azulfidine (Pharmacia Labs, Piscataway, NJ)	Sulfapyridine, 5-ASA	Colon	Tablets
Olsalazine			
Dipentum (Pharmacia Labs, Piscataway, NJ)	5-ASA dimer	Colon	Gelatin capsules
Mesalamine			
Asacol (Tillotts Labs, Henlow, Bedfordshire, UK; Proctor & Gamble Pharmaceuticals, Norwich, NY)	5-ASA	Ileum, colon pH > 7	Eudragit S cover
Pentasa (Ferring AB, Malmö, Sweden, Marion Merrell Dow, Kansas City, MO)	5-ASA (pH- and time-dependent)	Duodenum, jejunum ileum, colon	Ethylcellulose microgranules
Claversol* (SmithKline Beecham, Philadelphia, PA)	5-ASA	Ileum	Eudragit L cover
Salofalk* (Dr. Falk, GmbH & Co., Freiburg, Germany; Interfalk Canada, Mont-Saint-Hilaire, Quebec, Canada)		pH > 6	
Rowasa* (Reid-Rowell Labs, Baudette, MN; Interfalk Canada, Mont-Saint-Hilaire, Quebec, Canada)	5-ASA	Ileum pH > 6	Eudragit L 100 cover
Balsalazide*			
Colazide* (Biorex, UK; Salix Pharmaceuticals, Palo Alto CA)	5-ASA + 4-amino-benzoyl + B-alanine	Colon	Capsule
Ipsalazide* (Biorex, UK)	4-aminobenzoyl-glycine + 5-ASA	Colon	Capsule
Poly-ASA* (Wellcome, UK)	Sulfanilamidoethyl polymer + 5-ASA	Colon	Capsule

*Currently not available in the United States.
ASA—aminosalicylate.

The data from recent studies in which oral 5-aminosalicylate compounds are used as maintenance therapy for Crohn's disease are encouraging. Four studies have demonstrated that oral 5-aminosalicylate decreases recurrence by approximately 40% when given on a long-term basis to patients with inactive Crohn's disease [10–13]. Those patients who seem to derive the most benefit are those with previous ileitis and those who have had resections prior.

The discovery that the mesalamine (5-aminosalicylate) was the active moiety responsible for the beneficial effect seen with sulfasalazine led to the development of other derivatives of 5-aminosalicylate with attempts to deliver the 5-aminosalicylate to the proximal colon and small bowel. Several principles have been used to deliver the 5-aminosalicylate to the bowel, including the following: 1) enema formulation that allows the direct application of 5-aminosalicylate topically to the left colon (up to the splenic flexure), 2) foam formulation that permits the delivery of 5-aminosalicylate to the colon, 3) the linkage of 5-aminosalicylate to either a molecule that is less toxic to patients than sulfapyridine via an azo bond, or 4) oral delayed release preparations of 5-aminosalicylate that either permit absorption of the 5-aminosalicylate in the proximal intestinal tract (*eg*, Pentasa), or they allow delivery of the compound to the ileum and or colon (*eg*, Asacol) for absorption.

Topical 5-aminosalicylate compounds

Topical mesalamine is currently firmly established as therapy for treatment of acute disease and maintenance of remission in left-side ulcerative colitis or ulcerative proctitis. Mesalamine enemas (Rowasa, Reid-Rowell Labs, Baudette, MN; Interfalk Canada, Mont-Saint-Hilaire, Quebec, Canada) have been shown to reach up to the splenic flexure in most patients. This was demonstrated in 22 of 24 patients (approximately 92%) in a study by Chapman *et al.* [8]. Mesalamine enemas are thus efficacious in the treatment of ulcerative colitis up to the descending colon/splenic flexure level. Topical therapy currently in use in the United States has been in the form of mesalamine enemas or mesalamine suppositories. Other medications have been used topically (not currently available in the United States) and include 5-aminosalicylate products such as mesalamine foam, olsalazine enemas, Salofalk (Dr. Falk, GmbH & Co., Freiburg, Germany) suppositories, Asacol suppositories, and sulfasalazine enemas and 4-aminosalicylate products such as paraminosalicylic acid and Balsalazide (Biorex, UK).

Patients with left-sided colitis using mesalamine enemas have a typical response rate of 80% during treatment of active disease, owing to the ability of the mesalamine to travel to the level of the splenic flexure. The typical onset of action for mesalamine enemas in patients with new, uncomplicated ulcerative colitis is 3 to 21 days [9]. Usually the time of treatment necessary for an acute flare of ulcerative colitis requires 3 to 6 weeks. When evaluating patients with refractory distal colitis, anywhere from 50% to 75% of these patients will respond but it may take 4 to 6 months. Few side effects are seen with the topical 5-aminosalicylate. Eighty percent to 90% of patients who are intolerant of or allergic to sulfasalazine are able to tolerate topical 5-aminosalicylate.

Topical 5-aminosalicylate has been demonstrated to be effective as a prophylactic agent for ulcerative colitis in remission; however, the relapse rate is high if the drug is discontinued once the patient is in remission. The best maintenance dose has yet to be determined, but patients do well on every-other-night or every-third-night enemas. The role of combination therapy (*eg*, steroid enemas, sulfasalazine, or oral corticosteroids) is not clear. Another form of topical mesalamine, the mesalamine suppository, has been used in the United States. The suppositories are felt to be as efficacious as sulfasalazine in the treatment of acute ulcerative proctitis. One 500-mg suppository is typically given on a twice daily or three times a day basis.

The use of mesalamine foam has not been approved in the United States, but preliminary studies indicate that its distribution is similar to mesalamine enemas in about 90% of patients when tested via scintigraphic evaluation [14]. Additionally, the foam has a more uniform distribution and has a longer persistence in the descending and sigmoid colon. These characteristics suggest that the 5-aminosalicylate foam demonstrates more favorable characteristics than enema for the local treatment of left-sided ulcerative colitis. In a recent follow-up trial to this initial study [15], the efficacy, tolerance and acceptance of 5-aminosalicylate foam versus 5-aminosalicylate liquid enemas was evaluated for the treatment of active ulcerative colitis in a 3-week multicenter, randomized, prospective, investigator-blind study in 233 patients. The study suggested that 5-aminosalicylate foam may provide prompter remission of symptoms compared with liquid enema and it improves the quality of topical therapy in ulcerative colitis.

Omega-3 fatty acids

Several studies [16–19] have documented elevated levels of leukotriene B_4 and prostaglandin E_2 in rectal dialysates of patients with active ulcerative colitis. Levels in the rectal dialysates have been shown with approximate tissue levels. The exact source of the elevated levels of arachidonic acid pathway metabolites is unknown; however, they may arise from the neutrophils that are characteristic of the acute inflammatory response in ulcerative colitis. It is known that leukotriene B_4, a powerful chemoattractant, is involved in the recruitment of neutrophils with the site of inflammation. Leukotriene B_4 levels in rectal dialysates have been shown with decrease in patients when their ulcerative colitis is in remission. Animal studies [16,20–22] have suggested that prostaglandin E_2 may have a cytoprotective effect on the intestinal mucosa. The inhibition of cyclooxygenase (with associated decrease in levels of the cytoprotective agent, prostaglandin E_2) by nonsteroidal anti-inflammatory drug use has been

shown to be associated with colitis flaring. In light of the elevated leukotriene concentrations in rectal dialysates and in rectal mucosa in patients with active IBD and because the concentrations reflect the disease activity, the development of compounds that either inhibit the production of leukotriene B_4 or block its effect is the next logical step.

Patients with IBD have been treated with fish oil, a material that contains large amounts of eicosapentanoic acid (EPA) and is structurally similar to arachidonic acid. EPA is metabolized by the enzyme 5′-lipoxygenase with form leukotriene B_5 and prostaglandin E_3 with subsequent reduction of leukotriene B_4 levels. Leukotriene B_5 does not possess most of the proinflammatory properties of leukotriene B_4, thus making its production theoretically more desirable.

In order to test the effect of EPA on leukotriene generation *in vivo*, Ikehata *et al.* [23] infused intravenous EPA into ten patients with active Crohn's disease. The patients had polymorphonuclear leukocytes isolated with measure leukotriene levels. Leukocyte leukotriene B_5 levels prior to administration of EPA were notably lower in patients with Crohn's than in normal controls. The amount of leukotriene B_5 increased whereas the amount of leukotriene B_4 did not change significantly after administration of EPA.

In an attempt to determine if oral EPA is effective therapy for ulcerative colitis, Stenson *et al.* [24] conducted a multicenter, randomized, double-blind, placebo-controlled, crossover trial with 4-month treatment periods (EPA and placebo) separated by a 1-month washout in 24 patients (18 completed the study). EPA supplementation with 18 Max-EPA capsules daily (EPA 3.24 and docosahexanoic acid 2.16) resulted in a significant reduction in rectal dialysate levels of leukotriene B_4 and a similar histologic improvement. Aslan *et al.* [25] performed a similar study, giving patients either 15 Max-EPA tablets or placebo in an 8-month, double-blind, placebo-controlled, crossover trial. The patients who received EPA had a decrease in disease activity without a significant change in leukotriene B_4 levels or change on histology. The lack of change in leukotriene B_4 levels may be due to inadequate duration of treatment, too short a duration of washout periods, too low a dose of EPA, or to the effect of the placebo (which was corn oil compared with vegetable oil in the study by Stenson *et al.* [24]). In an effort to assess effect on maintenance therapy, Hawthorne *et al.* [26] investigated EPA in a controlled, randomized, blinded study and compared this with olive oil (placebo) for a period of 1 year. They concluded that EPA provides no benefit in maintenance therapy treatment. Similar findings were noted in a recent study evaluating the efficacy of fish oil compared with primrose oil for treatment of ulcerative colitis [27].

It should be noted that like any other material, fish oil may have multiple mechanisms whereby it exerts its effects. EPA has also been demonstrated to decrease production of interleukin-1 in peripheral circulating monocytes of normal subjects [28]. Interleukin-1 is a pivotal mediator that is released by monocyte macrophages in inflammatory and immunologic responses. It has also been hypothesized to stabilize lysosomal membranes. It remains unclear which if any of these mechanisms are responsible for the clinical improvement seen in active ulcerative colitis patients treated with supplemental EPA in the form of fish oil.

Corticosteroids

Treatment of immunologically mediated and inflammatory diseases is frequently achieved with the administration of pharmacologic doses of corticosteroids. It is well established that oral corticosteroids are efficacious for the treatment of active ulcerative colitis and Crohn's disease regardless of the disease distribution; however, corticosteroids have not been shown to be effective for maintenance of remission in either disease. The beneficial effects are counterbalanced, though, by the side effects that are often seen in conjunction with their use and thus, corticosteroids are often avoided and other medications with less toxic effects are chosen as initial therapy.

Several irreversible side effects, however, can be seen with the use of corticosteroids including:

1) Osteonecrosis. Nontraumatic bone necrosis, otherwise known as aseptic, avascular necrosis is relatively common, accounting for a significant percentage of all joint replacements. Osteonecrosis has been seen in patients with IBD either before or subsequent to therapy with corticosteroids [29–33].

2) Posterior subcapsular cataracts.

3) Abdominal striae.

4) Osteoporosis. Multiple bone fracture and bone pain may ensue in some patients. Limitation of long-term administration of corticosteroids is one of the most helpful measures available to the clinician. The use of assessment of bone densitometry may help to determine which patients are at high risk for this complication. Ribs and vertebrae, bones with a high degree of trabecular bone structure, are generally more severely affected. Glucocorticocorticoids appear to inhibit the activities of osteoblasts directly; they cause an increased secretion of parathyroid hormone, causing decreased formation and increased resorption of bone. Hormone replacement therapy has been demonstrated to be efficacious for prevention of bone loss in patients with IBD [34].

5) Growth retardation. Inhibition or arrest of growth in children can result from the administration of relatively small amounts of corticosteroids in children. This effect is not overcome with the exogenous administration of human growth hormone.

6) Myopathy. The finding of weakness of the proximal musculature of the arms and legs and of their associated shoulder and pelvic musculature can occasion-

ally be seen in patients taking large doses of corticosteroids. It may occur soon after treatment initiation and may be severe enough to prevent ambulation. Recovery after steroid withdrawal may be slow and incomplete.

In light of this, several strategies have been used to help reduce the incidence of side effects in individuals using corticosteroids, including 1) employment of rapid, well-defined tapering regimens, 2) use of every-other day steroid schedules, 3) use of topically applied corticosteroids in the form of suppositories, foam, and enemas, and 4) use of new, rapidly metabolized, first-pass corticosteroids.

Because corticosteroids are associated with many side effects, especially with prolonged use, there have been research efforts to develop rapidly metabolized steroids in efforts to limit availability of active components to the serum, thus minimizing the usual steroid side effects. Budesonide, tixocortol pivalate, beclomethasone diproprionate, and prednisolone metasulphobenzoate are examples of steroids rapidly metabolized by erythrocytes or the liver. Topically applied tixocortol pivalate, beclomethasone, and budesonide are at least as effective as hydrocortisone and 5-aminosalicylate enemas in the treatment of acute distal ulcerative colitis. Danielsson *et al.* [35] compared budesonide enemas in the dose of 2 g/100 mL with placebo for the treatment of distal colitis or proctitis for a 4-week period. No drug side effects were seen and there was no decrease in the endogenous morning plasma cortisol levels. Budesonide was more effective than placebo, and sigmoidoscopy and biopsy scores improved significantly in patients treated with budesonide. In a study to determine the optimal dose for budesonide enemas, doses of 1, 2, and 4 mg were used for 2 weeks and compared with prednisolone disodium phosphate enemas for patients with distal ulcerative colitis [36]. Patients treated with the 1-mg dose of budesonide had less benefit than those in all other treatments. Plasma cortisol did not change in any of the budesonide-treated patients; however, patients treated with prednisolone had a mean reduction of 30%. At present, placebo-controlled trials are being performed in the United States before Food and Drug Administration approval.

Several trials investigating the efficacy and safety of poorly absorbed, rapidly metabolized, potent oral corticosteroid therapy are currently ongoing. There is preliminary data to suggest that oral budesonide is efficacious in ileocecal Crohn's [37–39]. Currently, multicenter trials evaluating slow-release formulation for the treatment of ileocolitis are in progress. In a double-blind clinical trial, oral fluticasone proprionate in a dose of 5 mg orally four times a day was compared with placebo for the treatment of active distal ulcerative colitis for a period of 4 weeks [40]. There was no significant difference among patients taking placebo or those taking fluticasone, suggesting that fluticasone is not effective treatment for distal ulcerative colitis.

Another trial, however, compared the efficacy of fluticasone proprionate with prednisolone in the management of active left-sided or total ulcerative colitis [41]. Two hundred fifty patients were evaluated in a 4-week, double-blind, multicenter study. Prednisolone was administered orally in a dose of 40 mg daily, reduced over 4 weeks to 10 or 20 mg. Fluticasone was given in a dose of 20 mg orally. There was no statistical difference in clinical response observed between the two groups; however, there was no suppression of the corticoadrenal axis by fluticasone proprionate. Another trial comparing fluticasone proprionate (20 mg daily for 4 weeks) and prednisolone (40, 30, 20, and 15 mg daily in divided doses over 4 successive weeks) yielded similar results [42]. Perhaps higher doses of fluticasone proprionate would be more efficacious in patients? Another trial by Ford *et al.* [43] evaluated the effect of coating prednisolone metasulphabenzoate, a steroid with poor colonic absorption, with a pH-dependent acrylic resin, Eudragit S. Twelve patients with active ulcerative colitis were then administered the medication orally for a period of 12 weeks. All patients demonstrated symptomatic, sigmoidoscopic, and histologic improvement without any evidence of adrenal suppression on formal testing.

Immunosuppressants

Azathioprine and 6-mercaptopurine

The use of immunosuppressant agents such as azathioprine and 6-mercaptopurine have been received with enthusiasm by some proponents and with reservation by others. Currently, however, these two similar agents are considered to be efficacious in the treatment of both ulcerative colitis and Crohn's disease. The rationale for their use is derived from the findings that multiple immunologic abnormalities have been described in patients with IBD. The exact mechanism of action of 6-mercaptopurine or azathioprine remains unknown, although it is known that azathioprine is metabolized to 6-mercaptopurine *in vivo*, which is subsequently metabolized to 6-thioinosinic acid, the presumed active metabolite that becomes incorporated into developing strands of DNA. In lymphocytes, this substitution "acts to block critical gene activation of effector lymphocyte clones, thus inhibiting their proliferation" [44]. Other anti-inflammatory effects may be derived from their action on leukocyte cell membranes. At a low dosage there is mild decrease in T-, K- and natural killer-mediated cytotoxicity, whereas at higher doses there is inhibition of T-cell activation and cytokine production [45]. The majority of clinical investigators believe that 6-mercaptopurine and azathioprine have similar actions, efficacy and toxicity [46,47]. Typically 6-mercaptopurine and azathioprine have been used to treat patients with active Crohn's disease with particular interest in their potent effect on steroid-sparing effects, fistula healing, treatment of perineal disease, and remission maintenance. Their role in the treatment of ulcerative colitis is emerging. The onset of action may require 3 to 6 months and thus patients may require treatment with other agents for acute symptoms until the immunosuppressive agents begin to demonstrate benefit.

In an attempt to ascertain whether azathioprine is effective in preventing disease relapse in patients with ulcerative colitis who were in remission, Hawthorne *et al.* [48] conducted a 1-year, placebo-controlled, double-blind trial of withdrawal or continuation of azathioprine in 79 patients who had been taking azathioprine for 6 months prior to the trial and were in remission for a period of 2 months or more. This is the only published controlled trial for maintenance of remission in ulcerative colitis. A relapse rate of 36% was found in the azathioprine group, whereas a 59% relapse rate was seen for those patients on placebo, suggesting that azathioprine maintenance treatment in patients with ulcerative colitis is beneficial if patients have achieved remission while taking the drug.

In assessing the efficacy of 6-mercaptopurine in the treatment of patients with Crohn's disease, Kortelitz *et al.* [49] recently reviewed their experience in a retrospective fashion in 148 patients who had not responded to steroids or other medications. Sixty-six percent of patients eliminated steroids, 65% (32 of 49) healed or improved internal fistulas (rectovaginal: six of seven, ileorectal and ileosigmoid: 11 of 15, enteroenteric: two of five, ileocutaneous: six of 10, colocutaneous: two of two, ileovesical: five of 10), and 87% had healing or improvement by elimination of pain, tenderness and discharge of perirectal fistulas and abscesses. Other goals such as healing or marked improvement of Crohn's disease of the stomach and duodenum (three of three), permitting surgery to performed electively after 6-mercaptopurine allowed margins for surgical resection to be delineated (five of five). Similarly, overall clinical improvement rates of 68% have been observed in pediatric patients treated with these agents [50].

Similar results were observed in the only placebo-controlled randomized study evaluating the efficacy of 6-mercaptopurine in Crohn's disease performed by Present *et al.* [51]. The study was performed in a double-blind crossover design consisting of 1 year on 6-mercaptopurine and 1 year on placebo. The crossover data showed a 67% response to 6-mercaptopurine as compared with an 8% placebo response rate. The mean response time was 3.1 months with 81% responding at 4 months and the remaining 19% responding within 6 months. Fifty percent of patients were able to discontinue corticosteroids and another 23% were able to significantly reduce the dosage. Approximately 25% of fistulas healed with 6-mercaptopurine, whereas another 50% demonstrated improvement (including perianal, abdominal wall, ileosigmoid, gastrocolic, and colovesical fistulas) [52]. Recently, the combined treatment with azathioprine and prednisolone in 42 patients with active Crohn's disease has been shown to be more efficacious than treatment with prednisolone alone for the induction of remission [53•]. At the end of the trial (4 months), 16 of 21 (76%) of patients treated with combination therapy achieved remission whereas only eight of 21 (38%) treated with prednisolone alone achieved remission ($P=0.03$). No major side effects were seen in this trial.

The long-term toxicity of 6-mercaptopurine and azathioprine has been demonstrated to be less than that of corticosteroids [54]. Only about 10% of patients are intolerant of these medications with approximately 90% being able to use the medications. Side effects commonly seen include bone marrow toxicity (2%), allergic reactions (2%), an allergic-type pancreatitis (≈3%), infections (2%), and rare hepatitis. There have been two reports of lymphoma in patients with IBD on immunosuppressants. Myelosuppression can take the form of leukopenia, thrombocytopenia, and rarely pancytopenia. Leukopenia is the most common form of myelosuppression and the most important hematologic complication. Regular monitoring of the complete blood count is recommended during treatment [55].

Cyclosporin A

Cyclosporin A is an immunosuppressant that has been extensively used in the arena of organ transplantation. It has recently been used for treatment of IBD and has the advantage of a rapid onset of action (about 2 weeks) as compared with the 3 to 6 months that is seen with azathioprine and 6-mercaptopurine. The benefit of such a rapid onset of action is that the medication needs only to be tested for a short period of time to determine if it will be clinically efficacious. Cyclosporin A, an undecapeptide extracted from the soil fungus *Tolypocladium infatum gams*, acts by binding to an endogenous extracellular peptide, cyclophilin, which blocks the entry of activated T lymphocytes into the S phase of the cell cycle [56]. It selectively inhibits cellular immunity. In addition to its effect on T lymphocytes it alters B-cell function by inhibiting the production of B-cell activating factors and interferon-γ by T-helper cells. Granulocyte, monocyte, and macrophage function remain unaltered by cyclosporin A therapy.

In a comprehensive review, Brynskov [57••] discusses the utility of cyclosporin A in ulcerative colitis and Crohn's disease. He reviews the only controlled trial assessing cyclosporin A in Crohn's disease, which he published in 1989 in the *New England Journal of Medicine* [58], noting this is the only published controlled trial performed for treatment of active Crohn's disease. Seventy-one patients with active Crohn's involving the terminal ileum, colon or both were randomly assigned to receive either oral placebo or cyclosporin A (5 to 7.5 mg/kg/d) for 3 months. After 3 months, 59% of the cyclosporin A group responded in comparison to 32% in the placebo group ($P<0.05$). Patient response to treatment occurred within 2 weeks. During the study, malabsorption of cyclosporin A was suspected in 27% of patients, among whom 8% had complete and 19% had partial malabsorption. Although the placebo response rate of 32% may at first glance appear to be rather high compared with the 8% placebo response rate in the 6-mercaptopurine study of Present *et al.* [51], this is consistent with the average value of 25% to 40% in a recent survey of several clinical Crohn's disease trials [59].

In their article on cyclosporin A use in fistulous Crohn's disease, Hanauer and Smith [60] note that cyclosporin A has also been used for treatment of fistulous Crohn's disease that has not responded to corticosteroids, metronidazole, or antimetabolites. They review the eight published studies in the literature and demonstrate that 28 of 39 patients (72%) had fistula closure initially with 18 of 39 (46%) remaining closed in long-term follow-up. These studies, however are uncontrolled case reports and thus further randomized placebo-controlled assessment is needed.

Currently, there is one published controlled study on the efficacy of cyclosporin A in severe ulcerative colitis [61••]. The study was a randomized placebo controlled multicenter trial evaluating treatment of patients with active severe ulcerative colitis. Sixteen patients failed 10 days of intravenous hydrocortisone at a dose of 300 mg intravenously daily. Fourteen of 16 (88%) responded favorably within a mean time of 7.1 days. Of the 11 initial patients receiving cyclosporin A, nine improved whereas two did not. Of the nine patients initially receiving placebo, four required colectomy and five were medically stable and were switched to cyclosporin A with a response. The initial study protocol was for 42 patients but was halted after 20 patients were treated because outside reviewers noted a significant difference between treatment and placebo. Uncontrolled literature suggests that cyclosporin A is beneficial acutely in 81% of patients with severe ulcerative colitis and is effective for approximately 69% to maintain remission (the mean follow-up was 2.6 years) [62].

There have been four uncontrolled studies evaluating the use of cyclosporin A enemas for refractory proctosigmoiditis [63–66]. Twenty-one of 36 patients (58%) responded to initial therapy with 13 of 36 patients (36%) remaining in remission after therapy. There is only one controlled study published in abstract form suggesting that cyclosporin A enemas at a daily dose of 350 mg are not efficacious in the treatment of mildly to moderately active left-sided ulcerative colitis [67••]. This study evaluated clinical symptoms and histology in 38 patients with left-sided colitis.

If cyclosporine is going to be used for long-term treatment of patients, then the potential long-term toxicity needs to be evaluated carefully. A multitude of side effects have been noted in patients including hypertension, seizures (especially when patients have low serum cholesterol), paresthesias, tremor, gingival hyperplasia, hypertrichosis and renal damage. The most typical renal side effects are an increase in serum blood urea nitrogen and creatinine with a decrease in the glomerular filtration rate subsequent to a decrease in renal blood flow. Tubular dysfunction has also been found with subsequent hypomagnesemia and or hyperkalemia. Dose reduction may decrease toxicity in some patients, however, some may develop irreversible renal dysfunction. Also, therapeutic levels do not protect against renal dysfunction [68].

Short-chain fatty acids

There is evidence to suggest that short-chain fatty acids (SCFAs), mainly proprionate, butyrate, and acetate, derived from bacterial breakdown of starch polysaccharides, oligosaccharides, degradable fibers, and oligopeptides in the colon, are important regulators of the colonic milieu. Regional differences in large bowel SCFA metabolism, absorption, and utilization have been identified, but their implications related to pathologic conditions have not been established. Studies on isolated human colonocytes have shown a greater degree of *n*-butyrate utilization in distal than in proximal colon, despite similar rates of absorption. This observation suggests a greater dependence of the distal colonocyte on the utilization of *n*-butyrate for metabolic fuel.

Various alterations of SCFA metabolism have suggested a nutritionally deficient state in colonocytes of patients with ulcerative colitis. Colonocyte cells have demonstrated an inhibition of SCFA β-oxidation and an inability to oxidize *n*-butyrate to CO_2 and ketones, resulting in metabolic inefficiency. A lowered intraluminal pH and high concentration of *n*-butyrate has been correlated with the severity of inflammation within the colon of patients with ulcerative colitis. This observation may be explained by ineffective *n*-butyrate absorption, possibly reflecting diminished cellular utilization of butyrate [69]. It is also interesting to note that colonocytes of patients with ulcerative colitis have been demonstrated to have enhanced β-oxidation of glutamine compared with normal controls. This finding may reflect the ability of the colonocyte to utilize alternate fuel sources under conditions of ineffective SCFA metabolism.

Based on these data, Scheppach *et al.* [70] investigated the effect of the administration of butyrate, the major energy yielding substrate to colonocytes, in the form of enemas on the colonic mucosa in patients with distal ulcerative colitis. A randomized, single-blind study with crossover design was used. Ten patients with distal ulcerative colitis unresponsive to standard therapy were treated for 8 weeks with 100 mmol/L sodium butyrate enemas or with sodium chloride placebos (100 mL per rectum twice daily). They were treated with active medication for 2 weeks and with placebo for 2 weeks in random order with an intervening 2-week washout period. All patients improved with some (three patients) requiring an additional 2 weeks (total of 4 weeks). The authors thus suggest that "butyrate deficiency may play a role in the pathogenesis of distal ulcerative colitis and that butyrate irrigation ameliorates this condition."

In a similar study, Senagore *et al.* [71] performed a randomized, prospective comparison of corticosteroid enemas (100 mg of hydrocortisone/60 mL per rectum each bedtime), mesalamine enemas (4 g of 5-aminosalicylate in 60 mL twice daily), and SCFA enemas (sodium acetate 60 mmol/L, sodium *n*-butyrate 40 mmol/L, sodium proprionate 30 mmol/L mixed to pH 7 via NaOH and an osmolality of 280 to 290 was achieved by use of NaCl; 60 mL per rectum twice daily was instilled) in patients with proctosigmoiditis. There was no significant difference in response rate among the three groups. It is important to note that the butyrate concentration in this study was only 40 mmol/L compared with the study by Scheppach *et al.* [70] where it was 100 mmol/L. The ideal concentration of butyrate necessary for effective treatment is unknown. The authors do point out that there is a significant cost savings when SCFAs are used for treatment compared with the other modalities. Six weeks of therapy with corticosteroid enemas are noted to cost $71.82, mesalamine enemas $347.28, and SCFA enemas $31.50.

Another study has demonstrated similar efficacy of SCFAs for treatment of patients with ulcerative colitis. In a 6-week study, Breuer demonstrated clinical, endoscopic and histologic improvement in nine of 10 patients [72].

5′-Lipoxygenase inhibitors

Several studies have demonstrated increased levels of leukotriene B_4 and prostaglandin E_2 in rectal dialysates of patients with active ulcerative colitis. Rectal dialysate levels of leukotriene B_4 and prostaglandin E_2 have been shown to parallel disease activity and correspond to tissue levels. Leukotriene B_4 levels in rectal dialysates have been shown to decrease in patients when their ulcerative colitis is in remission. Animal studies have suggested that prostaglandin E_2 may have a cytoprotective effect on the intestinal mucosa. Inhibition of cyclooxygenase by nonsteroidal anti-inflammatory drug use has been shown to be associated with colitis flaring. Some authors have additionally suggested that the use of cyclooxygenase inhibitors may actually perhaps shunt the arachidonic acid cascade toward the 5′-lipoxygenase pathway to increase the production of leukotriene B_4.

Azulfidine and other 5-aminosalicylate products have been shown to inhibit the production of both prostaglandin E_2 and leukotriene B_4, thus "losing" the cytoprotective effect of prostaglandin E_2. In light of the elevated leukotriene concentrations in rectal dialysates and in rectal mucosa in patients with active IBD and because the concentrations reflect the disease activity, the development of selective 5′-lipoxygenase inhibitors and leukotriene receptor antagonists is the next logical step. Many different 5′-lipoxygenase inhibitors are currently being developed and evaluated. In a phase 2 trial, Zileuton (Abbott Laboratories, Abbott Park, IL) at a dose of 800 mg daily was given for 28 days to 11 patients with active ulcerative colitis [73]. All patients experienced a decrease in the discomfort of their disease and eight of the 11 patients improved endoscopically. Publications of further randomized, placebo controlled trials are necessary to evaluate this new class of compounds.

Antimycobacterial agents

Since the initial report from 1978 by Burnham and Lennard-Jones [74] of a Mycobacterium species (*Mycobacterium kansasi*) cultured from tissues of a patient with Crohn's disease, there have been several reports that suggest that mycobacteria may play a role in IBD [75]. Several reports [76,77] have documented positive cultures for mycobacteria in patients with Crohn's disease, the first being by Chiodini *et al.* [78] in 1984 from four patients with Crohn's disease, who had positive cultures for *Mycobacterium paratuberculosis. M. paratuberculosis* is an organism that is not often found in the environment and in animals it produces a Crohn's-like disease, termed *Johne's disease.* In animals, *M. paratuberculosis* replicates only in intestinal tissues. Thus, there have been several trials performed to attempt to treat patients who have Crohn's disease with antituberculous medications.

In 1984, Thayer *et al.* reported on an enzyme-linked immunoassay attached to the protoplasmic antigen of *M. paratuberculosis.* They noted a markedly raised level of antibodies to this antigen in the serum of patients with Crohn's disease when compared with control patients. Other investigators were unable to duplicate these findings. In another investigation, Brenello *et al.* [79] searched for the presence of these antibodies in patients with Crohn's disease, ulcerative colitis, active pulmonary tuberculosis, past pulmonary tuberculosis, and in healthy controls. Positive values were identified in 50% of patients with active pulmonary tuberculosis, 20% of ppd positive individuals with past pulmonary tuberculosis. These results were expected due to the antigenic sharing that occurs with different strains of mycobacteria. In the control group, 2% of people were positive with similar numbers being positive in ulcerative colitis (5%) and Crohn's disease (3.7%). They note that their data did not suggest a causal role for *M. paratuberculosis* and Crohn's disease, but "occasional patients with IBD show unexpected positivities for these mycobacterial antibodies."

Ibbotson *et al.* [80] investigated the proliferative responses of both peripheral blood mononuclear cells and mesenteric lymph node mononuclear cells to a range of mycobacterial and nonmycobacterial antigens. There was no evidence of specific sensitization in the responses of the patients with IBD to the mycobacterial antigens. In this study, anergy to *M. paratuberculosis* could not, however, be excluded. These results do not support the proposed role of mycobacteria in the pathogenesis of Crohn's disease.

Another argument suggesting that *M. paratuberculosis* is not the etiologic agent in Crohn's disease is the finding that treatment with antituberculous agents does not help recurrent Crohn's disease in the neoterminal ileum. Rutgeerts *et al.* [81] tested the efficacy of rifabutin and ethambutol in combination for their ability to heal severe recurrent Crohn's disease at the neoterminal ileum. Sixteen patients with recurrent severe Crohn's were given rifabutin at a dose of 5 mg/kg together with ethambutol at a dose of 20 mg/kg. Six patients dropped out due to adverse events and 10 patients received treatment. Of the 10 who received treatment, only five received therapy for 12 months whereas the other five received therapy for 6 months. No patients who received treatment demonstrated improvement either endoscopically or clinically.

Elsaghier *et al.* [82] recently examined the possible role of *M. paratuberculosis* in the pathogenesis of Crohn's disease. They found that 57% of their patients with Crohn's had antibodies to *M. paratuberculosis* antigens, whereas only 18% concurrently had raised titers to three different *M. paratuberculosis* antigens. The authors thus suggest that their findings support the notion that infection with *M. paratuberculosis* could cause Crohn's disease. They did not, however, include controls with other small bowel disorders nor did they do assays for other bacterial antigens making their data hard to interpret.

Stainsby *et al.* [83] did not determine any significant difference between serum concentrations of antibodies to various mycobacteria, including *M. paratuberculosis*, between patients with Crohn's disease, ulcerative colitis and healthy controls. This argues against the hypothesis that Crohn's disease is caused by *M. paratuberculosis.*

Recently, the use of specific DNA probes with polymerase chain reaction amplification has been performed because it is difficult to culture mycobacteria from tissues affected by Crohn's disease. Hermon-Taylor's group [84] identified IS900, a DNA repetitive element, in an uncharacterized mycobacterial agent from a patient with Crohn's disease. This was demonstrated by DNA fingerprinting to be indistinguishable from *M. paratuberculosis.* Recently, a related insertion sequence, called IS901 has been found in the wood pigeon strain of *Mycobacteria avium*, described as *Mycobacteria avium columbae* by some investigators. Another insertion sequence designated *Mycobacteria avium RFLP A* is indistinguishable from *M. avium* complex organisms. Recently McFadden *et al.* [85] described probes that were able to identify the wood pigeon strain of *M. avium* and *M. paratuberculosis* from human tissue. This report demonstrates the first time that the wood pigeon strain of *M. avium* was isolated from human tissue. The authors speculate that perhaps this organism, wood pigeon strain of *M. avium* and *M. paratuberculosis* are each responsible for some cases or IBD in humans. A similar study by Wall *et al.* [86] demonstrated the presence of DNA from *M. paratuberculosis* in four of 28 tissue samples of patients with Crohn's disease.

The role of mycobacteria in the pathogenesis of Crohn's disease is thus not firmly established based on published data to date because there is a failure to find evidence for organisms in all tissues examined and there is a variable response of the condition to antituberculous drugs. Perhaps future studies will improve detection and treatment techniques and change our current management strategies for patients with Crohn's disease.

Antibiotics

There are two possible uses of antibiotics for treatment of IBD: 1) as primary therapy for the IBD and 2) as treatment of intercurrent infection. Both of these will be assessed; however, it should also be stressed that intercurrent infections may lead to flares of the underlying IBD.

There is no evidence to suggest that use of metronidazole is of benefit for treatment of either mild to moderate acute ulcerative colitis or in severe colitis. There is some evidence to suggest that it might be effective as a prophylactic agent. Thus far there have been a total of four controlled studies evaluating efficacy of metronidazole in ulcerative colitis. Chapman *et al.* [87] found no advantage to the addition of 1.5 g of intravenous metronidazole to corticosteroids in the treatment of severe ulcerative colitis. Similarly, a study by Gilat *et al.* [88] demonstrated that 1.3 g of metronidazole was less effective than 4.5 g of azulfidine in patients with mild to moderately active acute ulcerative colitis. In a 12-month trial of metronidazole and azulfidine for maintenance of remission in ulcerative colitis, it was found that metronidazole at a dose of 600 mg daily was superior to azulfidine at a dose of 2 g daily with 25% of patients remaining in remission compared with 50% on metronidazole [89]. Finally, Davies *et al.* [90] found that 500 mg of metronidazole suppositories three times daily was not more efficacious than placebo in a 28-day crossover study for treatment of patients with ulcerative proctitis.

In general, it is felt that antibiotics are only indicated for patients with ulcerative colitis who have infectious complications such as *Clostridium difficile* or those undergoing emergency surgery. Enteric infections are uncommon in patients who present with active ulcerative colitis [91]. There are few studies examining the efficacy of antibiotics in managing ulcerative colitis. Peppercorn [92•] reports on the efficacy of antibiotics in managing nontoxic severe ulcerative colitis. He reports on seven patients who avoided colectomy subsequent to initiation of broad spectrum antibiotics. All had not responded to an initial dose of prednisolone 60 mg daily for 7 days. He thus recommends that "severely ill patients with ulcerative colitis deserve a trial of antibiotics before being considered failures of medical therapy."

The effect of antibiotic treatment on maintenance of remission was evaluated recently by Lobo *et al.* [93] using oral tobramycin for 7 days. It has been demonstrated that oral tobramycin has been an adjunct to conventional medication in the treatment of ulcerative colitis. There was no significant benefit seen for maintenance of remission. The authors thus hypothesize that the short-lived benefit from tobramycin may reflect short-term changes in the fecal flora. Finally, the role of *B. hominis* as it relates to IBD is unclear. In a retrospective analysis, Nagler *et al.* [94] analyzed the course of patients with stool isolates specifically related to treatment. They conclude that *Blastocystic hominis* is not a significant pathogen in IBD and treatment should be directed at the underlying disorder.

Metronidazole has been demonstrated to be efficacious for the treatment of Crohn's disease. Its use has been demonstrated to be useful for treatment of perineal disease and for treatment of refractory colitis or treatment of patients intolerant to other therapies. There are four controlled trials to date [95–98] following the initial report by Ursing [99] evaluating efficacy of metronidazole in Crohn's disease. A trial by Blichfeldt *et al.* [95] demonstrated no significant benefit to adding metronidazole to corticosteroids and azulfidine in patients with Crohn's disease. The Cooperative Crohn's Disease Study from Sweden [96] evaluated 78 patients randomized to either metronidazole or azulfidine. Both agents were equally effective for producing clinical improvement but metronidazole was superior to azulfidine in decreasing an acute phase reactant that closely parallels disease activity, orosomucoid levels. A study by Ursing *et al.* [97] demonstrated that in Crohn's colitis and ileocolitis metronidazole (400 mg twice a day) is as effective as azulfidine (3 g daily) and more effective than placebo for treatment of active Crohn's disease.

Recently, the Flagyl-Crohn's study was completed by 14 centers in the United States and Canada [98]. In this study metronidazole was demonstrated to be significantly superior to placebo for treatment of patients with moderately active Crohn's disease. The efficacy of metronidazole at 10 mg/kg and 20 mg/kg was assessed versus placebo in patients with active Crohn's disease. Crohn's disease activity index scores were significantly improved in both metronidazole groups (*ie*, the 10 mg/kg group and the 20 mg/kg group) over placebo, however there was no difference in remission rates between metronidazole and placebo. In patients with disease confined to the small bowel, metronidazole was superior to placebo, but the difference did not reach statistical significance.

Metronidazole has also been effective for treatment of perineal Crohn's disease. In an open trial in 21 patients with severe perineal Crohn's disease, patients received 20 mg/kg daily [100]. All patients noted improvement of drainage, erythema and induration. Ten of 18 who completed the trial had complete healing. Often after discontinuation of the drug, relapse of disease occurs. This can be managed with reinstitution of metronidazole [101].

Finally, metronidazole has been efficacious for treatment of patients who develop pouchitis. This clinical syndrome of pouchitis is characterized by symptoms indistinguishable for the original ulcerative colitis is treated effectively in most cases with metronidazole.

Other agents

Although the use of corticosteroids, aminosalicylates, antibiotics, and immunosuppressants are well established as effective therapy for IBD there are some agents that are not as well established and are being investigated for treatment of IBD. I will highlight some of these exciting new findings.

The production of reactive oxygen metabolites (ROMs) has been shown to be increased in the intestine in patients with colitis. Granulocytes and macrophages comprise significant components of the inflammatory infiltrate of intestines of patients with IBD. Investigators have demonstrated increased production of reactive oxygen metabolites in IBD patients' peripheral circulating monocytes and granulocytes. Verspaget *et al.* [102] note that there are very few studies assessing ROMs in IBD at the intestinal level. They point out that intestinal macrophages from IBD patients have been shown to be more responsive to O_2 production than peripheral blood monocytes.

In patients with Crohn's disease, Baldassano *et al.* [103••] had demonstrated that peripheral blood monocytes are primed by lipopolysaccharide for enhancement of the respiratory burst with subsequent increased release of toxic oxygen metabolites. As a direct result of this study, it has been suggested that bacterial cell wall products may be important proinflammatory molecules involved in the initiation or perpetuation of Crohn's disease. Also, intestinal macrophages from patients with IBD have been shown to have increased spontaneous and stimulated ROM production. Sulfasalazine and 5-aminosalicylate have been shown to have reactive oxygen metabolite scavenging activity thus explaining some of their anti-inflammatory activity in IBD. Superoxide dismutase, an enzyme that functions to accelerate the conversion of O_2 to hydrogen peroxide, which is subsequently metabolized to water either by catalase or glutathione peroxidase, has been administered to IBD patients encapsulated in liposomes or as a free enzyme, subcutaneously or intramuscularly. Most of the 34 patients in this study improved, suggesting that ROM may play a significant clinical role in IBD.

Additionally, in an acetic acid model of colitis [104], Catalase, WR-2721, or Cu(II)2(3,5-DIPS)4 were shown to decrease histologic evidence of experimental colitis suggesting that ROMs, particularly superoxide, hydrogen peroxide, or one of its secondarily derived species may play a role in acetic acid–derived colitis. Before any conclusion can be reached, randomized, placebo-controlled, double-blind studies need to be performed in humans in a prospective fashion.

Of similar interest, NO (nitric oxide) has received recent press. NO is produced in tissues by the enzyme NO synthetase with the release of equimolar amounts of citrulline. Middleton *et al.* [105•] have demonstrated increased NO production in patients with active ulcerative colitis by measuring the concentrations of L-citrulline in rectal biopsy specimens. Also, L-citrulline synthesis was inhibited by incubation with Ng-monomethyl-L-arginine, a competitive inhibitor of NO synthetase. NO has been postulated to be an immunomodulator with many activities during inflammation. NO synthetase activity in ulcerative colitis patients was demonstrated to be elevated, whereas in Crohn's patients NO synthetase activity did not differ from control values and activity in the colonic mucosa was low. It is suggested that perhaps the induction of NO synthetase may be involved in the mucosal vasodilation and increased vascular permeability of active ulcerative colitis, and may also contribute to the impaired motility that accompanies toxic dilation. Other investigators

[106] note, however, that NO synthetase is elevated as well in patients with Crohn's disease. They also note that NO is probably generated by other tissues in the body, as well as in inflamed mucosa, because high levels of endotoxin, and tumor necrosis factor are seen in patients with IBD. The NO increase in ulcerative colitis correlates with disease activity; but not in Crohn's disease. These differences are hypothesized to be related to different cytokine profiles in these disorders. The authors suggest that "further studies are needed to better define the role of NO in the pathogenesis of IBD and the possible protective effect of inhibitors of NO synthetase."

Despite our ignorance regarding the etiology of the initiating events in IBD, we have made a considerable amount of progress in understanding the presumably common, nonspecific events that culminate in tissue destruction and the associated clinical manifestations. Production of soluble mediators of inflammation has been felt to coordinate the inflammatory attack by recruitment of inflammatory cells (neutrophils, lymphocytes, and monocytes and to a lesser extent eosinophils and mast cells) from the vasculature to the specific sites of inflammation. Blockade of this cascade is felt to likely attenuate the production of these specific agents responsible for the production of the end organ damage and tissue injury. Recently, research has uncovered specific protein sites of interaction between leukocyte membranes and vascular endothelium. An array of these proteins have been discovered and are members of the selectin, integrin and immunoglobulin protein superfamilies. Several cytokines, specifically, interleukin-1, tumor necrosis factor, and interferon, have been shown to evoke production of several important adhesion molecules (endothelial leukocyte adhesion molecule-1 [E-selectin], vascular cell adhesion molecule-1, and intercellular adhesion molecule-1) located on the vascular endothelium at sites of inflammation. Recent studies have identified the presence of E-selectin and intercellular adhesion molecule-1 at sites of inflammation in both ulcerative colitis and Crohn's disease. The Cotton-top Tamarin model [107••] and anti-$\alpha 4$ integrin monoclonal antibody was administered and resulted in a significant reduction of the intestinal inflammation compared with the pretreatment level. This provides support to the notion that interference with the binding endothelial adhesion molecules may provide therapeutic benefit to help abate the inflammatory component in IBD.

Conclusions

The assortment of therapies currently available and under investigation for treatment of IBD emphasize the progress we have made in the understanding of these disease processes over the recent years. Despite the great strides of advancement that have transpired, we still have a vast repository of knowledge that has not been unearthed. Further progress will evolve if understanding of the basic disease process is emphasized and therapy is targeted at the abnormal physiology. Selective inhibition of a single mediator of the inflammatory cascade seems unlikely to be successful rather it seems likely that an agent which is inhibitory to multiple mediators would be more beneficial unless the specific mediator is pivotal to the inflammatory response. Future success requires the continued close collaboration between the basic scientist and the clinical investigator. It is hoped that these close working relationships will lead to the cure for both Crohn's disease and ulcerative colitis.

References and recommended reading

Papers of particular interest, published within the annual period of review, have been highlighted as:
- • Of special interest
- •• Of outstanding interest

1. Svartz N: **Salazopyrin, a New Sulfanilamide Preparation: A. Therapeutic Results in Rheumatic Polyarthritis. B. Therapeutic Results in Ulcerative Colitis. C. Toxic Manifestations in Treatment With Sulfanilamide Preparation.** *Acta Med Scandinavia* 1942, **110**:557–590.
2. Azad Khan AK, Piris J, Truelove SC: **An Experiment to Determine the Active Therapeutic Moiety in Sulphasalazine.** *Lancet* 1977, 2:892–895.
3. Bachrach WH: **Sulfasalazine. An Historical Perspective.** *Am J Gastorenterol* 1988, **83**:487–496.
4. Peppercorn MA: **Sulfasalazine.** *Ann Intern Med* 1984, **101**:377–386.
5. Dick AP, Grayson MJ, Carpenter RG, Petrie A: **Controlled Trial of Sulphasalazine in the Treatment of Ulcerative Colitis.** *Gut* 1964, **5**:437–442.
6. Baron JH, Connell PM, Lennard-Jones JE, Jones FA: **Sulphasalazine and Salicylazosulphadimidine in Ulcerative Colitis.** *Lancet* 1962, 1:1094–1096.
7. Margolin ML, Krumholz MP, Fochios SE, Korelitz BI: **Clinical Trials in Ulcerative Colitis.** *Am J Gastroenterol* 1988, **83**:227–243.
8. Chapman NJ, Brown ML, Phillips SF, Tremaine WJ, Schroeder KW, Dewanjee MK, Zinmeister AR: **Distribution of Mesalamine Enemas in Patients With Active Distal Ulcerative Colitis.** *Mayo Clin Proc* 1992, 67:245–248.
9. Linn FV, Peppercorn MA: **Drug Therapy for Inflammatory Bowel Disease: Part I.** *Am J Surg* 1992, 164:85–89.
10. Thomson ABR: **International Mesalazine Study Group. Coated Oral 5-Aminosalicylic Acid Versus Placebo in Maintaining Remission of Inactive Crohn's Disease.** *Aliment Pharamacol Ther* 1990, 4:55–64.
11. Prantera C, Pallone F, Brunetti G, Cottone M, Miglioli M, and the Italian IBD Study Group: **Oral 5-Aminosalicylic Acid (Asacol) in the Maintenance Treatment of Crohn's Disease.** *Gastroenterology* 1992, **103**:363–368.
12. Gendre J-P, Mary J-Y, Florent C. Modigliani R, Colombel J-F, Soule J-C, *et al.*: **Oral Mesalamine (Pentasa) as Maintenance Treatment in Crohn's disease: A Multicenter Placebo-Controlled Study.** *Gastroenterology* 1993, 104:435–439.
13. Caprilli R, Andreoli A, Capurso L, D'Albasio G, D'Agostino L, Ferretti P, *et al.*: **5-ASA in the Prevention of Crohn's Disease Postoperative Recurrence: An Interim Report of the Italian Study Group of the Colon (GISC) [Abstract].** *Gastroenterology* 1992, **102**:A601.
14. Campieri M, Corbelli C, Gionchetti P, Brignola C, Belluzzi A, Di Febo G, Zagni P, Brunetti G, Miglioli M, Barbara L: **Spread and Distribution of 5-ASA Colonic Foam and 5-ASA

Enema in Patients With Ulcerative Colitis. *Dig Dis Sci* 1992, 37:1890–1897.

15. Campieri M, Paoluzi P, D'Albasio G, Brunetti G, Pera A, Barbara L: **Better Quality of Therapy With 5-ASA Colonic Foam Inactive Ulcerative Colitis: A Multicenter Comparative Trial With 5-ASA Enema.** *Dig Dis Sci* 1993, **38**:1843–1850.

16. Hawkey CJ, Rampton DS: **Prostaglandins and the Gastorintestinal Mucosa: Are They Important in its function, Disease, or Treatment.** *Gastroenterology* 1985, **89**:1162.

17. Sharon P, Ligumsky M, Rachmilewitz D, Zor U: **Role of Prostaglandins in Ulcerative Colitis: Enhanced Production During Active Disease and Inhibition by Sulfasalazine.** *Gastroenterology* 1978, **75**:638.

18. Ligumsky M, Karmpli F, Sharon P, Zor U, Cohen F, Rachmilewitz D: **Enhanced Production During Active Disease and Inhibition by Sulfasalzine..** *Gastroenterology* 1981, **81**:444–449.

19. Sharon P, Stenson WF: **Enhanced Synthesis of Leukotriene by Colonic Mucosa in Inflammatory Bowel Disease.** *Gastroenterology* 1984, **86**:453–460.

20. Hawkey CJ, Truelove SC: **Inhibition of Prostaglandin Synthesis in Human Rectal Mucosa.** *Gut* 1983, **24**:213.

21. Hoult JRS, Page H: **5-Aminosalicylic Acid A Cofactor for Prostacyclin Synthesis.** *Lancet* 1981, **2**:255.

22. Gould SR: **Studies of Prostaglandins and Suphasalazine in Ulcerative Colitis..** *Prostaglandins Med* 1981, **6**:165.

23. Ikehata A, Hiwatashi N, Kniouchi Y, Yamazaki H, Kumagai Y, Ito K, Kayaba Y, Toyota T: **Effect of Intravenous Infused Eicosapentanoic Acid on the Leukotriene Generation in Patients With Active Crohn's.** *Am J Clin Nutr* 1992, **56**:938–942.

24. Stenson WF, Cort D, Rodgers J, Burakoff R, DeSchryver-Kecskemeti K, Gramlich TL, Beeken W: **Dietary Supplementation With Fish Oil in Ulcerative Colitis.** *Ann Intern Med* 1992, **116**:609–614.

25. Aslan A, Triadafilopoulos G: **Fish Oil Fatty Acid Supplementation in Active Ulcerative Colitis: A Double-Blind, Placebo-Controlled, Crossover Study.** *Am J Gastroenterol* 1992, **87**:432–437.

26. Hawthorne AB, Daneshmend, Hawkey CJ, Belluzzi A, Everitt SJ, Holmes GKT, Malkinson C, Shaheen MZ, Willars JE: **Treatment of Ulcerative Colitis With Fish Oil Supplementation: A Prospective 12 Month Randomised Controlled Trial.** *Gut* 1992, **33**:922–928.

27. Greenfield SM, Green AT, Teare JP, Jenkins AP, Punchard NA, Ainley CC, Thompson RPH: **A Randomized Controlled Study of Evening Primrose Oil and Fish Oil in Ulcerative Colitis.** *Aliment Pharmacol Ther* 1993, **7**:159–166.

28. Lee TH, Hoover RL, Williams JD, Sperling RI, Ravalese J III, Spur BW, Robinson DR, Corey EJ, Lewis RA, Austen KF: **Effect of Dietary Enrichment With Eicosapentanoic Acid and Docosahexanoic Acid on In Vitro Neutrophil and Monocyte Leukotriene Generation and Neutrophil Function.** *N Engl J Med* 1988, **312**:1212–1224.

29. Brom B, Bank S, Marks IN, Cobb JJ: **Periostitis, Aseptic Necrosis and Arthritis Occurring in a Patient With Crohn's Disease.** *Gastroenterology* 1971, **60**:1106–1109.

30. Shapiro SC, Rothstein FC, Newman AJ, Fletcher B, Halpin TC Jr: **Multifocal Osteonecrosis in Adolescents With Crohn's Disease: A Complication of Therapy?** *J Pediatr Gastroenterol Nutr* 1985, 4:502–506.

31. Vakil N, Sparberg M: **Steroid-Related Osteonecrosis in Inflammatory Bowel Disease.** *Gastroenterology* 1989, **96**:62–67.

32. Culp RW, Schaffer JL, Osterman AL, Bora FW Jr: **Kienbock's Disease in a Patient With Crohn's Enteritis Treated With Corticosteroids.** *J Hand Surg [Am]* 1989, **14**:294–296.

33. Freeman HJ, Kwan WCP: **Brief Report: Non-Corticosteroid-Associated Osteonecrosis of the Femoral Heads in Two Patients With Inflammatory Bowel Disease.** *N Engl J Med* 1993, **329**:1314–1316.

34. Clements D, Compston JE, Evand WD, Rhodes J: **Hormone Replacement Therapy Prevents Bone Loss in Patients With Inflammatory Bowel Disease.** *Gut* 1993, **34**:1543–1546.

35. Danielsson A, Lofberg R, Persson T, Salde L, Schioler R, Suhr O, Willen R: **A Steroid Enema, Budesonide, Lacking Systemic Effects for the Treatment of Distal Ulcerative Colitis or Proctitis.** *Scand J Gastroenterol* 1992, **27**:9–12.

36. The Danish Budesonide Study Group: **Budesonide Enema in Distal Ulcerative Colitis. A Randomized Dose-Response Trial With Prednisolone Enema as Positive Control.** *Scand J Gastroenterol* 1991, **26**:1225–1230.

37. Wolman SL: **Use of Oral Budesonide in a Patient With Small Bowel Crohn's Disease and Previous Pseudotumor Cerebri Secondary to Steroids.** *Scand J Gastroenterol* 1989, **24**:146–147.

38. Lofberg R, Danielsson A, Salde L: **Oral Budesonide in Active Ileocaecal Crohn's Disease—a Pilot Trial With a Topically Acting Steroid [Abstract].** *Gastroenterology* 1991, **100**:A226

39. Roth M, Ueberschaer, Ewe K, Gross V, Scholmerich J: **Oral Slow Release Budesonide Induces Remission in Active Crohn's Disease With Little Effect on Adrenal Function.** *Gastroenterology* 1992, **102**:A688.

40. Angus P, Snook JA, Reid M, Jewell DP: **Oral Fluticasone Proprionate in Active Distal Ulcerative Colitis.** *Gut* 1992, **33**:711–714.

41. Hawthorne AB, Record CO, Holdsworth CD, Giaffer MH, Burke DA, Keech ML, Hawkey CJ: **Double Blind Trial of Oral Fluticasone Proprionate Versus Prednisolone in the Treatment of Active Ulcerative Colitis.** *Gut* 1993, **34**:125–128.

42. Wright JP, Jarnum S, Muckadell OS, Keech ML, Lennard-Jones JE: **Oral Fluticasone Proprionate Compared With Prednisolone in Treatment of Active Crohn's Disease: A Randomized Double-blind Multicentre Study.** *Eur J Gastroenterol Hepatol* 1993, **5**:499–503.

43. Ford GA, Oliver PS, Shepherd NA, Wilkinson SP: **An Eudragit-Coated Prednisolone Preparation for Ulcerative Colitis: Pharmacokinetics and Preliminary Therapeutic Use.** *Aliment Pharmacol Therap* 1992, **6**:31–40.

44. Linn FV, Peppercorn MA: **Drug Therapy for Inflammatory Bowel Disease. Part I and Part II.** *Am J Surg* 1992, 164:85–89 and 178–185.

45. Brogan M, Hiserodt J, Oliver M, Stevens R, Korelitz B, Targan S: **The Effect of 6-Mercaptopurine on Natural Killer Cell Activities in Crohn's Disease.** *J Clin Immunol* 1985, **5**:204–211.

46. Lennard-Jones JE: **Azathioprine and 6-Mercaptopurine Have a Role in the Treatment of Crohn's Disease.** *Dig Dis Sci* 1981, **26**:364–368.

47. Mackay IR, Weiden S, Ungar B: **Treatment of Active Chronic Hepatitis and Lupoid Hepatitis With 6-Mercaptopurine and Azathioprine.** *Lancet* 1964, **1**:899–902.

48. Hawthorne AB, Logan RFA, Hawkey CJ, Foster PN, Axon ATR, Swarbrick ET, Scott BB, Lennard-Jones JE: **Randomized Controlled Trial of Azathioprine Withdrawal in Ulcerative Colitis.** *Brit Med J* 1992, **305**:20–22.

49. • Korelitz BI, Adler DJ, Mendelsohn RA, Sacknoff AL: **Long-Term Experience With 6-Mercaptopurine in the Treatment of Crohn's Disease.** *Am J Gastroenterol* 1993, **88**:1198–1205.

A retrospective analysis of use of 6-mercaptopurine in 148 patients with Crohn's disease. Indications for use and efficacy are discussed. Overall, 68% of patients achieved therapeutic goals.

50. Markowitz J, Grancher K, Mandel F, Daum F: **Immunosuppressive Therapy in Pediatric Inflammatory Bowel Disease: Results of a Survey of the North American Society for Pediatric Gastroenterology and Nutrition.** *Am J Gastroenterol* 1993, **88**:44–48.

51. Present DH, Korelitz BI, Wisch N, Glass JL, Sachar DB, Pasternack BS: **Treatment of Crohn's Disease With 6-Mercaptopurine. A Long-Term Randomised Double-Blind Study.** *N Engl J Med* 1980, **302**:981–987.

52. Korelitz BI, Present DH: **Favorable Effect of 6-Mercaptopurine on Fistulas of Crohn's Disease.** *Dig Dis Sci* 1985, **30**:58–64.

53. • Ewe K, Press AG, Singe C, Stufler M, Ueberschaer B, Hommel G, Buschenfelde KMZ: **Azathioprine Combined With Prednisolone or Monotherapy With Prednisolone in Active Crohn's Disease.** *Gastroenterology* 1993, **105**:367–372.
Forty-two patients with active Crohn's disease (CDAI > 150) were treated with azathioprine (2.5 mg/kg body weight) and prednisolone (60 mg daily in a tapering regimen to a maintenance dose of 10 mg) for 4 months—Group I or a placebo and prednisolone (60 mg daily in a tapering regimen to a maintenance dose of 10 mg) for 4 months—Group II. Sixteen of 21 (76%) in Group I achieved remission whereas only 8 of 21 (38%) in group II achieved remission (p=0.03). No significant side effects were observed in either group.

54. Present DH, Meltzer SJ, Krumholz MP, Wolke A, Korelitz BI: **6-Mercaptopurine in the Management of Inflammatory Bowel Disease: Short and Long Term Toxicity.** *Ann Intern Med* 1989, **111**:641–649.

55. Connell WR, Kamm MA, Ritchie JK, Lennard-Jones JE: **Bone Marrow Toxicity Caused by Azathioprine in Inflammatory Bowel Disease: 27 Years of Experience.** *Gut* 1993, **34**:1081–1085.

56. Marsh JW, Vehe KL, White HM: **Immunosuppressants.** *Gastro Clinics North Am* 1992, **21**:679–693.

57. •• Brynskov J: **Review: Cyclosporin for Inflammatory Bowel Disease: Mechanisms and Possible Actions.** *Scand J Gastroenterol* 1993, **28**:849–857.
Excellent review of the mechanisms and summary of clinical trials using cyclosporin A for treatment of IBD.

58. Brynskov J, Freund L, Rasmussen SN, Lauritsen K, De Muckadell OS, Williams N, MacDonald AS, Tanton R, Moling F, Campianini MC, *et al*: **A Placebo-Controlled, Double clind, Randomized Trial of Cyclosporine Therapy in Active Chronic Crohn's Disease.**. *N Engl J Med* 1989, **321**:845–850.

59. Meyers S, Janowitz HD: **'Natural History' of Crohn's Disease. Analytic Review of the Placebo Lesson.** *Gastroenterology* 1984, **87**:1189–1192.

60. Hanauer SB, Smith MB: **Rapid Closure of Crohn's Disease Fistulas With Continuous Intravenous Cyclosporin A.** *AmJ Gastroenterol* 1993, **88**:646–649.

61. •• Lichtiger S, Present DH, Kornbluth A, Hanauer S: **Cyclosporin A in the Treatment of Severe Refractory Ulcerative Colitis: A Double Blinded Placebo Controlled Trial [Abstract].** *Gastroenterology* 1993, **104**:A732.
A randomized, placebo controlled trial in patients with severe ulcerative colitis refractory to 10 days of high dose intravenous steroids demonstrated an 82% response rate with a mean time of 7.1 days to response.

62. Lichtiger S, Present DH: **Cyclosporin A in the Treatment of Severe Ulcerative Colitis [Abstract].** *Gastroenterology* 1992, **102**:A653.

63. Sandborn WJ, Tremaine WJ, Schroeder KW, Steiner BL, Batts KP, Lawson GM: **Cyclosporine Enemas for Treatment-Resistant Mildly to Moderately Active, Left-Sided Ulcerative Colitis.** *Am J Gastroenterol* 1993, **88**:640–645.

64. Winter TA, Dlaton HR, Merrett MN, Campbell A, Jewell DP: **Cyclosporin A Retention Enemas in Refractory Distal Ulcerative Colitis and 'Pouchitis.'** *Scand J Gastroenterol* 1993, **28**:701–704.

65. Brynskov J, Freund L, Thomsen OO, Andersen CB, Rasmussen SN, Binder V: **Treatment of Refractory Ulcerative Colitis With Cyclosporin Enemas [Letter to the Editor].** *Lancet* 1989, **1**:721–722.

66. Ranzi T, Campanini MC, Velio P, di Palo FQ, Bianchi P: **Treatment of Chronic Proctosigmoiditis With Cyclosporin Enemas [Letter to the Editor].** *Lancet* 1989, **2**:97.

67. •• Sandborn WJ, Tremaine WJ, Schroeder KW, Batts KP, Lawson GM, Steiner BL: **A Randomized, Double-Blind, Placebo-Controlled Trial of Cyclosporine Enemas for Mildly to Moderately Active Left-Sided Ulcerative Colitis [Abstract].** *Gastroenterology* 1993, **104**:A775
The only controlled study for cyclosporin enema treatment of left-sided ulcerative colitis. Response rate for CyA enema treated patients and placebo treated patients were similar; suggesting that CyA enemas are not efficacious in the treatment of mildly to moderately active left-side ulcerative colitis.

68. Lobo AJ, Juby LD, Smith AH, Foster PN, Rothwell J, Pentith J, Poole TW, Axon ATR: **Effect of Oral Cyclosporin on Renal Function in Crohn's Disease.** *Dig Dis Sci* 1993, **38**:1624–1630.

69. Ellestad-Sayed JJ, Nelson RA, Adson MA, Palmer WM, Soule EH: **Pantothenic Acid, Coenzyme A, and Human Chronic Ulcerative Colitis and Granulomatous Colitis.** *Am J Clin Nutrit* 1976, **29**:1333–1338.

70. Scheppach W, Sommer H, Kirchner T, Paganelli G, Bartram P, Christl S, Richter F, Dusel G, Kasper H: **Effect of Butyrate Enemas on the Colonic Mucosa in Distal Ulcerative Colitis.** *Gastroenterology* 1992, **103**:51–56.

71. Senagore AJ, MacKeigan JM, Scheider M, Ebrom S: **Short Chain Fatty Acid Enemas: A Cost Effective Alternative in the Treatment of Nonspecific Proctosigmoiditis.** *Dis Colon Rectum* 1992, **35**:923–927.

72. Breuer RI, Buto SK, Christ MI, Bean J, Vernia P, Paoluzi P, *et al.*: **Rectal Irrigation With Short Chain Fatty Acids for Distal Ulcerative Colitis. Preliminary Report.** *Dig Dis Sci* 1991, **36**:185–187.

73. Collawn C, Rubin P, Perez N, Bohadilla J, Cabrera G, Reyes E, Borovoy J, Kershenobich D: **Phase II Study of the Safety and Efficacy of a 5-Lipoxygenase Inhibitor in Patients With Ulcerative Colitis.** *Am J Gastroenterol* 1992, **87**:342–346.

74. Burnham WR, Lennard-Jones JE: **Mycobacteria as a Possible Cause of Inflammatory Bowel Disease.** *Lancet* 1978, **ii**:693–696.

75. Burnham WR, Lennard-Jones JE: **Mycobacteria as a Possible Cause of Inflammatory Bowel Disease.** *Lancet* 1978, **2**:693–696.

76. Graham DY, Markesich DC, Estes MK, Yoshimura HH: **Mycobacteriae and Inflammatory Bowel Disease: Culture and DNA Hybridization.** *Gastroenterology* 1985, **90**:1436.

77. Hermon-Taylor J, Moss M, Tizard M, Malik Z, Sanderson J: **Molecular Biology of Crohn's Disease Mycobacteria.**. *Bailleve's Clin Gastroenterol* 1990, **4**:23–42.

78. Chiodini RJ, Kruininyen HJ, Thayer WR, Merkal RS, Coutu JA: **Possible role of Mycobacteria in Inflammatory Bowel Disease. 1. An Unclassified Mycobacterium Species Isolated From Patients With Crohn's Disease.**. *Dig Dis Sci* 1984, **29**:1073–1079.

79. Brunello F, Pera A, Martini S, Marino L, Astegiano M, Barletti C, Gastaldi P, Verme G, Emanuelli G: **Antibodies to *Mycobacterium Paratuberculosis* in Patients With Crohn's Disease.** *Dig Dis Sci* 1991, **36**:1741–1745.

80. Ibbotson JP, Lowes JR, Chahal H, Gaston JSH, Life P, Kumararaine DS, Sharif H, Alexander-Williams J, Allan RN: **Mucosal Cell-Mediated Immunity to Mycobacterial, Enterobacterial and Other Microbial Antigens in Inflammatory Bowel Disease.** *Clin Exp Immunol* 1992, **87**:224–230.

81. Rutgeerts P, Geboes K, Vantrappen G, Van Isveldt J, Peeters M, Penninckx F, Hiele M: **Rifabutin and Ethambutol Do Not**

Help Recurrent Crohn's Disease in the Neoterminal Ileum. *J Clin Gastroenterol* 1992, **15**:24–28.

82. Elsaghier A, Prantera C, Moreno C, Ivanyi J: **Antibodies to Mycobacterium Paratuberculosis-Specific Protein Antigens in Crohn's Disease.** *Clin Exp Immunol* 1992, **90**:503–508.

83. Stainsby KJ, Lowes JR, Allan RN, Ibbotson JP: **Antibodies to Mycobacterium Paratuberculosis and Nine Species of Environmental Mycobacteria in Crohn's Disease and Control Subjects.** *Gut* 1993, **34**:371–374.

84. Moss MTG, Green, EP, Tizard ML, Malik ZP, Hermon-Taylor J: **Specific detection of Mycobacterium Paratuberculoris by DNA Hyridisation With a Fragment of the Insertion Element IS 900.** *Gut* 1991, **32**:395–398.

85. McFadden J, Collins J, Beaman B, Arthur M, Gitnick G: **Mycobacteria in Crohn's Disease: DNA Probes Identify the Wood Pigeon Strain of Mycobacterium Avium and Mycobacterium Paratuberculosis From Human Tissue.** *J Clin Microbiol* 1992, **30**:3070–3073.

86. Wall S, Kunze ZM, Saboor S, Soufleri I, Seechurn P, Chiodini R, McFadden JJ: **Identification of Spheroblast-Like Agents Isolated From Tissues of Patients With Crohn's Disease and Control Tissues by Polymerase Chain Reaction.** *J Clin Microbiol* 1993, **31**:1241–1245.

87. Chapman RW, Selby WS, Jewell DP: **Controlled Trial of Metronidazole as an Adjunct to Corticosteroids in Severe Ulcerative Colitis.** *Gut* 1986, **27**:1210–1212.

88. Gilat T, Sussa A, Leichtman G, Delpre G, Pavlotzky M, Grossman A, Firearm Z: **A Comparative Study of Metronidazole and Sulfasalazine in Active, Not Severe, Ulcerative Colitis. An Israeli Multicenter Study.** *J Clin Gastroenterol* 1987, **9**:415–417.

89. Gilat T, Leichtman G, Delpre G, Eschar J, Bar Meir S, Firearm Z: **A Comparison of Metronidazole and Sulfasalazine in the Maintenance of Remission in Patients With Ulcerative Colitis.** *J Clin Gastroenterol* 1989, **11**:392–395.

90. Davies PS, Rhodes J, Heatley RV: **Metronidazole in the Treatment of Chronic Proctitis: A Controlled Trial.** *Gut* 1977, **18**:680–681.

91. Brown WJ, Hudson MJ, Patrick S, Matthews SCW, Hill MJ, Gent AE, Grace RH, Hellier MD, Swarbrick ET: **Search for Enteric Microbial Pathogens in Patients With Ulcerative Colitis.** *Digestion* 1992, **53**:121–128.

92. • Peppercorn MA: **Are Antibiotics Useful in the Management of Nontoxic Severe Ulcerative Colitis?** *J Clin Gastroenterol* 1993, **17**:14–17.

The use of broad spectrum antibiotics in 7 patients who initially failed to respond to intravenous high dose corticosteroids helped to avoid colectomy. It is thus recommended that severely ill patients with ulcerative colitis deserve a trial of antibiotics before being considered failures of medical therapy.

93. Lobo AJ, Burke DA, Sobala GM, Axon ATR: **Oral Tobramycin in Ulcerative Colitis: Effect on Maintenance of Remission Aliment.** *Pharmacol Ther* 1993, **7**:155–158.

94. Nagler J, Brown M, Soave R: **Blastocystis Hominis in Inflammatory Bowel Disease.** *J Clin Gastroenterol* 1993, **16**:109–112.

95. Blichfeldt P, Blomhoff JP, Myhre E, Gjone E: **Metronidazole for Crohn's Disease: A Double Blind Cross-Over Clinical Trial.** *Scand J Gastroenterol* 1978, **13**:123–127.

96. Ambrose NS, Allan RN, Keighley MRB, Burdon DW, Youngs D, Barnes P, Lennard Jones JE: **Antibiotic Therapy for Treatment in Relapse of Intestinal Crohn's Disease.** *Dis Colon Rectum* 1985, **28**:81–85.

97. Ursing B, Alm T, Barany F, Bergelin I, Ganrot-Norlin K, Hoevels J, Hitfeldt B, Jarnerot G, Krause U, Krook A, *et al.*: **A Comparative Study of Metronidazole and Sulfasalazine for Active Crohn's Disease: The Cooperative Crohn's Disease Study in Sweden.** *Gastroenterology* 1982, **83**:550–562.

98. Jacobvitz J, Schuster MM: **Metronidazole Therapy for Crohn's Disease and Associated Fistulae.** *Am J Gastroenterol* 1984, **79**:533–540.

99. Ursing B, Kamme C: **Metronidazole for Crohn's Disease.** *Lancet* 1975, **1**:775–777.

100. Bernstein LH, Frank MS, Brandt LJ, Boley SJ: **Healing of Perineal Crohn's Disease With Metronidazole.** *Gastroenterology* 1980, **79**:357–365.

101. Brandt LJ, Bernstein LH, Boley SJ, Frank MS: **Metronidazole Therapy for Perineal Crohn's Disease: A Followup Study.** *Gastroenterology* 1982, **83**:383–387.

102. Verspaget HW, Multer TPJ, Van der Sluys Veer A, Pena AS, Lamers CBHW: **Reactive Oxygen Metabolites and Colitis: A Disturbed Balance Between Damage and Protection: A Selective Review.** *Scand J Gastroenterol* 1991, **26**:44–51.

103. •• Baldassano RN, Schrieber S, Johnston RB, Fu RD, Muraki T, MacDermott RP: **Crohn's Disease Monocytes Are Primed for Accentuated Release of Toxic Oxygen Metabolites.** *Gastroenterology* 1993, **105**:60–66.

Freshly isolated monocytes from active untreated Crohn's disease patients demonstrated enhanced stimulated release of superoxide anion compared with normal monocytes. The hypothesis that the monocyte priming factor in Crohn's disease serum was Lipopolysaccharide. This was shown by demonstrating that Crohn's disease serum lost its ability to prime monocytes after lipopolysaccharide was removed. The authors suggest that these studies indicate that bacterial cell wall products may be important proinflammatory molecules involved in the initiation and/or perpetuation of Crohn's disease.

104. Keshavarzian A, Haydek J, Zabihi R, Doria M, D'Astice M, Sorenson JRJ: **Agents Capable of Eliminating Reactive Oxygen Species: Catalase, WR-2721, or Cu(II)2(3,5-DIPS)4 Decrease Experimental Colitis.** *Dig Dis Sci* 1992, **37**:1866–1873.

105. • Middleton SJ, Shorthouse M, Hunter JO: **Increased Nitric Oxide Synthesis in Ulcerative Colitis.** *Lancet* 1993, **341**:465–466.

It was demonstrated that there is increased NO production in patients with active ulcerative colitis by measuring the concentrations of L-citrulline in rectal biopsy specimens. Also, L-citrulline synthesis was inhibited by incubation with N_G-monomethyl-L-arginine, a competitive inhibitor of NO synthetase. The authors suggest that NO may play a role in ulcerative colitis.

106. Tran DD, Visser JJ, Pool MO, Cuesta MA, Hoekman K, Pena AS, Meuwissen SGM: **Enhanced Systemic Nitric Oxide Production in Inflammatory Bowel Disease.** *Lancet* 1993, **341**:1150.

107. •• Podolsky DK, Lobb R, King N, Benjamin CD, Pepinsky B, Sehgal P, de Beaumont M: **Attenuation of Colitis in the Cotton-Top Tamarin by Anti-Alfa 4 Integrin Monoclonal Antibody.** *J Clin Invest* 1993, **92**:372–380.

Using the Cotton-top Tamarin model an Anti-alpha4 integrin monoclonal antibody was administered and resulted in a significant reduction of the intestinal inflammation compared with the pretreatment level. This provides support to the notion that interference with the binding endothelial adhesion molecules may provide therapeutic benefit to help abate the inflammatory component in IBD.

Gary R. Lichtenstein, MD, Assistant Professor of Medicine, Director, Inflammatory Bowel Disease Center, Hospital of the University of Pennsylvania, University of Pennsylvania School of Medicine, Gastrointestinal Division, Department of Internal Medicine, 8th Floor, Gates Building, 3400 Spruce Street, Philadelphia, PA 19104-4283, USA.

Pediatric inflammatory bowel disease

Ian D.A. D'Agata, MD,* and Harland S. Winter, MD*†

*Massachusetts General Hospital and †Boston City Hospital, Boston, Massachusetts, USA

This manuscript highlights recent advances relevant to pediatric patients with inflammatory bowel disease. Four areas are presented: growth failure, diagnosis and pathobiology, therapy, and clinical associations. Articles most likely to affect investigators and clinicians working on issues of importance to children and adolescents with Crohn's disease and ulcerative colitis were selected. Growth failure is a common and frequently serious problem in the pediatric population affected by inflammatory bowel disease. In 1993, both prospective and retrospective studies evaluated the effects of various treatment regimens. The role of pharmacotherapy and hormones in modifying alterations of growth were determined. Cytokines were studied as possible diagnostic tools in the clinical evaluation of disease and their role in the pathogenesis of mucosal inflammation became somewhat better defined, but much more complicated. The relationship between immunology, genetics, and clinical disease became clearer with the introduction of antineutrophil cytoplasmic antibodies in differentiating between Crohn's disease and ulcerative colitis. Therapy with immunosuppressive agents and reassessment of the role of surgical management of inflammatory bowel disease in children were the major therapeutic advances, although new agents appropriate for children are on the horizon. An interesting series of case reports highlighted aspects of the disease that are unique to the pediatric population.

Current Opinion in Gastroenterology 1994, **10**:404–408

Growth failure

Malnutrition in inflammatory bowel disease (IBD) has always been a problem for patients of all ages. Of particular concern to the pediatric gastroenterologist is the resulting delay in linear growth and sexual maturation observed in children with Crohn's disease and ulcerative colitis. Indeed, growth failure is thought to be the single most common extraintestinal complication of Crohn's disease in childhood. The prevention of malnutrition and ensuing growth failure for these individuals is the cornerstone of therapy for these individuals.

In a recent review by Markowitz *et al.* [1], the records of 48 adults diagnosed with IBD in childhood were analyzed to assess if permanent impairment of linear growth had occurred. Final adult heights were predicted by use of height-for-age percentiles and the Bailey-Pinneau and Roche-Wainer-Thissen methods. The predicted height was then compared with the final stature of each individual. It was found that 31% of subjects had adult height deficiencies as identified by two or more methods, and this was particularly true of those patients with Crohn's disease as opposed to those with ulcerative colitis. Growth impairment did not correlate with either the extent of disease in ulcerative colitis patients or the intestinal segment affected by Crohn's disease. Of all the patients reviewed, 60% had transient growth failure whereas 19% to 35% had permanent growth deficit, depending on the method of analysis. Interestingly, growth curves were the least sensitive of the methodologies employed. Growth failure using the NCHS charts was defined as a fall in height for age of more than two major channels, a definition that requires severe growth failure to be present. The authors conclude that meaningful deficits of adult height are common in patients who acquire IBD in childhood or adolescence.

In an accompanying editorial, Kirschner [2•] commented that assessment of skeletal age by a pediatric endocrinologist might provide better prediction of

Abbreviations

ANCA—antineutrophil cytoplasmic antibodies; **IBD**—inflammatory bowel disease; **IGF**—insulin-like growth factor; **TNF**—tumor necrosis factor.

 ISBN 1-85922-609-4 ISSN 0267–1379

adult height. Clearly, physicians caring for children and adolescents with growth retardation must be cognizant of long-term outcomes when planning intervention.

In another retrospective study, Griffiths *et al.* [3] reviewed the records of 100 children with Crohn's disease and analyzed the influence of sex, anatomic location of disease, severity of symptoms, surgery, and steroids on growth by uni- and multivariate regression analysis. The authors found that the severity of disease symptoms was the major factor in delaying linear growth velocity, and that the duration of daily prednisone therapy also negatively affected height velocity when analyzed independently by simple linear regression. However, after adjusting for severity of symptoms, length of corticosteroid administration did not significantly predict height velocity. Of interest, the 67 children who had been followed to their completion of linear growth ultimately maintained their height percentile. The authors point out, however, that because height percentiles had not been uniformly available prior to the onset of disease, the impact of IBD on genetically determined growth potential remained undetermined. Nonetheless, 50% of children below the third percentile for height at time of diagnosis failed to reach the third percentile for adult height. This observation suggests that stunted patients at time of presentation may require a different long-term therapeutic approach.

Recently, Motil *et al.* [4] published one of the first reports to detail growth failure prospectively in a large number of children. In this study, growth failure and its relationship to disease activity versus steroid therapy were analyzed. Sixty-nine children with IBD were enrolled and their height was monitored for 3 years. The authors found that there was a significant negative association between linear growth and disease activity but not steroid therapy. They also confirmed previous observations that growth is impaired more in Crohn's disease than in ulcerative colitis. Height deficits were independent of Tanner stage and linear growth delay persisted throughout puberty and did not reverse after surgery. The authors conclude that in some children, growth failure represents an early, "pre-patterned" manifestation of IBD and that it is the inflammatory process itself, and not the steroids, that predominantly affects growth.

Previous discussions suggested that growth failure associated with IBD may be attributed to hormonal factors, but current data does not support hormonal deficits as a cause of growth failure in IBD. Children with Crohn's disease or ulcerative colitis with or without growth retardation, appear to have normal thyroid, adrenal, and hypothalamic-pituitary function. Braeggar *et al.* [5] measured urinary growth hormone concentrations in 36 children with IBD and 51 healthy controls. No statistically significant difference was found between the IBD patients and the control group. Furthermore, there was no significant difference in urinary growth hormone concentration between stunted patients with IBD and IBD patients with normal growth. It was concluded that growth retardation in children with IBD was not related to growth hormone defects. However, insulin-like growth factor (IGF)-1 levels correlated with growth rates in children and adolescents with IBD.

Recently, Thomas *et al.* [6] studied 29 children with Crohn's disease before and after steroid or an elemental diet therapy to assess the effect of disease activity and therapy on serum concentrations of IGF-1, IGF binding protein, and insulin. Levels measured at the onset revealed that the insulin and IGF binding protein concentrations were not significantly different between groups, whereas the median serum IGF-1 concentration was lower in patients with active disease as opposed to matched controls. The latter finding may simply be a reflection of decreased energy intake in this subset of children. The authors found that after 4 weeks of either therapy, there was an increase in the median IGF-1 concentration. In the steroid-treated group, the median serum insulin level increased and the median serum IGF blood protein level decreased respectively. These changes were not observed in the elemental diet group. Surprisingly, the IGF-1 concentration increase was higher in the steroid-treated group than in the elemental diet group, despite better growth in the latter group.

Thomas *et al.* [7] also recently performed a randomized controlled trial comparing high-dose steroids to an elemental diet. Twenty-four children with Crohn's disease were enrolled and sex- and height-matched with healthy siblings of other patients. The authors found that growth velocity was better in the elemental diet group but there was greater and more sustained energy intake in the steroid group. This data led to the recommendation that elemental diets should be the therapy of choice in acute childhood Crohn's disease.

Polk *et al.* [8] attempted to determine the effect of a defined formula diet on growth and disease activity in children with Crohn's disease and growth failure. An isotonic, hydrolyzed, medium-chain triglyceride formula was administered by nasogastric tube infusion, followed by 2 weeks of an exclusion diet and 2 weeks of a low-residue diet. Both height and weight velocity significantly increased, with a significant decrease in disease activity as demonstrated by an improvement in the Crohn's Disease Activity Index. In view of the cost and risks of total parenteral nutrition, it is increasingly apparent that enteral nutrition may represent one possible solution to the malnutrition issue in IBD. As was the case in the above study, exclusion diets are used by some clinicians in the management of IBD, as food sensitivity is of concern in some patients. Consequently, it is noteworthy that Pearson *et al.* [9] reported that exclusion of foods after therapy with an elemental diet did not prolong remission in patients with Crohn's disease, although the authors state that reintroduction of food must be done with caution. Clinicians should be cautious in overinterpreting results of nutritional studies that follow patients for relatively short periods of time.

Diagnosis and pathobiology

The hallmark of IBD, chronic inflammation responsible for progressive tissue destruction, has led researchers to investigate the role of the enteric immune system in pathogenesis. Efforts directed at characterization of the cellular and humoral mechanisms in IBD and in particular the role of proinflammatory and immunoregulatory cytokines, antibodies and autoantibodies, has been the subject of recent investigations. A clearer understanding of specific molecular mechanisms involved in IBD may lead to the development of better or novel diagnostic and therapeutic modalities.

A number of studies in the pediatric population continued to provide insight in the past year. Youngman *et al.* [10••] showed that substantial amounts of interleukin-1α and interleukin-β are produced by lamina propria mononuclear cells and are increased in cells obtained from patients with IBD. Breese *et al.* [11] were able to demonstrate an increase in inflammatory mediator production (such as interleukin-1 and interferon-γ) in patients with Crohn's disease, but not in those with ulcerative colitis. Olson *et al.* [12] used an immunohistochemical staining technique to determine the specific cells that synthesize tumor necrosis factor (TNF)-α and interleukin-1β. Mononuclear cells stained brightly for both TNF and interleukin-1β, whereas small lymphocytes, macrophages, polymorphonuclear leukocytes, and epithelial cells did not.

Interleukin-6 is an immunoregulatory cytokine that stimulates hepatic acute-phase reactants and activates other immune cells. Investigators have shown an increased production of both intestinal mucosa and peripheral blood mononuclear cell interleukin-6 in patients with IBD. In particular, elevated serum levels of interleukin-6 have been documented in adult patients with Crohn's disease, but not in those with ulcerative colitis.

Recently, Hyams *et al.* [13•] attempted to examine the relationship of serum interleukin-6 levels to clinical and laboratory parameters of IBD. The sera from 26 children with ulcerative colitis, 49 with Crohn's disease, and 29 healthy controls were collected and circulating interleukin-6 levels were measured. Although increased levels of serum interleukin-6 were found in all patients with IBD, interesting differences were noted between the two measurement systems (bioassay and enzyme-linked immunosorbent assay) and clinical and laboratory parameters. Functional and antigenic levels were highest in Crohn's patients, but higher in children with ulcerative colitis than in controls. Both functional and antigenic interleukin-6 levels were greater in Crohn's disease affecting the colon than in disease involving the small bowel only. It is noteworthy that in both Crohn's and ulcerative colitis, antigenic interleukin-6 levels correlated with acute-phase reactants in both diseases, and again, functional levels did not. There was a significant negative correlation between both serum functional and antigenic interleukin-6 and serum albumin. Previous studies in adults using either the bioassay or enzyme-linked immunosorbent assay technique have failed to show a relationship between disease activity and interleukin-6 levels. It may be that both the functional and antigenic assays are necessary in order to establish a relationship between serum interleukin-6 and the clinical parameters of IBD. Justly, the authors point out that as interleukin-6 acts in concert with other cytokines in the context of the inflammatory response, further studies need to address if other cytokines play a significant role.

Ever since antineutrophil cytoplasmic antibodies (ANCAs) have been associated with certain inflammatory diseases, numerous studies have been conducted in adults in an effort to determine their role in IBD. In particular, investigators have concentrated on ANCAs that exhibit a perinuclear fluorescence pattern as these have particularly been associated with IBD. Although most researchers have failed to show any relationship between titer of perinuclear-ANCA and disease activity, it has been reported recently that perinuclear-ANCA measurement may be both sensitive and specific for the diagnosis of ulcerative colitis in adults. There have been few studies in children.

Proujansky *et al.* [14] examined the sera of children with ulcerative colitis and Crohn's disease, as well as the sera of a control group for the presence of ANCAs. ANCAs were detected in the serum of 66% of patients with ulcerative colitis, 19% of patients with Crohn's disease, and none of the control patients. Therefore, the sensitivity and specificity of ANCA in ulcerative colitis in this group of pediatric patients was only of 66% and 84%, respectively. Furthermore, perinuclear-ANCAs were found in only 46% of the ulcerative colitis patients studied, and this differs from series where perinuclear-ANCAs were found in over 60% of adult patients with ulcerative colitis. In this study, no relationship was established between a positive ANCA value and disease activity, and it was not felt to be of clinical relevance in distinguishing between ulcerative colitis and Crohn's disease. Other studies suggest that ANCA may be beneficial in the pediatric population [15].

Therapy

There has been an increasing interest in the application of immunosuppressive agents such as azathioprine and cyclosporine for the treatment of IBD. Efficacy of these agents for this indication remains controversial, and published reports in pediatric patients are extremely limited. Regardless, anecdotal experience reveals that immunosuppressives are in fact being used with increasing frequency by pediatric gastroenterologists, especially in those IBD patients whose disease is refractory to standard therapy.

Markowitz *et al.* [16] published the results of a survey polling physician members of the North American Society for Pediatric Gastroenterology and Nutrition on the subject of immunosuppressive use in the IBD patient. As is usually the case (and problem) with medical surveys, response rate was low (only 27% of physicians polled responded), rendering it difficult to draw truly meaningful conclusions from these results. Also, the questionnaire was sent out in 1990, and in the intervening years attitudes towards these agents has changed. Nonetheless, the results indicated some trends: 1) immunosuppressives were used approximately twice as often in patients with Crohn's disease; 2) the most commonly used agents were 6-mercaptopurine and azathioprine, although cyclosporine and methotrexate were also used; 3) 66 of 105 physicians using the agents found them to be effective; 4) no consensus was obtained on the use of these agents in female patients; and 5) the most common indications for immunosuppressive use were either intractable disease not responding to usual methods of management or as a corticosteroid-sparing alternative.

For patients not responding to immunosuppressive therapy and bowel rest, surgery remains the primary option. A scholarly review was published by Lester Martin [17], the surgeon who pioneered the continence-preserving colectomy technique that is now used in both children and adolescents.

Clinical associations

The risk that active and passive smoking pose to IBD patients remains controversial. In a recent case-control study by Lashner *et al.* [18], it appears that passive smoke exposure at birth was significantly associated with the development of IBD, although the effect was greater in patients with Crohn's disease than in those with ulcerative colitis. In adults, it seems that the risk of developing ulcerative colitis is greater in former smokers and reduced in current smokers, so that the effect of passive smoking in children reflects the "former smoking" effect seen in adults. The mechanism by which this may occur is unclear and further research is needed on the issue.

Gryboski [19] presented an interesting report of three patients with IBD who also had an established eating disorder. Two patients had bulimia and one was presumed to have anorexia and bulimia. All three presented because of failed treatment for IBD. The author suggests that an abnormal eating behavior should be considered in patients whose IBD symptoms do not correlate with their disease state or whose disease increases in severity despite seemingly adequate therapy.

A rare case of isolated Crohn's jejunitis was reported by Mendelsohn and Korelitz [20] in a 19-year-old who had been diagnosed with ulcerative colitis at 7 years of age. An upper gastrointestinal and small bowel series at that time were normal, whereas a rectal biopsy confirmed ulcerative colitis. He responded well to sulfasalazine and prednisone. Years later he re-presented with abdominal pain and emesis, and work-up revealed a thickened wall of the proximal jejunum on upper gastrointestinal series. A subsequent laparotomy showed a 45-cm long strictured jejunal segment. Pathology was consistent with Crohn's. The coexistence of Crohn's disease and ulcerative colitis in the same patient remains an area of controversy.

Abscess and fistula formation is a debilitating complication of Crohn's disease. Both inflammation and increased intraluminal pressure from intestinal stenoses secondary to the inflammatory process have been implicated as a cause of fistula formation. In a retrospective study, Kahn *et al.* [21] reviewed 55 surgically resected specimens obtained from patients with Crohn's. Of these, 31 contained fistulae: 16 of 31 specimens had stenoses and 12 of 24 did not. Because all fistulae were associated with the presence of inflammation, the authors conclude that inflammation is of primary importance in the pathogenesis of fistulae in Crohn's disease.

In what is believed to be the first reported case in the literature, Smith *et al.* [22] report the association of epidermolysis bullosa simplex and ulcerative colitis in a 3-week-old infant. As is often the case when ulcerative colitis presents early in life, the course of the disease was severe and a subtotal colectomy was required at 6 months of age. Treem *et al.* [23] reported the association between alopecia areata and ulcerative colitis in a mother and son.

Advances in pediatric IBD have occurred in clinical diagnosis and therapeutic intervention, but most importantly, immunologic and genetic factors are being studied in this population. These areas of investigation are most likely to provide fertile ground for progress in the pathogenesis of IBD.

References and recommended reading

Papers of particular interest, published within the annual period of review, have been highlighted as:
- • Of special interest
- •• Of outstanding interest

1. Markowitz J, Grancher K, Rosa J, Aiges H, Daum F: **Growth Failure in Pediatric Inflammatory Bowel Disease.** *J Pediatr Gastroenterol Nutr* 1993, **16**:373–380.

2. • Kirschner BS: **Permanent Growth Failure in Pediatric Inflammatory Bowel Disease.** *J Pediatr Gastroenterol Nutr* 1993, **16**:368–369.

A good discussion of growth issues in pediatric IBD.

3. Griffiths A, Koletzko S, Sylvester F, Marcon M, Sherman P: **Slow-Release 5-Aminosalicylic Acid Therapy in Children With Small Intestinal Crohn's Disease.** *J Pediatr Gastroenterol Nutr* 1993, **17**:186–192.

4. Motil KJ, Grand RJ, Davis-Kraft L, Ferlic LL, Smith EO: **Growth Failure in Children With Inflammatory Bowel Disease: A Prospective Study.** *Gastroenterology* 1993, **105**:681–691.

5. Braegger CP, Torresani T, Murch SH, Savage MO, Walker-Smith JA, MacDonald TT: **Urinary Growth Hormone in Growth-Impaired Children With Chronic Inflammatory Bowel Disease.** *J Pediatr Gastroenterol Nutr* 1993, **16**:49–52.

6. Thomas AG, Holly JM, Taylor F, Miller V: **Insulin Like Growth Factor-I, Insulin Like Growth Factor Binding Protein-1, and Insulin in Childhood Crohn's Disease.** *Gut* 1993, **34**:944–947.

7. Thomas AG, Taylor F, Miller V: **Dietary Intake and Nutritional Treatment in Childhood Crohn's Disease.** *J Pediatr Gastroenterol Nutr* 1993, **17**:75–81.

8. Polk DB, Hattner JA, Kerner JA: **Improved Growth and Disease Activity After Intermittent Administration of a Defined Formula Diet in Children With Crohn's Disease.** *JPEN J Parenter Enteral Nutr* 1992, **16**:499–504.

9. Pearson M, Teahon K, Levi AJ, Bjarnason I: **Food Intolerance and Crohn's Disease.** *Gut* 1993, **34**:783–787.

10. •• Youngman KR, Simon PL, West GA, Cominelli F, Rachmilewitz D, Klein JS, Fiocchi C: **Localization of Intestinal Interleukin 1 Activity and Protein and Gene Expression to Lamina Propria Cells.** *Gastroenterology* 1993, **104**:749–758.

Discusses the role of immunoregulation in IBD.

11. Breese E, Braegger CP, Corrigan CJ, Walker-Smith JA, MacDonald TT: **Interleukin-2 and Interferon-Gamma-Secreting T Cells in Normal and Diseased Human Intestinal Mucosa.** *Immunology* 1993, **78**:127–131.

12. Olson AD, Ayass M, Chensue S: **Tumor Necrosis Factor and IL-1 Beta Expression in Pediatric Patients With Inflammatory Bowel Disease.** *J Pediatr Gastroenterol Nutr* 1993, **16**:241–246.

13. • Hyams JS, Fitzgerald JE, Treem WR, Wyzga N, Kreutzer DL: **Relationship of Functional and Antigenic Interleukin 6 to Disease Activity in Inflammatory Bowel Disease.** *Gastroenterology* 1993, **104**:1285–1292.

Relates immunoregulatory abnormalities to clinical state of disease in children.

14. Proujansky R, Fawcett PT, Gibney KM, Treem WR, Hyams JS: **Examination of Anti-Neutrophil Cytoplasmic Antibodies in Childhood Inflammatory Bowel Disease.** *J Pediatr Gastroenterol Nutr* 1993, **17**:193–197.

15. Winkelstein A, Winter HS, Landers C, Targan S: **Antineutrophil Cytoplasmic Antibody as Measured by Elisa is Sensitive and Specific for Childhood Ulcerative Colitis.** *Gastroenterology* 1993, **104**:A802.

16. Markowitz J, Grancher K, Mandel F, Daum F: **Immunosuppressive Therapy in Pediatric Inflammatory Bowel Disease: Results of a Survey of the North American Society for Pediatric Gastroenterology and Nutrition.** *Am J Gastroenterol* 1993, **88**:44–48.

17. Martin LW: **Current Surgical Management of Patients With Chronic Ulcerative Colitis [Review].** *J Pediatr Gastroenterol Nutr* 1993, **17**:121–131.

18. Lashner BA, Shaheen NJ, Hanauer SB, Kirschner BS: **Passive Smoking is Associated With an Increased Risk of Developing Inflammatory Bowel Disease in Children.** *Am J Gastroenterol* 1993, **88**:356–359.

19. Gryboski JD: **Ulcerative Colitis in Children 10 Years Old or Younger.** *J Pediatr Gastroenterol Nutr* 1993, **17**:24–31.

20. Mendelsohn RA, Korelitz BI: **Crohn's Disease Presenting as Isolated Jejunitis Years After Childhood Colitis.** *Am J Gastroenterol* 1993, **88**:105–108.

21. Kahn E, Markowitz J, Blomquist K, Daum F: **The Morphologic Relationship of Sinus and Fistula Formation to Intestinal Stenoses in Children With Chrohn's Disease.** *Am J Gastroenterol* 1993, **88**:1395–1398.

22. Smith PK, Davidson GP, Moore L, Clapton W, Jaunzems A, Little KE, Moore DJ: **Epidermolysis Bullosa and Severe Ulcerative Colitis in an Infant.** *J Pediatr* 1993, **122**:600–603.

23. Treem WR, Veligati LN, Rotter JI, Targan SR, Hyams JS: **Ulcerative Colitis and Total Alopecia in a Mother and Her Son.** *Gastroenterology* 1993, **104**:1187–1191.

Harland S. Winter, MD, Children's Hospital, 454 Brookline Avenue, Suite 29, Boston, MA 02215, USA.

Surgical and nutritional treatment of inflammatory bowel disease

John L. Rombeau, MD, and Yevgeniy Gincherman, BA

University of Pennsylvania, Philadelphia, Pennsylvania, USA

Patients with ulcerative colitis who undergo an ileal-anal pouch operation without ileostomy have increased morbidity. The quality of life after ileal-anal pouch procedure is comparable to patients with ulcerative colitis treated medically. The number of anastomoses is an important prognostic indicator for early symptomatic recurrence after Crohn's disease. Diversion of the fecal stream for patients with Crohn's disease of the colon produces a high incidence of sustained idsease remission, but the prospect of future restoration of intestinal continuity is limited. The energy requirements for patients with active Crohn's disease is similar (30 to 35 kcal/kg body weight/d) to other hospitalized patients. Polymeric diets are as effective as steroids in inducing short-term remission in patients with active Crohn's disease. Food sensitivities in patients with Crohn's disease are of insufficient importance to warrant routine trials of elimination diets.

Current Opinion in Gastroenterology 1994, **10**:409–416

Surgical treatment

Ulcerative colitis

The majority of reports of the surgical treatment for ulcerative colitis concern the ileal-anal pouch (IAP) operation. Similar to other technical innovations in surgery, the IAP technique continues to evolve as to its perioperative management and intraoperative technique. This section summarizes recent publications on the IAP operation with reference to general overview, technical aspects, and short- and long-term sequelae.

Several reviews of the IAP procedure were published during 1993. An extensive review of 221 patients [1••] focused on the clinical outcome of 73 patients less than 21 years of age at the time of surgery. Fifty-six consecutive surviving pediatric patients were followed for at least 1 year and up to 17 years after surgery. Fifty (89%) were leading normal lives with an acceptable stool frequency and complete fecal continence. Crohn's disease was the most important finding in patients with unsatisfactory postoperative outcomes. Improved methods of preoperative screening are needed to differentiate between Crohn's colitis and ulcerative colitis in pediatric patients. In a subsequent report [2••], 168 IAP operations were performed without mortality during 9 years. Postoperative morbidity included pelvic sepsis (12%), ileoanal stricture (15%), and pouch-related fistulas (16%). This morbidity decreased with increasing operative experience. Pouch excision was necessary in 30% of the first 50 patients, but in only 4% of the last 68 patients. Intestinal obstruction is a significant postoperative complication occurring in 18% of patients. Similar to the previous report, the failure to identify Crohn's disease preoperatively continues to be a significant factor of adverse outcome. In the six patients identified with Crohn's disease, three required pouch excision. Ten women had children after IAP procedure and eight uncomplicated vaginal deliveries occurred without impaired continence. Seven of the nine patients over 60 years of age in whom the operation was performed had a successful outcome.

Surgical technique

Studies have questioned whether a concomitant temporary ileostomy is needed in all patients undergoing IAP surgery. A recent report compared 50 IAP patients without ileostomy with 50 patients undergoing an IAP operation with a diverting ileostomy during the same time period [3••]. The patients were closely matched for age, gender, surgeon, diagnosis, extent, and duration of ulcerative colitis prior to colectomy. All patients had a stapled IAP without mucosectomy. Anastomic leaks and pelvic abscesses were more common in patients without ileostomy (14% vs 4%); eight of the nine patients with postoperative pelvic abscesses were taking more than 20 mg of prednisone daily. Septic complications requiring relaparotomy (6% vs 0%), prolonged ileus, and fever of unknown origin (10%

Abbreviations

IAP—ileal-anal pouch; **IBD**—inflammatory bowel disease; **IGF**—insulin-like growth factor.

 ISBN 1-85922-609-4 ISSN 0267–1379

vs 4%) were also more common in patients without ileostomy. Additionally, patients without ileostomy had a poorer quality of life index. The IAP operating without ileostomy is not as safe as the same operation with diversion, especially in patients taking more than 20 mg of prednisone daily.

Controversy continues as to whether pouch function is improved if the IAP procedure is performed without mucosectomy. In a report of 45 patients with the double-stapled IAP without mucosectomy for ulcerative colitis, 19 (35%) had ulcerative colitis at the distal margin of resection and six had persistent ulcerative colitis at the time of subsequent biopsy [4]. However, only one patient (1.8%) with evidence of ulcerative colitis at the distal margin of resection or of biopsy experienced symptoms referable to active ulcerative colitis. None of the specimens examined had any evidence of dysplasia. A subsequent study in patients with mucosectomies determined whether the epithelium of the anal transitional zone was involved by chronic ulcerative colitis and whether preserving this zone preserved the disease [5••]. Proctocolectomy specimens from 50 patients with ulcerative colitis and 50 patients with rectal cancer, serving as controls, were examined. The mean inflammation score of the rectal mucosa within the anal transition zone was significantly increased in ulcerative colitis when compared with controls. Although the double staple without mucosectomy technique appears to be safe, periodic monitoring is recommended. Preserving the anal transitional zone may preserve the disease in the majority of patients with ulcerative colitis.

Short-term and long-term sequelae

Anastomotic stricture after IAP procedure is an important postoperative complication. A consecutive series of 115 patients were reviewed retrospectively at a median of 34 months after operation or ileostomy closure [6•]. Of the 102 patients available for review, 39 (38%) developed an ileoanal anastomotic stricture, which was severe and persistent in 16%. Significant factors that predisposed to the development of anastomotic stricture were the 25-mm diameter (small) stapling gun, the quadruplicated reservoir, defunctioning ileostomy, anastomotic dehiscence, and pelvic sepsis. The functional outcome after dilatation of stricture was as good as the outcome in the patients who did not develop a stricture. In a subsequent report [7•], 144 consecutive patients who underwent either a handsewn or stapled anastomoses were reviewed between 1983 and 1991. Ninety-six patients had handsewn and 48 patients had stapled anastomoses. Significant differences in outcome between groups occurred in the length of operation (greater in the handsewn group) and in the incidence of stenosis at the anastomosis (greater in the handsewn group). It was concluded that the stapled anastomoses gave superior results, but it remains to be seen whether other differences will emerge as the length of follow-up increases.

Methods to improve the adaptation and function of the IAP before ileostomy closure have been investigated. Increasing volumes of liquid nutrients were injected into the pouch through an ileal-mucous fistula proximal to the pouch twice daily for 2 months before closing the temporary ileostomy [8•]. With this method, the number of evacuations per 24 hours was significantly reduced during the first few weeks following the reestablishment of intestinal continuity, compared with a control group (average 8.5 vs 18.2). Patients receiving nutrient infusion into the pouch also had better continence and less urgency to defecate.

Proctectomy is often deferred at the time of urgent colectomy because of severe illness and the difficulty in differentiating between ulcerative colitis and Crohn's disease. Definitive diagnosis of either ulcerative colitis or Crohn's disease is often difficult in the retained rectal stump following subtotal colectomy with ileostomy. The pathology of 15 defunctioned rectal stumps was investigated [9•]. All patients had previously undergone urgent total colectomy for presumed ulcerative colitis and rectal stumps had been left *in situ* prior to IAP procedure. All rectal stumps had mucosal disease, but there were additional features such as florid lymphoid follicular hyperplasia (12 patients), transmural inflammation (nine patients), granulomas, fissures, and changes akin to ischemia or to pseudo obstruction colitis. Many of these histologic changes in the retained rectum mimicked Crohn's disease; nevertheless, all of the 15 colectomy specimens showed unequivocal ulcerative colitis and none of the patients had subsequent clinical, radiologic, or pathologic evidence of Crohn's disease. Histologic changes in the retained rectal stump in ulcerative colitis may lead to an erroneous diagnosis of Crohn's disease and the patient may subsequently be denied an IAP operation.

Investigators have evaluated the quality of life after IAP when compared with ulcerative colitis patients treated medically. A detailed questionnaire and the hospital anxiety and depression tests were completed by 103 patients who had undergone IAP operation and by 95 patients with ulcerative colitis in remission on medical treatment [10••]. Patients with IAP had a greater frequency of bowel action but less urgency of defecation than medically treated patients. Efficiency of evacuation, discrimination between flatus and feces, use of perianal pads, and perianal soreness were similar. Use of antidiarrheal medication was more common in the pouch group, whereas use of topical steroids was more common in medically treated patients. Limitation of social activity and anxiety and depression scores were significantly higher in medically treated patients. It was concluded that quality of life for patients with a pouch was as good as that for patients with medically treated colitis. A similar quality of life and functional analysis was published in 240 randomly selected patients from an 8-year period [11]. Patients undergoing cholecystectomy during each of the same years served as controls (20 patients/y; total, 160 patients). In spite of the altered bowel habits, 90% of the IAP patients had an excellent overall quality of life, 76% enjoyed good health, and 91% had good performance scores in the areas examined. Interestingly, quality of life and performance were similar between IAP patients and cholecystectomy patients. Moreover, quality of life and bowel habits remained steady in both groups of patients during the 8-year follow-up. It was concluded that functional results were satisfactory and quality of life was excellent after IAP anastomosis; neither deteriorated as patients aged over an 8-year period after surgery.

Crohn's disease

Investigations of the prevalence and pathogenesis of anastomotic recurrence after surgical treatment of Crohn's disease continue to be reported. Additionally, improved operative techniques continue to decrease postoperative morbidity and mortality.

Postoperative anastomotic recurrence

The early symptomatic recurrence after intestinal resection in Crohn's disease continues to be high. One hundred sixty-four patients undergoing intestinal resection for Crohn's disease between 1976 and 1989 were studied prospectively [12••]. Early recurrence was defined as happening within 36 months of surgery. Multivariant analysis revealed that the number of anastomoses was the most important prognostic indicator ($P=0.001$), followed by inflammation at the resection margins ($P<0.05$). Patients requiring an ileostomy had a significantly lower early recurrence rate than those having single or multiple anastomoses. There was no significant correlation between inflammation at the margins and early recurrence in patients requiring an ileostomy or a single anastomosis. When the margins were examined in the 28 patients with two or more anastomoses, 10 of 11 (91%) with inflammation at either margin experienced early recurrence. Patients having multiple anastomoses with normal margins had the same recurrence rate as patients with single anastomoses. It was concluded that patients with extensive Crohn's disease requiring multiple resections with anastomoses, especially when microscopic inflammation is present at the margins, are at very high risk for symptomatic early recurrence. Further study is needed to determine whether avoidance of multiple anastomoses or adjuvant medical treatment can alter the course of the disease after intestinal resection in patients at high risk for early symptomatic recurrence.

The pathogenesis of anastomic recurrent disease continues to be investigated in animal preparations. The mechanisms of recurrence were investigated in a ferret model of multifocal intestinal infarction [13••]. It was concluded that the combination of two self-limiting, ischemic insults produces a pattern of intestinal inflammation similar to that seen in anastomotic recurrence in Crohn's disease. The relationship between suppression of macrophage function by six different suture materials and anastomotic, recurrent Crohn's disease was investigated in a rat model [14•]. All suture materials significantly impaired macrophage function.

Intraoperative and perioperative endoscopy of the small intestine are used to identify early postoperative recurrent Crohn's disease. Intraoperative small bowel endoscopy was performed in 31 patients with Crohn's disease [15•]. The extent of mucosal inflammation was compared with that of intraoperative examinations of the external bowel wall for findings such as serositis, fat wrapping, and mural thickening. Endoscopic findings influenced surgical decisions on 20 of the 33 occasions, limiting planned resection in 14, identifying strictures for repair in one and deciding against resection in two cases and for extended resection in three. The results suggested that external inflammatory changes are unreliable guides as to the extent of intestinal mucositis and requirements for resection in Crohn's disease. Intraoperative enteroscopy provided information for more precise surgery, thereby limiting resection. In a subsequent report [16•], perioperative endoscopy was performed in 20 patients operated on for Crohn's disease. A total retrograde exploration to the ligament of Treitz during an ileal colectomy or a colonic or ileoresection was performed. Endoscopic exploration was completed, through an enterotomy, from the surgical area to the ligament of Treitz. Periendoscopic biopsies were taken on microscopic lesions and every 20 cm systematically. In 13 of 20 patients, different lesions distributed throughout the entire small intestine were identified. In seven patients, none of the lesions detected at perioperative endoscopy had been recognized by preoperative evaluation or surgical inspection of the serosal surface. Thus, 65% of patients operated on for Crohn's disease had lesions of the small intestine detected by endoscopy that were unrecognized before surgery in more than half of the cases. Whether these lesions predispose to early symptomatic recurrence is unknown.

Surgical technique

Because of the apparent association between mucosal contact with the fecal stream and recurrence of Crohn's disease, the clinical course of 44 patients undergoing elective proximal fecal diversion for Crohn's disease of the colon was reported [17•]. Sustained disease remission occurred in 31 patients (70%). Diversion was associated with a significant reduction in steroid requirements and a significant improvement in hemoglobin, erythrocyte sedimentation rate, and albumin. Sixteen patients (36%) required a proctocolectomy, 19 patients (43%) remained defunctioned, and four patients (9%) died. It was concluded that fecal diversion for Crohn's disease of the colon produces a high incidence of sustained disease remission, but for the majority of patients the prospect of future restoration of intestinal continuity is limited.

The value of strictureplasty for the treatment of selected patients with partially obstructing Crohn's disease continues to be reported. A recent report [18•] reviewed the use of both Heineke-Mikulicz and Finney strictureplasties in 12 patients with long strictures. An innovative technique incorporating both of these techniques into a single strictureplasty was described. An additional report [19••] reviewed the long-term follow-up of strictureplasty in patients with Crohn's disease. One hundred sixteen patients with obstructive Crohn's disease undergoing 452 primary strictureplasties were reviewed. The median number of strictureplasties was three (range, one to 15). There was no postoperative mortality, septic complications occurred in seven patients (6%), and reoperation for sepsis was needed in two patients. Relief of obstructive symptoms was achieved in nearly all patients. The postoperative median weight gain was 4 kg and two thirds of the patients were weaned off steroids. Rates of restricture and new stricture or perforation disease were 2.8% and 24%, respectively. Strictureplasty remains a useful adjunct in the treatment of Crohn's disease, especially when short-bowel syndrome is a possibility.

Ileorectal anastomoses for Crohn's colitis continues to be a good operation in selected patients. One hundred thirty-one patients who underwent ileorectal anastomosis for Crohn's colitis were reviewed [20]. The mean duration of function was 9.2 years and there was a mean follow-up of 9.5 years. Seventy-two patients (61%) had a functioning anastomosis with 44 being free of disease and 28 being treated with steroids or antidiarrheal medication. The mean stool frequency was 4.7/d. Ileorectal anastomosis is an acceptable alternative to proctocolectomy if the rectum is not severely diseased and sphincter function is not compromised.

Proctectomy for patients with severe anorectal Crohn's disease is associated with a high incidence of unhealed perineal wounds. To prevent this problem, the use of the low Hartmann procedure for severe anorectal Crohn's disease was investigated [21]. Twenty-five patients with severe anorectal Crohn's disease, perineal fistulas, and colitis necessitating colectomy, underwent a low Hartmann's procedure in lieu of a standard proctocolectomy. Fifteen of the 25 (60%) patients had a completely healed perineum and required no further surgery. Although perineal disease persisted in the other 10 patients, their perinea were much improved when compared with the initial presentation. If a proctectomy became necessary, a perineal intersphincteric approach was used without a laparotomy because only a 3- to 5-cm cuff of rectum was retained from the initial surgery. Three of the 10 patients who subsequently underwent perineal proctectomies had unhealed perinea. Thus, 22 of the 25 (88%) patients had a completely healed perineum (mean follow-up, 61.9 months). It was concluded that the problem of the unhealed perineal wound can be reduced by this approach, thereby reducing long-term morbidity.

Nutrition and metabolic treatment

Recent advances have been made in the nutritional-metabolic treatment of patients with inflammatory bowel disease (IBD). New approaches to the treatment of patients with growth failure continue to be reported. Innovative enteral and parenteral nutritional regimens effective in Crohn's disease and ulcerative colitis are being identified. This section briefly reviews the results of recent publications with particular emphasis upon controlled clinical studies.

Growth failure

Growth retardation is a significant problem in prepubertal patients with IBD. Investigations have been performed to accurately determine nutrient requirements for these patients. The use of a combined body scan technique to determine the total energy expenditure was described in a recent report [22••]. This technique combines new energy balance studies as an alternative to classic direct calorimetry. Dual energy x-ray absorptiometry is used in combination with *in vivo* neutron activation analysis and tritiated water dilution. These combined techniques produce accurate measurements of changes in body fat, protein, and glycogen stores, thereby accurately calculating total energy expenditure. Thirteen patients with Crohn's disease who required nutritional support for at least 14 days were studied. Decreased activity energy expenditure was positively correlated with the increased activity of the disease. Thus, resting metabolic expenditure increases and activity energy expenditure decreases while the diet-induced thermogenesis remains constant with the increasing severity of the disease. As a result, total energy expenditure remains relatively stable. These data provide additional evidence that patients with Crohn's disease have energy requirements (30 to 35 total kcal/kg body weight/d) similar to other hospitalized patients.

Three different methods (height-for-age percentiles, the Bailey-Pinneau, and the Roche-Wainer-Thissen methods) were used to study the permanent impairment of linear growth in children with IBD [23•]. Forty-eight young adults were enrolled in the study. The authors documented permanent growth failure in 19 to 35 percent of subjects depending on the method used. Permanent growth failure was more common in patients with Crohn's disease (37%) than in patients with ulcerative colitis (10%). Duration of corticosteroid use was an important contributor to permanent growth impairment ($P<0.05$). Growth impairment was independent of age of onset and site of Crohn's disease, or extent of disease in ulcerative colitis. The small numbers of patients involved in each study subgroup could explain the differences between the data obtained in this report and other studies [24,25] as to the importance of the onset, site, and extent of disease on growth impairment.

Growth factors

As many as 30% of the children with chronic IBD have growth failure [26]. Chronic dietary insufficiency is the most important cause for this growth failure, but its pathogenetic mechanism is unclear. Abnormal growth hormone production and end-organ resistance have both been implicated in the pathogenesis of IBD-associated cachexia [27]. Twenty-nine children with Crohn's disease, treated with either steroids or elemental diet, were studied [28••]. The effects of disease activity and treatment on the serum levels of insulin-like growth factor (IGF)-1, IGF-1 binding protein-1, and insulin were determined. The authors found lower median levels of IGF-1 in patients with active disease, as compared with matched controls, and lower median levels of IGF-1 in patients with stunted growth, as compared with well-grown individuals. There were no significant differences in binding protein and plasma insulin levels. Both treatments resulted in increased IGF-1 serum levels. Patients receiving steroids sustained their increase in energy intake whereas those treated with elemental diet had greater median height velocity scores. The authors suggested that the growth suppressant effects of steroids "override" any benefits from increased energy intake, increased IGF-1 concentration, and reduced IGF binding protein-1 concentration.

Urinary growth hormone concentration was measured in 36 children with chronic IBD (24 patients with Crohn's disease and 12 patients with ulcerative colitis) and 51 normal controls [29•]. The median urinary growth concentration in patients with stunted growth was 15.8 ng/g creatinine and 11.7 ng/g creatinine in children with normal growth. There was no significant difference between urinary growth hormone concentrations in patients with IBD versus normal controls. Eighty percent of the patients with low urinary concentrations of growth hormones were receiving steroids. The authors concluded that administration of physiologic amounts of growth hormone to the patients with IBD is unlikely to improve growth failure.

Epidermal growth factor increases DNA synthesis, enhances crypt cell production rate [30–32], promotes migration of intestinal epithelial cells [33], and stimulates the growth of cultured fibroblasts [34]. Each of these effects could result in increased rates of healing of colonic ulcers in IBD. Epidermal growth factor administrated both systemically and intracolonically was investigated in rats with artificially induced colitis [35••]. The authors noted reduced colonic ulceration and inflammation after systemic administration of epidermal growth factor; however, intracolonic administration was ineffective.

Further research is needed to elucidate the possible roles that growth factors might play in the pathogenesis and treatment of patients with IBD. Moreover, the compiled interactions among IGF-1, IGF binding protein-1, and insulin in patients with IBD need to be elucidated. Further studies are needed to define the role of growth hormone in the IBD-associated growth retardation, because conflicting data have been reported.

Enteral and parenteral feeding

Crohn's disease

The effectiveness of elemental diet (Vivonex [Norwich Eaton, Norwich, NY] total enteral nutrition 2.1 L/d) and steroid treatment (prednisolone 0.75 mg/kg/d) was compared in 42 patients with active Crohn's disease [36••]. Forty-one percent of patients receiving the elemental diet were intolerant of the diet. Disease activity decreased in both groups. However, the elemental diet was less effective than steroids in maintaining long-term remission. The elemental diet and prednisolone treatment induced comparable short-term remissions.

A prospective randomized controlled trial of polymeric diet versus steroids as primary treatment in active Crohn's disease was recently reported [37••]. Thirty-two patients randomly received either polymeric diet (2800 kcal/d) or prednisone (1 mg/kg/d). Polymeric diet induced remission in 80% of the patients. Percentiles reduction in disease activity indices (Van Hees index) were comparable in both groups. Relapse rates within a 1-year period were higher in the steroid group (66.6%) than in the polymeric diet group (41.6%). The authors concluded that polymeric diets are as effective as steroids in inducing short-term remission in patients with active Crohn's disease.

Food intolerance in 42 patients with Crohn's disease was investigated [38•]. Thirty-three percent of the patients dropped out of the study for various reasons. Twenty patients identified food sensitivities, and 17 had an open rechallenge with recurrence of symptoms in 10. Food sensitivity was confirmed in only three of these patients on double-blind rechallenge. The authors concluded that food sensitivities in patients with Crohn's disease are of insufficient importance to warrant routine trials of elimination diets.

Ulcerative colitis

Few studies have investigated the relative effectiveness of enteral and parenteral nutrition as adjunct therapies in active ulcerative colitis. Forty-two patients randomly received either polymeric enteral diet or total parenteral nutrition given isocalorically [39•]. Remission rates were almost identical in the two groups. Median increase in serum albumin was much greater in the enteral group than in the parenteral group (4.6%). Patients receiving enteral nutrition had a much lower rate of nutrition-related complications (9%) than the patients receiving total parenteral nutrition (35%). The authors concluded that enteral nutrition is more clinically effective, safer, and cost-effective than total parenteral nutrition in patients with active ulcerative colitis.

Increased levels of inflammatory mediators derived from arachidonic acid have been implicated in the etiology of ulcerative colitis. Gamma-linolenic acid contained in evening primrose oil is converted *in vivo* to dihomogamma-linoleic acid, which competes with arachidonic acid for the cyclooxygenase enzyme. Eicosapentaenoic acid, present in fish oils, competes with arachidonic acid for the cyclooxygenase and lipoxygenase enzymes. Administration of dihomogamma-linoleic acid and eicosapentaenoic acid can therefore result in decreased levels of proinflammatory prostaglandins, leukotrienes, and cytokines. Several trials have confirmed the benefits of polyunsaturated fatty acids derived from fish oil on the disease activity in IBD. In a randomized, controlled study of the effects of oils on disease activity in ulcerative colitis [40••], 42 patients received max-eicosapentaenoic acid oil, evening primrose oil, or olive oil as placebo in addition to their regular regimens. Treatment with evening primrose oil and max eicosapentaenoic acid increased the concentrations of eicosapentaenoic acid and dihomogamma-linoleic acid. Administration of olive oil decreased the production of anti-inflammatory substances and arachidonic acid concentrations. The use of olive oil as a placebo is questionable because arachidonic acid is the main proinflammatory precursor in the body. Administration evening primrose oil significantly improved stool consistency as compared with other oils. All substances were ineffective in reducing stool frequency, rates of rectal bleeding, rates of disease relapse, sigmoidoscopic appearance, or rectal inflammation. The authors concluded that max-eicosapentaenoic acid was ineffective in patients with ulcerative colitis, whereas further research is needed to study the possible role of evening primrose oil in the treatment of this disease.

In conclusion, elemental diet is an effective adjunct in the short-term treatment of active Crohn's disease. Polymeric enteral diet is an effective alternative to steroids in the short- and long-term management of active Crohn's disease. Food intolerance is uncommon in Crohn's disease and does not warrant routine trials of elimination diets. Total enteral nutrition is an effective alternative to other modes of treatment in patients with acute ulcerative colitis. Further research is needed to examine the possible roles of polyunsaturated fatty acids in the treatment of ulcerative colitis.

References and recommended reading

Papers of particular interest, published within the annual period of review, have been highlighted as:

• Of special interest
•• Of outstanding interest

1. •• Martin LW: **Current Surgical Management of Patients With Chronic Ulcerative Colitis.** *J Pediatr Gastroenterol Nutr* 1993, 17:121–131.

An excellent overview of the experience with the IAP operation in a large pediatric population. The importance of differentiating Crohn's disease from ulcerative colitis in this population is emphasized.

2. •• Keighley MRB, Grobler S, Bain I: **An Audit of Restorative Proctocolectomy.** *Gut* 1993, 34:680–684.

An extensive review of 168 patients receiving restorative proctocolectomies during 9 years. Emphasis is placed upon the improved results with enhanced experience. Undiagnosed Crohn's disease was a frequent indication for pouch excisions.

3. •• Tjandra JJ, Fazio VW, Milsom JW, Lavery IC, Oakley JR, Fabre JM: **Omission of Temporary Diversion in Restorative Proctocolectomy - Is it Safe?** *Dis Colon Rectum* 1993, 36:1007–1014.

A retrospective comparison of two well-matched groups of patients undergoing IAP operation either with or without a proximal diverting ileostomy. It was concluded that restorative proctocolectomy without diversion was not as safe as the inclusion of diversion, especially in patients taking more than 20 mg of prednisone daily.

4. Schmitt SL, Wexner SD, Lucas FV, James K, Nogueras JJ, Fagelman DG: **Retained Mucosa After Double-Stapled Ileal Reservoir and Ileoanal Anastomosis.** *Dis Colon Rectum* 1992, 35:1051–1056.

5. •• Ambroze WL, Jr, Pemberton JH, Dozois RR, Carpenter HA, O'Rourke JS, Ilstrup DM: **The Histological Pattern and Pathological Involvement of the Anal Transition Zone in Patients With Ulcerative Colitis.** *Gastroenterology* 1993, 104:514–518.

A detailed evaluation of 50 patients with ulcerative colitis and 50 control patients with rectal cancer to determine if the anal transition zone was involved by ulcerative colitis following restorative proctocolectomy. Retaining the anal transitional zone preserved the anal inflammation in the majority of patients with ulcerative colitis.

6. • Lewis WG, Kuzu A, Sagar PM, Holdsworth PJ, Johnston D: **Stricture at the Pouch-Anal Anastomosis After Restorative Proctocolectomy.** *Dis Colon Rectum* 1994, 37:120–125.

A retrospective review of 102 patients receiving an IAP operation. Anastimotic stricture was present in 38% and was severe and persistent in 16%.

7. • Wettergren A, Jorgen H, Grosmann E, Svendsen LB, Hjortrup A, Stadil F, Kirkegaard P: **Complications After J-Pouch Ileoanal Anastomosis: Stapled Compared With Handsewn Anastomosis.** *Eur J Surg* 1993, 159:121–124.

A retrospective evaluation of 144 patients who underwent either handsewn or stapled j-pouch ileoanal anastomoses. The rate of stenosis requiring dilatation was significantly lower in the stapled group than the handsewn group. Patients who developed anastomotic breakdown lost significantly more blood during operation. Women were more likely to develop anastomotic leaks than men.

8. • Kuster GG, Andree G: **Attempts to Aid the Adaptation of Pelvic Pouch Before Temporary Ileostomy Closure.** *Dis Colon Rectum* 1993, 36:1022–1025.

Increasing volumes of liquid nutrients were injected twice daily for 2 months into the pelvic pouch through a mucous ileal fistula proximal to the pouch before closing the temporary ileostomy. Patients having the infusions had significantly reduced number of evacuations, better continence, and less urgency to defecate.

9. • Warren BF, Shepherd NA, Bartolo DCC, Bradfield JWB: **Pathology of the Defunctioned Rectum in Ulcerative Colitis.** *Gut* 1993, 34:514–516.

The pathology of 15 defunctioned rectal stumps in patients undergoing subtotal colectomy prior to an IAP were investigated. Many of the findings of Crohn's disease were noted in the rectal stump despite unequivocal confirmation of ulcerative colitis in the resected colon.

10. •• Sagar PM, Lewis W, Holdsworth PJ, Johnston D, Mitchell C, MacFie J: **Quality of Life After Restorative Proctocolectomy With a Pelvic Ileal Reservoir Compares Favorably With That of Patients With Medically Treated Colitis.** *Dis Colon Rectum* 1993, 36:584–592.

An extensive quality of life survey in 103 patients who had undergone restorative proctocolectomy was compared with 95 patients with ulcerative colitis on medical treatment. The quality of life for patients with a pouch appeared to be as good as that for patients with medically treated colitis.

11. Kohler LW, Pemberton JH, Hodge DO, Zinsmeister AR, Kelly KA: **Long-Term Functional Results and Quality of Life After Ileal Pouch-Anal Anastomosis and Cholecystectomy.** *World J Surg* 1992, **16**:1126–1132.

12. •• Heimann TM, Greenstein AJ, Lewis B, Kaufman D, Heimann DM, Aufses AH: **Prediction of Early Symptomatic Recurrence After Intestinal Resection in Crohn's Disease.** *Ann Surg* 1993, **218**:294–299.
An extensive review of 164 patients undergoing intestinal resection for Crohn's disease at Mt. Sinai hospital was examined prospectively. The number of anastomoses was the most important prognostic indicator of recurrent disease.

13. •• Osborne MJ, Hudson M, Piasecki C, Dhillon AP, Lewis AAM, Pounder RE, Wakefield AJ: **Crohn's Disease and Anastomotic Recurrence: Microvascular Ischaemia and Anastomotic Healing in an Animal Model.** *Br J Surg* 1993, **80**:226–229.
A model of microvascular intestinal ischemia in ferrets was created to simulate anastomotic recurrence of Crohn's disease. The combination of two self-limiting ischemic insults produced a pattern of intestinal inflammation similar to that seen in anastomotic recurrence in Crohn's disease.

14. • Scott ADN, Uff C, Phillips RKS: **Suppression of Macrophage Function by Suture Materials and Anastomotic Recurrences of Crohn's Disease.** *Br J Surg* 1993, **80**:387–391.
The influence of six suture materials on the function of macrophages obtained from rat peritoneal cavity and human intestinal mucosa was evaluated. All materials significantly impaired macrophage function.

15. • Smedh K, Olaison G, Nyström PO, Sjödahl R: **Intraoperative Enteroscopy in Crohn's Disease.** *Br J Surg* 1993, **80**:897–900.
Intraoperative small bowel endoscopy was performed in 31 patients with Crohn's disease. It was suggested that visualizing the mucosa provided information for more precise surgery, thereby limiting resection.

16. • Lescut D, Vanco D, Bonniére P, Lecomte-Houcke, Quandalle P, Wurtz A, Colobel JF, Delmotte JS, Paris JC, Cortot A: **Perioperative Endoscopy of the Whole Small Bowel in Crohn's Disease.** *Gut* 1993, **34**:647–649.
Perioperative endoscopy of the whole small bowel was performed in 20 patients with Crohn's disease. Sixty-five percent of patients had lesions of the small intestine detected by endoscopy, which were unrecognized before surgery in more than half of the cases.

17. • Winslet MC, Andrews H, Allan RN, Keighley MRB: **Fecal Diversion in the Management of Crohn's Disease of the Colon.** *Dis Colon Rectum* 1993, **36**:757–762.
A retrospective review of 44 patients undergoing proximal fecal diversion for Crohn's disease of the colon. A high incidence of sustained disease remission occurred, but the majority of the patients were not candidates for reestablishment of intestinal continuity.

18. • Fazio VW, Tjandra JJ: **Strictureplasty for Crohn's Disease With Multiple Long Strictures.** *Dis Colon Rectum* 1993, **36**:71–72.
The principles of the Heineke-Mikulicz and Finney surgical techniques were combined to treat patients with Crohn's disease and multiple long strictures. Successful results were observed in 12 patients.

19. •• Fazio VW, Tjandra JJ, Lavery IC, Church JM, Milsom JW, Oakley JR: **Long-Term Follow-up of Strictureplasty in Crohn's Disease.** *Dis Colon Rectum* 1993, **36**:355–361.
Rates of restricture and new stricture-perforative disease were 2.8% and 24%, respectively, in a retrospective review of 116 patients with obstructive Crohn's disease undergoing 452 primary strictureplasties.

20. Longo WE, Oakley JR, Lavery IC, Church JM, Fazio VW: **Outcome of Ileorectal Anastomosis for Crohn's Colitis.** *Dis Colon Rectum* 1992, **35**:1066–1071.

21. Sher ME, Bauer JJ, Gorphine S, Gelerni I: **Low Hartmann's Procedure for Severe Anorectal Crohn's Disease.** *Dis Colon Rectum* 1992, **35**:975–980.

22. •• Stokes MA, Hill GL: **Total Energy Expenditure in Patients With Crohn's Disease: Measurement by Combined Body Scan Technique.** *JPEN J Parenter Enteral Nutr* 1993, **17**:3–7.
The combined *in vivo* neutron activation-energy technique was used to measure total energy expenditure in patients with Crohn's disease. The measurements confirmed that total energy expenditure was not raised and that 30 to 35 kcal/kg/day was sufficient to achieve energy balance in such patients.

23. • Markowitz J, Grancher K, Rosa J, Aiges H, Daum F: **Growth Failure in Pediatric Inflammatory Bowel Disease.** *J Pediatr Gastroenterol Nutr* 1993, **16**:373–380.
Records from 48 young adults who had IBD during childhood or early adolescence were analyzed. Permanent impairment of linear growth leading to ultimate deficits in adult height was a common finding.

24. Castille RG, Telander RL, Coney DR, Struppin IL, Perrault J, Van Murclen J, Stickler GB: **Crohn's Disease in Children: Assessment of Progression of Disease, Growth, and Prognosis.** *J Pediatr Surg* 1980, **15**:462–469.

25. Gryboski JD, Spiro HM: **Prognosis in Children With Crohn's Disease.** *Gastroenterology* 1978, **74**:807–817.

26. Jackson WD, Grand RJ: **Crohn's Disease** In *Pediatric Gastrointestinal Disease.* Editedy by Walker WA, Peter MD, Durre M, *et al.*. Philadelphia: BC Decker; 1991:592–608.

27. McCaffery TD, Nasr K, Lawrence AM, Kirsher JB: **Effects of Administered Human Growth Hormone on Growth Retardation in Inflammatory Bowel Disease.** *Dig Dis* 1974, **19**:411–416.

28. •• Thomas AG, Holly JMP, Taylor F, Miller V: **Insulin Like Growth Factor-I, Insulin Like Growth Factor Binding Protein-I, and Insulin in Childhood Crohn's Disease.** *Gut* 1993, **34**:944–947.
Twenty-nine children with Crohn's disease were assigned to receive steroids or an elemental diet to assess the disease activity or effect of treatment on serum IGF-1, IGF binding protein-1, and insulin concentration. Both treatments results in increased IGF-1 levels.

29. • Braegger CP, Torresani T, Murch SH, Savage MO, Walker-Smith JA, MacDonald TT: **Urinary Growth Hormone in Growth-Impaired Children With Chronic Inflammatory Bowel Disease.** *J Pediatr Gastroenterol* 1993, **16**:49–52.
Urinary growth hormone concentrations were measured in 36 children with chronic IBD and 51 normal controls. There was no significant difference between urinary growth hormone concentrations between groups. The authors concluded that administration of growth hormone to patients with chronic IBD was unlikely to improve growth failure.

30. Sheving LA, Yeh YC, Tsai TH, Sheving LE: **Circadian Phase-Dependent Stimulatory Effects of Epidermal Growth Factor on Deoxyribonucleic Acid Synthesis in the Duodenum, Jejunum, Ileum, Caecum, Colon, and Rectum of the Adult Male Mouse.** *Endocrinology* 1980, **106**:1498–1503.

31. Al-Nafussi AI, Wright NA: **The Effect of Epidermal Growth Factor (EGF) on Cell Proliferation of the Gastrointestinal Mucosa in Rodents.** *Virch Arch* 1982, **40**:63–69.

32. Goodlad RA, Raja KB, Peters TJ, Wright NA: **Effects of Urogastrone-Epidermal Growth Factor on Intestinal Brush Border Enzymes and Mitotic Activity.** *Gut* 1991, **32**:994–998.

33. Blay J, Brown KD: **Epidermal Growth Factor Promotes the Chemotactic Migration of Cultured Rat Intestinal Epithelial Cells.** *J Cell Physiol* 1985, **124**:107–112.

34. Carpenter G, Cohen S: **Human Epidermal Growth Factor and the Proliferation of Human Fibroblast.** *J Cell Physiol* 1976, **88**:227–238.

35. •• Luck MS, Bass P: **Effect of Epidermal Growth Factor on Experimental Colitis in the Rat.** *J Pharm Exp Ther* 1993, **264**:984–990.

Reduced colonic ulceration and inflammation after systemic administration of epidermal growth factor was noted in a model of experimental colitis.

36. •• Gorard DA, Hunt JB, Payne-James JJ, Palmer KR, Rees RG, Clark ML, Farthing MJ, Misiewicz JJ, Silk DB: **Initial Response and Subsequent Course of Crohn's Disease Treated With Elemental Diet or Prednisolone.** *Gut* 1993, 34:1198–1202.

A randomized, prospective comparison of corticosteroids and elemental diet in 42 patients with active Crohn's disease. Elemental diet was as effective as prednisolone in the short term treatment of active Crohn's disease.

37. •• Gonzalez-Huix F, de Leon R, Fernandez-Banares F, Esteve M, Cabre E, Acero D, Abad-Lacruz A, Figa M, Guilera M, Planas R, *et al.*: **Polymeric Enteral Diets As Primary Treatment of Active Crohn's Disease: A Prospective Steroid Controlled Trial.** *Gut* 1993, 34:778–782.

Thirty-two patients with active Crohn's disease were randomly assigned to receive polymeric enteral nutrition or steroids. Polymeric enteral nutrition was as effective as steroids in inducing short-term disease remission.

38. • Pearson M, Teahon K, Levi AJ, Bjarnason I: **Food Intolerance and Crohn's Disease.** *Gut* 1993, 34:783–787.

The occurrence of food intolerance was investigated in 42 patients with Crohn's disease. The authors concluded that food sensitivities in patients with Crohn's disease were of insufficient importance to warrant routine trials of elimination diets.

39. • Gonzalez-Huix F, Fernandex-Banares F, Esteve-Comas M, Abad-Lacruz A, Cabre E, Acero D, Figa M, Guilera M, Humbert P, de Leon R, *et al.*: **Enteral Versus Parenteral Nutrition As Adjunct Therapy in Acute Ulcerative Colitis.** *Am J Gastroenterol* 1993, **88**:227–232.

Forty-two patients were randomly assigned to receive either enteral or parenteral nutrition as adjunct therapies in active ulcerative colitis. Enteral nutrition was more clinically efficacious, safer and cost-effective than total parenteral nutrition.

40. •• Greenfield SM, Green AT, Teare JP, Jenkins AP, Punchard NA, Ainley CC, Thompson RP, *et al.*: **A Randomized Controlled Study of Evening Primrose Oil and Fish Oil in Ulcerative Colitis.** *Aliment Pharmacol Ther* 1993, 7:159–166.

Forty-three patients with stable ulcerative colitis were randomly assigned to receive evening primrose oil, fish oil, or olive oil in this placebo-controlled study. Fish oil was ineffective in patients with ulcerative colitis, whereas the role of evening primrose oil in the treatment of this disease could not be clearly established.

John L. Rombeau, MD, and Yevgeniy Gincherman, BA, Department of Surgery, 4 Silverstein Pavillion, Hospital of the University of Pennsylvania, 3400 Spruce Street, Philadelphia, PA 19104, USA.

Esophagus

Commentary

G.N.J. Tytgat, MD

Academic Medical Center, Amsterdam, the Netherlands

Current Opinion in Gastroenterology 1994, **10**:417–418

Esophageal cancer, both squamous cell carcinoma and adenocarcinoma, remains a devastating disease with a very poor ultimate outcome. The only hope for improvement is through detection of the lesions at an earlier stage. It is clear that novel approaches to the prevention, early detection, and treatment of esophageal cancer are necessary. To accomplish these goals, an accurate understanding of the interaction between environmental factors and the genetics and biology of this cancer is required. Identification of relevant environmental factors may lead to future preventive strategies. Moreover, better understanding of the cellular and genetic abnormalities may inspire new screening tests, new markers of disease severity, and novel therapies.

The past year has seen a major output of manuscripts related to the molecular biological abnormalities in the malignant process. One is struck with some of the similarities between malignancies in different areas of the gastrointestinal tract, such as stomach or colon, and the abnormalities present at the esophageal level. The *p53* tumor-suppressor gene is considered a pivotal influence on cell proliferation. The loss of a normal *p53* allele in the presence of mutations within the remaining allele has been demonstrated not only in established esophageal cancer, but also in high-degree dysplasia. Genetic aberrations or different protein expression profiles will have diagnostic importance, but how useful they will be in routine clinical practice in the years to come is still difficult to envisage. However, studies such as these must continue because molecular alterations may be discovered that indicate those patients at risk who might profit from a meticulous follow-up.

The output of manuscripts on columnar metaplasia, dysplasia, and cancer remains fascinating. At the last OESO meeting in Paris in September 1993, this topic was analyzed in depth by world authorities. There is a growing consensus that columnar metaplasia should be redefined as any length of "intestinal" or "specialized-type" metaplastic mucosa in the distal esophagus because only this type of mucosa carries the risk for malignant degeneration, regardless of its extent in the distal esophagus. Some physicians feel that several cancers of the esophagogastric junction are related to short-segment columnar metaplasia and that the behavior of those tumors and the traditional Barrett cancers is quite similar. Whether the rapid rise of cancer of the cardia, at least in the United States, is related to a high frequency of short-segment columnar metaplasia remains to be proven.

Still controversial is the issue of the value of endoscopic bioptic screening for the detection of high-grade dysplasia c.q. early columnar metaplasia-associated carcinoma. The cost of preventing one death from cancer, as calculated by Dr. Cameron from the Mayo Clinic, is truly astronomical. Moreover, the advice of the Seattle Group to take four quadrant biopsies at 1- to 2-cm intervals, preferably with a large caliber biopsy forceps, is impossible as a routine practice for many physicians. There is, however, consensus that the risk of malignant degeneration is surprisingly high. The critical question of whether or not endoscopic-bioptic surveillance for dysplasia is a cost-effective practice for reducing cancer mortality has remained controversial. If endoscopy plus repetitive biopsy is not cost-effective, do we then have to look for other modalities as suggested by Dr. Richter, namely abrasive balloon cytology? Can we use some of the currently detected molecular aberrations at the cytologic level to detect those patients who are at alarming risk and who need expert endoscopy and biopsy?

Further progress is being made with endosonographic staging of esophageal malignancies. As new information becomes available, the data seem to be congruent; yet there are still limitations, especially in case of stricturing and with respect to lymph node detection and analysis. I believe that the use of high frequencies (20 MHz) might further facilitate the accuracy of detecting cancer at the epithelial-mucosal level versus submucosal cancer, as the level of the muscularis mucosae can be detected when using those high frequencies. I tend to agree with the Japanese authors that we have to redefine superficial or early esophageal cancer. As the risk of metastasis is very substantial and as the long-term follow-up is already quite poor for submucosal cancer, we should limit early or superficial malignancies to cancer limited to the epithelium or the mucosal layer. This may require that in the future the TNM classification for esophageal cancer be redesigned, because now T1 means cancer at the epithelial, mucosal, and submucosal level. Early epithelial-mucosal cancers, especially, can be removed by endo-

 ISBN 1-85922-609-4 ISSN 0267–1379

scopic resection, photodynamic therapy, and so forth. Undoubtedly, Japanese endoscopists are leading in this area and we all can benefit from their expertise.

A multimodality approach is obviously the way to improve the overall results obtainable in esophageal cancer. This requires a close collaboration between gastroenterologist, surgeon, oncologist-radiotherapist, and imaging specialist. With respect to the surgical approach, it is still uncertain and debatable whether extensive lymph node dissection truly improves the outcome, except for very select patients. Progress is being made with combined intraluminal and external radiotherapy, but it would be advantagous if extensive, slow-healing ulceration could be prevented by better dosing and monitoring of the tissue reaction.

Of significant importance is the availability of self-expanding metal stents. Currently, four types are commercially available. Especially for malignant fistulas, coating is absolutely essential. Moreover coating may well prevent the rapid tumor ingrowth that otherwise occurs in uncoated stents. Currently only the Wallstent, the Wilson Cook Gianturco stent, and the Korean Song stent have an outer membrane. More data need to be gathered to find out how stable those prostheses are once inserted.

Progress in gastroesophageal reflux disease during the past year was rather limited. The excellent results with longstanding profound acid inhibition and the usefulness of prokinetics in long-term management have been consolidated. A major problem is the lack of consensus in defining the degree of damage in the esophageal mucosa as a consequence of excessive reflux. It is hoped that the medical community will come up with a worldwide acceptable grading scheme for esophageal reflux–induced damage. Many patients with severe reflux disease require long-term therapy. The alterations of the gastric mucosa during 5-year nonstop proton pump inhibitor therapy have been published. Beyond a doubt, in some of these individuals there was progression of atrophic changes in the corpus mucosa. This observation deserves further follow-up over a 10-year or more period to find out what the ultimate outcome is of these morphologic changes.

As new technology for computer-assisted analysis of both motor and pH patterns in the esophagus becomes available, new data are being gathered in patients with obscure esophageal pain. Although the latter information has become more accurate, it has not as yet led to a more refined understanding of the various pathogenic events that may lead to motor disturbances or esophageal pain.

The molecule of the year, nitric oxide, was also extensively evaluated at the level of the esophagus. Inhibitory nonadrenergic, noncholinergic nerves play an important role in the coordination of peristalsis in the esophageal body and in the relaxation of the lower esophageal sphincter. Nitric oxide generated by an enzymatic process from L-arginine was found to be the mediator of nonadrenergic, noncholinergic transmission in circular muscle of both the esophageal corpus and the lower esophageal sphincter. The effect of nitric oxide is mediated by an increase in cyclic GMP content and perhaps also by a cyclic GMP–independent mechanism. It may very well be that disturbed control of nitric oxide formation is significant in disorders like achalasia, diffuse esophageal spasm, and even reflux esophagitis. Modulation of the formation and degradation of nitric oxide and cyclic GMP is possible and these principles will probably be of major importance for future therapeutic approaches to various esophageal diseases.

Finally, a new journal on esophageal diseases was created called *Diseases of the Esophagus*, which is a merger of two previous journals: *Gullet* and *Diseases of the Esophagus*. *Diseases of the Esophagus* was the journal of the International Society for Diseases of the Esophagus. The directors of that society said that nothing seemed more appropriate than to merge the two journals so that they can become even more successful together in disseminating knowledge about esophageal diseases. As in any good partnership, each journal had to give up some of its own identity and format in order to achieve a new and better journal together. Such a reduction in the number of scientific journals can only be applauded and undoubtedly the quality of the new journal *Diseases of the Esophagus* will gain from such a merger.

G.N.J. Tytgat, MD, Academic Medical Center, University of Amsterdam, Department of Gastroenterology-Hepatology, P.O. Box 22700, 1100DE Amsterdam, the Netherlands.

Esophageal motility

M. Brian Fennerty, MD, and Harinder S. Garewal, MD, PhD

Arizona Health Sciences Center and Veterans Affairs Medical Center, Tucson, Arizona, USA

Animal studies continue to show the importance of nitric oxide as a mediator of lower esophageal tone. It may act directly on or in conjunction with vasoactive intestinal polypeptide. Human studies show little evidence that would support the notion that swallowing function is significantly affected by age. Esophageal motility studies differ between swallowing liquids versus solids. The findings of "nutcracker" esophagus may simply be a marker for gastroesophageal reflux, as symptoms can resolve with treatment of the latter, although a nutcracker esophagus motility pattern may persist. Using a graded pneumatic regimen, dilation in achalasia can be performed safely and successfully in the majority of patients on an outpatient basis. Nonspecific motor disorder is associated with selective impairment of semisolid emptying and is thus a "real" clinical disorder of motility. Esophageal manometry is a useful and cost-effective test leading to diagnostic and management decisions in more than half of patients.

Current Opinion in Gastroenterology 1994, **10**:419–425

Physiology

Animal studies

Lower esophageal sphincter

Animals continue to provide a reliable model in the investigation of neurologic and muscle function of the esophagus, especially in the region of the lower esophageal sphincter (LES). Much of the interest remains centered on the role of NO (nitric oxide) as a nonadrenergic, noncholinergic neurotransmitter controlling LES tone and relaxation. Studies in the opossum model revealed that a NO-like compound is responsible for relaxation of LES [1]. Activation of nonadrenergic, noncholinergic nerves of the LES hyperpolarizes the sphincter and thus causes relaxation of the circular smooth muscle.

Conklin *et al.* found that NO or a NO-like compound mediated the hyperpolarization of the opossum LES, resulting in relaxation [2•]. Further study in opossum esophagus of the pharmacologic characteristics of LES relaxation induced by swallowing, vagal nerve efferent stimulation, and esophageal distention demonstrated that NO inhibited LES relaxation and that this effect could be reversed by the NO synthetase substrate, L-arginine [3]. In the LES of the cat, however, vasoactive intestinal polypeptide (VIP) may also be a nonadrenergic, noncholinergic inhibitory neurotransmitter [4]. Additionally, in a rat colon muscle model during neurally induced relaxation, NO was produced in muscle cells by the action of VIP; thus, relaxation represented the combined effects of VIP and NO via the enhancement of VIP release by NO [5]. These studies indicate that NO plays a pivotal role in relaxation of the LES via an inhibitory effect on tone, but this effect may be augmented by other nonadrenergic, noncholinergic neurotransmitters, such as VIP.

Body

Esophageal muscle function was studied in sheep using m-mode ultrasound attached by a suction device [6]. During periods of contraction, the inner circular muscle layer increased from 0.2 to 2.2 mm and with dilation, the full thickness of the esophageal wall decreased from 3.6 to 2.9 mm. This technique may be applicable to similar study of esophageal muscle function in humans.

Human studies

Pharyngeal motility

Oropharyngeal swallowing has been difficult to study because of the complexity of this act as well as the brevity of the response (< 1 s). In an elegantly designed study using high-speed computed tomography scanning (17 images/s), Ergun *et al.* [7•] demonstrated that the deglutitive chamber increased in size during tongue loading and was 15 cc greater than the bolus volume, implying swallowing an obligatory 15 cc of air (trapped

Abbreviations

GERD—gastroesophageal reflux disease; **LES**—lower esophageal sphincter;
NEMD—nonspecific esophageal motility disorder; **VIP**—vasoactive intestinal polypeptide.

 ISBN 1-85922-609-4 ISSN 0267–1379

during closure of the pharynx and larynx) during swallowing. Normal deglutitive tongue function was also studied [8•] using biplane video fluoroscopy synchronized with intraluminal manometry in eight normal subjects. Deglutitive tongue function includes bolus containment and volume accommodation, and is a major contributor to bolus propulsion.

Age and bolus variables on glottal and upper esophageal sphincter coordination during swallowing were studied by concurrent video endoscopy, upper esophageal manometry, spirography, and submental surface electromyography [9]. Coordination was the same in young and old persons. Shaker *et al.* [10] demonstrated that hypopharyngeal wave amplitude and duration increased with age, whereas pharyngeal peristaltic wave amplitude and duration modulation by bolus consistency and upper esophageal sphincter pressure decreased with age, but the response to esophageal distention was preserved. Thus, there is little evidence supporting the notion that age significantly affects swallow function.

Body

Whereas conventional or perfused manometry has traditionally been used to study the phasic contractile activity of the esophagus, little is known about tonic activity of the esophagus. Mayrand and Diamant [11] used a computerized isobaric recording system measuring both compliance as well as resting tone, and determined that smooth muscle is more compliant than striated muscle. Orvar *et al.* [12] showed there was no tone in the esophageal wall before inflation of a balloon, but that inflation produced induced contractions once the pressure of the balloon reached 15 cm of water or balloon diameter reached 14 mm. Williams *et al.* [13] studied 30 volunteers to clarify the contractile and propulsive forces generated in response to intraluminal distention of the esophagus. In the lower esophagus, injection of more than 5 mL of air resulted in a proximal contractile activity and a distal quiescent esophagus; the effect increased with increasing volume. This study demonstrates that the quiescent distal esophagus represents a true descending inhibitory response.

Clinical studies have indicated a difference in esophageal motility between swallowing solids versus liquids. Although classic clinical manometric testing measures liquid swallows, solid food has been reported to demonstrate an increase in nonconducted and nonperistaltic contractions. Johnson *et al.* [14] studied 20 healthy volunteers. Peristaltic amplitude, duration of contraction, and nonconducted and nonperistaltic contractions were greater in the proximal esophagus with solids. Therefore, when solids are used during manometry in studying patients with dysphagia, wider limits of normality will need to be set.

Nondeglutitive simultaneous contractions have been widely reported. An ambulatory motility study of 25 fasted healthy subjects, by Janssens *et al.* [15•], demonstrated frequent nonsequential pressure peaks seen in esophageal smooth muscle, usually immediately before phase 3 of the migrating motor complex. Therefore, previously reported nondeglutitive simultaneous contractions may represent the esophageal body component of the phase 3 of the migrating motor complex and are not necessarily a sign of an esophageal motor abnormality.

The effect of diet on ambulatory pressure monitoring was studied in 17 volunteers [16]. Contraction characteristics and propagation patterns were identical for different meal types. However, meal periods revealed a higher percentage of peristaltic contractions and a lower percentage of simultaneous contractions when compared with supine periods. Therefore, with ambulatory motility, standardization of meals does not appear to be necessary.

The response of esophageal motility to exercise was tested in eight cyclists [17]. Duration, amplitude, and frequency of esophageal contractions decreased with graded exercise intensity. This effect was not hormonally mediated.

The effect of the menstrual cycle on esophageal emptying of liquids and solids was studied in 30 healthy females [18]. ^{99m}Tc sulfur colloid scintigraphy was used to quantify emptying. There was no difference between emptying of liquids or solids during the follicular versus the luteal phase.

Lower esophageal sphincter

The LES has been intensively studied. However, the effects of prostaglandin inhibitors on LES tone are controversial. Cagossi *et al.* [19] used three structurally unrelated prostaglandin E inhibitors in 20 volunteers. LES pressure tone was increased transiently with either intravenous or rectal prostaglandin installation. Thus, prostaglandins physiologically exert some inhibitory influence on LES pressure (*eg,* VIP and NO in animal studies).

Crookes *et al.* [20] used manometry of LES segments to study resting pressure and total length, as well as the intra-abdominal segment length. The LES is asymmetrical, secondary to its configuration and external structures such as the diaphragmatic crura. This study compared standard analysis (averaging the measurements from each radial channel) to segment analysis. The authors found that segmental analysis offered no advantage over standard analysis in motility interpretation.

Gastroesophageal junction competence and the influence of the LES versus hiatal hernia on competence was studied in 34 patients with a hiatal hernia and 16 normal subjects [21]. A hiatal hernia increased the reflux score and decreased LES pressure. Sphincter competence was most dependent on the length of the hernia, although it also depended on the LES pressure as well as the combination of the length of the hernia and sphincter pressure.

Motility disorders of the esophagus

Noncardiac chest pain

Chest pain of uncertain origin (or noncardiac chest pain) may have an esophageal cause in up to 50% of patients. Paterson *et al.* [22•] studied 25 patients with 24-hour pH, ambulatory motility, and electrocardiography, as well as standard manometry with provocative testing. There was a poor correlation between the results of testing and symptoms. Therefore, other stimuli must trigger esophageal-type pain, perhaps suggesting dysfunction of visceral pain sensory mechanisms. Costantini *et al.* [23] studied 30 patients with irritable bowel syndrome. Decreased pain threshold to esophageal balloon distention was seen, but no difference in LES pressure, esophageal body motility, or bethanechol-induced motility abnormalities were detected. These data suggest an altered visceral receptor sensitivity may exist throughout the gut, including the esophagus.

Detection of esophageal dysmotility in patients with noncardiac chest pain has traditionally relied on esophageal manometry. Kao *et al.* [24] used radionucleotide scintigraphy with ^{99m}Tc phytate in 31 patients and 25 healthy subjects [24]. In the 31 patients, mean transit time was increased 48%, and residual fraction increased 39%. Thus, radionucleotide esophageal transit test may be a simple noninvasive screening method to detect dysmotility in patients with noncardiac chest pain. Scintigraphy was performed in 60 normal patients with ^{99m}Tc to establish normal ranges as well as reproducibility [25]. The mean transit time had low variability, whereas residual activity had high variability. Therefore, in the study of esophageal transit, mean transit time may be more reliable.

Nutcracker esophagus

Segmental nutcracker esophagus is an intermittent motility pattern referring to segmental, high-amplitude peristaltic contractions, as opposed to *nutcracker esophagus,* where the abnormality is diffuse. Achem *et al.* [26] reported that 53% of nutcracker esophagus and 20% of segmental, high-amplitude peristaltic contraction esophagus retained the original diagnosis over time. Thirty-three percent of nutcracker esophagus cases and 40% of segmental cases permutated into each other. Thus, segmental, high-amplitude peristaltic contractions are not an early process evolving into nutcracker esophagus, but both clinical situations represent a labile marker associated with noncardiac chest pain.

Noncardiac chest pain and nutcracker esophagus have often been considered synonymous. Both entities are associated with gastroesophageal reflux disease (GERD). In 14 of 20 patients with nutcracker esophagus, GERD was found [27•]. Twelve patients were put on an open label trial with a proton pump inhibitor. Healing and symptomatic relief occurred in 10 of 12. However, only two of these patients normalized their motility. Therefore, nutcracker esophagus may simply be a marker of GERD in some patients with noncardiac chest pain.

Trospium chloride, a muscarinergic antagonist like atropine and scopolamine but without central nervous side effects, was studied in 16 healthy men [28]. Decreased contractile activity, duration, and amplitude in all parts of the esophageal body were noted. Trospium chloride's potency and mild side effects make it a promising agent in hypercontractile esophageal disorders.

Achalasia

The use of balloon dilation in the treatment of achalasia has withstood the test of time. However, not all patients respond to balloon dilation and perforation rates as high as 10% have been reported. In an attempt to improve efficacy and minimize complications, Kadakia *et al.* [29•] studied graded pneumatic dilation in 29 patients receiving 47 dilations with a polyethylene balloon catheter (Rigiflex, Microvasive Corp., Watertown, MA). Patients initially underwent a 3-cm balloon dilation and after 4 to 8 weeks, if they remained symptomatic, underwent a 3.5-cm balloon dilation followed by another 4-week observation period. Continued symptomatic patients were dilated with a 4-cm balloon. Success was seen in 27 of 29 patients (93%) and there were no complications.

Parkman *et al.* [30] reported on a 10-year study of 123 patients undergoing pneumatic dilation. Fifty-eight percent required no further treatment and 12% underwent a surgical esophagomyotomy (two for perforation, and 13 for persistent symptoms). Patients over 45 years of age did better with balloon dilation and subsequent dilations were less successful than initial attempts. The surgical cost was 2.5 times higher than pneumatic dilation. Pneumatic dilation will be the only treatment needed in the majority of patients, but need for subsequent treatment may favor surgery.

Risk factors, characteristics, and outcome of complications for pneumatic balloon dilation in achalasia or esophageal spasm in 178 patients undergoing 236 dilations with a Brown-McHardy dilator were retrospectively evaluated by Nair *et al.* [31]. Sixteen (9%) had complications, including perforation, hematoma, fever, and angina. Prior dilation and pressure over 11 psi were independent risk factors for complications. An esophagram immediately after the procedure identified three of four perforations and perforation risk was associated with blood on the dilator, tachycardia, or chest pain within 4 hours of the procedure. All complications were recognized within 5 hours and there was no long-term morbidity.

Outpatient dilation of achalasia was reported by Ciarolla *et al.* [32•] in a study of 110 dilations performed over 6 years. Seventy-one of these patients were outpatients who received 5 to 8 hours of monitoring following dilation. Fifteen underwent contrast studies because of fever or pain and seven of these had perforations resulting in an operation. Overall, good results were noted in 82%. Therefore, pneumatic dilation can be performed on an outpatient basis without the routine use of contrast studies.

An objective means of quantifying the success of pneumatic dilation for achalasia would be useful. The Cohen test has been proposed by some as an objective means of measuring the effect of dilation. Lee *et al.* [33] prospectively studied 28 patients over a 6-year period and found no association between dysphagia relief and the findings on the Cohen test.

Return of peristalsis in patients with achalasia has been reported after balloon dilation as well as surgical myotomy. Coccia *et al.* [34] studied the return of peristalsis in patients receiving nifedipine as a medical therapy for achalasia. Thirty-two patients received 10 to 20 mg of sublingual nifedipine before meals. At 6 months of follow-up, six patients had return of peristalsis. The only clinical characteristics defining these patients were that they had had a shorter history of dysphagia and less esophageal dilation, *eg,* probable earlier achalasia. Medical, balloon, or surgical therapy early in the course of achalasia may result in the return of motility.

The effects of the clostridium botulinum toxin on the LES were studied by Pasricha *et al.* [35•]. Botulinum toxin inhibits release of acetylcholine from the nerve terminals, causes paralysis of skeletal muscle, and may have similar effects on gastrointestinal smooth muscle. The effects of botulinum toxin on LES pressure was studied on five piglets. No pressure change in the LES was seen with the injection of sodium chloride; however, there was a 40% decrease in LES pressure with the injection of botulinum toxin. A case report [36] describes a 71-year-old woman, who had failed balloon dilation, treated with botulinum toxin. Injection of 2 ng (80 mouse units) of botulinum toxin by a sclerotherapy needle resulted in better swallowing at 1 day and complete lack of symptoms by 1 week without side effects. Manometry at 1 week revealed a decreased LES pressure of 50% and a decrease in esophageal diameter of 40%. Further human studies with botulinum toxin are presently being conducted.

Motility and gastroesophageal reflux

Gastroesophageal reflux disease occurs in the setting of esophageal motility abnormalities. Whether these motility abnormalities are an epiphenomenon or a primary mechanism resulting in GERD has been controversial. It has been shown that patients with severe esophagitis have altered motility, but whether lesser degrees of esophagitis also have abnormal motility is unknown.

Timmer *et al.* [37] studied 27 patients with Savory grade I and II changes and 24 age- and sex-matched control subjects. Patients with mild GERD had an increase in the number of nontransmitted contractions. However, amplitude and number of contractions were equal. Therefore, impaired peristalsis does not appear to be a major etiologic factor in mild gastroesophageal reflux.

Barham [38] reported that in a healthy volunteer population, physiologic gastroesophageal reflux is associated with peristaltic waves of increased amplitude and duration. These studies would indicate that a primary motility abnormality (other than diminished LES pressure) plays little role in gastroesophageal reflux. However, Singh *et al.* [39] studied 43 patients with esophagitis, before and after healing, versus 34 healthy control subjects. Pretreatment findings demonstrated decreased LES pressure, decreased distal and middle amplitude of contraction waves, and increased duration, with decreased velocity of contraction waves in esophagitis patients. After healing, there were no significant changes in these manometric findings. This would indicate that motor dysfunction is a primary phenomenon and not secondary to esophagitis.

Scleroderma

Esophageal motor function in scleroderma patients has been previously described, including decreased peristaltic amplitude progressing to aperistalsis. This esophageal motility abnormality is associated with gastroesophageal reflux. However, the severity of the reflux and its relationship to motility is unknown. Thirty-six scleroderma patients were studied by solid state manometry and ambulatory dual pH monitoring [40]. Findings included decreased LES pressure and distal esophageal aperistalsis in 70%. In those with distal aperistalsis, there was increased acid exposure. However, there was a poor correlation between LES pressure and esophageal acid exposure. High-resolution endoluminal sonography was also used to study the esophagus in scleroderma patients [41]. Hypoechoic muscularis propria, corresponding to fibrosis seen on histologic specimens, was observed and correlated with the manometric abnormalities previously described.

Sjögren's syndrome

Motor function of the esophagus in 20 patients with Sjögren's syndrome was studied [42]. Seventy-five percent of these patients had dysphagia. No specific motility pattern was found or correlated with dysphagia.

Chronic cord injury

Esophageal motility was studied in 46 patients with spinal cord injury [43]. Thirty percent had intermittent dysphagia and 30% had esophageal chest pain. Ten patients had motility studies revealing low amplitude, slowly propagating, and double-peaked contraction waves. Esophageal motor abnormalities may be frequent in patients with spinal cord injuries.

Heart-lung transplant patients

The vagus nerve can be injured during heart-lung transplantation and this may affect esophageal motility. Ten patients underwent esophageal manometry as well as radio isotope tracer studies; two patients had esophageal dysmotility, neither of whom were symptomatic [44].

Plummer-Vinson syndrome

A patient with Plummer-Vinson syndrome presented with dysphagia. Manometry revealed 20% simultaneous contractions, low amplitude, and high interbolus pressures. After treatment with iron therapy, dysphagia disappeared and repeat manometry revealed increased contraction amplitude, decreased interbolus pressure, and only 5% simultaneous contractions [45].

Simultaneous contractions

Pathogenesis of simultaneous contractions was studied by Behar and Biancani [46]. A defective deglutitive inhibitory reflux was seen that may result in the shorter latency seen with simultaneous contractions. Spontaneous contractions appear to be generated by swallowing, independent of discharges of acetylcholine.

Nonspecific esophageal motility disorder

Nonspecific esophageal motility disorder (NEMD) is a catch-all term to describe manometric findings that do not meet other manometric criteria. In one study [47•], 10 symptomatic patients, 26 healthy control subjects, and disease controls (achalasia, scleroderma, and diffuse esophageal spasm) underwent esophageal transit with liquid and solids. Patients with NEMD had no impairment of liquid emptying. However, there was impairment of solid emptying equal to that seen in disease controls. Therefore, NEMD represents a real disorder characterized by selective impairment of solid and semisolid emptying.

Esophageal manometry

The clinical utility and cost effectiveness of esophageal motility has been questioned by some authors. Between 1988 and 1991, 276 consecutive manometries were performed (dysphagia 50%, noncardiac chest pain 23%, GERD 14%, connective tissue disease 11%, and other 1%) [48•]. Results were as follows: normal 49%, achalasia 18%, diffuse esophageal spasm 13%, connective tissue disease 8%, hypertensive LES 4.5%, nutcracker esophagus 2.6%, and other 4.5%. Patients with dysphagia had a positive diagnosis of 66% versus 35% for other indications (30% noncardiac chest pain, 21% GERD). Management changed in 49% based on manometric findings, including 20% of those with noncardiac chest pain or GERD and 60% of those with dysphagia. Therefore, esophageal manometry is both a useful and cost-effective test.

References and recommended reading

Papers of particular interest, published within the annual period of review, have been highlighted as:

- • Of special interest
- •• Of outstanding interest

1. Murray JA, Du C, Ledlow A, Manternach PL, Conklin JL: **Guanylate Cyclase Inhibitors: Effect on Tone, Relaxation, & cGMP Content of Lower Esophageal Sphincter.** *Am J Physiol* 1992, **263**:G97–G101.

2. • Conklin JL, Du C, Murray JA, Bates JN: **Characterization and Mediation of Inhibitory Junction Potentials From Opossum Lower Esophageal Sphincter.** *Gastroenterology* 1993, **104**:1439–1444.

NO or NO-like compounds mediate nonadrenergic, noncholinergic nerve activation and hyperpolarization (and thus, relaxation) of LES smooth muscle. This study confirmed that NO (or a NO-like compound) was responsible for this effect and that sphincteric muscle behaved differently than body muscle (*ie*, longer duration and no depolarization following hyperpolarization) in response to NO.

3. Paterson WG, Anderson MAB, Anand N: **Pharmacological Characterization of Lower Esophageal Sphincter Relaxation Induced by Swallowing, Vagal Efferent Nerve Stimulation, and Esophageal Distention.** *Can J Physiol Pharmacol* 1992, **70**:1011–1015.

4. Mao YK, Wang YF, Daniel EE: **Distribution and Characterization of Vasoactive Intestinal Polypeptide Binding in Canine Lower Esophageal Sphincter.** *Gastroenterology* 1993, **150**:1370–1377.

5. Grider JR: **Interplay of VIP and Nitric Oxide in Regulation of the Descending Relaxation Phase of Peristalsis.** *Am J Physiol* 1993, **264**:G334–G340.

6. Taniguchi DK, Martin RW, Trowers EA, Dennis MB, Odegaard S, Silverstein FE: **Changes in Esophageal Wall Layers During Motility: Measurements With a New Miniature Ultrasound Suction Device.** *Gastrointest Endosc* 1993, **39**:146–152.

7. • Ergun GA, Kahrilas PJ, Lin S, Logemann JA, Harig JM: **Shape, Volume, and Content of the Deglutitive Pharyngeal Chamber Imaged by Ultrafast Computerized Tomography.** *Gastroenterology* 1993, **105**:1396–1403.

This manuscript adds to the understanding of the complex act of deglutition. This more complete understanding should aid in the evaluation and treatment of patients with deglutitive dysfunction.

8. • Kahrilas PJ, Lin S, Logemann JA, Ergun GA, Facchini F: **Deglutitive Tongue Action: Volume Accommodation and Bolus Propulsion.** *Gastroenterology* 1993, **104**:152–162.

This manuscript adds to the understanding of the complex act of deglutition. This more complete understanding should aid in the evaluation and treatment of patients with deglutitive dysfunction.

9. Ren J, Shaker R, Zamir Z, Dodds WJ, Hogan WJ, Hoffmann RG: **Effect of Age and Bolus Variables on the Coordination of the Glottis and Upper Esophageal Sphincter During Swallowing.** *Am J Gastroenterol* 1993, **88**:665–669.

10. Shaker R, Ren J, Podvrsan B, Dodds WJ, Hogan WJ, Kern M, Hoffman R, Hintz J: **Effect of Aging and Bolus Variables on Pharyngeal and Upper Esophageal Sphincter Motor Function.** *Am J Physiol* 1993, **264**:G427–G432.

11. Mayrand S, Diamant NE: **Measurement of Human Esophageal Tone In Vivo.** *Gastroenterology* 1993, **105**:1411–1420.

12. Orvar KB, Gregersen H, Christensen J: **Biomechanical Characteristics of the Human Esophagus.** *Dig Dis Sci* 1993, **38**:197–205.

13. Williams D, Thompson DG, Heggie L, Bancewicz J: **Responses of the Human Esophagus to Experimental Intraluminal Distension.** *Am J Physiol* 1993, **265**:G196–G203.

14. Johnston BT, Collins JSA, McFarland RJ, Blackwell JN, Love AHG: **A Comparison of Esophageal Motility in Response to Bread Swallows and Water Swallows.** *Am J Gastroenterol* 1993, **88**:351–355.

15. Janssens J, Annese V, Vantrappen G: **Bursts of Non-Deglutitive Simultaneous Contractions May Be a Normal Oesophageal Motility Pattern.** *Gut* 1993, **34**:1021–1024.
•
Many motility patterns considered pathologic or abnormal have later proved to not be associated with a symptom complex or indeed are found to be part of the normal motility spectrum. Nondeglutitive simultaneous contractions previously thought to be a sign of disordered motility may represent the esophageal body component of phase 3 of the migrating motor complex.

16. Langevin S, DeNuna SF, Castell DO: **Does Diet Affect Values Obtained During Prolonged Ambulatory Pressure Monitoring?** *Dig Dis Sci* 1993, **38**:225–232.

17. Soffer EE, Merchant RK, Duethman G, Launspach DJ, Gisolfi C, Adrian TE: **Effect of Graded Exercise on Esophageal Motility and Gastroesophageal Reflux in Trained Athletes.** *Dig Dis Sci* 1993, **38**:220–224.

18. Hsu JJ, Kim CH, O'Connor MK, Brown ML: **Effect of Menstrual Cycle on Esophageal Emptying of Liquid and Solid Boluses.** *Mayo Clin Proc* 1993, **68**:753–756.

19. Cagossi M, Salgarello M, Patrignani P, Salgarello G: **Effects of Various Prostaglandin Synthesis Inhibitors on the Tone of the Lower Esophageal Sphincter in Man.** *Eur J Clin Pharmacol* 1992, **43**:303–305.

20. Crookes PF, Kaul BK, DeMeester TR, Stein HJ, Oka M: **Manometry of Individual Segments of the Distal Esophageal Sphincter.** *Arch Surg* 1993, **128**:411–415.

21. Sloan S, Rademaker AW, Kahrilas PJ: **Determinants of Gastroesophageal Junction Incompetence: Hiatal Hernia, Lower Esophageal Sphincter, or Both?** *Ann Int Med* 1992, **117**:977–982.

22. Paterson WG, Abdollah H, Beck IT, DaCosta LR: **Ambulatory Esophageal Manometry, pH-Metry, and Holter ECG Monitoring in Patients With Atypical Chest Pain.** *Dig Dis Sci* 1993, **38**:795–802.
•
The esophageal trigger and mechanism producing cardiac chest pain has been presumed to be a reflux or dysmotility event. This study casts doubt on a direct relationship between these events and suggests that chest pain in these patients results from dysfunction of visceral sensation.

23. Costantini M, Sturniolo GC, Zaninotto G, D'Inca R, Polo R, Naccarato R, Ancona E: **Altered Esophageal Pain Threshold in Irritable Bowel Syndrome.** *Dig Dis Sci* 1993, **38**:206–212.

24. Kao CH, Wang SJ: **Radionuclide Esophageal Transit Test: Detection of Esophageal Dysmotility and Reflux in Noncardiac Chest Pain.** *Abdom Imaging* 1993, **18**:220–222.

25. Jörgensen F, Hesse B, Tromholt N, Höjgaard L, Stubgaard M: **Esophageal Scintigraphy: Reproducibility and Normal Ranges.** *J Nucl Med* 1992, **33**:2106–2109.

26. Achem SR, Kolts BE, Burton L: **Segmental vs Diffuse Nutcracker Esophagus: An Intermittent Motility Pattern.** *Am J Gastroenterol* 1993, **88**:847–851.

27. Achem SR, Kolts BE, Wears R, Burton L, Richter JE: **Chest Pain Associated With Nutcracker Esophagus: A Preliminary Study of the Role of Gastroesophageal Reflux.** *Am J Gastroenterol* 1993, **88**:187–192.
•
Cardiac-type chest pain associated with "nutcracker esophagus" was presumed to be the result of the dysmotility event. These investigators demonstrate that GERD was present in 35% of these patients and treatment of their reflux improved symptoms, yet dysmotility (nutcracker) persisted in most. Thus, nutcracker may not be the cause of chest pain when present and may function only as a marker of other causal events.

28. Frieling T, Enck P, Dohmann R, Weinbeck M, Lübke HJ: **The Effect of Trospium Chloride on Oesophageal Motility.** *Aliment Pharmacol Ther* 1993, 7:75–80.

29. Kadakia SC, Wong RKH: **Graded Pneumatic Dilation Using Rigiflex Achalasia Dilators in Patients With Primary Esophageal Achalasia.** *Am J Gastroenterol* 1993, **88**:34–38.
•
There is no standardization to balloon type, inflation pressure, or duration in the treatment of achalasia by pneumatic dilation. These investigators demonstrated that the use of a "graded" approach was successful in 93% without complication. This technique may represent a more effective and safer approach to pneumatic dilation.

30. Parkman HP, Reynolds JC, Ouyang A, Rosato EF, Eisenberg JM, Cohen S: **Pneumatic Dilation or Esophagomyotomy Treatment for Idiopathic Achalasia: Clinical Outcomes and Cost Analysis.** *Dig Dis Sci* 1993, **38**:75–85.

31. Nair LA, Reynolds JC, Parkman HP, Ouyang A, Strom BL, Rosato EF, Cohen S: **Complications During Pneumatic Dilation for Achalasia or Diffuse Esophageal Spasm.** *Dig Dis Sci* 1993, **38**:1893–1904.

32. Ciarolla DA, Traube M: **Achalasia. Short-Term Clinical Monitoring After Pneumatic Dilation.** *Dig Dis Sci* 1993, **10**:109. **Monitoring After Pneumatic Dilation.** *Dig Dis Sci* 1993, 10:1905–1908.
•
Pneumatic dilation to treat achalasia is frequently followed by routine contrast fluoroscopy and hospital monitoring. These authors demonstrate the safety of outpatient dilation without routine radiologic contrast study.

33. Lee JD, Cecil BD, Brown PE, Wright RA: **The Cohen Test Does Not Predict Outcome in Achalasia After Pneumatic Dilation.** *Gastrointest Endosc* 1993, **39**:157–160.

34. Coccia G, Bortolotti M, Michetti P, Dodero M: **Return of Esophageal Peristalsis After Nifedipine Therapy in Patients With Idiopathic Esophageal Achalasia.** *Am J Gastroenterol* 1992, **87**:1705–1708.

35. Pasricha PJ, Ravitch WJ, Kalloo AN: **Effects of Intrasphincteric Botulinum Toxin on the Lower Esophageal Sphincter in Piglets.** *Gastroenterology* 1993, **105**:1045–1049.
•
This seminal paper describes what may become the therapy of choice in the treatment of achalasia: botulinum toxin injected intrasphincterically.

36. Pasricha PJ, Ravich WJ, Kalloo AN: **Botulinum Toxin for Achalasia [Letter].** *Lancet* 1993, **34**:1.

37. Timmer R, Breumelhof R, Nadorp JHSM, Smout AJPM: **Esophageal Motility in Low-Grade Reflux Esophagitis, Evaluated by Stationary and 24-Hour Ambulatory Manometry.** *Am J Gastroenterol* 1993, **88**:837–841.

38. Barham CP, Gotley DC, Miller R, Alderson D: **Pressure Events Surrounding Oesophageal Acid Reflux Episodes and Acid Clearance in Ambulant Healthy Volunteers.** *Gut* 1993, **34**:444–449.

39. Singh P, Adamopoulos A, Taylor RH, Colin-Jones DG: **Oesophageal Motor Function Before and After Healing of Esophagitis.** *Gut* 1992, **33**:1590–1596.

40. Yarze JC, Varga J, Stampfi D, Castell DO, Jimenez SA: **Esophageal Function in Systemic Sclerosis: A Prospective Evaluation of Motility and Acid Reflux in 36 Patients.** *Am J Gastroenterol* 1993, **88**:870–876.

41. Miller LS, Lui JB, Klenn PJ, Holahan MP, Varga J, Feld RI, Troshinsky M, Jimenez SA, Castell DO, Goldberg BB: **Endoluminal Ultrasonography of the Distal Esophagus in Systemic Sclerosis.** *Gastroenterology* 1993, **105**:31–39.

42. Grande L, Lacima G, Ros E, Font J, Pera C: **Esophageal Motor Function in Primary Sjögren's Syndrome.** *Am J Gastroenterol* 1993, **88**:378–381.

43. Stinneford JG, Keshavarzian A, Nemchausky BA, Doria MI, Durkin M: **Esophagitis and Esophageal Motor Abnormalities**

in Patients With Chronic Spinal Cord Injuries. *Paraplegia* 1993, 31:384–392.

44. Au J, Hawkins T, Venables C, Morritt G, Scott CD, Gascoigne AD, Corris PA, Hilton CJ, Dark JH: **Upper Gastrointestinal Dysmotility in Heart-Lung Transplant Recipients.** *Ann Thorac Surg* 1993, **55**:94–97.

45. Dantas RO, Villanova MG: **Esophageal Motility Impairment in Plummer-Vinson Syndrome. Correction by Iron Treatment.** *Dig Dis Sci* 1993, **38**:968–971.

46. Behar J, Biancani P: **Pathogenesis of Simultaneous Esophageal Contractions in Patients With Motility Disorders.** *Gastroenterology* 1993, **105**:111–118.

47. • Hsu JJ, O'Connor MK, Kang YW, Kim CH: **Nonspecific Motor Disorder of the Esophagus: A Real Disorder or a Manometric Curiosity?** *Gastroenterology* 1993, **104**:1281–1284.
As mentioned previously dysmotility events are not always associated with a disease or symptom complex. NEMD of the esophagus was found to result in a selective impairment of semisolid emptying. Thus, NEMD represents a real disorder of motility.

48. • Johnston PW, Johnston BT, Collins BJ, Collins JSA, Love AHG: **Audit of the Role of Oesophageal Manometry in Clinical Practice.** *Gut* 1993, **34**:1158–1161.
Is manometry helpful clinically and is it cost effective? This important sutdy not only reveals manometry's clinical utility, but at little cost versus other "tests of esophageal disease."

Harinder S. Garewal, MD, PhD, Section of Hematology-Oncology and Gastroenterology, Veterans Affairs Medical Center, 3601 South 6th Avenue, Tucson, AZ 85723, USA.

Gastroesophageal reflux disease, pH monitoring, and treatment

David Armstrong, MB, BChir, MA, MRCP, FRCPC, and Gervais Tougas, MD, CM, FRCPC

McMaster University Medical Center, Hamilton, Ontario, Canada

Research into the causes of gastroesophageal reflux disease continues to cover a broad base. It ranges from the roles of transient relaxations of the lower esophageal sphincter, neural control mechanisms, nitric oxide, and impairment of the crural diaphragm in the production of reflux, to the roles of mucosal bicarbonate secretion, mucosal blood flow, and epithelial cell acid handling in the protection of the esophageal mucosa. Impaired esophageal acid clearance is also likely to be a major factor, although current manometric techniques have not been able to identify a clear abnormality in mild to moderate reflux disease. It is still unclear whether episodes of esophageal alkalinization signal the reflux of noxious pancreaticobiliary secretions or whether they indicate the presence of esophageal mucosal and salivary bicarbonate. There is increasing interest in the central and peripheral mechanisms responsible for the genesis of esophageal symptoms and also in the relationship between reflux and respiratory tract symptoms. Esophageal pH monitoring is used widely but there is continuing debate regarding its clinical utility; concomitant monitoring of other modalities, including esophageal motility and electrocardiography, remains a research tool. It is clear that the proton pump inhibitors, omeprazole and lansoprazole, are highly effective therapy for reflux esophagitis but the comparison of healing rates achieved by different medical modalities and by surgery remains thwarted by the absence of a generally accepted classification system for reflux esophagitis. Controlled studies comparing the latest treatment options, including laparoscopic fundoplication and proton pump inhibitors, are needed urgently.

Current Opinion in Gastroenterology 1994, **10**:426–438

Gastroesophageal reflux disease (GERD), in its protean manifestations, remains an affliction of great importance to patients, clinicians, and researchers. In 1993, as in previous years, it generated a host of publications including excellent reviews covering GERD and its treatment in adults [1•] and in children [2•], as well as specific reviews of peptic esophageal strictures [3•] and the therapeutic role of prokinetic agents [4•].

Epidemiology

The absolute prevalences of GERD and reflux esophagitis remain conjectural because neither condition can be diagnosed solely on the basis of symptoms. Reports from Sweden [5•] and Italy [6] indicate that severe esophagitis is more prevalent in older patients, consistent with reports that older patients have more acid reflux than younger patients [6,7•]. A prospective study has confirmed the authors' previous report that cholecystectomy is associated with increased acid reflux and a twofold increase in the frequency of esophagitis [8•], although the postulated cause—compromised lower esophageal sphincter (LES) competence—remains unproven.

Pathophysiology

In most cases, GERD is thought to be related to disordered upper gastrointestinal tract motility but, un-

Abbreviations
GERD—gastroesophageal reflux disease; **LES**—lower esophageal sphincter.

 ISBN 1-85922-609-4 ISSN 0267–1379

like peptic ulcer disease, GERD is not a *Helicobacter pylori*–related condition [9•].

Structural abnormalities

In some patients, reflux can be attributed to structural abnormalities such as hiatal herniation, which facilitates reflux and then impairs clearance of refluxate. In one study, hiatus hernia was more prevalent in older patients without being related to esophagitis severity [5•], whereas a study in children indicated that hiatal herniation was associated with a higher incidence of prolonged reflux episodes and endoscopically proven esophagitis [10•]. Other structural abnormalities are also associated, particularly in children, with GERD. Hypertrophic pyloric stenosis is associated with excessive acid reflux and erosive esophagitis; interestingly, corrective surgery decreased esophageal acid exposure despite a fall in the resting LES pressure and an accompanying rise in intragastric pressure [11•]. In other cases, corrective surgery for esophageal atresia, tracheoesophageal fistula [12,13], or congenital diaphragmatic hernia [14] is associated with an increased incidence of GERD and esophagitis.

The role of esophageal transection or terminal esophagoproximal gastrectomy [15•] in the induction of GERD is unclear because reflux has been reported in 64% of cirrhotic patients not operated upon, regardless of etiology or variceal size [16•]. Postoperative changes in esophageal motility are minor and mucosal damage may be due to reduced esophageal mucosal blood flow [15•].

Lower esophageal sphincter

It is now accepted that inappropriate transient LES relaxations are associated with most reflux episodes, particularly in healthy subjects. The finding that 69% of reflux episodes in healthy volunteers are associated with manometric features of belching [17••] suggests that transient LES relaxations may not be "inappropriate"; they may rather be an appropriate mechanism for regulating intragastric pressure and volume. A study of 24 children with GERD, 14 with esophagitis, showed that most reflux episodes were, indeed, associated with transient LES relaxations although the proportion of transient LES relaxations associated with reflux was similar regardless of whether the patients had esophagitis [18•]. All reflux episodes in patients without esophagitis were associated with transient LES relaxations, whereas 22.9% of reflux episodes in esophagitis patients were associated with a gradual decline in resting LES pressure [18•].

The control of LES function remains a topic of keen interest particularly since the recognition of NO (nitric oxide) as a neurotransmitter able to hyperpolarize and relax gastrointestinal smooth muscle. Studies in the opossum suggest that NO, or an NO-like compound, mediates nonadrenergic-noncholinergic nerve-induced hyperpolarization of LES muscle strips, while producing a more transient hyperpolarization and depolarization of circular muscle from the esophageal body [19•]. These data help to elucidate mechanisms coordinating esophageal and LES activity, but NO is ubiquitous in humans and it will be difficult to target the LES specifically. Furthermore, LES function in health may be altered by inflammation; experimental esophagitis in cats decreased basal LES pressure and increased the inhibitory response to cholecystokinin and esophageal balloon distension [20•], suggesting that esophagitis may induce a vicious cycle of esophageal inflammation and LES incompetence. Clearly, the LES is a potential target for antireflux therapy but, although current prokinetic drugs can modify LES function, it is not clear that this explains their therapeutic effect [4•].

Crural diaphragm

Crural myotomy in cats increases acid reflux and abolishes the increase in esophagogastric junction pressure induced by airway obstruction without affecting the increase induced by abdominal compression [21••]. The potential importance of the crural diaphragm is underscored in a study of 10 patients who had undergone esophagogastrectomy [22••]. Resection of the smooth muscle LES notwithstanding, these patients retained a thoracoabdominal junction high-pressure zone that relaxed partially on swallowing and contracted in response to increased intra-abdominal pressure. Although the crural diaphragm appears to contribute to the antireflux barrier, it is not, on its own, sufficient to prevent reflux [22••].

Esophageal body

Clearance of refluxed gastric contents and propulsion of swallowed saliva, able to neutralize refluxed acid, are important mechanisms for the prevention of esophageal damage. Ambulatory monitoring of esophageal pH and motility has provided further evidence that acid clearance in healthy volunteers [17••] and esophagitis patients [23•] is achieved by primary peristalsis initiated by a pharyngeal swallow; secondary contractions are infrequent and they clear acid only rarely [23•]. Defective peristalsis, leading to impaired acid clearance [24•] is thought to be responsible for the increased prevalence of esophagitis in scleroderma [24•,25•]. As distal esophageal aperistalsis is associated with greater acid exposure [26•] and symptoms correlate poorly with GERD severity in scleroderma [24•,25•], it has been suggested that pH monitoring is necessary in all patients to assess the need for antisecretory therapy [25•]. Severe esophageal dysmotility, seen in scleroderma patients, is not generally a major pathogenetic factor in adults [27•] or children with mild esophagitis [28•]. Furthermore, distal esophageal contraction amplitudes are not predictive of increased esophageal acid exposure [7•] and the esophageal motor response to acid reflux is not impaired in esophagitis patients [29•].

Effective bolus transport occurs consistently only if the esophagus generates a peak intrabolus pressure that is 20 mm Hg greater than the baseline pressure at the midpoint of the bolus [30••]. However, intrabolus pressure is dependent, in part, on the volume of the swallowed bolus and it may, therefore, be difficult to define an absolute threshold contraction amplitude below which peristalsis is ineffective, particularly during ambulatory manometry because of diurnal variations in bolus size. Prokinetics increase esophageal contraction amplitude, area under the pressure-time curve, and propagation velocity [31•] but the interpretation of esophageal motility studies must also consider concomitant medical therapy. Nifedipine, for example, decreases esophageal contractility and LES pressure in healthy subjects and esophagitis patients [32•].

Diet, exercise, and stress

The management of GERD often includes advice about lifestyle and dietary modifications, although there are relatively few data to support such recommendations. Replacement of a triglyceride meal by a nondigestible fat substitute can reduce esophageal acid exposure markedly [33•] and the consumption of beer or an alcohol solution of comparable strength rather than white wine has a similar effect (Fig. 1) [34•]. Graded increases in exercise produce steady increases in esophageal acid exposure in trained athletes accompanied by progressive decreases in the amplitude, duration, and frequency of esophageal contractions [35•]. However, psychological stress has no effect on esophageal acid exposure in patients with documented GERD, despite an increase in the severity of symptoms [36••].

Toxicity of refluxed material

Refluxed gastric acid is responsible directly, or indirectly, for many of the symptoms and signs of GERD, despite controversy about the role of gastric acid hypersecretion [37•]. The importance of "alkaline reflux," however, remains unclear. In one study, esophageal alkaline exposure, determined by pH monitoring in patients with Barrett's esophagus, was greater in patients with complications [38•] and, in another study, reflux of duodenal contents, determined by measuring esophageal total bile acid concentrations, was increased in 15 of 30 patients with Barrett's esophagus [39•]. However, in the latter study, there was no overall difference between controls and patients with esophagitis or Barrett's esophagus with respect to esophageal bile acid concentrations [39•]. Thus, the magnitude of alkaline reflux in esophageal disease remains unclear, as does its etiology. Salivary stimulation with a Breath Saver (Hershey Foods Corp., Hershey, PA) lozenge produces esophageal pH rises suggestive of alkaline reflux [40•], whereas pH monitoring of the proximal esophagus, distal esophagus, and proximal stomach suggests that distal esophageal alkalinization is attributable to swallowed saliva and mucosal bicarbonate secretion [41•] rather than duodenogastroesophageal reflux [42•].

Protection of esophageal mucosa

Prevention of acid-induced esophagitis is dependent in part on neutralization of refluxed acid by swallowed saliva [40•,42•]. Patients with reflux esophagitis or Barrett's esophagus did not show the expected fall in distal esophageal pH when supine and this relative alkalinization was attributed, not to alkaline reflux [40•,42•], but rather to bicarbonate secretion by the esophageal mucosa [42•], which produces up to two thirds of the bicarbonate measured in the esophagus of healthy subjects [41•]. Mucosal blood flow may also be an impor-

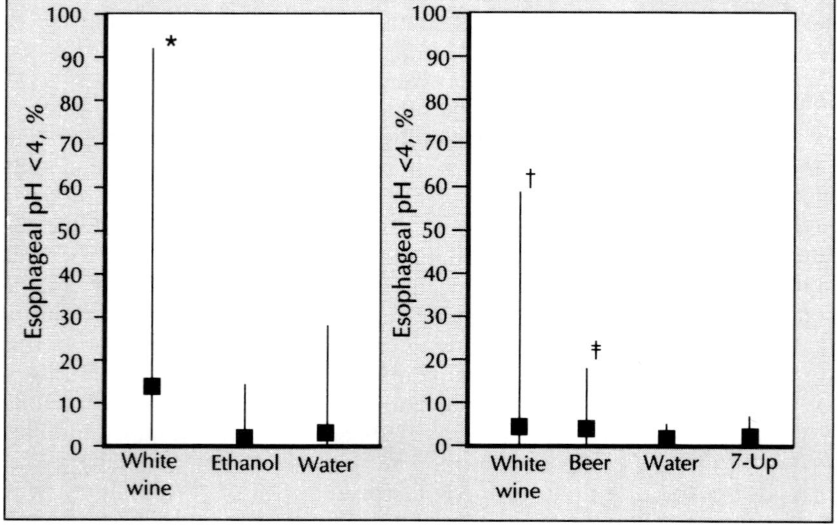

Fig. 1. Median percentages (range) of the 1-hour post-prandial period during which esophageal pH was less than 4.0 related to the ingestion of various beverages. *Asterisk* indicates $P<0.001$ white wine versus ethanol and water; *dagger* indicates $P<0.05$ white wine versus 7-Up, (Pepsi Cola, Offenbach, Germany) $P<0.01$ white wine versus beer, $P<0.001$ white wine versus water; *double dagger* indicates $P<0.01$ beer versus water. (*Adapted from* Pehl *et al.* [34•]; with permission.)

tant protective mechanism [15•] which can be attenuated experimentally by the NO synthesis antagonist, *N*-nitro-L-arginine methyl ester [43•].

There is increasing evidence that esophageal epithelial cells can respond directly to luminal acid. Rabbit esophageal epithelial cells have three exchangers that regulate intracellular pH: two (an Na^+/H^+ exchanger and an Na^+-dependent Cl^-/HCO_3^- exchanger) restore intracellular pH after intracellular acidification and a third (an Na^+-independent Cl^-/HCO_3^- exchanger), which responds to intracellular alkalinization [44•] is implicated in the intracellular acidification that follows exposure of esophageal cell cultures to an extracellular acid load [45•]. Intracellular acidification is associated, in turn, with inhibition of the regulatory volume decrease that follows hyperosmolar stress, suggesting that acid-induced cell swelling and injury may be due to inhibition of a basolateral Cl^-- and pH-dependent K^+ channel responsible for cell volume regulation [46•,47•].

Symptoms and sequelae

In many patients, symptoms can be attributed without difficulty to excessive gastroesophageal reflux but GERD symptoms are not invariably related directly to esophageal acid exposure or to esophagitis severity [24•,25•]; this may be due to variations in esophageal sensitivity, to variations in pain perception [36••,48•], or to the existence of multiple pathologies. In these cases, some form of symptom index may be helpful [49•,50•], particularly if there is more than one possible cause for the patient's symptoms. For example, chest pain attributed to a motility disorder, *ie*, nutcracker esophagus, improved with acid antisecretory therapy (Fig. 2) [51••]. In another study, esophageal acid instillation produced typical angina and reduced coronary artery blood velocity in 11 of 20 patients with syndrome X [52••]. That said, simultaneous Holter electrocardiographic monitoring, esophageal pH-metry, and manometry have again proven disappointing in elucidating the cause of atypical chest pain [48•].

The importance of central mechanisms is supported by the finding that stress increases reflux symptoms without modifying objective measures of acid reflux [36••] and that stress is a risk factor for esophagitis relapse [53•]. The relative importance of central and peripheral mechanisms will require further studies of putative peripheral chemonociceptive neurotransmitters, as well as studies of central responses to peripheral stimuli such as vagal and esophageal stimulation [54•].

A study of 36 children with poorly controlled asthma found evidence of GERD in 27 (75%) [55•]. Treatment with cisapride decreased asthma symptoms and reflux in 19 and 11 patients, respectively, who were available for follow-up. The relationship between acid reflux and asthma was investigated in 3 patients with asthma and GERD by monitoring esophageal and tracheal pH simultaneously; a pH electrode, inserted

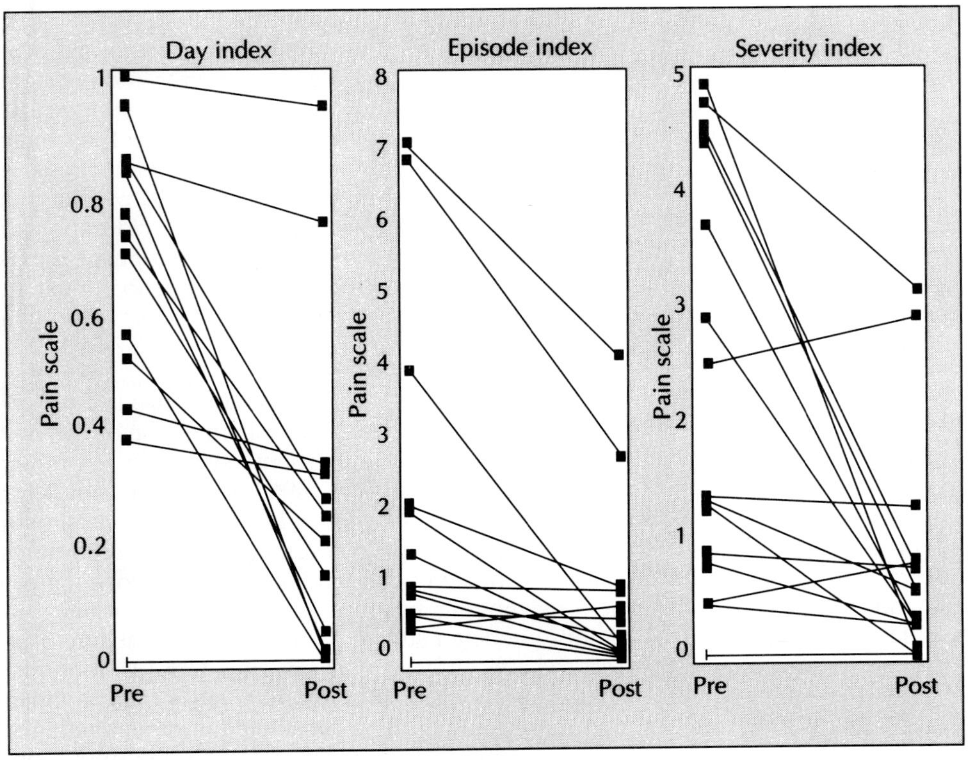

Fig. 2. Change in pain indices produced by intensive antireflux therapy in 12 patients with manometric evidence of nutcracker esophagus and pH-monitoring evidence of gastroesophageal reflux. "Day index" is the proportion of study days with pain, "Episode index" is the mean number of pain episodes per study day, and "Severity index" is the mean daily total pain score. (*Adapted from* Achem *et al.* [51••]; with permission.)

through the cricothyroid membrane, recorded pH falls associated with episodes of esophageal acidification and wheezing [56•]. Surgery prevented tracheal but not esophageal acidification, improved asthmatic symptoms, and decreased medication requirements in two patients. In 13 patients with persistent laryngitis and concomitant GERD, fundoplication produced resolution of symptoms and laryngeal inflammation in eight of the 11 patients available for follow-up [57•]. However, factors other than reflux must also be considered because acid reflux times were similar, regardless of whether the patients had symptoms of laryngitis [57•]. Recordings using two pH electrodes, 5 and 20 cm above the LES, indicate that acidification of the proximal esophagus depends on acidification of the distal esophagus [58•] and that it is associated with lower contraction amplitudes, lower resting pressures in the upper esophageal sphincter and a higher incidence of pulmonary aspiration [59•]. However, manometric studies suggest that pathologic esophagopharyngeal reflux in children is attributable to transient relaxations of the upper esophageal sphincter following distension of the esophageal body, rather than to a decrease in resting upper esophageal sphincter tone [60•].

Diagnosis

Endoscopy

Endoscopy remains the preeminent investigation in patients suspected of having esophageal disease, despite a report that it is possible to identify patients with GERD using a validated questionnaire [61•]. The high prevalence of reflux esophagitis and its chronicity preclude endoscopic examination in all symptomatic subjects. Fortunately, recurrent erosive disease is uncommon (1.5%) in asymptomatic patients [62•] and repeat endoscopy is unlikely, therefore, to modify management in an asymptomatic patient with uncomplicated reflux esophagitis. Endoscopy is, however, important for assessing the effect of treatment in clinical trials. Unfortunately, the proliferation of grading systems and diversity of endpoints used in treatment studies hampers any attempt to summarize the literature. It is hoped that clinicians, researchers, and the pharmaceutical industry can adopt a standardized, universally acceptable grading system in the near future.

In an important study of interobserver variation, Bytzer *et al.* [63••] reported good agreement between three endoscopists for diagnosing moderate to severe esophagitis but poor agreement for mild esophagitis. This study provides further evidence that "soft signs" such as diffuse erythema, edema, and mucosal friability are nonspecific markers of GERD.

Esophageal pH monitoring

Despite its widespread use, there is continuing uncertainty as to the utility of ambulatory pH monitoring in the diagnosis and management of GERD [64•]. Customarily, GERD is diagnosed if esophageal acid exposure exceeds a certain predetermined threshold and much effort has been expended over the last quarter century in attempts to define a universally acceptable threshold. The proposition that a reflux time of 18% identifies children who will fail medical treatment (sensitivity 70%; specificity 92%) must be verified prospectively [65•].

In another study, asymptomatic males had greater esophageal acid exposure than females but older (>65 y of age) subjects did not differ from younger subjects [66•]. The finding that nine (30%) of 30 subjects had markedly elevated reflux times again illustrates how difficult it is to establish clear diagnostic criteria for GERD. This is due, in part, to the traditional assumption that reflux is defined by an esophageal pH below 4, a definition that may exclude up to 50% of reflux episodes [67•]. The development of other measures of esophageal acid exposure, such as the mean hydrogen ion concentration (mmol/L) [68•] does not appear, on present evidence, to offer any advantage over the established "percentage reflux time." Other explanations for the absence of a generally applicable diagnostic threshold for esophageal pH monitoring include variations in technique [35•,58•,59•,69•] or diet [33•,34•], differences in study population demographics [6,7•,65•,66•], differences in the definition of GERD [49•,64•], and the use of different measures of esophageal acid exposure [64•,69•].

Difficulties with the establishment of diagnostic criteria do not, however, indicate that esophageal pH monitoring is necessarily a flawed technique; in many cases, the quantification of esophageal acid exposure cannot be expected to provide an answer to the question posed by the investigator. By analogy, hypertension can be associated with an increased risk of ischemic heart disease, but the finding of high blood pressure does not prove that an individual's chest pain is due to angina. Thus, increased esophageal acid exposure is associated with an increased risk of esophageal mucosal damage and heartburn, but the duration or extent of reflux is often a poor predictor of disease severity in any given subject.

Endoscopy, with or without histology, has the advantage that it can detect mucosal inflammation or damage but it cannot prove that a patient's symptoms are reflux related. Symptom indices [49•,50•] show promise for evaluating the significance of heartburn and chest pain during esophageal pH recordings [50•]; such recordings should be made under conditions that provoke the patient's symptoms whereas standardized recording conditions are better suited to investigations that aim to assess the effect of treatment on reflux time. A report that stationary monitoring is more reliable than ambulatory monitoring must be considered unproven until the two procedures are compared in the same study population [69•]. Provocation tests, such as the Bernstein test, have the advantages of brevity and financial economy, but they may be less accurate in identifying patients with reflux-related symptoms and they may not distinguish esophageal pain from angina [52••]. Dual point esophageal pH monitoring allows more accurate identification of reflux episodes associated with upper esophageal or respiratory tract symptoms [58•,59•], as do simultaneous tracheal and esophageal pH monitoring [56•], but normal values for proximal esophageal or tracheal acidity must be validated and symptom indices are again important in determining the mechanisms responsible for respiratory symptoms.

Esophageal pH monitoring and other modalities

Simultaneous monitoring of several modalities is increasingly common in the investigation of GERD, chest pain, and respiratory disease but for the present, ambulatory combined pH and pressure monitoring [31•,35•,49•,65•] remains a research tool for investigating reflux-related symptoms and motor abnormalities [27•,29•], their response to treatment [31•], and the etiology of chest pain [48•,49•].

Alternatives to esophageal pH monitoring

To elucidate the role of refluxed gastric contents other than acid in the pathogenesis of GERD, investigators have monitored the presence of other, nonacidic substances in the esophagus. Simultaneous pH monitoring and scintigraphy studies indicate that the two techniques detect different events, although the optimal duration of the image acquisition periods is still unclear [70•]. Scintigraphy has potential utility in patients who secrete little acid but, in patients who can secrete acid, scintigraphy is more sensitive than pH-metry during the first postprandial hour, perhaps because acid is buffered by food. Thereafter, pH monitoring is more sensitive, perhaps because much of the marker has left the stomach [71•]. Not surprisingly, there was no correlation between the total numbers of reflux episodes detected by the two techniques [71•]. A new ambulatory technique, using a small external gamma detector, also showed a poor correlation between the reflux of acid and the reflux of ^{99m}Tc-labeled omelet in the postprandial period [72•]. This said, analysis of carefully synchronized data from pH monitoring and gamma camera scintigraphy has demonstrated a significant temporal correlation between reflux episodes detected by the two techniques during the postprandial period, provided that the patients did not have rapid gastric emptying [70•]. There was no correlation between the results of scintigraphy and 24-hour pH studies. The conclusion to be drawn from these studies is not that one technique is invariably superior to the other but rather that neither test is better than the question it has to answer.

Treatment

Medical therapy

Acid antisecretory agents

Initial studies indicate that the proton pump inhibitors, omeprazole and lansoprazole, are comparably effective [73•] and that both are more effective than ranitidine at standard doses (Table 1) [74•,75•]. Furthermore, recent studies suggest that little is to be gained by using histamine H_2-receptor antagonists at higher daily doses (Table 1) [76–79]. Omeprazole has been used with circumspection in children but an uncontrolled study in 15 children with reflux esophagitis resistant to histamine H_2-receptor antagonists and prokinetic agents reported complete healing of erosive esophagitis by 6 months in all cases [80•].

Prokinetic agents

Omeprazole is clearly superior to the combination of ranitidine and metoclopramide (Table 1) [81•]. However, metoclopramide is not the most effective prokinetic [4•] and it would be more realistic to compare omeprazole or lansoprazole with the combination of an H_2-receptor antagonist and cisapride, which is more effective than placebo at healing esophagitis [82] and comparable in efficacy to H_2-receptor antagonists [83•,84•] (Table 1).

Preventing relapse

Esophagitis often relapses rapidly once treatment has stopped, but a multicenter French study suggests that many patients with mild disease will remain relapse-free using only conservative measures and alginate therapy as necessary [53•]. Esophagitis severity before healing was a risk factor for relapse in a double-blind study showing that 12-month relapse rates were lower with cisapride maintenance therapy (cisapride 20 mg daily: 32%–34%) than with placebo (51%) [62•].

Complications

Endoscopic stricture dilation with bougies is facilitated by the use of a graduated guide wire [85•] and it is rarely necessary to check the position of the guidewire fluoroscopically. Retrospective reviews confirm that stricture dilation with a "through-the-scope" balloon is effective in children [86] and adults [87]. In the event of acute bolus impaction, an aerated drink may be the real thing and clear the obstruction before endoscopic evaluation [88•]. Isolated reports that Barrett's esophagus can regress are supported by the finding that a 2-year course of omeprazole reduced the length of esophagus covered by Barrett's epithelium [89••].

Surgical therapy

Effective antireflux surgery has been attributed largely to an increase in basal LES pressure [90••], but recent studies suggest that fundoplication also decreases the frequency of transient and swallow-associated LES

Table 1. Esophagitis healing rates reported in 1993 for proton pump inhibitors, H_2-receptor antagonists, and prokinetic agents

	Healing rates, %			
Study and therapy	4 wk	6 wk	8 wk	12 wk
Hatlebakk *et al.* [73•]				
Lansoprazole (30 mg od)	63	–	85	–
Omeprazole (20 mg od)	65	–	87	–
Petite *et al.* [Unpublished observations]*				
Lansoprazole (30 mg od)	81	–	83	–
Omeprazole (20 mg od)	74	–	77	–
Feldman *et al.* [74•]				
Lansoprazole (30 mg od)	80	–	89	–
Ranitidine (150 mg bid)	33	–	38	–
Bardhan *et al.* [97]				
Lansoprazole (30 mg od)	82	–	91	–
Ranitidine (150 mg bid)	38	–	48	–
Robinson *et al.* [98]				
Lansoprazole (30 mg od)	83	–	92	–
Ranitidine (150 mg bid)	52	–	70	–
Petite *et al.* [Unpublished observations]*				
Lansoprazole (30 mg od)	80	–	91	–
Ranitidine (150 mg bid)	40	–	53	–
Robinson *et al.* [81•]				
Omeprazole (20 mg od)	68	–	82	–
Ranitidine (150 mg bid plus metoclopramide, 10 mg qid)	30	–	46	–
Euler *et al.* [76]				
Ranitidine (150 mg qid)	45	–	69	–
Ranitidine (300 mg qid)	47	–	62	–
Placebo	19	–	28	–
Simon *et al.* [78]				
Ranitidine (150 mg bid)	–	42	–	60
Famotidine (20 mg bid)	–	52	–	68
Famotidine (40 mg bid)	–	48	–	71
Wesdorp *et al.* [77]				
Famotidine (20 mg bid)	–	43	–	67
Famotidine (40 mg bid)	–	58	–	76
Baldi *et al.* [79]				
Nizatidine (150 mg tid)	–	81	–	–
Nizatidine (150/150/300 mg)	–	79	–	–
Nizatidine (300 mg bid)	–	68	–	–
Geldof *et al.* [83•]				
Ranitidine (150 mg bid)	–	–	45	–
Cisapride (10 mg qid)	–	–	47	–
Cisapride (20 mg bid)	–	–	63	–
Arvanitakis *et al.* [84•]				
Cisapride (10 mg qid)	–	–	89	–
Cisapride (20 mg bid)	–	–	100	–
Robertson *et al.* [82]				
Placebo	–	–	–	20
Cisapride (10 mg qid)	–	–	–	69

*Reported in Berstad and Hatlebakk [75•].
bid—twice a day; od—once a day; qid—four times a day; tid–three times a day.

relaxations [91•]. Antireflux procedures are legion although the Nissen fundoplication and its variants remain the most widely used. The choice of procedure is clearly important; a prospective, randomized comparison indicates unequivocally that teres cardiopexy is inferior to Nissen fundoplication [92•], but an interesting paper attributes the good outcome of surgery (77% healed at 2 years) to the fact that all surgeons followed predefined guidelines for fundoplication [93••]. In another study, 21 patients were available for follow-up from a group of 46 who underwent Nissen fundoplication 20 years earlier; 15 had an intact wrap and 19 were free of esophagitis [90••]. Meanwhile, Johansson *et al.* [94••] reporting on 40 patients who underwent fundoplication, found that all 33 available for review were free of esophagitis at 5-year follow-up. Thus, medium- and long-term outcome data are available for open fundoplication but it is now imperative that optimal surgical and medical therapies be compared prospectively, particularly with the advent of new techniques, including laparoscopic surgery [95•].

Surgery performed in children with GERD is often difficult because of associated neurological impairment or abnormalities related to earlier surgery; it remains to be seen whether proton pump inhibitors [80•] will improve medical management and supplant fundoplication in the short- and medium-term. The role of surgery in the treatment of peptic strictures is also ripe for reevaluation. A recent report recommends fundoplication unless there is prior gastric surgery, esophageal shortening, or severe concomitant esophageal disease [96•].

References and recommended reading

Papers of particular interest, published within the annual period of review, have been highlighted as:

- • Of special interest
- •• Of outstanding interest

1. • Sontag SJ: **Rolling Review - Gastro-Oesophageal Reflux Disease.** *Aliment Pharmacol Ther* 1993, 7:293–312.

A characteristically thorough review covering predominantly the epidemiology and therapy of GERD.

2. • Vandenplas Y: **The Diagnosis and Treatment of Gastro-Oesophageal Reflux Disease in Infants and Children.** *Ann Med* 1993, **25**:323–328.

A useful review highlighting some of the areas where childhood gastroesophageal reflux disease differs from adult disease.

3. • Marks RD, Richter JE: **Peptic Strictures of the Esophagus.** *Am J Gastroenterol* 1993, **88**:1160–1173.

A comprehensive review of the pathophysiology, diagnosis, and therapy of peptic strictures.

4. • Ramirez B, Richter JE: **Review Article: Promotility Drugs in the Treatment of Gastro-Oesophageal Reflux Disease.** *Aliment Pharmacol Ther* 1993, 7:5–20.

A detailed review of prokinetic drugs, their possible site of action, and their clinical efficacy in GERD.

5. • Lööf L, Götell P, Elfberg B: **The Incidence of Reflux Oesophagitis. A Study of Endoscopy Reports From a Defined Catchment Area in Sweden.** *Scand J Gastroenterol* 1993, **28**:113–118.

A detailed analysis of all patients presenting with reflux esophagitis over a 2-year period; severe esophagitis was seen more frequently in the elderly and in men.

6. Zhu H, Pace F, Sangaletti O, Bianchi Porro G: **Features of Symptomatic Gastroesophageal Reflux in Elderly Patients.** *Scand J Gastroenterol* 1993, **28**:235–238.

7. • Johnson BT, McFarland RJ, Collins JSA, Love AHG: **Predictors of Oesophageal Acid Exposure in Gastro-Oesophageal Reflux Disease.** *Eur J Gastroenterol Hepatol* 1993, **5**:875–879.

Acid reflux increases with age. Epigastric pain is a negative predictor for acid reflux and neither LES pressure nor distal esophageal contraction amplitude are correlated with acid reflux.

8. • Jazrawi S, Walsh TN, Byrne PJ, Hill AD, Li H, Lawlor P, Hennessy TPJ: **Cholecystectomy and Oesophageal Reflux - A Prospective Evaluation.** *Br J Surg* 1993, **80**:50–53.

Important confirmation of a prior observation that cholecystectomy increases acid reflux; the suggestion that this is due to LES incompetence is based on the authors' sphincter index, which decreased despite the fact that the individual components of the index did not change.

9. • Rosioru C, Glassman MS, Halata MS, Schwartz SM: **Esophagitis and *Helicobacter pylori* in Children: Incidence and Therapeutic Implications.** *Am J Gastroenterol* 1993, **88**:510–513.

Biopsy-proven esophagitis was equally common in the presence or absence of *H. pylori* and the proportion of children whose esophagitis responded to antisecretory therapy was unaffected by *H. pylori* positivity.

10. • Stewart RJ, Johnston BT, Boston VE, Dodge J: **Role of Hiatal Hernia in Delaying Acid Clearance.** *Arch Dis Child* 1993, **68**:662–664.

Hiatal hernia, present in 39% of children with symptoms of gastroesophageal reflux, was associated with a significantly higher incidence of prolonged reflux episodes and esophagitis.

11. • Takeuchi S, Tamate S, Nakahira M, Kadowaki H: **Esophagitis in Infants with Hypertrophic Pyloric Stenosis - A Source of Hematemesis.** *J Pediatr Surg* 1993, **28**:59–62.

Description of esophagitis as a cause of hematemesis associated with pyloric stenosis. This paper is notable for the interesting observation that surgery decreased acid reflux despite an increase in intragastric pressure and a decrease in LES pressure.

12. Lindahl H, Rintala R, Sariola H: **Chronic Esophagitis and Gastric Metaplasia Are Frequent Late Complications of Esophageal Atresia.** *J Pediatr Surg* 1993, **28**:1178–1180.

13. Wheatley MJ, Coran AG, Wesley JR: **Efficacy of the Nissen Fundoplication in the Management of Gastroesophageal Reflux Following Esophageal Atresia Repair.** *J Pediatr Surg* 1993, **28**:53–55.

14. Koot VCM, Bergmeijer JH, Bos AP, Molenaar JC: **Incidence and Management of Gastroesophageal Reflux After Repair of Congenital Diaphragmatic Hernia.** *J Pediatr Surg* 1993, **28**:48–52.

15. • Tamura S, Shiozaki H, Kobayashi K, Yano T, Yano H, Tahara H, Mori T: **Postoperative Motor Function and Mucosal Blood Flow of Lower Esophagus - Comparison Between Terminal Esophagoproximal Gastrectomy and Esophageal Transection for Esophageal Varices.** *Am J Gastroenterol* 1993, **88**:1065–1070.

Esophageal mucosal blood volume, measured by reflectance spectrometry, was lower after terminal esophagogastrectomy but there was no difference between the groups with respect to the occurrence of esophagitis or anastomotic ulcers.

16. • Ahmed AM, Alkarawi MA, Shariq S, Mohamed AE: **Frequency of Gastroesophageal Reflux in Patients With Liver Cirrhosis.** *Hepatogastroenterology* 1993, **40**:478–480.

16 of 25 cirrhotics had increased acid reflux, a proportion comparable to that seen in patients with reflux symptoms but no cirrhosis; the mechanism is not known but reflux may predispose to variceal bleed.

17. •• Barham CP, Gotley DC, Miller R, Mills A, Alderson D: **Pressure Events Surrounding Oesophageal Acid Reflux Episodes and Acid Clearance in Healthy Ambulant Volunteers.** *Gut* 1993, **34**:444–449.

Ambulatory esophageal pH and pressure monitoring, including the esophageal body and LES, shows that two thirds of reflux episodes in healthy subjects were related to belching and that swallow-related primary peristalsis is responsible for virtually all acid clearance from the esophagus.

18. • Cucchiara S, Bortolotti M, Minella R, Auricchio S: **Fasting and Postprandial Mechanisms of Gastroesophageal Reflux in Children With Gastroesophageal Reflux Disease.** *Dig Dis Sci* 1993, **38**:86–92.

Evidence that transient LES relaxations are the predominant mechanism leading to reflux in children with reflux disease; however, some reflux episodes are associated with a gradual loss of LES resting pressure, the mechanism of which is unknown.

19. • Conklin JL, Du C, Murray JA, Bates JN: **Characterization and Mediation of Inhibitory Junction Potentials From Opossum Lower Esophageal Sphincter**. *Gastroenterology* 1993, **104**:1439–1444.

NO, or a NO-like compound, produces differing neurophysiologic responses in circular muscle from the esophageal body and the LES, suggesting that it may be important in the coordinated control of the LES.

20. • Salapatek AMF, Diamant NE: **Assessment of Neural Inhibition of Lower Esophageal Sphincter in Cats with Esophagitis**. *Gastroenterology* 1993, **104**:810–818.

Acid-induced esophageal inflammation is associated with diminished basal LES tone, an increased inhibitory response to cholecystokinin and a maintained inhibitory response to esophageal luminal distension.

21. •• Mittal RK, Sivri B, Schirmer BD, Heine KJ: **Effect of Crural Myotomy on the Incidence and Mechanism of Gastroesophageal Reflux in Cats**. *Gastroenterology* 1993, **105**:740–747.

Experimental evidence that the crural diaphragm contributes to, but is not solely responsible for, the maintenance of esophagogastric junction pressure and prevention of gastroesophageal reflux.

22. •• Klein WA, Parkman HP, Dempsey DT, Fisher RS: **Sphincterlike Thoracoabdominal High Pressure Zone After Esophagogastrectomy**. *Gastroenterology* 1993, **105**:1362–1369.

Ten patients who had undergone esophagogastrectomy, with loss of the smooth muscle LES had a persistent high pressure zone at the thoracoabdominal junction, attributable to the crural diaphragm which was not, however, sufficient to prevent reflux disease in half of the patients.

23. • Bremner RM, Hoeft SF, Costantini M, Crookes PF, Bremner CG, DeMeester TR: **Pharyngeal Swallowing. The Major Factor in Clearance of Esophageal Reflux Episodes**. *Ann Surg* 1993, **218**:364–370.

Primary, not secondary, peristalsis is responsible for esophageal acid clearance.

24. • Basilisco G, Barbera R, Molgora M, Vanoli M, Bianchi P: **Acid Clearance and Oesophageal Sensitivity in Patients With Progressive Systemic Sclerosis**. *Gut* 1993, 34:1487–1491.

Development of esophagitis is associated with impaired peristalsis assessed by manometry and manifest as delayed clearance of acid instilled into the esophagus.

25. • Shoenut JP, Wieler JM, Micflikier AB: **The Extent and Pattern of Gastro-Oesophageal Reflux in Patients with Scleroderma Oesophagus: The Effect of Low-Dose Omeprazole**. *Aliment Pharmacol Ther* 1993, 7:509–514.

The absence of heartburn does not preclude increased gastroesophageal reflux in scleroderma patients; the authors recommend ambulatory esophageal pH monitoring in all scleroderma patients to identify those who will respond to antisecretory therapy with a proton pump inhibitor.

26. • Yarze JC, Varga J, Stampfl D, Castell DO, Jimenez SA: **Esophageal Function in Systemic Sclerosis: A Prospective Evaluation of Motility and Acid Reflux in 36 Patients**. *Am J Gastroenterol* 1993, **88**:870–876.

Detailed characterization of the esophageal motility changes in systemic sclerosis; acid exposure is correlated with distal aperistalsis and not with LES dysfunction.

27. • Timmer R, Breumelhof R, Nadorp JHSM, Smout AJPM: **Esophageal Motility in Low-Grade Reflux Esophagitis, Evaluated by Stationary and 24-hour Ambulatory Manometry**. *Am J Gastroenterol* 1993, **88**:837–841.

Mean LES pressure is lower in adults with mild (Savary-Miller grades 1 and 2) erosive esophagitis but esophageal body motility is not significantly different from that of healthy controls.

28. • Berezin S, Halata MS, Newman LJ, Glassman MS, Medow MS: **Esophageal Manometry in Children With Esophagitis**. *Am J Gastroenterol* 1993, **88**:680–682.

Children with mild esophagitis do not differ from controls with respect to basal LES pressure and esophageal body contraction characteristics.

29. • Timmer R, Breumelhof R, Nadorp JHSM, Smout AJPM: **Oesophageal Motor Response to Reflux Is Not Impaired in Reflux Oesophagitis**. *Gut* 1993, **34**:317–320.

Patients with reflux esophagitis (Savary-Miller grades 1 to 4) had greater acid reflux than controls and, if anything, they also had a higher number of contractions that were of greater amplitude and duration.

30. •• Ren JL, Massey BT, Dodds WJ, Kern MK, Brasseur JG, Shaker R, Harrington SS, Hogan WJ, Arndorfer RC: **Determinants of Intrabolus Pressure During Esophageal Peristaltic Bolus Transport**. *Am J Physiol* 1993, **264**:G407–G413.

Bolus transport depends on the intrabolus pressure developed at the tail end of a bolus and not on the luminal pressure generated in the absence of a bolus; if the differential between the peak intrabolus pressure and the baseline pressure at the midpoint of the bolus is less than 20 mm Hg, ineffective peristalsis may ensue.

31. • Inauen W, Emde C, Weber B, Armstrong D, Bettschen HU, Huber T, Scheurer U, Blum AL, Halter F, Merki HS: **Effects of Ranitidine and Cisapride on Acid Reflux and Oesophageal Motility in Patients with Reflux Oesophagitis - A 24-hour Ambulatory Combined pH and Manometry Study**. *Gut* 1993, 34:1025–1031.

Ambulatory monitoring of esophageal pH and motility shows that the addition of cisapride to ranitidine therapy further decreases esophageal acid exposure in esophagitis patients, perhaps by virtue of an increase in the amplitude, duration, and propagation velocity of esophageal body contractions.

32. • Mehta AJ, De Caestecker JS, Northfield TC: **Effects of Nifedipine and Atenolol on Gastro-Oesophageal Reflux**. *Eur J Gastroenterol Hepatol* 1993, **5**:627–629.

Nifedipine but not atenolol decreases LES pressure and provokes acid reflux compared with placebo in normal controls and in esophagitis patients.

33. • Just R, Katz L, Verhille M, Schlagheck T, Castell DO: **Comparison of the Effect of Olestra and Triglyceride on Postprandial Esophageal Acid Exposure**. *Am J Gastroenterol* 1993, **88**:1734–1737.

Potato chips fried in a nondigestible fat substitute, Olestra, produce significantly less acid reflux than the same quantity of chips fried in triglyceride.

34. • Pehl C, Wendl B, Pfeiffer A, Schmidt T, Kaess H: **Low-Proof Alcoholic Beverages and Gastroesophageal Reflux**. *Dig Dis Sci* 1993, **38**:93–96.

Beware of white wine: it provokes reflux to a greater extent than beer, water, 7-Up, or an ethanol solution of comparable strength.

35. • Soffer EE, Merchant RK, Duethman G, Launspach J, Gisolfi C, Adrian TE: **Effect of Graded Exercise on Esophageal Motility and Gastroesophageal Reflux in Trained Athletes**. *Dig Dis Sci* 1993, **38**:220–224.

Increasing exercise levels were associated with progressive decreases in the duration, amplitude, and frequency of esophageal contractions, leading to progressive increases in acid reflux in four of the 8 cyclists.

36. •• Bradley LA, Richter JE, Pulliam TJ, Haile JM, Scarinci IC, Schan CA, Dalton CB, Salley AN: **The Relationship Between Stress and Symptoms of Gastroesophageal Reflux - The Influence of Psychological Factors**. *Am J Gastroenterol* 1993, **88**:11–19.

Stressful tasks increased reflux symptoms in GERD patients who scored highly on a gastrointestinal susceptibility scale; increased symptoms were accompanied by rises in blood pressure and pulse but not by increased reflux, suggesting that some patients are more sensitive to low intensity esophageal stimuli.

37. Zhu H, Pace F, Sangaletti O, Bianchi Porro G: **Gastric Acid**
• **Secretion and Pattern of Gastroesophageal Reflux in Patients with Esophagitis and Concomitant Duodenal Ulcer. A Multivariate Analysis of Pathogenetic Factors**. *Scand J Gastroenterol* 1993, **28**:387–392.

There is no correlation between gastric acid output and esophagitis severity in patients with esophagitis and concomitant duodenal ulceration.

38. Attwoood SEA, Ball CS, Barlow AP, Jenkinson L, Norris
• TL, Watson A: **Role of Intragastric and Intraoesophageal Alkalinisation in the Genesis of Complications in Barrett's Columnar-Lined Oesophagus**. *Gut* 1993, **34**:11–15.

Patients with complicated Barrett's esophagus had more prolonged alkaline exposure (percentage recording with pH > 7; antimony pH electrodes) than did patients with uncomplicated Barrett's, but acid exposure was similar in the two groups. It is still unclear whether "alkaline reflux" is due to pancreaticobiliary secretions, esophageal and salivary bicarbonate, or a technical artefact.

39. Iftikhar SY, Ledingham S, Steele RJC, Evans DF, Lendrum
• K, Atkinson M, Hardcastle JD: **Bile Reflux in Columnar-Lined Barrett's Oesophagus**. *Ann R Coll Surg Engl* 1993, **75**:411–416.

Fifteen of 30 patients with Barrett's esophagus had a median 18-hour total bile acid concentration that was higher than the 95th percentile value for control subjects.

40. DeVault KR, Georgeson S, Castell DO: **Salivary Stimulation**
• **Mimics Esophageal Exposure to Refluxed Duodenal Contents**. *Am J Gastroenterol* 1993, **88**:1040–1043.

Salivary stimulation with a Breath Saver lozenge produces esophageal pH rises characteristic of "alkaline reflux" episodes attributed by some authors to the duodenogastroesophageal reflux of pancreaticobiliary secretions.

41. Brown CM, Snowdon CF, Slee B, Sandle LN, Rees WDW:
• **Measurement of Bicarbonate Output From the Intact Human Oesophagus**. *Gut* 1993, **34**:872–880.

Human esophageal bicarbonate secretion rates are comparable to gastric bicarbonate secretion rates and esophageal bicarbonate accounts for about 70% to 80% of the bicarbonate measured in the esophagus.

42. Singh S, Bradley LA, Richter JE: **Determinants of Oe-**
• **sophageal 'Alkaline' pH Environment in Controls and Patients With Gastro-Oesophageal Reflux Disease**. *Gut* 1993, **34**:309–316.

Esophageal and gastric pH monitoring studies suggest that "alkaline reflux" episodes are not due to duodenogastresophageal reflux and they are not explicable solely by swallowed saliva: esophageal secretion of alkali is postulated as a possible cause.

43. Sandler AD, Schmidt CD, Richardson K, Murray JA, Maher
• JW, Donahue PC, Bass BL, Mulvihill SJ: **Regulation of Distal Esophageal Mucosal Blood Flow - The Roles of Nitric Oxide and Substance-P**. *Surgery* 1993, **114**:285–294.

Increases in esophageal mucosal blood flow, produced by application of hydrochloric acid, are mediated by a lidocaine-insensitive mechanism that appears to be dependent, at least in part, on a paracrine effect of nitric oxide.

44. Tobey NA, Reddy SP, Khalbuss WE, Silvers SM, Cragoe EJJ,
• Orlando RC: **Na^+-Dependent and -Independent Cl^-/HCO_3-Exchangers in Cultured Rabbit Esophageal Epithelial Cells**. *Gastroenterology* 1993, **104**:185–195.

Demonstration of three ion exchangers able to regulate intracellular pH in cultured rabbit esophageal epithelial cells.

45. Tobey NA, Reddy SP, Keku TO, Cragoe EJ Jr., Orlando RC:
• **Mechanisms of HCl-Induced Lowering of Intracellular pH in Rabbit Esophageal Epithelial Cells**. *Gastroenterology* 1993, **105**:1035–1044.

Extracellular acid loading produces intracellular acidification by means of a basolateral 4,4′ -di-isothiocyanatostilbene-2,2′ -disulfonic acid-sensitive, chloride-dependent mechanism; esophageal epithelial cell acidification may, therefore, be due to increased absorption of hydrochloric acid rather than to impaired acid extrusion.

46. Goldstein JL, Fogelson BG, Snow JC, Schmidt LN, Mozwecz
• H, Layden TJ: **Rabbit Esophageal Cells Possess K+ Channels: Effect of Hyposmotic Stress on Channel Activity**. *Gastroenterology* 1993, **104**:417–426.

Rabbit esophageal cells have basolateral potassium channels that may correspond to potassium channels activated by external hyperosmolarity: these may, therefore, play a part in the protective mechanism of regulatory volume decrease.

47. Snow JC, Goldstein JL, Schmidt LN, Lisitza P, Layden
• TJ: **Rabbit Esophageal Cells Show Regulatory Volume Decrease: Ionic Basis and Effect of pH**. *Gastroenterology* 1993, **105**:102–110.

Demonstration that isolated rabbit esophageal epithelial cells possess regulatory volume decrease mechanisms mediated by potassium channels that are inhibited by decreased extracellular pH.

48. Paterson WG, Abdollah H, Beck IT, Dacosta LR: **Ambulatory**
• **Esophageal Manometry, pH-metry and Holter ECG Monitoring in Patients With Atypical Chest Pain**. *Dig Dis Sci* 1993, **38**:795–802.

Simultaneous ambulatory Holter monitoring, esophageal pH monitoring, and esophageal manometry detected an abnormality in only 35% of pain events. Atypical chest pain may, in many cases, reflect disordered visceral pain perception.

49. Weusten BLAM, Akkermans LMA, Van Berge Henegouwen
• GP, Smout AJPM: **Ambulatory Combined Oesophageal Pressure and pH Monitoring: Relationships Between Pathological Reflux, Oesophageal Motility and Symptoms of Oesophageal Dysfunction**. *Eur J Gastroenterol Hepatol* 1993, **5**:1055–1060.

There is poor correlation between symptoms and global assessments of esophageal acid exposure or contractility; the authors describe the use of a symptom index to look for a temporal correlation between the symptoms and recorded abnormalities.

50. Singh S, Richter JE, Bradley LA, Haile JM: **The Symptom In-**
• **dex. Differential Usefulness in Suspected Acid-Related Complaints of Heartburn and Chest Pain**. *Dig Dis Sci* 1993, **38**:1402–1408.

Retrospective review of patients undergoing pH-monitoring and endoscopy shows that a heartburn symptom index of 50% or more is sensitive (93%) for the the detection of acid reflux disease.

51. Achem SR, Kolts BE, Wears R, Burton L, Richter JE: **Chest**
•• **Pain Associated with Nutcracker Esophagus - A Preliminary Study of the Role of Gastroesophageal Reflux**. *Am J Gastroenterol* 1993, **88**:187–192.

Esophageal manometric abnormalities are not necessarily the cause of chest pain: 14 of 20 patients with a manometric diagnosis of nutcracker esophagus had concurrent reflux disease; aggressive antireflux therapy produced marked symptomatic improvement with little change in the manometric findings.

52. Chauhan A, Petch MC, Schofield PM: **Effect of Oesophageal**
•• **Acid Instillation on Coronary Blood Flow**. *Lancet* 1993, **341**:1309–1310.

Instillation of acid into the esophagus of 20 syndrome X patients produced typical angina in 11 and a significant reduction in left anterior descending coronary artery blood flow. This indicates that cardiac and esophageal pain may be closely interrelated; it suggests also that Bernstein's test is not specific for esophageal pain.

53. Poynard T, and a French Co-Operative Group: **Relapse Rate**
• **of Patients After Healing of Oesophagitis - A Prospective Study of Alginate As Self-Care Treatment for 6 Months**. *Aliment Pharmacol Ther* 1993, **7**:385–392.

Six-month relapse rates after endoscopically confirmed healing of erosive esophagitis were related to initial grade of esophagitis (grade I 15%; grade III 44%) and stress.

54. Tougas G, Hudoba P, Fitzpatrick D, Hunt RH, Upton ARM:
• **Cerebral-Evoked Potential Responses Following Direct Vagal and Esophageal Electrical Stimulation in Humans**. *Am J Physiol* 1993, **264**:G486–G491.

This exciting report details a method for assessing vagal afferent gastrointestinal pathways. It has great potential for the investigation of chest pain in the presence and absence of objective peripheral abnormalities.

55. Tucci F, Resti M, Fontana R, Novembre E, Lami CA, Vierucci
• A: **Gastroesophageal Reflux and Bronchial Asthma - Prevalence and Effect of Cisapride Therapy**. *J Pediatr Gastroenterol Nutr* 1993, **17**:265–270.

Further evidence for an association between asthma and reflux disease. Pathologic reflux was found in 27 of 36 asthmatic children. Three months' therapy with cisapride decreased acid reflux and improved asthmatic symptoms.

56. Donnelly RJ, Berrisford RG, Jack CIA, Tran JA, Evans CC:
• **Simultaneous Tracheal and Esophageal pH Monitoring: Investigating Reflux-Associated Asthma**. *Ann Thorac Surg* 1993, **56**:1029–1034.

The gold standard for detecting tracheal aspiration of acid is an intratracheal pH electrode. Larger studies, with evaluation of outcome will be necessary to assess the utility of this approach.

57. Deveney CW, Benner K, Cohen J: **Gastroesophageal Reflux**
• **and Laryngeal Disease**. *Arch Surg* 1993, **128**:1021–1027.

GERD should be considered in patients with upper respiratory tract symptoms unresponsive to standard therapy. If GERD is demonstrated, antireflux surgery will produce symptomatic improvement in a proportion of patients.

58. Dobhan R, Castell DO: **Normal and Abnormal Proximal**
• **Esophageal Acid Exposure - Results of Ambulatory Dual-Probe pH Monitoring**. *Am J Gastroenterol* 1993, **88**:25–29.

Study to determine normal values for acid exposure in the proximal esophagus (20 cm above the LES). Proximal esophageal acid exposure is minimal (< 1%) in normal subjects and, when present, it is proportional to distal esophageal acid exposure.

59. Patti MG, Debas HT, Pellegrini CA: **Clinical and Functional**
• **Characterization of High Gastroesophageal Reflux**. *Am J Surg* 1993, **165**:163–168.

Patients who have acid reflux detectable in the proximal esophagus also have lower basal pressures in the upper and lower esophageal sphincters and lower contraction amplitudes in the esophageal body.

60. Willing J, Davidson GP, Dent J, Cook I: **Effect of Gastro-Oe-**
• **sophageal Reflux on Upper Oesophageal Sphincter Motility in Children**. *Gut* 1993, **34**:904–910.

Incompetence of the upper esophageal sphincter and ensuing esophagopharyngeal reflux are probably due to transient relaxations of the sphincter rather than to a decrease in resting tone.

61. Johnsson F, Roth Y, Pedersen NED, Joelsson B: **Cimetidine**
• **Improves GERD Symptoms in Patients Selected by a Validated GERD Questionnaire**. *Aliment Pharmacol Ther* 1993, 7:81–86.

Presentation of a GERD questionnaire that had a positive predictive value of 85% for the diagnosis of objectively-verified GERD.

62. Blum AL, Adami B, Bouzo MH, Brandstätter G, Fumagalli
• I, Galmiche JP, Hebbeln H, Hentschel E, Hüttemann W, Schütz E, Verlinden M, and the Italian Eurocis Trialists: **Effect of Cisapride on Relapse of Esophagitis. A Multinational, Placebo-Controlled Trial in Patients Healed With an Antisecretory Drug**. *Dig Dis Sci* 1993, **38**:551–560.

Maintenance therapy with cisapride, 20 mg daily, reduces the 1-year relapse rate for erosive reflux esophagitis healed with antisecretory therapy. Recurrence was rare in the absence of recurrent symptoms.

63. Bytzer P, Havelund T, Møller Hansen J: **Interobserver Vari-**
•• **ation in the Endoscopic Diagnosis of Reflux Esophagitis**. *Scand J Gastroenterol* 1993, **28**:119–125.

Three endoscopists were in substantial agreement when diagnosing and grading the severity of erosive and ulcerative esophageal lesions, but agreement was poor for grade 1 esophagitis. Diffuse erythema, edema, mucosal friability and non–fibrin-covered erythematous lesions are nonspecific markers of GERD.

64. Ferreira C, Lohoues MJ, Bensoussan A, Yazbeck S, Brochu P,
• Roy CC: **Prolonged pH Monitoring Is of Limited Usefulness for Gastroesophageal Reflux**. *AJDC* 1993, **147**:662–664.

Esophageal pH monitoring cannot be used to detect esophagitis in children. Endoscopy with or without histology should be the initial investigation and pH monitoring should then be used to seek objective evidence that a child's symptoms are due to acid reflux.

65. Varty K, Evans D, Kapila L: **Paediatric Gastro-Oesophageal**
• **Reflux: Prognostic Indicators from pH Monitoring**. *Gut* 1993, 34:1478–1481.

Retrospective review of 24-hour pH monitoring data from children with primary or secondary GERD suggests that a reflux time of 18% is the optimal threshold for deciding whether a child will require surgical therapy.

66. Fass R, Sampliner RE, Mackel C, McGee D, Rappaport W:
• **Age- and Gender-Related Differences in 24-hour Esophageal pH Monitoring of Normal Subjects**. *Dig Dis Sci* 1993, 38:1926–1928.

There was no apparent effect of age on gastroesophageal reflux, but study numbers were limited. Notwithstanding, males were found to have significantly more reflux than females.

67. Wyman JB, Dent J, Holloway RH: **Changes in Oesophageal**
• **pH Associated With Gastro-Oesophageal Reflux - Are Traditional Criteria Sensitive for Detection of Reflux?** *Scand J Gastroenterol* 1993, **28**:827–832.

The traditional definition of a reflux episode (pH <4 for >15 s) may miss up to 50% of reflux events and will complicate considerably the assessment of reflux-related symptoms and motor events.

68. Schindlbeck NE, Klauser AG, Voderholzer WA, Müller-Liss-
• ner SA: **Mean Acidity or Percentage Reflux Time in Oesophageal pH-Monitoring**. *Eur J Gastroenterol Hepatol* 1993, 5:155–159.

The use of mean acidity as an index of esophageal acid exposure does not improve the diagnostic accuracy of esophageal pH monitoring for GERD.

69. Grande L, Culell P, Ros E, Lacima G, Pujol A, Garciavalde-
• casas JC, Fuster J, Visa J, Pera C: **Comparison of Stationary vs Ambulatory 24-hour pH Monitoring Systems in Diagnosis of Gastroesophageal Reflux Disease**. *Dig Dis Sci* 1993, 38:213–219.

The conclusion that ambulatory pH monitoring is less reliable than stationary monitoring is not justified: the two techniques used different types of pH electrodes and were tested in different groups of patients.

70. Orenstein SR, Klein HA, Rosenthal MS: **Scintigraphy Versus**
• **pH Probe for Quantification of Pediatric Gastroesophageal Reflux - A Study Using Concurrent Multiplexed Data and Acid Feedings**. *J Nucl Med* 1993, **34**:1228–1234.

Scintigraphy and pH monitoring often detect different events; scintigraphy may be preferable for the detection of neutral reflux immediately after meals whereas pH monitoring is better in later periods when gastric acidity increases.

71. Tolia V, Kuhns L, Kauffman RE: **Comparison of Simultane-**
• **ous Esophageal pH Monitoring and Scintigraphy in Infants With Gastroesophageal Reflux**. *Am J Gastroenterol* 1993, **88**:661–664.

There was no correlation between the two techniques for the detection of reflux episodes; scintigraphy detects more reflux in the postprandial hour, whereas pH monitoring is more sensitive thereafter.

72. Washington N, Moss HA, Washington C, Greaves JL, Steele
• RJC, Wilson CG: **Non-Invasive Detection of Gastro-Oesophageal Reflux Using an Ambulatory System**. *Gut* 1993, 34:1482–1486.

Novel development of scintigraphy techniques that permits the detection of radiolabeled, nonacidic reflux in ambulatory subjects. Again, gamma scintigraphy and pH monitoring did not always detect the same reflux events.

73. Hatlebakk JG, Berstad A, Carling L, Svedberg S-E, Unge P,
• Ekström P, Halvorsen L, Stallemo A, Hovdenak N, Trondstad R, Kittang E, Lange OJ: **Lansoprazole Versus Omeprazole in Short-Term Treatment of Reflux Oesophagitis. Results of a Scandinavian Multicentre Trial**. *Scand J Gastroenterol* 1993, **28**:224–228.

Double-blind, controlled 8-week trial in 229 patients with reflux esophagitis. Lansoprazole produced greater relief from heartburn at 4 weeks, but there was no difference in healing rates at 4 or 8 weeks.

74. Feldman M, Harford WV, Fisher RS, Sampliner RE, Murray
• SB, Greski-Rose PA, Jennings DE, and Other Members of the

Lansoprazole Study Group: **Treatment of Reflux Esophagitis Resistant to H_2-Receptor Antagonists With Lansoprazole, a New H+/K+-ATPase Inhibitor: A Controlled, Double-Blind Study**. *Am J Gastroenterol* 1993, **88**:1212–1217.
Double-blind, controlled 8-week trial in 103 patients with reflux esophagitis resistant to H_2-receptor antagonist therapy. Lansoprazole was significantly more effective than ranitidine with respect to healing and symptom relief at 2, 4, 6, and 8 weeks although it was not, perhaps, unexpected that H_2-receptor antagonist–resistant disease was unresponsive to an H_2-receptor antagonist.

75. • Berstad A, Hatlebakk JG: **Lansoprazole in the Treatment of Reflux Oesophagitis: A Survey of Clinical Studies**. *Aliment Pharmacol Ther* 1993, **7(Suppl 1)**:34–36.
A preliminary review of lansoprazole in the treatment of reflux esophagitis.

76. Euler AR, Murdock RH, Wilson TH, Silver MT, Parker SE, Powers L: **Ranitidine Is Effective Therapy for Erosive Esophagitis**. *Am J Gastroenterol* 1993, **88**:520–524.

77. Wesdorp ICE, Dekker W, Festen HPM: **Efficacy of Famotidine 20 mg Twice a Day Versus 40 mg Twice a Day in the Treatment of Erosive or Ulcerative Reflux Esophagitis**. *Dig Dis Sci* 1993, **38**:2287–2293.

78. Simon TJ, Berlin RG, Tipping R, Gilde L, For the Famotidine Erosive Esophagitis Study Group: **Efficacy of Twice Daily Doses of 40 or 20 Milligrams Famotidine or 150 Milligrams Ranitidine for Treatment of Patients With Moderate to Severe Erosive Esophagitis**. *Scand J Gastroenterol* 1993, **28**:375–380.

79. Baldi F, Longanesi A, Ferrarini F, Morselli-Labate AM, Voi M, Camarri F, Italian Gord Study Group: **Nizatidine in the Treatment of Reflux Oesophagitis: Italian Multicentre Study**. *Eur J Gastroenterol Hepatol* 1993, **5**:475–478.

80. • Gunasekaran TS, Hassall EG: **Efficacy and Safety of Omeprazole for Severe Gastroesophageal Reflux in Children**. *J Pediatr* 1993, **123**:148–154.
Uncontrolled trial reporting efficacy and safety of omeprazole in the short-term treatment of children with severe gastroesophageal reflux unresponsive to other medical therapy.

81. • Robinson M, Decktor DL, Maton PN, Sabesin S, Roufail W, Kogut D, Roberts W, McCullough A, Pardoll P, Saco L, Rustgi V, Kovacs T: **Omeprazole Is Superior to Ranitidine Plus Metoclopramide in the Short-Term Treatment of Erosive Oesophagitis**. *Aliment Pharmacol Ther* 1993, 7:67–73.
Omeprazole 20 mg (1 capsule daily) produced better healing, better symptom relief, and lower treatment-related withdrawals than the combination of ranitidine and metoclopramide (6 tablets daily).

82. Robertson CS, Evans DF, Ledingham SJ, Atkinson M: **Cisapride in the Treatment of Gastro-Oesophageal Reflux Disease**. *Aliment Pharmacol Ther* 1993, 7:181–190.

83. • Geldof H, Hazelhoff B, Otten MH: **Two Different Dose Regimens of Cisapride in the Treatment of Reflux Oesophagitis: A Double-Blind Comparison With Ranitidine**. *Aliment Pharmacol Ther* 1993, 7:409–415.
A double-blind study in 165 patients compared the effects of cisapride, 40 mg daily in divided doses, and ranitidine, 150 mg twice daily. The treatments did not differ significantly at 8 to 12 weeks.

84. • Arvanitakis C, Nikopoulos A, Theoharidis A, Giannoulis E, Vagios I, Anthopoulou H, Michailidis D, Tourkantonis A: **Cisapride and Ranitidine in the Treatment of Gastro-Oesophageal Reflux Disease - A Comparative Randomized Double-Blind Trial**. *Aliment Pharmacol Ther* 1993, 7:635–641.
Cisapride 10 mg, four times a day, and ranitidine, 150 mg twice daily, did not differ with respect to healing, symptom relief or numbers of adverse drug events.

85. • Kadakia SC, Parker A, Carrougher JG, Shaffer RT: **Esophageal Dilation With Polyvinyl Bougies, Using a Marked Guidewire Without the Aid of Fluoroscopy: An Update**. *Am J Gastroenterol* 1993, **88**:1381–1386.
A progress report on 197 dilation sessions in 138 patients, 114 of whom had benign strictures. In eight patients, fluoroscopy was necessary to monitor safe passage of the guidewire; in the remaining 130 patients, the guidewire was passed endoscopically and dilation was achieved without any procedure-related complications.

86. Shah MD, Berman WF: **Endoscopic Balloon Dilation of Esophageal Strictures in Children**. *Gastrointest Endosc* 1993, 39:153–156.

87. Jönsson P, Högström H: **Non-Operative Treatment of Benign Oesophageal Strictures - Results After Endoscopic Balloon Dilatation and H_2 Antagonists**. *Eur J Surg* 1993, **159**:405–407.

88. • Karanjia ND, Rees M: **The Use of Coca-Cola in the Management of Bolus Obstruction in Benign Oesophageal Stricture**. *Ann R Coll Surg Engl* 1993, **75**:94–95.
Administration of an aerated drink was very effective at clearing acutely impacted food boluses in this uncontrolled trial.

89. •• Gore S, Healey CJ, Sutton R, Eyre-Brook IA, Gear MWL, Shepherd NA, Wilkinson SP: **Regression of Columnar Lined (Barrett's) Oesophagus With Continuous Omeprazole Therapy**. *Aliment Pharmacol Ther* 1993, 7:623–628.
Convincing data to show that Barrett's epithelium can revert to squamous epithelium and that this can be achieved with continuous omeprazole therapy for 2 years. Regression comprises a reduction in the longitudinal extent of columnar epithelium and the appearance of squamous islands in the midst of the columnar epithelium.

90. •• Luostarinen M, Isolauri J, Laitinen J, Koskinen M, Keyriläinen O, Markkula H, Lehtinen E, Uusitalo A: **Fate of Nissen Fundoplication After 20 Years. A Clinical, Endoscopical and Functional Analysis**. *Gut* 1993, **34**:1015–1020.
Important endoscopic follow-up of patients who had undergone a Nissen fundoplication up to 20 years before. Six of 21 patients had a defective, wrap, two had erosive oesophagitis, and seven had Barrett's esophagus. Only 14 of 25 patients had a good or excellent results from surgery.

91. • Ireland AC, Holloway RH, Toouli J, Dent J: **Mechanisms Underlying the Antireflux Action of Fundoplication**. *Gut* 1993, 34:303–308.
The efficacy of fundoplication may be due to more than a simple increase in basal LES pressure. Surgery reduces the frequency of transient LES relaxations and prevents complete abolition of sphincter tone when the LES does relax.

92. • Janssen IMC, Gouma DJ, Klementschitsch P, Van Der Heyde MN, Obertop H: **Prospective Randomized Comparison of Teres Cardiopexy and Nissen Fundoplication in the Surgical Therapy of Gastro-Oesophageal Reflux Disease**. *Br J Surg* 1993, **80**:875–878.
Teres cardiopexy was clearly a worse antireflux procedure than Nissen fundoplication. Is there any reason to expect that it will be better when performed laparoscopically?

93. •• Dunnington GL, DeMeester TR, Department Of Veterans Affairs Gastroesophageal Reflux Disease Study Group: **Outcome Effect of Adherence to Operative Principles of Nissen Fundoplication by Multiple Surgeons**. *Am J Surg* 1993, **166**:654–659.
An interesting and potentially influential paper. Nissen fundoplication gave a 2-year healing rate of 77% in a multicenter trial. The good results are attributed to compliance with operative principles by the surgeons involved. Should all physicians document their adherence to therapeutic principles in the future? Should these data not be analysed to determine which operative principles contributed most to the satisfactory outcome?

94. •• Johansson J, Johnsson F, Joelsson B, Floren CH, Walther B: **Outcome Five Years After 360-Degrees Fundoplication for Gastro-Oesophageal Reflux Disease**. *Br J Surg* 1993, **80**:46–49.
Important, comprehensive follow-up documenting good results from antireflux surgery. Endoscopy was performed at 5-year follow-up in

33 of 40 patients who underwent fundoplication; three patients had persistent Barrett's esophagus but none had erosive esophagitis.

95. • Cuschieri A: **Laparoscopic Antireflux Surgery and Repair of Hiatal Hernia**. *World J Surg* 1993, **17**:40–45.
Technical description of the principles of laparoscopic antireflux surgery.

96. • Bonavina L, Fontebasso V, Bardini R, Baessato M, Peracchia A: **Surgical Treatment of Reflux Stricture of the Esophagus**. *Br J Surg* 1993, **80**:317–320.
In the absence of esophageal shortening or other structural abnormalities, fundoplication is the procedure of choice if surgery is necessary.

97. Bardhan KD, Long R, Haukey CJ, Wormsley KG, Brocklebank D, Moules I (for the UK Lansoprazole Clinical Research Group): **Lansoprazole, a New Proton Pump Inhibitor, vs Ranitidine in Treatment of Reflux Erosive Esophagitis [Abstract]**. *Gastroenterology* 1991, **100**:A30.

98. Robinson M, Kogut O, Jennings D, Levy C, Greski-Rose P, and the Lansprazole Study Group: **Lansoprazole Heals Erosive Reflux Esophagitis Better Than Ranitidine [Abstract]**. *Gastroenterology* 1992, **102**:A153.

David Armstrong, MB, BChir, MA, MRCP, FRCPC, Division of Gastroenterology, McMaster University Medical Center, 1200 Main Street West, Hamilton, Ontario L8N 3Z5, Canada.

Vascular lesions of the esophagus

Whitney F. Jones, MD, and Norman E. Marcon, MD

The Wellesley Hospital, the University of Toronto, Toronto, Ontario, Canada

The world's literature regarding vascular lesions of the esophagus is focused again on the diagnosis, management, and clinical outcome of patients with varices secondary to portal hypertension. Novel diagnostic modalities, in addition to endoscopic visualization, are described for gastroesophageal varices. Reports of medical management with infusion of vasoactive agents, minimally invasive management with endoscopy, or radiologic techniques continue to expand. Orthotopic liver transplantation is the surgical procedure of choice in patients with varices and end-stage liver disease; portal systemic shunting and devascularization procedures are declining but continue to be studied in some centers and remain a treatment alternative. Only small descriptive accounts are found in the literature regarding endoscopically identified esophageal vascular lesions, other than varices.

Current Opinion in Gastroenterology 1994, **10**:439–447

Diagnosis and natural history of gastroesophageal varices

Minimally invasive measurement of esophageal varices and portal hemodynamics were the focus of several articles. An endoscopically placed manometric balloon to determine size and intravariceal pressure, by measuring the collapse of esophageal varices, was demonstrated by Gertsch *et al.* [1] to be equivalent to direct needle puncture (regression analysis $r = 0.8$) without complications or bleeding. If confirmed, this technique would provide a minimally invasive and indirect outcome measurement of pharmacologic therapy. Another described technique was the use of catheter-based endoscopic ultrasound utilizing a high frequency (12.5 or 20 MHz) transducer mounted on a 6.2F catheter, which can be placed endoscopically or transnasally, as in the study by Liu *et al.* [2], to image the bowel wall. Catheter-based sonographic imaging with a 20-MHz probe effectively demonstrated both submucosal and periesophageal-gastric varices and was superior to endoscopic imaging alone in determining the presence of gastric varices (27 of 29 vs 11 of 29) and periesophageal varices (27 of 29 vs 0 of 29) (Fig. 1). Catheter-based endoscopic ultrasound will likely prove useful to distinguish varices from other prominent folds in the upper gastrointestinal tract, and to evaluate variceal changes following therapeutic interventions.

Portal flow, both direction and quantity, are important determinants of intravariceal hemodynamics. Three studies, using noninvasive technology for determining portal hemodynamics, demonstrated an increased frequency of variceal hemorrhage in patients with hyperdynamic portal flow [3•,4,5]. In the first study by Matsutani *et al.* [3•], high left gastric vein flow velocity, determined by transcutaneous Doppler ultrasound, was strongly associated with variceal bleeding ($P < 0.01$). Schmassmann *et al.* [4] were unable to demonstrate a predictive value of hyperdynamic portal vein flow characteristics by duplex sonography in cirrhotic patients who had not bled; however, the study did demonstrate a predictive value for rebleeding after first variceal hemorrhage in patients with a high-risk sonoscore. The third study by Burkart *et al.* [5] demonstrated an increased incidence of bleeding ($P = 0.006$) in patients with high or "hyperdynamic" portal flow rates, as determined by the cine-phase contrast magnetic resonance imaging. These noninvasive modalities could improve the identification of patients with portal hypertension and gastroesophageal varices, who are at highest risk for variceal hemorrhage, and thereby, assist in selecting the optimal treatment plan. The role of these new technologies in selecting patients for prophylactic management remains to be determined.

Although endoscopy remains the standard for the diagnosis of varices of the esophagus and proximal stomach, descriptive classifications alone are inadequate to predict future hemorrhage [6]. However, an excellent description of the natural progression of gastroesophageal varices was provided by Sarin *et al.* [7],

Abbreviations

EBL—endoscopic band ligation; **EVS**—endoscopic variceal sclerotherapy;
IGVs—isolated gastric varices; **TIPS**—transjugular intrahepatic portosystemic shunting.

 ISBN 1-85922-609-4 ISSN 0267–1379

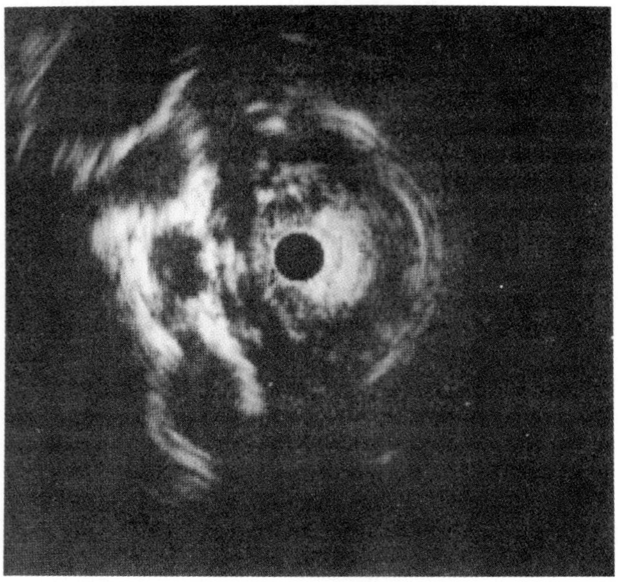

Fig. 1. 12.5-MHz catheter-based endoscopic ultrasound (Endosound probe, Microvasive, Watertown, MA) image of large periesophageal and minute submucosal esophageal varices following ablative endoscopic band ligation.

who reported a simplified grading system in a prospective follow-up of 568 patients with gastroesophageal varices. The gastric extensions of esophageal varices into the proximal stomach are divided into two groups: varices extending 2 to 5 cm below the gastroesophageal junction along the lesser curve (gastroesophageal varices 1); and, varices extending from the gastroesophageal junction along the lesser curve into the fundus (gastroesophageal varices 2). Isolated gastric varices (IGVs) were also classified into two groups: varices located solely in the fundus (IGV1); and, varices present in any other part of the stomach or duodenum (IGV2). Endoscopic injection sclerotherapy, with absolute alcohol, was performed for acute hemorrhage and was performed electively for management of both esophageal varices and gastric varices that had bled. Although the mean number of bleeding episodes prior to inclusion in the study were similar between esophageal varices and gastric varices, the risk for first episode of bleeding, among 31% of patients who had not bled, was twice as high for esophageal varices than for gastric varices. However, gastric varices bled more severely than esophageal varices, as reflected by an increased transfusion requirement. The authors concluded that gastroesophageal varices 1 and 2 be treated with sclerotherapy, followed by, or in combination with, the obliteration of esophageal varices. IGV1's may be managed endoscopically or with surgical devascularization procedures if endoscopic expertise is unavailable. IGV2's should be managed expectantly and should be treated only for acute bleeding episodes.

The study by Sarin *et al.* [7] was an encouraging report on the endoscopic management of bleeding gastric varices, which have long been the nemesis of endoscopists. Sarin, in response to a review by Chey and Elta [8], quotes a previous study that reported successful control of acute gastric variceal hemorrhage with absolute alcohol injection in 88% (14 of 16), rebleeding in 19% of patients, and elective obliteration in 25 of 37 (68%) with a rebleeding rate of 24% (9 of 37). Additionally, Soehendra *et al.* [9] have previously reported superior results using intravariceal injection of cyanoacrylate (Histoacryl, Braun, Melsungen, Germany), achieving hemostasis in all 23 (100%) active bleeders, with no recurrent bleeding within 30 days, and a late recurrence rate of bleeding in only 5.5%. Unfortunately, Histoacryl currently is not approved in the United States for use endoscopically.

Pharmacologic management of variceal hemorrhage

Several trials reported the results of pharmacologic management of variceal hemorrhage, either as primary therapy compared with emergent sclerotherapy for acute bleeding, or as preventative therapy for rebleeding. Sung *et al.* [10••] compared an infusion of octreotide, a long acting somatostatin analogue (50-μg bolus, followed by 50 μg/h over 48 hours, $n=49$), to emergency sclerotherapy ($n=49$) for the management of acute variceal hemorrhage. After 48 hours of infusion, patients in the octreotide group received sclerotherapy. Patients included had evidence of active bleeding or stigmata of recent hemorrhage. Despite an increased percentage of active bleeders in the octreotide group (51% vs 37%), there were no statistical differences with regard to initial control of bleeding, early rebleeding, mean number of blood transfusions, hospital stay, or in-hospital mortality between the two treatment groups. Treatment-related complications in the octreotide group were minor. Although not strongly stated in the paper, it is important to note that *both* sclerotherapy and octreotide frequently either failed to control acute bleeding or to prevent rebleeding within 48 hours. Consequently, rescue with balloon tamponade was required in approximately 50% of cases.

Terlipressin is the long-acting analogue of lysine-vasopressin that is activated by enzymatic cleavage to vasopressin [11]. In a multicenter trial by Silvain *et al.* [12], patients with endoscopically proven actively bleeding esophageal or cardiac varices, were randomly assigned to receive either terlipressin infusion (7 mg/24 h) plus transdermal nitroglycerin (10 mg/12 h) ($n=41$); or octreotide infusion (25 μg/h for 12 h then 100 μg subcutaneously at 12 and 18 h) ($n=46$). Control of bleeding was assessed by hemodynamic stability and hematocrit levels. There was no statistically significant difference between the two groups in terms of control of bleeding (59% terlipressin plus nitroglycerin vs 78% octreotide, $P=0.064$), rebleeding within 48 hours (20% terlipressin plus nitroglycerin vs 27% octreotide), or 1-

month mortality (28% terlipressin plus nitroglycerin vs 22% octreotide). Two serious adverse events reported in the terlipressin plus nitroglycerin group, including left ventricular failure followed by death and severe bradycardia, prompted early cessation of the trial.

Finally, in a small study by Stanciu *et al.* [13], intravenous metoclopramide lowered the intravariceal pressure in 10 of 12 patients with cirrhosis, as measured by direct variceal puncture, from 21.5±5.0 mm Hg to 14.0±3.4 mm Hg (P<0.001). Whether the primary mechanism of action is a decrease in portal-systemic circulation, or an increase in lower esophageal sphincter tone that reduces variceal blood flow across the gastroesophageal junction, remains to be proven.

The future role of pharmacologic infusion therapy will be to temporize a patient's condition until definitive endoscopic therapy can be performed or to improve endoscopic visualization during active bleeding. Octreotide appears to be safe and well tolerated, although the additional cost to endoscopic management must be considered.

Endoscopic therapy of varices

The endoscopic assessment and treatment of varices, both acutely and on a long-term basis, have undergone a rapid evolution [14••]. Endoscopic band ligation (EBL) is increasingly supported in the literature as a comparable, and in some aspects, a superior, alternative to endoscopic variceal sclerotherapy (EVS). In practice, however, EVS still remains the most widely used and foremost studied technique.

Endoscopic variceal sclerotherapy

Whereas it is generally accepted and proven that obliteration of varices with sclerotherapy reduces rebleeding, the beneficial effect on long-term survival remains disputed. Teres *et al.* [15••] attempted to address this issue by comparing sclerotherapy with propranolol in patients surviving their first variceal hemorrhage. Sclerotherapy was superior to propranolol in preventing rebleeding (P = 0.02), although the beneficial effect was established within the first month. No other significant differences were demonstrated in hospitalization requirements, long-term survival, or cause of death. Treatment-related complications were both more common and more severe in the sclerotherapy group. Future studies are needed to clarify the role of β-adrenergic blockade after first variceal hemorrhage, with or without endoscopic intervention.

Chan *et al.* [16] compared the efficacy of 3% sodium tetradecyl sulfate and 5% ethanolamine oleate in a double-blind, randomized controlled trial for the treatment of esophageal variceal hemorrhage. The two agents were equally effective in controlling acute variceal hemorrhage (87.5%) and inducing ulceration and stricture formation. The number of sessions required to obliterate the varices was fewer with sodium tetradecyl sulfate (3.3 vs 4.5), but sodium tetradecyl sulfate injection was accompanied by an increased incidence of post injection pyrexia (42% vs 30%). In another study from Bombay [17], absolute alcohol caused pleural effusions in six of 31 patients undergoing both acute and ablative EVS. Effusions were associated with the development and persistance of chest pain. An excellent review article by Heaton and Howard [18•] concluded that although small differences existed, all sclerosants were equally effective in the management of variceal hemorrhage and were associated with similar complications.

A question that confronts clinicians is the determination of the optimal endoscopic endpoint for variceal obliteration. Miyoshi *et al.* [19] suggested two additions to the already complicated Japanese Research Society's classification system for esophageal varices [20], attempting to determine the optimal outcome following EVS. The F0 category describes the complete absence of local venous dilatations representing varices in the esophagus. Previously, F1 to F3 designated the form of the variceal columns. They designated the absence of any mucosal red color signs, including even small superficial vessels, as RC(2-), whereas before, only RC(-) and RC(+) were used when describing the mucosal red color sign. They concluded that a more aggressive ablation of small superficial vessels to the F0, RC(2-) state resulted in an increased incidence of stricture formation with no decrease in the incidence of rebleeding, when compared with the F0, RC(-) state. This study sheds new light on the difficulty of determining what is an appropriate endoscopic endpoint, but it does not completely answer the question of how much is enough.

Two studies examined the factors that influence the long-term outcome in patients treated with EVS. Pugh *et al.* [21] followed 53 consecutive patients with alcoholic cirrhosis for 7 years and found a significantly higher incidence of recurrent symptomatic bleeding in patients who continued to imbibe alcohol compared with abstainers (P<0.0001). Kokawa *et al.* [22] concluded from a 6-year study that incomplete eradication of varices and the presence of coexisting hepatoma were predictors of rebleeding and decreased survival. As expected, both studies confirmed that the worst outcomes occurred in patients with poor hepatic reserve as predicted by the Child-Pugh class.

Endoscopic band ligation

Endoscopic band ligation involves placing small rubber bands around portions of esophageal mucosa and submucosa that have been entrapped by a suction device placed on the end of an endoscope. Since EBL's introduction in 1986 [23], the technique has gained increasing attention as an alternative to EVS. Variceal obliteration occurs by strangulation-induced necrosis of the entrapped tissue, followed by ulceration and fibrosis, as was well demonstrated in a case report by Marks *et al.* [24]. Already EBL is undergoing experimental modifications, including a transparent ligation device to improve visualization [25] and combination treatment with EVS [26].

The popularity of EBL is understandable considering its easier application, equal or higher efficacy rate, and possibly fewer treatment-related complications, when compared to EVS [27]. As expected with any new technique, as its usage has increased, so have the reports of EBL-associated complications. The majority of complications are related to pressure-induced damage to the proximal esophagus during placement of the overtube, varying from minor mucosal damage (Fig. 2) to variceal laceration with massive hemorrhage and esophageal perforation [28,29]. Massive variceal hemorrhage from the *distal* esophagus also has been described after overtube placement. Finally, a single case of refractory bleeding from an EBL-induced ulceration requiring balloon tamponade, was reported [30]. Patients should be advised to remain on a soft or liquid diet to prevent food bolus obstruction for 1 to 2 days following the procedures to prevent this complication.

Endoscopic variceal sclerotherapy versus endoscopic band ligation trials

A summary of two randomized controlled trials published in 1993 is presented in Table 1 [31••,32••].

Although having a smaller number of patients, the study by Laine *et al.* [31••] provided the most convincing data because no patients were withdrawn from the study for alternative treatments. Both groups received overtube placement during the treatment sessions, which essentially eliminated the complication of pulmonary aspiration. Findings included fewer complications and more rapid variceal eradication, and a tendency toward decreased rebleeding in the EBL-treated group. The incidence of complications in the EVS group was extremely high when compared with previous studies, primarily as a result of esophageal stricture formation.

The study by Gimson *et al.* [32••] from London, demonstrated similar results in variceal eradication, but had a statistically significant reduction in rebleeding in EBL-treated patients compared with EVS ($P<0.05$). No difference in the incidence of complications was found. For unstated reasons, treatment-induced ulcerations, which occur in all patients receiving EBL, were considered complications. Several patients were withdrawn for alternative treatments for a variety of reasons (14 of 49 for EVS vs five of 54 for EBL, $P=0.023$), which also interferes with the data interpretation. The authors of these two studies, concluded that EBL has significant advantages over EVS, although survival was not affected by treatment group. Both studies excluded patients with gastric varices.

Hashizume *et al.* [33] studied EVS versus EBL in the initial treatment session for patients treated prophylacticly and electively, followed by EVS until variceal eradication was achieved. Procedure-related pyrexia, retrosternal pain, and pleural effusion were significantly more common in the EVS-treated group ($P<0.05$). A study of treatment-induced ulcerations by Young *et al.* [34], found EBL-induced ulcerations, compared with those induced by EVS, were shallower (0.6 vs 1.8 mm), had larger surface areas (85.4 vs 13.3 mm^2), and healed

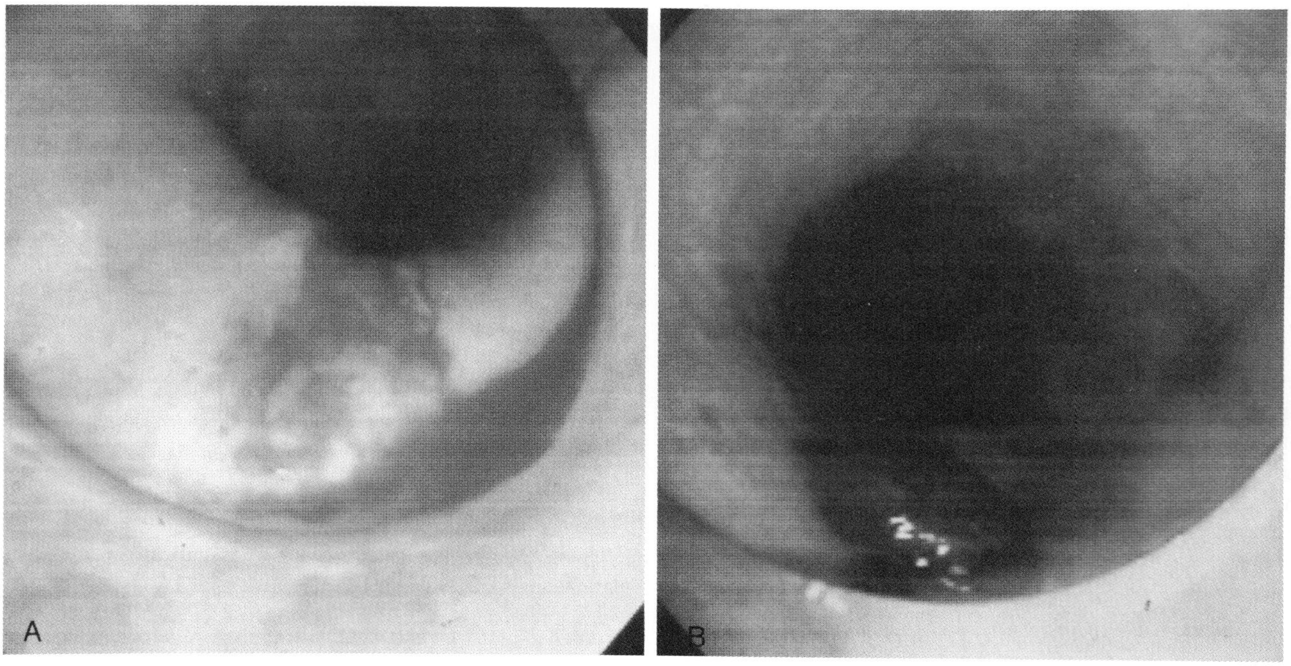

Fig. 2. Minor overtube-induced injury to the esophageal mucosa. **Left**, mucosal laceration; **Right**, submucosal hematoma.

Table 1. Endoscopic band ligation versus endoscopic variceal sclerotherapy

	Laine *et al.* [31••] (*n*=77)		Gimson *et al.* [32••] (*n*=103)	
	EBL	EVS (1.5% sodium tetradecylsulfate)	EBL	EVS (ethanolamine)
Patients, *n*	38	39	54	49
Initial hemostasis, *n/n (%)**	8/9 (89)	8/9 (89)	19/21 (91)	21/23 (92)
Recurrent bleeding, *n (%)*	10 (26)	17 (44)	16 (30)†	26 (53)
Variceal obliteration, *n/n (%)*	22/38 (59)	27/39 (69)	32/54 (59)	27/49 (55)
Endoscopy sessions to obliteration, *n*	4.1†	6.2	3.4†	4.9
Total complications, *n (%)*	9 (24)†	22 (56)	NA	NA
Esophageal stricture, *n (%)*	0 (0)†	13 (33)	0 (0)	0 (0)

*Actively bleeding varices.
†Statistically significant to at least $P \leq 0.05$.
EBL—endoscopic band ligation; EVS—endoscopic variceal sclerotherapy; NA—not available.

in fewer days (14.4 vs 20.9 d). These favorable characteristics of EBL-treatment–induced ulcers compared with EVS help to explain the increased effectiveness and decreased complications associated with EBL.

Despite the increased reporting of associated complications, the past year's literature provided strong support for the safety and efficacy of EBL in the acute and long-term management of esophageal varices. We predict that in the future, EBL will become the treatment of choice for esophageal varices. Future comparative trials must address the role of EBL versus the various injection modalities, such as Histoacryl. Furthermore, all three major published trials comparing EBL with EVS have excluded bleeding gastric varices, for which subsequent research will be needed.

Transjugular intrahepatic portal-systemic shunts

The creation of self-expanding metallic stents for nonselective, portal-systemic, radiographic shunt placement through the hepatic parenchyma has been a significant advance in the minimally invasive therapy of patients with variceal hemorrhage. Three studies reported on this technique in 1993 [35••,36••,37]. LaBerge *et al.* [35••] described the results of 100 patients who underwent transjugular intrahepatic portal-systemic shunting (TIPS), the majority for variceal bleeding ($n=97$). The overall success rate was 96%, and active variceal bleeding was controlled in 29 of 30 patients. Variceal bleeding recurred in 10 patients, all owing to shunt thrombosis or stenosis, which was subsequently controlled by shunt revision in nine of 10. Fourteen of 17 patients developed new or worsening encephalopathy following TIPS, which was controlled with oral administration of lactulose. Twenty-two patients underwent orthotopic liver transplantation and 26 patients died within 90 days. Primarily these were patients with Child's class C and had multiple coexisting medical problems prior to TIPS. The excellent results and acceptable complication rates reflect the experience and expertise of the medical center.

Two additional studies described a somewhat different appraisal of TIPS [36••,37]. In a retrospective study by Helton *et al.* [36••], 59 consecutive patients undergoing TIPS with excellent follow-up were reviewed. Active bleeding was strongly correlated with mortality ($P<0.0001$) and in six of 23, active bleeding was not controlled. Thirty percent required placement of a second stent during the initial hospitalization because of technical problems, stent thrombosis, or stenosis. Procedural complications occurred in eight of 59 patients with an associated mortality of 25%. The overall cost per TIPS procedure was $14,200 (US$). A smaller study (n=22) by Simpson *et al.* [37] demonstrated the effectiveness of TIPS in patients with hemorrhage secondary to portal hypertension, including portal hypertensive gastropathy. The problems encountered in the early application of the new technique were also described.

Transjugular intrahepatic portosystemic shunting is an exciting new alternative to surgical, portal systemic shunting. Like all new procedures, the learning curve is substantial, the resources required are accessible only at tertiary care hospitals, and the procedure costs are higher. Repeat interventions are frequently required and complications are not insignificant. Randomized controlled trials are needed to compare its efficacy with endoscopic therapy.

Surgical management of variceal hemorrhage

The current surgical procedure of choice for refractory variceal hemorrhage associated with end-stage liver disease is orthotopic liver transplantation [38]. The use of surgical portal-systemic shunts, selective or nonselective, has continued to decrease in favor of minimally invasive therapy. However, in centers without the benefit of advanced therapeutic endoscopy or TIPS capability, operative intervention remains the only life-saving alternative, especially in patients bleeding from portal hypertensive gastropathy or gastric fundal varices.

Rikkers *et al.* [39] studied patients (n=60) randomly assigned to either EVS or shunt surgery (26 distal splenorenal, 4 nonselective) in a 6-year study. Nonoperative control of variceal bleeding was required before randomization. Similar to previous studies, rebleeding episodes were more common in the EVS group (60% vs 17%, $P<0.001$). The bleeding etiology of two thirds of sclerotherapy failures was either portal hypertensive gastropathy or gastric varices. Unlike other studies, 6-year survival was longer in the surgical group (53% vs 26%, $P<0.05$) because of increased mortality in the EVS group. A likely explanation for this is the variability of endoscopist expertise in executing variceal hemostasis and the limited availability of endoscopic options, which were not described in the manuscript. In contrast, all shunt procedures were performed by a single expert surgeon.

The results of a prospective trial of EVS versus esophageal transection and gastric devascularization in the long-term management (4.5 years) of patients with variceal hemorrhage was reported by Triger *et al.* [40]. After urgent treatment with EVS, 92 patients were evaluated. Three-month mortality was greater in the surgery group (20% vs 1%), but survival curves merged by 2 years and thereafter were similar. Rebleeding occurred in 31% of patients randomly assigned to surgery and in 49% of patients in the EVS group (P= not significant). The overall costs to manage patients surgically was four times greater than for EVS ($P<0.0001$). Mercado *et al.* [41] described the results of an alternate technique for esophageal transection involving mucosal exclusion, which may reduce the risks of fistula formation and postoperative esophageal stricture.

Other studies worth noting are summarized below. Advanced age increases the risks associated with portal systemic shunt surgery. However, a report by Gusberg [42] of 19 selected patients (14 of 17 Child's A or B class) more than 60 years of age, who successfully underwent selective portal systemic shunting, demonstrated its feasibility in this age group. There was only one in-hospital death and 14 of 17 patients were alive at a mean follow-up of 44 months. Patients with a hypertrophied caudate lobe or vascular anatomy, precluding traditional operations, may be candidates for the relatively unknown surgical procedure of portal vein to left renal vein anastomosis, which is described by Lewis *et al.* [43] as an alternative to the side-to-side shunt. Finally, Ho *et al.* [44] reported that EVS or placement of portal systemic shunts prior to orthotopic liver transplantation did not alter survival following transplant, suggesting that previous variceal hemorrhage should not adversely affect patient selection for transplantation.

Prophylaxis for variceal hemorrhage

The use of β-adrenergic blockade in the prevention of variceal hemorrhage reduces the long-term risk of bleeding and possibly mortality [45,46]. Angelico *et al.* [47] compared isosorbide-5-mononitrate with propranolol in the prevention of first variceal bleed in cirrhotic patients with high-risk esophageal varices. Rates of first bleeding and actuarial survival were no different between groups, suggesting that nitrates are an effective, safe alternative to β-adrenergic blockers in patients with contraindications or drug intolerance.

Prophylactic EVS remains controversial despite numerous clinical trials. This year, a 6-year study follow-up was presented by Potzi *et al.* [48], which demonstrated no beneficial effect to either rebleeding or mortality in patients treated with prophylactic EVS compared with controls. However, results from a trial of prophylactic EVS from a major liver transplantation center yielded markedly contrasting results [49•]. The patients studied had end-stage liver disease with large varices, and were accepted for liver transplantation. They were nonrandomly admitted to either the medical service (n=648) or surgical service (n=628). Patients on the medical service received prophylactic EVS, whereas patients on the surgery service received EVS only for acute hemorrhage (n=172 of 628). Thirty-eight of the patients treated with prophylactic EVS went on to bleed, requiring emergent EVS. Those not receiving prophylactic EVS had an increased relative risk (4.6-fold, $P<0.001$) of requiring emergency EVS for acute bleeding and an increased risk of pretransplant hemorrhage-associated liver failure (6.1-fold, $P<0.025$). Complications of EVS were markedly increased in patients who required emergent EVS versus elective EVS (19.6% vs 1.9%, $P<0.001$). In the pretransplantation population, prophylactic EVS reduced the short-term (3 months to 1 year) risk of acute variceal bleeding—the exact time period overlapping with the mean waiting list time prior to transplantation—resulting in a higher percentage of patients surviving to transplantation. Results this impressive should be easily replicated in a randomized controlled trial.

Miscellaneous vascular lesions of the esophagus

Non-ulcer/nonvariceal vascular lesions of the esophagus remain uncommon, but are increasingly reported with improvements in endoscopic recognition and therapeutic intervention. Two reports [50,51] of a Dieulafoy's lesion of the esophagus described the typical visible vessel without associated ulceration, one treated successfully with injection of 1:10,000 epinephrine [50]. In the second report [51], two cases had early rebleeding despite injection therapy with ethanolamine, eventually requiring balloon tamponade in one case and angiographic embolization in the other. These articles "complete the loop" for the description of Dieulafoy-like lesions throughout the gastrointestinal tract.

A lesion described as idiopathic acute esophageal necrosis is reported by Moreto *et al.* [52] in 10 patients, as a well-demarcated, black discoloration of the mucosa viewed endoscopically. Diabetes or hyperglycemia was present in the majority of cases (as is the authors' experience), as were other significant underlying medical problems. The pathology demonstrated ischemia with variable depths of wall involvement, including full thickness esophageal necrosis, perforation and death. All patients except one improved with supportive care. Four patients experienced serious complications and two patients had new, long esophageal stenosis after recovery. If this entity is suspected at endoscopy, biopsies should be taken, oxygenation and perfusion maximized, and careful observation conducted for signs of perforation or mediastinitis.

The Lusorian artery is a variant of the right subclavian artery that arises from the left-sided descending aortic arch and usually crosses the midline behind the esophagus. A case of massive esophageal bleeding, secondary to duodenal tube-induced erosion of a Lusorian artery requiring surgical repair, was described by Vehling-Kaiser *et al.* [53]. Vascular-enteric fistulas should be included in the differential diagnosis for any patient with massive gastrointestinal bleeding following recent surgical procedures or instrumentation. A more common complaint is chest pain or dysphagia secondary to esophageal compression.

Spontaneous esophageal hematomas occur in the absence of trauma, previous ingestions, or interventions. A total of four cases were reported by Sen and Lea [54] and by Furukawa *et al.* [55]. Patients presented with chest pain or minimal hematemesis. The diagnosis was made after identifying a bulging intramural esophageal mass, with or without abnormal overlying mucosa, that resolves with conservative treatment over time. Computerized tomographic scanning is helpful in making the correct diagnosis.

Conclusions

The reported novel diagnostic modalities for esophageal varices may help the endoscopist to predict which patients are at risk for future bleeding. The endoscopist has a multitude of options from which to choose to treat the acute bleeding patient or for preventative therapy of rebleeding. These new options include a variety of pharmacologic agents useful in temporizing patients with variceal hemorrhage. Reports of endoscopic therapy give increasing support for EBL as an equal, and in some aspects possibly superior, alternative to EVS, regardless of which sclerosant is used. TIPS and surgical procedures are a viable option for patient management, particularly in the absence of therapeutic endoscopic availability. Whether the endoscopist chooses to pursue prophylactic treatment of varices remains controversial. Therefore, continuing studies of the current treatment modalities are necessary to determine if any one method is superior, or if a particular combination of treatment modalities are preferred for control of acute esophageal bleeding, prevention of esophageal rebleeding, or prophylatic endoscopic intervention.

Acknowledgments

The authors wish to thank Meliessa Siemens, R.N. for her careful and thoughtful assistance in preparing the manuscript.

References and recommended reading

Papers of particular interest, published within the annual period of review, have been highlighted as:
- • Of special interest
- •• Of outstanding interest

1. Gertsch P, Fischer G, Klebler G, Wheatley AM, Geigenberger G, Sauerbruch T: **Manometry of Esophageal Varices: Comparison of an Endoscopic Balloon Technique With Needle Puncture.** *Gastroenterology* 1993, **105**:1159–1166.

2. Liu JB, Miller LS, Feld RI, Barbarevech CA, Needleman L, Goldberg BB: **Gastric and Esophageal Varices: 20-MHz Transnasal Endoluminal US.** *Radiology* 1993, **187**:363–366.

3. • Matsutani S, Furuse J, Ishii H, Mizumoto H, Kimura K, Ohto M: **Hemodynamics of the Left Gastric Vein in Portal Hypertension.** *Gastroenterology* 1993, **105**:513–518.
Study correlates the use of transcutaneous Doppler sonography in determining left gastric vein flow characteristics associated with esophageal variceal hemorrhage.

4. Schmassmann A, Zuber M, Livers M, Jager K, Jenzer HR, Fehr HF: **Recurrent Bleeding After Variceal Hemorrhage: Predictive Value of Portal Venous Duplex Sonography.** *AJR Am J Roentgenol* 1993, **160**:41–47.

5. Burkart DJ, Johnson CD, Ehman RL, Weaver AL, Ilstrup DM: **Evaluation of Portal Venous Hypertension With Cine Phase-Contrast MR Flow Measurements: High Association of Hyperdynamic Portal Flow With Variceal Hemorrhage.** *Radiology* 1993, **188**:643–648.

6. Rico G, Merighi A, Chahin NJ, Mastronardi M, Codeluppi PL, Ferrari A, Armocida C, Zanasi G, Christani A, Cioni G, Manenti F: **A Prospective Study of the Ability of Three Endoscopic Classifications to Predict Hemorrhage From Esophageal Varices.** *Gastrointest Endosc* 1992, **38**:425–429.

7. Sarin SK, Lahoti D, Saxena SP, Murthy NS, Makwana UK: **Prevalence, Classification and Natural History of Gastric Varices.** *Hepatology* 1992, **16**:1343–1349.

8. Chey WD, Elta GH: **Natural History of Gastric Varices.** *Gastroenterology* 1993, **105**:599–602.

9. Soehendra N, Grimm H, Maydeo A, Nam VCh, Eckmann B, Bruckner M: **Endoscopic Obliteration of Fundal Varices.** *Can J Gastroenterol* 1990, 4:643–646.

10. Sung JJY, Chung SCS, Lai CW, Chan FKL, Leung JWC, Yung
•• MY, Kassianides C, Li AKC: **Octreotide Infusion of Emergency Sclerotherapy for Variceal Haemorrhage.** *Lancet* 1993, 342:637–641.
A prospective, randomized controlled trial that demonstrates equivalent efficacy, safety, and survival of patients treated for acute variceal hemorrhage with octreotide infusion compared with emergent sclerotherapy.

11. Soederlund C: **Terlipressin (Glypressin) in the Treatment of Bleeding Esophageal Varices. State of the Art.** *Regul Pept* 1993, 45:299–302.

12. Silvain C, Carpentier S, Sautereau D, Czernichow B, Metreau JM, Fort E, Ingrand P, Boyer J, Pillegand B, Doffel M, Dhumeaux D, Beauchant M: **Terlipressin Plus Transdermal Nitroglycerin Vs. Octreotide in the Control of Acute Bleeding Form Esophageal Varices: A Multicenter Randomized Trial.** *Hepatology* 1993, 18:61–65.

13. Stanciu C, Cijevschi C, Stan M, Sandulescu E: **Endoscopic Intravascular Esophageal Pressure Measurements in Cirrhotic Patients: Response to Metoclopramide.** *Hepatogastroenterology* 1993, 40:173–175.

14. Brewer TG: **Treatment of Acute Gastroesophageal Variceal**
•• **Hemorrhage.** *Med Clin North Am* 1993, 77:993–1014.
A comprehensive review of the treatment of acute variceal hemorrhage including pharmacologic, endoscopic, and surgical management strategies.

15. Teres J, Bosch J, Bordas JM, Pagan JCG, Feu F, Cirera I,
•• Rhodes J: **Propranolol Versus Sclerotherapy in Preventing Variceal Rebleeding: A Randomized Controlled Trial.** *Gastroenterology* 1993, 105:1508–1514.
This excellent trial confirmed the efficacy of sclerotherapy in preventing rebleeding after first variceal hemorrhage versus propranolol but demonstrated no other differences in important outcomes such as hospitalization, survival, or causes of death.

16. Chan AWC, Chung SCS, Sung JY, Leung JWC, Li AKC: **A Double-Blind Randomized Controlled Trial Comparing Sodium Tetradecyl Sulfate and Ethanolamine Oleate in the Sclerotherapy of Bleeding Oesophageal Varices.** *Endoscopy* 1993, 25:513–517.

17. Parikh SS, Amarapurkar DN, Dhawan PS, Kalro RH, Desai HG: **Development of Pleural Effusion After Sclerotherapy With Absolute Alcohol.** *Gastrointest Endosc* 1993, 39:404–405.

18. Heaton ND, Howard ER: **Complications and Limitations of**
• **Injection Sclerotherapy in Portal Hypertension.** *Gut* 1993, 34:7–10.
An overview of the previous trials utilizing EVS and the numerous sclerotherapy-associated complications.

19. Miyoshi H, Matasumoto A, Umegaki E, Oka M, Hirata I, Oshhiba S: **Endoscopic Evaluation of the Therapeutic Effect of Sclerotherapy for Esophageal Varices.** *Gastrointest Endosc* 1993, 39:37–42.

20. Japanese Research Society for Portal Hypertension: **The General Rules for Recording Endoscopic Finding on Esophageal Varices.** *Jpn J Surg* 1980, 10:84–86.

21. Pugh S, Lewis S, Smith PM: **Bleeding Oesophageal Varices in Alcoholic Cirrhosis: Long-Term Follow-Up of Endoscopic Sclerotherapy.** *Q J Med* 1993, 86:241–245.

22. Kokawa H, Shijo H, Kubara K, Nakaoka K, Toriya H, Shirai Z, Okazaki M: **Long-Term Risk Factors for Bleeding After First Course of Endsocopic Injection Sclerotherapy: A Univariate and Multivariate Analysis.** *Am J Gastroenterol* 1993, 88:1206–1211.

23. Van Steigmann G, Cambre T, Sun JH: **A New Endoscopic Elastic Band Ligating Device.** *Gastrointest Endosc* 1986, 32:230–233.

24. Markes RD, Arnold MD, Baron TH: **Gross and Microscopic Findings in the Human Esophagus After Esophageal Variceal Band Ligation: A Postmortem Analysis.** *Am J Gastroenterol* 1993, 88:272–274.

25. Hashizume M, Ohta M, Ueno K, Tomikawa M, Kitano S, Sugimachi K: **A Transparent Endoscopic Elastic Band Ligating Device.** *Gastrointest Endosc* 1993, 39:686–688.

26. Reveille RM, Goff JS, Stiegmann GV, Stauffer JT: **Combination Endoscopic Variceal Ligation (EVL) and Low Volume Endoscopic Sclerotherapy (ES) for Bleeding Esophageal Varices: A Faster Route to Variceal Eradication? [Abstract]** *Gastrointest Endosc* 1991, 37:243.

27. Stiegmann GV, Goff JS, Michaeltz-Onody PA, Korula J, Lieberman D, Saeed ZA, Reveille M, Sun JH, Lowenstein SR: **Endoscopic Sclerotherapy as Compared With Endoscopic Ligation for Bleeding Esophageal Varices.** *N Engl J Med* 1992, 326:1527–1532.

28. Berkelhammer C, Madhav G, Lyon S, Roberts J: **"Pinch" Injury During Overtube Placement in Upper Endoscopy.** *Gastrointest Endosc* 1993, 39:186–198.

29. Johnson PA, Campbell DR, Antonson CW, Weston AP, Schuler FN, Lozoff RD: **Complications Associated With Endoscopic Band Ligation of Esophageal Varices.** *Gastrointest Endosc* 1993, 39:181–185.

30. Saltzman JR, Arora S: **Complications of Esophageal Band Ligation.** *Gastrointest Endosc* 1993, 39:185–186.

31. Laine L, El-Newihi HM, Migokovshy B, Sloane R, Garcia F:
•• **Endoscopic Ligation Compared With Sclerotherapy for the Treatment of Bleeding Esophageal Varices.** *Ann Intern Med* 1993, 119:1–7.
The second randomized controlled trial comparing EVS to EBL that demonstrated fewer complications and more rapid variceal eradication and a tendency toward less frequent rebleeding in patients treated with EBL versus EVS. There were no differences between the treatment groups regarding patient survival.

32. Gimson AES, Ramage JK, Panos MZ, Hayllar K, Harrison
•• PM, Williams R, Westaby D: **Randomized Trial of Variceal Banding Ligation Versus Injection Sclerotherapy for Bleeding Esophageal Varices.** *Lancet* 1993, 342:391–394.
The third randomized controlled trial comparing EVS to EBL that demonstrated lower rebleeding rates and more rapid variceal eradication with EBL. Efficacy, complications, and survival were similar between the two groups; however 19 of 103 patients were withdrawn from the study for a variety of reasons including orthotopic liver transplantation [n=8].

33. Hashizume M, Masayuki O, Ueno K, Tanoeu K, Kitano S, Sugimachi K: **Endoscopic Ligation of Esophageal Varices Compared With Injection Sclerotherapy: A Prospective Randomized Trial.** *Gastrointest Endosc* 1993, 39:123–126.

34. Young MF, Sanowski RA, Rasche R: **Comparison and Characterization of Ulcerations Induced by Endoscopic Ligation of Esophageal Varices Versus Endoscopic Sclerotherapy.** *Gastrointest Endosc* 1993, 39:119–122.

35. LaBerge JM, Ring EJ, Gordon RL, Lake JR, Doherty MM,
•• Somberg KA, Roberts JP, Ascher NL: **Creation of Transjugular Intrahepatic Portosystemic Shunts With the Wallstent Endoprosthesis: Results in 100 Patients.** *Radiology* 1993, 187:413–420.
Report on the first 100 patients undergoing TIPS, including 97 patients with variceal bleeding. Successful shunt placement was possible in 96%. Variceal rebleeding occurred in 10 patients and was always associated with either stent thrombosis or stenosis. New or worsened encephalopathy was controlled with lactulose in 14 of 17 patients.

36. Helton WS, Belshaw A, Althaus S, Park S, Coldwell D, Jo-
•• hansen K: **Critical Appraisal of the Angiographic Portacaval Shunt (TIPS).** *Am J Surg* 1993, 165:566–571.

An extensive retrospective review of 59 patients undergoing TIPS including well-documented complications, failures, and economic impact. Active bleeding at the time of TIPS was strongly associated with in-hospital mortality [$P<0.0001$].

37. Simpson KJ, Chalmers N, Redhead DN, Finlayson NDC, Bouchier IAD, Hayes PC: **Transjugular Intrahepatic Portosystemic Shunting for Control for Acute and Recurrent Upper Gastrointestinal Haemorrhage Related to Portal Hypertension.** *Gut* 1993, **34**:968–973.

38. Iwatsuki S, Starzl TE, Todo S, Gordon RD, Tzakis AG, Marsh JW, Makowka L: **Liver Transplantation in the Treatment of Bleeding Esophageal Varices.** *Surgery* 1988, **104**:697–705.

39. Rikkers LF, Jin G, Burnett DA, Buchi KN, Cormier RA: **Shunt Surgery Versus Sclerotherapy for Variceal Hemorrhage: Late Results of a Randomized Trial.** *Am J Surg* 1993, **165**:27–33.

40. Triger DR, Johnson AG, Brazier JE, Johnston GW, Spencer EFA, McKee R, Anderson JR, Carter DC: **A Prospective Trial of Endoscopic Sclerotherapy v Oesophageal Transection and Gastric Devascularization in the Long Term Management of Bleeding Oesophageal Varices.** *Gut* 1992, **33**:1553–1558.

41. Mercado MA, Takahashi T, Orozco H: **An Alternative Low Risk Technique for Esophageal Transection in the Sugiura-Futagawa Procedure.** *Am Surgeon* 1993, **59**:461–464.

42. Gusberg RJ: **Selective Shunts in Selected Older Cirrhotic Patients With Variceal Hemorrhage.** *Am J Surg* 1993, **166**:274–278.

43. Lewis WD, Sanchez H, Jenkins RL: **Indications and Technique for the Use of the Porto-Renal Shunt in the Treatment of Variceal Hemorrhage.** *Am J Surg* 1993, **165**:336–340.

44. Ho KS, Lashner BA, Emond JC, Baker AL: **Prior Esophageal Bleeding Does Not Adversely Affect Survial After Orthotropic Liver Transplantation.** *Hepatology* 1993, **18**:66–72.

45. Hayes PC, Davis JM, Lewis JA, Bouchier IAD: **Meta-Analysis of the Value of Propranolol in Prevention of Variceal Haemorrhage.** *Lancet* 1990, **336**:153–156.

46. Poynard T, Cales P, Pasta L, Ideo G, Pascal J-P, Pagliaro L, Lebrec D, Franco-Italian Multicentric Study Group: **Beta-Adrenergic-Antagonist Drugs in the Preventions of Gastrointestinal Bleeding in Patients With Cirrhosis and Esophageal Varices. An Analysis of Data and Prognostic Factors From 589 Patients From Four Randomized Clinical Trials.** *N Engl J Med* 1991, **324**:1532–1538.

47. Angelico M, Carli L, Piat C, Gentile S, Rinaldi V, Bologna E, Capocaccia L: **Isosorbide-5-Mononitrate Versus Propranolol in the Prevention of First Bleeding in Cirrhosis.** *Gastroenterology* 1993, **104**:1460–1465.

48. Potzi R, Bauer P, Schofl R, Reichel W, Kerstan E, Renner F, Gangl A: **Prophylactic Endoscopic Sclerotherapy of Esophageal Varices in Liver Cirrhosis - Long Term Follow-Up of a Multicenter Prospective Controlled Trial in Vienna.** *Endoscopy* 1993, **25**:287–289.

49. • Van Thiel DH, Dindzans VJ, Schade RR, Rabinovitz M, Gavalier JS: **Prophylactic Versus Emergency Sclerotherapy of Large Esophageal Varices Prior to Liver Transplantation.** *Dig Dis Sci* 1993, **38**:1505–1510.

A large study suggesting that prophylactic EVS in patients with large esophageal varices improves the patients chances of surviving to liver transplant by preventing variceal hemorrhage and resulting liver failure.

50. Anireddy D, Timberlake G, Seibert D: **Dieulafoy's Lesion of the Esophagus.** *Gastrointest Endosc* 1993, **39**:604.

51. Rabago L, Mora P, Gea F, Martinez P, Ruiperez J, Campos R: **An Unusual Source of Gastrointestinal Bleeding From the Esophagus: Two New Cases of Esophageal Visible Vessel.** *Endoscopy* 1993, **25**:197–198.

52. Moreto M, Ojembarrena E, Zabella M, Tanago JG, Ibanez S: **Idiopathic Acute Esophageal Necrosis: Not Necessarily a Terminal Event.** *Endoscopy* 1993, **25**:534–538.

53. Vehling-Kaiser U, Schleuning M, Kueffer G, Jauch KW, Kaiser E: **Lusorian Artery Lesion as a Rare Cause of Severe Upper Gastrointestinal Tract Bleeding.** *Dig Dis Sci* 1993, **38**:178–180.

54. Sen A, Lea RE: **Spontaneous Esophageal Hematoma: A Review of the Difficult Diagnosis.** *Ann R Coll Phys Surg* 1993, **75**:293–295.

55. Furukawa H, Hara T, Taniguchi T, Tetsu O: **A Case of Spontaneous Intramural of the Esophagus.** *Gastroenterol Jpn* 1993, **28**:81–87.

Whitney F. Jones, MD, and Norman E. Marcon, MD, Division of Gastroenterology, The Centre for Advanced Therapeutic Endoscopy and Endoscopic Oncology, The Wellesley Hospital, 160 Wellesley Street East, Toronto, Ontario, M4Y 1J3, Canada.

Barrett's esophagus

Stuart Jon Spechler, MD

Beth Israel Hospital and Harvard Medical School, Boston, Massachusetts, USA

Barrett's esophagus is the major recognized risk factor for adenocarcinoma of the gastroesophageal junction, a tumor whose incidence has been increasing dramatically in the United States and Europe. Carcinogenesis in Barrett's esophagus involves genetic alterations that may activate protooncogenes and disable tumor suppresoor genes. Unlike the colon, in which losss of chromosome 5q is an early event in carcinogenesis that usually precedes deletion of chromosome 17p, recent data suggest that 17p loss usually precedes 5q deletion during the development of adenocarcinoma in Barrett's epithelium. In an attempt to prevent these tumors, several groups of investigators have used laser irradiation to obliterate Barrett's epithelim. The irradiated mucosa heals with the regrowth of squamous epithelium, provided acid reflux is controlled by the administration of omeprazole. Further studies are necessary before laser photoablation of Barrett's epithelium can be recommended for widespread clinical application.

Current Opinion In Gastroenterology 1994, **10:**448–454

Pathogenesis

In most tissues that exhibit epithelial metaplasia, such as the uterine cervix and respiratory tract, stratified squamous mucosa replaces an inflamed columnar epithelium. Contrary to this common pattern, epithelial metaplasia in the esophagus usually involves the replacement of damaged squamous mucosa by columnar epithelium. The resulting condition is called Barrett's esophagus. In the transformation zone of the uterine cervix, the area that undergoes squamous metaplasia, scanning electron microscopy has revealed a distinctive cell that has surface characteristics of both squamous and columnar cells. Shields *et al.* [1•] have discovered a similar cell at the squamo-columnar junction in Barrett's esophagus. Scanning electron microscopic evaluation of endoscopic biopsies obtained from the junction area revealed a distinctive cell that had both microvilli (a feature of columnar cells) and intercellular ridges (a feature of squamous cells) on its surface. The distinctive cell was not found in any biopsy specimen taken from the squamo-columnar junctions of 14 patients who had no Barrett's epithelium. The authors speculated that the distinctive cell might represent an intermediate step in either the development or regression of Barrett's epithelium.

Barrett's esophagus usually develops in the setting of chronic gastroesophageal reflux disease (GERD). Some reports have alleged that Barrett's metaplasia also is a frequent consequence of long-term chemotherapy with drugs that injure the esophageal squamous epithelium such as cytoxan, methotrexate, and 5-fluorouracil. This contention has been challenged by Peters *et al.* [2•], who performed endoscopic examinations looking for Barrett's esophagus in 20 men who had been treated with combination chemotherapy for testicular cancer, and in 18 women who had received combination chemotherapy for the treatment of breast cancer. Only one of the men and none of the women had Barrett's esophagus apparent on endoscopic examination. Although further investigations are needed to determine the precise frequency and importance of chemotherapy-induced Barrett's esophagus, this study and others suggest that Barrett's metaplasia is not a common sequela of long-term chemotherapy.

In some cases, Barrett's esophagus appears to be a familial disorder. Fahmy and King [3•] have described four families with a high prevalence of Barrett's esophagus. In at least three of the four families, the pattern of involvement was consistent with an autosomal dominant mode of inheritance. The frequency of familial Barrett's esophagus remains to be determined.

Barrett's esophagus and even adenocarcinoma clearly can affect children. Hassall *et al.* [4•] have reported the case of a 17-year-old, neurologically handicapped boy who had an esophagectomy for adenocarcinoma in a Barrett's esophagus lined extensively by special-

Abbreviations

EGF-r—epidermal growth factor receptor; **GERD**—gastroesophageal reflux disease.

 ISBN 1-85922-609-4 ISSN 0267–1379

ized columnar epithelium. Hassall has also written two excellent review articles on Barrett's esophagus in children [5•,6•].

Alkaline reflux

The reflux of duodenal contents such as bile and pancreatic enzymes may contribute to esophagitis in patients with Barrett's esophagus. Some investigators have used esophageal pH monitoring to estimate the frequency of duodenoesophageal reflux, assuming that a rise in esophageal pH above 7 might indicate the reflux of alkaline duodenal contents.

Attwood *et al.* [7•] used esophageal pH monitoring to seek alkaline reflux in 26 patients with Barrett's esophagus, 10 of whom had complications of GERD, including esophageal ulceration and stricture. Esophageal acid exposure (the percent of the monitoring period that esophageal pH was <4) in the 10 patients with complicated disease (19.2%) did not differ significantly from that in the 16 patients without complications (19.3%). In contrast, esophageal alkaline exposure (the percent of the monitoring period that esophageal pH was >7) was significantly greater in the patients with GERD complications (24.2%) than in the uncomplicated cases (8.4%). The temporal correlation observed between gastric and esophageal alkaline events suggested that the material raising the esophageal pH was not swallowed saliva, but duodenal juice that passed through the stomach on its way to the esophagus. The authors concluded that reflux of duodenal contents may contribute to the inflammatory complications of GERD in Barrett's esophagus.

A similar study by Stein *et al.* [8•] concluded as well that patients with Barrett's esophagus had significantly more "alkaline reflux" than control subjects without Barrett's epithelium. A contrary opinion was expressed by Singh *et al.* [9•], however, who also used esophageal pH monitoring to study "alkaline reflux" in 10 patients with Barrett's esophagus. Although esophageal pH rose to levels above 7 in study patients during the day, no such pH elevations occurred during sleep when salivation ceased. These observations and others suggest that most episodes of "alkaline reflux" in patients with Barrett's esophagus were not due to the reflux of duodenal contents, but were rather the result of swallowing alkaline saliva. Presently, esophageal pH monitoring appears to be an insensitive and nonspecific test for duodenoesophageal reflux. The contribution of such reflux to the pathogenesis of Barrett's esophagus and its complications remains unclear.

A report by Pera *et al.* [10•] suggests that the reflux of pancreatic and biliary secretions may contribute to carcinogenesis in Barrett's esophagus. These investigators previously had shown that rats treated with the carcinogen 2,6-dimethylnitrosomorpholine developed esophageal adenocarcinomas only when the esophagus was exposed chronically to duodenal contents containing both pancreatic and biliary secretions [11]. To study the relative contribution of these elements to carcinogenesis, the investigators observed the effects of 2,6-dimethylnitrosomorpholine in rats treated surgically so that their esophagi were exposed to pancreatic secretions alone, to biliary secretions alone, or to both pancreatic and biliary secretions. Carcinoma of the esophagus was observed in three of 22 rats (13%) exposed to pancreatic secretions alone and in nine of 27 rats (33%) exposed to both pancreatic and biliary secretions. In contrast, none of 28 rats exposed only to biliary secretions developed esophageal cancer. These findings suggest that exposure to pancreatic secretions may be necessary to induce esophageal cancer in this animal preparation. Exposure to biliary secretions alone may not be sufficient to induce carcinogenesis, but these secretions seem to exert a co-carcinogenic effect.

A report by Jankowski *et al.* [12•] supports the possibility that alkaline reflux contributes to carcinogenesis in Barrett's esophagus. These investigators described two patients with Barrett's esophagus in whom gastric secretory studies documented the development of achlorhydria over a period of years. Both patients also developed high-grade dysplasia in Barrett's epithelium. Flow-cytometric analyses for epidermal growth factor receptor (EGF-r) revealed increased EGF-r expression in the dysplastic Barrett's epithelium compared with normal gastric cardiac epithelium and with Barrett's epithelium without dysplasia. The authors speculated that the reflux of bile and pancreatic juice in these achlorhydric patients somehow contributed to the pathogenesis of dysplasia in the Barrett's epithelium.

Expression of sucrase-isomaltase

Barrett's specialized columnar epithelium appears to be a form of incomplete intestinal metaplasia. The metaplastic epithelium contains a heterogeneous population of columnar cells that can resemble intestinal absorptive cells morphologically. Ultrastructurally, biochemically, and functionally, however, the specialized columnar cells of Barrett's esophagus have been shown to differ from normal intestinal absorptive cells. One earlier study [13] found that specialized columnar cells lacked the disaccharidase activity characteristic of normal intestinal absorptive cells.

Wu *et al.* [14•] used reverse transcription polymerase chain reaction techniques to seek expression of the messenger RNA for the intestinal sucrase-isomaltase disaccharidase in Barrett's epithelium and in Barrett's adenocarcinomas. Messenger RNA for sucrase-isomaltase was identified in 76% of specimens of Barrett's epithelium and in 82% of specimens of adenocarcinoma. Immunohistochemical study showed that sucrase-isomaltase protein was located primarily on the apical membrane of the specialized columnar cells, whereas the protein was found primarily in the cytoplasm of Barrett's adenocarcinoma cells. This study shows that columnar cells of Barrett's specialized epithelium and adenocarcinoma do express sucrase-isomaltase, contrary to the popular notion.

Epidemiology of adenocarcinoma

Adenocarcinoma of the gastroesophageal junction continues to increase in frequency at an alarming rate. Blot *et al.* [15••] analyzed data from the Surveillance, Epidemiology, and End Results program of the National Cancer Institute on adenocarcinoma of the gastroesophageal junction in the United States for the years 1988 to 1990. The annual age-adjusted incidence rate for esophageal adenocarcinoma in white men during this period was 2.5 per 100,000, a rate threefold higher than that observed during the years 1976 to 1978. In contrast, the incidence rate for esophageal squamous cell carcinoma declined by 23% over the same period. Adenocarcinoma of the esophagus affected white men four times more frequently than black men (4:1), and white men were affected seven times more often than white women (7:1). The annual incidence rate for adenocarcinoma of the gastroesophageal junction (including adenocarcinoma of the esophagus and adenocarcinoma of the gastric cardia) was 5.8 per 100,000. Adenocarcinoma of the esophagus now accounts for 50% of all esophageal malignancies in the United States, and adenocarcinoma of the gastroesophageal junction now ranks among the top 15 cancers affecting white men in this country.

A report from the Mayo Clinic [16•] also documents a dramatic rise in the incidence of adenocarcinomas of the gastroesophageal junction. Pera *et al.* reviewed medical records and histology slides on patients with these tumors who resided in Olmsted County, Minnesota. The incidence of adenocarcinoma of the gastroesophageal junction during the years 1974 to 1989 was more than sixfold greater than that found during the period from 1935 to 1971. During this same interval, the incidence of squamous cell carcinoma in this predominantly white population declined.

The cause of the dramatic rise in the frequency of adenocarcinomas in Barrett's esophagus is not known. Two groups recently have tried to identify risk factors for these tumors [17•,18•]. Menke-Pluymers *et al.* [17•] conducted a retrospective, case-control study in 96 patients with benign Barrett's esophagus and 62 patients with Barrett's adenocarcinoma to evaluate the importance of cigarette smoking, alcohol consumption, and extent of Barrett's epithelium as risk factors for malignancy. The risk of adenocarcinoma was associated significantly with the extent of Barrett's epithelium and with cigarette smoking, but not with alcohol consumption.

Gray *et al.* [18•] compared the cigarette smoking and alcohol consumption histories of 58 patients with benign Barrett's esophagus, 23 patients with adenocarcinoma in Barrett's esophagus, and 24 patients who had severe esophagitis without Barrett's epithelium. The smoking and drinking habits of the patients with adenocarcinoma in Barrett's esophagus did not differ significantly from those of the patients with severe esophagitis. Interestingly, however, tobacco and alcohol use were significantly less common in patients with benign Barrett's esophagus than in patients with Barrett's adenocarcinomas. The authors concluded that neither cigarette smoking nor alcohol use predisposed to the development of Barrett's esophagus in patients with reflux esophagitis. In patients with established Barrett's esophagus, however, both cigarettes and alcohol appeared to be risk factors for the development of adenocarcinoma.

Carcinogenesis

In a number of tissues, cancers appear to evolve through a sequence of genetic alterations that disable tumor suppressor genes such as the *APC* (adenomatous polyposis coli), *MCC* (mutated in colon cancer), and *p53* genes. The *APC* and *MCC* genes are located on chromosome 5q, whereas chromosome 17p harbors the *p53* gene. Allelic losses of 5q and 17p often are found in adenocarcinomas of the colon and esophagus. During carcinogenesis in the colon, loss of a 5q allele appears to be a relatively early event that usually precedes 17p allelic deletions.

The study of Blount *et al.* [19•] suggests that carcinogenesis in Barrett's esophagus involves the opposite sequence of allelic losses. The investigators studied esophageal specimens obtained from 29 patients who had Barrett's esophagus with high-grade dysplasia, adenocarcinoma, or both. DNA-content cell-sorting techniques were used to isolate 38 aneuploid cell populations (cells with an abnormal amount of DNA) from 14 patients, and the aneuploid cells were evaluated for losses of the 5q and 17p alleles using polymerase chain reaction techniques. Only 17p allelic losses (without 5q losses) were detected in aneuploid cells from three patients, whereas four patients exhibited both 17p and 5q allelic losses in all of their aneuploid cell populations. The remaining seven patients had two types of aneuploid cell populations: those with 17p losses only, and those with losses of both 17p and 5q. No aneuploid cell population from any patient had only 5q allelic deletions without loss of 17p. These findings suggest that 17p allelic losses usually precede 5q losses during carcinogenesis in Barrett's esophagus.

When cells that have an unstable genome enter the cell cycle and proliferate, clones of cells can emerge having acquired genetic errors endowing them with proliferative advantages. Cancers can evolve when these cells proliferate and acquire further genetic abnormalities that enable them to invade adjacent tissues and proliferate in unnatural locations. The nature of the abnormalities in the cell cycle that contribute to carcinogenesis in Barrett's esophagus have not been well defined.

Reid *et al.* [20•] studied cell cycle abnormalities in Barrett's epithelium using a multiparameter flow cytometric assay that assessed DNA content in cells recognized by Ki67, a monoclonal antibody that labels proliferating cells. Biopsy specimens of control gastric epithelia had low fractions of proliferating cells. In contrast, Ki67-positive G_1 fractions were increased in specimens of Barrett's specialized columnar epithelium. Biopsy specimens of Barrett's epithelium with dysplasia and adenocarcinoma often had aneuploid cell populations, increased S-phase fractions, or both. The authors concluded that carcinogenesis in Barrett's esophagus involves at least three types of cell cycle abnormalities: 1) mobilization of cells from the quiescent G_0 phase into the active G_1 phase of the cell cycle, 2) loss of control of the transition from the G_1 phase to the S phase wherein DNA is synthesized, and 3) accumulation of cells in the G_2 phase from where they can undergo mitosis.

In order for cells to progress through the cell cycle, there must be an adequate supply of polyamines such as putrescine, spermidine, and spermine. These polyamines facilitate DNA replication, and appear to enhance both the transcription of DNA to messenger RNA and the translation of messenger RNA to protein. Increased mucosal activity of ornithine decarboxylase, the rate-limiting enzyme in polyamine synthesis, has been described in patients with dysplasia in Barrett's epithelium.

Gray *et al.* [21•] studied polyamine content in endoscopic biopsy specimens obtained from the esophagus and stomach of patients with Barrett's epithelium and Barrett's adenocarcinoma. Nondysplastic, dysplastic, and malignant Barrett's epithelium could not be distinguished by the total mucosal content of polyamines, or by the mucosal content of individual polyamines. This study suggests that mucosal polyamine content is not a useful biomarker for malignant potential in Barrett's epithelium.

Dysplasia

As discussed, cancers in Barrett's esophagus evolve through a sequence of genetic alterations in the cells of the metaplastic epithelium. Before these genetic alterations render the cells frankly malignant, the DNA abnormalities often cause morphologic changes recognizable on histologic examination as dysplasia. In patients found to have Barrett's esophagus with high-grade dysplasia on initial endoscopic examination, a number of earlier reports have suggested that esophageal resection might reveal an invasive malignancy (missed by endoscopic biopsy) in approximately one third.

Levine *et al.* [22••] have reported that they can differentiate high-grade dysplasia from early adenocarcinoma in Barrett's esophagus by adherence to a rigorous endoscopic biopsy protocol. The investigators obtained four-quadrant "jumbo" biopsy specimens at 2-cm intervals throughout the columnar-lined esophagus, and took many additional samples from sites of known dysplasia. After preoperative evaluation by this protocol, none of seven patients who had an esophageal resection for high-grade dysplasia in Barrett's epithelium was found to have invasive cancer in the resected specimens. For each of those seven patients, 29 to 185 preoperative biopsy specimens were available for review. One patient had 185 biopsy specimens obtained during 5 preoperative endoscopies in a period of 10 months from a segment of Barrett's epithelium that spanned only 3 cm, *ie,* more than 60 biopsies per centimeter of metaplastic mucosa. The authors also described 29 patients with high-grade dysplasia who had no esophageal resection and were followed for 2 to 46 months. Seven of those 29 patients (24%) were found to have invasive cancer during the follow-up period, whereas the other 22 had no apparent progression to malignancy. This study shows that adherence to a very rigorous biopsy protocol for patients with high-grade dysplasia might exclude a synchronous malignancy with reasonable certainty, but the risk for developing invasive cancer appears to remain high.

Laser therapies

Two groups of investigators have used laser irradiation to obliterate Barrett's epithelium while administering omeprazole to inhibit gastric acid secretion [23••,24•]. With no acid reflux to stimulate metaplastic repair, they reasoned, the damaged esophageal tissue might heal normally, *ie,* by regeneration of squamous mucosa. Berenson *et al.* [23••] tested this hypothesis in 10 men with longstanding Barrett's esophagus. During multiple endoscopic examinations, one to 8 segments of Barrett's epithelium with areas ranging from 0.25 cm^2 to 4.00 cm^2 were irradiated using an argon laser until the treated segments turned white. Omeprazole therapy (40 mg every day) was begun 2 weeks before the first laser treatment, and was continued for the duration of the study (6 to 38 weeks). In 38 of 40 laser-treated segments, squamous mucosa completely or partially replaced the photoablated Barrett's epithelium. To achieve these results, patients had three to 12 endoscopic examinations during which each treated segment was irradiated on one to 6 occasions. Except for transient pain in the retrosternal area, there were no complications of the laser treatments. Using a neodymium:yttrium-aluminum garnet laser, Sampliner *et al.* [24•] also described successful photoablation of Barrett's epithelium in a 76-year-old man.

Although these reports document the feasibility of laser ablation of Barrett's epithelium, they do not establish the benefit of the technique. In an editorial, Spechler [25•] pointed out that the procedure is costly and entails some risk, and it is not clear that photoablation reduces the incidence of esophageal cancer. Also, it is not known whether life-long, intensive acid suppression will be necessary to prevent the return of columnar epithelium. Further studies addressing these issues are necessary before laser ablation of Barrett's epithelium can be recommended for clinical application.

Another potential application for laser treatment in Barrett's esophagus is for photodynamic therapy of neoplasms. In this therapy, patients are given a systemic dose of a light-activated drug (porphyrin) that is concentrated in the neoplastic tissues. These tissues then are irradiated with laser light, stimulating the porphyrin to produce singlet oxygen that can destroy the neoplastic cells.

Overholt *et al.* [26•] have described two patients with early adenocarcinomas in Barrett's esophagus who were treated with photodynamic therapy. In one patient, photodynamic therapy seemed to obliterate the primary adenocarcinoma, but cancer appeared 15 months later in a region 5 cm above the treated area. Another course of photodynamic therapy seemed to eradicate the second neoplasm, but the treatment was complicated by the development of an esophageal stricture. Another patient had photodynamic therapy without complication and with apparent obliteration of the adenocarcinoma, but high-grade dysplasia was noted in the remaining Barrett's epithelium. The duration of follow-up in both cases was too short to allow meaningful conclusions regarding whether photodynamic therapy was curative.

Cancer surveillance

Patients with Barrett's esophagus commonly are advised to have regular endoscopic surveillance under the assumption that early detection of esophageal neoplasia will reduce their morbidity and mortality from esophageal cancer. This assumption is unproved, however, and the cost-effectiveness of endoscopic surveillance is hotly debated. The study of Streitz *et al.* [27•] provides some support for the practice of endoscopic surveillance in Barrett's esophagus. These investigators reviewed their experience with 77 patients who had adenocarcinoma in Barrett's esophagus. In 58 patients, Barrett's esophagus was discovered when they came to the hospital for the evaluation of esophageal cancer. The other 19 patients had adenocarcinoma discovered during endoscopic surveillance for known Barrett's esophagus. The patients whose cancer was discovered during endoscopic surveillance had tumors in an earlier stage of development (58% stages 0 or 1) than those who presented to the hospital with esophageal cancer (17% stages 0 or 1, $P=0.006$). The 5-year actuarial survival in the surveillance group (62%) also was significantly better than in the patients who presented with cancer (20%, $P=0.007$). Although this retrospective study does not prove that endoscopic surveillance reduces the morbidity and mortality from cancer in Barrett's esophagus, it does show that surveillance can detect early, curable esophageal neoplasms.

In an editorial, Richter [28•] suggests an alternative to costly endoscopic surveillance for patients with Barrett's esophagus. He reviews data indicating that brush cytology is a useful diagnostic test for neoplasia in Barrett's epithelium, and suggests that blind (not endoscopically directed) cytologic sampling of the esophagus might be an inexpensive and effective alternative to endoscopic surveillance. Data on the efficacy of cytology as a test for neoplasia in Barrett's esophagus are derived primarily from studies that used endoscopically directed brush cytology techniques, however. It is not clear that these data can be extrapolated reliably to predict the efficacy of blind cytologic sampling of Barrett's esophagus. Nevertheless, Richter's proposal clearly warrants investigation.

References and recommended reading

Papers of particular interest, published within the annual period of review, have been highlighted as:
- • Of special interest
- •• Of outstanding interest

1. • Shields HM, Zwas F, Antonioli DA, Doos WG, Kim S, Spechler SJ: **Detection by Scanning Electron Microscopy of a Distinctive Esophageal Surface Cell at the Junction of Squamous and Barrett's Epithelium.** *Dig Dis Sci* 1993, **38**:97–108.

Scanning electron microscopic evaluation of biopsies obtained from the squamocolumnar junction in Barrett's esophagus revealed a distinctive cell that had both microvilli (a feature of columnar cells) and intercellular ridges (a feature of squamous cells) on its surface.

2. • Peters FTM, Sleijfer DT, Imhoff GWV, Kleibeuker JH: **Is Chemotherapy Associated With Development of Barrett's Esophagus?** *Dig Dis Sci* 1993, **38**:923–926.

This study suggests that Barrett's metaplasia is not a common sequela of chronic chemotherapy.

3. • Fahmy N, King JF: **Barrett's Esophagus: An Acquired Condition With Genetic Predisposition.** *Am J Gastroenterol* 1993, **88**:1262–1265.

Four families with a high prevalence of Barrett's esophagus are described. The pattern of involvement suggests that Barrett's esophagus may have been inherited as an autosomal dominant trait.

4. • Hassall E, Dimmick JE, Magee JF: **Adenocarcinoma in Childhood Barrett's Esophagus: Case Documentation and the Need for Surveillance in Children.** *Am J Gastroenterol* 1993, **88**:282–288.

This report describes a 17-year-old, neurologically handicapped boy who underwent an esophagectomy for adenocarcinoma in a Barrett's esophagus.

5. • Hassall E: **Barrett's Esophagus: New Definitions and Approaches in Children.** *J Pediatr Gastroenterol Nutr* 1993, **16**:345–364.

An excellent review article on pediatric Barrett's esophagus.

6. • Hassall E: **Barrett's Esophagus: Congenital or Acquired?** *Am J Gastroenterol* 1993, **88**:819–824.

This report reviews published data that support either a congenital or acquired pathogenesis for Barrett's esophagus. The author concludes that Barrett's esophagus is usually acquired as a sequela of GERD, but that there may be a congenital predisposition to develop Barrett's epithelium in response to reflux esophagitis.

7. • Attwood SEA, Ball CS, Barlow AP, Jenkinson L, Norris TL, Watson A: **Role of Intragastric and Intraesophageal Alkalinisation in the Genesis of Complications in Barrett's Columnar Lined Lower Oesophagus.** *Gut* 1993, **34**:11–15.

In 26 patients with Barrett's esophagus, esophageal alkaline exposure (the percent of the pH monitoring period that esophageal pH was greater than 7) was significantly greater in the 10 patients with GERD complications (24.2% of the monitoring period) than in the 16 uncomplicated cases (8.4% of the monitoring period).

8. • Stein HJ, Hoeft S, DeMeester TR: **Functional Foregut Abnormalities in Barrett's Esophagus.** *J Thorac Cardiovasc Surg* 1993, **105**:107–111.

By 24-hour esophageal pH monitoring, patients with Barrett's esophagus were found to have increased esophageal exposure to acid and alkali compared with subjects who had reflux esophagitis without Barrett's epithelium.

9. • Singh S, Bradley A, Richter JE: **Determinants of Oesophageal "Alkaline" pH Environment in Controls and Patients With Gastro-oesophageal Reflux Disease.** *Gut* 1993, 34:309–316.

Most elevations of esophageal pH greater than 7 in patients with Barrett's esophagus appeared to be due to the swallowing of alkaline saliva rather than the reflux of duodenal contents.

10. • Pera M, Trastek VF, Carpenter HA, Fernandez PL, Cardesa A, Mohr U, Pairolero PC: **Influence of Pancreatic and Biliary Reflux on the Development of Esophageal Carcinoma.** *Ann Thorac Surg* 1993, **55**:1386–1393.

After treatment with a carcinogen, carcinoma of the esophagus was observed in three of 22 rats (13%) exposed to pancreatic secretions alone, and in nine of 27 rats (33%) exposed to both pancreatic and biliary secretions. In contrast, none of 28 rats exposed only to biliary secretions developed esophageal cancer.

11. Pera M, Cardesa A, Bombi JA, Ernst H, Pera C, Mohr U: **Influence of Esophagojejunostomy on the Inudction of Adenocarcinoma of the Distal Esophagus in Sprague-Dawley rats by Subcutaneous Injection of 2,6-Dimethylnitrosomorpholine.** *Cancer Res* 1989, 49:6803–6808.

12. • Jankowski J, Hopwood D, Pringle R, Wormsley KG: **Increased Expression of Epidermal Growth Factor Receptors in Barrett's Esophagus Associated With Alkaline Reflux: A Putative Model for Carcinogenesis.** *Am J Gastroenterol* 1993, **88**:402–408.

Two patients with Barrett's esophagus are described in whom gastric secretory studies documented the development of achlorhydria over a period of years. Both patients also developed high-grade dysplasia in Barrett's epithelium.

13. Berenson MM, Herbst JJ, Freston JW: **Enzyme and Ultrastructural Characteristics of Eophageal Columnar Epithelium.** *Dig Dis* 1974, **19**:895-907.

14. • Wu GD, Beer DG, Moore JH, Orringer MB, Appelman HD, Traber PG: **Sucrase-Isomaltase Gene Expression in Barrett's Esophagus and Adenocarcinoma.** *Gastroenterology* 1993, **105**:837–844.

Messenger RNA for sucrase-isomaltase was identified in 76% of biopsy specimens of Barrett's epithelium, and in 82% of specimens of Barrett's adenocarcinoma.

15. •• Blot WJ, Devesa SS, Fraumeni JF Jr: **Continuing Climb in Rates of Esophageal Adenocarcinoma: An Update.** *JAMA* 1993, **270**:1320.

Adenocarcinoma of the esophagus now accounts for 50% of all esophageal malignancies in the United States, and adenocarcinoma of the gastroesophageal junction now ranks among the top 15 cancers affecting white men in this country.

16. • Pera M, Cameron AJ, Trastek VF, Carpenter HA, Zinsmeister AR: **Increasing Incidence of Adenocarcinoma of the Esophagus and Esophagogastric Junction.** *Gastroenterology* 1993, **104**:510–513.

The incidence of adenocarcinoma of the gastroesophageal junction in Olmsted County, Minnesota during the years 1974 to 1989 was more than sixfold greater than that during the period from 1935 to 1971.

17. • Menke-Pluymers MBE, Hop WCJ, Dees J, van Blankenstein M, Tilanus HW, the Rotterdam Esophageal Tumor Study Group: **Risk Factors for the Development of an Adenocarcinoma in Columnar-Lined (Barrett) Esophagus.** *Cancer* 1993, 72:1155–1158.

The risk of adenocarcinoma in patients who had Barrett's esophagus was associated significantly with the extent of Barrett's epithelium and with cigarette smoking, but not with alcohol consumption.

18. • Gray MR, Donnelly RJ, Kingsnorth AN: **The Role of Smoking and Alcohol in Metaplasia and Cancer Risk in Barrett's Columnar Lined Oesophagus.** *Gut* 1993, 34:727–731.

Neither cigarette smoking nor alcohol use appeared to predispose to the development of Barrett's esophagus in patients with reflux esophagitis. In patients with established Barrett's esophagus, however, both cigarettes and alcohol were associated with the development of adenocarcinoma.

19. • Blount PL, Meltzer SJ, Yin J, Huang Y, Krasna MJ, Reid BJ: **Clonal Ordering of 17p and 5q Allelic Losses in Barrett Dysplasia and Adenocarcinoma.** *Proc Natl Acad Sci* 1993, **90**:3221–3225.

DNA-content cell-sorting techniques were used to isolate aneuploid cell populations from patients with high-grade dysplasia and adenocarcinoma in Barrett's esophagus, and the aneuploid cells were evaluated for losses of the 5q and 17p alleles using polymerase chain reaction techniques. 17p allelic losses appeared to precede 5q allelic losses during carcinogenesis in Barrett's esophagus.

20. • Reid BJ, Sanchez CA, Blount PL, Levine DS: **Barrett's Esophagus: Cell Cycle Abnormalities in Advancing Stages of Neoplastic Progression.** *Gastroenterology* 1993, **105**:119–129.

Cell cycle abnormalities in Barrett's epithelium were studied using a multiparameter flow cytometric assay that assessed DNA content in cells recognized by Ki67 monoclonal antibody. Biopsy specimens of control gastric epithelia had low fractions of proliferating cells, whereas Ki67-positive G_1 fractions were increased in specimens of Barrett's specialized columnar epithelium. Biopsy specimens of Barrett's epithelium with dysplasia and adenocarcinoma often had aneuploid cell populations, increased S phase fractions, or both.

21. • Gray MR, Wallace HM, Goulding H, Hoffman J, Kenyon WE, Kingsnorth AN: **Mucosal Polyamine Metabolism in the Columnar Lined Oesophagus.** *Gut* 1993, 34:584–587.

Nondysplastic, dysplastic, and malignant Barrett's epithelium could not be distinguished by the total mucosal content of polyamines or by the mucosal content of individual polyamines.

22. •• Levine DS, Haggitt RC, Blount PL, Rabinovitch PS, Rusch VW, Reid BJ: **An Endoscopic Biopsy Protocol Can Differentiate High-Grade Dysplasia from Early Adenocarcinoma in Barrett's Esophagus.** *Gastroenterology* 1993, **105**:40–50.

This study shows that adherence to a very rigorous biopsy protocol for patients with high-grade dysplasia in Barrett's esophagus might exclude a synchronous malignancy with reasonable certainty, but the risk for developing invasive cancer appears to remain high.

23. •• Berenson MM, Johnson TD, Markowitz NR, Buchi KN, Samowitz WS: **Restoration of Squamous Mucosa After Ablation of Barrett's Esophageal Epithelium.** *Gastroenterology* 1993, **104**:1686–1691.

Ten patients with Barrett's esophagus receiving long-term omeprazole therapy had endoscopic examinations during which segments of Barrett's epithelium were irradiated with laser light. In 38 of 40 laser-treated segments, squamous mucosa completely or partially replaced the photoablated Barrett's epithelium.

24. • Sampliner RE, Hixson LJ, Fennerty B, Garewal HS: **Regression of Barrett's Esophagus by Laser Ablation in an Anacid Environment.** *Dig Dis Sci* 1993, **38**:365–368.

Successful photoablation of Barrett's epithelium using an neodymium:yttrium-aluminum-garnet laser in a 76-year-old man is described.

25. Spechler SJ: **Laser Photoablation of Barrett's Epithelium:**
• **Burning Issues About Burning Tissues.** *Gastroenterology* 1993, **104**:1855–1858.

This editorial discusses the pros and cons of laser photoablation therapy for Barrett's epithelium and concludes that further studies are necessary before the technique can be recommended for clinical application.

26. Overholt B, Panjehpour M, Tefftellar E, Rose M: **Photody-**
• **namic Therapy for Treatment of Early Adenocarcinoma in Barrett's Esophagus.** *Gastrointest Endosc* 1993, 39:73–76.

Two patients with early adenocarcinomas in Barrett's esophagus who were treated with photodynamic therapy are described.

27. Streitz JM Jr, Andrews CW Jr, Ellis FH Jr: **Endoscopic Surveil-**
• **lance of Barrett's Esophagus. Does It Help?** *J Thorac Cardiovasc Surg* 1993, **105**:383–388.

Nineteen patients whose Barrett's adenocarcinoma was discovered during endoscopic surveillance had tumors in an earlier stage of development (58% stages 0 or 1) than those patients who presented to the hospital with esophageal cancer (17% stages 0 or 1, $P=0.006$). The 5-year actuarial survival in the surveillance group (62%) also was significantly better than in the patients who presented with cancer (20%, $P=0.007$).

28. Richter JE: **Endoscopic Surveillance of Barrett's Esophagus:**
• **Another Viewpoint.** *Am J Gastroenterol* 1993, **88**:630–632.

This editorial reviews data indicating that brush cytology is a useful diagnostic test for neoplasia in Barrett's epithelium, and suggests that blind (not endoscopically directed) cytologic sampling of Barrett's esophagus might be an inexpensive and effective alternative to endoscopic surveillance.

Stuart Jon Spechler, MD, Director, Center for Swallowing Disorders, Beth Israel Hospital, 330 Brookline Avenue, Boston, MA 02215, USA.

Esophageal cancer

G.N.J. Tytgat, MD

Academic Medical Center, University of Amsterdam, Amsterdam, the Netherlands

In this paper, the most important publication of 1993 with respect to all facets of esophageal cancer are summarized and put in perspective with the current state of knowledge. Columnar metaplasia and esophageal surgery, chemotherapy, and radiotherapy will not be covered as they are the subject of separate chapters. Undoubtedly, a major emphasis was given to the further unraveling at the molecular level of the complex genetic aberrations that ultimately lead to esophageal carcinogenesis. Understanding these molecular abnormalities becomes increasingly complex for the clinician. However, clinicians should be aware, albeit superficially, of these new insights because they may lead to clinically useful diagnostic and prognostic elements. It has become clear that there is an increasing need for a better subclassification of the superficial or early esophageal cancers. Currently, these cancers encompass epithelial, mucosal, and submucosal tumors. As there is already a high percentage of lymph node metastasis for submucosal tumors, true progress can only be made if malignancies are detected at the stage of epithelial or mucosal cancer. In the future, this may require an adaptation of the T system, as T1 now equals mucosal and submucosal cancer. As new techniques are being developed to treat malignancy at the level of the mucosa by nonsurgical means, it will become essential to accurately detect tumors with high-frequency endoluminal ultrasound.

Current Opinion in Gastroenterology 1994, **10**:455–464

Tumorigenesis

The nuclear phosphoprotein p53 is believed to regulate entry into and progression through the normal cell cycle, being induced during the transition from phase G0 to G1 in the cell cycle. In most adult tissues, p53 is expressed at low levels and has a very short half-life. The human *p53* gene is located on chromosome 17P13 and encodes a nuclear protein that may be vital in the regulatory control of cell proliferation. Loss of wild-type *p53* function is considered to be a key event in the induction of malignant transformation in many cancers. Frequent mutation of the *p53* gene at Exon's 5, 6, 7, and 8 have been found in a wide variety of human cancers, including esophageal squamous cell carcinoma.

Immunolocalization of the nuclear protein *p53* tumor-suppressor gene product is considered one of the best methods of detecting a mutated form of *p53*. Immunoreactive *p53* is often observed in the nuclei of tumor cells and is closely correlated with the malignant phenotype, including dysplasia; *p53* expression is not observed in histologically normal mucosa. The strong correlation of *p53* with the expression of ki67 and proliferating cellular nuclear antigen in carcinoma and in dysplastic cells, but not in normal mucosa, suggests involvement of the mutated form of *p53* in the cell cycle of malignant cells [1].

Protein p53 accumulates with increasing frequencies in proliferating cells in basal cell hyperplasia, dysplasia, carcinoma *in situ*, and ultimately full-blown carcinoma. Diffuse immunostaining occurs more frequently in more advanced lesions. The failure to detect p53 positively immunostained cells in some precancerous or cancerous lesions suggests that *p53* alteration is not an obligatory process in esophageal carcinogenesis [2•].

Allelic deletions are not exclusive to *p53* tumor-suppressor genes, but occur in a variety of other tumor-suppressor genes. Esophageal cancers frequently lose the heterozygosity within *Rb* (13q), *p53* (17p), *APC*, or *MCC* (5q) and less frequently within *DCC* (18q) loci. Deletion of at least one of these four loci takes place in 93% of tumors. These data suggest the hypothesis that loss at one locus potentiates loss at other loci sites or

Abbreviations

EGF—epidermal growth factor; **TGF**—transforming growth factor.

 ISBN 1-85922-609-4 ISSN 0267–1379

that additive deletions confer a greater growth advantage than do single losses alone. Presumably, loss of *MCC* heterozygosity will occur only if deletions of *p53*, *Rb*, or *DCC* have already occurred. Deletions of tumor-suppressor genes other than *MCC* may occur independently. Unexpectedly, there does not seem to be a significant correlation between loss of heterozygosity of *APC* and of *MCC*, even though these are closely linked loci on chromosome 5q. These findings suggest that loss of heterozygosity of *APC* occurs independently of loss of heterozygosity involving *MCC*. Why some tumors do not lose heterozygosity at any of the tumor suppressor gene loci examined awaits further study [3].

Normal function of tumor suppressor genes is thought to control growth and differentiation of cells. Because mutations of these genes are supposed to be recessive, both alleles of a particular gene should be inactivated during tumorigenesis. Whereas the first allele may be inactivated by any type of mutation of deletion, a second allele often is inactivated by chromosomal mechanisms such as chromosome loss or mitotic recombination. The *p53* gene on chromosome 17p13 may be the most frequent target of such genetic changes. The majority of point mutations of the *p53* gene thus far reported are clustered in highly conserved domains of the p53 protein, usually resulting in abnormal proteins with a prolonged half-life and an accumulation in the cells. In 75% of esophageal cancers with a deletion of 17p, mutations in the remaining *p53* allele were also observed [4•].

Like the gene *p53*, *Rb* also encodes a nuclear protein that plays a role in the regulation of normal cell growth. In addition to abnormalities of *p53*, abnormalities in *Rb* are found in the majority of esophageal cancers including point mutations, microdeletions, allelic deletions of DNA, and abnormal size of quantity of messenger RNA. Half of the *p53* mutations are nonsense mutations that create premature stop codons. This suggests a unique mutation profile for esophageal cancer with involvement of both *p53* and *Rb* in tumorigenesis [5•]. Although mutation in the *p53* tumor-suppressor gene gives rise to a different protein conformation compared with the wild type, the antibodies or the anti-p53 response in cancer patients recognize both mutant and wild-type p53 proteins equally well. Yet, mutant p53 molecules may contain dominant antigenic epitopes that are not present in the wild-type p53 protein [6•].

Oncogenic transformation is often associated with changes in glycosylation in either glycolipids or glycoproteins in cell membranes. Among the variety of changes in glycosylation, Sialyl-Tn antigen, which is a mucin-associated antigen, is a result of premature sialylation of the Tn antigen by a sialyl-transferase. Sialyl-Tn antigen is not only expressed in cancer, but may also be expressed in esophageal submucosal glands, although not in normal squamous epithelium. The expression of the antigen in squamous cancer cells indicates that the malignant transformation is accompanied by the appearance of premature sialylation of the O-linked carbohydrate core. It may also be possible to think that some carcinomas do originate from esophageal glands. The sensitivity of Sialyl-Tn antigen for esophageal cancer is low and even in positive cases, expression is seen in less than half of the malignant cells. Furthermore, the expression is not a useful indicator of tumor progression or metastatic potential [7•].

Proteolytic enzymes, in particular matrix metalloproteinases, play an important role in tumor invasion and metastasis (collagenases, gelatinases, and stromelysin). The production of metalloproteinases can be increased by epidermal growth factor (EGF), transforming growth factor (TGF)-α, and platelet-derived growth factor. Esophageal carcinoma cells are known to express a large number of EGF receptors. Matrix metalloproteinases, a gene family of zinc enzymes capable of degrading almost all of the extracellular matrix macromolecules, have also been observed in cancer nests of invading esophageal cancer and along the margins of the tumor. A good correlation may be seen among the histologic stage, tumor invasion, lymph node metastasis, and expression of matrix metalloproteinases. In all probability, they affect tumor invasion and metastasis [8]. Presumably, EGF stimulates matrix metalloproteinases to produce large amounts of prometalloproteinase-9, which then results in destruction of the stromal tissue [9•].

Transforming growth factor–α, one of the ligands of EGF receptor, that is overexpressed in esophageal cancers, may act as an autocrine growth factor through hyperproducing EGF receptor and stimulating its expression. EGF receptor overexpression may prove useful as a prognostic indicator of esophageal cancer. The survival rate is significantly lower in patients with TGF-α positivity and in patients with EGF receptor positivity compared with those in whom these are negative. The survival is lowest in the groups of patients who have both TGF-α and EGF receptor expression [10•].

Tumor invasiveness is affected by three major factors: enzymatic proteolysis, cell motility, and cell adhesion. Various molecules including integrins, selectins, CD44, and cadherins are involved in cell adhesion. E-cadherin is a member of the cadherin family, which plays a major role in intercellular adhesion of normal epithelial cells. Many cancer cells, including esophageal cancer cells, have reduced or no E-cadherin expression *in situ*. Such impaired expression is frequently observed in tumors with aggressive histopathology characterized by dedifferentiation, high degree of invasiveness, and lymph node involvement. Cell clones from human esophageal cancer with positive E-cadherin expression are round and form cobblestone colonies. In contrast, negative clones have spindle shaped cells and form dispersed colonies. E-cadherin–positive cells form complete stratified epithelium, whereas negative cells do not. Importantly, positive cells do not invade a collagen fibroblast gel, whereas negative cells do. Both translational disorders or allelic losses may interfere with the E-cadherin expression [11•].

Urokinase-type plasminogen activator plays a major role in extracellular matrix breakdown. Most malignant cells produce urokinasetype plasminogen activator. The latter is also significantly enhanced in esophageal cancer, but not expressed in normal squamous mucosa [12•].

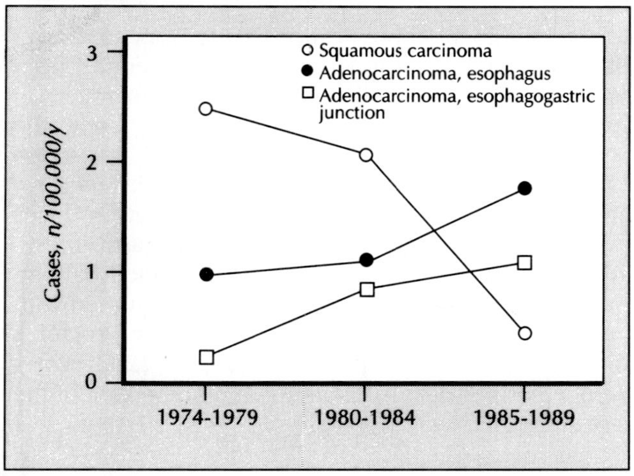

Fig. 1. Changing incidence of different types of cancer in Olmstead County from 1974 to 1989. (*From* Pera *et al.* [13••]; with permission.)

Clinical characteristics

One of the striking features in digestive oncology is the rapid rise in frequency of cancer at the level of the gastroesophageal junction. In a detailed study from Olmstead County, Minnesota [13••], the incidence of esophageal adenocarcinoma rose from 0.13 (1935–1971) to 0.74 (1974–1989), whereas the incidence of adenocarcinoma of the esophagogastric junction rose from 0.25 to 1.34 per 100,000 person-years for those periods. Interestingly, intestinal-type columnar metaplasia was detectable in five of nine specimens of esophagogastric adenocarcinoma. For both locations, the incidence of adenocarcinoma increased five- to sixfold. The authors suggest that adenocarcinoma of the esophagus and of the esophago-gastric junction are related disorders. This would mean that many of the so-called cancers of the cardia might be related to short-segment columnar metaplasia with intestinal type mucosa (Fig. 1, Fig. 2) [13••]. Obviously, these data should be confirmed in other geographic areas. If true the consequences would be enormous, as clinicians must take biopsy samples of any minute columnar mucosal extension in the distal esophagus to detect intestinal type mucosa with or without dysplasia.

We are reminded that members of those families afflicted with tylosis have at least a 90% risk of esophageal carcinoma by age 65 years. This condition has an autosomal dominant mode of transmission and probably is controlled at a single genetic locus. The actual pathologic state might be mediated through an increase in EGF receptors in the abnormal tissues. EGF is known to increase messenger RNA production by the *myc* oncogene via activation of the protein kinases, and increased EGF-receptor levels are correlated with greater expression of the *erb*-B-oncogene. These oncogenes, themselves, can encode directly for growth factors and their receptors as well as the regulatory kinases, conferring further growth autonomy on cancer cells via an autocrine mechanism of growth regulation. Of note, there has been a suggestion in the literature that tylosis may be related to abnormal vitamin A metabolism. Vitamin A and its derivatives can alter epithelial growth and differentiation. It may affect cancer initiation by absorption of free radicals such as singlet oxygen or it may have an antipromotion effect by blocking the effects of TGF [14•].

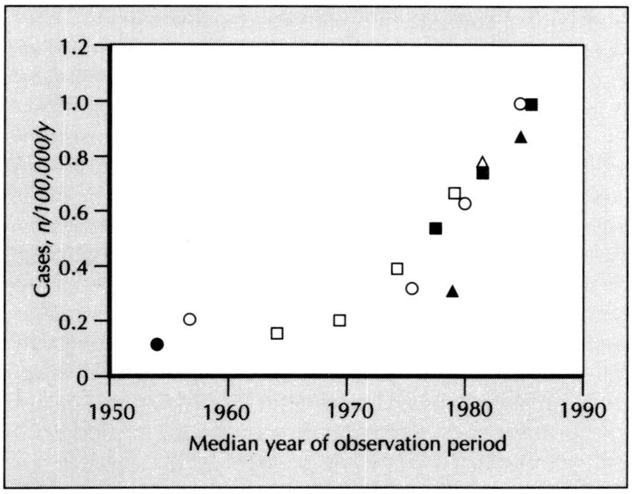

Fig. 2. The incidence of adenocarcinoma of the esophagus in population-based studies. Symbols represent the following studies: *solid circle*, Olmsted County; *open circle*, Connecticut Cancer Registry; *solid square*, National Cancer Institute, Surveillance, Epidemiology, and End Results program, approximately 10% of the US population; *open square*, Birmingham, England; *solid triangle*, Canton Vaud, Switzerland; and *open triangle*, Olmsted County (most recent report). (*From* Pera *et al.* [13••]; with permission.)

The histogenesis of small cell carcinoma of the esophagus is still rather controversial. Most probably, a primitive cell possessing capabilities towards multidirectional differentiation in the esophageal mucosa is the origin, because foci of squamous, glandular, or carcinoid differentiation have been frequently observed in small cell carcinoma. To characterize esophageal neuroendocrine tumors, a spectrum composed of typical carcinoid, atypical carcinoid, and small cell anaplastic carcinoma has been proposed.

Esophageal small cell carcinoma is usually considered a highly malignant tumor because of early dissemination and rapidly fatal outcome. The calculated tumor doubling time has been estimated to be approximately two days. In line with the neuroendocrine nature is the ectopic hormone production that has been reported in those patients. These hormones include adrenocorticotrophic hormone, calcitonin, and vasoactive intestinal peptide. An interesting case [15•] was published by Japanese authors on primary small cell carcinoma of the esophagus with ectopic gastrin production. The tumor showed intracytoplasmic argyrophilia, neurosecretory granules, stained positive for neuron-specific enolase with Grimelius stain.

Esophageal cancers are being detected at earlier stages. The terminology is confusing. Superficial esophageal cancer includes epithelial, mucosal, and submucosal carcinoma. Looking for clinical characteristics that might improve the detection rate of early esophageal cancer, a Japanese group carefully analyzed 46 afflicted patients (three epithelial, 13 mucosal, and 30 submucosal carcinomas) [16•]. Endoscopic detection was 100% for epithelial, 92% for mucosal, and 73% for submucosal carcinomas. It was intriguing to note that more than half of the patients with early esophageal cancer were symptomatic, including mild dysphagia and retrosternal pain or discomfort on swallowing. The authors even state that a piercing sensation in swallowing hot or pungent food was diagnostic for protruded-type early tumors. The more superficial type, however, was rarely associated with symptoms. Radiology often failed to detect early lesions, especially when the lesion was of the superficial type. In asymptomatic patients, most early cancers were detected during the follow-up therapy for gastric diseases, during mass screening or medical examination for gastric cancer, or in the evaluation of abdominal pain due to other causes. The authors stress that in order to detect early carcinomas, it is important to perform lugol staining combined with endoscopy [16•].

The destruction of the basement membrane, which is made up of glycoproteins such as laminin, fibronectin, entactin, and collagens, is considered to be an initial step of cancer progression. The first step in tumor invasion is the attachment of the cancer cells to the basement membrane. In the second step, the attached cells secrete hydrolytic enzymes that locally degrade the basement membrane such as plasmin, which disrupts laminin, fibronectin, and entactin. The third step is the migration of the cancer cells into the matrix modified by proteolysis. According to a detailed Japanese study [17•], most superficial esophageal cancers continue to progress while destroying the basement membrane. Proteolytic activity produced by cancer cells might be one of the causes of the destruction of the basement membrane and lymphocytes tend to infiltrate as a host immune reaction to regions where the basement membrane has been destroyed [17•].

Adenomas of the esophagus are rare. A tubulovillous adenoma lined by two layers of cuboidal cells within the submucosa and lamina propria was described in a patient with squamous cell carcinoma. The histology suggested that this adenoma had originated from the ducts of the esophageal glands. Therefore, adenomas do not only occur in patients with columnar metaplasia, but can occur also in patients with squamous carcinoma [18].

Staging esophageal cancer

A large number of publications have appeared over the past year with respect to the role of endosonography in staging esophageal cancer summarized in several overviews [19,20•–22•] (Fig. 3). Currently, the most popular instrument is the Olympus EUS-M3 scope (Olympus Corp., Lake Success, NY), which has a rotating crystal at the tip of the endoscope that produces a 360° view. Acoustical coupling to the gastrointestinal wall occurs either by using a water-filled balloon that surrounds the scanner or by filling the lumen with water. A 7.5-MHz frequency is used to view structures up to 18 cm from the probe, whereas a 12-MHz frequency permits detailed examination of the wall of the gastrointestinal tract.

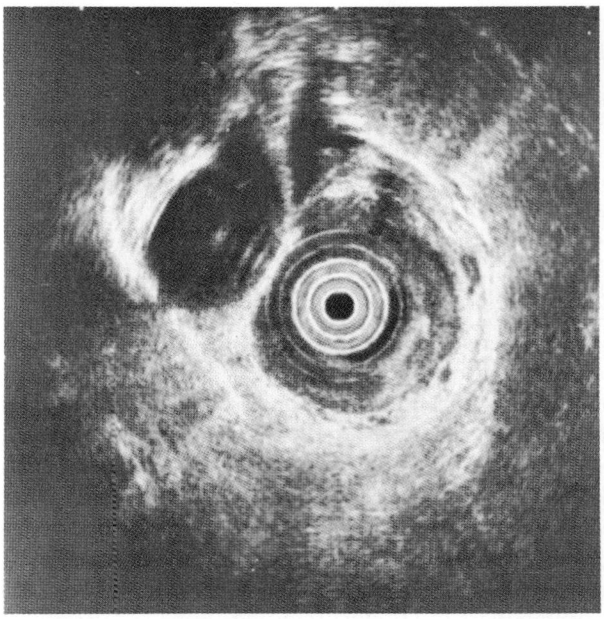

Fig. 3. Endosonography in a patient with T3 esophageal cancer. The tumor invades through the muscularis propria (between 5 and 6 o'clock position). The aorta (from 3 to 5 o'clock) is not invaded.

A phased-array instrument is available, designed by Hitachi Denshi America, Woodbury, NY, in cooperation with Pentax Precision Instrument Corp., Orangeburg, NY, that has a phased-array ultrasound in front of the optical bundle and produces a sector scan that is sagittal to the endoscope. This configuration permits ultrasonic viewing of a biopsy needle during puncture. In addition, the instrument has a color Doppler option for assessing blood flow. For esophageal cancer, accurate staging and detection of the tumor and of nodal metastasis is generally high (≈80%–90%), despite failure to pass the instrument through the stenotic tumor in roughly 30% of patients.

Lymph node micrometastasis is difficult to distinguish from inflammatory changes [20•]. Dittler and Siewert [21•] analyzed 167 patients with esophageal cancer. The T stage and N stage were correctly determined in 86% and 73%, respectively. Prediction of resectability was correct in 89% for adenocarcinoma but in only 64% for esophageal cancer. This is due to a high incidence of submucosal microscopic tumor spread of squamous cell cancer not detectable at endosonography, which the authors call *lymphangiosis carcinomatosa.* Furthermore, there was a tendency to overstage T1 and T2 tumors, which was best explained by peritumorous inflammation. Similarly gratifying results were obtained by Grimm *et al.* [22•]. The accuracy of T staging was 86% and the detection of regional lymph node metastasis was 90%. Again, the most frequent causes of misdiagnosis were microscopic tumor invasion and peritumorous inflammatory changes.

In a Dutch study [23•], endosonography was compared with computed tomography scanning. The overall accuracy of T staging was 76%, compared with 49% for computed tomography. T staging was excellent in easily traversable (92%) or nontraversable stenosis (87%). The latter high accuracy was due to the fact that almost all tumors that were nontraversable were in advanced stage T3 or T4. In contrast, cancers that could be passed, albeit with difficulty, had a lower accuracy for T staging of 46%.

The criteria for diagnosing lymph node metastasis remain the most problematic. Many investigators still use the criteria of hypoechoic pattern, roundish configuration, and sharp demarcation as indicators of malignant invasion. Yet, these are still rather unsatisfactory. Heintz *et al.* [24•] analyzed 90 regional lymph nodes *in vitro* by endosonography. The rate of visualization of regional lymph nodes by endosonography in resection specimens was only 30% under *in vitro* conditions, which may be explained by the use of the high frequency 12-MHz transducer of which the ultrasound waves have limited penetration depth. Only a few of the nodes with a diameter of 5 mm or less were visualized. Lymph nodes with a diameter of over 10 mm were metastatic in 72% of the cases, confirming previous results that node size over 10 mm increases the probability of metastasis. Surprisingly, echogenicity evaluation was not accurate. Lymph nodes evaluated as poorly or highly echogenic by the examiners actually revealed quite different gray scale values on objective computer analysis, stressing the subjective nature of visual assessment. Appreciation of the internal echostructure and the margins of the nodes permitted diagnosis of metastasis by an experienced examiner, but the value was rather impaired by the high proportion of false-positive. The authors conclude that the accuracy of endosonography in diagnosis regional lymph node metastasis is overestimated. There is need for improvement or refinement of endosonographic criteria for accurate lymph node analysis.

It is often said in the literature that endosonography is of limited value in the detection of T1 esophageal cancer. However, endosonography is of vital importance in detecting those malignancies that are truly limited to the epithelial layer or the mucosa. Indeed lymph node metastasis and vascular invasion is present respectively in more than 30% and 58% if the tumor infiltrates into the submucosa. This explains the high recurrence rate and the unsatisfactory 5-year survival for submucosal cancer. Therefore, it is repeatedly stressed that new criteria for early carcinoma of the esophagus are necessary that include epithelial and mucosal cancer only, regardless of the presence or absence of lymph node metastasis, but that exclude submucosal carcinoma. Epithelial and mucosal carcinomas of the esophagus are considered to have a much better prognosis than cancers with submucosal extension, although both are currently classified as superficial or early carcinomas.

Toh *et al.* [25•] tried to distinguish epithelial or mucosal carcinoma from submucosal carcinoma with endosonography. They analyzed 26 patients (two epithelial, 11 mucosa, and 13 submucosal carcinomas). Of the 13 epithelial or mucosal carcinomas, 10 were correctly diagnosed with endosonography (77%) whereas the remaining three were overdiagnosed as being submucosal. Of the 13 submucosal carcinomas, 12 were correctly diagnosed (92%) and one was overestimated. The overall accuracy of endosonography was therefore 82% in truly superficial cancers. It is rather surprising that these excellent results were obtained with a 12-MHz frequency and certainly they need to be confirmed by other groups. Furthermore, particularly for the detection of epithelial or mucosal cancer, the 20-MHz small probes that are currently being evaluated may prove to be superior.

Siewert and Dittler [26•] published an interesting overview on the impact of staging on therapy (Fig. 4). According to the authors, it is important to differentiate between tumors located at or above the tracheal bifurcation and tumors below the tracheal bifurcation. The suprabifurcal tumors are considered unresectable, even in less advanced stages, because of their close vicinity to, and therefore possible invasion of, the tracheobronchial system. The infrabifurcal carcinomas are usually resectable, owing to a more favorable anatomic location [26•].

According to Siewert and Dittler [26•], surgery is primarily indicated for suprabifurcal tumors in stages T1 and T2. The more advanced tumors (T3 to T4) should undergo preoperative chemoradiotherapy and should only be operated on in response to treatment. A resection is much more likely to be successful in tu-

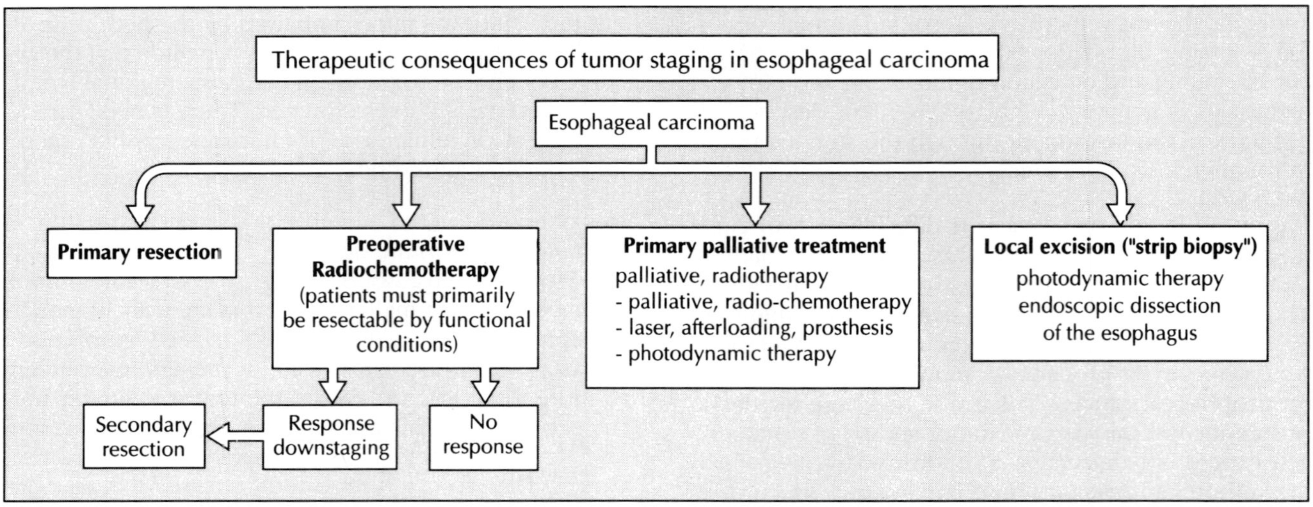

Fig. 4. Therapeutic consequences of tumor staging in esophageal carcinoma. (*From* Siewert and Dittler [26•]; with permission.)

mors below the tracheal bifurcation. These tumors are therefore primarily treated surgically except for those already infiltrating in surrounding structures. If endosonography indicates infiltration of vital structures or metastasis in the area of the celiac trunk or perigastrically, preoperative chemoradiotherapy should be performed with subsequent esophagectomy only in the event of response to treatment. It would be helpful if there were surgical consensus on this issue.

The significance of supraclavicular lymph node imaging in patients with carcinoma of the esophagus and gastroesophageal junction was confirmed [27•]. Both ultrasonography and computed tomography scanning are clearly superior to palpation in the assessment of supraclavicular metastasis. The relatively high number of false-positives in that study were due to the fact that lymph nodes were considered abnormal when they had a short axis of 5 mm or more. When nodes were considered abnormal only when they had a short axis of 10 mm or more, the number of false-positives decreased from six to one on ultrasound. The authors recommend performing fine needle aspiration of supraclavicular nodes with a short axis of 5 mm or more to confirm or to exclude the presence of metastasis by cytology. Ultrasound and, to a lesser degree, computed tomography were limited in the assessment of celiac lymph node metastasis. Only a minority of the metastatic nodes were detected on ultrasound and normal-sized nodes were invariably not seen. The relatively low sensitivity of computed tomography in detecting those nodes has been reported previously and may be explained by the fact that normal size nodes may harbor metastasis.

State of the art overviews were published on the role of endoscopy in staging esophageal cancer [28•] and the role of radiology in the preoperative staging of esophageal malignancies [29•]. A major problem in using computed tomography is understaging due to the inability to define the individual layers of the esophageal wall, the problems in cachectic patients, or the changes induced by prior surgery or radiotherapy. Another limitation of computed tomography is the inability to detect involvement of periesophageal lymph nodes. For staging cervical cancer or cancer at the cardia, computed tomography seems to be less accurate and less reliable than for staging mediastinal cancers. Magnetic resonance imaging provides not only transversal but also sagittal and coronal sections, thus representing quite accurate topographic relationships of lesions and surrounding tissues. Magnetic resonance imaging might therefore become useful in the future provided there is further standardization of the scanning criteria, further improvement of the definition of the diagnostic signs and further refinement of the imaging technique perhaps through contrast enhancement.

The limitations of computed tomography scanning were also stressed by two further studies. In a study from Norway, computed tomography was found to be unreliable in diagnosing the depth of infiltration or the presence of lymph node metastasis. The accuracy for staging of the growth was 88% and 55% for lymph node metastasis [30]. However, operative findings were not consistent with the histologic findings and this reduced the accuracy for the growth to 54%. Roughly 7% were overstaged and 38% were understaged. Suspicious lymph node size was defined differently by the authors as 2 cm or 1 cm or 0.5 cm, whereas some authors did not even define the size of metastatic nodes. Moreover lymph nodes closer than 3 cm to the tumor were usually indistinguishable from the tumor itself. Understaging lymph node metastasis is indeed a great problem that may amount to 43%. Moreover, lymph nodes below the diaphragm are poorly visualized by computed tomography. Similar results were published from the Netherlands [31•]. Computed tomography correctly staged 57% of the patients. Understaging (31%) occurred more often than overstaging (11%). Computed tomography was accurate in diagnosing tracheo-broncheal involvement, but was limited in diagnosing invasion of other adjacent structures. Furthermore, computed tomography was limited in detecting diaphragmatic invasion of lymph node involvement.

Nonsurgical destruction of early esophageal cancer

Photodynamic therapy has been used for the treatment of superficial adenocarcinoma associated with Barrett's esophagus [32•]. Photodynamic therapy involves the administration of a light-sensitive drug, such as a hematoporphyrin derivative, which is concentrated in malignant tissue and activated to produce local cell death caused by the release of cytotoxic singlet oxygen. Two patients (three lesions) remained free of malignancy for 6 to 24 months after photodynamic therapy, although one patient developed severe ulceration after the first course of therapy followed by a severe stricture after the second course. This technique needs to be refined to allow a more controlled delivery of light to the lesion and to allow protection of normal mucosa.

Inoue *et al.* [33•] described endoscopic mucosal resection of early esophageal cancer with a cap-fitted endoscope. Their technique involves the production of a submucosal bleb by injecting up to 10 mL of saline and epinephrine; the mucosal bleb is then aspirated into a cap fitted to the tip of the endoscope, allowing diathermy snare resection of the lesion. The cap is identical to the one used for variceal ligation. In principle, this procedure permits relatively atraumatic removal of superficial esophageal lesions but, like other luminally based techniques, it does not address the problem of early lymphatic metastases.

Palliation of malignant dysphagia

There is consensus that esophageal carcinoma is a distressing condition with a dismal prognosis, however, there is no consensus as to the best way to manage this disease. Unfortunately many patients will be suitable only for palliation of dysphagia because of old age, frailty, or advanced disease. The options for palliative treatment have proliferated with the introduction of endoscopic intubation, intraluminal radiotherapy, laser recanalization, bipolar diathermy coagulation, alcohol injection, and so forth.

Of a large group of cancers from the Nottingham area, only 34% were suitable for surgery and in a quarter of them only palliation was possible because of advanced disease detected at operation [34]. The patients treated surgically had a small but significant survival advantage and probably the best palliation of dysphagia. Hospital mortality was 9%. Two thirds were considered unsuitable for surgery; when fit enough they began receiving radical radiotherapy, but only two thirds completed a full course of radiotherapy. The results of survival in the radiotherapy group were obviously disappointing. Interestingly, these patients spent approximately 37% of their survival time in hospital and had a similar readmission rate to those undergoing surgery. Endoscopic intubation alone usually resulted in reasonable palliation but mortality (15%) was high. There was little difference in survival between squamous carcinoma and adenocarcinoma.

In the past, all discussion on the management of cancer centered around maximizing surviving time and debate was dominated by the continuing controversy over the role of radical radiotherapy or surgery for squamous cell cancer. As this study emphasizes, this debate is irrelevant to the management of two thirds of the patients not suitable for surgery [34]. According to the authors, intubation alone is a reasonable option in those not suitable for surgery, but randomized trials are needed to compare intubation with other methods of palliation [34].

Obvious progress is being made in intubation with the introduction of self-expanding stents. Swedish authors published their initial experience with self-expanding esophageal nitinol Strecker stent (Boston Scientific Corp., Watertown, MA) [35•]. This stent is knitted of 0.15–mm nitinol wire in the form of a tube with a diameter of 18 mm when fully expanded. (Nitinol is an alloy of nickel and titanium that has thermal as well as shape memory.) An important factor in the construction of this stent is the superelastic behavior of nitinol, which is almost rubberlike. To maximize the lumen of the stent directly after insertion, a 15-mm dilatation balloon can be used. Sixteen of 40 stents were self-expanded to maximum diameter within 24 hours and the other stents expanded to a maximum diameter during further observation. There were no serious stent-related complications and the dysphagia was reduced considerably in all patients immediately after stent insertion. Persisting bleeding occurred in two and ingrowth of tumor into the stent was seen in eight patients. Two stents occluded because of tumor ingrowth but were successfully recanalized with endoscopic laser coagulation [35•].

It is still debatable whether self-expanding stents may also be used for benign lesions. The reaction of the normal esophageal wall to the inserted self-expanding nitinol stent was studied in pigs [36•]. An inflammatory reaction with increasing fibrosis and degeneration of the muscular layers of the esophageal wall was readily demonstrable. Stents were also inserted in five patients with truly difficult benign stricturing. In one patient, the esophagus was lateron resected. There was deep implantation of the stent mesh work in the esophageal wall and significant stenosis secondary to tissue hyperplasia located at the edges of the stent occurred in two patients. Because of the observed reactions in the esophageal wall, such stents should be restricted to selected patients with very severe dysphagia until more experience is gained. The stents indeed expose the wall to severe forces. Further research and construction of removable stent for short-term treatment of benign esophageal strictures should be performed in an effort to extend the current therapeutic possibilities.

A major problem with all currently uncoated expandable stents is the possibility for tumor ingrowth through the mesh work; therefore, coating the stent is important. A group of Korean doctors presented and evaluated a new silicon-covered, modified Gianturco stent tube [37•]. The proximal and distal end of the stent is 4 mm wider in diameter than the middle portion. The barrel is 18 mm in diameter when fully expanded. A 100% nylon mesh is wrapped around the outside of the stent and covered with silicon rubber. The stent is inserted over an introducing tube and a pusher catheter (Myung Sung, Medi-tech, Korea). Eight patients with a malignant fistula were treated and all were symptomatically improved and capable of normal food and fluid intake. In a few patients with malignant fistula, we could confirm those gratifying results. A major advantage of the various kinds of self-expandable stents is that in the majority of the patients, no prior dilatation is necessary and that the insertion procedure is often easy [37•].

Maunoury *et al.* [38] published a 4-year prospective study using dilatation, laser photocoagulation or bipolar coagulation, and eventually radiotherapy in 128 patients with nonresectable or inoperable esophageal or gastroesophageal cancer. A limited dilatation was performed initially when a small caliber endoscope was unable to pass the stricture. Prompt and significant relief of dysphagia without complications was achieved in 83% of patients. Patients that were improved were retreated monthly during follow-up. Whenever possible, radiotherapy was recommended. Symptomatic relief of obstruction lasted 4.2 months on average and 76% of patients remained palliated until death. Monthly retreatment using the most appropriate endoscopic procedure depended on the tumor configuration. Radiotherapy after endoscopic relief of the obstruction seemed to give the best palliation. For laser therapy the authors used noncontact fibers and low irradiance. They confirmed that tumor length larger than 5 cm, a complex stricture at the gastroesophageal junction, predominantly submucosal location of the tumor, and upper third location of the malignancy, adversely affect the outcome of laser application [38].

References and recommended reading

Papers of particular interest, published within the annual period of review, have been highlighted as:
- • Of special interest
- •• Of outstanding interest

1. Sasano H, Miyazaki S, Gooukon Y, Nishhira T, Sawai T, Nagura H: **Expression of p53 in Human Esophageal Carcinoma: An Immunohistochemical Study With Correlation to Proliferating Cell Nuclear Antigen Expression.** *Hum Pathol* 1992, 23:1238–1243.

2. • Wang L-D, Hong J-Y, Qiu S-L, Gao H, Yang CS: **Accumulation of p53 Protein in Human Esophageal Precancerous Lesions: A Possible Early Biomarker for Carcinogenesis.** *Cancer Res* 1993, 53:1783–1787.

This paper discusses how p53 accumulates with invasing frequencies in the proliferating cells of basal cell hyperplasia, dysplasia, and carcinoma *in situ*. Yet *p53* alteration is not an obligatory process in esophageal carcinogenesis.

3. Huang Y, Boynton RF, Blount PL, Silverstein RJ, Yin J, Tong Y, McDaniel TK, Newkirk C, Resau JH, Sridhara R, Reid BJ, Meltzer SJ: **Loss of Heterozygosity Involves Multiple Tumor Suppressor Genes in Human Esophageal Cancers.** *Cancer Res* 1992, 52:6525–6530.

4. • Wagata T, Shibagaka I, Inamura M, Shimada Y, Toguchida J, Yandell DW, Ikenaga M, Tobe T, Ishizaki K: **Loss of 17p, Mutation of the p53 Gene, and Overexpression of p53 Protein in Esophageal Squamous Cell Carcinomas.** *Cancer Res* 1993, 53:846–850.

Loss of 17p is closely associated with mutation of *p53* gene in esophageal cancer. In 75% of tumors with a deletion of 17p, mutations in the remaining *p53* allele are observed.

5. • Huang Y, Meltzer SJ, Yin J, Tong Y, Change EH, Srivastava S, McDaniel T, Boynton RF, Zou Z-Q: **Altered Messenger RNA and Unique Mutational Profiles of p53 and Rb in Human Esophageal Carcinomas.** *Cancer Res* 1993, 53:1889–1894.

Abnormalities of *p53* and *Rb* are found in the majority of esophageal cancers. Allelic deletion of *p53* occurs in virtually all cases that have *p53* point mutation. Half of the mutations are nonsense mutations that create premature stop codons, a unique mutational profile.

6. • Labrecque S, Naor N, Thomson D, Matlashewski G: **Analysis of the Anti-p53 Antibody Response in Cancer Patients.** *Cancer Res* 1993, 53:3468–3471.

The antibody response in cancer patients directed against p53 recognizes both mutant and wild-type p53 proteins. Mutant p53 proteins do not express other dominant antigenic epitopes not present on the wild-type p53 protein.

7. • Ikeda Y, Kuwano H, Baba K, Ikebe M, Matushima T, Adachi Y, Mori M, Sugimachi K: **Expression of Sialyl-Tn Antigens in Normal Squamous Epithelium, Dysplasia, and Squamous Cell Carcinoma in the Esophagus.** *Cancer Res* 1993, 53:1706–1708.

Sialyl-Tn Antigen, a mucin-associated antigen, is expressed in roughly half the patients with esophageal carcinoma. The expression does not predict the velocity of tumor progression or metastatic potential.

8. Shima I, Sadaguri Y, Kusukawa J, Yamana H, Fujita H, Kakegawa T, Morimatsu M: **Production of Matrix Metalloproteinase-2 and Metalloproteinase-3 Related to Malignant Behavior of Esophageal Carcinoma. A Clinicopathologic Study.** *Cancer* 1992, 70:2747–2753.

9. • Shima I, Sasaguri Y, Kusukawa J, Nakano R, Yamana H, Fujita H, Kakegawa T, Morimatsu M: **Production of Matrix Metalloproteinase 9 (92-kDa Gelatinase) by Human Oesophageal Squamous Cell Carcinoma in Response to Epidermal Growth Factor.** *Br J Cancer* 1993, 67:721–727.

Esophageal carcinoma cell lines may be stimulated by EGF to produce large amounts of proMMP-9 which may result in pronounced destruction of stromal tissue.

10. • Iihara K, Shiozaki H, Tahara H, Kobayashi K, Inoue M, Tamura S, Miyata M, Oka H, Doki Y, Mori T: **Prognostic Significance of Transforming Growth Factor-α in Human Esophageal Carcinoma.** *Cancer* 1993, 71:2902–2909.

Patients with TGF-α–positive esophageal cancers have a substantially worse prognosis. In case of simultaneous expression of TGF-α and TGF-receptor, the prognosis is even worse. TGF-α may act as an autocrine growth factor through hyperproduction of TGF-R multivariate analysis indicates TGF-α as the only significant prognostic factor.

11. • Doki Y, Shiozaki H, Tahara H, Inoue M, Oka H, Iihara K, Kadowaki T, Takeichi M, Mori T: **Correlation Between**

E-Cadherin Expression and Invasiveness *In Vitro* in a Human Esophageal Cancer Cell Line. *Cancer Res* 1993, **53**:3421–3426.
Loss or dysfunction of E-cadherin, which plays a major role in cell-cell adhesion of normal epithelium, diminishes intercellular adhesion and results in the acquisition of invasive capacity.

12. • Sier CFM, Verspaget HW, Griffioen G, Ganesh S, Vloedgraven HJM, Lamers CGHW: **Plasminogen Activators in Normal Tissue and Carcinomas of the Human Oesophagus and Stomach.** *Gut* 1993, **34**:80–85.
Urokinase-type plasminogen activator was found in squamous cell carcinoma.

13. •• Pera M, Cameron AJ, Trastek VF, Carpenter HA, Zinsmeister AR: **Increasing Incidence of Adenocarcinoma of the Esophagus and Esophagogastric Junction.** *Gastroenterology* 1993, **104**:510–513.
There is a striking rise of both esophageal and esophagogastric junction adenocarcinomas, especially in white males. Both malignancies may well represent the same disorder.

14. • Marger RS, Marger D: **Carcinoma of the Esophagus and Tylosis. A Lethal Genetic Combination.** *Cancer* 1993, **72**:17–19.
Members with tylosis (autosomal dominantly inherited) have at least a 90% risk of esophageal cancer by age 65. There may be enhanced expression of EGF-receptors.

15. • Nishimaki T, Suzuki T, Fukuda T, Aizawa K, Tanaka O, Muto T: **Primary Small Cell Carcinoma of the Esophagus With Ectopic Gastrin Production. Report of a Case and Review of the Literature.** *Dig Dis Sci* 1993, **38**:767–771.
A small cell esophageal carcinoma is described with gastrin production.

16. • Adachi Y, Kitamura K, Tsutsui S, Ikeda Y, Matsuda H, Sugimachi K: **How to Detect Early Carcinoma of the Esophagus.** *Hepatogastroenterology* 1993, **40**:207–211.
Endoscopy is the best method to detect superficial esophageal cancer. Half of these patients are symptomatic. Otherwise their detection is an incidental finding either during mass screening or endoscopic evaluation of gastric disorders.

17. • Baba K, Kuwano H, Kitamura K, Sugimachi K: **Carcinomatous Invasion and Lymphocyte Infiltration in Early Esophageal Carcinoma With Special Regard to the Basement Membrane. An Immunohistochemical Study.** *Hepatogastroenterology* 1993, **40**:226–231.
Superficial esophageal cancer progresses while destroying the basal lamina. Proteolytic activity (urokinase type plasminogen activator?) produced by the cancer cells may be one of the destroying factors. Lymphocytes tend to infiltrate as a host immune reaction especially in areas where the basal lamina has been destroyed.

18. • Takubo K, Esaki Y, Watanabe A, Umehara M, Sasajima K: **Adenoma Accompanied by Superficial Squamous Cell Carcinoma of the Esophagus.** *Cancer* 1993, **71**:2435–2438.
Rarely, submucosal adenomas can develop from the ducts of the esophageal glands in the absence of columnar metaplasia.

19. Rankin S, Mason R: **Staging of Oesophageal Carcinoma. Review.** *Clin Radiol* 1992, **46**:373–377.

20. • Wang KK, DiMagno EP: **Endoscopic Ultrasonography: High Technology and Cost Containment. Editorials.** *Gastroenterology* 1993, **105**:283–296.
A critical overview is given of the technique and usefulness of endosonography, mainly for staging of malignancy.

21. • Dittler HJ, Siewert JR: **Role of Endoscopic Ultrasonography in Esophageal Carcinoma.** *Endoscopy* 1993, **25**:156–161.
In 167 patients, the T and N stage were correctly determined respectively in 86% and 73%. Resectability was correctly predicted by endoscopic ultrasonography in 82% of adenocarcinomata but only in 64% of squamous cell cancer due to lymphangiosis carcinomatosa.

22. • Grimm H, Binmoeller KF, Hamper K, Koch J, Henne-Bruns D, Soehendra N: **Endosonography for Preoperative Locoregional Staging of Esophageal and Gastric Cancer.** *Endoscopy* 1993, **25**:224–230.
Endosonography is accurate in determining the depth of invasion of esophageal cancer and in detecting regional lymph node metastasis confirming previous results. Microinvasion is the most important cause of understaging. Overstaging is mainly due to peritumoral inflammation and scarring.

23. • Hordijk ML, Zander H, Van Blankenstein M, Tilanus HW: **Influence of Tumor Stenosis on the Accuracy of Endosonography in Preoperative T Staging of Esophageal Cancer.** *Endoscopy* 1993, **25**:171–175.
The usefulness of endosonography in staging esophageal cancer is confirmed. Overall accuracy in T staging was 76%. All nontraversable stenoses were T3 to T4. No N staging is given.

24. • Heintz A, Mildenberger P, Georg M, Graunstein S, Junginger TH: **Endoscopic Ultrasonography in the Diagnosis of Regional Lymph Nodes in Esophageal and Gastric Cancer - Results of Studies In Vitro.** *Endoscopy* 1993, **25**:231–235.
Size, echogenicity, internal echopattern, and distinctness of margins were analyzed *in vitro* in 90 regional lymph nodes. Only 30% of the nodes could be visualized. The majority of the nodes larger than 10 mm were metastatic. Echogenicity was not contributory. There was a high proportion of false-positives.

25. • Toh Y, Baba K, Ikebe M, Adachi Y, Kuwano H, Sugimachi K: **Endoscopic Ultrasonography in the Diagnosis of an Early Esophageal Carcinoma.** *Hepatogastroenterology* 1993, **40**:212–216.
Endoscopic ultrasonography allows precise staging of early or superficial esophageal cancer. Seventy-seven percent of 13 patients with epithelial-mucosal esophageal cancer and 92% of 12 submucosal cancers were correctly staged with endosonography.

26. • Siewert JR, Dittler H-J: **Esophageal Carcinoma: Impact of Staging on Treatment.** *Endoscopy* 1993, **25**:28–32.
The authors give a detailed overview of the surgical strategy based upon the accurate preoperative staging of the malignancy (T) and of the presence or absence of suspicious lymph nodes.

27. • Van Overhagen H, Laméris JS, Berger MY, Tilanus HW, Van Pel R, Klooswijk AIJ, Schütte HE: **Improved Assessment of Supraclavicular and Abdominal Metastases in Oesophageal and Gastro-Oesophageal Junction Carcinoma With the Combination of Ultrasound and Computed Tomography.** *Br J Radiol* 1993, **66**:203–208.
The authors recommend systematically performing fine-needle aspiration cytology of supraclavicular lymph nodes with a short axis length of at least 5 mm.

28. • Caletti GC, Ferrari A, Fiorino S, Bocus P, Barbara L: **Staging of Esophageal Carcinoma by Endoscopy.** *Endoscopy* 1993, **25**:2–9.
A state of the art overview is presented of the role of endoscopy and endosonography in staging esophageal cancer.

29. • Reeders JWAJ, Bartelsman JFWM: **Radiological Diagnosis and Preoperative Staging of Oesophageal Malignancies.** *Endoscopy* 1993, **25**:10–27.
Excellent overview on the role of radiology (barium meal, computed tomography scanning) and magnetic resonance imaging in staging esophageal cancer.

30. Sondenaa K, Skaane P, Nygaard K, Skjennald A: **Value of Computed Tomography in Preoperative Evaluation of Resectability and Staging in Oesophageal Carcinoma.** *Eur J Surg* 1992, **158**:537–540.

31. • Van Overhagen H, Laméris JS, Berger MY, Klooswijk AIJ, Tilanus HW, Van Pel R, Schütte HE: **CT Assessment of Resectability Prior to Transhiatal Esophagectomy for Esophageal/Gastroesophageal Junction Carcinoma.** *J Comput Assist Tomogr* 1993, **17**:367–373.
Computed tomography correctly staged 57% of patients (31% understaging; 11% overstaging). Computed tomography was accurate in diagnosing tracheobronchial involvement but was limited in detection of invasion of other organs, of the diaphragm, or of regional lymph nodes.

32. Overholt B, Panjehpur M, Tefftellar B, Rose M: **Photodynamic Therapy for Treatment of Early Adenocarcinoma in Barrett's Esophagus.** *Gastrointest Endosc* 1993, 39:73–76.
•
Photodynamic therapy is effective in the treatment of superficial adenocarcinoma in patients who are not suitable for surgery.

33. Inoue H, Takeshita K, Hori H, Muracka Y, Yoneshima H, Endo M: **Endoscopic Mucosal Resection With a Cap-Fitted Panendoscope for Esophagus, Stomach and Colon Mucosal Lesions.** *Gastrointest Endosc* 1993, 39:58–62.
•
Full-thickness endoscopic resection of mucosal malignancies is possible allowing detailed examination of the resection specimen.

34. Oliver SE, Robertson CS, Logan RFA: **Oesophageal Cancer: A Population-Based Study of Survival After Treatment.** *Br J Surg* 1992, 79:1321–1325.

35. Cwikiel W, Stridbeck H, Tranberg K-G, Von Holstein ChS, Hambraeus G, Lillo-Gil R, Willén R: **Malignant Esophageal Strictures: Treatment With a Self-Expanding Nitinol Stent.** *Radiology* 1993, 187:661–665.
•
The insertion of an ultraflex self-expanding stent knitted of nitinol wire is rather easy and less traumatic than the insertion of a plastic stent. Stent migration is rare. Occlusion due to tumor ingrowth can occur but recanalization with laser coagulation is possible.

36. Cwikiel W, Willén R, Stridbeck H, Lillo-Gil R, Von Holstein ChS: **Self-Expanding Stent in the Treatment of Benign Esophageal Strictures: Experimental Study in Pigs and Presentation of Clinical Cases.** *Radiology* 1993, 187:667–671.
•
An expandable stent exposes the esophageal wall to severe forces. The mucosa proximal to the stent herniates into the stent, causing ulceration and fibrosis. Laterally the mucosa is pressed through the meshwork, with subsequent ulceration and fibrosis involving the muscle coat. The distal end is also forced into the wall causing ulceration.

37. Do YS, Song H-Y, Lee BH, Byun HS, Kim KH, Chil SY, Park JH: **Esophagorespiratory Fistula Associated With Esophageal Cancer: Treatment With A Gianturco Stent Tube.** *Radiology* 1993, 187:673–677.
•
A new type of silicone membrane covered expandable Gianturco stent was successfully used in malignant esophagorespiratory fistula.

38. Maunoury V, Brunetaud JM, Cochelard D, Boniface B, Cortot A, Paris JC: **Endoscopic Palliation for Inoperative Malignant Dysphagia: Long Term Follow Up.** *Gut* 1992, 33:1602–1607.

G.N.J. Tytgat, MD, Academic Medical Center, University of Amsterdam, Department of Gastroenterology-Hepatology, P.O. Box 22700, 1100DE Amsterdam, the Netherlands.

Surgery, radiotherapy, and chemotherapy for esophageal cancer

J. Jan B. van Lanschot, MD, Joke G.J. Letschert, MD, and Cees H.N. Veenhof, MD

Academic Medical Center, Amsterdam, the Netherlands

Current surgical research addresses the optimal approach to potentially curative resection. Several retrospective studies indicate that the transhiatal procedure is technically safe. It is still unclear, however, whether long-term survival can be improved by using more extensive, transthoracic procedures, including two-regional or three-regional lymph node dissection. Minimally invasive techniques have been described with impressive preliminary results both for preoperative staging and for operative resection of esophageal cancer. For locally irresectable tumors, effective palliation can be achieved with combined intraluminal and external radiotherapy. A slight improvement in local control is achieved by addition of intraluminal radiotherapy to conventional external radiotherapy, but long-term survival is poor. If life expectancy is short, single intraluminal radiotherapy can offer effective relief of dysphagia. As of yet, no data are available comparing this approach with pertubation. Finally, the efficacy of multimodality treatment to improve long-term surgical results has been extensively investigated. After neoadjuvant chemotherapy and/or radiotherapy, pathologically complete remission rates vary widely in several retrospective studies. Sterile surgical specimens seem to be associated with better survival results, although patients with microscopical residual disease may have long-term survival. In conclusion, the data on combined approaches are promising, but more randomized studies are needed to establish their exact role in the treatment of esophageal carcinoma.

Current Opinion in Gastroenterology 1994, **10**:465–472

Esophageal cancer is an increasing problem in Western countries. Whereas the incidence of squamous cell carcinoma remains stable, a steady rise has been suggested in the incidence of adenocarcinoma of the esophagus and the esophagogastric junction [1]. In a well-defined study population, the incidence of adenocarcinoma increased five- to sixfold during the past 60 years [2••].

Most institutions consider operative therapy an essential part of potentially curative treatment. The 1993 literature mainly focused on two aspects of curative treatment of esophageal cancer: the selection of the correct surgical approach and whether surgery should be combined with (neo)adjuvant chemotherapy and/or radiotherapy [3,4•]. Furthermore, the role of intraluminal radiotherapy has more clearly been defined in the palliative treatment of esophageal cancer.

Surgical therapy

Transthoracic versus transhiatal esophagectomy

Although a transthoracic approach is most frequently chosen for resection of an esophageal tumor and its adjacent lymph nodes, transhiatal resection without thoracotomy has been advocated to minimize the perioperative morbidity and mortality. However, with this technique an extensive intrathoracic lymphadenectomy cannot be performed. It has been suggested that wide local excision in combination with radical lymphadenectomy can improve locoregional tumor control and long-term survival [5]. So far, very little randomized data are available comparing the different surgical approaches.

In a randomized French study, 67 patients with squamous cell carcinoma underwent either transthoracic re-

 ISBN 1-85922-609-4 ISSN 0267–1379

section or blind transhiatal resection [6•]. No difference in postoperative morbidity or mortality was shown, including pulmonary complications. Long-term survival was not affected by the type of operation. Within the limited number of patients in this study, the traditional transthoracic and the transhiatal esophagectomy seem to be equally effective surgical options. However, it is not clear which patients received neoadjuvant chemotherapy or radiotherapy and whether this neoadjuvant therapy influenced the outcome of the study.

In three retrospective studies, transthoracic and transhiatal esophagectomy were compared. A group from Turkey analyzed 238 patients treated between 1983 and 1991 [7•]. After transhiatal resection and cervical esophagogastrostomy, early and late respiratory complications were significantly less frequent than after transthoracic resection with intrathoracic anastomosis; vocal cord paralysis was the major complication in the transhiatal group. Anastomotic tumor recurrence and late gastroesophageal reflux were less frequently observed after transhiatal resection than after transthoracic resection. Neither in-hospital mortality nor long-term survival was significantly different. The authors conclude that transhiatal resection is the safest of the two operations.

Comparable results were published by the Rotterdam Esophageal Tumor Study Group [8•]. Over a period of 10 years, 293 patients were operated on, receiving either right-sided thoracotomy with an intrathoracic anastomosis or blunt transhiatal resection with a cervical anastomosis. Vocal cord paralysis and anastomotic leakage occurred significantly more often in the transhiatal group; pulmonary complications were less frequent in the transhiatal group. In-hospital mortality and long-term survival did not differ between the two groups. It was concluded that transhiatal resection is technically safe and oncologically justifiable.

A German study identified the surgical procedure (thoraco-abdominal versus blunt transhiatal) as a significant perioperative risk factor in a multivariate analysis of 127 consecutive patients [9]. In-hospital mortality after transthoracic and transhiatal resection was 29.2% and 11.6%, respectively. Long-term survival was not correlated with the surgical procedure.

In a noncomparative retrospective study from the Mayo Clinic [10], the postoperative complications of 131 patients, who underwent transhiatal resection for carcinoma of the esophagus were analyzed. The majority of the tumors (91%) were located in the lower half of the intrathoracic esophagus or involved the gastroesophagal junction. One hundred twenty-six patients (97%) were extubated within 24 hours and in-hospital mortality was only 2.3%. However, anastomotic leakage occurred in 32 patients (24%) and unilateral vocal cord paralysis developed in 15 patients (11%). Only 37 patients (28%) had an uneventful postoperative course. Based on these data, the authors favor the tranthoracic approach.

While some authors try to define the surgical standard with minimal perioperative complications, others focus on more extensive procedures, including lymph node dissection to improve long-term survival. Lerut *et al.* [11] retrospectively analyzed the outcome after surgery for adenocarcinoma or squamous cell carcinoma of the esophagus in 257 patients [11]. Over the years 1975 to 1988, the surgical procedure changed substantially. The role of radical lymphadenectomy was gradually more emphasized. The procedures were classified according to the type of resection as palliative, curative without radical lymphadenectomy, or curative with radical lymphadenectomy. The overall in-hospital mortality rate was 9.6%; perioperative morbidity and mortality did not differ between the three groups. Radical curative resection was shown to have a significant beneficial effect on survival as compared with a less radical curative resection, the 2-year survival rate was 81% versus 46% and the 5-year survival rate was 49% versus 41% (Fig. 1). However, this benefit of extensive resections only concerned patients with positive lymph nodes.

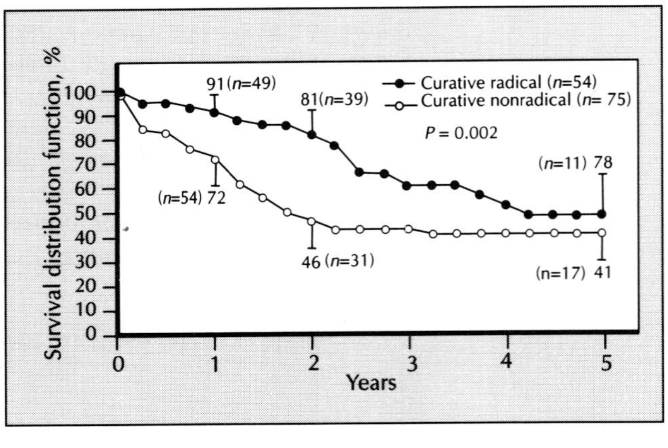

Fig. 1. Survival curves according to radicalness of resection for thoracic esophageal carcinoma. (*From* Lerut *et al.* [11]; with permission.)

In a Japanese series of 68 patients who underwent three-region lymph node dissection for intrathoracic esophageal cancer, 20 patients (29%) had cervical metastasis [12]. The 4-year survival rates of patients with and patients without positive cervical lymph nodes were 30% and 43%, respectively (difference statistically not significant). Six of the seven patients with positive nodes along the recurrent laryngeal nerve were still alive 3 years after the operation. Based on these (small) numbers, the authors suggest to classify positive recurrent laryngeal nerve nodes as N1 instead of M1(according to the TNM classification of the International Union Against Cancer).

Minimally invasive techniques

Thoracoscopic, mediastinoscopic, and laparoscopic techniques can be applied for both diagnostic and therapeutic purposes in esophageal cancer patients. *Diagnostic* thoracoscopy allows evaluation of the mediastinum with lymph node biopsy and assessment of local tumor extension. Krasna and McLaughlin [13•] reported on the results in 14 patients who underwent thoracoscopic lymph node staging. In 13 out of 14 patients the procedure could be completed; all had correct thoracic lymph node staging confirmed at surgical exploration. The major disadvantage is that the procedure requires general anesthesia. In addition, the mediastinal pleura must be opened and the esophagus largely mobilized, which makes subsequent resection more difficult [14,15].

Data have become available suggesting that long-term survival after surgery can be improved by neoadjuvant therapy, but that this more aggressive therapy should be tailored to the preoperative stage of the tumor. In this respect, the high accuracy of diagnostic thoracoscopy is more promising than that of computed tomography scanning. In a group of 71 patients who underwent transhiatal esophagectomy, only 40 tumors (56%) were correctly staged by computed tomography-scan. In assessing mediastinal lymph node metastases, computed tomography had a sensitivity of only 30% [16]. Recently, Fok *et al.* [17] have demonstrated that endoscopic ultrasonography has a sensitivity and a specificity for lymph node metastasis of 85% and 86%, respectively.

Therapeutic endodissection of the thoracic esophagus can be performed either through mediastinoscopy or through thoracoscopy. A group from Munich [18••] reported on 30 patients in whom a distal tumor was resected under direct transhiatal vision while the normal esophagus proximal to the tumor was mobilized by mediastinoscopic dissection. Compared with matched historical controls, these patients had significantly less postoperative pulmonary complications, possible because of reduced aspiration and more efficient coughing owing to the low incidence of vocal cord paralysis.

If, on the contrary, the tumor itself and the intrathoracic lymph nodes are to be dissected, the mediastinoscopic approach is not helpful because it does not allow a sufficient view of the surrounding mediastinal structures. For this purpose, thoracoscopy seems to be superior. Azagra *et al.* [19] published preliminary data on thoracoscopic esophagectomies in eight patients. The procedure was successfully completed in seven patients, whereas conversion to transhiatal digital mobilization was necessary in one. The mean time required to perform thoracoscopy was 180 minutes. In a group of 15 patients from Paris, the thoracoscopic dissection was successful in 12, whereas in three cases the procedure had to be converted [15]. Comparable results were reported by Collard *et al.* [20•], who added an extensive lymph node dissection to the thoracoscopic procedure. Further experience is required to define the safety of this new approach.

Other technical aspects

Despite all technical advances, anastomic healing is still a critical part of esophageal surgery. Early leakage and late stricture formation are two important complications. In a Dutch study [21•], 81 patients were followed after cervical esophagogastrostomy. Twenty-four patients (30%) developed a benign anastomotic stricture that required endoscopic dilation. During operation, poor vascularization of the gastric tube was noticed in 14 patients (17%). Postoperative anastomotic leakage occurred in 12 patients (15%). Poor vascularization and postoperative leakage were statistically significant risk factors for stricture formation.

In a randomized clinical trial, one-layer and two-layer anastomoses were compared following subtotal esophagectomy and gastric tube substitution [22•]. With equal leakage rates (19% in both groups), one-layer anastomosis appeared to be superior because of a lower incidence of fibrotic stricture (22% vs 48%).

After subtotal esophagectomy, the interposed esophageal substitute can either be placed in the anatomic, prevertebral position (*ie*, the posterior mediastinum) or in the extra-anatomic retrosternal position (*ie*, the anterior mediastinum). Extra-anatomic reconstruction allows postoperative irradiation of the esophageal bed without damaging the neoesophagus. Furthermore, it prevents ingrowth of intrathoracic, peripheral tumor recurrence into the neoesophagus. In a randomized study, the postoperative complications after prevertebral and retrosternal gastric tube reconstruction were compared [23•]. Because the prevertebral reconstruction was associated with a significantly shorter stay in the intensive care unit, fewer cardiopulmonary complications, and lower in-hospital mortality, the authors recommend the prevertebral route, particularly for patients with cardiopulmonary risk factors.

Results on two new methods for composite reconstruction of the esophagus have been published [24,25]. In one patient with a short gastric tube after laryngo-pharyngo-esophagectomy, a free jejunal autograft was successfully interposed between the pharyngeal stump and the mobilized stomach [24]. In a series of 14 consecutive patients from Japan [25], pedicled and revascularized jejunal interposition were combined. In this upward extension of the jejunal interposition, the internal thoracic artery and vein were used as recipient vessels. All extended jejunal grafts survived.

Radiotherapy

Radiotherapy with curative intent

The combination of external beam and intraluminal radiotherapy is an attractive treatment option for patients with irresectable tumors. Intraluminal brachytherapy enables the administration of a high dose to the exophytic part of the tumor, without exceeding the tolerance dose to the adjacent normal tissues. Radioactive elements with high specific activity (cesium-137, iridium-192) have reduced the treatment time of the intraluminal procedure to 1 to 2 hours. With external radiotherapy, the deeper part of the tumor and adjacent lymph nodes are treated.

Hareyama *et al.* [26] reported on 161 patients with squamous cell carcinoma of the esophagus treated with combined external beam and intraluminal radiotherapy. External beam radiotherapy (55 to 60 Gy in 5.5 to 6 weeks) was followed by intraluminal radiotherapy (4 to 10 Gy, dose rate 2 Gy/h). Intraluminal radiotherapy was repeated three times at most. One month after treatment, clinical response was assessed by barium-esophagography and endoscopy. A complete remission was observed in 53% of patients. At 5 years, local control was achieved in 31% of patients and 5-year survival was 43% and 21% for stage I and II, and 0% for stage III and IV, respectively. Eighteen percent of long-term survivors developed benign ulcerations or strictures.

Clearly, with this treatment, no improvement in long-term survival for patients with advanced stages has yet been determined when compared with conventional external beam radiotherapy. Although a complete response occurs in 29% to 53% of patients, and up to 100% of patients can swallow at least soft food after treatment, local recurrence is a cause of failure in 49% to 68% of patients [26,27]. Benign strictures or ulcers occur infrequently (7% to 18%) if low dose rate intraluminal radiotherapy (<2 Gy/h) is used. Under these conditions, the optimal dose of intraluminal therapy is 12 Gy in one to two fractions, combined with external beam treatment of 50-55 Gy in 5 weeks [28]. High dose rate intraluminal radiotherapy (>6 Gy/h) in combination with external beam radiotherapy (60 Gy in 6 weeks) has resulted in a high rate of esophageal ulcers (58%) [29].

The prophylaxis of esophageal ulceration by potential mucosal protective agents is currently being investigated in patients treated with high dose rate intraluminal radiotherapy [29].

Palliative radiotherapy

Jager *et al.* [30] observed a good palliative effect for a single intraluminal treatment with a dose of 15 Gy, in 36 patients who had mainly advanced (stage III and IV) disease. In 67% of these patients dysphagia improved, and in 27% retreatment was necessary. Sixteen percent of all patients needed insertion of an endoprosthesis. Median survival was 4 months.

One fraction of high dose rate intraluminal radiotherapy (12.5 Gy) was compared with low dose rate intraluminal radiotherapy (20 Gy in three fractions) with respect to palliation of symptoms by Harvey *et al.* [31]. Dysphagia was relieved in nine of 10 low dose rate patients and in 11 of 12 high dose rate patients. High dose rate patients experienced more esophagitis than low dose rate patients (80% vs 30%, respectively).

The value of external beam radiotherapy or chemotherapy as additive treatment to endoprosthesis has been investigated by Schmid *et al.* [32••] in a randomized trial. Radiotherapy was given as split-course treatment (2 courses of 5×4 Gy), and chemotherapy consisted of trimetrexate, ifosfamide, or 5-fluorouracil. No difference in palliative effect or treatment tolerance was observed between patients treated with pertubation (46 patients), or additional chemotherapy or radiotherapy (40 and 41 patients, respectively). Median survival was 13 weeks for the whole group of patients.

Radiotherapy in patients with malignant tracheoesophageal fistula

Radiotherapeutic treatment of malignant tracheoesophageal fistula is considered controversial because the treatment might compromise healing, and even increase the size of the fistula. A recent report on 10 patients treated with radiotherapy for malignant tracheoesophageal fistula has shown no enlarging of the fistula nor aggravation of symptoms [33•]. Four of these patients died of local disease and seven required a second palliative procedure for persistent symptoms. Considering the poor survival observed in these patients (on average 1.4 and 4 months respectively for patients with recurrent cancer, and tracheoesophageal fistula as first symptom of disease), the role of radiotherapy as palliative treatment is questionable.

Adjuvant radiotherapy

The aim of postoperative radiotherapy is reducing locoregional recurrences by sterilizing microscopic or macroscopic residual disease. Postoperative radiotherapy has the advantages of tailoring treatment to tumor stage and adjusting the treatment volume based on pathologic findings.

In a randomized study [34••], an unacceptably high rate of life-threatening complications have been observed in patients treated with postoperative radiotherapy with a high dose per fraction. One hundred ten patients were stratified after surgery, based on curative or palliative resection, and randomly allocated to receive either no adjuvant therapy or postoperative radiotherapy (49 to 52.6 Gy). Radiotherapy was given three times weekly, with 3.5 Gy per fraction. Complications in the intrathoracic stomach occurred in 24 out of 65 patients (37%) who received radiotherapy (five of whom died of gastric bleeding), versus four out of 65 patients (6%) in the control group. The median survival of patients treated with or without postoperative radiotherapy was 8.7 months and 15.2 months, respectively ($P = 0.002$). Local recurrences occurred less frequently in patients receiving radiotherapy (20% vs 46%, $P = 0.04$). In patients with residual disease after surgery (palliative resection), fewer patients died of tracheobronchial obstruction in the radiotherapy group (7%) than in the control group (33%, $P = 0.03$). The authors conclude that the poorer survival for patients treated with radiotherapy was mainly due to radiation-induced fatal complications.

New developments in intraoperative radiotherapy

Arimoto *et al.* [35•] have investigated the feasibility of intraoperative radiotherapy combined with esophagectomy and modified three-region lymph node dissection in patients with locally advanced disease [35•]. Theoretically, the advantage of intraoperative radiotherapy is two-fold: 1) by delivering radiotherapy during the operative procedure, the treatment volume is directly visualized; and 2) retraction of mobile organs and lead shielding result in maximal sparing of normal structures. All patients underwent transthoracic resection, followed by intraoperative radiotherapy with 11 or 13 MeV electrons to a dose of 20 or 25 Gy. Postoperative radiotherapy was added with 6-Mv X-rays (45 Gy in 4 weeks). Seventeen out of 62 patients developed tracheal or pulmonary complications, two of whom died of complications. Tracheal ulceration was an important late complication and was observed only in the high intraoperative radiotherapy dose group. The actuarial 2-year survival rate was 62.5%; no local recurrences were observed. The authors conclude that intraoperative radiotherapy combined with esophagectomy is feasible, if the dose of intraoperative radiotherapy does not exceed 20 Gy.

Chemotherapy

To improve treatment results of patients with esophageal carcinoma, new combined treatment modalities are developed focusing on (neo)adjuvant chemotherapy-radiotherapy [36•]. The most important drugs used are cisplatin, 5-fluorouracil, etoposide, bleomycin, vindesine, and vinblastin.

Metastatic disease

Few drugs have recently been studied in metastatic disease. The response rate to cytotoxic drugs is low (15% to 20%), with responses of short duration and no effect on survival. Wadler *et al.* [37] described a phase 2 trial with the combination of 5-fluorouracil and interferon [37]. Twenty previously untreated patients were included with measurable locally advanced or metastatic disease. In two patients, a pathologically confirmed complete response was observed; three patients had a partial response. The approach with modulation of well-known drugs and the use of biologic response modifiers is subject of study in ongoing trials.

Locoregional disease

Chemoradiation without resection

Herskovic *et al.* [38] have published a randomized trial comparing chemoradiotherapy (61 patients) with radiotherapy (60 patients), as potentially curative treatments in localized disease. Treatment consisted of four courses of combined 5-fluorouracil and cisplatin with 50 Gy of radiation therapy, as compared with 64 Gy in patients treated with radiation alone. Survival rates at 2 years were 38% and 10% for patients with combined and radiation alone treatment, respectively. This study, however, has several drawbacks. The gain in median survival of 3.6 months was still disappointing (with a treatment duration of 3 months), and side-effects were severe and life-threatening in 44% and 20% of patients, respectively. Twenty-seven patients in the neoadjuvant treatment group (44%) developed a recurrence in the radiation field at a short median follow-up duration.

Two studies have addressed the palliative effect of chemoradiotherapy on dysphagia in locally advanced disease. Coia *et al.* [39] have described rapid improvement of long duration in dysphagia by concurrent high-dose radiation and chemotherapy (mitomycin C and 5-fluororacil, two courses) in 120 patients with esophageal cancer [39]. Of 102 evaluable patients, improved swallowing was experienced in 46 at 2 weeks after the initiation of treatment and in 84 patients at treatment completion (6 weeks).

The study of Izquierdo *et al.* [40] showed an improvement of dysphagia in 16 of 25 patients treated with sequential chemotherapy (cisplatin and bleomycin, three courses) followed by radiotherapy (50 to 60 Gy).

Chemoradiation (neo)adjuvant to resection

Wolfe *et al.* [41] published a retrospective study comparing the treatment outcome in 165 patients treated with preoperative chemoradiotherapy followed by resection, with results obtained in 64 patients treated with chemoradiation alone. Chemotherapy consisted of three courses cisplatin plus etoposide for squamous cell carcinoma (72 patients) and cisplatin plus 5-fluororacil for adenocarcinoma (93 patients). Five-year survival was 25% versus 18% for resected and nonresected patients, respectively. Patients with a sterile surgical specimen had the best treatment outcome.

Forastiere *et al.* [42•] reported on the long-term results of preoperative chemoradiation (cisplatin, vinblastin, and 5-fluororacil) in 43 patients. Two treatment-related deaths were observed before surgery. Twenty of 41 patients assessable for response to chemoradiation had stable disease and 18 patients had a reduction in tumor mass. Thirty-six patients (84%) underwent resection; in 10 of these patients a pathologically complete response was confirmed. In these 10 patients, median survival was 70 months and 5-year survival was 60%, versus median survival of 26 months and 5-year survival of 32% in 26 patients with residual tumor in the surgical specimen (Fig. 2). Analysis of the pattern of failure revealed excellent local control for patients treated with this regimen (no local recurrences, 26% regional recurrences). Distant metastasis was the major cause of failure, underlining the need for more effective systemic treatment.

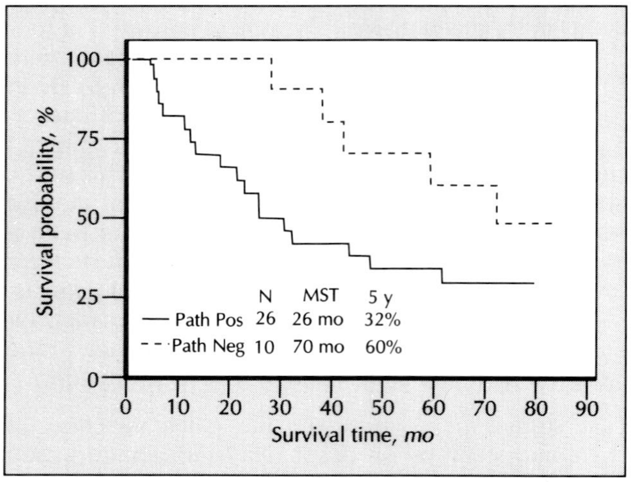

Fig. 2. Survival of 36 patients treated with preoperative chemoradiation and potentially curative resection according to pathology result ($P = 0.114$ log-rank test, $P = 0.04$ Wilcoxon test). MST—median survival time; N—number; 5 y—5-year survival rate. (*From* Forastiere [42•]; with permission.)

In the study by Terz *et al.* [43], no benefit in survival was observed in 22 patients treated with cisplatin 5-fluororacil and concurrent radiotherapy followed by resection, if compared with a historical group of patients treated with surgery alone. Median survival was 18 months. An important finding was that the clinical staging before resection overestimated the complete response to chemoradiotherapy.

Carey *et al.* [44] treated 70 patients suffering from squamous cell carcinoma with preoperative 5-fluororacil and cisplatin followed by resection. Patients with involvement of regional lymph nodes or positive resection margins received postoperative radiotherapy. Four additional courses of postoperative chemotherapy were given to patients who responded to chemotherapy. Of 68 patients evaluated for clinical response to chemotherapy, 28 responded completely, 17 responded partially, and 23 had no response. Of 55 resected patients, 50 showed residual tumors and one necrotic tumor; in only four patients a pathologically complete response was observed. Five-year survival in the resected patients was 39%, demonstrating the fact that patients with residual disease may experience long-term survival.

This observation was confirmed by the results of Hoff *et al.* [45] who tested 68 patients with two cycles of cisplatin, 5-fluororacil plus leucovorin, etoposide, and radiation (30 Gy), followed by resection. In 12 out of 51 resected patients, a complete response to preoperative therapy was observed. Median survival was 36 and 15 months in patients with adenocarcinoma and squamous cell carcinoma, respectively. The overall median survival was 24 months compared with 9 months in historical controls. Pathologically complete response was not associated with improved survival.

Peddada *et al.* [46] reported preliminary results of two courses of cisplatin/5-fluororacil combined with high dose rate intraluminal radiation (12.5 Gy) followed by resection in 13 patients. Only two patients had a pathologically complete remission. In the 2 year follow-up, nine patients developed distant recurrent disease.

Postoperative chemotherapy and/or radiotherapy was investigated in three prospective studies. In the study by Saito *et al.* [47], adjuvant concurrent chemoradiotherapy (50 Gy; cisplatin, vindesine, and pepleomycin) in 35 resected patients was associated with a 5-year survival of 31% compared with 5% in 26 historical controls treated with postoperative radiotherapy alone. These encouraging results need to be confirmed in larger randomized studies. In a prospective randomized trial, the Japanese Esophageal Oncology Group [48••] compared radiotherapy (50 Gy) with two courses of cisplatin/vindesine after curative resection in 258 patients at nine institutions. There was no statistically significant difference in the survival rates of the two groups.

Leucopenia is encountered more frequently and is more severe after chemoradiation than after radiotherapy alone. In the study by Sakata *et al.* [49] of 12 patients with postoperative successive chemotherapy-radiotherapy-chemotherapy, hG-CSF (human granulocyte colony–stimulating factor) remarkably reduced the decrease of the neutrophil counts as well as decreasing the duration of the neutropenic state. The application of this growth factor should be considered when developing trials with potentially severe myelosuppression.

References and recommended reading

Papers of particular interest, published within the annual period of review, have been highlighted as:
- • Of special interest
- •• Of outstanding interest

1. Mayer RJ: **The Changing Nature of Esophageal Cancer**. *Chest* 1993, **103(Suppl)**:404S–405S.

2. •• Pera M, Cameron AJ, Trastek VF, Carpenter HA, Zinsmeister AR: **Increasing Incidence of Adenocarcinoma of the Esophagus and Esophagogastric Junction**. *Gastroenterology* 1993, **104**:510-513.

This population-based study shows a five- to sixfold increase in the incidence of adenocarcinoma of the esophagus and the esophagogastric junction over the past 60 years.

3. Sugarbaker DJ, DeCamp MM: **Selecting the Surgical Approach to Cancer of the Esophagus**. *Chest* 1993, **103 (Suppl)**:410S-414S.

4. • Orringer MB: **Multimodality Therapy for Esophageal Carcinoma-Update**. *Chest* 1993, **103(Suppl)**:406S-409S.

Over a 15-year period, the treatment results of transhiatal resection in esophageal cancer patients are summarized. A phase II neoadjuvant chemoradiotherapy trial suggests a beneficial effect on long-term survival in comparison to historical controls.

5. Kato H, Tachimori Y, Wantanabe H, Iizuka T, Terui S, Itabashi M, Hirota T: **Lymph Node Metastasis in Thoracic Esophageal Carcinoma.** *J Surg Oncol* 1991, **48**:106-111.

6. • Goldminc M, Maddern G, le Prise E, Meunier B, Campion JP, Launois B: **Oesophagectomy By a Transhiatal Approach or Thoracotomy:A Prospective Randomized Trial.** *Br J Surg* 1993, **80**:367-370.

Within the limited number of patients in this randomized study, the traditional transthoracic esophagectomy and the transhiatal esophagectomy are equally effective with respect to postoperative recovery and long-term survival.

7. • Paç M, Başoglu A, Koçak H, Yekeler I, Yediyildiz S, Aydin NE, Yilmaz A, Okçu N, Keles M: **Transhiatal Versus Transthoracic Esophagectomy for Esophageal Cancer.** *J Thorac Cardiovasc Surg* 1993, **106**:205-209.

In this retrospective study, early and late complications were less frequently observed after transhiatal resection than after transthoracic resection. Long-term survival was comparable.

8. • Tilanus HW, Hop WCJ, Langenhorst BLAM, van Lanschot JJB: **Esophagectomy With or Without Thoractomy. Is There Any Difference?** *J Thorac Cardiovasc Surg* 1993, **105**:898-903.

Retrospective analysis of 293 patients suggests that transhiatal resection without thoracotomy is technically safe and oncologically justifiable when compared with traditional transthoracic resection.

9. Imadhl A, Munzar T, Schulte-Monting J, Ruckauer KD, Kirchner R, Farthmann EH: **Perioperative Risikofaktoren Beim Osophaguskarzinom: Eine Retrospektive Studie Zur Analyse von Unabhangigen Faktoren.** *Zentralbl Chir* 1993, **118**:190-196.

10. Vigneswaran WT, Trastek VF, Pairolero PC, Deschamps C, Daly RC, Allen MS: **Transhiatal Esophagectomy for Carcinoma of the Esophagus.** *Ann Thorac Surg* 1993, **56**:838-846.

11. Lerut T, de Leyn P, Coosemans W, van Raemdonck D, Scheys I, LeSaffre E: **Surgical Strategies in Esophageal Carcinoma With Emphasis on Radical Lymphadenectomy.** *Ann Surg* 1992, **216**:583-590.

12. Okama T, Kaneko H, Yoshioka M, Torigoe Y, Miyauchi Y: **Prognosis in Esophageal Carcinoma With Cervical Lymph Node Metastases.** *Surgery* 1993, **114**:513-518.

13. • Krasna MJ, McLaughlin JS: **Thoracoscopic Lymph Node Staging for Esophageal Cancer.** *Ann Thorac Surg* 1993, **56**:671-674.

Preliminary experience of thoracoscopic lymph node with impressive results.

14. LoCicero III J: **Laparoscopy/Thoracoscopy for Staging. II. Pretherapy Nodal Evaluation in Carcinoma of the Esophagus.** *Semin Surg Oncol* 1993, **9**:56-58.

15. Gossot D, Fourquier P, Celerier M: **Thoracoscopic Esophagectomy: Technique and Initial Results.** *Ann Thorac Surg* 1993, **56**: 667-670.

16. van Overhagen H, Laméris JS, Berger MY, Klooswijk AIJ, Tilanus HW, van Pel R, Schutte HE: **CT Assessment of Resectability Prior to Transhiatal Esophagectomy for Esophageal/Gastroesophageal Junction Carcinoma.** *J Comput Assist Tomogr* 1993, **17**:367-373.

17. Fok M, Cheng SWK, Wong J: **Endosonography in Patient Selection for Surgical Treatment of Esophageal Carcinoma.** *World J Surg* 1992, **16**:1098-1103.

18. •• Bumm R, Holscher AH, Feussner H, Tachibana M, Bartels H, Siewert JR: **Endodissection of the Thoracic Esophagus; Technique and Clinical Results in Transhiatal Esophagectomy.** *Ann Surg* 1993, **218**:97-104.

Mediastinoscopic endodissection was compared with conventional transhiatal resection, using a matched pair algorithm. Endodissection prevented recurrent nerve damage and reduced pulmonary complications.

19. Azagra JS, Ceuterick M, Goergen M, Jacobs D, Gilbar, E, Zaouk G, Carlier E, Lejeune P, Alle JL, Mathys M: **Thoracoscopy in Oesophagectomy for Oesophageal Cancer.** *Br J Surg* 1993, **80**:320-321.

20. • Collard JM, Lengele B, Otte JB, Kestens PF: **En Bloc and Standard Esophagectomies by Thoracoscopy.** *Ann Thorac Surg* 1993, **56**:675-679.

Feasibility study of extensive esophagectomies by thoracoscopy with impressive results.

21. • Pierie JPEN, de Graaf PW, Poen H, van der Tweel I, Obertop H:**Incidence and Management of Benign Anastomotic Stricture After Cervical Oesophagogastrostomy.** *Br J Surg* 1993, **80**:471-474.

Poor vascularization of the gastric tube and postoperative anastomotic leakage are significant risk factors for stricture formation in patients with cervical esophagogastrostomy.

22. • Zieren HU, Muller JM, Pichlmaier H: **Prospective Randomized Study of One- or Two-Layer Anastomosis Following Oesophageal Resection and Cervical Oesophago-Gastrostomy.** *Br J Surg* 1993, **80**:608-611.

In patients with cervical esophagogastrostomy one-layer anastomosis is superior to the two-layer procedure because of the lower incidence of fibrotic stricture.

23. • Bartels H, Thorban S, Siewert JR: **Anterior Versus Posterior Reconstruction After Transhiatal Oesophagectomy: A Randomized Controlled Trial.** *Br J Surg* 1993, **80**:1141-1144.

In a randomized study, prevertebral gastric tube reconstruction after subtotal esophagectomy is associated with less postoperative complications as compared with extra-anatomical, retrosternal reconstruction.

24. Omura K, Misake T, Urayama H, Ishida F, Watanabe Y: **Composite Reconstruction of the Esophagus.** *J Surg Oncol* 1993, **52**:18-20.

25. Hirabayashi S, Miyate M, Shoji M, Shibusawa H: **Reconstruction of the Thoracic Esophagus, With Extended Jejunum Used as a Substitute, With the AID of Microvascular Anastomosis.** *Surgery* 1993, **113**:515-519.

26. Hareyama M, Nishio M, Kagami Y, Narimatsu N, Saito A, Sakurai T: **Intracavitary Brachytherapy Combined With External-Beam Irradiation for Squamous Cell Carcinoma of the Thoracic Esophagus.** *Int J Radiat Oncol Biol Phys* 1992, **24**:235-240.

27. Caspers RJL, Zwinderman AH, Griffioen G, Welvaart K, Sewsingh EN, Davelaar J and Leer JWH: **Combined External Beam and Low Dose Rate Intraluminal Radiotherapy in Oesophageal Cancer.** *Radiother Oncol* 1993, **27**:7-12.

28. Udaya Kumar M, Swamy K, Supe S, Anantha N: **Influence of Intraluminal Brachytherapy Dose on Complications in the Treatment of Esophageal Cancer.** *Int J Radiat Oncol Biol Phys* 1993, **27**:1069-1072.

29. Hishikawa Y, Izumi M, Kurisu K, Taniguchi M, Kamikonya N: **Esophageal Ulceration Following High-Dose Rate Intraluminal Brachytherapy for Esophageal Cancer.** *Radiother Oncol* 1993, **28**:252-254.

30. Jager JJ, Pannebakker M, Rijken J, de Vos J, Vismans FJFE: **Palliation in Esophageal Cancer With a Single Session of Intraluminal Irradiation.** *Radiother Oncol* 1992, **25**:134-136.

31. Harvey JC, Fleischman EH, Bellotti JE, Kagan AR: **Intracavitary Radiation in the Treatment of Advanced Esophageal Carcinoma: A Comparison of High Dose Rate Vs. Low Dose Rate Brachytherapy.** *J Surg Oncol* 1993, **52**:101-104.

32. •• Schmid EU, Alberts AS, Greeff F, Terblanche APS, Schoeman L, Burger W, Shiels RA, Friediger D, Van der Hoven A, Falkson G: **The Value of Radiotherapy or Chemother-**

apy **After Intubation for Advanced Esophageal Carcinoma-A Prospective Randomized Trial**. *Radiother Oncol* 1993, **28**:27-30.

No benefit with respect to palliation or survival was demonstrated for additional chemo- or radiotherapy after pertubation in patients with locally advanced tumors.

33. • Gschossmann JM, Bonner JA, Foote RL, Shaw EG, Martenson JA, Su J: **Malignant Tracheoesophageal Fistula in Patients with Esophageal Cancer**. *Cancer* 1993, 72:1513-1521.

In 10 of 41 patients with malignant fistula treated with radiotherapy, no deterioration of symptoms was observed, but survival was poor.

34. •• Fok M, Sham JST, Chow D, Cheng SWK, Wong J: **Postoperative Radiotherapy for Carcinoma of the Esophagus: A Prospective, Randomized Controlled Study**. *Surgery* 1993, **113**:138-147.

Postoperative radiotherapy with a high dose per fraction resulted in a high rate of severe complications in the intrathoracic stomach and a poorer survival in the radiotherapy group, although less local recurrences occurred.

35. • Arimoto T, Takamura A, Tomita M, Suzuki K, Hosokawa M, Kaneko Y: **Intraoperative Radiotherapy for Esophageal Carcinoma-Significance of IORT Dose for the Incidence of Fatal Tracheal Complications**. *Int J Radiat Oncol Biol Phys* 1993, **27**:1063-1067.

In patients treated with esophagectomy and electron beam intraoperative radiotherapy followed by postoperative external beam radiotherapy, tracheal ulceration occurred only in the 25-Gy intraoperative radiotherapy–dose group.

36. • LoCicero J: **Will Multimodality Therapy Solve the Enigma of Long-Term Survival for Squamous Cell Carcinoma of the Esophagus?** *Semin Surg Oncol* 1993, 9:14-18.

An overview of a variety of combined-treatment studies clarifies that phase III trials are required to establish the best multimodality therapy for esophageal cancer. Suggestions are made for the design of such trials.

37. Wadler S, Fell S, Haynes H, Katz HJ, Rozenblit A, Kaleya R, Wiernik PH:**Treatment of Carcinoma of the Esophagus with 5-Fluorouracil and Recombinant Alfa-2a-Interferon**. *Cancer* 1993, **71**:1726-1730.

38. Herskovic A, Martz K, Al-Sarraf M, Leichman L, Bridle J, Vaitkevicius V, Cooper J, Byhardt R, Davis L, Emami B: **Combined Chemotherapy and Radiotherapy Compared With Radiotherapy Alone in Patients With Cancer of the Esophagus**. *N Engl J Med* 1992, **326**:1593-1598.

39. Coia LR, Soffen EM, Schultheiss TE, Martin EE, Hanks GE: **Swallowing Function in Patients With Esophageal Cancer Treated With Concurrent Radiation and Chemotherapy**. *Cancer* 1993, **71**:281-286.

40. Izquierdo MA, Marcuello E, Gomez de Segura G, Blanco R, Canals E, Gomez A, Sampedro F: **Unresectable Nonmetastatic Squamous Cell Carcinoma of the Esophagus Managed by Sequential Chemotherapy (Cisplatin and Bleomycin) and Radiation Therapy**. *Cancer* 1993, **71**:287-292.

41. Wolfe WG, Vaughn AL, Seigler HF, Hathorn JW, Leopold KA, Duhaylonsod FG: **Survival of Patients With Carcinoma of the Esophagus Treated With Combined-Modality Therapy**. *J Thorac Cardiovasc Surg*, 1993, **105**:749-756.

42. • Forastiere AA, Orringer MB, Perez-Tamayo C, Urba SG, Zahurak M: **Preoperative Chemoradiation Followed by Transhiatal Esophagectomy for Carcinoma of the Esophagus: Final Report**. *J Clin Oncol*, 1993, **11**:1118-1123.

Preoperative chemoradiation showed a doubling of the 5-year survival rate compared with surgery alone (historical controls). The value of a pathologically complete remission is discussed.

43. Terz JJ, Leong LA, Lipsett JA, Wagman LD: **Preoperative Chemotherapy and Radiotherapy for Cancer of the Esophagus**. *Surgery*, 1993, **114**:71-75.

44. Carey RW, Hilgenberg AD, Wilkins EW, Choi NC, Mathisen DJ, Grillo HC, Wain JC, Logan DL, Bromberg C: **Long-Term Follow-Up of Neoadjuvant Chemotherapy With 5-Fluorouracil and Cisplatin with Surgical Resection and Possible Postoperative Radiotherapy and/or Chemotherapy in Squamous Cell Carcinoma of the Esophagus**. *Canc Invest* 1993, **11**:99-105.

45. Hoff SJ, Stewart JR, Sawyers JL, Murray MJ, Merrill WH, Adkins RB, Johnson DH: **Preliminary Results With Neoadjuvant Therapy and Resection for Esophageal Carcinoma**. *Ann Thorac Surg* 1993, **56**:282-287.

46. Peddada AV, Harvey JC, Anderson PJ, Davidson W, Smith DE, Kagan R: **High Dose Rate Intraluminal Radiation in a Combined Modality Treatment Plan for Carcinoma of the Esophagus**. *J Surg Oncol* 1993, **52**:160-163.

47. Saito T, Shigemitsu Y, Kinoshita T, Shimoda K, Abe T, Nakamura A, Chikuba K, Kobayashi M: **Cisplatin, Vindesine, Pepleomycin and Concurrent Radiation Therapy Following Esophagectomy With Lymphadenectomy for Patients With an Esophageal Carcinoma**. *Oncology* 1993, **50**:293-297.

48. •• Japanese Esophageal Oncology Group. **A Comparison of Chemotherapy and Radiotherapy As Adjuvant Treatment to Surgery for Esophageal Carcinoma**. *Chest* 1993, **104**:203-207.

A randomized study did not show any difference in survival between patients treated with adjuvant chemotherapy or radiotherapy.

49. Sakata K, Aoki Y, Muta N, Therahara A, Karasawa K, Onogi Y, Nakagawa K, Hasezawa K, Sasaki Y, Akanuma A:**Effect of Human Granulocyte Colony-Stimulating Factor on Neutropenia Induced by Radiotherapy and Chemotherapy**. *Oncology* 1993, **50**:238-240.

J. Jan B. van Lanschot, Joke G. J. Letschert, and Cees H. N. Veenhof, Academic Medical Center, Meibergdreef 9, 1105 AZ Amsterdam, the Netherlands.

Esophageal therapeutic endoscopy, laser, and prosthesis

Horst Neuhaus, MD

II. Medizinische Klinik und Poliklinik, Klinikum rechts der Isar der Technischen Universität München, München, Germany

Recent work in therapeutic endoscopy of nonvascular diseases of the esophagus continues to focus on dilatation or stenting of stenoses and ablation of metaplastic or neoplastic tissue. For individual indications, the selection of the optimal treatment can be difficult in view of a plethora of alternative procedures and a limited number of comparative trials. Dilatation can be considered the first-line method for achalasia because of excellent long-term results and a low number of major complications that can be safely and durably treated by surgery. Bougienage and pneumatic dilatation seem to be equally effective for various types of benign strictures. The latest techniques do not require routine fluoroscopic control. Laser photoablation of Barrett's epithelium leading to restoration of squamous mucosa is an exciting new tool for research. Photodynamic therapy can achieve complete ablation of early esophageal adenocarcinoma in selected cases, but it does not seem to offer major advantages over thermal laser therapy for advanced tumor stages. Self-expandable metal stents rapidly achieve recanalization of obstructing esophageal malignancies with a minimally invasive approach. Considerable long-term complications may be overcome by covered stents, which are especially useful for occlusion of esophagorespiratory fistulas.

Current Opinion in Gastroenterology 1994, **10**:473–480

Removal of foreign bodies

Retained esophageal foreign bodies should be rapidly removed to avoid complications such as perforation or aspiration. Berggreen *et al.* [1•] reviewed the efficacy of various extraction methods in 76 adults and 116 children. Intravenous application of glucagon or nifedipine showed a failure rate of 75%, so its use should be restricted to selected cases. Young children, who do not tolerate endoscopic maneuvers well, underwent rigid endoscopy under general anesthesia for removal of sharp or pointed objects. In contrast, flexible endoscopy was performed in the majority of the adults. Both endoscopic approaches achieved success rates of more than 96%, but rigid esophagoscopy carried a higher complication rate (10% vs 5.1%).

The Foley catheter technique was exclusively used in children, particularly for extraction of coins, with a success rate of 95% and no major complications [1•].

Kelley *et al.* [2] recommended Foley catheters or bougienage for simple removal of esophageal coins in children with no history of esophageal disease, no respiratory distress, and a duration of ingestion of less than 24 hours. These methods succeeded in all 38 cases and were considerably less expensive than rigid endoscopy. However, for the majority of older children and adults with foreign esophageal bodies, flexible endoscopy is now the preferable procedure in many centers because it allows a safe extraction with inspection of the mucosa and does not require general anesthesia. Even sharp objects can be removed with overtubes or a protector hood that can be positioned at the end of almost any endoscope [3]. Tsutsui *et al.* [4] reported on a removal of a press-through package with sharp edges from the esophagus using two flexible endoscopes for forceps extraction.

Dilatation for achalasia

Owing to a lack of appropriate randomized trials, the choice between pneumatic dilatation and cardiomyotomy as the initial treatment for achalasia is still controversial. Recent studies [5–9] suggest that a treatment regimen starting with dilatation is usually effective and has a shorter recovery and less overall costs than initial cardiomyotomy. Perforations are rare and can be managed by surgery with an excellent clinical outcome.

Parkman *et al.* [5••] reviewed 123 patients undergoing initial pneumatic dilatation for achalasia using the Browne-McHardy dilatator (Narco Scientific, Fort Washington, PA). Perforation was seen in 1.6% of the

 ISBN 1-85922-609-4 ISSN 0267–1379

patients who subsequently underwent surgery. An additional 11% of the patients underwent elective cardiomyotomy for persistent or recurrent symptoms during a mean follow-up period of 4.7 years. All other patients were successfully managed with a single session or repeated sessions of dilatation in 58% and 42%, respectively. Each subsequent dilatation had less benefit. In agreement with previous studies, youthful age unfavorably affected the efficacy of the procedure. Initial cardiomyotomy performed in an additional six patients achieved comparable clinical results as initial dilatation and subsequent surgery. However, the overall costs of surgery were 2.4 times greater than the nonsurgical approach including subsequent treatments of symptomatic patients.

Many endoscopists now prefer the Rigiflex balloon dilatator (Microvasive, Watertown, MA) for achalasia because it can be inserted over a guidewire, which is particularly helpful in patients with a markedly dilated esophagus. The correct position of the dilatator can be controlled by fluoroscopy or by means of an endoscope that is inserted beside the catheter with the tip proximal to the transparent balloon. The Rigiflex balloon has a noncompliant characteristic so that inflation is restricted to its designated diameter. In contrast, the final diameter of many other devices depends on the inflation pressure, which is associated with the risk of perforation [5••].

Kadakia and Wong [6•] reported on 47 dilations in 29 patients using Rigiflex dilatators. A 3.0-cm balloon was used first with a symptomatic response in 62% of the patients over a mean follow-up period of 47 months. The overall success rate increased to 93% when balloons of 3.5 cm to 4.0 cm were used after failure of the smaller dilatator. The type of the balloon and the strategy of gradual dilatation may explain why there were no perforations. However, because procedure-related complications can be serious, careful clinical monitoring is mandatory.

Nair *et al.* [7••] retrospectively analyzed risk factors, clinical characteristics, and outcome of pneumatic dilatation with a Browne-McHardy balloon in 178 patients with achalasia or esophageal spasm. Nine major complications, including four perforations, occurred. A prior pneumatic dilatation and an inflation pressure of at least 11 psi were determined as independent risk factors. The incidence of chest pain during the procedure had no influence on the development of complications. In contrast, subsequent chest pain, blood on the dilatator, and tachycardia were indicators of patients with an increased risk of having developed a complication. In all cases with a major complication, one of these indicators or the complication itself was recognized within 5 hours of the procedure. In view of these results, an esophagogram could be restricted to symptomatic cases but this may cause a delay of detection and treatment.

Ciarolla and Traube [8•] reported on a short-term clinical monitoring after pneumatic dilatation with no routine hospitalization. Esophagram was performed in only 15 of 100 patients because of pain, fever, or retching and revealed a perforation in seven patients, all of whom successfully underwent surgery. The complication rate is higher than in other recent series, despite a comparable technique of dilatation apart from an initial use of the 40-mm Rigiflex balloon in more than half of the cases. Schwartz *et al.* [9•] compared the outcome of the seven patients with perforations undergoing surgery for repair, usually supplemented by myotomy, with five patients treated by elective myotomy during the same period. There was no significant difference in duration of operation, hospitalization, and long-term outcome between both groups. These results and comparable data of Nair *et al.* [7••] favor pneumatic dilatation as initial treatment because even if perforation occurs, rapid surgical treatment leads to results similar to elective cardiomyotomy. Surgical repair without cardiomyotomy seems to be as effective as the combined approach because adequate myotomy has usually been performed by the endoscopist [10]. In view of these excellent results of emergency surgery, conservative treatment of perforation should be restricted to small lesions with minimal symptoms.

In the future, laparoscopic cardiomyotomy may offer a minimally invasive alternative treatment. Local injection of the toxin of *Clostridium botulinum* seems to be another promising and simple form of treatment of achalasia. Animal studies showed that this agent has a relatively specific anticholinergic effect and is a potent inhibitor of resting the baseline lower esophageal sphincter [11••]. Preliminary clinical data showed a complete response in four of five patients undergoing endoscopic intrasphincteric injection of botulinum toxin over a follow-up period of up to 6 months [12•]. No major side effects were observed.

Management of benign esophageal strictures

Esophageal dilatation has become the method of choice for treating most benign strictures. Balloon dilatation guided over a wire or through the scope offers theoretic advantages over bougienage because only axial and no shear forces are applied to the stricture, which may increase the efficacy and safety of the procedure. However, a recent trial [13] showed no significant difference in the clinical outcome between the two techniques. Tucker [14] performed Maloney dilatation of benign strictures of the esophagus in 145 patients. Fluoroscopy altered the dilatation technique in every fourth patient and was in particular needed for patients with peptic strictures or larger hiatal hernias. Blind Maloney dilatation should therefore be restricted to selected cases with a straight and well-defined esophageal anatomy. Using the same type of dilatator, Burdick *et al.* [15•] treated 75 patients with a lower esophageal ring. The procedure failed in only seven patients, who subsequently underwent endoscopic electrocautery incision with excellent long-term results in six of these cases.

Kadakia *et al.* [16•] reported on bougienage with American endoscopy dilatators passed over an endoscopically inserted guidewire in 138 patients with predominately benign strictures. In 41 of these cases, the marked guidewire had to be advanced blindly through an endoscopically impassable stenosis. A fluoroscopic control of the procedure was needed in only eight patients. There were no method-related complications. Preliminary results of a randomized trial [17•] indicate that in patients with peptic esophageal strictures, less frequent bougie dilatations are needed and better clinical results can be expected when steroids are injected into the lesions. Broor *et al.* [18•] compared the efficacy and safety of bougienage of corrosive strictures ($n=52$) with peptic strictures ($n=39$). Comparably high initial success rates of more than 93% were obtained in both groups with a higher number of procedures and recurrences in patients with corrosive strictures. These results could be expected because corrosive lesions are frequently very tight, long, and multiple. However, the need for further dilatations decreased over time and the difference in the recurrence rates between the two groups was not more significant after 36 months. All patients could be managed without surgery during the study period, but on average 15 dilatations were required per patient. Nine perforations could be conservatively treated.

In children, stenoses of the esophagus are predominately due to a repair of esophageal atresia, fundoplication, and caustic or peptic lesions. Two studies [19•,20] report on bougienage or dilatation in a total of 65 cases. During a mean follow-up period of 1.2 years, 94% of the children responded to the treatment after a mean number of five dilatation sessions. Only one perforation was observed.

Endoscopic insertion of self-expandable metal stents can theoretically reduce the incidence of recurrence of benign stenoses after dilatation. Cwikiel *et al.* [21•] reported on esophageal implantation of Ultraflex stents (Boston Scientific, Jyllinge, Denmark) in 10 healthy pigs and five patients with benign strictures. This stent is a mesh tube made of memory nitinol filaments that is inserted with a delivery catheter with a diameter of 8 mm and expands to 18 mm after release. Autopsy and histologic examinations of the animals indicated severe necrosis of the mucosa and granulation in the submucosa after 1 to 2 weeks of stent placement. Severe fibrosis and degeneration of the muscular tissue was seen after 4 to 8 weeks. These findings corresponded to the clinical results, which showed significant stenoses due to hyperplastic tissue infiltration in two of the five patients. Esophageal resection was required in one case. In view of these results and a lack of further trials, esophageal insertion of metal stents for benign stenoses does not seem to be justified at present, particularly in view of the irremovability of uncovered devices. In the future, removable or absorbable expanding stents may be available for this indication.

Laser photoablation of Barrett's epithelium

Barrett's esophagus is widely regarded as a risk factor for adenocarcinoma of the esophagus. Theoretically, a regression of Barrett's metaplastic epithelium might prevent the development of dysplasia and cancer. This goal cannot usually be achieved by antireflux therapy alone but by additional ablation of the metaplastic tissue. Berenson *et al.* [22••] performed argon laser photoablation of columnar tissue in 10 patients having longstanding Barrett's esophagus who received 40 mg of omeprazol daily. Reepthelialization of squamous tissue was seen in 38 of 40 laser-treated segments. Surprisingly, squamous regrowth did not occur only from contiguous squamous borders but also from areas surrounded by columnar epithelium alone. This observation suggests that there are progenitor cells within Barrett's mucosa that can differentiate normally under suppression of acid reflux. Regression of Barrett's esophagus was also seen after neodymium:yttrium-aluminum-garnet laser ablation or photodynamic therapy in combination with acid suppression [23,24]. Further studies are needed before this exciting treatment can be used for clinical purposes [25•]. Endoscopic biopsy surveillance of Barrett's esophagus has been recommended and the results of a recently reported biopsy protocol [26•] indicated that high-grade dysplasia can be accurately detected and differentiated from early adenocarcinoma. Clinical management of high-grade dysplasia in Barrett's esophagus is controversial. Photodynamic therapy of severe dysplasia or early adenocarcinoma [27•] may offer an alternative to surgery. Endoscopic ultrasound could be helpful in staging and selection of patients.

Endoscopic treatment of esophageal carcinoma

Endoscopic destruction of early esophageal carcinoma with a curative objective can be achieved in selected cases, in particular by photodynamic therapy [27•,28]. However, all of four recently published trials [29•,30–32] on this exciting method aimed at palliation in patients with advanced tumor stages. Endoscopic local injection of anticancer drugs is another option for radical treatment of early cancer of the esophagus. Hagiwara *et al.* [33••] developed a drug-delivery format comprising activated carbon particles absorbing peplomycin. Experiments with rats showed that local injection of this format achieves high levels of peplomycin to the injection site and regional lymph nodes and low levels to blood plasma. Five of 6 patients with superficial esophageal cancer undergoing this treatment have survived to the present or died without cancer after 27 to 72 months.

Because the majority of the few patients with T1, N0 tumor stages undergo surgery, endoscopic procedures are predominately performed for palliation of advanced obstructing tumors. For this purpose, endoscopic local tumor debulking and intubation are more complementary than competitive methods, which should both be available in endoscopic centers. A combination of these procedures with chemotherapy or radiation offers several theoretic advantages, but the benefit of appropriate treatment protocols must be confirmed in randomized trials.

Palliative tumor ablation

Sclerosant injection is a simple and inexpensive measure for local tumor debulking. However, there are little data on its efficacy and safety and a comparison to laser treatment is not available. Fiorini *et al.* [34] performed endoscopic injection of ethanol in 37 patients with malignant dysphagia. Symptomatic relief was seen in 95% of the cases for a mean period of 47 days after one to two procedures. There were no complications. Of numerous studies on laser treatment only two previous trials compared this procedure directly with endoscopic intubation or additional insertion of tubes in a randomized fashion [35,36].

Recently, another controlled study [37] was performed in 40 patients with malignant dysphagia who were randomly assigned to laser recanalization or endoscopic intubation. Patency was achieved in all patients except one failed intubation. The quality of swallowing was significantly better with laser treatment than with intubation, which was associated with less loss of weight. Surprisingly, there was no significant difference in the in-patient stay as a proportion of survival time between both groups, although patients treated by laser required on average 2.5 times more admissions. The authors claim that, in contrast to a previous report [35], the advantage of laser recanalization would be independent of the tumor length, but appropriate data were not reported. Enhancement of laser treatment by external radiotherapy is a promising approach for effective irradiation of the whole tumor. In addition to laser application, a 30-Gy dose was well tolerated and achieved a mean prolongation of a dysphagia-controlled interval from 5 to 13 weeks compared with historical controls of laser treatment only. Based on these uncontrolled observations, a randomized trial is underway [38].

Nonthermal tumor ablation can be achieved by photodynamic therapy, another expensive procedure, after injection of a photosensitizing agent with affinity for tumor tissue. At present most studies are performed with hematoporphyrin, but new drugs promising less side effects are under investigation. Recent animal studies [39•] indicated that 630 nm of continuous wave light from an argon laser was as effective as pulsed light from a KTP/532 dye laser at the same wavelength. Laser application by a cylindrical diffuser inserted through the instrumentation channel of an endoscope may result in a noncircumferential and unpredictable photodynamic therapy response. According to an animal study, a recently developed balloon holding a diffuser in the centrum of the lumen can overcome this problem [40]. Lightdale *et al.* [29•] reported on a randomized controlled multicenter trial of photodynamic therapy versus neodymium:yttrium-aluminum-garnet laser therapy for palliation of malignant dysphagia in 236 patients. Response, improvement in dysphagia, procedure-related complications, median time to treatment failure, and median survival were comparable between both groups. A tendency toward fewer treatment endoscopies and a shorter treatment course was noted in patients undergoing photodynamic therapy, but the statistical relevance was not published until now. These minor advantages of photodynamic therapy over thermal laser destruction for tumor palliation were achieved at the expense of photosensitivity reactions in every fifth patient. The usually recommended time for avoidance of sunlight after photodynamic therapy is 1 month, which is a long period considering the short life-expectancy in this group of patients.

Tubes and stents

In many centers endoscopic intubation is still the most commonly used method for palliation of malignant dysphagia, as this inexpensive procedure can be performed rapidly and provides immediate and durable relief of dysphagia. A variety of self-expandable metal stents have been introduced to overcome drawbacks of conventional plastic tubes such as an invasive implantation procedure requiring large-bore dilatation and a significant risk of migration. In contrast, esophageal dilatation to a diameter of 10 to 12 mm is usually sufficient for insertion of a delivery device with a compressed metal stent. General anesthesia, which is preferred for endoscopic intubation in some centers, is not required for insertion of metal stents. Most previous small clinical series were performed with uncovered Wallstents (Schneider Europe, Bülach, Switzerland). The Wallstent is made from stainless steel alloy wires formed into a tubular mesh with a diameter of 16 to 20 mm when fully expanded.

Knyrim *et al.* [41••] reported on the first randomized controlled trial on Wallstents versus plastic tubes in 42 patients. Technical success rate, improvement and recurrence of dysphagia, postprocedural Karnofsky index, 30-day mortality, number of reinterventions, and survival were not significantly different between both groups (Table 1). The total hospital stay was longer in the plastic group, which can outweigh the initial costs of metal stents depending on the cost of hospitalization. Complications defined as perforation, aspiration pneumonia, and migration were significantly less with the metal stents than with the plastic prostheses. The incidence of perforation of 14% in the plastic tube group was high compared with other controlled trials on endoscopic intubation [35,37], which may be due to a single-stage dilatation with a 20-mm balloon under general anesthesia [42•]. Surprisingly, recurrent dysphagia caused by bolus impaction, tumor ingrowth or overgrowth, and occurrence of a fistula was not regarded as a complication in this study. If so, there would have been only minor differences in the total number of complications between both groups. In a recent uncontrolled trial, esophageal Wallstent implantation was associated with complications in every second patient [43] (Table 1).

Cwikiel *et al.* [44•] reported on esophageal implantation of self-expanding Ultraflex stents in 40 patients with malignant dysphagia. This nitinol stent is released after contact with fluid that dissolves a gelatin encasing the compressed device on a delivery catheter (Fig. 1). All stents expanded completely, but the capacity of the self-expanding mechanism is difficult to determine because postprocedural balloon dilatation was performed to a diameter of up to 15 mm, which is 3 mm less than the maximal width of the stent. Most of the patients received a normal diet thereafter. The complication rate was lower than in other recent trials on esophageal metal stents, perhaps because of a less strict follow-up protocol of the Ultraflex study (Table 1).

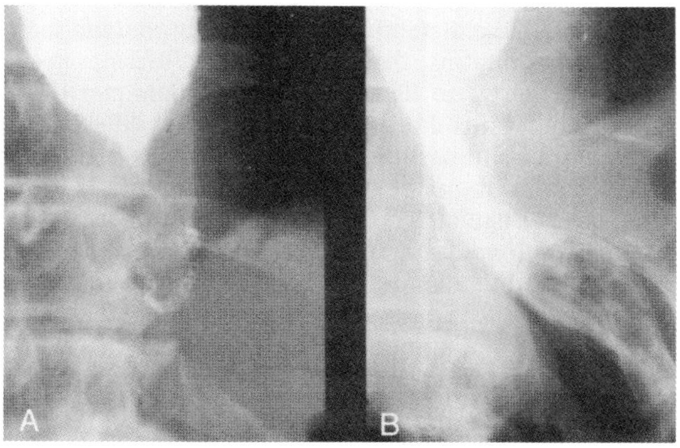

Fig. 1. A, Complete obstruction of a esophagojejunal anastomosis after gastrectomy. **B**, Passage of contrast medium after insertion of an Ultraflex (Boston Scientific, Jyllinge, Denmark) stent; note the sweeping shape of the stent adapting to the lumen of the jejunum. The clinical relevance of the different characteristics between various types of metal stents is undetermined owing to lack of comparative trials.

Two case reports described a successful treatment of a strictured malignant esophagojejunostomy by uncovered Gianturco stents [45,46]. All manufactures of self-expanding stents test covered devices to overcome the problem of tissue infiltration. At present, little experimental and clinical uncontrolled data are available.

Table 1. Recent trials on use of self-expanding metal stents for malignant dysplasia

	Study outcomes				
	Knyrim *et al.* [41••]		Vermeijden *et al.* [43]	Cwikiel *et al.* [44•]	Wu *et al.* [47•]
Stent used	Plastic tube	Wallstent†	Wallstent†	Ultraflex‡	Gianturco-Rösch-Z
Coating	—	No	No	No	Yes
Patients, *n*	21	21	25	40	24 with stenosis, 8 with fistula
Short-term improvement, %	95	95	NR	100	84
Total complication, %	52	33*	55	25	31
Complications, *n*					
Perforation	3	—	2	–	1
Fistula	1	2	3	—	—
Migration	5	—	—	1	4
Reobstruction					
Bolus impaction	1	3	1	1	2
Tissue ingrowth or overgrowth	—	5	5	3	2
Undetermined	—	—	—	3	—
Aspiration	1	—	—	—	—
Bleeding	—	—	—	2	1
30-day mortality, %	29	14	5	8	3

*Three patients had two complications at a different period of time.
†Wallstent (Schneider Europe, Bülach, Switzerland).
‡Ultraflex (Boston Scientific, Jyllinge, Denmark).
NR—not reported.

Wu *et al.* [47•] reported on modified Gianturco stents and covered by the same group. Anchoring hooks at the midportion of the stent should prevent migration, which is a major problem of covered tubes. These stents were implanted in 24 patients with malignant esophageal stenoses and in eight patients with esophagorespiratory fistulas (Table 1). Before insertion, stenoses were dilated to a mean diameter of 14 mm, which does not seem to be very different to conventional endoscopic intubation. In the dysphagia group, 88% of the patients clinically improved. A complete seal of fistulas could be achieved in six of eight patients. As expected, tumor ingrowth was no major problem for this technique and was seen in only one case, due to a disruption of the stent membrane. On the other hand, migration, a rare complication of uncovered stents, occurred in 13% of all cases and required laparotomy in one patient.

Do *et al.* [48•] treated eight patients with malignant esophagorespiratory fistulas by insertion of a covered Gianturco-Song stent (Sooho Medi-Tech Co., Seoul, Korea) (Fig. 2). Details of this type of stent were previously reported by the same group [49]. All fistulas could be occluded with subsequent relief of aspiration. Tumor overgrowth was observed in one case. Late esophageal perforation occurred in another patient but did not seem to be related to the stent. There was no further complication. These preliminary results suggest that covered stents are effective and safe for sealing of esophagorespiratory fistulas, which require a rapid treatment. Because there is no optimal therapy for this indication, the new devices should be considered as a nonsurgical alternative to cuffed plastic tubes, conventional plastic tubes plus tracheo-bronchial metal stents, or injection of cyanoacrylate [50–52].

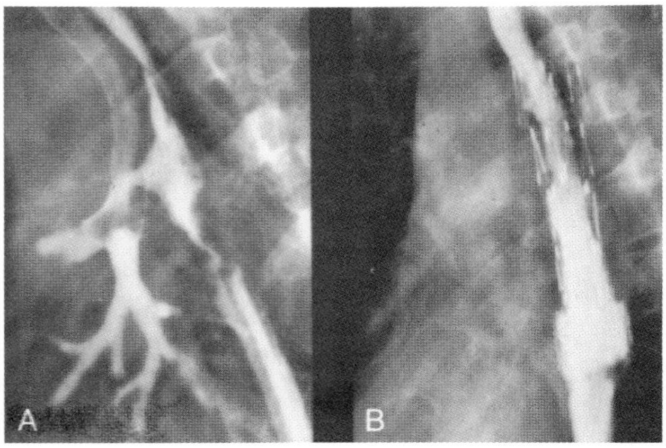

Fig. 2. A, Esophagogram indicating a large esophagorespiratory fistula. **B**, Complete sealing of the fistula after implantation of a covered Gianturco-Song stent (Sooho Medi-Tech Co., Seoul, Korea).

The recent studies on esophageal metal stents demonstrate that their major advantage is the minimally invasive implantation procedure associated with a low rate of early complications. However, in the long-term, various stent-related problems indicate that further improvement of self-expanding stents is required to justify considerably higher initial costs compared with alternative palliative procedures in patients with a short life-expectancy.

References and recommended reading

Papers of particular interest, published within the annual period of review, have been highlighted as:
• Of special interest
•• Of outstanding interest

1. • Berggreen PJ, Harrison ME, Sanowski RA, Ingebo K, Noland B, Zierer S: **Techniques and Complications of Esophageal Foreign Body Extraction in Children and Adults.** *Gastrointest Endosc* 1993, **39**:626–630.
Large retrospective analysis of the efficacy and safety of different methods for removal of esphageal foreign bodies. Owing to a higher complication rate, rigid endoscopy should be reserved for failures of flexible endoscopy. The Foley catheter technique can be recommended for proximally located blunt objects in young children to avoid general anesthesia for endoscopy.

2. Kelley JE, Leech MH, Carr MG: **A Safe and Cost-Effective Protocol for the Management of Esophageal Coins in Children.** *J Pediatr Surg* 1993, **28**:898–900.

3. Bertoni G, Pacchione, Sassatelli R, Ricci E, Mortilla MG, Gumina C: **A New Protector Device for Safe Endoscopic Removal of Sharp Gastroesophageal Foreign Bodies in Infants.** *J Pediatr Gastroenterol Nutr* 1993, **16**:393–396.

4. Tsutsui S, Masuda T, Matsuda H, Harada N, Sonoda T, Takada K: **Removal of a Press-through Package in the Thoracic Esophagus Using Two Flexible Endoscopes.** *Endoscopy* 1993, **25**:374–375.

5. •• Parkman HP, Reynolds JC, Ouyang A, Rosato EF, Eisenberg JM, Cohen S: **Pneumatic Dilatation or Esophagomyotomy Treatment for Idiopathic Achalasia: Clinical Outcomes and Cost Analysis.** *Dig Dis Sci* 1993, **38**:75–85.
Detailed retrospective comparison between balloon dilatation or surgery for achalasia. A single dilatation achieved long-term improvement in 58% of 123 cases. A further 30% could be managed by subsequent dilatation. Only 15 patients with failure of this approach successfully underwent esophagomyotomy. These results support pneumatic dilatation as the first-line treatment for achalasia.

6. • Kadakia SC, Wong RKH: **Graded Pneumatic Dilation Using Rigiflex Achalasia Dilatators in Patients with Primary Esophageal Achalasia.** *Am J Gastroenterol* 1993, **88**:34–38.
Dilatation with the noncompliant Rigiflex balloon was performed in 29 patients with no complications and a overall success rate of 93%. These excellent results may be due to the protocol of graded dilatation in 4- to 8-week intervals if there was no initial symptomatic response to a 3.0-cm balloon.

7. •• Nair LA, Reynolds JC, Parkman HP, Ouyang A, Strom BL, Rosato EF, Cohen S: **Complications During Pneumatic Dilation for Achalasia or Diffuse Esophageal Spasm. Analysis of Risk Factors, Early Clinical Characteristics, and Outcome.** *Dig Dis Sci* 1993, **38**:1893–1904.
Major complications of balloon dilatation are rare and can be detected within 5 hours suggesting that an outpatient procedure is practicable. Previous dilatation and inflation pressures of at least 11 psi are independent risk factors. Surgical repair of perforation plus cardiomyotomy has a comparable long-term outcome as elective cardiomyotomy.

8. • Ciarolla DA, Traube M: **Achalasia; Short-Term Clinical Monitoring After Pneumatic Dilatation.** *Dig Dis Sci* 1993, **38**:1905–1908.

A review of 100 dilatations without routine postprocedural esophagogram or hospitalization. All seven patients with perforations had pain within 3 hours of the dilatation and successfully underwent surgery.

9. • Schwartz HM, Cahow CE, Traube M: **Outcome After Perforation Sustained During Pneumatic Dilatation for Achalasia.** *Dig Dis Sci* 1993, **38**:1409–1413.

Emergency surgery for repair of perforation caused by dilatation has a comparable outcome as elective myotomy for achalasia. These results suggest that rapid detection of perforation is mandatory and conservative treatment should be restricted to selected cases.

10. Pricolo VE, Park CS, Thompson WR: **Surgical Repair of Esophageal Perforation Due to Pneumatic Dilatation for Achalasia. Is Myotomy Really Necessary?** *Arch Surg* 1993, **128**:540–544.

11. •• Pasricha PJ, Ravich WJ, Kalloo AN: **Effects of Intrashincteric Botulinum Toxin on the Lower Esophageal Sphincter in Piglets.** *Gastroenterology* 1993, **105**:1045–1049.

Endoscopic injection of botulinum toxin significantly decreases the lower esophageal pressure. This agent promises to be an exciting tool for further studies on cholinergic and anticholinergic pathways in the regulation of gastrointestinal sphincters.

12. • Pasricha PJ, Ravich WJ, Hendrix TR, Kalloo AN: **Treatment of Achalasia With Intrasphincteric Injection of Botulinum Toxin - Results of a Pilot Study.** *Gastroenterology* 1993, **104**:A168.

Preliminary data on local injection of botulinum toxin demonstrate excellent clinical response and improvement of objective parameters in four of five patients with achalasia. A placebo-controlled trial is underway.

13. Yamamoto H, Hughes RW, Schroeder KW, Viggiano TR, DiMagno EP: **Treatment of Benign Esophageal Stricture by Eder-Puestow or Balloon Dilatators: A Comparison Between Randomized and Prospective Nonrandomized Trials.** *Mayo Clin Proc* 1992, 67:228–236.

14. Tucker LE: **The Importance of Fluoroscopic Guidance for Maloney Dilation.** *Am J Gastroenterol* 1992, **87**:1709–1711.

15. • Burdick JS, Venu RP, Hogan WJ: **Cutting the Defiant Lower Esophageal Ring.** *Gastrointest Endosc* 1993, **39**:616–619.

Endoscopic needle-knife incision of a lower esophageal ring is safe and effective in patients refractory to dilatation.

16. • Kadakia SC, Parker A, Carrougher JG, Shaffer RT: **Esophageal Dilation With Polyvinyl Bougies, Using a Marked Guidewire Without the Aid of Fluoroscopy: An Update.** *Am J Gastroenterol* 1993, **88**:1381–1386.

Bougie dilatation of malignant or benign esophageal stenoses was performed in 197 sessions without fluoroscopic control. This approach seems to be safe even when a guidewire must be advanced blindly through tight strictures. A marker on the guidewire is helpful for prevention of dislocation.

17. • Rupp T, Earle D, Dick P, Hawes R, Rex D, Wiersema M, Crabb D, Rathgaber S, Lumeng L, Lehmann G: **Randomized Trial of Dilation Plus Intralesional Steroids Vs. Dilation Alone for Benign Gastroesophageal Strictures [Abstract].** *Gastrointest Endosc* 1993, **39**:A287.

Ongoing study that indicates a trend toward less frequent procedures and better dysphagia improvement in patients with benign esophageal stenoses treated with endoscopic injection of steroids in addition to dilatation compared with those treated with dilatation alone.

18. • Broor SL, Raju GS, Bose PP, Lahoti D, Ramesh GN, Kumar A, Sood GK: **Long Term Results of Endoscopic Dilatation for Corrosive Oesophageal Strictures.** *Gut* 1993, **34**:1498–1501.

Large series on bougienage of corrosive and peptic esophageal strictures that shows how repeated dilatations are justified even in difficult corrosive lesions because the initially high recurrence rate decreases over time and the procedure related complication rate is 1% or less.

19. • Shah MD, Berman WF: **Endoscopic Balloon Dilation of Esophageal Strictures in Children.** *Gastrointest Endosc* 1993, **39**:153–156.

On average, 6.6 sessions of balloon dilatation achieved symptomatic long-term response in 15 out of 17 children with various types of benign esophageal stenoses. A through-the-scope Rigiflex balloon was used under direct visual control so that radiation exposure could be avoided. Only one perforation was observed.

20. Goenka AS, Dasilva MS, Cleghorn GJ, Patrick MK, Shepherd RW: **Therapeutic Upper Gastrointestinal Endoscopy in Children: An Audit of 443 Procedures and Literature Review.** *J Gastroenterol Hepatol* 1993, **8**:44–51.

21. • Cwikiel W, Willén R, Stridbeck H, Lillo-Gil R, Stael von Holstein C: **Self-Expanding Stent in the Treatment of Benign Esophageal Strictures: Experimental Study in Pigs and Presentation of Clinical Cases.** *Radiology* 1993, **187**:667–671.

Preliminary data demonstrate that esophageal metal stents cause severe pressure-induced lesions in animals as well as in clinical cases. Because uncovered stents usually can not be removed, esophagectomy had to be performed in one patient for treatment of stent obstruction. These results should be a reminder for over-enthusiastic endoscopists.

22. •• Berenson MM, Johnson TD, Markowitz NR, Buchi KN, Samowitz WS: **Restoration of Squamous Mucosa After Ablation of Barrett's Esophageal Epithelium.** *Gastroenterology* 1993, **104**:1686–1691.

This paper detailed documentation of successful laser ablation of columnar tissue with subsequent replacement by squamous epithelium in 10 patients with Barrett's esophagus. Omeprazol was applied during the time the esophageal epithelium healed. Data on the duration of remission have not yet been reported.

23. Sampliner RE, Hixson LJ, Fennerty MB, Garewal HS: **Regression of Barrett's Esophagus by Laser Ablation in an Anacid Environment.** *Dig Dis Sci* 1993, **38**:365–368.

24. Laukka MA, Wang KK, Cameron AJ, Alexander GL: **The Use of Photodynamic Therapy in the Treatment of Barrett's Esophagus: Preliminary Results [Abstract].** *Gastrointest Endosc* 1993, **39**:A291.

25. • Spechler SJ: **Laser Photoablation of Barrett's Epithelium: Burning Issues About Tissues.** *Gastroenterology* 1993, **104**:1855–1858.

Interesting editorial review of the present role of an exciting but still experimental new treatment of Barrett's esophagus with suggestions for further studies.

26. • Levine DS, Haggitt RC, Blount PL, Rabinovitch PS, Rusch VW, Reid BJ: **An Endoscopic Biopsy Protocol Can Differentiate High-Grade Dysplasia From Early Adenocarcinoma in Barrett's Esophagus.** *Gastroenterology* 1993, **105**:40–50.

Multiple biopsies taken at different areas of Barrett's esophagus allow accurate differentiation between severe dysplasia and early adenocarcinoma. Therefore, surgical resection does not seem to be required to rule out an undiagnosed cancer. The biopsy protocol is also useful for studies on endoscopic treatment of dysplastic lesions in Barrett's esophagus.

27. • Overholt B, Panjehpour M, Tefftellar E, Rose M: **Photodynamic Therapy for Treatment of Early Adenocarcinoma in Barrett's Esophagus.** *Gastrointest Endosc* 1993, **39**:73–76.

A further report on successful photodynamic therapy in two patients with early esophageal adenocarcinoma who were no candidates for surgery. Biopsies remained negative for cancer during a follow-up of 6 and 24 months.

28. Lambert R: **Endoscopic Therapy of Esophago-Gastric Tumors.** *Endoscopy* 1992, **24**:24–33.

29. • Lightdale C, Heier S, Marcon N, McCaughan J, Naya H, Overholt B, Sobel R, Grose M, Reisman A, Dugan M and the PDT Esophageal Study Group: **A Multicenter Phase III Trial of Photodynamic Therapy (PDT) Vs Nd:YAG Laser in the Treatment (RX) of Malignant Dysphagia [Abstract].** *Gastrointest Endosc* 1993, **39**:A283.

Large randomized controlled trial on palliative photodynamic therapy versus thermal laser treatment, which showed no major benefit of photodynamic therapy.

30. Heier SK, Rothman K, Heier LM, Rosenthal WS: **Final Results of a Randomized Trial: Photodynamic Therapy Vs. Nd:YAG Laser Therapy [Abstract]**. *Gastroenterology* 1993, **104**:A408.

31. Marcon N, Siemens M, Haber G, Kandel G, Kortan P: **Palliation of Partially Obstructing Esophageal Carcinoma With Photodynamic Therapy [Abstract]**. *Gastrointest Endosc* 1993, 39:A283.

32. Herman LL, Gerdes H, Mendis R, Likier H, Lightdale CJ: **Photodynamic Therapy for Completely Obstructing Esophageal Cancer [Abstract]**. *Gastrointest Endosc* 1993, **39**:A278.

33. •• Hagiwara A, Takahashi T, Kojima O, Kitamura K, Sakakura C, Shoubayashi S, Osaki K, Iwamoto A, Lee M, Fujita K: **Endoscopic Injection of a New Drug-Delivery Format of Peplomycin for Superficial Esophageal Cancer: A Pilot Study**. *Gastroenterology* 1993, **104**:1037–1043.

This is an interesting and detailed report on a new endoscopic injection treatment that provides a selective and longlasting distribution of high levels of the anticancer drug to the injection site and regional lymph nodes.

34. Fiorini AB, Roca E, Valero J, Bai J: **Ethanol-Induced Tumor Necrosis (EITN) for Palliation of Dysphagia Caused by Esophageal Adenocarcinoma and Squamous Cell Carcinoma [Abstract]**. *Gastrointest Endosc* 1993, **39**:A275.

35. Alderson D, Wright PD: **Laser Recanalization Versus Endoscopic Intubation in the Palliation of Malignant Dysphagia**. *Br J Surg* 1990, 77:1151–1153.

36. Barr H, Krasner N, Raouf A, Walker RJ: **Prospective Randomized Trial of Laser Therapy Only and Laser Therapy Followed by Endoscopic Intubation for the Palliation of Malignant Dysphagia**. *Gut* 1990, **31**:252–258.

37. Carter R, Smith JS, Anderson JR: **Laser Recanalization Versus Endoscopic Intubation in the Palliation of Malignant Dysphagia: A Randomized Prospective Study**. *Br J Surg* 1992, 79:1167–1170.

38. Sargeant IR, Loizu LA, Tobias JS, Blackman G, Thorpe S, Bown SG: **Radiation Enhancement of Laser Palliation for Malignant Dysphagia: A Pilot Study**. *Gut* 1992, **33**:1597–1601.

39. • Panjehpour M, Overholt BF, DeNovo RC, Petersen MG, Sneed RE: **Comparative Study Between Pulsed and Continuous Wave Lasers for Photofrin Photodynamic Therapy**. *Lasers Surg Med* 1993, **13**:296–304.

Gross and histologic examinations in dogs treated with photodynamic therapy showed that both pulsed KTP/532-pumped dye-laser and continuous wave argon-pumped dye-laser tuned at 630 nm were equally effective.

40. Panjehpour M, Overholt BF, DeNovo RC, Sneed RE, Petersen MG: **Centering Balloon to Improve Esophageal Photodynamic Therapy**. *Lasers Surg Med* 1992, **12**:631–638.

41. •• Knyrim K, Wagner HJ, Bethge N, Keymling M, Vakil N: **A Controlled Trial of an Expansile Metal Stent for Palliation of Esophageal Obstruction Due to Inoperable Cancer**. *N Engl J Med* 1993, **329**:1302–1307.

First randomized study on Wallstents versus plastic tubes with complete follow-up in 36 of 42 patients. Results indicate less complications and shorter hospitalization for insertion of metal stents than for plastic tube implantation under general anesthesia. When interpretating these data, one should consider the uncommon definition of complications, which included tube migration but excluded bolus obstruction, tumor ingrowth, or occurrence of tracheoesophageal fistulas.

42. • Boyce HW: **Stents for Palliation of Dysphagia Due to Esophageal Cancer**. *N Engl J Med* 1993, **329**:1345–1346.

Well-balanced editorial on the pros and cons of esophageal metal stents and plastic tubes which concludes that one of both options should be considered at an early stage in the palliation of malignant dysphagia.

43. Vermeijden JR, Bartelsman JFWM, Fockens P, Meijer RCA, Tytgat GNJ: **Self-Expanding Metal Stents for Palliation of Esophagocardial Malignancies [Abstract]**. *Gastrointest Endosc* 1993, **39**:A291.

44. • Cwikiel W, Stridbeck H, Tranberg KG, Stael von Holstein C, Hambraeus G, Lillo-Gil R, Willén R: **Malignant Esophageal Strictures: Treatment With a Self-Expanding Stent**. *Radiology* 1993, **187**:661–665.

Excellent early results of nitinol Ultraflex stent insertion for palliation of malignant dysphagia. Long-term outcome seems comparable to other studies on uncovered metal stents.

45. Iwasaki T, Hayashi N, Kimoto T, Murashima S, Nakashima T, Odori T, Ishii Y, Noriki S, Yoshioka T, Uchida H: **Application of a Self-Expanding Metallic Stent to a Strictured Esophagojejunostomy**. *Cardiovasc Intervent Radiol* 1993, **16**:98–101.

46. Iguchi H, Kimura Y, Yanada J, Murasawa M: **Treatment of a Malignant Stricture after Esophagojejunostomy by a Self-Expanding Metallic Stent**. *Cardiovasc Intervent Radiol* 1993, **16**:102–104.

47. • Wu WC, Katon RM, Saxon RR, Barton RE, Uchida BT, Keller FS, Rösch J: **Silicone-Covered Self-Expanding Metallic Stents for the Palliation of Malignant Esophagel Obstruction and Esophagorespiratory Fistulas: Experience in 32 Patients and a Review of the Literature**. *Gastrointest Endosc* 1994, **40**:22–33.

Promising design of a covered Gianturco stent with modifications for reduction of the risk of migration. Dysphagia improved in 88% of 24 patients with malignant dysphagia. In addition this type of stent is a promising new tool for occlusion of esophagorespiratory fistula which succeeded completely in 6 of 8 patients. Migration and pressure necrosis were the most common late complications.

48. • Do YS, Song HJ, Lee BH, Byun HS, Kim KH, Chin SY, Park JH: **Esophagorespiratory Fistula Associated With Esophageal Cancer: Treatment With a Gianturco Stent Tube**. *Radiology* 1993, **187**:673–677.

Another promising report on minimally invasive treatment of high-risk patients with recurrent aspiration due to esophagorespiratory fistulas. The design of the presented stent is different from the Gianturco-Rösch-Z Stent. The influence of the stent construction on the clinical results is difficult to determine without comparative trials.

49. Song HJ, Choi KC, Kwon HC, Yang DH, Cho BH, Lee ST: **Esophageal Strictures: Treatment With a New Design of Modified Gianturco Stent**. *Radiology* 1992, **184**:729–734.

50. Sargeant IR, Thorpe S, Bown SG: **Cuffed Esophageal Prosthesis: A Useful Device in Desperate Situations in Esophageal Malignancy**. *Gastrointest Endosc* 1992, **38**:669–675.

51. Colt HG, Meric B, Dumon JF: **Double Stents for Carcinoma of the Esophagus Invading the Tracheo-Bronchial Tree**. *Gastrointest Endosc* 1992, **38**:485–489.

52. Vandenplas Y, Helven R, Derop H, Malfroot A, De Backer T, Beyens T, Vandevelde A, Desprechins B, Laureys W, Devis G, Deconinck P: **Endoscopic Obliteration of Recurrent Tracheoesophageal Fistula**. *Dig Dis Sci* 1993, **38**:374–377.

Horst Neuhaus, MD, Medizinische Klinik und Poliklinik der Technischen Universität München, Ismaninger Street 22, D-81675, München, Germany.

Pancreatic diseases

Editorial overview

Fred S. Gorelick, MD

West Haven VA Hospital, West Haven, Connecticut, USA

Current Opinion in Gastroenterology 1994, **10**:481–484

The review of the past year's publications on pancreatic physiology and pancreatic diseases is introduced by Steve Pandol's article (pp 485–490) on pancreatic acinar cell function. He has reviewed aspects of acinar cell receptors, phospholipid and calcium signaling, protein phosphorylation, and zymogen granule physiology. It has been difficult to demonstrate a direct effect of somatostatin on acinar cell enzyme secretion. However, during this past year, two groups have found that although somatostatin does not inhibit the secretory response to secretagogues that act when cyclic AMP or calcium-dependent pathways are used alone, it does inhibit the augmented secretory response observed when these two classes of agents are combined. The mechanism of this inhibition is unknown. A number of studies are now examining the complex phosphorylation of the cholecystokinin receptors, but the physiologic importance of these phosphorylation events remains unclear. The cloning of the cholecystokinin receptors may allow investigators to study the effects of phosphorylation by performing site-directed mutagenesis. Studies of calcium signaling within the acinar cell have demonstrated that after neurohumoral stimulation the initial rise in intracellular calcium occurs in the apical region of the cell and propagates towards the base. Similarly, intracellular injection of inositol 1,4,5-trisphosphate or calcium results in the release of intracellular calcium in the apical domain of the cell. The apical localization of the type 3 inositol 1,4,5-trisphosphate receptor in the acinar cell may explain the polarity of the initial calcium signal [1].

Several studies of the physiology of pancreatic duct cells deserve special note. It has been observed that pancreatic acinar cells lose their phenotype when placed in culture. It has now been shown that these cells differentiate to an epithelial cell type that closely resembles pancreatic duct cells [2]. Further, when a pancreatic acinar cell line tumor is placed in tissue culture, it too assumes the characteristics of ductular epithelium [3]. When the duct-like tissues are returned to an *in vivo* host, they maintain the ductular phenotype. These systems may provide useful models for examining the regulation of epithelial differentiation and for studies of duct cell physiology.

It has become popular to introduce antisense oligonucleotides into cells in culture to inhibit the production of a specific protein. This approach often fails, however, because the probe does not enter the cytoplasm. The structure of the antisense probe and its mechanism of cell entry are among the factors that determine the success of this approach. Expression of cystic fibrosis transmembrane conductance regulator (CFTR), in the PANC 1 human pancreatic duct cell line has been blocked using an antisense technique [4]; this may be a useful model for examining CFTR function. The physiologic role of CFTR has also been studied in transgenic mice. Surprisingly, animals that are homozygous for a disruption of the CFTR gene show little evidence of pancreatic disease. A recent study suggests that the pancreas may be spared in transgenic mice because some wild-type CFTR is generated even in *null* animals and that calcium-dependent chloride channels may substitute for the missing CFTR [5].

In a survey of neurohumoral control of pancreatic secretion, Chung Owyang (pp 491–495) details studies involving neurohumoral regulation, feedback regulation of pancreatic secretion, endocrine-exocrine interactions and the effects of nitric oxide, and regulation of pancreatic growth. Although the pancreatic acinar cell has a rich endowment of cell surface receptors, many stimulatory neurohumoral agents appear to indirectly regulate secretion primarily through neural pathways. These include cholecystokinin, neurotensin, and adenylate cyclase activating peptide, which stimulate secretion, and somatostatin which suppresses secretion. These indirect effects are observed under physiologic conditions. It is likely that some of these agents influence pancreatic acinar cell function both directly and indirectly depending on the level of the neurohumoral agent and the stimulatory state of the acinar cell. Whether acinar cell receptors for cholecystokinin and other ligands are directly involved in the physiologic regulation of pancreatic growth and differentiation remains unclear. The regulation of cholecystokinin synthesis and release is complex. Administration of the cholecystokinin antagonist L364,718 in the fasting state increases cholecystokinin synthesis, but not its release. This suggests that cholecystokinin may have an autocrine or paracrine effect that results in the feedback regulation of its synthesis. It would be interest-

Abbreviations

CFTR—cystic fibrosis transmembrane conductance regulator; **ERCP**—endoscopic retrograde cholangiopancreatography; **IAPP**—islet amyloid polypeptide.

© 1994 Current Science ISBN 1-85922-610-8 ISSN 0267–1379

ing to examine this question using the cholecystokinin-containing gut endocrine cell system developed by Liddle *et al.*

The role of nitric oxide in regulating pancreatic function has been an area of active study. It appears that in the acinar cell, the generation of nitric oxide is linked to the cytoplasmic levels of calcium and intracellular calcium stores. The working model is that calcium released from internal stores stimulates nitric oxide generation, which leads to increased cyclic GMP production; cyclic GMP subsequently stimulates calcium entry. Immunohistochemical studies demonstrate that one form of nitric oxide synthase was detectable in pancreatic vascular endothelium and neurons but not in acinar cells. Thus, the major physiologic site of nitric oxide action in the pancreas may be vascular or neuronal. However, the presence of another isoform of nitric oxide synthase in the acinar cell must be considered.

In his review of acute pancreatitis, C. W. Imrie (pp 496–501) comments on studies of experimental pancreatitis, and the diagnosis, prognosis, and treatment of acute pancreatitis. Models that describe the pathophysiology of acute pancreatitis are primarily based on experimental animal systems. These studies have led to the portrayal of pancreatitis as a complex cascade of interrelated pathologic events [6]. Changes in pancreatic blood flow and acute inflammation appear to contribute to this process. Nitric oxide may play a role in the pathogenesis through its effect on blood flow; increasing nitric oxide levels have been reported to reduce the severity of some forms of acute experimental pancreatitis. The effects of decreased pancreatic blood flow during bile salt–induced pancreatitis has been reported by Kusterer *et al.* [7]. A dramatic decrease in blood flow was observed within minutes of applying bile salts. Further, prominent leukocyte adherence to vascular endothelium was also observed in the same time frame. The vasoconstriction and leukocyte adherence were blocked by pretreating animals with either a leukotriene antagonist or free radical scavengers. If these changes are related to the pathogenesis of pancreatitis they may be very early events. It is accepted that pancreatitis is associated with increased vascular permeability; it has recently been demonstrated that intestinal epithelial paracellular permeability is also increased during experimental pancreatitis [8]. The mechanism of this increased permeability, its effect on other epithelial tissues, and its role in the pathogenesis of pancreatitis remain unclear.

Bradley *et al.* have established a modified classification of acute pancreatitis that eliminates some of the confusing terminology that has been used in our field; its greatest utility will be to provide a consistent framework for describing pancreatitis in the literature. Studies continue to support the contention that lipase assays provide diagnostic sensitivity and specificity near 100% (when an abnormal value is set at three times the upper limit of normal) and thus may be the preferred test for the diagnosis of acute pancreatitis. Several groups have observed that obesity is a major prognostic factor in acute pancreatitis. The tendency for the disease to be more severe in these patients may be due to limited respiratory excursion secondary to obesity and the enhanced generation of free fatty acids that are enzymatically released from necrotic peritoneal fat stores. A large study from Hong Kong evaluated the use of urgent endoscopic papillotomy in patients with pancreatitis. Notably, this population had a high incidence of biliary parasitism and were not treated with antibiotics even when there was evidence of cholangitis. The benefit of urgent intervention was a reduction of biliary sepsis. These findings are consistent with previous studies and suggest that a population that should be considered for urgent endoscopic retrograde cholangiopancreatography (ERCP) are patients with biliary pancreatitis and evidence of cholangitis. In my estimation, this intervention should be reserved for those patients with severe disease or those who deteriorate.

The topic of chronic pancreatitis has been reviewed by Murray Korc and Wolff Schmiegel (pp 502–506). In their article they comment on studies of the pathogenesis of chronic pancreatitis, its clinical course, treatment with pancreatic enzymes, octreotide, endoscopy, and surgery, and finally the resulting complications including cancer. Topics of considerable discussion are the indications and benefits of pancreatic decompression for patients with chronic pancreatitis who are operated on for pain. An important study by Nealon and Thompson [9] has examined the effect of pancreatic duct decompression on the natural history of the disease. The functional status of patients was scored preoperatively using the criteria of signs of chronic pancreatitis by ERCP, abnormal hyperglycemia, lipid-stimulated pancreatic polypeptide release, 72-hour fecal fat, and the Benteromide test. The findings of the study suggest that 1) early pancreatic decompression may delay the progression to endocrine and exocrine dysfunction, and 2) patients having dilated pancreatic ducts and elevated intraductal pressures are more likely to experience pain relief from decompression than those with nondilated ducts and normal intraductal pressures. This study should be viewed as a preliminary investigation; a larger multicenter study might help to address questions such as the benefit of decompression in patients with little pain but with a dilated pancreatic duct.

Nealon and Thompson [9] reported that the fat-stimulated release of pancreatic polypeptide may be a good marker for pancreatic insufficiency. Pancreatic polypeptide is released by the islets in response to a meal and inhibits pancreatic secretion by interacting with intrapancreatic neural pathways. Pancreatic polypeptide release is a multistep process that involves intestinal lipid hydrolysis, intact neural pathways, and intact pancreatic neuroendocrine function. Thus, a failure of any step along this pathway will compromise pancreatic polypeptide release and potentially make this a very sensitive test. It would be valuable to establish the sensitivity and specificity of this test prospectively. In a well documented study from France by Levy *et al.* [10], chronic pancreatitis was reported to follow abdominal radiation (average dose, 4100 rads) for lymphoma. None of these patients were alcoholics and most presented with abdominal pain. The salient features in these patients with endocrine and exocrine dysfunction were 1) presentation of chronic pancreatitis from 6 to 24 years after radiation, 2) paucity of pancreatic calcifications and little pancreatic inflammation, and 3) a pancreatic duct that has strictures with occasional regions of dilation. Because we are now seeing more long-term survivors of lymphoma therapy, it is useful to keep this diagnosis in mind.

Publications from the past year on pancreatic cancer were surveyed by Carlos Fernández-del Castillo and Andrew Warshaw (pp 507–512). The specific areas of review include the epidemiology, etiology, and pathobiology of pancreatic cancer, and its diagnosis and treatment. Two studies in the past year, one from the United States and Europe by Lowenfels *et al.* and a second from India by Chari *et al.* have firmly established a relationship between chronic pancreatitis and pancreatic cancer. This relationship holds whether the pancreatitis is alcoholic, tropical fibrocalcific, hereditary, or idiopathic in origin. Although the risk of pancreatic cancer is small with alcoholic disease, it appears to be more appreciable when associated with the fibrocalcific disease. Specific mutations of oncogenes such as c-Ki-*ras* that occur during chronic pancreatitis may predispose to the development of cancer. Smokers with pancreatic carcinoma frequently have mutations in this *ras* gene. Although mutations in the tumor suppressor gene *p53* are frequently seen in pancreatic cancer, they have not been associated with chronic pancreatitis.

Decreased endocrine function during the course of chronic pancreatitis can be attributed to loss of islet mass. However, this mechanism does not appear to account for the development of diabetes associated with pancreatic carcinoma. Permert *et al.* from Sweden have observed that patients with pancreatic carcinoma and diabetes usually have normal insulin release and that diabetes sometimes disappears after the resection of a pancreatic cancer. Further, extracts of the pancreas have been found to contain a factor that inhibits muscle glycogen synthesis. This factor appears to be islet amyloid polypeptide (IAPP) produced by the β-cell. Pancreatic cancer appears to lead to enhanced IAPP release from islets and is associated with elevated plasma levels of IAPP. This peptide can also cause anorexia. Thus, enhanced IAPP release may be related to the diabetes associated with pancreatic cancer and contribute to weight loss. Increased serum levels of IAPP may be specific for the form of diabetes associated with pancreatic cancer and may serve as a useful diagnostic test. The diagnosis of pancreatic cancer may be aided by the use of endoscopic ultrasonography; it appears to be particularly useful in detecting small tumors (<25 mm). However, it remains to be proven whether application of this challenging technique will lead to any improvement in survival.

In an interesting study from Japan, Kayahara *et al.* examined the sites of pancreatic cancer reoccurrence after resection. Using either postmortem or antemortem examinations, they discovered that the most common site of recurrence was retroperitoneal (>80%), followed by hepatic (>50%). This pattern of recurrence was observed for small and large tumors. These findings indicate that an extensive retroperitoneal dissection should be considered even when pancreatic tumors appear to be small and limited in extent.

Michael Steer (pp 513–516) has reviewed the most recent literature on pancreatic surgery and includes sections on pancreatic pseudocysts, cystic tumors, endocrine and exocrine tumors, and pancreatic transplantation. The treatment of pancreatic pseudocysts has evolved over the past 5 years. There is a consensus that asymptomatic pseudocysts less than 6 cm that are not enlarging usually resolve without surgery. Despite initial enthusiasm for percutaneous drainage of pseudocysts, many clinicians have experienced a high incidence of infectious complications and now favor surgical drainage. Pseudocysts that are impinging on the gastric or duodenal wall have been drained endoscopically, but the published experience with the technique is limited. To guide intervention and avoid vascular structures, some clinicians advocate the use of endoscopic ultrasonography. It seems prudent to avoid endoscopic approaches to drain pseudocysts until this technique can be prospectively evaluated by experienced clinical investigators. The localization of neuroendocrine tumors has been problematic and often leads to extensive diagnostic and therapeutic interventions that can generate considerable morbidity. The recognition that somatostatin dramatically reduces secretion from many of these tumors provided a clue that led to a novel method of localizing neuroendocrine tumors. The plasma membranes of such tumors are rich in somatostatin receptors and can be localized using radiolabeled somatostatin and three-dimensional radionuclide imaging. It appears that a high percentage of gastrinomas including those involving the duodenal wall can be imaged using this technique. Unfortunately, lesser numbers of other neuroendocrine tumors can be imaged using this technique. The somatostatin scan will be useful both for localizing resectable neuroendocrine tumors and may be a sensitive method for detecting metastatic disease.

Michael Steer provides some guidance for the evaluation and treatment of patients with pancreatic adenocarcinoma. He suggests that angiography be reserved to evaluate patients with pancreatic body and tail tumors who have been deemed resectable using computed tomographic criteria. Although discussion and studies continue on the use of endoscopic versus surgical approaches for the drainage of the biliary tract, I agree with his suggestion that the most reasonable approach is surgical drainage for patients with early localized disease and endoscopic drainage for patients with extensive and advanced disease or significant comorbidity.

In the final paper, Gary Leavitt and Morton Burrell (pp 517–522) provide a review of radiologic advances over the past year. In their paper they comment on new techniques that are being used to image the pancreas, studies on specific forms of pancreatic neoplasms, studies of acute and chronic pancreatitis, and interventional radiology. They provide a useful summary on the present methods used to distinguish between benign and malignant pancreatic cystic lesions. Pancreatic tumors and cystic lesions are frequently biopsied using percutaneous approaches. In a summary of cases from the Mayo Clinic seen between 1985 and 1989, Brandt *et al.* reported that the use of real-time ultrasonographic guidance was superior to contrast-enhanced computed tomography for obtaining malignant tissue. Although more than one-fourth of the biopsies passed through the gastrointestinal tract, there were no adverse effects. I would agree with the suggestion by Warshaw *et al.* and the position taken in an editorial by Mueller that because pancreatic biopsy can lead to peritoneal tumor seeding, percutaneous biopsy should be avoided when a surgical cure is being contemplated. Focal hypoechogenic regions in the ventral aspect of the pancreatic head often raise concerns about the presence of neoplasm. In an interesting study by Atri *et al.*, the appearance of these sonographic changes was correlated with pathology specimens. It was found that these changes were caused by focal deposition of fat restricted to the uncinate region. The restricted distribution of this change when detected by ultrasonography and computed tomography density measurements should allow one to distinguish this form of limited fat deposition from pancreatic neoplasia.

Acknowledgments

The author wishes to thank Lisa Matovcik, PhD, and Chris Marino, MD, for their helpful comments. Dr. Gorelick is a recipient of a VA Merit Research Award and Clinical Investigator Career Development Award.

References

1. Nathanson MH, Fallon MB, Padfield PJ, Maranto AR: **Localization of the Type 3 Inositol 1,4,5-Triphosphate Receptor in the Ca^{2+} Wave Trigger Zone of Pancreatic Acinar Cells.** *J Biol Chem* 1994, **269**:4693–4696.

2. Arias AE, Bendayan M: **Differentiation of Pancreatic Acinar Cells Into Duct-Like Cells In Vitro.** *Lab Invest* 1993, **69**:518–530.

3. Pettengill OS, Faris RA, Bell RH, Kuhlmann ET, Longnecker DS: **Derivation of Duct-Like Cell Lines From a Transplantable Acinar Cell Carcinoma of the Rat Pancreas.** *Am J Pathol* 1993, **143**:292–303.

4. Kopelman H, Gauthier C, Bornstein M: **Antisense Oligonucleotide to the Cystic Fibrosis Transmembrane Conductance Regulator Inhibits Cyclic AMP-Activated but Not Calcium-Activated Cell Volume Reduction in a Human Pancreatic Duct Cell Line.** *J Clin Invest* 1993, **91**:1253–1257.

5. Gray MA, Winpenny JP, Porteous DJ, Dorin JR, Argent BE: **CFTR and Calcium-Activated Chloride Currents in Pancreatic Duct Cells of a Transgenic CF Mouse.** *Am J Physiol* 1994, **266**:C213–C221.

6. Lerch MM, Adler G: **Acute Pancreatitis.** *Curr Opin Gastroenterol* 1992, **8**:817–823.

7. Kusterer K, Poschmann T, Friedemann A, Enghofer M, Zendler S, Usadel KH: **Arterial Constriction, Ischemia-Reperfusion, and Leukocyte Adherence in Acute Pancreatitis.** *Am J Physiol* 1993, **265**:G165–G171.

8. Ryan CM, Schmidt J, Lewandrowski K, Compton CC, Rattner DW, Warshaw AL, Tompkins RG: **Gut Macromolecular Permeability in Pancreatitis Correlates With Severity of Disease in Rats.** *Gastroentrology* 1993, **104**:890–895.

9. Nealon WH, Thompson JC: **Progressive Loss of Pancreatic Function in Chronic Pancreatitis Is Delayed by Main Pancreatic Duct Decompression.** *Ann Surg* 1993, **217**:458–468.

10. Levy P, Menzelxhiu A, Paillot B, Bretagne JF, Flejou JF, Bernades P: **Abdominal Radiotherapy Is a Cause for Chronic Pancreatitis.** *Gastroenterology* 1993, **105**:905–909.

Fred S. Gorelick, MD, Gastrointestinal Research Laboratory, Building 27, West Haven VA Hospital, West Spring Street, West Haven, CT 06516, USA.

Pancreatic acinar cell signaling mechanisms

Stephen J. Pandol, MD

University of California, San Diego, California, USA

Significant progress has been made in several areas of pancreatic acina cell physiology. Further evidence has been developed indicating that cholecystokinin's effect *in vivo* on the acinar cell is mediated through neural pathways. A direct effect of somatostatin on secretion from the pancreatic acinar cell has been demonstrated. The acinar cell continues to be a model system for investigating the phospholipid and Ca^{2+} pathways activated by agonists. Cholecystokinin was found to have phospholipase D effect on membrane phosphatidylcholine. New insights into the mechanisms of agonist-stimulated Ca^{2+} signaling were presented. These include a role for Ca^{2+} stores, Ca^{2+} ATPase, intercellular gap junctions, cyclic GMP, and functional heterogeneity of intracellular Ca^{2+} stores in mediating the complex patterns of $[Ca^{2+}]i$ changes in the cell, including waves and oscillations. Studies directed at understanding the roles of agonist-stimulated phosphorylation and dephosphorylation of cellular proteins, including the cholecystokinin receptor, continue to indicate that regulation of phosphorylation states of specific proteins is necessary for several cellular functions including enzyme secretion. In total, these results demonstrate a rapid pace of discovery in elucidating the signaling pathways underlying acinar cell physiology.

Current Opinion in Gastroenterology 1994, **10**:485–490

The pancreatic acinar cell continues to be a model system for studies elucidating stimulus-response pathways in cellular physiology. This review covers studies demonstrating progress delineating the *in vivo* neurohumoral pathways that lead to the secretory response of the cell, followed by key papers investigating mechanisms of Ca^{2+} signaling and roles of protein phosphorylation states in cell function. The combined works covered herein indicate rapid advances in our understanding of the physiology of the pancreatic acinar cell. This review is organized into topics starting with neurohumoral control of exocrine secretion followed by receptor function, intracellular signaling by Ca^{2+}, and phosphoproteins and zymogen granule functions.

Neurohumoral control of pancreatic enzyme secretion

Cholecystokinin is the major secretagogue of pancreatic enzyme secretion. The pancreatic acinar cell has receptors for cholecystokinin as well as receptors for acetylcholine, gastrin-releasing peptide (or bombesin), and vasoactive intestinal polypeptide. It has been assumed that cholecystokinin has a direct action on the acinar cell to cause enzyme secretion. However, over the past few years, evidence has been accumulating from *in vivo* experiments that cholecystokinin may be acting to cause secretion through cholinergic pathways. That is, atropine can block the effects of cholecystokinin on secretion.

In an elegant study, Li and Owyang [1••] demonstrated that bilateral vagotomy, atropine, or hexamethonium blocked enzyme secretion stimulated by physiologic concentrations of intravenously infused cholecystokinin-8 in the rat. Furthermore, the gastroduodenal mucosal application of the sensory neurotoxin, capsaicin, abolished the pancreatic secretory response to physiologic concentrations of cholecystokinin-8. Supraphysiologic concentrations of cholecystokinin-8 caused enzyme secretion that was not blocked by atropine, vagotomy, or hexamethonium. These results indicate that at physiologic levels, cholecystokinin causes pancreatic secretion via activation of capsaicin-sensitive afferent vagal pathways originating from the gastroduodenal mucosa. Greater concentrations of cholecystokinin cause secretion by interacting with intrinsic pancreatic neurons or directly with pancreatic acinar cells. These findings revolutionize our concepts of the mechanism action of cholecystokinin and indicate that under physiologic situations, the pancreatic acinar cell is not the direct target of cholecystokinin in mediating secretion.

Somatostatin is a potent inhibitor of pancreatic exocrine secretion in humans as well as rats and dogs.

Abbreviations

CGRP—calcitonin gene-related peptide; **IP_3**—inositol 1,4,5-trisphosphate; **PACAP**—pituitary adenylate cyclase activating polypeptide.

 ISBN 1-85922-610-8 ISSN 0267–1379

Although specific somatostatin receptors have been demonstrated on pancreatic acinar cells, until recently, *in vitro* studies have not found them active in regulating enzyme secretion. The general consensus has been that somatostatin regulates enzyme secretion via nerves. However, two recent publications [2•,3•] identified specific actions for somatostatin analogues in pancreatic acini prepared from mice and rats. In acini from both species, somatostatin abolished the augmented response observed with a combination of an agonist that acts by increasing cyclic AMP (*eg*, secretin or vasoactive intestinal peptide) and an agonist that acts by increasing $[Ca^{2+}]i$ (*eg*, cholecystokinin, acetylcholine analogues, or bombesin analogues). In acini from mice [2•], somatostatin also inhibited the augmented enzyme secretion that occurred with a combination of cholecystokinin-8 and dibutyryl cyclic AMP or the calcium ionophore, A23187, and secretin, suggesting that the effect of somatostatin occurs at a step beyond the generation of the second messengers, cyclic AMP and Ca^{2+}. In contrast, in acini from the rat [3•], the augmented response with 8-bromo cyclic AMP and cholecystokinin-8 was not inhibited by somatostatin. Thus, although the intracellular mechanism of action of somatostatin is not established, these papers present clear evidence that somatostatin regulates pancreatic secretion at least in part by a direct effect on the pancreatic acinar cell.

Acinar cell receptors

Over the past several years, there has been significant interest in the mechanisms underlying both homologous and heterologous desensitization of pancreatic acinar cell responses with cholecystokinin, carbachol, and bombesin. Homologous desensitization indicates that exposure of a cell to an agonist attenuates the response of the cell to the same agonist. Heterologous desensitization indicates that exposure of the cell to one agonist attenuates the response of the cell to other agonists operating through distinct receptors. For the pancreatic acinar cell, both cholecystokinin and acetylcholine analogues cause homologous and heterologous desensitization whereas bombesin analogues cause only homologous desensitization. The heterologous desensitization with cholecystokinin and acetylcholine analogues is intriguing because it suggests that intracellular signals activated one agonist effect on the receptor function of another agonist. The mechanism of heterologous desensitization is not known.

Although cholecystokinin, carbachol, and bombesin cause similar changes in cell Ca^{2+} and inositol 1,4,5-trisphosphate during cell activation, the increases in 1,2-diacylglycerol are much greater with cholecystokinin and carbachol than with bombesin. Because 1,2-diacylglycerol activates protein kinase C, it seems possible that 1,2-diacylglycerol or protein kinase C is involved in the heterologous desensitization process observed with cholecystokinin and acetylcholine analogues.

Recent studies [4•,5,6•] demonstrate that cholecystokinin and carbachol regulate the phosphorylation states of the pancreatic cholecystokinin and muscarinic receptor, the phosphorylation is mediated at least in part by protein kinase C, and that the phosphorylation state may be involved in the mechanism of heterologous desensitization.

Two of the papers [4•,5] included direct measurements of both phosphorylation and dephosphorylation of the cholecystokinin receptor molecule. The receptor was phosphorylated by a variety of homologous and heterologous secretogogues and the phosphorylation events represented action by more than one protein kinase. One group of kinases included one or more isoforms of protein kinase C. The other group of kinases were inhibited by heparin. The nature of the kinases inhibited by heparin are not known but they may be related to B-adrenergic receptor kinase and rhodopsin kinase that are inhibited by heparin in other systems.

The phosphorylated state of the cholecystokinin receptor was transient, decreasing toward control levels after 20 minutes of incubation with cholecystokinin. The mechanism of the decreased phosphorylation was found to be a result of activation of phosphatase during stimulation [4•]. Characterization of the phosphatase activity indicated that it was due to serine- and threonine-specific protein phosphatase of the PP-2A type.

In an evaluation of the effects of cholecystokinin on heterologous desensitization of muscarinic cholinergic receptors another paper [6•] demonstrated that cholecystokinin-8 and the phorbol ester TPA caused desensitization of the carbachol response and prevented the decreased binding capacity of the muscarinic receptors induced by carbachol. The effect of TPA was blocked by the protein kinase C inhibitor, staurosporine. These results suggested that protein kinase C or the maintenance of binding sites was related to the heterologous desensitization process.

The studies described above provide us with a hypothesis that receptor phosphorylation and dephosphorylation are involved in receptor function and the heterologous desensitization process. Further studies will be needed both to establish the relationship between specific receptor phosphorylation states and receptor function and to determine specific effects of the receptor phosphorylation states on intracellular signaling.

Other recent papers related to acinar cell receptors characterized vasoactive intestinal peptide/pituitary adenylate cyclase activating polypeptide (PACAP)-2 receptors [7], calcitonin gene-related peptide (CGRP) receptors [8] and endothelin receptors [9•]. PACAP receptors have been described in two forms. One interacts specifically with PACAP (PACAP-1 receptor). The other is closely related to the previously described high affinity vasoactive intestinal peptide receptor. Characterization of these receptors on both rat pancreatic acini and pancreas-derived AR 4-2J cells indicated that acini contained predominantly vasoactive intestinal peptide/PACAP-2 receptors whereas the AR 4-2J cells expressed mainly PACAP-1 receptors.

Characterization of the CGRP receptor in guinea pig gastric smooth muscle and pancreatic acini indicated that it has a M_r of 57,000 and that it is an N-linked sialoglycoprotein.

Analysis of pancreatic acini for endothelin receptors indicated that they contain two classes of receptors for endothelin. One has a high affinity for endothelin-1 and a low affinity for endothelin-3. The other has equal affinities for both endothelin-1 and endothelin-3. Occupation of either receptor by ligand resulted in rapid internalization, which was regulated by phospholipase C-activating agonists such as cholecystokinin. Endothelins had no effect on enzyme secretion, inositol phosphate metabolism, or calcium metabolism. Thus, the function of the endothelin receptors on pancreatic acinar cells is unknown. Because endothelins act as mitogens and growth factors in other tissues, such functions should be considered for them in pancreatic acinar cells.

Acinar phospholipid and calcium signaling

The pancreatic acinar cell continues to be a model system for elucidating the effects of agonists on cellular phospholipid and calcium metabolism. For nearly a decade we have known that agonists such as cholecystokinin, acetylcholine analogues, and bombesin analogues cause a phospholipase C–mediated breakdown of the phosphatidylinositols to 1,2-diacylglycerol and inositol phosphates and phosphatidylcholine to 1,2-diacylglycerol and phosphorylcholine. One of the inositol phosphates, inositol 1,4,5-trisphosphate (IP_3), has been established as the messenger mediating intracellular calcium mobilization caused by these agonists. 1,2-diacylglycerol activates protein kinase C.

In the past year, one report demonstrated that cholecystokinin also causes a phospholipase D–mediated breakdown of phosphatidylcholine [10••]. This reaction leads to the formation of phosphatidic acid and choline. Although the role of this effect of cholecystokinin is not known, the authors speculated that phospholipase D may mediate the trophic effects of cholecystokinin. This suggestion came from the findings that in contrast to cholecystokinin, carbachol has no pancreatic trophic effects and it does not have a phospholipase D effect on phosphatidylcholine. Whether or not this pathway is involved in the trophic effect of cholecystokinin, it represents a signaling system unique for cholecystokinin and probably mediates cholecystokinin-specific effects.

Using AR 4-2J cells, Menniti *et al.* [11] demonstrated the presence of pyrophosphate derivatives of both inositol 1,3,4,5,6 pentakisphosphate and inositol hexakisphosphate. These pyrophosphates were observed when cellular pyrophosphatase were inhibited by fluoride. Although there is no information about what these very polar inositol phosphates might be doing, the results are provocative.

Studies over the past few years suggest that the agonist-sensitive intracellular stores of calcium are a heterogenous group. In an elegant study, Kasai *et al.* [12••] used confocal Ca^{2+} imaging and injections of IP_3 and Ca^{2+} to localize stores responsive to each of these signals. Using these techniques they found three zones of Ca^{2+} stores in the rat pancreatic acinar cell. One zone, termed the trigger or T zone, located in the apical or zymogen granule area of the cell responded to low doses of IP_3 to release Ca^{2+}. This same area was the first to show a $[Ca^{2+}]$ increase during agonist stimulation. Injections of Ca^{2+} demonstrated Ca^{2+}-induced Ca^{2+} release channels in the apical area of the cell. Finally, the basolateral regions of the cell responded with Ca^{2+} release to greater concentrations of IP_3. These results not only established the heterogeneity of agonist-sensitive Ca^{2+} stores, they provided important information that must be used in models to explain the mechanism of Ca^{2+} waves and oscillations. The results of this study certainly explain the finding that with agonist stimulation, $[Ca^{2+}]i$ increases first in the apical region of the cell followed by a wave of $[Ca^{2+}]i$ spreading toward the basolateral region of the cell.

Although the mechanism of agonist-stimulated intracellular Ca^{2+} release has been established, the pathways involved in agonist-stimulated influx of Ca^{2+} have been unknown. It has been known for several years that Ca^{2+} mobilizing agonists increase cellular cyclic GMP. The role of cyclic GMP in acinar cells as well as many other cell types has been unknown. More recently it has been shown that cyclic GMP has a role in mediating some of the Ca^{2+} transports activated during agonist stimulation. During the past year, using patch-clamp recordings Bahnson *et al.* [10••] demonstrated that intracellular injections of cyclic GMP activated the same Ca^{2+} entry pathway that is activated by agonists. Furthermore, intracellular application of IP_3 activated the Ca^{2+} entry pathway. These results suggest a model in which intracellular Ca^{2+} release leads to formation of cyclic GMP which, in turn, activates a plasma membrane Ca^{2+} influx transport. One would suspect that nitric oxide formation results from intracellular Ca^{2+} release via activation of nitric oxide synthase and that the nitric oxide mediates cyclic GMP formation through activation of soluble guanylyl cyclase. The mechanism by which cyclic GMP regulates Ca^{2+} influx may be directly through a cyclic GMP-gated cation channel or through cyclic GMP-dependent protein kinases.

Several papers during the past year dealt with aspects of agonist-stimulated $[Ca^{2+}]i$ oscillations [13•,14•,15–17, 18••]. It has been known for several years that low concentrations of agonists as well as a constant infusion of IP_3 into the acinar cell cytoplasm will stimulate $[Ca^{2+}]i$ oscillations. Furthermore, each oscillation causes enzyme secretion. The mechanism of $[Ca^{2+}]i$ oscillations are not established. However, there is a general consensus that Ca^{2+}-induced Ca^{2+} release is involved. Ca^{2+}-induced Ca^{2+} release is best described in skeletal muscle where Ca^{2+} causes release of further Ca^{2+} by interacting with a specific receptor on the sarcoplasmic reticulum of the muscle cell. The receptors in muscle are referred to as ryanodine receptors because the plant alkaloid, ryanodine, was found to interact with this receptor.

Two papers illustrated the roles for both the Ca^{2+} ATPase on the agonist-sensitive stores and gap junctions between cells in regulating the frequency of oscillations [13•,14•]. Ca^{2+} ATPases on the stores are necessary to reduce $[Ca^{2+}]i$ toward resting levels after Ca^{2+} is released from the store. The cycle of release and resequestration account for a single spike in $[Ca^{2+}]i$. In the recent paper [13•], decreasing the activity of the stores Ca^{2+} ATPases with the specific inhibitor, thapsigargin, led to a shorter interspike interval and thus a high spiking (oscillatory) frequency. Furthermore, the duration of each spike increased. If fully activated, the Ca^{2+} ATPases prevented $[Ca^{2+}]i$ spikes by rapidly resequestering released Ca^{2+}. These results point out the critical role of Ca^{2+} ATPases in the duration of $[Ca^{2+}]i$ increases and the frequency of $[Ca^{2+}]i$ oscillations. One might imagine endogenous regulators of the Ca^{2+} ATPases in the cell that have functions of regulating these aspects of $[Ca^{2+}]i$ oscillations.

The cells of the acini are both electrically and chemically coupled by gap junctions. A Ca^{2+} imaging microscopic study by Stauffer *et al.* [14•] demonstrated that the gap junctions coordinate the amplitude and frequency of agonist-stimulated $[Ca^{2+}]i$ oscillations within the cells of an acinus. The coordination was demonstrated by reducing gap junction permeability with octanol and increasing permeability with NO_2^-. Furthermore, the focal application of an agonist (cholecystokinin JMV-180 or bombesin) to a few cells of the acinus led to spread of increased $[Ca^{2+}]i$ to other cells of the acinus. These results point to an important role for the gap junction in coordinating Ca^{2+} signaling in the acinus. The signals that traverse the gap junctions to affect the coordination are not known. Both IP_3 and Ca^{2+} traverse gap junctions and could act to transmit signals between cells.

In a further demonstration that IP_3 is necessary to sustain $[Ca^{2+}]i$ oscillations, one report demonstrated that $[Ca^{2+}]i$ oscillations induced by the partial cholecystokinin agonist, JMV-180, were blocked by the intracellular application of heparin [15]. Heparin specifically blocks IP_3 receptors. This result suggested that activation of IP_3 receptors is necessary to sustain Ca^{2+}-induced Ca^{2+} release in these cells. The finding is of particular interest because several laboratories have been unable to measure increases in IP_3 with JMV-180 stimulation. Thus, either the increases in IP_3 are too small to measure or there is a change in sensitivity of the Ca^{2+} release mechanisms to IP_3 with JMV-180 stimulation.

One paper demonstrated that sphingosine and sphingosylphosphorylcholine cause $[Ca^{2+}]i$ oscillations in pancreatic acinar cells [16]. These molecules are derived from metabolism of cellular sphingomyelin. Enzymes do exist in the cell to accomplish this metabolism but experiments to demonstrate their activation during agonist stimulation have not been performed in the pancreatic acinar cell.

The mechanism by which sphingosine caused $[Ca^{2+}]i$ oscillations was not due to interaction with IP_3 receptors because the oscillations were not inhibited by heparin. Thus, the exact mechanism of the sphingosine action is not known. Because of the experiments demonstrating that stores of Ca^{2+} ATPases are involved in the mechanism of $[Ca^{2+}]i$ oscillations, further experiments to characterize the mechanism of sphingosine action should evaluate uptake as well as release mechanisms. In addition, experiments demonstrating whether or not pancreatic agonists regulate sphingomyelin metabolism should be performed. In other tissues sphingomyelin metabolism has been observed with growth-promoting hormones. It is possible that such a role for sphingomyelin metabolism exists in the exocrine pancreas.

Role of protein phosphorylation signaling acinar cell responses

Several studies have demonstrated that agonist stimulation of acinar cells result in multiple serine/threonine phosphorylation events. However, missing from this body of work has been the demonstration of a role for these phosphorylation events in the stimulation-secretion coupling pathway. In order to determine the role of protein tyrosine phosphorylation in the secretory pathway of pancreatic acinar cells, Lutz *et al.* [18••] measured both tyrosine phosphorylation and enzyme secretion with cholecystokinin in the presence of phosphorylation inhibitors. They found that cholecystokinin stimulated tyrosine phosphorylation of several cellular proteins. All of these phosphorylation events were inhibited by genistein, an inhibitor of tyrosine kinases. By contrast, H-7, a specific inhibitor of protein kinase C, and staurosporine, an inhibitor of both protein kinase C and tyrosine kinase, affected different subsets of tyrosine phosphorylated proteins. Genistein inhibited enzyme secretion caused by cholecystokinin but not by the phorbol ester, TPA. H-7 did not inhibit cholecystokinin-stimulated enzyme secretion whereas staurosporine did. These results indicated that tyrosine kinase activity is essential for cholecystokinin activation of the secretory pathway whereas protein kinase C is not. In another study [19], inhibition of tyrosine kinase activity resulted in growth inhibition in three human pancreatic cancer lines. The results of these studies are important because they demonstrate that there are a few tyrosine kinase–mediated events that are necessary in the stimulus-secretion coupling pathway in normal acinar cells as well as in the growth stimulation pathways of pancreatic cancer cells. The tyrosine phosphorylated proteins necessary for each pathway may be different. Hopefully, future studies will demonstrate specific functions for tyrosine phosphorylated proteins.

The zymogen granule

In addition to storing digestive enzymes, the zymogen granule is actively involved in the process of regulated secretion or exocytosis. That is, with the appropriate stimulus, the granule moves to the apical membrane of the acinar cell, fuses with that membrane and opens and discharges its contents. Although significant information has accumulated about the signals that regulate secretion, little is known about mechanisms of the exocytosis process. Presumably the membrane of the granules has specializations that are involved.

Three papers present findings of zymogen granule membrane characteristics that may play a role in the exocytosis process. In one [20•], an ATP-sensitive K^+ channel is described that is inhibited by both ATP and a product of phospholipase A action, lysophosphatidylcholine. Although the role of this transport was not identified, together with the Cl^- transport previously described in the granule membrane it may serve to promote granule swelling associated with exocytosis or to solubilize the condensed,macromolecular product and aid in flushing it along the secretory duct.

Two papers provide characterization of granule membrane proteins [21•,22•]. This membrane contains about 10 proteins. Three of the more abundant being glycoproteins 1, 2, 3. Glycoprotein-2 is the most abundant of the glycoproteins and has been studied in the greatest detail. Although its function is unknown, it is known to be linked to the inner surface of the zymogen membrane via a glycosyl phosphatidylinositol moiety. Glycoprotein-2 possesses amino acid sequence homology with uromodulin/Tamm-Horsfall kidney protein. One paper [21•] described organelle targeting of glycoprotein-2 in secretory cells. Complementary DNA for glycoprotein-2 was transfected into exocrine (AR 4-2J) tumor cells as well as endocrine (AtT20 anterior pituitary and Rin5F insulinoma-derived) tumor cells. Expressed protein was targeted to zymogen granule membranes in AR 4-2J cells but not the endocrine cell lines. Although the mechanism of targeting was not established, the results indicate that glycoprotein-2 is not necessary for the exocytotic process.

The second paper on membrane glycoproteins, using complementary DNA cloning, demonstrated that glycoprotein-3 revealed a predicted protein sequence with strong homology to a triacylglycerol lipase expressed in cytotoxic T lymphocytes and a lesser homology to various pancreatic lipases. Specific functions in exocytosis or digestion for this lipase are not known.

Although not established, it has been suggested for several years that the subapical actin web in the pancreatic acinar cell is involved in transport of zymogen granules toward the apical membrane during exocytosis. Previous studies have shown that supramaximal concentrations of cerulein that cause inhibition of enzyme secretion and heterologous desensitization also cause disruption and dissolution of the apical actin web. One paper this past year [23] demonstrated that JMV-180 prevented the supramaximal inhibition of enzyme secretion and disruption of the subapical actin web caused by supramaximal concentrations of cerulein, presumably by blocking the interaction of cerulein with the low affinity cholecystokinin receptor. These results support a role for the subapical actin web in the exocytotic process and may explain some of the observations attributed to desensitization.

References and recommended reading

Papers of particular interest, published within the annual period of review, have been highlighted as:

- • Of special interest
- •• Of outstanding interest

1. •• Li Y, Owyang C: **Vagal Afferent Pathway Mediates Physiological Action of Cholecystokinin on Pancreatic Enzyme Secretion.** *J Clin Invest* 1993, 92:418–424.

In rats, infused cholecystokinin-8 to give postprandial plasma concentrations caused pancreatic secretion that was abolished by atropine, hexamethonium, bilateral vagotomy, and gastroduodenal application of the sensory neurotoxin, capsaicin. These results indicated that at physiologic concentrations cholecystokinin stimulates pancreatic enzyme secretion via a capsaicin-sensitive afferent vagal pathway originating from the gastroduodenal mucosa.

2. • Ishiguro H, Hayakawa T, Kondo T, Shibata T, Kitagawa M, Sakai Y, Sobajima H, Nakae Y, Tanikawa M: **The Effect of Somatostatin Analogue Octreotide on Amylase Secretion From Mouse Pancreatic Acini.** *Digestion* 1993, 54:207–212.

Findings demonstrated that somatostatin inhibited the augmented secretory response in pancreatic acini incubated with a combination of an agent that increased cellular cyclic AMP and an agent that increased cellular $[Ca^{2+}]$. These results indicate that somatostatin has a direct effect on the acinar cell to regulate secretion.

3. • Matushita K, Okabayashi Y, Hasegawa H, Koide M, Kido Y, Okutani T, Sugimoto Y, Kasuga M: **In Vitro Inhibitory Effect of Somatostatin on Secretin Action in Exocrine Pancreas of Rats.** *Gastroenterology* 1993, 104:1146–1152.

Findings demonstrated that somatostatin inhibited the augmented secretory response in pancreatic acini incubated with a combination of an agent that increased cellular cyclic AMP and an agent that increased cellular $[Ca^{2+}]$. These results indicate that somatostatin has a direct effect on the acinar cell to regulate secretion.

4. • Lutz MP, Pinon DI, Gate LK, Shenolikar S, Miller LJ: **Control of Cholecystokinin Receptor Dephosphorylation in Pancreatic Acinar Cells.** *J Biol Chem* 1993, 268:12136–12142.

This study demonstrates that cholecystokinin causes dephosphorylation as well as phosphorylation of the cholecystokinin receptor. Dephosphorylation was mediated by serine-threonine-specific protein phosphatase of the PP-2A type. The role of the phosphatase in receptor function was not determined.

5. Gates LK, Ulrich CD, Miller LJ: **Multiple Kinases Phosphorylate the Pancreatic Cholecystokinin Receptor in an Agonist-Dependent Manner.** *Am J Physiol* 1993, 264:G840–G847.

6. • Doi R, Chowdhury P, Rayford PL: **Agonist-Regulated Alteration of the Affinity of Pancreatic Muscarinic Cholinergic Receptors.** *J Biol Chem* 1993, 268:22436–22443.

This study examined the mechanisms of heterologous desensitization of cholinergic stimulated enzyme secretion by cholecystokinin in pancreatic acini. The results indicated that cholecystokinin decreased the affinity of the muscarinic receptor for its ligand and prevented the sequestration of muscarinic receptors caused by carbachol. Both effects were mediated at least in part by activation of protein kinase C.

7. Schmidt WE, Seebeck J, Höcker M, Schwarzhoff R, Schäfer H, Fornefeld H, Morys-Wortmann C, Fölsch UR, Creutzfeldt W: **PACAP and VIP Stimulate Enzyme Secretion in Rat Pancreatic Acini via Interaction With VIP/PACAP-2 Receptors: Additive Augmentation of CCK/Carbachol-Induced Enzyme Release.** *Pancreas* 1993, 8:476–487.

8. Honda T, Zhou Z-C, Gu Z-F, Kitsukawa Y, Mrozinski JE, Jensen RT: **Structural Analysis of CGRP Receptors on Gastric Smooth Muscle and Pancreatic Acinar Cells.** *Am J Physiol* 1993, 264:G1142–G1152.

9. • Hildebrand P, Mrozinski JE, Mantey SA, Patto RJ, Jensen RT: **Pancreatic Acini Possess Endothelin Receptors Whose Internalization Is Regulated by PLC-Activating Agents.** *Am J Physiol* 1993, 264:G984–G993.

This study demonstrated the presence of two types of endothelin receptors on pancreatic acini. Occupation of both resulted in rapid internalization that was regulated by phospholipase C–activating secretagogues. Occupations of neither resulted in changes in intracellular Ca^{2+}, cyclic AMP, or enzyme secretion.

10. •• Bahnson TD, Pandol SJ, Dionne VE: **Cyclic GMP Modulates Depletion-Activated Ca2+ Entry in Pancreatic Acinar Cells.** *J Biol Chem* 1993, 268:10808–10812.

Using patch-clamp recording methods, this study demonstrated that the intracellular application of cyclic GMP mimics the Ca^{2+} entry activated by carbachol. These results indicated that cyclic GMP mediates agonist-stimulated Ca^{2+} influx.

11. Menniti FS, Miller RN, Putney JW, Shears SB: **Turnover of Inositol Polyphosphate Pyrophosphates in Pancreatoma Cells.** *J Biol Chem* 1993, 268:3850–3856.

12. Kasai H, Li Y, Miyashita Y: **Subcellular Distribution of Ca2+ Release Channels Underlying Ca2+ Waves and Oscillations in Exocrine Pancreas.** *Cell* 1993, 74:669–677.
•• Using confocal Ca^{2+} imaging and injections of inositol 1,4,5-trisphosphate and Ca^{2+} into pancreatic acinar cells, this study demonstrated three specific zones of Ca^{2+} storage organelles in the pancreatic acinar cells. The heterogenous localization of these stores underlie the mechanism of Ca^{2+} waves and oscillations.

13. Petersen CJH, Petersen OH, Berridge MJ: **The Role of Endoplasmic Reticulum Calcium Pumps During Cytosolic Calcium Spiking in Pancreatic Acinar Cells.** *J Biol Chem* 1993, **268**:22262–22264.
• This study demonstrated that regulation of endoplasmic reticulum Ca^{2+} ATPases may be involved in the mechanism of $[Ca^{2+}]i$ oscillations.

14. Stauffer PL, Zhao H, Luby-Phelps K, Moss RL, Star RA, Muallem S: **Gap Junction Communication Modulates [Ca2+]i Oscillations and Enzyme Secretion in Pancreatic Acini.** *J Biol Chem* 1993, **268**:19769–19775.
• The results demonstrated that gap junctions coordinate $[Ca^{2+}]i$ oscillations between individual cells of an acinus. Stimulation of one cell in an acinus resulted in synchronized $[Ca^{2+}]i$ oscillations in the entire acinus.

15. Thorn P, Petersen OH: **Calcium Oscillation in Pancreatic Acinar Cells, Evoked by the Cholecystokinin Analogue JMV-180, Depend on Functional Inositol 1,4,5-Trisphosphate Receptors.** *J Biol Chem* 1993, **268**:23219–23221.

16. Yule DI, Wu D, Essington TE, Shayman JA, Williams JA: **Sphingosine Metabolism Induces Ca2+ Oscillations in Rat Pancreatic Acinar Cells.** *J Biol Chem* 1993, **268**:12353–12358.

17. Yule DI, Essington TE, Williams JA: **Pilocarpine and Carbachol Exhibit Markedly Different Patterns of Ca2+ Signaling in Rat Pancreatic Acinar Cells.** *Am J Physiol* 1993, **264**:G786–G791.

18. Lutz MP, Sutor SL, Abraham RT, Miller LT: **A Role for Cholecystokinin-Stimulated Protein Tyrosine Phosphorylation in Regulated Secretion by the Pancreatic Acinar Cell.** *J Biol Chem* 1993, **268**:11119–11124.
•• Agonist-stimulated tyrosine phosphorylation occurred via both calcium-dependent and protein kinase C–dependent pathways. Only the calcium-dependent tyrosine phosphorylation was involved in triggering enzyme secretion.

19. Gillespie J, Dye JF, Schachter M, Guillou PJ: **Inhibition of Pancreatic Cancer Cell Growth In Vitro by the Tyrphostin Group of Tyrosine Kinase Inhibitors.** *Br J Cancer* 1993, **68**:1122–1126.

20. Gasser KW, Holda JR: **ATP-Sensitive Potassium Transport by Pancreatic Secretory Granule Membrane.** *Am J Physiol* 1993, **264**:G137–G142.
• This study demonstrated the presence of an ATP and phospholipase A_2–regulated K^+ transport on the zymogen granule membrane. Together with previously described Cl^- channels, these transports may be involved in granule swelling and flushing during exocytosis.

21. Hoops TC, Ivanov I, Cui Z, Colomer-Gould V, Rindler MJ: **Incorporation of the Pancreatic Membrane Protein GP-2 Into Secretory Granules in Exocrine but Not Endocrine Cells.** *J Biol Chem* 1993, **268**:25694–25705.
• The pancreatic zymogen granule membrane protein, glycoprotein-2, was targeted to secretory granule membranes of exocrine pancreatic derived AR 425 cells, but not the secretory granule membrane of cells of anterior pituitary, or insulinoma origin. Thus, flycoprotein-2 is targeted to secretory granule membranes by cell-type–specific mechanisms.

22. Wishart MJ, Andrews PC, Nichols R, Blevins GT, Lodgsdon CD, Williams JA: **Identification and Cloning of GP-3 From Rat Pancreatic Acinar Zymogen Granules As a Glycosylated Membrane-Associated Lipase.** *J Biol Chem* 1993, **268**:10303–10311.
• This study demonstrated that the zymogen granule embrane glycoprotein, GP-3, is a lipase.

23. O'Konski MS, Pandol SJ: **Cholecystokinin JMV-180 and Caerulein Effects on the Pancreatic Acinar Cell Cytoskeleton.** *Pancreas* 1993, **8**:638–646.

Stephen J. Pandol, MD, 3350 La Jolla Village Drive 111-D, San Diego, CA 92161, USA.

Neurohormonal control of the exocrine pancreas

Chung Owyang, MD

The University of Michigan Medical Center, Ann Arbor, Michigan, USA

Increasing numbers of peptide hormones appear to stimulate pancreatic enzyme secretion via vagal cholinergic pathways. Studies in rats indicated that cholecystokinin at physiologic levels stimulates pancreatic secretion via a capsaicin-sensitive afferent vagal pathway. Similar cholinergic dependency was observed in other stimulatory peptides such as neurotensin and adenylate cyclase activating polypeptide. Recent human studies further confirmed the existence of a feedback mechanism between cholecystokinin release and pancreatico-biliary secretion. Cholecystokinin receptor blockade resulted in enhancement of postprandial plasma cholecystokinin levels but had no effect on basal plasma cholecystokinin levels. Under fasting conditions, however, cholecystokinin receptor blockade increased cholecystokinin synthesis but not its release. Further studies in rats indicated that dietary problems in the intestine modulate feedback regulation of cholecystokinin release by luminal trypsin inhibitors. Endocrine and exocrine pancreatic interaction has important functional and clinical significance. Studies in rats showed that insulin exerted a direct potentiating effect on pancreatic acinar cells by increasing Na^+,K^+-ATPase activity. In isolated rat pancreas, somatostatin-enhanced arginine evoked pancreatic secretion by inhibiting the release of glucagon under hypoglycemic conditions. However, in euglycemic conditions somatostatin inhibited pancreatic secretion by acting at a central vagal site. Two separate laboratories provided convincing evidence that NO (nitric oxide) produced by NO synthase mediated the stimulation by carbachol of cyclic GMP formation, which in turn evoked Ca^{2+} influx in pancreatic acinar cells. The activity of NO synthase was regulated by internal Ca^{2+} stores. This provides a novel mechanism to explain Ca^{2+} transport in pancreatic acinar cells. In the field of pancreatic growth and proliferation, the demonstration that concomitant expression of high levels of fibroblast growth factors (FGFs) and FGF receptors in pancreatic cancer cells was associated with advanced clinical stages and poor prognosis suggests that these growth factors may contribute to progression of the pancreatic cancer by allowing excessive autocrine and paracrine growth stimulation.

Current Opinion in Gastroenterology 1994, **10**:491–495

Over the past several years, there has been considerable progress in our knowledge of neurohormonal regulation of pancreatic enzyme secretion. Many peptide hormones are now believed to act via vagal cholinergic mechanisms to modulate pancreatic secretion. This renders the separation of neural versus hormonal control of pancreatic secretion as somewhat artificial. The advances of cellular and molecular biology provide better tools to elucidate the mechanisms of action of neurotransmitters and hormones on pancreatic secretion. In this review, important observations published over the past year that enhance our understanding of the neurohormonal control of pancreatic secretion are discussed.

Vagal mediation of pancreatic action of hormones

Recent human studies indicated that under physiologic conditions, cholinergic pathways rather than pancreatic acinar cells represent the primary targets on which cholecystokinin acts as a major mediator of postprandial pancreatic enzyme secretion. This was reviewed in a previous issue of *Current Opinion in Gastroenterology* [1]. Additional studies showed that the inhibitory effect of atropine can be attributed to M_1-muscarinic receptor blockade, because a comparable inhibition of pancreatic secretion was achieved with pirenzepine, a selective M_1-receptor antagonist [2•]. However, re-

Abbreviations

FGF—fibroblast growth factor; **FGFR-1**—fibroblast growth factor receptor-1.

 ISBN 1-85922-610-8 ISSN 0267–1379

peated administration of the M_1-selective, muscarinic antagonist telenzepine in a therapeutic dose over 1 week led to an increased volume and pancreatic enzyme secretion stimulated by secretin and ceruletide. This suggests that the adaptation of physiologic mechanisms governing the exocrine pancreas may occur after 1 week of receptor blockade by telenzepine to the extent that M_1-blockade no longer inhibits secretion.

To further investigate the mechanisms and sites of the physiological action of cholecystokinin, Li and Owyang [3••] have shown that in an anesthetized rat, treatment with atropine or hexamethonium completely abolished pancreatic protein responses to cholecystokinin-8 given at 40 pmol/kg/h, a dose that produced plasma levels closely approximating proprandial plasma cholecystokinin levels. Bilateral truncal vagotomy also abolished the pancreatic responses to this dose of cholecystokinin-8. Similarly, perivagal or mucosal treatment with a sensory neurotoxin, capsaicin, caused a complete inhibition of cholecystokinin-stimulated pancreatic protein secretion. These observations indicate that cholecystokinin at physiologic levels stimulates pancreatic enzyme secretion via a capsaicin-sensitive afferent vagal pathway originating from the gastroduodenal mucosa. In contrast, doses of cholecystokinin-8 that produce supraphysiologic plasma cholecystokinin levels act on intrapancreatic neurons and, to a lesser degree, on pancreatic acini. These findings have important physiologic ramifications. Not only to they explain the discrepancies in previous *in vivo* versus *in vitro* studies but they revolutionize our current concept on the mechanisms of action of cholecystokinin on pancreatic exocrine secretion. Similar observations were made by Ami *et al.* [4•] who showed that vagotomy induced a decrease and delay in postprandial responses to pancreatic volume and protein outputs. The observation that postprandial pancreatic secretion was reduced but not abolished may reflect the differential effects of vagotomy on secretion stimulated by cholecystokinin and enteropancreatic reflexes.

Cholinergic dependency of stimulatory effectors of hormones is not limited to cholecystokinin. Shinozaki *et al.* [5•] showed that neurotensin-stimulated pancreatic enzyme secretion in conscious rats could be completely inhibited by atropine, suggesting mediation via the cholinergic pathway. In addition, it has been shown that galanin inhibits pancreatic enzyme secretion via the modulation of cholinergic transmission [6]. These observations suggest that the exocrine pancreas is under complex neurohormonal control.

Feedback regulation of pancreatic enzyme secretion

In rats, intraluminal pancreatic proteases appear to play an important role in regulating cholecystokinin release and pancreatic enzyme secretion. Diversion of pancreatic juice from the duodenum stimulates cholecystokinin release and pancreatic enzyme secretion. On the other hand, intraduodenal administration of trypsin or chymotrypsin inhibits the release of cholecystokinin and pancreatic secretion. The increased plasma cholecystokinin levels following diversion of pancreatic juice appear to be mediated by a trypsin-sensitive "cholecystokinin-releasing peptide" secreted by the proximal small intestine [7]. Several laboratories have shown a protease-specific negative feedback mechanism to exist in humans that appears to be mediated via cholecystokinin [8]. However, the role of cholecystokinin as the mediator of this feedback regulation of pancreatic secretion in humans remains controversial because elevated plasma cholecystokinin levels in patients with chronic pancreatitis have not been consistently observed. Recently it was shown that stimulation of cholecystokinin release by bombesin in humans was augmented by cholecystokinin receptor blockade with loxiglumide [9]. It was hypothesized that this augmented cholecystokinin release results from the inhibition of the pancreatico-biliary response to bombesin during cholecystokinin receptor blockade. To test this hypothesis, Jebbink *et al.* [10••] showed that in humans, intraduodenal perfusion of pancreatico-biliary juice resulted in a significant inhibition of bombesin-stimulated plasma cholecystokinin concentrations during infusion of loxiglumide, a cholecystokinin A receptor antagonist. These observations support the concept of a feedback mechanism between cholecystokinin release and pancreatico-biliary secretion as previously demonstrated [8].

In an attempt to further elucidate the mechanisms regulating feedback regulation of pancreatic enzyme secretion in rats, Otsuki *et al.* [11••] investigated the effects of an oral dose of a synthetic trypsin inhibitor camostat on pancreatic exocrine function in fed and fasted rats. This study demonstrated that oral administration of camostat has an immediate and delayed effect on pancreatic exocrine secretion. The former was seen within 30 minutes in both fed and fasted rats, whereas the latter was observed only in fed rats at 12 hours after the feeding of camostat. It was hypothesized that the dietary protein in the duodenum in the fed state competed for the trypsin and chemotrypsin and prevented proteolytic inactivation of the cholecystokinin-releasing peptide. This may be responsible for the delayed effect of camostat observed in the fed animals. These observations indicate that the presence of dietary protein in the intestine may modulate the feedback regulation of cholecystokinin release and pancreatic secretion by a luminal trypsin inhibitor.

In a related study, Playford *et al.* [12•] evaluated the effects of diet and the cholecystokinin antagonist devazepide (L364,718) on cholecystokinin messenger RNA, tissue, and plasma cholecystokinin concentrations in rats. This study showed that diets such as raw soya, which stimulated high plasma cholecystokinin levels, also produced the highest cholecystokinin tissue and messenger RNA concentrations. On the other hand, foods rich in carbohydrate but low in protein cause little or no change in plasma cholecystokinin and cholecystokinin tissue and messenger RNA concentration.

Administration of devazepide produced a different pattern of responses [12•]. In the fasted state, treatment with devazepide caused an increase in the amount of cholecystokinin messenger RNA and tissue cholecystokinin, but no significant effect on the plasma concentrations of cholecystokinin. This suggests that devazepide increases the synthesis of cholecystokinin but not its release into the circulation. In the fed state, treatment with devazepide increased plasma cholecystokinin and tissue cholecystokinin messenger RNA levels above control values.

These results confirm and extend those of Liddle *et al.* [13] who showed that ingested proteins and proteinase inhibitors released cholecystokinin with differing potency, depending on the ability of the proteins to inhibit proteolytic activities in the duodenum. According to this model, the cholecystokinin receptor antagonist increases postprandial cholecystokinin release by diminishing the secretion of pancreatic enzymes, causing an increase in the amount of cholecystokinin-releasing peptide present in the duodenal lumen. The results of the study by Playford *et al.* [12•] are consistent with this hypothesis except that treatment with the cholecystokinin receptor antagonist did not increase plasma cholecystokinin levels in fasted rats. Under fasting conditions, pancreatic enzyme secretion in rats is quite low and is not under the control of cholecystokinin. Therefore, it is not surprising that devazepide did not increase fasting plasma cholecystokinin levels. However, the demonstration that devazepide stimulated the synthesis but not the release of cholecystokinin suggests that devazepide may exert its action on cholecystokinin synthesis independent of cholecystokinin-releasing peptide. Therefore, it appears that the relationship between rates of cholecystokinin synthesis and circulating plasma levels is complex and requires further investigation.

Endocrine-exocrine pancreatic interaction

It is well known that complex interactions occur between the exocrine and endocrine pancreas. Of the pancreatic islet hormones, glucagon, somatostatin, and pancreatic polypeptide inhibit pancreatic exocrine secretion. Insulin, on the other hand, has a stimulatory effect on pancreatic enzyme secretion. *In vivo* studies and secretory studies using isolated perfused rat pancreas showed that insulin potentiated pancreatic secretion stimulated by secretin and cholecystokinin. In these studies, neurohormonal interaction was not eliminated and hence it is not known if insulin has a direct effect on pancreatic exocrine secretion. To address this question, Matsushita *et al.* [14••] showed that in isolated rat pancreatic acini, insulin potentiated the secretory response to secretin plus cholecystokinin but not to secretin or cholecystokinin alone. This stimulatory action of insulin was abolished by ouabain, an inhibitor of Na^+, K^+-ATPase activity. In addition, these investigators also showed that insulin potentiated the stimulatory action of secretin on Na^+,K^+ATPase activity without affecting ^{125}I-secretin binding to pancreatic acini. This is the first demonstration that insulin exerts a direct effect on pancreatic acinar cells. It potentiated exocrine secretion elicited by secretin plus cholecystokinin in part by increasing Na^+,K^+-ATPase activity.

In a separate study, the role of somatostatin in the regulation of insular-acinar axis was investigated. Müller *et al.* [15•] showed that in the isolated rat pancreas, cystemine released somatostatin but has no effect on cholecystokinin-stimulated amylase secretion. On the other hand, in the presence of arginine, which stimulates the release of glucagon, cysteamine enhanced cholecystokinin-stimulated amylase secretion via the release of somatostatin, which inhibits arginine-evoked glucagon secretion. In a companion paper [16•], it was shown that endogenously released somatostatin by cysteamine inhibited insulin secretion under hyperglycemic conditions and this in turn reduced amylase secretion stimulated by cholecystokinin. It was thus proposed that somatostatin may play a role in the regulation of pancreatic exocrine secretion via its paracrine effects on pancreatic B and A cells. These observations are interesting but they do not explain the physiologic action of circulating somatostatin, which is known to inhibit pancreatic secretion even under euglycemic conditions.

In an effort to examine the sites and mechanisms responsible for the inhibitory action of somatostatin on pancreatic enzyme secretion, Li and Owyang [17••] investigated the effects of physiologic doses of somatostatin on pancreatic secretion evoked by stimulants that act on different sites. It was demonstrated that in rats, somatostatin-14 produced a dose-related inhibition of pancreatic protein secretion evoked by 2-deoxy-D-glucose, a central vagal stimulant that acts by stimulating the dorsal vagal nuclei. Similarly, somatostatin-14 also inhibited pancreatic protein secretion in response to a physiologic concentration of cholecystokinin-8, which acts via a vagal afferent pathway. In contrast, pancreatic secretions evoked by bethanechol, which directly stimulates pancreatic muscarinic receptors, or electrical stimulation of the vagal trunk, which activates the vagal efferent pathway, were unaffected by somatostatin-14. In addition, it was also shown that perivagal treatment with the sensory neurotoxin capsaicin impaired pancreatic responses to cholecystokinin-8 but had no effect on the inhibitory action of somatostatin-14 on pancreatic secretion evoked by 2-deoxy-D-glucose, ruling out an effect of somatostatin on the vagal afferent pathway. These studies demonstrated that somatostatin inhibits 2-deoxy-D-glucose- and cholecystokinin-8–evoked pancreatic enzyme secretion via a vagal pathway. Somatostatin does not act on peripheral vagal afferent or efferent pathways or directly on pancreatic acini but exerts its inhibitory action at a central vagal site.

Nitric oxide and pancreatic exocrine secretion

The activation of Ca^{2+} influx is required for the secretory response to cholecystokinin and carbachol in pancreatic acinar cells. The mechanisms by which these agonists cause Ca^{2+} influx is unknown. Gukovskaya and Pandol [18••] provided convincing evidence that NO (nitric oxide) produced by NO synthase mediated the stimulation by carbachol of cyclic GMP formation, which in turn evoked Ca^{2+} influx in pancreatic acinar cells from both rats and guinea pigs. These investigators showed that carbachol increased ^{3}H-arginine conversion to ^{3}H-citrulline. NO was produced by NO synthase during this biochemical reaction. Blocking NO production by inhibitors of NO synthase, N^G-monomethyl-L-arginine, abolished carbachol-induced cyclic GMP formation and $^{45}Ca^{2+}$ uptake. Because cyclic GMP has previously been shown to mediate Ca^{2+} influx, it was concluded that the NO production regulates cyclic GMP formation and calcium influx in pancreatic acinar cells during carbachol stimulation.

In a related study, Xu *et al.* [19••] showed that depletion of intracellular Ca^{2+} stores activated NO synthase to generate cyclic GMP and regulate Ca^{2+} influx in rat pancreatic acinar cells. Similar to results of Gukovskaya and Pandol [18••], this study demonstrated that the carbachol-activated Ca^{2+} entry was inhibited by L-NMMA (N^G-monomethyl-L-arginine), a specific inhibitor of NO synthase, and by LY33583, an inhibitor of guanylyl cyclase. Increasing cyclic GMP up to 10-fold above control activated Ca^{2+} entry. Using SLO-permeabilized cells, it was further demonstrated that when the internal Ca^{2+} stores were maintained loaded with Ca^{2+}, increasing medium [Ca^{2+}] only modestly increased NO synthase activity. On the other hand, the depletion of Ca^{2+}, from internal stores markedly increased NO synthase activity independent of medium [Ca^{2+}]. Thus it appears that NO synthase senses both cystosolic [Ca^{2+}] and internal Ca^{2+} stores. During carbachol stimulation, Ca^{2+} released from internal stores activates a Ca^{2+}-dependent constitutive NO synthase to generate NO from L-arginine. The activity of NO synthase is regulated by Ca^{2+} content present in internal stores. The NO production stimulates cyclic GMP formation that modulates Ca^{2+} entry. This attractive hypothesis provides a novel mechanism to explain Ca^{2+} transport in pancreatic acinar cells.

To provide a morphologic basis for understanding the role of NO in the pancreas, Shimosegawa *et al.* [20•] characterized the localization and distribution of NADPH diaphorase activity in the pancreas, because recent studies indicate that NADPH diaphorase activity corresponds to neuronal NO synthase. NADPH diaphorase activity was found in the neurons and vascular endothelium of the pancreas of the rat, guinea pig, dog, and human, and some of the nerve fibers and cell bodies coexpressed NADPH-diaphorase activity and vasoactive intestinal peptide-immunoreactivity. It is interesting to note that no NADPH-diaphorase activity was found in pancreatic islet and acinar cells. This potentially may argue against a functional role of endogenous NO in pancreatic acinar cells. However, it is conceivable that in nonneural tissue, staining of NADPH-diaphorase activity and NO synthase activity may be different and should not negate the potential importance of the observations made by Gukovskaya and Pandol [18••].

Pancreatic growth

The fibroblast growth factor (FGF) family consists of a number of homologous polypeptide growth factors that are mitogenic, promote angiogenesis, and participate in the regulation of cellular differentiation and tissue repair. Recently it has been shown that aFGF and bFGF are overexpressed in a significant proportion of pancreatic cancers. To determine the significance of aFGF and bFGF expression in the pancreatic cancer cells, immunohistochemical analyses of 78 human pancreatic carcinomas were performed [21••]. It was found that aFGF and bFGF immunoreactivity was present in 60% and 56% of the tumors. The presence of either aFGF or bFGF in the cancer cells correlated with a more advanced clinical stage. In addition, patients whose tumors contained cancer cells that were positive for bFGF had a shorter postoperative survival period than patients with bFGF-negative cancer. These observations suggest that aFGF and bFGF may contribute to progression of the pancreatic cancer. However, the reasons for the association of bFGF and shorter patient survival are not clear. It is conceivable that bFGF is a more potent mitogen than aFGF in these tumors, as reported in Chinese hamster lung fibroblasts or alternatively, bFGF may be released from pancreatic cancer cells more efficiently than aFGF, thus allowing for more potent autocrine and paracrine effects on cancer cell growth.

In a separate study from the same laboratory [22••], it was reported that the pattern of distribution of FGF receptor-1 (FGFR-1) was quite different in normal and malignant tissues. In the normal pancreas, FGFR-1 immunostaining was observed mainly in the acinar cells, whereas in the pancreatic cancers intense FGFR-1 immunostaining was evident in the ductal-like tumor cells. These cells were also shown to exhibit strong immunoreactivity with specific anti-aFGF and anti-bFGF antibodies and to overexpressed aFGF and bFGF messenger RNA by *in situ* hybridization. Thus there is concomitant expression of high levels of FGFs and FGFR-1 in pancreatic cancer cells, which may allow for excessive autocrine and paracrine growth-stimulation. Furthermore, analysis by the polymerase chain reaction and ribonuclease protection revealed that the 2-immunoglobulin-like and the 3-immunoglobulin-like forms of FGFR-1 were expressed in pancreatic tissue samples, but the 2-immunoglubulin-like form was overexpressed in the cancer tissues in comparison with the normal tissues. It is conceivable that this aberrant expression of FSFR-1 may contribute to excessive activation of pancreatic cancer cells by FGF and other growth factors.

References and recommended reading

Papers of particular interest, published within the annual period of review, have been highlighted as:

- • Of special interest
- •• Of outstanding interest

1. Owyang C: **Neurohormonal control of the exocrine pancreas.** *Curr Opin Gastroenterol* 1993, 9:747–751.

2. • Malfertheiner P, Nelson DK, Kemmer TP, Glasbrenner B, Schneider A, Ditschuneit H: **Exocrine Pancreatic Secretion in Man Following One Week of M_1-Muscarinic Receptor Blockade.** *Aliment Pharmacol Ther* 1993, 7:423–428.

Human studies demonstrate that the inhibitory effect of atropine on cholecystokinin-stimulated pancreatic enzyme secretion is mediated by M_1-muscarinic receptor and adaptative mechanisms occur after 1 week of M_1-blockade.

3. •• Li Y, Owyang C: **Vagal Afferent Pathway Mediates Physiological Action of Cholecystokinin on Pancreatic Enzyme Secretion.** *J Clin Invest* 1993, 92:418–424.

This is the first demonstration that cholecystokinin at physiologic levels stimulates pancreatic secretion via a capsaicin-sensitive afferent vagal pathway originating from the gastroduodenal mucosa.

4. • Ami M, Doi R, Inoue K, Chowdhury P, Rayford PL: **The Influence of Vagotomy on Basal and Postprandial Pancreatic Secretion and Plasma Levels of Gastrointestinal Hormones in Conscious Rats.** *Surg Gynecol Obstr* 1993, 177:577–582.

This paper provides further evidence that postprandial pancreatic secretion in rats is affected by vagotomy.

5. • Shinozaki H, Miyasaka K, Funakoshi A: **Cholinergic Dependency of Stimulatory Effects of Neurotensin on Exocrine Pancreas in Rats.** *Regul Pept* 1993, 47:205–211.

Rat studies show cholinergic dependency of the stimulatory action of neurotensin on pancreatic enzyme secretion.

6. •• Herzig KH, Brunke G, Schon I, Schaffer M, Folsch UR: **Mechanism of Galanin's Inhibitory Action on Pancreatic Enzyme Secretion: Modulation of Cholinergic Transmission - Studies *In Vivo* and *In Vitro*.** *Gut* 1993, 34:1616–1621.

In vivo and *in vitro* rat studies show that galanin modulates pancreatic enzyme secretion by inhibiting cholinergic transmission.

7. Lu L, Louie DS, Owyang C: **A Cholecystokinin Releasing Peptide Mediates Feedback Regulation of Pancreatic Secretion.** *Am J Physiol* 1989, 256:G430–G435.

8. Owyang C, Louie DS, Tatum D: **Feedback Regulation of Pancreatic Enzyme Secretion: Suppression of Cholecystokinin Release by Trypsin.** *J Clin Invest* 1986, 77:2042–2047.

9. Jansen JBMJ, Jebbink MCW, Douglas BR, Lamers CBHW: **Effect of Loxiglumide (CR 1505) on Bombesin and Meal Stimulated Plasma CCK in Man.** *Eur J Clin Pharmacol* 1990, 38:367–370.

10. •• Jebbink MCW, Jansen JBMJ, Van Der Kleu FGH, Mooy DM, Rovati LC, Lambers CBHW: **Effect of Duodenal Juice on Bombesin-Stimulated CCK Release During Loxiglumide Administration in Man.** *Eur J Clin Invest* 1993, 23:529–533.

Additional evidence supports the concept of a feedback mechanism between cholecystokinin release and pancreatico-biliary secretion in humans.

11. •• Otsuki M, Tani S, Fujii M, Nakamura T, Okabayashi Y, Koide M: **Differential Effects of Proteinase Inhibitor Camostat on Exocrine Pancreas in Fed and Fasted Rats.** *Am J Physiol* 1993, 265:R896–R901.

Administration of camostat produces a delayed stimulatory effect on cholecystokinin release and pancreatic secretion. This suggests that the presence of a dietary protein in the intestine may modulate feedback regulation of cholecystokinin release.

12. • Playford RJ, King AW, Deprez PH, Debelleroche J, Freeman TC, Calam J: **Effects of Diet and the Cholecystokinin Antagonist; Devazepide (L364,718) on CCK mRNA, and Tissue and Plasma CCK Concentrations.** *Eur J Clin Invest* 1993, 23:641–647.

Rat studies show that devazepide, a cholecystokinin receptor antagonist, increases the synthesis of cholecystokinin but not its release into the circulation.

13. Liddle RA, Green GM, Conrad CK, Williams JA: **Proteins but Not Amino Acids, Carbohydrates or Fats Stimulate Cholecystokinin Secretion in Rats.** *Am J Physiol* 1986, 251:G243–G248.

14. •• Matsushita K, Okabayashi Y, Koide M, Hasegawa H, Otsuki M, Kasuga M: **Potentiating Effect of Insulin on Exocrine Secretory Function in Isolated Rat Pancreatic Acini.** *Gastroenterology* 1994, 106:200–206.

The first demonstration that insulin exerts a direct stimulatory effect on rat pancreatic acini by increasing Na^+, K^+-ATPase activity.

15. • Müller MK, Von Schonfeld J, Singer MV: **Role of Somatostatin in Regulation of Insula-Acinar Axis.** *Dig Dis Sci* 1993, 38:1537–1542.

In isolated rat pancreas, somatostatin enhances arginine-evoked pancreatic secretion by inhibiting the release of glucagon under hypoglycemic conditions.

16. • Von Schonfeld J, Müller MK, Augustin M, Runzi M, Goebell H: **Effect of Cysteamine on Insulin Release and Exocrine Pancreatic Secretion In Vitro.** *Dig Dis Sci* 1993, 38:28–32.

In isolated rat pancreas, somatostatin inhibits pancreatic enzyme secretion by inhibiting the release of insulin under hyperglycemic conditions.

17. •• Li Y, Owyang C: **Somatostatin Inhibits Pancreatic Enzyme Secretion at a Central Vagal Site.** *Am J Physiol* 1993, 265:G251–G257.

Rat studies clarify the mechanism by which somatostatin inhibits pancreatic enzyme secretion.

18. •• Gukovskaya A, Pandol S: **Nitric Oxide Production Regulates cGMP Formation and Calcium Influx in Pancreatic Acinar Cells.** *Am J Physiol* 1994, 266:G350–G356.

This is the first demonstration that NO produced by NO synthase mediates the stimulation by carbachol of cyclic GMP formation, which in turn evokes Ca^{2+} influx in pancreatic acini.

19. •• Xu X, Star RA, Tortorici G, Muallem S: **Depletion of Intracellular Ca^{2+} Stores Activates Nitric Oxide Synthase to Generate cGMP and Regulate Ca^{2+} Influx.** *J Biol Chem* 1994, 269:12643–12653.

This elegant study shows that depletion of intracellular Ca^{2+} stores activates NO synthase to generate cyclic GMP and regulate Ca^{2+} influx in rat pancreatic acinar cells.

20. • Shimosegawa T, Abe T, Satoh A, Abe R, Kikuchi Y, Koizumi M, Toyota T: **NADPH-Diaphorase Activity in Neurons of the Mammalian Pancreas: Coexpression With Vasoactive Intestinal Polypeptide.** *Gastroenterology* 1993, 105:999–1008.

An immunohistochemical study characterizes the distribution of NADPH-diaphorase activity in the pancreas.

21. •• Yamanaka Y, Friess H, Buchler M, Beger HG, Uchida E, Onda M, Kobrin MS, Korc M: **Overexpression of Acidic and Basic Fibroblast Growth Factors in Human Pancreatic Cancer Correlates With Advanced Tumor Stage.** *Cancer Res* 1993, 53:5289–5296.

An interesting study suggesting that acidic and basic FGFs may contribute to progression of pancreatic cancer.

22. •• Kobrin MS, Yamanaka Y, Friess H, Lopez ME, Korc M: **Aberrant Expression of Type 1 Fibroblast Growth Factor Receptor in Human Pancreatic Adenocarcinoma.** *Cancer Res* 1993, 53:4741–4744.

This is the first report of expression of high levels of aberrant FGFR-1 in human pancreatic cancer cells.

Chung Owyang, MD, 3912 Taubman Center Box 0362, 1500 E. Medical Center Drive, Division of Gastroenterology, Department of Internal Medicine, The University of Michigan, Ann Arbor, MI 48109, USA.

Acute pancreatitis

C.W. Imrie, FRCS

Royal Infirmary, Glasgow, UK

There has been a movement away from the study of protease-antiprotease interactions in both experimental and clinical acute pancreatitis. Increasingly, the focus of the basic pathologic mechanism in acute pancreatitis reveals strong parallels with that of septic shock. Elevated levels of endotoxin, decreased levels of endogenous antiendotoxic core antibody, and elevated local levels (and less often, peripheral blood levels) of various cytokines are found in both conditions. Therapy to modify this response may prove valuable. Emphasis on new early methods of assessing prognosis continues and marked obesity has been shown as a significant marker of poor prognosis. Despite the lack of a specific large clinical trial categorically proving the place of early endoscopic retrograde cholangiopancreatography sphincterotomy, the trend of results in all studies indicates the value of this in those with severe acute pancreatitis. A consensus of experts has strongly suggested dropping confusing terminology such as "pancreatic phlegmon" and "infected pseudocyst" while clarifying the disease description.

Current Opinion in Gastroenterology 1994, **10**:496–501

Experimental acute pancreatitis

Many studies using the cerulein hyperstimulation model on male Wistar rats have been published over the past year and indicate a better understanding of pathophysiology, as well as potential therapy. Thus one Polish study [1•] investigating the effects of nitric oxide synthase blockade by means of *N*-nitro-L-arginine (L-NNA) found a significant reduction in basal pancreatic protein secretion as well as that induced by infusion of cholecystokinin. L-NNA also reduced pancreatic blood flow, particularly in acute pancreatitis. The provision of L-arginine enhanced the pancreatic blood flow and improved the pancreatitis status. The authors concluded that nitric oxide is involved in the stimulation of pancreatic secretion and has a beneficial effect on pancreatitis, possibly by favorably affecting pancreatic blood flow.

A research group from Salamanca, Spain showed the fascinating effects of cholecystokinin receptor antagonist L-364,318 on cerulein-induced acute pancreatitis. This agent given both prophylactically and therapeutically had a markedly beneficial effect on this type of pancreatitis. Cholecystokinin may play an important role in the development of this form of pancreatitis [2•].

In another study [3•] utilizing retrograde injection of 6% taurocholate in male Wistar rats, an inhibitor of 5-lipoxygenase (simply designated AA-861) was shown to ameliorate the histologically massive tissue necrosis that occurs in this model. Lipoxygenases metabolize arachidonic acid (released from the phospholipid of cell membranes) to form leukotrienes. Leukotriene C4 and leukotriene D4 are known to induce changes in tone of small vessels and to induce tissue edema, myocardial depression, and bronchoconstriction. The authors suggest that the lipoxygenase inhibitor AA-861 may prove useful in the clinical treatment of acute pancreatitis [3•].

In a similar way, another research group from Japan [4•] has shown that tumor necrosis factor (TNF)-α is produced in rats with cerulein-induced pancreatitis at a much higher level from the peritoneal macrophages than in control rats. The stimulus to the release of TNF was the customary one of lipopolysaccharide. This increased TNF production by the peritoneal macrophages may be of potential importance in the evolution of the disease.

The taurocholate duct injection model has been utilized in two studies [5,6] by the same group, with each showing TNF to be of probable importance as an inflammatory mediator in acute pancreatitis. Pretreatment with a polyclonal antibody to TNF modified disease outcome favorably [6].

Another cytokine, platelet-activating factor (PAF), has been further studied using the cerulein hyperstimulation model of pancreatitis by the research group from San Antonio who has published several papers on this subject. Their most recent contribution [7••] provides further evidence that PAF is a mediator of pancreatic inflammation in this type of pancreatitis. Their work suggests that the pancreatic accumulation of PAF coupled with ionized calcium overload comprises important

Abbreviations

APS—acute physiology score; **ERCP**—endoscopic retrograde cholangiopancreatography; **L-NNA**—*N*-nitro-L-arginine; **PAF**—platelet-activating factor; **TNF**—tumor necrosis factor.

 ISBN 1-85922-610-8 ISSN 0267–1379

biochemical components in the unfolding of cerulein-induced pancreatitis. Previous studies have indicated that PAF is important in changes of vascular permeability [8] and that the injection of this cytokine along the pancreatic artery of rabbits induces acute pancreatitis [9]. Furthermore, the administration of antagonists of PAF suggests that this cytokine is greatly involved in the inflammatory process in immune complex–induced pancreatitis as well as cerulein-induced pancreatitis in rats [10,11]. Finally Zhou *et al.* [12] showed that the lung pathology of experimental acute pancreatitis involves PAF whereas a Spanish group showed the same cytokine greatly involved in hemodynamic derangements [13].

All of these findings have prompted the investigation of the potential clinical benefit of PAF inhibitors, although the delay from onset of disease to the appearance in hospital and institution of therapy may be a limiting factor as it has been for many other proposed therapies in acute pancreatitis patients.

Clinical acute pancreatitis

Diagnosis

A potentially important paper from New York [14••] has suggested that blood lipase measurements would be a more suitable method of diagnosis of acute pancreatitis than the traditional measurement of amylase. In a study of 95 patients with nonpancreatic abdominal pain and 75 with acute pancreatitis, Gumaste *et al.* found lipase measurements more accurate. Whereas an overlap of results between the two groups of patients was found for amylase measurements at a rate of 27%, the overlap in results taking a cut-off of serum lipase of 680 U/L (three times the upper limit of normal) resulted in no overlap. The authors suggest, on the basis of a 100% sensitivity and 99% specificity of lipase, that much better diagnostic accuracy could be obtained from such a change-over using the suggested cut-off at three times the upper limit of normal. This is now a practical suggestion because the cost difference and rapidity of results using the two methods are not great and the increased efficiency of lipase measurements has much to commend it.

Prognosis

The simplest advance in terms of prognosis has been the emphasis on the importance of obesity as a predictor of poor outcome. In a well documented paper from Capetown, Funnell *et al.* [15••] quantified obesity using a body mass index. When this figure exceeded 30 kg/m^2 it was found that 12 of 19 obese patients in this category developed severe pancreatitis (five deaths and seven abscesses). A comparison with 80 nonobese patients showed a significantly greater risk of severe pancreatitis, abscess formation, and death in the overweight group. The rather simple single prognostic factor of obesity had a sensitivity of 63% and a specificity of 95% in predicting severe disease. The ability to predict severity was enhanced when the nongallstone patients were considered a separate entity. It is postulated that the peripancreatic fat deposits are particularly prone to necrosis by activated enzymes during acute pancreatitis and hence the poorer outcome.

Another simple approach to grading severity has come from a prospective study from Hong Kong. Fan *et al* [16•] have shown that the presence of urea levels above 7.4 mmol/L and blood glucose levels of 11.0 mmol/L or greater, indicated the presence of severe disease with a sensitivity of 79% and a specificity of 67%. They found that the overall accuracy of this system was comparable to the APACHE (Acute Physiology and Chronic Health Evaluation) II system (using a cut-off level of >11) and also to the Ranson scoring system, although the latter comparison was probably unfair as the original Ranson criteria were specifically designed for a population with an alcohol predominance, whereas gallstones were the predominant pathology in Hong Kong.

Our own group in Glasgow has not been able to verify the value of the Hong Kong criteria in an assessment of 125 patients [17•]. We found a sensitivity of only 33% and a specificity of 83% for detecting clinically severe attacks of acute pancreatitis. In the same group of patients using the Glasgow scoring system, a sensitivity of 78% and a specificity of 86% was found.

In a good review of prognostic factors in acute pancreatitis, Malfertheiner and Dominquez-Munoz [18•] lead the reader to believe that plasma polymorph nuclear elastase is a simple measurement with great sensitivity and specificity, but they [19,20] and others [21] only analyzed their polymorph nuclear elastase results in batches after storage at low temperature, so that in no instance has polymorph nuclear elastase been truly used in a clinical setting for the prospective assessment of severity. In a similar way, the same problem exists with interleukin-6 [22,23] where batch measurements after the initial management of acute pancreatitis were again performed. The simplicity that is claimed for the biochemical measurement of polymorph nuclear elastase using a commercial kit is not always realized in practice, whereas interleukin-6 is still very expensive and currently an impractical cytokine to measure in the clinical setting for individual patients.

It is reckoned by most workers in the field that endotoxemia (probably arising from the gut) in patients with acute pancreatitis is the initial stimulus to many of the changes that develop. The paper of Windsor *et al.* [24••] provides considerable support for this view. They found that a combination of a rising of acute physiology score (APS) in the first 48 hours of hospital admission and a significant fall in endogenous IgG antibody level was observed in all seven patients who developed multiple organ failure from a group of 33 with acute pancreatitis who were studied. The same changes in APS and IgG were only observed in one of 16 patients without multiple organ failure. These workers from Edinburgh suggest that measuring the initial trend in APS and the concentration of endogenous IgG antiendotoxin core antibody provides a good means of identifying patients with severe acute pancreatitis at high risk of developing multiorgan failure. They further suggest that this group may benefit from passive immunotherapy with antiendotoxin antibodies. Again, they do not go into the practicality of whether such information could be readily available to the clinician at the time of immediate management of the patient or whether this is simply a research tool at the present time.

Table 1. Effect of early sphincterotomy on outcome of severe acute pancreatitis*

Treatment	Patients, *n*	Complications, *n*(%)	Deaths, *n*
Endoscopic sphincterotomy within 72 hours	25	6(24)	1
Conventional management	28	17(61)	5

**Adapted from* Neoptolemos *et al.* [31]; with permission.

A prospective multicenter study from Spain evaluated the clinical usefulness of APACHE II and the simplified APS system in the initial prognostic classification of acute pancreatitis [25]. They were disappointed to find that the sensitivity was in the range of 70% and specificity 80% for each of those approaches. These results were poorer than those obtained by Larvin and McMahon [26] using the same cut-off points for both systems. They compared these more complex approaches with the simpler Glasgow scoring system [27] and concluded that the practical usefulness of APACHE II and simplified APS was limited and did not represent an advantage.

Most recently, a prospective study of different methods of prediction of outcome in acute pancreatitis was studied in 82 patients in Barcelona [28]. As in previous studies, the occurrence of death or major clinical complications put the patients into the group graded to have severe disease. An evaluation of three multifactorial systems (Ranson, Glasgow, and APACHE II) and C-reactive protein was performed. Most of the patients had a gallstone etiology and the original Ranson criteria were never intended for such a group. The percentage of such correct assessments that was most successful was 77% for C-reactive protein (at 48 hours) and 82% for the Glasgow prognostic score. Combining these two resulted in a figure of 85% and the authors suggest that this combination is a practical method of assessment. Adding the obesity index would probably help further pinpoint the high-risk patient [15••].

New developments

Vitamin C levels in patients with acute pancreatitis have been examined by Scott *et al.* [29•] in Manchester. They found that levels of both vitamin C and its immediately bioavailable form, ascorbic acid, were much lower in patients with a number of acute abdominal problems and in patients with acute pancreatitis compared with a control group (approximately 30 patients in each group). They showed not only that acute abdominal pathology causes a depletion of this key antioxidant (indicating a nonspecific decrease in plasma levels of vitamin C), but that the problem is more severe in acute pancreatitis. The reason for the much lower levels in acute pancreatitis was suggested to be denaturing of available vitamin. Although this oxidant-antioxidant imbalance may play a role in the initial mechanism of acute pancreatitis, the observation of these low levels suggests a possible place for the parenteral administration of ascorbic acid to bolster the antioxidant defense in acute pancreatitis. Clinical trials of this concept are necessary and are now planned.

A recent experimental study using isolated pancreatitic acinar cells also suggests that intracellular oxidative stress is an early phenomenon in cerulein induced pancreatitis that is significantly attenuated by the application by allopurinol and also of hyperbaric oxygen [30].

Treatment

The major change in treatment of acute pancreatitis to be introduced in the past few years is the switch from great concern at even diagnostic endoscopic retrograde cholangiopancreatography (ERCP) in 1984 to an acceptance that therapeutic ERCP probably has a very important place in the management of gallstone-induced acute pancreatitis. The paper that changed the overall approach was by Neoptolemos *et al.* [31] in 1988. They showed a statistically significant benefit in terms of morbidity and found fewer deaths (but not statistically significant) in the patients who had objectively graded severe acute pancreatitis and were treated by ERCP sphincterotomy within 72 hours of admission [31].

Table 2. Effect of early endoscopic sphincterotomy on outcome of all grades of gallstone acute pancreatitis*

Treatment	Patients, *n*	Complications, *n*(%)	Deaths, *n*
Endoscopic sphincterotomy within 24 hours	64	10(16)	1
Conventional management	63	21(33)	5

**Adapted from* Fan *et al.* [32••]; with permission.

A group from Hong Kong [32••] published results of a more rapid intervention, within 24 hours of admission, in a total of 195 patients who predominantly had gallstone acute pancreatitis. They demonstrated a marked reduction in biliary sepsis but not a statistically significant improvement in morbidity or mortality. There is an identical trend in this paper and the study mentioned above [31], with one death in the early interventional group and five deaths in the standard management group of both studies (Tables 1 and 2). If one combines the information from the two studies (allowing that intervention was at a different time), the trend in mortality would certainly not discourage the early application of ERCP sphincterotomy, provided a skilled endoscopist was available (Table 3). The data from both Leicester in the United Kingdom and Hong Kong derive from controlled clinical studies [31,32••]. Nowak [33] from Katowice in Poland has a similar trend of re-

Table 3. Early sphincterotomy for gallstone acute pancreatitis*

Treatment	Patients, *n*	Complications, *n*	Deaths, *n(%)*
Early endoscopic sphincterotomy	89	16	2(2.1)
Conventional management	91	38	10(11.0)

**Data from* Neoptolemos *et al.* [31] and Fan *et al.* [32••].

sults with uncontrolled studies indicating both freedom from the risk of further attacks of acute pancreatitis and a lower mortality where early endoscopic sphinctero-tomy is used (Table 4). It is important to be aware that undue delay in attempting ERCP, especially in severe pancreatitis, may make it very difficult (or even impossible) to identify the ampulla because of the marked duodenal edema that develops.

In older patients, ERCP sphincterotomy may be sufficient therapy in itself and removal of gallbladder not considered an essential part of therapy, whereas in younger patients it is a safe and sensible procedure to proceed with laparoscopic cholecystectomy in the same admission, provided there is an awareness of the wider cystic duct that is likely to be encountered in such patients. Tate *et al.* [34•] found that laparoscopic cholecystectomy performed a median of 7 days after admission was successful in 21 of 24 patients, but that the operation was more difficult when compared with 40 controls. They used an operative difficulty score and showed that the major difficulty was in the dissection of Calot's triangle. A wide cystic duct is to be expected in such patients and this group found that metal clips were unsafe and so recommend externally tied ligature in continuity to secure the cystic duct. Their conclusion was that early surgery is safe but technical difficulty is increased. Soper *et al.* [35] also found laparoscopic cholecystectomy valuable early in the first admission of gallstone acute pancreatitis.

A new paper on the influence of native somatostatin in the evolution of acute pancreatitis suggests that 250 μg/h administered for only 48 hours had a beneficial effect on outcome in 100 patients randomly divided in a prospective controlled study [36]. The patients were evenly divided in terms of age, sex, etiology, and objective grading of severity, although only 22 of the 100 patients had severe disease. There was one death in each group but more operations and a longer hospital stay in the control group. In addition, there was some evidence from computed tomography scans favoring a milder evolution of disease in the patients treated with synthetic somatostatin. Earlier studies with native somatostatin have suggested a beneficial trend, but no more [37–39].

The synthetic analogue octreotide has also been utilized in the management of patients and in an uncontrolled study it was suggested that this was beneficial in a group of 19 sequential patients, few of whom had severe disease [40]. A randomized, prospective controlled clinical study by our own group assessing octreotide not only showed no benefit in terms of mortality, but a trend in favor of the control group for morbidity in 56 patients with moderate and severe acute pancreatitis was found [41]. The patients were given continuous octreotide (50 μg/h) and it had been our concept that octreotide might prove beneficial because of its stimulatory effect on the reticulo-endothelial system rather than its ability to close down pancreatic secretion. This did not prove to be the case and this is the largest clinical study excluding patients with mild disease in which octreotide has been assessed and found to be wanting.

Outcome of acute necrotizing pancreatitis

A group from Helsinki has analyzed the long-term results in patients surviving severe acute pancreatitis and found that they are generally good [42•]. A qualitative analysis was performed of the outcomes in a predominantly alcohol-related group of 37 survivors at average follow-up of over 6 years. A rating of "good general condition" was given for 30 of the 37 and 24 were working normally. More than half the patients were diabetic (predominantly insulin dependent). Although many had reduced their alcohol intake and 11 of 28 became abstinent, 10 were still considered to have a serious drinking problem. The overall assessment was that treatment of this group was worthwhile.

In an attempt to quantify the cost of the management of acute necrotizing pancreatitis, 10 consecutive patients admitted within 1 year to one hospital were studied [43]. The etiology was gallstones in seven and alcohol

Table 4. Effect of early endoscopic sphincterotomy on outcome of all grades of biliary acute pancreatitis*

Treatment	Patients, *n*	Recurrent acute pancreatitis, *n*	Deaths, *n(%)*
Endoscopic sphincterotomy within 24 hours	178	0	3(1.6)
Conventional management	102	16	13(12.7)

**Adapted from* Nowak [33]; with permission.

abuse in three. Only one patient died and there was an average hospital stay of 74 days, with a range of 40 to 150 days. Patients underwent an average of two operations and four endoscopic procedures. The cost of management was a little under $28,000 broken into 65% for hospitalization, 20% for operations and endoscopic procedures, and 16% for laboratory investigations. A cost-utility analysis demonstrated a mean benefit per patient of 8.55 quality-adjusted life years at a cost of approximately $3250 each. This is comparable to that for coronary artery bypass grafting and less than the cost of renal transplantation. The authors conclude that the management of pancreatitic necrosis is expensive but justified by the excellent outcome in terms of quality of life [43•].

In September 1992, Bradley and members of the Atlanta International Symposium [44••] convened to clarify some of the more confusing nomenclature of acute pancreatitis. A group of 40 specialists from different aspects of medicine and surgery, as well as a diversity of countries specifically advocated the use of the term "acute fluid collection" for fluid in and around the pancreas in the early part of the disease process. It took about 4 weeks from the onset of pancreatitis for the nonepithelialized wall of a pseudocyst to develop. These experts recommend the term "infected pseudocyst" be replaced by "abscess" and "pancreatic phlegmon" by "inflammatory mass." It was also felt that "hemorrhagic pancreatitis" and "persistent acute pancreatitis" should be dropped from the current nomenclature as they also tended to cause confusion. The definitions described in the Atlanta classification are not mutually exclusive and the individual patient may develop complications of acute pancreatitis that fulfill two or more diagnostic criteria. The group endeavored to clarify nomenclature and to encourage careful description of disease, particularly in the area of severe acute pancreatitis and its complications [44••]. A book of the conclusions of the conference and various contributions from the participants have also been published [45••].

Finally, there have been an increasing number of drugs suspected of causing acute pancreatitis. This is again based on single case reports of reexposure to certain drugs resulting in further pancreatitis. Naproxen and diclofenac have been implicated [46,47]. There are also further reports of Didanosine either exacerbating or causing pancreatitis in patients with AIDS [48,49].

References and recommended reading

Papers of particular interest, published within the annual period of review, have been highlighted as:

- • Of special interest
- •• Of outstanding interest

1. • Konturek SJ, Szlachcic A, Dembinski A, Warzecha Z, Jaworek J, Stachura J: **Nitric Oxide in Pancreatitic Secretion and Hormone-Induced Pancreatitis in Rats.** *Int J Pancreatol* 1994, **15**:19–28.

The authors suggest that nitric oxide has a beneficial effect on the course of acute pancreatitis in this experimental model, mainly by improving pancreatic blood flow.

2. • Garcia-Montero AC, Manso MA, Rodriquez AI, De Dois I: **Therapeutic and Protective Effect of Subcutaneous Injections of L-364, 718 on Caerulein-Induced Acute Pancreatitis.** *Pancreas* 1994, 9:209–315.

Blockade of cholecystokin receptor sites had a beneficial effect on the course of pancreatitis in this experimental model.

3. • Kiriyama M, Izumi R, Miyazaki I: **Protective Effect of AA-861 (5-Lipoxygenase Inhibitor) on Experimental Acute Necrotizing Pancreatitis in Rats.** *Int J Pancreatol* 1993, **13**:201–208.

Inhibition of lipoxygenase had a beneficial effect on this taurocholate induced form of acute pancreatitis.

4. • Sameshima H, Ikei S, Mori K, Yamaguchi Y, Egami H, Misumi M, Moriyasu M, Ogawa M: **The Role of Tumor Necrosis Factor-α in the Aggravation of Cerulein-Induced Pancreatitis in Rats.** *Int J Pancreatol* 1993, **14**:107–115.

Peritoneal macrophages in rats with pancreatitis produced much more TNF than control animals.

5. Grewal HP, Koth M, El Din AM, Ohman M, Salem A, Gaber L, Gaber AO: **Induction of Tumor Necrosis Factor in Severe Acute Pancreatitis and Its Subsequent Reduction After Hepatic Passage.** *Surgery* 1994, 115:213–221.

6. Grewal HP, El Din AM, Gaber L, Kotb M, Gaber AO: **Amelioration of Physiologic and Biochemical Changes in Acute Pancreatitis Using an Anti-TNF-αPolyclonal Antibody.** *Am J Surg* 1994, 167:214–219.

7. •• Zhou W, Levine B, Olson M: **Platelet-Activating Factor: A Mediator of Pancreatitc Inflammation During Cerulein Hyperstimulation.** *Am J Pathol* 1993, **142**:1504–1511.

An excellent piece of experimental work showing that PAF functions as a mediator of pancreatitis.

8. Sirois MG, Jancar S, Braquet P, Plante GE, Sirois P: **PAF Increase Vascular Permeability in Selected Tissues: Effect of BN52021 and L-656.240.** *Prostaglandins* 1988, **36**:631–644.

9. Emanuelli G, Montrucchio G, Gaia E, Corvettii G, Gubatta L: **Experimental Acute Pancreatitis Induced by Platelet-Activating Factor in Rabbits.** *Am J Pathol* 1989, **134**:315–326.

10. Jancar S, Ciaccobi GD, Mariano M, Mencia-Huerta JM, Sirios P, Bracque P: **Immune Complex-Induced Pancreatitis: Effect on BN52021, a Selective Antagonist of Platelet-Activating Factor.** *Prostaglandins* 1988, 35:757–770.

11. Dabrowski A, Gabryelewicz A, Chyczewski L: **The Effects of Platelet Activating Factor Antagonist (BN52021) on Cerulein-Induced Acute Pancreatitis With Reference to Oxygen Radicals.** *Int J Pancreatol* 1991, 8:1–11.

12. Zhou W, McCollum MO, Levine BA, Olson MS: **Role of Platelet-Activating Factor in Pancreatitis-Associated Acute Lung Injury in the Rat.** *Am J Pathol* 1992, 140:971–979.

13. Lopez-Farre GAA, Gomez-Garre DN, Novo C, Romeo JM, Braquet P, Lopez-Novoa JM: **Role of Platelet-Activating Factor in Hemodynamic Derangements in an Acute Pancreatic Model.** *Gastroenterology* 1992, 102:181–187.

14. •• Gumaste VV, Roditis N, Mehta D, Dave PB: **Serum Lipase Levels in Non Pancreatic Abdominal Pain Versus Acute Pancreatitis.** *Am J Gastroenterol* 1993, **88**:2051–2055.

A strong case case is made for a change from routine blood amylase measurements to blood lipase because of the greater accuracy of this technique. It will be a bold move to change over for any hospital, but the evidence is very persuasive that the change should be made.

15. •• Funnell IC, Bornman PC, Weakley SP, Terblance J, Marks IN: **Obesity: An Important Prognostic Factor in Acute Pancreatitis.** *Br J Surg* 1993, **80**:484–486.

A simple, but good case, is made that measurement of body mass index is a very valuable prognostic factor in acute pancreatitis. Patients with more than 30 kg/m^2 fared badly and had many infective complications.

16. • Fan ST, Lai E, Mok F: **Prediction of the Severity of Acute Pancreatitis.** *Am J Surg* 1993, **166**:262–269.

These Hong Kong authors suggest that the simple measurement of either a blood urea greater than 7.4 mmol/L or a blood glucose greater than 11.0 mmol/L gives useful discrimination between mild and severe pancreatitis.

17. • Heath DI, Imrie CW: **The Hong Kong Criteria and Severity Prediction in Acute Pancreatitis.** *Int J Pancreatol* 1994, **15**:1–7.

These authors would refute the suggestion made in the previous reference that such a simple measurement of severity is accurate.

18. • Malfertheiner P, Dominguez-Munoz JE: **Prognostic Factors in Acute Pancreatitis.** *Int J Pancreatol* 1993, **14**:1–8.

A good review of the debate of prognostic factors in acute pancreatitis.

19. Dominguez-Munoz JE, Carballo F, Garcia MJ, De Diego JM, Rabago L, Simon MA, De la Morena J: **Clinical Usefulness of Polymorphononuclear Elastase in Predicting the Severity of Acute Pancreatitis: Results of a Multicentre Study.** *Br J Surg* 1991, **78**:1230–1234.

20. Uhl W, Buchler M, Malfertheiner P, Martina M, Beger HG: **PMN-Elastase in Comparison With CRP, Antiproteases, and LDH as Indicators of Necrosis in Human Acute Pancreatitis.** *Pancreas* 1991, 6:253–259.

21. Gross V, Scholmerich J, Leser HG, Salm R, Lensen M, Ruckaur K, Schoffel J, Lay L, Heinisch A, Farthmann EH, Gerok G: **Granulocyte Elastase in Assessment of Severity of Acute Pancreatitis. Comparison With Acute Phase Proteins C-Reactive Protein, ox2-Macroglobulin**, *Dig Dis Sci* 1990, **35**:97–105.

22. Viedma JA, Perez-Mateo M, Dominguez JE, Carballo F: **Role of Interleukin-6 in Acute Pancreatitis. Comparison With C-Reactive Protein and Phospholipase A.** *Gut* 1992, **33**:1264–1267.

23. Cruickshank A, Heath DI, Gudgeon M, Jehanli A, Shenkin A, Imrie CW: **Role of Interleukin-6 in Mediating the Acute Phase Protein Response and Potential as an Early Means of Severity Assessment in Acute Pancreatitis.** *Gut* 1993, **34**:41–45.

24. •• Windsor JA, Fearon KCH, Ross JA, Barclay GR, Smith E, Poxton I, Garden OJ, Carter DC: **Role of Serum Endotoxin and Anti-endotoxin Core Antibody Levels in Predicting the Development of Multiple Organ Failure in Acute Pancreatitis.** *Br J Surg* 1993, **80**:1042–1046.

A good piece of work not only showing endotoxaemia but significant falls in entogenous IgG antibody levels coinciding with arising acute physiology score in patients with severe acute pancreatitis.

25. Dominquez-Munoz JE, Carballo F, Garcia MJ, de Diego JM, Campos R, Yanguela J, de la Moreña J: **Evaluation of the Clinical Usefulness of APACHE II and SAPS Systems in the Initial Prognostic Classification of Acute Pancreatitis: A Multicenter Study.** *Pancreas* 1993, **8**:682–686.

26. Larvin M, McMahon MJ: **APACHE II Score for Assessment and Monitoring of Acute Pancreatitis.** *Lancet* 1989, **ii**:201–215.

27. Osborne DH, Imrie CW, Carter DC: **Biliary Surgery in the Same Admission for Gallstone-Associated Acute Pancreatitis.** *Br J Surg* 1981, **68**:758–761.

28. Bardaji M, Cugat E, Almenara R, Pierres M, Marco C: **Prediction of Outcome in Acute Pancreatitis: Three Multifactorial Scoring Systems and C-Reactive Protein.** *Inaugural World Congress of the International Hepato-Pancreatobiliary Association, Boston, 1994.*

29. • Scott P, Bruce C, Shofield D, Shiel N, Braganza JM, McCloy RF: **Vitamin C Status in Patients With Acute Pancreatitis.** *Br J Surg* 1993, **80**:740–754.

This study of vitamin C levels in patients with acute pancreatitis suggests there may be a specific depletion of this antioxident in acute pancreatitis that could even precede the onset of disease.

30. Suzuki H, Suematsu M, Miura S, Asako H, Kurose I, Ishii H, Houzawa S, Tsuchiya M: **Xanthine Oxidase-Mediated Intracellular Oxidative Stress in Response to Cerulein in Rat Pancreatic Acinar Cells.** *Pancreas* 1993, **8**:465–470.

31. Neoptolemos JP, Carr-Locke DL, London NJM: **Controlled Trial of Urgent ERCP and Endoscopic Sphincterotomy Versus Conservative Treatment for Acute Pancreatitis Due to Gallstones.** *Lancet* 1988, **ii**:989–983.

32. •• Fan ST, Lai Mok FPT, Lo C-M, Zheng S-S, Wong J: **Early Treatment of Acute Biliary Pancreatitis by Encoscopic Papillotomy.** *N Engl J Med* 1993, **328**:228–232.

In a randomized controlled trial involving 195 patients (most of whom had acute gallstone pancreatitis), ERCP with papillotomy, if indicated, performed within 24 hours of admission markedly reduced the frequency of biliary sepsis. However, there was no statistically significant improvement in survival or reduction in the number of local or systemic complications of pancreatitis.

33. Nowak A: **Results of Early Sphincterotomy in Gallstone Acute Pancreatitis.** *European Congress of Gastroenterology, Barcelona 1993.*

34. • Tate JJT, Lau WY, Li AKC: **Laparoscopic Cholecystectomy for Biliary Pancreatitis.** *Br J Surg* 1994, **81**:720–722.

Effective laparoscopic cholecystectomy in biliary pancreatitis in the same admission, but a warning as to greater care being required to deal with the larger than normal cystic duct.

35. Soper NJ, Brunt LM, Callery MP, Edmundowiez SA, Aliperti G: **Role of Laparoscopic Cholecystectomy in the Management of Acute Gallstone Pancreatitis.** *Am J Surg* 1994, **167**:42–51.

36. Luengo L, Vicente C, Gris F, Coronas JM, Escuder J, Gomez JR, Castellote JM: **Influence of Somatostatin in the Evolution of Acute Pancreatitis. A Prospective Randomized Study.** *Int J Pancreatol* 1994, **15**:139–144.

37. Usadel KH, Uberla KK, Leuschner U: **Treatment of Acute Pancreatitis With Somatostatin. Results of the Multicenter Double-Blind Trial (APTS Study) [Abstract].** *Dig Dis Sci* 1985, **30**:992.

38. Choi TK, Mok F, Zhian WH, Fan ST, Lai ECS: **Somastattin in the Treatment of Acute Pancreatitis: A Prospective Randomized Controlled Trial.** *Gut* 1989, **30**:223–237.

39. D'Amico D, Favia G, Biasiato R, Casaccia M, Falcome F, Fersini M, Marrano D, Napolitano F, Oliveriero S, Rodolico A: **The Use of Somatostatin in Acute Pancreatitis: Results of a Multicenter Trial.** *Hepatogastroenterology* 1990, **37**:92–98.

40. Beechey-Newman N: **Controlled Trial of High-Dose Octreotide in Treatment of Acute Pancreatitis. Evidence of Improvement in Disease Severity.** *Dig Dis Sci* 1993, **38**:644–647.

41. McKay C, Baxter JN, Imrie CW: **Randomised, Controlled Trial of Octreotide in Prognostically Severe Acute Pancreatitis.** *Inaugural World Congress of Internation Hepato-Biliary Association, Boston.*

42. • Doepel M, Eriksson J, Halme L, Kumpulainen T, Hockerstedt K: **Good Long-Term Results in Patients Surviving Severe Acute Pancreatitis.** *Br J Surg* 1993, **80**:1583–1586.

This is an unusual late review of patients surviving severe acute pancreatitis patients. On the whole they do well.

43. • Fenton-Lee D, Imrie CW: **Pancreatic Necrosis: Assessment of Outcome Related to Quality of Life and Cost of Management.** *Br J Surg* 1993, **80**:1579–1582.

This careful assessment of 10 consecutive patients with severe acute necrotising pancreatitis who came to surgery analyzes the total cost of management of each patient at 1991/1992 prices.

44. •• Bradley EL and Members of the Atlanta Internationl Symposium: **A Clinically Based Classification System for Acute Pancreatitis.** *Arch Surg* 1993, **128**:586–590.

An important attempt to simplify and make more accurate the nomenclature used in the description of patients with acute pancreatitis and complications of the disease.

45. •• Bradley EL: *Acute Pancreatitis, Diagnosis and Therapy*. New York: Raven Press; 1993.

This is the book based on the symposium reported in *Arch Surg* 1993, 128:586–590.

46. Duville L, Debeuckelcre S, Reynaert H, Devis G: **Pancreatitis Associated With Naproxen.** *Am J Gastroenterol* 1993, **88**:464.

47. Khan IH, Edward N: **Pancreatitis Associated With Diclofenac.** *Postgrad Med J* 1993, **69**:486–487.

48. Daniels M: **Pancreatitis in AIDS Patients Treated With Didanosine.** *Am J Gastroenterol* 1993, **88**:459–460.

49. Greenfield SM, Maxson C: **Pancreatitis in AIDS Patients Treated With Didanosine: Response.** *Am J Gastroenterol* 1993, **3**:460.

C.W. Imrie, FRCS, Department of Surgery, Glasgow Royal Infirmary, Glasgow, Scotland, UK.

Chronic pancreatitis

Murray Korc, MD, and Wolff Schmiegel, MD

University of California, Irvine, California, USA, and Ruhr University, Bochum, Germany

The clinical manifestations of chronic pancreatitis may be quite varied, ranging from a debilitating disease associated with excruciating pain and pancreatic exocrine and endocrine insufficiencies, to a relatively indolent course with intermittent episodes of abdominal discomfort. In the Western world, the majority of cases are due to chronic and excessive alcohol ingestion and to idiopathic forms of the disease. Additional causes may include trauma, hypercalcemia, cholelithiasis, pancreatic duct obstruction, hypertriglyceridemia, cystic fibrosis, hereditary factors, and congenital abnormalities. In some parts of the world, poorly understood nutritional dysfunctions contribute to a form of chronic pancreatitis in which pancreatic calcifications predominate. This review focuses on the natural history of chronic pancreatitis, an update on treatment modalities, new insights on the molecular alterations that occur in this condition, and the potential relationship between chronic pancreatitis and pancreatic cancer.

Current Opinion in Gastroenterology 1994, **10**:502–506

Pathophysiology

The molecular mechanisms that lead to the histological changes that occur in the pancreas in chronic pancreatitis are not known. A number of hypotheses have been suggested, including 1) decreased production of functional lithostathine in conjunction with increased production of an abnormal lithostathine that is incapable of inhibiting pancreatic stone formation; 2) accumulation of focal areas of necrosis, inflammation, and fibrosis as a result of recurrent episodes of acute pancreatitis; 3) failure of the pancreas to handle an excess of oxygen radicals; and 4) direct toxic effects of ethanol [1].

In all these models, inflammatory cell infiltrates may contribute to the fibrosis through the production of cytokines that recruit fibroblasts and enhance their intrapancreatic proliferation. However, the pancreas of transgenic mice that overexpress transforming growth factor (TGF)-α, a polypeptide that binds and activates the epidermal growth factor receptor, also exhibits extensive interstitial fibrosis in spite of the absence of inflammatory cells [2]. Thus, growth factors that are not classic cytokines can also contribute to pancreatic fibrosis. Bockman and Merlino [2] found that there is also aberrant presence of amylase and zymogen granules in the duct-like cells of TGF-α transgenes. They suggested that these duct-like cells may arise from redifferentiated acinar cells.

Wang *et al.* [3••] studied the effects of coexpression of human TGF-α and human gastrin in the pancreas of transgenic mice. In the TGF-α transgenes, there was a 10-fold increase in ductal cell mass, whereas the transgenes expressing gastrin did not exhibit altered pancreatic morphology. The double transgenes expressing both TGF-α and gastrin had a relatively normal pancreatic histology and a marked decrease in ductal cell mass, suggesting that differentiation signals initiated by gastrin in the double transgene model may abrogate the pathways activated by TGF-α.

The hypothesis that growth factors may play a role in the pathophysiology of chronic pancreatitis in humans was reinforced by a study by Friess *et al.* [4••], who reported that acidic and basic fibroblast growth factors are overexpressed in pancreatic ductal and acinar cells in chronic pancreatitis. Both growth factors are mitogenic and chemotactic towards fibroblasts, and have the potential to exert autocrine and paracrine effects in the pancreas. However, the mechanisms of their overexpression and their exact role in the pathobiology of chronic pancreatitis are yet to be determined.

Clinical course

Chronic pancreatitis is characterized by progressive destruction of the pancreatic parenchyma affecting the exocrine and endocrine components of the pancreas. This results in varying combinations of exocrine and endocrine insufficiency, abdominal pain, and a complex natural history [1]. Lankisch *et al.* [5••] reported on their experience with 335 patients having chronic pancreatitis. The 260 men and 75 women in this cohort were followed for a mean period of 11.3 years. The diagnosis was established on clinical grounds, with

Abbreviations

EPS—endoscopic pancreatic sphincterotomy; **ERCP**—endoscopic retrograde cholangiopancreatography; **ESWL**—extracorporeal shock-wave lithotripsy; **MPD**—main pancreatic duct; **TGF**—transforming growth factor.

 ISBN 1-85922-610-8 ISSN 0267–1379

at least one abnormal secretin-pancreozymin test in conjunction with fecal fat analysis, radiologic and ultrasound studies, and, in some cases, endoscopic retrograde cholangiopancreatography (ERCP). Most patients either abused alcohol (69%) or had idiopathic pancreatis (28%). Only 24 patients (7%) were pain-free throughout the study. At study's end, 202 (65%) of the other 311 patients still had episodes of pain. This group included 90 patients who underwent surgery for pancreatic pseudocysts or for pain relief. Thus, the majority of patients did not become pain-free. However, 47% of 152 patients who were followed for more than 10 years stopped having pain.

Only 66 (31%) of the patients who were classified as having painful alcohol-induced chronic pancreatitis were able to stop drinking alcohol, and 52% of these patients became pain-free [5••]. In contrast, 37% of the patients who did not abstain from alcohol became pain-free. The beneficial effects of alcohol abstinence on pain relief just failed achieving statistical significance, and there was no correlation between continued alcohol use and the incidence of pancreatic exocrine insufficiency. In contrast, discontinuing the use of alcohol led to a significant decrease in the incidence of diabetes mellitus. This study underscores the difficulty in coming to definitive conclusions about pain outcome in patients with established chronic pancreatitis. Such management difficulties are further compounded by the absence of specific tests to help distinguish between an initial episode of acute pancreatitis and the early stages of chronic pancreatitis presenting as an acute episode.

The high frequency of diabetes mellitus in the above study is consistent with previous findings. The etiology of this "pancreatic" diabetes has been attributed to the intense desmoplastic reaction and subsequent damage and destruction of pancreatic islets. However, it has also been suggested that some of these patients may have insulin resistance. To address this question, Cavallini *et al.* [6•] studied 66 patients with alcohol-induced chronic pancreatitis. Of the 66 patients, 29 had normal glucose tolerance, 12 had abnormal glucose tolerance, and 25 had overt diabetes requiring either insulin (n=9) or oral hypoglycemic agents (n=16). Only the patients with overt diabetes exhibited impaired insulin secretory dynamics, determined by measuring C-peptide secretion in response to glucagon. Insulin responsiveness, assessed by measuring glucose disposal rates following the intravenous administration of insulin, was impaired in all 66 patients by comparison with values obtained in 19 control subjects. Thus, chronic pancreatitis patients with overt diabetes may often have a dual defect consisting of diminished insulin secretory capacity in the face of peripheral resistance to insulin action.

Treatment modalities

Pancreatic enzymes

Pain in chronic pancreatitis may be related to elevated pancreatic tissue pressures and activation of secretory pathways. Theoretically, the intraluminal delivery of pancreatic proteases would act via a negative feedback loop to reduce cholecystokinin or cholinergic-mediated pancreatic secretion, thereby decreasing pain [1]. In a prospective placebo-controlled, double-blind multicenter study, Mossner *et al.* [7] examined the effects of digestive enzyme therapy in 47 patients with chronic pain and chronic pancreatitis. Patients were treated with acid-protected microtablets. The total daily dose of pancreatic proteases was 10,000 Pharmacopeia europaea units, administered for 2 weeks followed by placebo, or vice versa. No significant beneficial effect was observed. Nonetheless, it is generally accepted that a trial with pancreatic enzymes is justified because it improves the patient's nutritional status and ameliorates the steatorrhea.

Octreotide

The long-acting somatostatin analogue octreotide has increasingly found its way into clinical applications in gastroenterologic diseases [8•]. Its value in the treatment of pancreatic ascites and external pancreatic fistulas, leading to a more rapid recovery, has been confirmed in recent studies [9]. Progress has also been made in understanding the mechanisms of action of somatostatin in pancreatic cells, which directly inhibit secretion of pancreatic acinar cells by preventing secretin-induced cyclic AMP production *in vitro* [10]. Thus, somatostatin analogues may complement the effects of pancreatic enzyme supplementation in the treatment of chronic pancreatic pain by further suppressing pancreatic secretion.

Endoscopic treatment

There has been considerable progress in the use of endoscopic procedures in the diagnosis and management of patients with chronic pancreatitis. ERCP is extremely helpful in the diagnosis of chronic pancreatitis, and is a mandatory first step when endoscopic pancreatic sphincterotomy (EPS) is used to remove pancreatic calculi or protein plugs. When EPS can be performed, it can result in at least partial pain relief [11]. Recurrence of duct obstruction following EPS can also be treated endoscopically. Extracorporeal shock-wave lithotripsy (ESWL), performed in conjunction with endoscopic insertion of a pancreatic stent, has been used successfully to fragment pancreatic stones and to facilitate the deep cannulation of the main pancreatic duct (MPD) [12]. The authors treated 123 patients with ESWL, and noted a decrease in MPD diameter in 90% of the cases. However, complete clearance of the MPD was achieved in only 59% of the patients. Persistent pain relief was obtained in 45 patients during a mean follow-up of 14 months, whereas patients without a decrease in MPD diameter suffered recurrent attacks of pain. In some cases, there was progressive stricture formation and pancreatic stent obstruction or dislodgment. Clinically, 62% of the patients gained weight. Exocrine function was rarely documented, but steatorrhea was observed in 12 out of 22 tested patients and decreased in six patients, 1 year after treatment. Improvement of endocrine function was only observed in four of 41 patients. The authors concluded that endoscopic management, associated with ESWL, yielded results comparable to surgery. Moreover, endoscopic maneuvers can be repeated, are less invasive than surgery, and may be accompanied by a lower mortality rate.

Surgery

It has been proposed that operative drainage of the pancreatic duct may relieve pancreatic duct pressure, improve pancreatic function, and alleviate symptoms in many patients with chronic pancreatitis. To assess the effects of MPD decompression on pancreatic function, Nealon and Thompson [13••] carried out a comprehensive study prospectively in 143 patients. Severity of disease was determined by evaluating pancreatic morphology by ERCP, pancreatic exocrine function with a 72-hour fecal fat measurement and the bentiromide-*p*-aminobenzoic acid test performed in conjunction with a D-xylose test, and endocrine function with an oral glucose tolerance test and lipomul meal–stimulated release of pancreatic polypeptide. Interestingly, 41 patients required insulin for diabetes control. The presence of severe abdominal pain was an absolute requirement for surgery in the nonrandomized portion of the study.

Eighty-three of 143 patients had mild-to-moderate disease at initial evaluation, and 47 of these patients underwent MPD decompression by a longitudinal side-to-side Roux-en-Y pancreaticojejunostomy. In this group, 41 patients (87%) did not progress towards severe disease. An additional 40 patients with severe disease also underwent this surgical procedure. No patient in either the operated or nonoperated group who initially had severe chronic pancreatitis improved sufficiently to be reclassified into the mild-to-moderate group. However, regardless of the original grade, 74 of 87 (85%) patients operated on compared with one of 56 nonoperated patients experienced pain relief, which occurred in 58 patients with dilated MPD and elevated MPD pressure. In contrast, nine patients with normal pressure did not profit from decompression. Only 17 patients with mild-to-moderate disease were randomly assigned to a surgical and nonsurgical group. Seven of nine patients receiving an operation, and two of eight nonoperated patients remained in this category during the follow-up period. These observations support the hypothesis that elevated tissue pressure contributes to the pain in this disorder, and that early operative drainage performed before the appearance of irreversible functional impairment may be beneficial in patients with chronic pancreatitis.

Complications

Pancreatic pseudocysts occur with an incidence of 20% to 40% in chronic pancreatitis, accounting for many complications, including infection, obstruction of the pancreatic or bile duct, hemorrhage, and cyst rupture. Barthet *et al.* [14] reported their experiences based on a retrospective study of 143 patients with 170 cysts or pseudocysts. They compared conservative treatment with percutaneous puncture or drainage, endoscopic cystoenterostomy or transpapillary cyst drainage, and surgery. In the absence of marked MPD dilatation, pseudocysts spontaneously disappeared in 7.7% when they were small (average diameter of 28.6 mm), even when they communicated with the pancreatic duct system (60%). About one third of patients who underwent percutaneous puncture did not require further treatment. As expected, the recurrence rate was high (57%) and seemed to be accompanied by a communication of the cyst with the MPD. A total of 71% of patients were initially treated by endoscopic cystoenterostomy; 55% of these patients did not require further treatment and overall 72% were healed after an additional endoscopic procedure.

Grace and Williamson [15••] reported that acute pseudocysts were more often small and tended to resolve spontaneously, whereas chronic ones did not resolve. Instead, the chronic pseudocysts tended to grow above 6 cm in diameter, causing serious complications. Therefore, these pseudocysts should be treated as soon as possible. Smaller asymptomatic chronic pseudocysts could be kept under observation. However, endoscopic drainage of chronic pseudocysts impinging the gastric or duodenal wall is a challenging procedure for securing permanent internal drainage, especially in high-risk patients. Furthermore, it is still associated with a troublesome rate of complications, including death.

As there are no reliable clinical and radiological criteria to ensure the benign origin of pancreatic pseudocysts, the cyst fluid should be carefully analyzed. Even biopsy specimens can fail to identify malignant cysts that mimic benign pseudocysts. Lewandrowski *et al.* [16•] outlined preoperative diagnostic indices to assist in the decision regarding therapy in pseudocysts, serous cystadenomas, mucinous cystadenomas and carcinomas, and mucinous ductal adenocarcinomas. Carcinoembryonic antigen levels were high in all benign and malignant mucinous cysts, but were low in pseudocysts and benign serous cystadenomas, allowing for the differentiation between mucinous and nonmucinous cysts. Elevated CA 125 values suggest malignant cysts whereas CA 19-9 levels were nondiscriminatory. The combination of viscosity, carcinoembryonic antigen, CA 125, and cytology helps distinguish malignant cystic tumors and premalignant mucinous cystic neoplasms from pseudocysts and serous cystadenomas.

Chronic pancreatitis and pancreatic cancer

The association between chronic pancreatitis and pancreatic cancer has been controversial, with the exception of the relatively rare condition of familial relapsing pancreatitis [1]. Nonetheless, there have been persistent reports linking chronic pancreatitis to an increased incidence of pancreatic cancer. To more firmly define this relationship, Lowenfels *et al.* [17••] conducted a multicenter cohort study of 2015 subjects with chronic pancreatitis who were recruited after 1946 from five European countries and the United States. A total of 56 patients were identified as having pancreatic cancer during a mean follow-up of 7.4±6.2 years. Assuming a possible misinterpretation at initial diagnosis, 29 patients with proven cancer discovered during the first 2 years of follow-up were excluded. This reduced the standardized incidence ratio from 26.3 to 16.5. There was an additional slight decrease in the standardized incidence ratio to 14.4 after the exclusion period was extended to the first 5 years of follow-up. Because it could be argued that the initial diagnosis of chronic pancreatitis is delayed by the late appearance of abdominal pain or is established only after the development of cancer-associated pain, this exclusion may underestimate the incidence of pancreatic cancer in chronic pancreatitis. Conversely, it is possible that the incidence of pancreatic cancer was spuriously elevated as a result of two factors. First, a selection bias may have occurred as a result of the inclusion of patients who developed pain from an occult pancreatic cancer. Similarly, patients with moderate chronic pancreatitis may lack symptoms that require hospitalization, resulting in a gross underestimation of the prevalence of chronic pancreatitis in the general population.

In response to the above criticism, Lowenfels [18] stated that the risk for pancreatic cancer among patients with chronic pancreatitis was nearly identical in subjects declared as having incident or prevalent disease with respect to the active recruitment period. Nonetheless, because recruitment of study patients dates back to 1946, only 27% and 12% of the patients underwent ERCP and computer tomography, respectively [17••], raising the possibility of a misdiagnosis. Because the incidence of chronic pancreatitis in the general population is probably underestimated, the incidence ratio has to be divided by an unknown factor and has to be corrected for the assumption that patients with low risk could be lost during follow-up. This kind of arithmetic would lead to a further decrease in the incidence ratio.

Carcinogenesis is a multistage process that involves numerous genetic and cellular alterations, including oncogene activation, loss of tumor suppressor gene function, and receptor-ligand overexpression. Therefore, to illuminate the evolution of pancreatic cancer it is necessary to investigate the prevalence of these alterations in premalignant tissues. The development of pancreatic cancer in humans is associated with a comparatively high rate (75% to 90%) of c-Ki-*ras* oncogene mutations. It has been suggested that these mutations are highly sensitive and specific for malignancy in the pancreas. However, Yanagisawa *et al.* [19••] studied a total of 16 mucous cell hyperplasias and 13 flat ordinary mucosa samples in 11 pancreatic tissues, resected for chronic pancreatitis. They pointed out that 62.5% of benign mucous hyperplasia lesions in the pancreas also displayed c-Ki-*ras* oncogene mutations. These results suggest c-Ki-*ras* activation may be an event occurring at an early stage in pancreatic carcinogenesis. Urban *et al.* [20•] detected c-Ki-*ras* in 11 of 12 percutaneous fine-needle aspiration of patients with proven pancreatic carcinomas. Two patients with definitive diagnosis of adenocarcinoma had samples of chronic pancreatitis without malignant cells, but harbored c-Ki-*ras* oncogene mutations. Again, this suggests that chronic pancreatitis leads to an increased susceptibility for pancreatic cancer. Conversely, mutations in the *p53* tumor suppressor gene are relatively common in pancreatic cancer but are absent in chronic pancreatitis [21•]. These types of studies should prove useful in elucidating the mechanisms that contribute to the increased risk of pancreatic cancer in chronic pancreatitis.

Acknowledgments

The authors wish to thank Jan Schmielau for his assistance.

References and recommended reading

Papers of particular interest, published within the annual period of review, have been highlighted as:

• Of special interest
•• Of outstanding interest

1. DiMagno EP, Layer P, Clain JE: **Chronic Pancreatitis.** In *The Pancreas, Pathology, and Disease*. Edited by Go VLW. New York:Raven Press; 1993:665–706.

2. Bockman DE, Merlino G: **Cytological Changes in the Pancreas of Transgenic Mice Overexpressing Transforming Growth Factor a.** *Gastroenterology* 1992, **103**:1883–1892.

3. •• Wang TC, Bonner-Weir S, Oates PS, Chulak M, Simon B, Merlino GT, Schmidt EV, Brand SJ: **Pancreatic Gastrin Stimulates Islet Differentiation of TGF α-Induced Ductular Precursor Cells.** *J Clin Invest* 1993, 1349–1356.

Molecular evidence in transgenic mice suggests that excessive production of TGF-α in the pancreas can cause pancreatic fibrosis, and that gastrin expression in the islets reverses this effect.

4. •• Friess H, Yamanaka Y, Buchler M, Beger HG, Do DA, Kobrin MS, Korc M: **Increased Expression of Acidic and Basic Fibroblast Growth Factors in Chronic Pancreatitis.** *Am J Pathol* 1994, **144**:117–128.

This study relies on immunohistochemical and molecular techniques to demonstrate that fibroblast growth factors are expressed at high levels in acinar and ductal cells in chronic pancreatitis.

5. •• Lankisch PG, Lohr-Happe A, Otto J, Creutzfeld W: **Natural Course in Chronic Pancreatitis.** *Digestion* 1993, **54**:145–155.

This paper details the frustrating outcome concerning the long-term results in the treatment of chronic pancreatitis, especially for the leading symptom—pain.

6. • Cavallini G, Vaona B, Bovo P, Cigolini M, Rigo L, Rossi F, Tasini E, Brunori MP, DiFrancesco V, Frulloni L: **Diabetes in Chronic Alcoholic Pancreatitis: Role of Residual Beta Cell Function and Insulin Resistance.** *Dig Dis Sci* 1993, **38**:497–501.

This interesting study emphasizes that many patients with chronic pancreatitis exhibit insulin resistance.

7. Mossner J, Secknus R, Meyer J, Niederau C, Adler G: **Treatment of Pain With Pancreatic Extracts in Chronic Pancreatitis: Results of a Prospective Placebo-Controlled Multicenter Trial.** *Digestion* 1992, **53**:54–66.

8. • Burroughs AK, Malagelada R: **Potential Indications for Octreotide in Gastroenterology: Summary of Workshop.** *Digestion* 1993, **54**:59–67.

A good review on the spreading indications for octreotide in gastroenterologic diseases.

9. Segal I, Parekh D, Lipschitz J, Gecelter G, Myburgh JA: **Treatment of Pancreatic Ascites and External Pancreatic Fistulas With Long-Acting Somatostatin Analogue (Sandostatin).** *Digestion* 1993, **54**:53–58.

10. Matsushita K, Okabayashi Y, Hasegawa H, Koide M, Kido Y, Okutani T, Sugimoto Y, Kasuga M: **In Vitro Inhibitory Effect of Somatostatin Action in Exocrine Pancreas of Rats.** *Gastroenterology* 1993, **104**:1146–1152.

11. Linder S, Engstrom C-F, Rosen AV, Wiechel K-L: **Endoscopic Clearance of the Pancreatic Duct in Chronic Pancreatitis With Severe Pain.** *Surg Endosc* 1993, 7:37–41.

12. Delhaye M, Vandermeeren A, Baize M, Cremer M: **Extracorporeal Shock-Wave Lithotripsy of Pancreatic Calculi.** *Gastroenterology* 1992, **102**:610–620.

13. Nealon WH, Thompson JC: **Progressive Loss of Pancreatic Function in Chronic Pancreatitis Is Delayed by Main Pancreatic Duct Decompression: A Longitudinal Prospective Analysis of the Modified Puestow Procedure.** *Ann Surg* 1993, **217**:458–468.
••
This elegantly conducted study provides convincing arguments for early operative intervention based on the assumption that increased main pancreatic duct pressures are responsible for both the pain and progression of the functional impairment.

14. Barthet M, Bugallo M, Moreira LS, Bastid C: **Management of Cyst and Pseudocysts Complicating Chronic Pancreatitis.** *Gastroenterol Clin Biol* 1993, **17**:270–276.

15. Grace PA, Williamson RCN: **Modern Management of Pancreatic Pseudocysts.** *Br J Surg* 1993, **80**:573–581.
••
This complete overview includes an algorithm for the management of patients with pancreatic pseudocysts and presentation of representative cases.

16. Lewandrowski KB, Southern JF, Pins MR, Compton CC, Warshaw AL: **Cyst Fluid Analysis in the Differential Diagnosis of Pancreatic Cysts: A Comparison of Pseudocysts, Serous Cystadenomas, Mucinous Cystic Neoplasm, and Mucinous Cystadenocarcinoma.** *Ann Surg* 1993, **217**:41–47.
•
This excellent study suggests a role for the use of the tumor markers carcinoemgbryonic antigen, CA 125 and CA 19-9 in the differential diagnosis of potentially malignant pancreatic cysts.

17. Lowenfels AB, Maisonneuve P, Cavallini G, Amman RW, Lankisch PG, Andersen JR, DiMagno EP, Andren-Sandberg A, Domellof L: **International Pancreatitis Study Group: Pancreatitis and the Risk of Pancreatic Cancer.** *N Engl J Med* 1993, **328**:1433–1437.
••
This large, retrospective cohort study supports the concept of an increased risk for malignant transformation in chronic inflammation of the pancreas.

18. Lowenfels AB: **Correspondence: Pancreatitis and the Risk of Pancreatic Cancer.** *N Engl J Med* 1993, **329**:1502–1503.

19. Yanagisawa A, Otake K, Ohashi K, Hori M, Kitagawa T, Sugano H, Kato Y: **Frequent c-Ki-ras Oncogene Activation in Mucous Cell Hyperplasia of Pancreas Suffering From Chronic Inflammation.** *Cancer Res* 1993, **53**:953–956.
••
This is the first report demonstrating the presence of Ki-*ras* mutations in intraductal benign hyperplasia in the pancreas, raising the possibility that regeneration in chronic pancreatitis may enhance the potential risk for pancreatic malignant transformation.

20. Urban T, Ricci S, Grange J-D, Lacave R, Boudghene F, Breittmayer F, Languille O, Roland J, Bernaudin J-F: **Detection of c-Ki-ras Mutation by PCR/RFLP Analysis and Diagnosis of Pancreatic Adenocarcinomas.** *J Natl Cancer Inst* 1993, **85**:2008–2012.
•
This study underscores the important role of Ki-*ras* mutation in pancreatic cancer but also suggests a role for Ki-*ras* in premalignant chronic pancreatitis.

21. Casey G, Yamanaka Y, Friess H, Kobrin MS, Lopez ME, Buchler M, Beger HG, Korc M: **p53 Mutations Are Common in Pancreatic Cancer and Are Absent in Chronic Pancreatitis.** *Cancer Lett* 1993, **69**:151–160.
•
This study provides preliminary evidence in a limited number of cases that indicates that *p53* mutations do not occur in chronic pancreatitis.

Murray Korc, MD, Division of Endocrinology and Metabolism, Medical Sciences I, C240, University of California, Irvine, CA 92717, USA.

Pancreatic carcinoma

Carlos Fernández-del Castillo, MD, and Andrew L. Warshaw, MD

Harvard Medical School and Massachusetts General Hospital, Boston, Massachusetts, USA

Epidemiologic studies have provided strong evidence linking chronic pancreatitis with pancreatic carcinoma. For patients with alcoholic and idiopathic chronic pancreatitis, the standardized incidence rate was 16.5; for those with tropical pancreatitis it was 100. The molecular events leading to the development of this cancer continue to be the subject of intense research, with mutations of the K-*ras* oncogene playing a major role. Although early diagnosis of pancreatic cancer continues to be elusive, better tools for the differential diagnosis of pancreatic and biliary strictures are becoming available. Surgery continues to offer the only possibility of cure; however, most patients still have local recurrence after resection. More aggressive treatment protocols combining preoperative chemoradiation and intraoperative radiation with surgery are being used.

Current Opinion in Gastroenterology 1994, **10:**507–512

Etiology and epidemiology

The incidence of pancreatic cancer has remained unchanged in the United States over the past 20 years, and currently stands at 9.1 per 100,000. Its etiology remains unknown. A multicenter historical cohort study involving over 2000 patients with chronic pancreatitis from five European countries and the United States found that the risk of developing pancreatic cancer is significantly elevated in this disease [1••]. Even after excluding all patients who had been followed for less than 2 years (some of which could have been misdiagnosed), the standardized incidence rate of pancreatic cancer was 16.5 (95% confidence interval, 11.1 to 23.7). The cumulative risk increased almost linearly and by 20 years the proportion of patients with chronic pancreatitis that developed pancreatic cancer was 4% (Fig. 1). Cigarette smoking, which is a well-established risk factor for pancreatic cancer, was present in 86% of the study population but was not found to be a significant variable with the Cox proportional-hazards model. The type of pancreatitis was alcoholic in 77%, idiopathic in 17%, and hereditary in 1.9%. All categories demonstrated similar rates of increased risk.

Another study from Madras, India, found the risk of pancreatic cancer in patients with tropical calcifying pancreatitis to be 100 times greater than expected [2]. The average age of diagnosis of the cancer was 45.6 years, which is at least two decades younger than that found in western populations. This confirms earlier reports on the malignant potential of this variety of chronic pancreatitis, which is prevalent in many countries of Asia and Africa.

Diabetes mellitus is also significantly associated with pancreatic cancer. Although some studies have suggested that diabetes may predispose to the development of cancer, in most cases it occurs within the 2 years preceding the diagnosis of pancreatic cancer or shortly thereafter. Replacement of endocrine pancreas by tumor is unlikely to be an explanation for this, because the relative proportion of neoplastic tissue is small. Permart *et al.* [3] have further confirmed this by demonstrating that glucose metabolism is actually improved after pancreatectomy for cancer. In another study they demonstrate that plasma levels of islet amyloid polypeptide (IAPP) are increased in patients with pancreatic cancer [4•]. IAPP is produced by the beta cell of the islets and has a diabetogenic effect by inhibiting glucose uptake in skeletal muscle and liver. Because IAPP levels are usually low in patients with non–insulin-dependent diabetes mellitus, these authors propose that measurement of IAPP could help identify those patients that develop non–insulin-dependent diabetes mellitus as a consequence of pancreatic cancer.

Pathology and molecular biology

The molecular events leading to the development of pancreatic cancer continue to be the subject of intense research. In a series of 82 adenocarcinomas of the pancreas, Hruban *et al.* [5••] found point mutations in codon 12 of the K-*ras* oncogene in 83% of specimens. Interestingly, the prevalence of these mutations was significantly higher in tumors of patients who were

Abbreviation

IAPP—islet amyloid polypeptide.

 ISBN 1-85922-610-8 ISSN 0267–1379

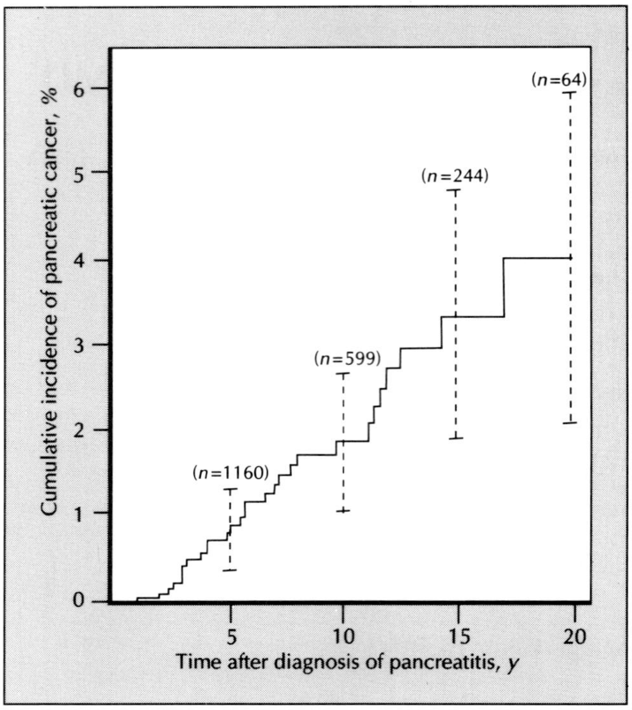

Fig. 1. Cumulative incidence of pancreatic cancer in 1552 subjects with chronic pancreatitis with a minimum of 2 years of follow-up. The vertical lines represent 95% confidence intervals and the number in parentheses the number of subjects at risk. (*From* Lowenfels *et al.* [1••]; with permission.)

or had been smokers (89%) compared with nonsmokers (68%).

The *ras* gene family codes for proteins involved as molecular switches in signal transduction, and mutations of K-*ras* can result in malignant transformation. These mutations have also been found in early pancreatic cancers [6], but not in benign tissue. The only exception is a study from Japan in which they were found in specimens of hyperplastic duct from chronic pancreatitis obtained by microdissection [7]. The *p53* tumor suppressor gene is involved in regulating both DNA repair and apoptotic cell death. Mutations of this gene or abnormal accumulation of this protein in the nucleus were described in 76% of pancreatic adenocarcinomas by another group [8]. In those tumors with mutations, coexistence with mutant K-*ras* was found in all. Understanding why and how these mutations occur and their consequences may ultimately help us in the prevention, early diagnosis, and treatment of this aggressive tumor.

Aberrations in the number and structure of chromosomes are frequent in pancreatic cancer, but not universal. Analysis of DNA content can determine presence of aneuploidy, which has been reported to be present in 15% to 94% of tumors in several studies and may have prognostic implications. Bose *et al.* [9] performed a comparative study between flow and absorption cytometry for measurement of DNA content, and found that flow cytometry vastly underestimates the number of aneuploid tumors (only one of 30 pancreatic cancers vs 21 of 30 when measured by absorption cytometry). This was felt to be due to the presence of the nonneoplastic fibroblastic stroma often present in this type of cancer.

Diagnosis

Freeney *et al.* [10•] reported on a series of 213 patients with pancreatic cancer in whom high-resolution dynamic abdominal computerized tomography was performed for diagnosis and staging [10•]. Scans were obtained using contiguous 5- to 10-mm collimated slices during rapid intravenous bolus infusion (2 to 2.5 mL/s of 150 mL 60% iodinated contrast). Computerized tomography was abnormal in 97% of patients and detected tumors as small as 1 to 1.5 cm in diameter. Criteria for unresectability included local tumor extension, contiguous organ invasion, vascular invasion, or liver metastases; 88% of patients had one or more of these signs. Of the 25 patients showing *resectable* tumors via computerized tomography only 18 were surgically explored and 13 found to be resectable (computerized tomography accuracy of 72%). Angiography was performed in 60 patients and contributed no additional or significant information to the staging of pancreatic cancer, although the authors acknowledged its value in displaying vascular anatomy before pancreatectomy.

In another report from the same institution [11], abnormal findings were found in 61% of 64 preoperative angiograms, with 30% being significant enough to alter preoperative or intraoperative management. We routinely perform laparoscopy in patients with pancreatic cancer who have no evidence of metastatic disease by computerized tomography. In our experience, 24% of patients will have positive findings (*ie*, liver or peritoneal implants). If laparoscopy is negative, we proceed with angiography both to rule out vascular invasion and to determine vascular anatomy.

Endoscopic ultrasound has rapidly evolved as a valuable tool for the differential diagnosis of pancreatic and peripancreatic malignancies. It is particularly useful in the detection of small tumors in patients with a clinical picture of pancreatic cancer and normal computerized tomography (Fig. 2). Palazzo *et al.* [12•] prospectively studied 64 patients with clinical suspicion of pancreatic cancer and independently performed endoscopic ultrasonography, ultrasonography, and computerized tomography [12•]. The accuracy of endoscopic ultrasonography to diagnose pancreatic cancer was significantly higher than the other two modalities (91% vs 64% and 66%, respectively), mostly because of the capacity to image all seven tumors less than 25 mm in diameter (only one was picked by computerized tomography and ultrasound). Endoscopic ultrasonography was also more sensitive in the detection of lymph node metastases and venous involvement.

Other developments in endoscopic instrumentation and techniques are also aimed at better defining the

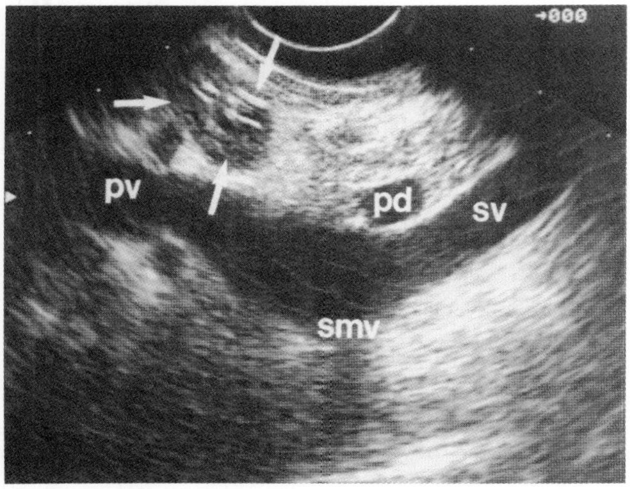

Fig. 2. Endoscopic ultrasound demonstrating a small pancreatic tumor producing obstructive jaundice. The tumor was not apparent by computed tomography. pd—pancreatic duct; pv—portal vein; smv—superior mesenteric vein; sv—splenic vein.

differential diagnosis of periampullary tumors, biliary, and pancreatic strictures. Examination with an intraductal ultrasound probe inserted via the papilla into the pancreatic duct was evaluated in 20 patients with pancreatic cancer, and was successfully performed in 85% of them [13]. It was particularly useful in delineating tumor spread in intraductal papillary carcinomas. Another group described flexible forceps for transpapillary biopsies of the pancreatic and biliary ducts [14]. Tissue samples were successfully obtained from 95% of 43 patients with pancreatobiliary strictures, with a sensitivity of 88% for cholangiocarcinomas and 71% for pancreatic cancers. There were no complications or false-positive results. This technique, together with endosonographically guided punctures [15], may allow for preoperative confirmation of malignancy while sparing the potential risks of intraperitoneal dissemination from percutaneous biopsies.

Another promising approach for the differentiation between benign and malignant strictures and potentially for the early detection of pancreatic cancer is the nonhistologic analysis of pancreatic juice or specimens obtained from brushings. Tada *et al.* [16•] report detection of mutant K-*ras* oncogene in a series of six patients with pancreatic carcinoma and one intraductal papillary neoplasm, and absence of the mutation in controls with chronic pancreatitis or choledocholithiasis. Their assay, which uses polymerase chain reaction, is extremely sensitive, being capable of detecting three to 30 copies of codon 12 mutations of the K-*ras* gene in the presence of 300,000 normal copies. They also describe the presence of the mutation in the peripheral blood of two patients with pancreatic cancer. In another report, Yeaton *et al.* [17] determined DNA content and proliferative index in 48 specimens obtained during cholangiopancreatography, and were able to distinguish malignant epithelium from normal or inflammatory epithelium with a 95% sensitivity and 100% specificity.

One of the fundamental problems in pancreatic cancer is the absence or nonspecific nature of symptoms in the early phase of the disease. In a provocative report, Ishikawa *et al.* [18•] describe the identification of eight patients with early pancreatic cancer, having normal computerized tomography and no evidence of tumor by cholangiopancreatography, who were diagnosed by the presence of malignant-appearing cells in pancreatic juice obtained before endoscopic retrograde cholangiopancreatography [18•]. All of these patients had nonspecific symptoms and had no evidence of tumor at the time of laparotomy. In order to locate the source of the malignant cells, the authors transected the pancreas at the level of the neck and cannulated both ends of the pancreatic duct. Stimulation with secretin yielded fluid for immediate intraoperative cytologic analysis, which then dictated the type of resection (three pancreatoduodenectomies, three distal pancreatectomies, and two total pancreatectomies). Histopathology revealed either *in situ* or minimally invasive carcinoma in all specimens.

The search for a serologic test useful in pancreatic cancer continues. A new tumor marker, CA 242, was compared with CA 19-9, CA 50, and carcinoembryonic antigen in 300 patients [19]. At a specificity level of 90%, its sensitivity was only 66% (and no different than that of the other markers). Although combination of the different tests improved sensitivity and specificity, the effect was rather modest and unlikely to have any application in clinical practice. We still must await symptoms to make a diagnosis. Another study [20] describes the role of CA 19-9 as a prognostic index following resection for pancreatic cancer. Patients with preoperative levels under 200 U/mL had a significantly better prognosis than those with higher levels. The same was true for patients whose CA 19-9 normalized after resection when compared with those with persistent elevation. CA 19-9 elevations after surgery predicted tumor recurrence 1 to 10 months prior to clinical and radiologic evidence.

Surgical treatment

Surgical resection of the tumor is attainable in about 15% of patients, and remains the only possibility of cure for pancreatic cancer. Because the majority of resectable tumors are in the head of the pancreas, a pancreatoduodenectomy is required. The morbidity and mortality of this surgical procedure have decreased markedly in the last decade. Cameron *et al.* [21•] reported on 145 consecutive pancreatoduodenectomies without mortality, including 37 patients 70 years of age or older. Despite improved operative outcomes, however, in most cases the disease recurs and patients die; only 15% to 20% of resected patients are alive 5 years after diagnosis. A study evaluating patterns of recurrence following macroscopically curative resection in 45 patients with pancreatic cancer demonstrated that local retroperitoneal recurrence is more common than liver metastases or peritoneal dissemination (83%, 60%, and 30%, respectively, of 30 patients who recurred) [22]. Seventeen of the 45 patients had microscopically positive margins, and not surprisingly their incidence of recurrence was significantly higher. In the Massachusetts General Hospital experience, positive margins were found in 51% of 72 patients [23]. The 5-year survival of patients with negative resection margins was 22%, compared with no survivors in the group having positive margins. The most commonly involved resection margin was the peripancreatic soft tissue (37%), followed by the pancreatic transection line (19%). These and other studies have prompted a more aggressive approach in the management of resectable pancreatic cancer, including more extensive surgical procedures, preoperative irradiation, and intraoperative radiation therapy. Evans *et al.* [24•] reported on the use of preoperative chemoradiation followed by pancreatoduodenectomy with intraoperative radiation therapy in 41 patients with periampullary malignancies, demonstrating that it can be done with a morbidity and mortality no different from that of pancreatoduodenectomy alone [24•]. Long-term results of this approach are not yet available.

For the remaining 85% of patients who are no longer resectable, palliation will be needed. Nonoperative approaches are commonly employed for jaundice with placement of endoscopic or percutaneous stents. Prospective studies have demonstrated that they are at least as equally effective as surgical bypass. Proponents of a surgical approach argue that a gastrojejunostomy will be needed in 13% of patients, and that a surgical biliary bypass has a lesser incidence of recurrent obstruction. Lillemoe *et al.* [25] reported on a series of 118 patients with unresectable pancreatic cancer who underwent surgical palliative procedures, most commonly combined biliary bypass and gastrojejunostomy. The hospital mortality was only 2.5%, which is less than the frequently cited 19% from older cumulative series, and the mean postoperative survival was 7.7 months. One drawback of the surgical approach for palliation is the need for hospitalization, which averaged 20 days in this study. Although endoscopic stenting is reported to be accompanied by the need for frequent rehospitalizations, this is not the case with newer expandable metallic stents, which have longer patency rates and are commonly placed in the outpatient setting.

In another study by Lillemoe *et al.* [26•], chemical splanchnicectomy with 50% alcohol was evaluated in a randomized, placebo-controlled, double-blind study. A total of 137 patients with pancreatic cancer who were found to be unresectable at the time of surgery underwent bilateral injections of the celiac ganglia with either 20 mL of alcohol or saline, in addition to having biliary and gastric bypass when indicated. The study showed no complications derived from the procedure, significant reduction in pain scores in patients with preoperative pain, and significant delay or prevention of pain in patients without preoperative pain. An intriguing finding was a marked improvement in survival ($P<0.0001$) in patients with preoperative pain treated with alcohol (Fig. 3).

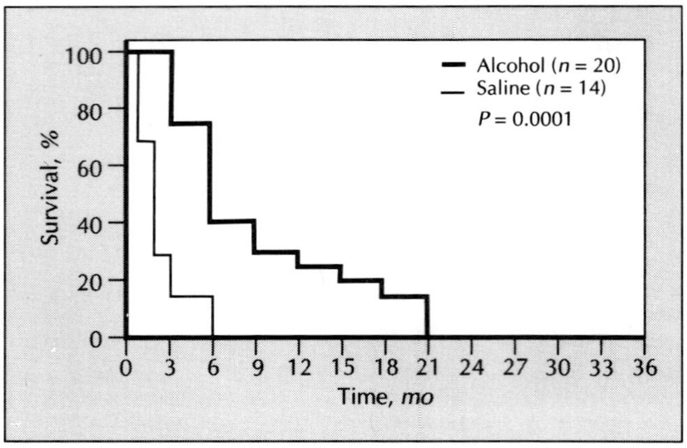

Fig. 3. Kaplan-Meier survival curves from the time of hospital discharge in 34 patients with pancreatic cancer and pain who underwent celiac ganglion infiltration with alcohol or placebo. (*From* Lillemoe *et al.* [26•]; with permission.)

Other forms of treatment

In a phase II trial, Bruckner *et al.* [27] treated 20 consecutive patients with unresectable, locally advanced pancreatic cancer with split courses of radiotherapy and continuous 5-fluorouracil infusion, streptozotozin, and cisplatin. Toxicity was acceptable and did not preclude completion of treatment for any patient. Median survival was 12 months, which was the same as that found in a contemporary cohort of successfully resected patients. This 12-month survival of unresectable patients, however is not different from that obtained with external radiotherapy with 5-fluorouracil alone, as reported by the Gastrointestinal Tumor Study Group 15 years ago.

Yeung *et al.* [28•] investigated the value of neoadjuvant chemoradiation (5040 cGy in 28 fractions with continuous 5-fluorouracil and mitomycin C as a bolus) in 26 patients with pancreatic cancer. There was one sepsis-related death and 18 patients ultimately underwent laparotomy 3 to 6 weeks after chemoradiation, 12 of whom were resected (the remaining six had liver or peritoneal metastases not detected by computed tomography). The overall 5-year actuarial survival was 16% for the entire group and 58% for the resected group. The authors concluded that neoadjuvant chemoradiation followed by pancreatectomy can be conducted safely and may lead to improved outcome in this disease. Interestingly, they also treated five patients with duodenal cancer in a similar fashion; four of them were resected and found to contain no residual tumor.

Patients with pancreatic cancer and metastatic disease continue to have a grim prognosis. The Southwest Oncology Group reported on a series of randomized phase II trials comparing combination chemotherapy with 5-fluorouracil, doxorubicin, mitomycin C, and streptozotozin, against three different single agents (methyl-glyoxal-bis-guanylhydrazone, dihydroxyanthracenedione, and aziridinylbenzoquinone) [29]. Response rates were 11% or less in all groups, and median survival was less than 5 months.

Clinical and experimental evidence suggest that pancreatic cancer may be sex steroid-hormone dependent, and preliminary reports describe a favorable effect of tamoxifen in patients with advanced disease. Two studies [30,31] evaluated the use of tamoxifen in unresectable pancreatic cancer. In a case-control study by Wong and Chan [30], 80 patients received tamoxifen (20 mg twice daily) and had a median survival of 7 months compared with 3 months in another group matched for age, sex, tumor, node, metastasis stage, and type of surgical procedure. The greatest benefit of tamoxifen was seen in women older than 60 years of age, whose median survival was 12 months. In a randomized placebo-controlled trial from the United Kingdom involving 44 patients, no difference was found with the use of tamoxifen (survival was less than 4.5 months in both groups) [31].

References and recommended reading

Papers of particular interest, published within the annual period of review, have been highlighted as:
- • Of special interest
- •• Of outstanding interest

1. •• Lowenfels AB, Maisonneuve P, Cavallini G, Ammann RW, Lankisch PG, Andersen JR, Dimagno EP, Andren-Sandberg A, Domellof L: **Pancreatitis and the Risk of Pancreatic Cancer.** *N Engl J Med* 1993, **328**:1433—1437.

A multinational epidemiologic study showed that the risk of pancreatic cancer is significantly elevated in subjects with chronic pancreatitis.

2. Chari ST, Mohan V, Pitchumoni CS, Viswanathan M, Madanagopalan N, Lowenfels AB: **Risk of Pancreatic Carcinoma in Tropical Calcifying Pancreatitis: An Epidemiological Study.** *Pancreas* 1994, 9:62–66.

3. Permert J, Ihse I, Jorfeldt L, von Schenck H, Arnquist HJ, Larsson J: **Improved Glucose Metabolism After Subtotal Pancreatectomy for Pancreatic Cancer.** *Br J Surg* 1993, **80**:1047–1050.

4. • Permert J, Larsson J, Westermark GT, Herrington MK, Christmanson L, Pour PM, Westermark P, Adrian TE: **Islet Amyloid Polypeptide in Patients With Pancreatic Cancer and Diabetes.** *N Engl J Med* 1994, **330**:313–318.

Diabetes in pancreatic cancer in many cases is probably related to increased levels of this peptide.

5. •• Hruban RH, van Mansfeld ADM, Offerhaus GJA, van Weering DH, Allison DC, Goodman SN, Kensler TW, Bose KK, Cameron JL, Bos JL: **K-ras Oncogene Activation in Adenocarcinoma of the Human Pancreas.** *Am J Pathol* 1993, **143**:545–554.

K-*ras* mutation was found in 83% of 82 ductal adenocarcinomas of the pancreas and the prevalence was significantly higher in smokers compared to nonsmokers.

6. Schaeffer BK, Glasner S, Kuhlmann E, Myles JL, Longnecker DS: **Mutated c-K-ras in Small Pancreatic Adenocarcinoma.** *Pancreas* 1994, 9:161–165.

7. Yanagisawa A, Ohtake K, Ohashi K, Hori M, Kitagawa T, Sugano H, Kato Y: **Frequent c-Ki-ras Oncogene Activation in Mucous Cell Hyperplasias of Pancreas Suffering From Chronic Inflammation.** *Cancer Res* 1993, **53**:953–956.

8. Scarpa A, Capelli P, Mukai K, Zamboni G, Oda T, Iacono C, Hirohashi S: **Pancreatic Adenocarcinomas Frequently Show p53 Gene Mutations.** *Am J Pathol* 1993, **142**:1534–1543.

9. Bose KK, Allison DC, Hruban RH, Piantadosi S, Zahurak M, Dooley WC, Lin P, Cameron JL: **A Comparison of Flow Cytometric and Absorption Cytometric DNA Values as Prognostic Indicators for Pancreatic Carcinoma.** *Cancer* 1993, **71**:691–700.

10. • Freeny PC, Traverso W, Ryan JA: **Diagnosis and Staging of Pancreatic Adenocarcinoma With Dynamic Computed Tomography.** *Am J Surg* 1993, **165**:600–606.

Computed tomography continues to be the single most useful diagnostic test for the diagnosis and staging of pancreatic cancer.

11. Biehl TR, Traverso W, Hauptmann E, Ryan JA: **Preoperative Visceral Angiography Alters Intraoperative Strategy During the Whipple Procedure.** *Am J Surg* 1993, **165**:607–612.

12. • Palazzo L, Roseau G, Gayet B, Vilgrain V, Belghiti J, Fekete F, Paolaggi JA: **Endoscopic Ultrasonography in the Diagnosis and Staging of Pancreatic Adenocarcinoma.** *Endoscopy* 1993, **25**:143–150.

Endoscopic ultrasound detects small lesions in the pancreatic head which are otherwise not identified by computed tomography.

13. Furukawa T, Tsukamoto Y, Naitoh Y, Hirooka Y, Katoh T: **Evaluation of Intraductal Ultrasonography in the Diagnosis of Pancreatic Cancer.** *Endoscopy* 1993, **25**:577–581.

14. Kubota Y, Takaoka M, Tani K, Ogura M, Kin H, Fujimura K, Muzuno T, Inoue K: **Endoscopic Transpapillary Biopsy for Diagnosis of Patients With Pancreatobiliary Ductal Strictures.** *Am J Gastroenterol* 1993, **88**:1700–1704.

15. Tio TL, Sie LH, Tytgat GNJ: **Endosonography and Cytology in Diagnosing and Staging Pancreatic Body and Tail Carcinoma.** *Dig Dis Sci* 1993, **38**:59–64.

16. • Tada M, Omata M, Kawai S, Saisho H, Ohto M, Saiki RK, Sninsky JJ: **Detection of Ras Gene Mutations in Pancreatic Juice and Peripheral Blood of Patients With Pancreatic Adenocarcinoma.** *Cancer Res* 1993, **53**:2472–2474.

Detection of the molecular changes of pancreatic cancer may help in its early diagnosis.

17. Yeaton P, Kiss R, Deviere J, Salmon I, Bourgeois N, Pasteels JL, Cremer M: **Use of Cell Image Analysis in the Detection of Cancer From Specimens Obtained During Endoscopic Retrograde Cholangiopancreatography.** *Am J Clin Pathol* 1993, **100**:497–501.

18. • Ishikawa O, Ohigashi H, Nakaizumi A, Uehara H, Kitamura T, Takenaka A, Sasaki Y, Imaoka S: **Surgical Resection of Potentially Curable Pancreatic Cancer With Improved Preservation of Endocrine Function: Further Evaluation of Intraoperative Cytodiagnosis.** *Hepatogastroenterology* 1993, **40**:443–447.

Pancreatic fluid cytology may help identify cases of early pancreatic cancer without morphologic changes, and intraoperative cytology can help decide the surgical treatment.

19. Rothlin MA, Joller H, Largiader F: **CA 242 is a New Tumor Marker for Pancreatic Cancer.** *Cancer* 1993, **71**:701–707.

20. Sperti C, Pasquali C, Catalani S, Cappellazzo F, Bonadimani B, Behboo R, Pedrazzoli S: **CA 19-9 as a Prognostic Index After Resection for Pancreatic Cancer.** *J Surg Oncol* 1993, **52**:137–141.

21. • Cameron JL, Pitt HA, Yeo CJ, Lillemoe KD, Kaufman HS, Coleman J: **One Hundred and Forty-Five Consecutive Pancreaticoduodenectomies Without Mortality.** *Ann Surg* 1993, **217**:430–438.

The current safety of pancreaticoduodenectomies in experienced hands is demonstrated in this remarkable achievement.

22. Kayahara M, Nagakawa T, Ueno K, Ohta T, Takeda T, Miyazaki I: **An Evaluation of Radical Resection for Pancreatic Cancer Based on the Mode of Recurrence as Determined by Autopsy and Diagnostic Imaging.** *Cancer* 1993, **72**:2118–2123.

23. Willett CG, Lewandrowski K, Warshaw AL, Efird J, Compton CC: **Resection Margins in Carcinoma of the Head of the Pancreas: Implications for Radiation Therapy.** *Ann Surg* 1993, **217**:144–148.

24. • Evans DB, Termuhlen PM, Byrd DR, Ames FC, Ochran TG, Rich TA: **Intraoperative Radiation Therapy Following Pancreaticoduodenectomy.** *Ann Surg* 1993, **218**:54–60.

Intraoperative radiotherapy can be safely combined with surgical resection and hopefully will improve survival in pancreatic cancer.

25. Lillemoe KD, Kal Sauter P, Pitt HA, Yeo CJ, Cameron JL: **Current Status of Surgical Palliation of Periampullary Carcinoma.** *Surg Gynecol Obstet* 1993, **176**:1–10.

26. • Lillemoe KD, Cameron JL, Kaufman HS, Yeo CJ, Pitt HA, Sauter PK: **Chemical Splanchnicectomy in Patients With Unresectable Pancreatic Cancer.** *Ann Surg* 1993, **217**:447–457.

This fine example of a prospective, randomized, double-blind study demonstrating that chemical splanchnicectomy with alcohol reduces or prevents pain in patients with unresectable pancreatic cancer.

27. Bruckner HW, Kanicki S, Dalton J, Snady H, Schwartz GK, Chesser MR, Lehrer D, Mandeli J, Harpaz N, Janus C: **Survival After Combined Modality Therapy for Pancreatic Cancer**. *J Clin Gastroenteol* 1993, 16:199–203.

28. • Yeung RS, Weese JL, Hoffman JP, Solin LJ, Paul AR, Engstrom PF, Litwin S, Kowalyshyn MJ, Eisenberg BL: **Neoadjuvant Chemoradiation in Pancreatic and Duodenal Carcinoma. A Phase II Study.** *Cancer* 1993, 72:2124–2133.

Intensive preoperative chemotherapy and radiation are feasible and may improve results in resection for pancreatic cancer.

29. Bukowski RM, Fleming TR, MacDonald JS, Oishi N, Taylor SA, Baker LH: **Evaluation of Combination Chemotherapy and Phase II Agents in Pancreatic Adenocarcinoma**. *Cancer* 1993, 71:322–325.

30. Wong A, Chan A: **Survival Benefit of Tamoxifen Therapy in Adenocarcinoma of Pancreas**. *Cancer* 1993, 71:2200–2203.

31. Taylor OM, Benson EA, McMahon MJ: **Clinical Trial of Tamoxifen in Patients With Irresectable Pancreatic Adenocarcinoma.** *Br J Surg* 1993, 80:384–386.

Carlos Fernández-del Castillo, MD, Massachusetts General Hospital, ACC/464, and Andrew L. Warshaw, MD, Massachusetts General Hospital, ACC/336, 15 Parkman Street, Boston, MA 02114, USA.

Pancreatic surgery

Michael L. Steer, MD

Harvard Medical School, Boston, Massachusetts, USA

Pancreatic pseudocysts should be managed selectively. Roux-en-Y cyst-jejunostomy may be the surgical procedure of choice, but some patients can be managed by observation alone or by endoscopic internal drainage procedures. The Peustow procedure may retard progression of exocrine and endocrine insufficiency in some patients with chronic pancreatitis. Preoperative studies, including somatostatin receptor scintigraphy, may be helpful in localizing neuroendocrine tumors of the pancreas. Cyst fluid analysis may aid preoperatively in determining whether cystic tumors of the pancreas are malignant or premalignant. Computed tomography can accurately stage most patients with pancreatic adenocarcinoma. For selected patients who are not candidates for curative resection, surgical biliary and gastric bypass procedures can successfully palliate symptoms with a perioperative mortality rate similar to that associated with endoscopic stenting procedures. Combined pancreas and kidney transplantation in diabetic patients with renal failure can be accomplished with a perioperative mortality rate similar to that following isolated kidney transplantation.

Current Opinion in Gastroenterology 1994, **10**:513–516

Chronic pancreatitis

The role of surgery in the modern management of pseudocysts was reviewed by Grace and Williamson [1•]. They noted that pseudocysts have been reported to occur in 16% to 50% of patients with acute pancreatitis and 20% to 40% of those with chronic pancreatitis. Obviously, this reported incidence must reflect sampling bias and patient selection because many patients with mild pancreatitis may not be extensively evaluated. Grace and Williamson concluded that asymptomatic chronic pseudocysts 6 cm or less in diameter do not require intervention, whereas those that are symptomatic, enlarging, or greater than 6 cm in diameter should be treated. They recommend treating such pseudocysts with internal drainage via a Roux-en-Y cyst-jejunostomy. I would also favor this procedure for individuals undergoing an operation.

Recently, a number of nonoperative options have attracted considerable interest [2–4]. My own experience with percutaneously placed drainage catheters has not been favorable because of the prolonged morbidity and repeated episodes of drain tract infection that these patients experience. For patients whose pseudocyst impinges on the duodenum and is closely adherent to the duodenum, endoscopic cystoduodenostomy may be the treatment of choice, particularly if these patients are poor surgical risks.

Intractable pain in patients with "large duct" pancreatitis is generally considered to be the prime indication for performance of a longitudinal pancreaticojejunostomy (modified Peustow procedure). Nealon and Thompson [5••] have suggested that this procedure may also retard the progressive loss of exocrine and endocrine function that is part of the chronic pancreatitis syndrome. As a result, they have suggested that preservation of function should also be considered an indication for the Peustow procedure. During the past year, they updated an earlier report [6] that described the postoperative course of a large group of patients undergoing the modified Peustow procedure and noted that the procedure did appear to arrest the progression of chronic pancreatitis. More importantly, however, they also described a prospective, randomized trial of surgery versus observation for patients with large duct mild-to-moderate chronic pancreatitis who had nondisabling pain. Nine patients underwent longitudinal pancreaticojejunostomy while eight patients were observed without operation. Mean follow-up was for 39 months. Progressive loss of exocrine or endocrine function or worsening of ductal morphology was noted in six of the eight nonsurgically treated patients but in only two of the nine patients undergoing a modified Peustow procedure (Table 1). They concluded that ductal drainage via a longitudinal pancreaticojejunostomy can preserve endocrine or exocrine function in patients with large duct chronic pancreatitis. Obviously, a larger study with more patients will be needed before this issue is completely resolved, but these results clearly indicate that pain relief may not be the only reason for performing a Peustow procedure.

Abbreviation

ERCP—endoscopic retrograde cholangiopancreatography.

 ISBN 1-85922-610-8 ISSN 0267–1379

Table 1. Prospective evaluation of patients having mild-to-moderate chronic pancreatitis with minimal pain*

Patient groups	Initial evaluation, *n/n(%)*	Improvement at follow-up, *n/n(%)*†
Operated	9/9(100)	7/9(78)
Nonoperated	8/8(100)	2/8(25)

**Modified from* Nealon and Thompson [5••]; with permission.
†Mean follow-up of 39 months. The change in severity grade from initial evaluation to follow-up for mild-to-moderate stage chronic pancreatitis in patients randomly assigned to operation or nonoperation was noted.

Endocrine tumors

The following three issues regarding surgical management of pancreatic endocrine tumors are the subject of important reports during the past year: 1) preoperative localization of endocrine tumors, 2) a surgical approach to removing endocrine pancreatic tumors, and 3) the use of somatostatin analogues to treat residual disease in patients with endocrine tumors of the pancreas. van Ecyk *et al.* [7•] evaluated the use of an indium-labeled somatostatin analogue for preoperative localization of pancreatic endocrine tumors in 25 patients. They found that the radiolabeled compound bound to and correctly identified the location of tumors in 20 of the 25 patients and aided in finding tumor metastases in many patients. In addition, preoperative labeling of the tumors *in situ* was useful in predicting the response to treating residual tumor with somatostatin analogues.

Weinel *et al.* [8•] evaluated the potential value of several types of preoperative localizing techniques for patients with neuroendocrine tumors of the pancreas. In nine patients, they noted correct localization by computed tomography in three, by ultrasound in four, and by somastatin receptor scintography in five. Taken together, this report and studies reported by others suggest that patients with functioning pancreatic endocrine tumors should undergo extensive preoperative attempts to localize and stage their tumor and that scans done after administration of radiolabeled somatostatin analogues may be particularly useful.

Udelsman *et al.* [9•] reported on a series of 12 patients who underwent pancreaticoduodenectomy for pancreatic endocrine tumors. They recommended that tumors of the body or tail of the pancreas be treated by distal pancreatectomy. Benign tumors of the head should, if possible, be enucleated. This would seem appropriate treatment for insulinomas that are frequently benign. Malignant tumors of the head, on the other hand, should be treated by pancreaticoduodenectomy.

Arnold *et al.* [10] describe a series of 21 patients with metastatic gastroenteropancreatic endocrine tumors (six gastrinomas, eight carcinoids, and seven nonfunctioning tumors) treated with a somatostatin analogue (200 μg three times a day). Tumor growth was halted in five patients whereas growth appeared to be slowed in another seven patients. Nine individuals failed to respond. Response and lack of response were not uniformly predicted by the presence or absence of somatostatin receptors. Clearly, further experiences with larger groups of patients, perhaps treated with larger doses of the somatostatin analogue, will be required before the ultimate role of this agent in the treatment of metastatic endocrine tumors of the pancreas and gastrointestinal tract can be clarified.

Cystic exocrine tumors

Cystic tumors of the pancreas, which must be distinguished from retention cysts and pseudocysts, may be either serous or mucinous. Serous tumors frequently comprise multiple small cysts (microcystic) and are almost always benign whereas mucinous tumors, which are often made up of several large cysts (macrocystic), are frequently malignant or capable of undergoing progressive changes eventually leading to the development of malignancy [11–13]. Because of these differences, correct preoperative diagnosis of these tumors may be particularly important in planning treatment. Iselin *et al.* [14•] reported that computed tomography correctly identified the nature of these lesions in only two thirds of patients whereas fine-needle aspiration cytology and staining for either intracellular glycogen (serous cystic tumors) or mucin (mucinous cystic tumors) correctly diagnosed only two of the four patients undergoing that procedure.

Gazelle *et al.* [15•] evaluated the use of preoperative endoscopic retrograde cholangiopancreatography (ERCP) in a series of 38 patients with cystic tumors (23 benign and 15 malignant). The ERCP was normal in nine patients (eight benign, one malignant), showed ductal narrowing or draping in 14 (11 benign, three malignant), showed duct-cyst communication in five (three benign, two malignant), and revealed ductal obstruction by the tumor in 10 (one benign, nine malignant). Thus, ductal obstruction, which was present in 60% of the patients with malignant disease and only 4% of those with benign disease, seems to be the best ERCP predictor of malignancy.

Lewandrowski *et al.* [16••] reported that cyst fluid analysis might be used to identify malignant cystic tumors. They evaluated 26 patients of whom nine had pseudocysts, five had serous cystadenomas, four had mucinous cystic neoplasms, seven had mucinous cystadenocarcinomas, and one had a mucinous ductal carcinoma with cystic degeneration. They evaluated carcinoembryonic antigen levels, CA-125 levels, CA 19-9 levels, amylase and lipase levels, viscosity, and cytology on cyst fluid samples and found that the amylase or lipase levels were usually high in pseudocysts but low in tumors (Table 2). Viscosity was usually high in mucinous tumors and cysts but low in pseudocysts and serous tumors. Cytology was helpful when positive but, because of sampling error, false-negatives made cytology by itself not a reliable test. The carcinoembryonic antigen and CA-125 were particularly valuable tests. A very high carcinoembryonic antigen was noted in all of the mucinous cystic neoplasms and mucinous cystadenocarcinomas, but in none of the pseudocysts or serous tumors. CA-125 was elevated in all seven of the mucinous cystadenocarcinomas but variably elevated in the mucinous cystic tumors and serous tumors. CA-125 was not elevated in any of the pseudocysts. These results suggest that cyst fluid analysis may be quite useful in evaluating patients with cystic tumors of the pancreas. In particular, fluid viscosity, cytology (if positive), and measurement of carcinoembryonic antigen as well as CA-125 may identify those individuals with mucinous tumors who warrant resection.

Exocrine tumors

Freeny *et al.* [17••] evaluated 60 patients to determine whether computed tomography alone would have served as well as computed tomography combined with angiography in staging patients with pancreatic cancer. They noted that the computed tomography and angiogram yielded the same results in 75% of patients whereas, in 20% of patients, the computed tomography detected invasion of the superior mesenteric artery or superior mesenteric vein, which was missed on the angiogram. On the other hand, the angiogram detected major vascular involvement missed on computed tomography in 5% of patients. In this latter group, however, the computed tomography revealed other lesions that indicated a curative resection could not be performed. Thus, the authors concluded that the angiogram contributed nothing to tumor staging or treatment planning that could not be obtained with a contrast-enhanced computed tomography. They recommended that patients with pancreatic cancer not be subjected to angiography. In general, I would agree with their conclusion and recommendation, especially in patients with periampullary and pancreatic head tumors. On the other hand, I usually obtain an angiogram in patients with cancer of the body or tail of the pancreas whose computed tomography suggests resectability because the vast majority of those individuals do, unfortunately, have vascular involvement that precludes a curative resection. Some, however, do have surgically resectable cancers of the body and tail of pancreas and, as reported by Johnson *et al.* [18•], some of those individuals may benefit greatly from resection. They describe 13 resections in a total of 105 patients (12%) with a median survival of 13 months. Five patients survived at least 2 years and three were still alive 30, 43, and 50 months following resection.

In 1989, Dowsett *et al.* [19] reported a randomized trial of endoscopic versus surgical biliary decompression for 127 patients with obstructive jaundice caused by an unresectable tumor. Although the morbidity for endoscopic stenting was significant (23%), they concluded that the endoscopic approach was preferable because the early mortality rate for surgical bypass was much higher than that for endoscopic stenting (15% vs 6%). Although this may be true for unselected patients, a recent report by Lillemoe *et al.* [20•] suggests that much better mortality rates can be achieved in properly selected patients. They performed surgical biliary bypass (combined with gastrojejunostomy in 75% of patients) in a group of 118 patients with unresectable periampullary cancer. In-hospital mortality in this group was only 2.5%. It would appear, therefore, that good surgical risk patients, particularly those with substantial life expectancy because of small tumor burden or minimal evidence of metastatic disease, may be best treated by surgical biliary bypass. Patients with more advanced disease and, therefore, shorter life expectancy and those whose co-morbid diseases make them poor surgical risks should continue to be treated with endoscopic techniques unless gastric outlet obstruction is also present.

Transplantation

The role and timing of pancreas transplantation in patients with type 1 diabetes mellitus continues to be a subject of considerable controversy. Many transplant centers offer simultaneous cadaver pancreas and kidney transplantation to diabetic patients with end-stage renal disease in the hope that a successful pancreas transplant in such individuals will limit the progression of diabetic complications and prevent diabetic nephropathy in the transplanted kidney. As noted by Stratta, *et al.* [21•], combined pancreas and kidney transplantation can be performed with roughly the same perioperative morbidity and mortality as simple cadaver kidney transplant. Because these patients will be receiving immunosuppressive treatment for their

Table 2. Cyst fluid indices useful in differential diagnosis*

Diagnosis	Cyst fluid levels: Viscosity	CEA	CA-125	Enzymes	Cytologic findings
Pseudocyst	Low	Low	Low	High (isoamylase diagnostic)	Negative
Serous cystadenoma	Low	Low	Variable	Variable	Negative
Mucinous cystic neoplasm	Usually high	High	Variable	Variable	Usually positive
Mucinous cystadenocarcinoma	High	High	High	Variable	Usually positive

*From Lewandrowski *et al.* [16••]; with permission.
CEA—carcinoembryonic antigen.

transplanted kidney in any event, the addition of a pancreas transplant does not greatly alter their postoperative management. From the standpoint of the operative risk and postoperative care, it would therefore appear that type 1 diabetic patients with endstage renal failure requiring kidney transplant might be well served by receiving a simultaneous kidney and pancreas transplant. On the other hand, this approach requires that those individuals receive a cadaver kidney-pancreas transplant as opposed to receiving a kidney obtained from a living, related donor. Because the latter is associated with a greater rate of transplant success [22•], the decision to perform a simultaneous kidney-pancreas transplant in all diabetic patients might certainly be questioned. Rather, it would appear to me to be most appropriate to perform combined kidney-pancreas transplants primarily in those individuals who cannot be given the kidney of a living, related donor.

References and recommended reading

Papers of particular interest, published within the annual period of review, have been highlighted as:

- • Of special interest
- •• Of outstanding interest

1. • Grace PA, Williamson RCN: **Modern Management of Pancreatic Psuedocysts.** *Br J Surg* 1993, **80**:573–581.

This excellent review covers natural history, timing of intervention, therapeutic options, and outcome for patients with pancreatic pseudocysts.

2. van Sonnenberg E, Wittich GR, Casola G, Stauffer AE, Polansky AD, Coons HG, Cabrera OA, Gerver PS: **Complicated Pancreatic Inflammatory Disease: Diagnostic and Therapeutic Role of Interventional Radiology.** *Radiology* 1985, **155**:335–340.

3. van Sonnenberg E, Wittich GR, Casola G, Brannigan TC, Karnel F, Stabile BE, Varney RR, Christensen RR: **Percutaneous Drainage of Infected and Non-Infected Pancreatic Pseudocysts:. Experience in 101 Cases.** *Radiology* 1989, **170**:757–761.

4. Sahel J, Bastid C, Pellat B, Schurgers P, Sarles H: **Endoscopic Cystoduodenostomy of Cysts of Chronic Calcifying Pancreatitis: A Report of 20 cases.** *Pancreas* 1987, **2**:447–453.

5. •• Nealon WH, Thompson JC: **Progressive Loss of Pancreatic Function in Chronic Pancreatitis Is Delayed by Main Pancreatic Duct Decompression.** *Ann Surg* 1993, **217**:458–468.

This retrospective study of patients either observed or decompressed suggests that a Peustow procedure delays progressive loss of exocrine and endocrine function in chronic pancreatitis. Data are also presented from a prospective randomized trial of observation versus operation that leads to the same conclusion.

6. Nealon WH, Townsend CM JR, Thompson JC: **Operative Drainage of the Pancreatic Duct Delays Functional Impairment in Patients With Chronic Pancreatitis: A Prospective Analysis.** *Ann Surg* 1988, **208**:321–329.

7. • van Eyck CHJ, Bruining HA, Reubi J-C, Bakker WH, Oei HY, Krenning EP, Lamberts SWJ: **Use of Isotope-Labeled Somatostatin Analogs for Visualization of Islet Cell Tumors.** *World J Surg* 1993, **17**:444–447.

Indium-labeled somatostatin analogue can be used to localize islet cell tumors of the pancreas.

8. • Weinel RJ, Neuhaus C, Stapp J, Klotter HJ, Trautmann ME, Joseph K, Arnold R, Rothmund M: **Preoperative Localization of Gastrointestinal Endocrine Tumors Using Somatostatin-Receptor Scintigraphy.** *Ann Surg* 1993, **218**:640–645.

A comparison was made of somatostatin-receptor scintography, computed tomography, and ultrasonography for localization of gastrointestinal endocrine tumors.

9. • Udelsman R, Yeo CJ, Hruban RH, Pitt HA, Niederhuber JE, Coleman J, Cameron JL: **Pancreaticoduodenectomy for Selected Pancreatic Endocrine Tumors.** *Surg Gynecol Obstet* 1993, 177:269–278.

Whipple resection versus distal pancreatectomy versus enucleation for pancreatic endocrine tumors is discussed.

10. Arnold R, Neuhaus C, Benning R, Schwerk WB, Trautmann ME, Joseph K, Bruns C: **Somatostatin Analog Sandostatin and Inhibition of Tumor Growth in Patients With Metastatic Endocrine Gastroenteropancreatic Tumors.** *World J Surg* 1993, **17**:511–519.

11. Compagno J, Oertel J: **Mucinous Cystic Neoplasms of the Pancreas With Overt and Latent Malignancy (Cystadenocarcinoma and Cystadenoma): A Clinicopathologic Study of 41 Cases.** *Am J Clin Pathol* 1978, **69**:573–580.

12. Compagno J, Oertel J: **Microcystic Adenomas of the Pancreas (Glycogen-Rich Cystadenoma): A Clinicopathologic Study of 34 Cases.** *Am J Clin Pathol* 1978, **69**:289–298.

13. Tarpila E, Borch K, Franzen L, *et al.*: **Cystic Neoplasms of the Pancreas: A Clinicopathological Study of 38 Cases.** *Dig Surg* 1989, **6**:138–141.

14. • Iselin CE, Meyer P, Hauser H, Kurt AM, Vermeulen BJM, Rohner A: **Computed Tomography and Fine-Needle Aspiration Cytology for Preoperative Evaluation of Cystic Tumours of the Pancreas.** *Br J Surg* 1993, **80**:1166–1169.

Malignant and premalignant cystic tumors of the pancreas can be identified by computed tomography and fine-needle aspiration.

15. • Gazelle GS, Mueller PR, Raafat N, Halpern EF, Cardenosa G, Warshaw AL: **Cystic Neoplasms of the Pancreas: Evaluation With Endoscopic Retrograde Pancreatography.** *Radiology* 1993, **188**:633–636.

Endoscopic retrograde cholangiopancreatography is not diagnostic in many patients with cystic tumors of the pancreas.

16. •• Lewandrowski KB, Southern JF, Pins MR, Compton CC, Warshaw AL: **Cyst Fluid Analysis in the DIfferential Diagnosis of Pancreatic Cysts.** *Ann Surg* 1993, **217**:41–47.

Cyst fluid analysis can be used to identify cystic pancreatic tumors that are either malignant or premalignant.

17. •• Freeny PC, Traverso W, Ryan JA: **Diagnosis and Staging of Pancreatic Adenocarcinoma With Dynamic Computed Tomography.** *Am J Surg* 1993, **165**:600– 606.

Angiography provides little or no information regarding the staging of pancreatic cancer that cannot be obtained by computed tomography.

18. • Johnson CD, Schwall G, Flechtenmacher J, Trede M: **Resection for Adenocarcinoma of the Body and Tail of the Pancreas.** *Br J Surg* 1993, **80**:1177–1179.

Up to 12% of patients with pancreatic body or tail cancers can undergo surgical resection and long-term survival can be achieved in some of these individuals.

19. Dowsett JF, Russell RCG, Hatfield ARW, *et al.*: **Malignant Obstructive Jaundice: A Prospective Randomized Trial of By-Pass Surgery Versus Endoscoic Stenting [Abstract].** *Gastroenterology* 1989, **96**:128.

20. • Lillemoe KD, Sauter PK, Pitt HA, Yeo CJ, Cameron JL: **Current Status of Surgical Palliation of Periampullary Carcinoma.** *Surg Gynecol Obstet* 1993, **176**:1–10.

21. • Stratta RJ, Taylor RJ, Ozaki CF, Bynon JS, Miller SA, Baker TL, Lykke C, Krobot ME, Langnas AN, Shaw BW: **The Analysis of Benefit and Risk of Combined Pancreatic and Renal Transplantation Versus Renal Transplantation Alone.** *Surg Gynecol Obstet* 1993, 177:163–171.

Combined pancreas and kidney transplantation can be performed with perioperative mortality and morbidity rates that are not greater than those associated with isolated kidney transplantation in diabetic patients.

22. • Sutherland DER: **Pancreas Transplants.** *Br J Surg* 1994, **81**: 2–4.

Excellent short review of the current status of pancreas transplantation.

Michael L. Steer, MD, Professor of Surgery, Harvard Medical School, Beth Israel Hospital, Boston, MA 02215, USA.

Pancreatic imaging

Gary D. Leavitt, MD, and Morton I. Burrell, MD

Yale University School of Medicine, New Haven, Connecticut, USA

New imaging techniques to diagnose pancreatic pathology and interventional procedures to treat disease continue to be developed. Of note is the investigation of new contrast agents for magnetic resonance to better delineate pancreatic tumors and endoscopic ultrasound to image tumors less than 25 mm. Nuclear isotopes to evaluate islet cell tumors are being investigated. The use of computed tomography to evaluate acute pancreatitis continues to grow. Investigators have examined lithotripsy and celiac ganglion blockade to treat chronic calcific pancreatitis and pancreatic neoplasms respectively. Finally, normal ultrasonographic and computed tomographic pancreatic anatomy has been further elucidated.

Current Opinion in Gastroenterology 1994, **10:**517–522

Technique

Magnetic resonance continues to hold promise for the evaluation of pancreatic neoplasm. Earlier studies have evaluated fat-suppression T_1-weighted spin-echo magnetic resonance [1] and T_1-weighted spin-echo with gadolinium [2]. More recent studies have looked at newer oral and intravenous contrast. Helical computed tomography, endoscopic ultrasound, and nuclear medicine were explored for pancreatic imaging. Angiography, though less widely used than before, was revisited.

Gehl *et al.* [3] report their clinical experience with intravenous manganese dipyridoxal diphosphate (Mn-DPDP)–enhanced magnetic resonance imaging (Fig. 1). Fifteen patients were imaged with T_1-weighted spin-echo and T_1-weighted gradient-echo, both Mn-DPDP enhanced and unenhanced. Superior delineation of the tumor was seen in both spin-echo and gradient-echo images enhanced with Mn-DPDP compared with the unenhanced images. Whereas Mn-DPDP shows promise as an intravenous agent, this study does not compare Mn-DPDP enhanced images with other modalities or other magnetic resonance techniques such as fat suppression or enhancement with gadolinium.

A paper by Bach-Gansmo *et al.* [4•] evaluated whether a negative oral contrast agent consisting of crystals of iron oxide with super paramagnetic properties improved the diagnostic utility of abdominal magnetic resonance images. In pancreatic imaging, the duodenum may obscure pathology. Forty patients with a variety of indications were evaluated with magnetic resonance before and after the administration of oral contrast. Proton density and T_2-weighted images were obtained. In their study, 41% of the diagnosis could not be established without the oral agent.

Helical (spiral) computed tomography of the abdomen continues to generate interest. Helical computed tomography provides the ability to rapidly scan a patient and perform reconstructions in different planes. In a nice review of helical computed tomography of the abdomen, Zeman *et al.* [5••] postulate that helical computed tomography may improve the ability to image pancreatic carcinoma and improve staging. Support for this view is provided by the same authors, who compared helical and nonhelical computed tomography in 60 patients. With reconstruction of overlapping images, small in-plane structures (Fig. 2), important in staging, were better seen on helical computed tomography [6••].

Several centers have reported excellent results with endoscopic ultrasound, both diagnosing and staging of pancreatic carcinoma [7•,8••,9•]. In a series of 64 patients in which endoscopic ultrasound was found to be superior to computed tomography and ultrasound [8••], sensitivity was 96% and specificity was 73%. Endoscopic ultrasound was found to be especially sensitive in detecting cancers less than 25 mm in diameter, imaging all seven cancers of this size (Fig. 3). However, the authors caution that reproducibility in other centers may be one of the major limitations of this technique.

The possible role of nuclear medicine in the evaluation of carcinoid and islet cell tumors was examined by Kvols *et al.* [10•]. Iodine-123 ocreotide (an analogue of somatostatin) was used to localize known carcinoid

Abbreviations

CCN—central cavitary necrosis; **ESWL**—extracorporeal shock wave lithotripsy; **Mn-DPDP**—manganese dipyridoxal diphosphate.

 ISBN 1-85922-610-8 ISSN 0267–1379

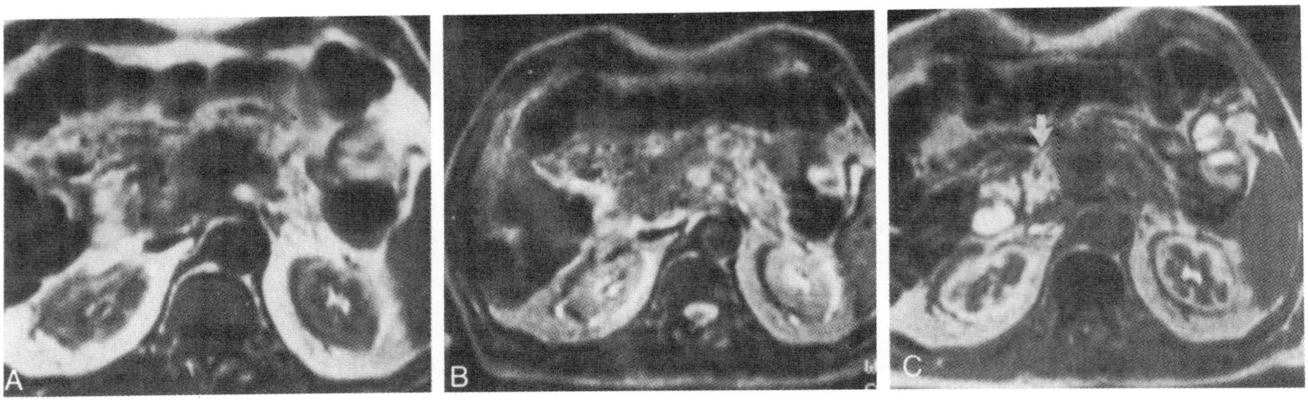

Fig. 1. Magnetic resonance images of a 61-year-old patient with adenocarcinoma of the pancreatic head and uncinate process, with invasion of the retropancreatic space toward the aorta. **A**, Mn-DPDP–enhanced T_1-weighted SE image (500/15). **B** T_2-weighted SE image (2000/70, 70° flip angle). **C** Mn-DPDP–enhanced T_1-weighted GRE image (100/6, 70° flip angle), which allows the most distinct separation between normal pancreas (*arrow*), tumor, and central hypointense necrosis. The Mn-DPDP–enhanced T_1-weighted SE image offers less distinct separation between the parenchyma and the tumor. The necrotic area may be mistaken for a tumor at T_2-weighted imaging. (*From* Gehl *et al.* [3]; with permission.)

and islet cell tumors. Of the 14 patients with known islet cell tumors, 10 had positive scans with one scan demonstrating an unsuspected lesion in the head confirmed by magnetic resonance (Fig. 4). The eventual clinical utility of this approach remains to be seen.

Pancreatic neoplasms

Ductal carcinomas

Preoperative angiography for staging of pancreatic neoplasms has largely been replaced by computed tomography as it is felt that there is little benefit in using angiography with no evidence of vascular involvement by dynamic computed tomography [11]. However, some still advocate its use to determine vascular invasion [12]. A prospective study of 52 patients by Murugiah *et al.* [13•] concludes that selective visceral angiography is not an accurate means of predicting resectability (based on findings of encasement of major vessels or hepatic metastasis). Angiography predicted resectability or unresectability correctly only 61% of the time, prompting the authors to conclude that selective visceral angiography is not indicated for preoperative staging of pancreatic carcinoma.

Endoscopic ultrasonography for staging of pancreatic neoplasms was investigated by Yasuda *et al.* [7•]. For 29 patients, endoscopic ultrasonography was 79% accurate in detecting vascular invasion, which was found to be more accurate than other modalities.

Islet cell neoplasms

The magnetic resonance appearance of islet cell carcinomas in 33 patients was reported by Carlson *et al.* [14••]. The tumors were 21% nonfunctioning with the rest hormonally active. The mean size was 7.1 cm. On

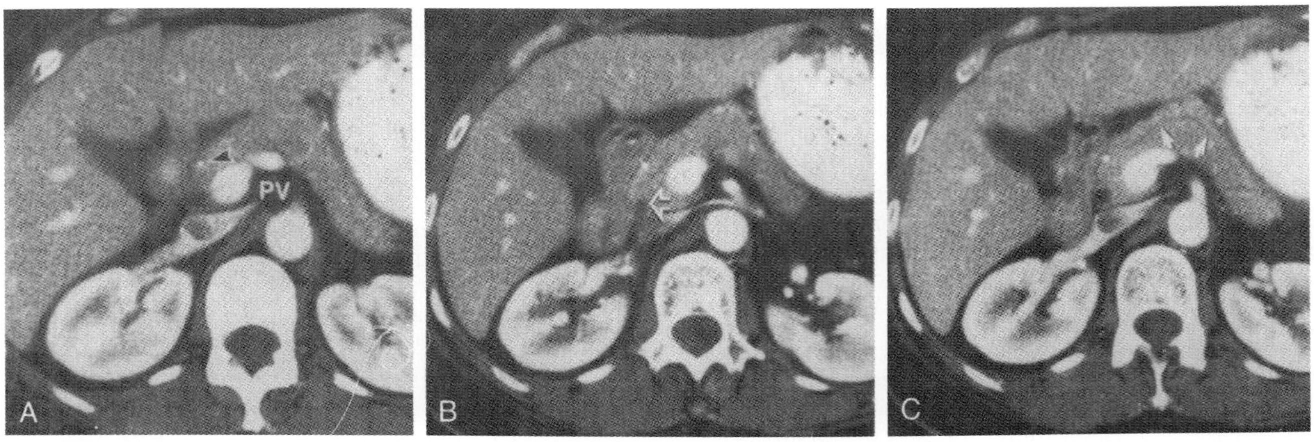

Fig. 2. Overlapping reconstruction at thinner slices using spiral computed tomography allows better visualization of smaller structures. **A,** Computed tomography section through the pancreas reveals normal glandular architecture, portal vein, and gastroduodenal artery (*arrowhead*). The pancreatic duct is not seen. **B,** Computed tomography scan (5 mm lower than in *panel A*) shows the common bile duct (*arrow*) in addition to the normal vessels. The pancreatic duct is not seen. **C,** Computed tomography section was retrospectively reconstructed 3 mm lower than in *panel A* (between those in *panels A* and *B*). This section shows similar anatomy, but unlike the sections reconstructed with 5-mm spacing, it also demonstrates the normal pancreatic duct (*arrows*). (*From* Zeman *et al.* [6••]; with permission.)

T_1-weighted imaging, the signal intensity was equal to or lower than that of the adjacent pancreas. On T_2-weighted imaging, 86% had the same or higher intensity than fat; mixed signal was seen in the remaining three lesions. Metastases generally mimicked the primary pancreatic tumor in appearance.

With effective medical management to control gastric hypersecretion of patients with Zollinger-Ellison syndrome, the malignant nature of the disease is becoming the primary determinant of long-term survival [15]. Investigators continue to examine the role of different surgical therapies in prolonging survival. Fishbeyn *et al.* [16••] have examined the data from 81 patients with Zollinger-Ellison syndrome who were treated with detailed exploration during surgery with removal of gastrinoma only. The authors questioned the role of imaging and laboratory data in determining freedom from disease. Disease-free was defined as improved symptoms, reduced acid output and antisecretory drug requirements, and normal imaging studies (computed tomography, ultrasound and magnetic resonance imaging). Follow-up was immediately after surgery, 6 months later, and yearly afterward. A total of 52% of patients were disease-free at immediate follow-up and 35% were at 5 years. All recurrences were detected by fasting serum gastrin levels and secretin provocative tests. No recurrences were detected by the imaging studies or calcium provocative test.

When the diagnosis of ectopic adrenocorticotrophic hormone syndrome is established, a search for a primary is undertaken. Doppman *et al.* [17•] question whether invasive studies such as pancreatic arteriography and portal venous sampling should be employed to exclude an occult islet cell tumor of the pancreas when laboratory and cross-sectional imaging studies fail to reveal a primary tumor. The authors studied 10 patients of theirs along with a literature review of 53 cases of adrenocorticotrophic hormone islet cell tumors. They found no occult islet cell tumor that was responsible for Cushing's syndrome. They conclude that in light of negative imaging studies, more invasive studies such as pancreatic arteriography and portal venous sampling are not necessary.

Cystic neoplasms

Cystic neoplasms of the pancreas range from being completely benign to aggressively malignant. Gazelle *et al.* [18••] analyzed images from endoscopic retrograde pancreatography in 38 patients with cystic pancreatic neoplasms to determine whether differentiation of benign from malignant lesions was possible. Twenty-three patients had histologically proven benign disease; 15 patients had frankly malignant lesions. Images were classified into four groups of findings: 1) normal, 2) narrowing or draping, 3) communicating with a cystic space, and 4) obstructing. The authors were not able to identify a group of findings that were reliable indicators of benign disease. The finding of obstruction, which was seen in 60% of malignant lesions, was considered virtually diagnostic of malignancy; one of the 23 patients with benign disease showed this finding.

Pancreatitis

Acute

The diagnosis of pancreatic necrosis on computed tomography is well established. However, opinions differ about appropriate treatment. In an excellent review about infection complicating acute pancreatitis, Widdison *et al.* [19••] recommend an aggressive approach. Computed tomography–guided fine-needle aspiration with gram stain and culture is recommended for areas of fluid collection and necrosis. Diagnosis of infection should lead to surgical intervention. Patients with sterile necrosis should be observed. Surgery is necessary in the face of deterioration despite intensive medical therapy.

An uncommon form of pancreatic necrosis is central cavitary necrosis (CCN). CCN is characterized by almost complete necrosis of pancreatic parenchyma with little or no peripancreatic necrosis. On contrast-enhanced computed tomography CCN appears as a well-defined

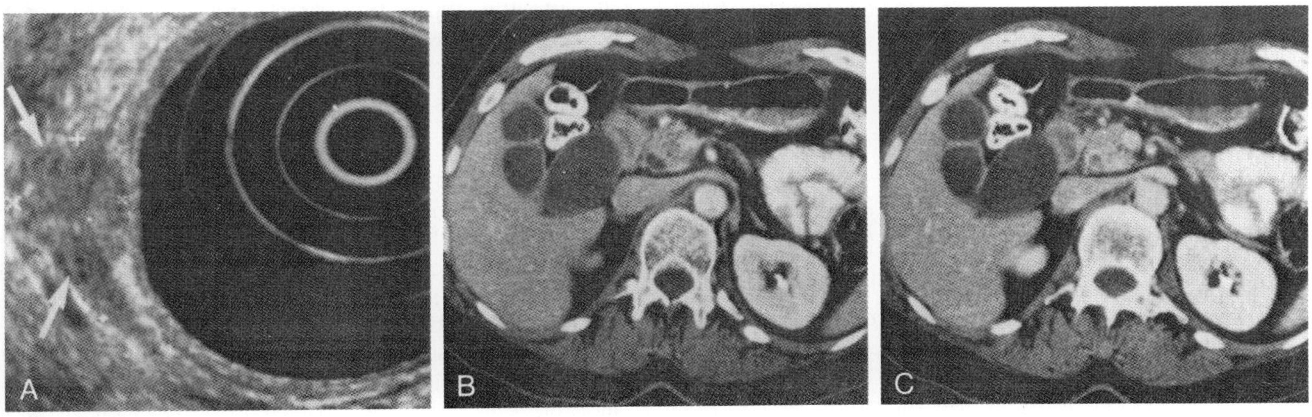

Fig. 3. T1 pancreatic adenocarcinoma. **A**, Endoscopic ultrasonographic scan demonstrates an inhomogenous hypoechoic tumor in the pancreatic head (*arrows*). The tumor is 2 cm in diameter. **B**, Computed tomographic scan shows dilatation of the gallbaldder and intrapancreatic common bile duct. **C**, Computed tomographic scan obtained adjacent to **panel B** shows the lumen of the common bile duct is abruptly diminished, without a discernible mass. (*From* Muller *et al.* [9•]; with permission).

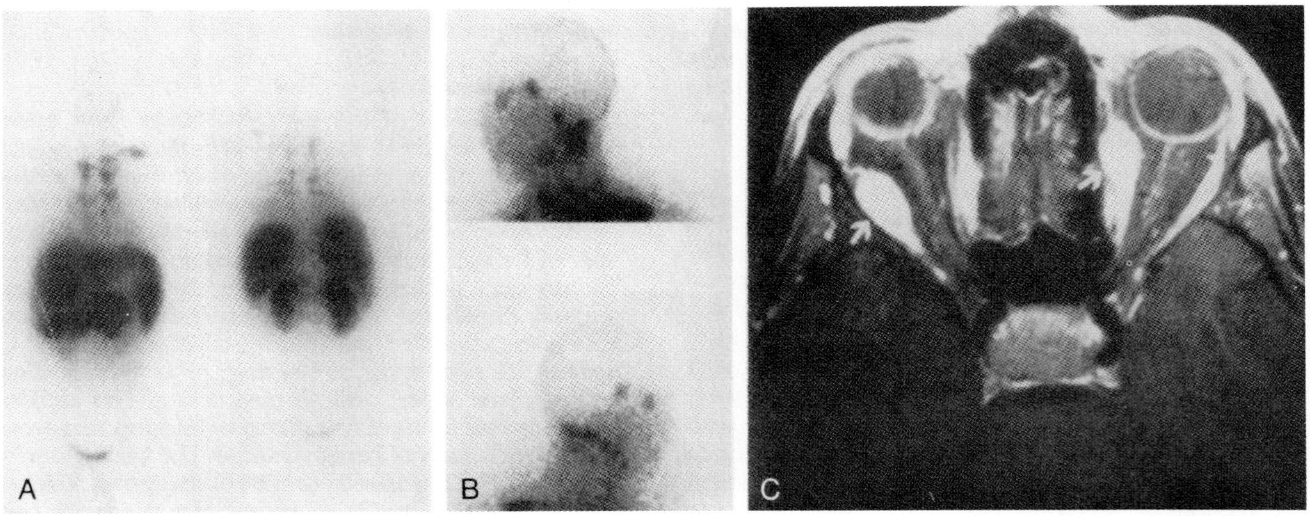

Fig. 4. A, Anterior (*left*) and posterior (*right*) whole-body scans obtained 2 hours after injection of I-123 octreotide demonstrate uptake in the pancreatic tumor and multiple areas of uptake in the mediastinum, both posterior cervical regions, and the head. **B,** Lateral spot views of I-123 octreotide activity seen retroorbitally and near the pituitary gland. Activity can also be seen in the cervical lymph nodes and in the left posterior auricular region. **C,** Magnetic resonance image of the head obtained with gadopentetate dimeglumine and fat-suppression techniques show small metastatic lesions involving the right lateral rectus and left medial rectus muscles. (*From* Kvols *et al.* [10•]; with permission.)

low-attenuation mass with convex borders, frequently conforming to the pancreatic contour [20]. The clinical features of CCN were looked at by Casey *et al.* [21•]. They report that in 10 patients with CCN, two developed infection and one died. These results were better than expected using standard clinical and radiologic scoring systems and the authors recommend medical treatment of patients with CCN in the absence of complications such as infection or unresolved pain.

Lewis *et al.* [22•] discuss 15 patients who developed pseudocysts following pancreatic trauma. None of the injuries were diagnosed during initial management. Endoscopic retrograde pancreatography was used to demonstrate the site of pancreatic duct injury in 11 of the patients. The authors found that pseudocysts following peripheral duct injury may resolve spontaneously, whereas those associated with proximal duct injuries require surgical intervention using resection or internal drainage. Distal duct injury can be treated by percutaneous aspiration or catheter drainage.

Chronic

Treatment of chronic calcific pancreatitis with extracorporeal shock wave lithotripsy (ESWL) was evaluated by van der Hul *et al.* [23••]. Seventeen patients were treated an average of 1.9 sessions. Thirteen (76%) of those treated had stone fragmentation and seven of the 13 had stone clearance. All patients with stone fragmentation experienced pain relief directly after ESWL. Patients with stone clearance remained free of pain at follow-up (6 to 41 months, median 22 months). Because of the good results and low mortality, the authors recommend ESWL as preferable to surgery for pain associated with chronic calcific pancreatitis.

Interventional radiology

There were a number of interesting observations in a 5-year review of 211 computed tomography–guided and 58 ultrasound-guided pancreatic biopsies on 251 patients performed at the Mayo Clinic [24••]. This study by Brandt *et al.* was a retrospective review of biopsies from 1985 to 1989. A total of 90% of the patients had a pancreatic malignancy, ductal adenocarcinoma being the predominant diagnosis (87% of the malignancies). The combined accuracy of computed tomography and ultrasonography biopsies in diagnosis of malignancy was 93% with computed tomography biopsy having an accuracy of 86% and ultrasonography guidance an accuracy of 95%. The average diameter of the lesions was 4.3 cm on computed tomography and 4.2 cm on ultrasonography and the authors postulate that the higher accuracy of ultrasonography was likely related to the continuous real time guidance of the needle into the hypoechoic mass. On computed tomography, the mass may become less obvious with intravenous contrast and continuous monitoring is not available. The possible selection bias that thinner patients with more accessible lesions were likely to have ultrasonography guided biopsy also was noted. Of interest is the fact that there were 66 documented needle passes through the gastrointestinal tract, including seven through the colon, with no evidence of adverse effect. In most cases a 21-gauge needle was used but in eight cases the needle was a larger 18 or 19 gauge. Minor complications included pain, vasovagal reaction, and small hemorrhage. The major complication rate was 1.1% and included two patients with adenocarcinoma who developed pancreatitis. The other major complication was a pancreatic duct leak necessitating emergency surgery.

Peter Mueller [25] in his editorial on the issue of pancreatic biopsy and the article by Brandt *et al.* [24••] comments that this is the largest series in the literature with the best results and that these results were obtained with more than 30 radiologists performing the biopsies. He commends the use of intravenous contrast in computed tomography–guided biopsies and notes that although it is accepted to traverse the bowel with small 21 gauge needles, the safety of this procedure with larger needles is not known. He also adds a word of caution about the potential of tumor spread by biopsy and noted that in a study by Warshaw [26] it was suggested that peritoneal washings were more likely to be positive in patients who underwent percutaneous biopsy than in patients with similar tumors who did not undergo biopsy. Based on this data, Warshaw argued for avoiding presurgical biopsy in patients in whom one is attempting surgical cure. Mueller [25] also points out that newer developments in fluid analysis of uncommon tumors may add more specificity to biopsy procedures.

An article by Lee *et al.* [27••] reviews the collective experience of computed tomography–guided celiac ganglion block at two medical centers. They injected 98% ethyl alcohol mixed with ether lidocaine to reduce pain or contrast to permit visualization. The results of a test block using long-acting anesthetic were difficult to evaluate and so its use was abandoned before injecting alcohol. The best results, 73% response, were seen in patients with malignant disease, particularly pancreatic and gastric carcinoma. It was about half as effective (37% response) in patients with benign disease. The transient severe hypotension that can result from loss of visceral and vascular tone and has been reported in up to 20% of patients did not occur in this series, although all patients were kept supine for 8 hours after the procedure because of the frequent occurrence of orthostatic hypotension.

Biopsy via the papilla during endoscopic retrograde cholangiopancreatography for patients with pancreaticobiliary ductal strictures seems a convenient technique and one that would eliminate the risk of intraperitoneal spread of tumor during the course of biopsy procedure. Its present limitation has been that stiff forceps have restricted its use. The authors describe an improved forceps for transpapillary tissue acquisition. They achieved successful tissue sampling in 41 of 43 patients (95%) without complications and had a diagnostic sensitivity of 88% for cholangiocarcinoma and 71% for pancreatic cancer [28••]. Because the overall sensitivity of brush cytology is considerably lower, use of these diagnostic forceps may considerably enhance the yield.

Anatomic considerations

Previous investigators have commented on a focal hypoechogenic appearance on ultrasound of the ventral aspect of the pancreatic head and have speculated that this may be due to uneven fat deposition [29]. Recognizing this normal variant is important so as not to mistake it with a pathologic process. To define the nature of this focal hypoechogenicity Atri *et al.* [30•] studied the ultrasonographic and histopathologic findings in 13 pancreatic autopsy specimens. The patients died from causes unrelated to pancreatic disease. They found that hypoechogenicity on ultrasound corresponded to focal fatty sparing. They suggest that differentiation from a pathologic process can be made because the hypoechoic zone is confined to the distribution of the embryologic ventral pancreas on transverse and sagittal views. Also the normal triangular appearance of the uncinate process and identification of normal pancreatic and common bile ducts help in differentiation from pathology. This normal variant of focal fatty sparing was also examined by Jacobs *et al.* [31•]. They reported ultrasonography, computed tomography, and magnetic resonance imaging findings in seven patients with focal fatty sparing and note that areas of focal fatty sparing are hyperdense on computed tomography (as opposed to the hypodense mass typically seen in adenocarcinoma). In addition, uniform contrast enhancement was seen on magnetic resonance imaging.

In computed tomography staging of pancreatic carcinoma, invasion of larger peripancreatic vessels is evaluated [11]. Crabo *et al.* [32•] investigated the efficacy of evaluating the smaller pancreaticoduodenal veins. The authors studied the appearance of the four pancreaticoduodenal veins on computed tomography scans of four cadavers in which the portal veins were injected with radiopaque solutions. After definition of the anatomy in the cadaveric specimens, dynamic bolus contrast abdominal computed tomography scans of 100 patients who had no evidence of pancreatic disease were analyzed. The anterior and posterior superior pancreaticoduodenal were seen on 98% and 88% of the scans respectively. The inferior pancreaticoduodenal veins were not definitely identified. The authors conclude that assessment of these veins may be useful in the staging of pancreatic carcinoma.

References and recommended reading

Papers of particular interest, published within the annual period of review, have been highlighted as:

- • Of special interest
- •• Of outstanding interest

1. Mitchell DG, Shapiro M, Schuricht A, Barbot D, Rosatto F: **Pancreatic Disease: Findings on State-of-the-Art MR Images.** *AJR Am J Roentgenol* 1992, **159**:533–538.
2. Semelka RC, Kroeker MA, Shoenut JP, Kroeker R, Yaffe CS, Micflikier AB: **Pancreatic Disease: Prospective Comparison of CT, ERCP, and 1.5-T MR Imaging with Dynamic Gadolinium Enhancement and Fat Suppression.** *Radiology* 1991, **181**:785–791.
3. Gehl HB, Vorwerk D, Klose KC, Gunther RW: **Pancreatic Enhancement After Low-Dose Infusion of Mn-DPDP.** *Radiology* 1991, **180**:337–339.
4. • Bach-Gansmo T, Dupas B, Gayet-Delacroix M, Lambrechts M: **Abdominal MRI Using a Negative Contrast Agent.** *Br J Radiol* 1993, **66**:420–425.

This paper examines oral contrast in improving diagnostic accuracy of magnetic resonance in a variety of pathologic conditions.

5. •• Zeman RK, Fox SH, Silverman PM, Davros WJ, Carter LM, Griego D, Weltman DI, Ascher AM, Cooper CJ: **Helical (Spiral) CT of the Abdomen.** *AJR Am J Roentgenol* 1993, **160**:719–725.

This paper gives an overview of helical computed tomography of the abdomen, including technical principles and initial clinical experience.

6. •• Zeman RK, Zeiberg AS, Davros WJ, Ascher SM, Cooper CJ, Weltman DI, Patt R, Garra BS, Griego DL, Silverman PM: **Routine Helical**

CT of the Abdomen: Image Quality Considerations. *Radiology* 1993, **189**:395–400.
This paper compares the image quality of helical and nonhelical abdominal computed tomography scans. The authors conclude that helical computed tomography is preferred to routine abdominal computed tomography images.

7. Yasuda K, Mukai H, Nakajima M, Kawai K: **Staging of Pancreatic Carcinoma by Endoscopic Ultrasonography.** *Endoscopy* 1993, **25**:290–293.
•
Favorable experience of staging pancreatic neoplasms using endoscopic ultrasonography is reported.

8. Palazzo L, Roseau G, Gayet B, Vilgrain V, Belghiti J, Fekete F, Paolaggi JA: **Endoscopic Ultrasonography in the Diagnosis and Staging of Pancreatic Adenocarcinoma: Results of a Prospective Study With Comparison to Ultrasonography and CT Scan.** *Endoscopy* 1993, **25**:143–150.
••
Endoscopic ultrasonography is compared favorably to computed tomography and conventional ultrasound. Examples of detection of tumors less than 25 mm are illustrated.

9. Muller MF, Meyenberger C, Bertschinger P, Schaer R, Marincek B: **Pancreatic Tumors: Evaluation With Endoscopic US, CT, and MR Imaging.** *Radiology* 1994, **190**:745–751.
•
Forty-nine patients with clinical suspicion of pancreatic carcinoma were evaluated with endoscopic ultrasonography, computed tomography, and magnetic resonance imaging. Endoscopic ultrasound was more accurate in the diagnosis of pancreatic tumor than computed tomography or magnetic resonance, especially for tumors less than 3 cm.

10. Kvols LK, Brown ML, OConnor MK, Hung JC, Reubi JC, Lamberts SWJ: **Evaluation of a Radiolabeled Somatostatic Analog (I-123 Octreotide) in the Detection and Localization of Carcinoid and Islet Cell Tumors.** *Radiology* 1993, **187**:129–133.
•
The usefulness of radiolabeled 123 ocreotide is evaluated in the detection of known carcinoid and islet cell tumors.

11. Freeny PC, Marks WM, Ryan JA, Traverso LW: **Pancreatic Ductal Adenocarcinoma: Diagnosis and Staging With Dynamic CT.** *Radiology* 1988, **166**:125–134.

12. Brambs HJ, Claussen CD: **Pancreatic and Ampullary Cancer: Ultrasound, Computed Tomography, Magnetic Resonance Imaging and Angiography.** *Endoscopy* 1993, **25**:58–68.

13. Murugiah M, Windsor JA, Redhead DN, Oneill JS, Suc B, Garden OJ, Carter DC: **The Role of Selective Visceral Angiography in the Management of Pancreatic and Periampullary Cancer.** *World J Surg* 1993, **17**:796–800.
•
A prospective study evaluating the accuracy of visceral angiography in assessing the resectability of pancreatic and periampullary cancer. The authors conclude that angiography is not useful for staging pancreatic and periampullary cancer.

14. Carlson B, Johnson CD, Stephens DH, Ward EM, Kvols LK: **MRI of Pancreatic Islet Cell Carcinoma.** *J Comput Assist Tomogr* 1993, **17**:735–740.
••
The authors report their magnetic resonance imaging findings in 33 patients with islet cell tumor.

15. Andersen DK: **Current Diagnosis and Management of Zollinger-Ellison Syndrome.** *Ann Surg* 1989, **210**:685–703.

16. Fishbeyn VA, Norton JA, Benya RV, Pisegna JR, Venson DJ, Metz DC, Jenson RT: **Assessment and Prediction of Long-Term Cure in Patients With the Zollinger-Ellison Syndrome: The Best Approach.** *Ann Intern Med* 1993, **119**:199–206.
••
Laboratory and imaging data is used to follow disease-free states in 81 patients with Zollinger-Ellison syndrome treated with surgical exploration and gastrinoma resection.

17. Doppman JL, Nieman LK, Cutler GB Jr, Chrousos GO, Fraker DL, Norton JA, Jensen RT: **Adrenocoticotropic Hormone-Secreting Islet Cell Tumors: Are They Always Malignant?** *Radiology* 1994, **190**:59–64.
•
A total of 63 cases of islet cell tumors producing ectopic adrenocorticotropic hormone were reviewed and it was found that none were occult tumors.

18. Gazelle GS, Mueller PR, Raafat N, Halpem EF, Cardenosa G, Warshaw AL: **Cystic Neoplasms of the Pancreas: Evaluation With Endoscopic Retrograde Pancreatography.** *Radiology* 1993, **188**:633–636.
••
Endoscopic retrograde pancreatography images were analyzed to see if characteristics could be found to distinguish benign from malignant neoplasms. The finding of obstruction was correlated with malignancy.

19. Widdison AL, Karanjia ND: **Pancreatic Infection Complicating Acute Pancreatitis.** *Br J Surg* 1993, **80**:148–154.
••
An excellent review recommending medical management for sterile necrosis in pancreatitis, with surgery reserved for infection.

20. Burrell M, Gold JA, Simeone J, Taylor K, Dobbins J: **Liquefactive Necrosis of the Pancreas.** *Radiology* 1980, **135**:157–160.

21. Casey JE, Porter KA, Langevin RE, Banks PA: **Clinical Features and Natural History of Central Cavitary Necrosis.** *Pancreas* 1993, **8**:141–145.
•
Features of 10 patients with central cavitary necrosis are examined and in the absence of complications, medical treatment is recommended.

22. Lewis G, Krige JEJ, Bomman PC, Terblanche J: **Traumatic Pancreatic Pseudocysts.** *Br J Surg* 1993, **80**:89–93.
•
Fifteen patients with traumatic psuedocysts are evaluated to determine outcome in relation to nature and site of pancreatic duct injury.

23. van der Hul RL, Plaisier PW, Terpstra OT, Bruining HA: **Role of Extracorporeal Shock Wave Lithotripsy in Hepato-Biliary-Pancreatic Surgery.** *World J Surg* 1993, 17:647–652.
••
Extracorporeal shock wave lithotripsy is evaluated for the treatment of calcific chronic pancreatitis and found to be preferable to surgery.

24. Brandt KR, Stephens DH, Welch TJ, Goellner JR: **CT-Guided and US-Guided Biopsy of the Pancreas.** *Radiology* 1993, **187**:99–104.
••
A retrospective review of 211 computed tomography– and ultrasonography-guided biopsies of pancreatic lesions is provided. High accuracy and low complications were found.

25. Mueller PR: **Pancreatic Biopsy: Striving for Excellence.** *Radiology* 1993, **187**:15–16.

26. Warshaw AL: **Implications of Peritoneal Cytology for Staging of Early Pancreatic Cancer.** *Am J Surg* 1991, **161**:26–30.

27. Lee MJ, Mueller PR, Vansonnenberg E, Dawson SL, Dagostino H, Saini S, Cats AM: **CT-Guided Celiac Ganglion Block With Alcohol.** *AJR Am J Roentgenol* 1993, **161**:633–636.
••
Experience with computed tomography–guided celiac ganglion block is examined; results are best with patients with malignant disease.

28. Kubota Y, Takaoka M, Tani K, Ogura M, Kin H, Fujimura K, Mizuno T, Inoue K: **Endoscopic Transpapillary Biopsy for Diagnosis of Patients With Pancreaticobiliary Ductal Strictures.** *Am J Gastroenterol* 1993, **88**:1700–1704.
••
An improved technique for transpapillary biopsy with flexible forceps is described. The authors demonstrate higher sensitivity for diagnosing cholangiocarcinoma and pancreatic carcinoma than that found with brush biopsy.

29. Donald JJ, Shorvon PJ, Lees WR: **A Hypoechoic Area Within the Head of the Pancreas: A Normal Variant.** *Clin Radiol* 1992, **41**:337–338.

30. Atri M, Nazarnia A, Mehio A, Reinhold C, Bret PM: **Hypoechogenic Embryologic Ventral Aspect of the Head and Uncinate Process of the Pancreas: In Vitro Correlation of US With Histopathologic Findings.** *Radiology* 1994, **190**:441–444.
•
Ultrasound and histology of pancreatic autopsy specimens are compared to establish that hypoechogenicity of the ventral aspect of the head of the pancreas is due to diminished fat content.

31. Jacobs JE, Coleman BG, Arger PH, Langer JE: **Pancreatic Sparing of Focal Fatty Infiltration.** *Radiology* 1994, **190**:437–440.
•
Computed tomography, magnetic resonance imaging, and ultrasonography findings, with illustrative examples, are described for fatty focal sparing of the head of the pancreas.

32. Crabo LG, Conley DM, Graney DO, Graney PC: **Venous Anatomy of the Pancreatic Head: Normal CT Appearance of Cadavers and Patients.** *AJR Am J Roentgenol* 1993, **160**:1039–1045.
•
The authors define the venous anatomy in cadaveric specimens injected with radioplaque solution. The frequency with which these vessels are seen in normal dynamic computed tomography scans is then assessed.

Gary D. Leavitt, MD, and Morton I. Burrell, MD, Department of Diagnostic Radiology, Yale University School of Medicine, 2-212, 333 Cedar Street, New Haven, CT 06510, USA.

Cholesterol gallstone disease: from pathogenesis to prevention

Commentary

J. Thomas LaMont, MD, and Nezam H. Afdhal, MD

Boston University School of Medicine, Boston, Massachusetts, USA

Current Opinion in Gastroenterology 1994, **10**:523–525

Gallstone disease is currently one of the most common and costly of all digestive diseases in the United States affecting 30 million Americans and costing in excess of $5 billion [1]. In Western societies, cholesterol gallstones account for the majority (>75%) of gallstones. The conventional wisdom has been to ignore gallstones until they become symptomatic and then to offer cholecystectomy as the standard treatment. With the advent of laparascopic cholecystectomy in the past 5 years, many physicians now opt for laparascopic cholecystectomy as the treatment of choice for permanent cure. When compared with the traditional open cholecystectomy, laparascopic cholecystectomy results in a shorter hospital stay with both decreased patient pain and an earlier return to work. However, this has not translated into a financial net gain to society because the immediate savings of this less invasive procedure have been offset by the greater than 20% increase in numbers of cholecystectomies performed [2]. Advances in understanding both the pathogenesis, natural history, and epidemiology of gallstones, as illustrated in this issue of *Current Opinion in Gastroenterology*, hold great promise for the prevention and treatment of gallstones. In this editorial we will highlight how advances in our understanding of gallstone formation can even now lead to studies to analyze the cost-benefit ratio of gallstone prevention in epidemiologically identified high-risk patient groups.

Cholesterol gallstone formation requires three simultaneous defects: 1) secretion of cholesterol supersaturated bile by the liver, 2) nucleation of cholesterol monohydrate crystals, and 3) stasis of gallbladder contents probably in a viscous mucus gel to allow crystal growth and gallstone formation. A unifying concept of gallstone formation is shown in Figure 1 and the available pharmacotherapeutic agents with their sites of action are listed in Table 1. However before we advocate any preventative therapy, we should first identify those groups of patients at highest risk and define the goals of prevention. Primary prevention of gallstones implies prevention of their formation and is the focus of this editorial. However, gallstone disease is so prevalent and only 1% to 2% of patients become symptomatic each year there is also the option of secondary prevention, which would focus on preventing symptoms or complications in patients with asymptomatic gallstones. Primary prevention can be achieved by both lifestyle modification and pharmacotherapy, whereas secondary prevention is predominantly dependent on the latter.

An increase in the risk of cholesterol gallstone formation is associated with multiple conditions (Table 2). Cholesterol supersaturation of bile is a prerequisite for gallstone formation and the majority of Americans even without gallstones will have nocturnal or fasting supersaturation of bile with cholesterol. The two major sources of cholesterol in the hepatocyte are from dietary lipoproteins or *de novo* synthesis. Together these two sources create a pool of "free" cholesterol within the hepatocyte that is closely regulated with any excess cholesterol either being converted into bile salts or lipoproteins or else excreted in bile as unesterified cholesterol. Studies on this "free" cholesterol pool in the hepatocyte have shown that it is predominantly dietary cholesterol derived from lipoproteins that is secreted into hepatic bile [3]. Thus, a reduction in dietary cholesterol should lead to a decrease in saturation of bile. Therefore, in countries such as Japan where a diet low in saturated fats is the norm, the incidence of gallstone disease is much reduced.

Decreased biliary cholesterol can be achieved by reducing cholesterol intake and by increasing dietary fiber. There is good evidence to suggest that increased dietary fiber not only decreases fat absorption but it also increases intestinal transit time resulting in a decrease in deoxycholate [4,5], an important potentially lithogenic bile salt. In addition to a high-fiber, low-cholesterol diet we should also take into account dietary factors that influence gallbladder emptying. Prolonged stasis of biliary contents results in formation of concentrated lithogenic bile and this is seen even during fasting in normal subjects. Therefore, regular meals three times a day will also help keep the gallbladder empty and at least one of the meals, probably break-

 ISBN 1-85922-610-8 ISSN 0267–1379

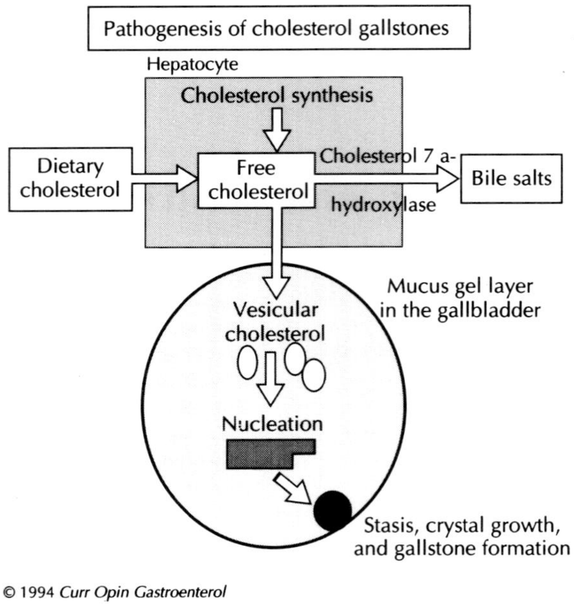

Fig. 1. Pathogenesis of cholesterol gallstones. The intrahepatic free cholesterol pool is contributed to by dietary cholesterol from lipoproteins and newly synthesized cholesterol. This pool is kept relatively constant by cholesterol secretion into bile as either bile salts or as free unesterified cholesterol. This cholesterol supersaturation of bile results in vesicular cholesterol nucleating into crystals within the gallbladder gel, which lead to stasis and growth of crystals into mature gallstones.

fast, should contain adequate fat (12 g) in the form of either cheese or butter, to ensure full emptying of the gallbladder after the overnight fast. Finally, increase in exercise will also improve both the cholesterol secretion in bile and may improve gallbladder emptying. These simple behavior and dietary modifications would be much more cost effective than either pharmacotherapy or cholecystectomy in prevention of gallstone disease but are much more difficult to implement in a society hooked on fat-laden snacks and fast food.

Two groups of patients are at high risk for gallstone formation for only brief periods of time: obese patients undergoing rapid weight reduction and women during the 3rd trimester of pregnancy and the puerperium. Obese patients during periods of weight loss on low calorie diets have an increase in gallbladder mucin and gallbladder hypomotility [6], resulting in a 25% incidence of gallstones [7]. Interestingly, the incidence of symptomatic gallstones is increased from a baseline of 1% to 2% per year up to 50% in this group resulting in significant clinical morbidity. Intervention with pharmacotherapy in this group during weight reduction may be both cost effective and clinically indicated. Several trials of ursodeoxycholic acid from 600 to 1200 mg/d have reported that this therapy almost completely abolishes gallstone formation in the obese patient during periods of low calorie dieting and weight reduction [8,9]. Other agents such as aspirin, nonsteroidal anti-inflammatory drugs and promotility agents such as cisapride or cholecystokinin analogues may also have a role in this situation. Because the clinical efficacy of ursodeoxycholic acid is proven, this can be recommended as a standard therapy for gallstone prevention in the obese while we await clinical data from trials on other potential antilithogenic agents.

Multiparity has always been associated with gallstone formation, probably through the effect of progesterones on diminishing gallbladder motility and an increase in cholesterol supersaturation of bile secondary to increased cholesterol synthesis [10]. Recent epidemiologic studies using ultrasonography during pregnancy have further defined the risks of gallstone formation [11,12]. In the 3rd trimester of pregnancy, up to 30% of women develop biliary sludge and a third of these patients will ultimately develop gallstones. In the remaining 60% of patients, sludge and small stones disappear during the puerperium, probably secondary to improvement in gallbladder emptying with ejection of this material through the cystic duct. Symptomatic gallstone disease in pregnancy correlates strongly to those patients with stones rather than sludge alone. Therefore, with each pregnancy up to 10% of women may develop gallstones and women who are overweight or have recently been dieting appear at increased risk of developing gallstones [13]. If epidemiologic studies could better define those at high risk for cholelithiasis during pregnancy, then the use of ursodeoxycholic acid, nonsteroidal anti-inflammatory drugs, antimucolytics, and prokinetic agents in controlled trials could be advocated in these patients. Again, therapy would be for a short, cost-effective period of time and

Table 1. Potential pharmacotherapeutic agents for gallstone prevention

Pharmacological agent	Action
Ursodeoxycholic acid	Decrease cholesterol supersaturation of bile. Stabilize vesicular cholesterol to decrease nucleation time.
Aspirin, NSAIDs	Decrease mucin synthesis, possibly prokinetic.
Fish oils, ω-3 fatty acids	Donate long-chain, unsaturated phospholipids to bile. Act as potential antinucleating agents.
Cholecystokinin agonists, cisapride, macrolides	Increase gallbladder emptying via pro-motility agents.
Future agents	Retard nucleation by phase transition inhibitors. Increase bile salt synthesis using up-regulators of cholesterol 7α-hydroxylase.
	Decrease bile viscosity and promote gel expulsion with antimucolytic agents.

NSAID—nonsteroidal anti-inflammatory drug.

all the above agents should be safe and nonteratogenic in the 3rd trimester of pregnancy.

Table 2. Risk factors for cholesterol cholelithiasis

Age
Female sex
Obesity and rapid weight loss in the obese
Pregnancy, estrogen therapy
Ethnic background (Pima Indians)
Ileal resection, jejunoileal bypass
Medications (clofibrate, octreotide)
Gallbladder dysmotility (diabetes, post vagotomy)
Spinal cord injury

The incidence of gallstone disease can be likened to the ocean in the Nordic fable of King Canute. The old King was master of his realm and believed he could control anything he wished. One day he went down to the beach to order the ocean to turn back from his commands. Unfortunately the tide continued to come in and the old king drowned. Unlike King Canute, our understanding of gallstone pathogenesis and epidemiology places us in a better position to stem the tide of gallstone formation. The physician today need not take such an expectant role in gallstone disease and merely wait for symptoms of disease to develop. The time has come to encourage educational initiatives into diet and exercise to prevent gallstone formation. The use of selective short term pharmacotherapy in high risk patients should become one of the focus points for prevention of gallstones in the new millenium.

Acknowledgment

This work was supported by NIH grant DK 45936 to NA.

References

1. Everhart JE: **Digestive Diseases in the United States.** *Epidemiology and Impact NIH, NIDDK Publication No: 94-1447,* 1994.
2. Steiner CA, Bass EB, Talamini MA, Pitt HA, Steinberg EP: **Surgical Rates and Operative Mortality for Open and Laparascopic Cholectomy.** *N Engl J Med* 1994, **330**:403–408.
3. Robins SJ, Fasulo JM, Collins MA: **Evidence of Separate Pathways of Transport of Newly Synthesized and Preformed Cholesterol Into Bile.** *J Biol Chem* 1985, **260**:6511–6518.
4. Marcus SN, Heaton KW: **Deoxycholic Acid and the Pathogenesis of Gallstones.** *Gut* 1988, **29**:522–533.
5. Carey MC, LaMont JT: **Cholesterol Gallstone Formation.** In *Progress in Liver Disease, Vol X.* Edited by Boyer JL, Ockner RK. Philadelphia:W.B. Saunders; 1993: 139–192.
6. Shiffman ML, Sugerman HJ, Kellum JM, Moore EW: **Changes in Gallbladder Bile Composition Following Gallstone Formation and Weight Reduction.** *Gastroenterology* 1992, **103**:214–221.
7. Everhart JE: **Contributions of Obesity and Weight Loss to Gallstone Disease.** *Ann Intern Med* 1993, **119**:1029–1035.
8. Broomfield PH, Chopra R, Sheinbaum RC, Bonorris CG, Silverman A, Schoenfeld LJ, Marks JW: **Effects of Ursodeoxycholic Acid and Aspirin on the Formation of Lithogenic Bile and Gallstones During Loss of Weight.** *N Engl J Med* 1988, **319**:1567–1572.
9. Shiffman ML, *et al.*: **A Multi-Center, Double-Blind, Placebo Controlled Trial of Ursodeoxycholic Acid for Prevention of Gallstone Formation in Obese Patients During Very Low Calorie Diet Induced Weight Reduction [Abstract].** *Gastroenterology* 1994, **106**:A982.
10. Everson GT: **Gallstones and Pregnancy.** *Hepatology* 1993, **17**:159–161.
11. Valdivieso V, Covarrubias C, Siegel F, Cruz F: **Pregnancy and Cholelithiasis: Pathogenesis and Natural Course of Gallstones Diagnosed in the Early Puerperium.** *Hepatology* 1993, **17**:1–4.
12. Maringhini A, Ciambra M, Baccelliere P, Raimondo M, Orlando A, Tine F, Grasso R, Randazzo MA, Barresi L, Gullo D, *et al.*: **Biliary Sludge and Gallstones in Pregnancy: Incidence, Risk Factors and Natural History.** *Ann Intern Med* 1993, **119**:116–120.
13. Basso L, McCollum PT, Darling MR, Tocchi A, Tanner WA: **A Descriptive Study of Pregnant Women With Gallstones: Relation to Dietary and Social Habits, Education, Physical Activity, Height and Weight.** *Eur J Epidemiol* 1992, **8**:629–633.

J. Thomas LaMont, MD, and Nezam H. Afdhal, MD, University Hospital 82 E. Newton Street, Boston, MA 02118, USA.

Pathobiology of biliary epithelia

Stuart K. Roberts, MD, and Nicholas F. LaRusso, MD

Mayo Medical School, Clinic, and Foundation, Rochester, Minnesota, USA

Recently, principally owing to the development of suitable experimental models, significant advances have been made in our understanding of the biological and pathobiological importance of intrahepatic biliary epithelial cells, or cholangiocytes. These advances include 1) the development of techniques to isolate and culture rodent and human cholangiocytes; 2) an appreciation of the mechanisms by which cholangiocytes contribute to bile formation via hormone-stimulated secretion of ions and water; and 3) a recognition that cholangiocytes are candidate target cells in several important chronic liver diseases. In this review, we first discuss the experimental models recently developed to study biliary epithelia then detail current concepts on the cellular mechanisms of hormone-induced ductal bile secretion. We then briefly summarize selected information on the pathophysiology of bile duct injury, emphasizing those liver diseases in which cholangiocytes appear to be the principal targets for immune-mediated destruction.

Current Opinion in Gastroenterology 1994, **10**:526–533

Cholangiocytes (*ie*, the epithelial cells that line the bile ductules and ducts inside the liver) account for about 3% of the total liver cell population [1,2] and form a three-dimensional network of interconnecting tributaries, termed the *intrahepatic biliary ductal system*, that extends from the canals of Hering to the porta hepatis. This system of progressively larger conduits includes ductules, interlobular and septal ducts (*ie*, the smallest ducts accompanied by branches of the hepatic artery), and segmental ducts [3]. Although it has been suspected for some time that cholangiocytes are important in modifying primary bile secreted by hepatocytes, efforts to delineate the functions of cholangiocytes have been hindered by a lack of suitable experimental models. However, the recent development of techniques to isolate and culture pure cholangiocytes from rodents and humans, and the availability of *in vivo* experimental models have led to significant advances in our understanding of cholangiocyte biology. These advances include the recognition that cholangiocytes 1) play an essential role in hormone-induced ductal bile secretion and 2) are candidate target cells in several immune-mediated liver diseases. This paper discusses the recent advances that have occurred in the rapidly evolving field of cholangiocyte biology.

Experimental models

The latest development of *in vitro* models of biliary epithelia including isolated bile ducts, isolated cholangiocytes, and primary cultures of cholangiocytes, has led to significant advances in our understanding of cholangiocyte biology. Recently, we developed a procedure for the isolation of intact, polarized intrahepatic bile duct units from normal rats that involves enzymatic digestion and microdissection [4•]. After isolation, rodent bile duct units retain their *in situ* morphology, polarity and cholangiocyte-specific phenotypes. Bile duct units appear as intact ducts with a lumen enclosed by a single layer of epithelial cells and a thin layer of connective tissue (Fig. 1*A* and 1*B*). Using this experimental model, we reported the direct demonstration of agonist-stimulated ductular HCO_3^- secretion [4•] Others have also isolated intrahepatic bile ducts by similar methods and have applied this model to study other ductal transport processes (*eg*, secretin-induced H^+ secretion or tubulovesicular transcytosis) [5•,6]. Most likely, this model will be increasingly used to study the physiology of intrahepatic bile ducts.

The isolation of purified cholangiocytes from normal rat liver has presented a technical challenge because of their low total number and the overlap of their physical properties (*ie*, size and density) with other liver cells. Nevertheless, several groups have recently reported isolating cholangiocyte-enriched cell populations from normal rat liver using several different separatory approaches, including isopycnic centrifugation [7, 8] and counterflow elutriation [9,10,11•]; the low degree of cholangiocyte purity achieved (*ie*, 20% to 68% from a normal rat) highlighted the limitation of these efforts. Alvaro *et al.* [11•] reported that overnight culture of such preparations increases cholangiocyte purity to 80%. Our group reported an alternative ap-

Abbreviations

CFTR—cystic fibrosis transmembrane conductance regulator; **CHIP**—channel-forming integral membrane protein of 28 kD; **ICAM**—intercellular adhesion molecule; **MHC**—major histocompatibility complex; **NSDC**—nonsuppurative destructive cholangitis; **PBC**—primary biliary cirrhosis; **PDC**—pyruvate dehydrogenase complex; **PSC**—primary sclerosing cholangitis.

 ISBN 1-85922-610-8 ISSN 0267–1379

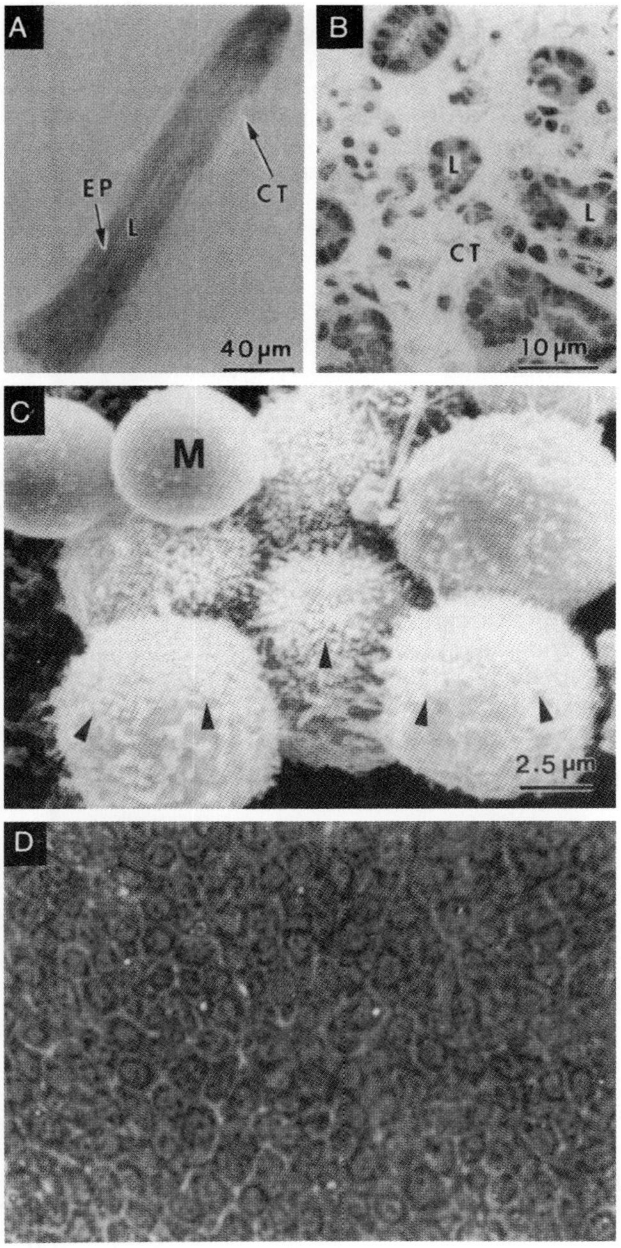

Fig. 1. Experimental *in vitro* models of biliary epithelia. **A,B**, Light micrographs of freshly isolated bile duct units showing structural morphology in an unstained whole-mount preparation (*panel A*) and in 1-μm cross-sections stained with methylene blue (*panel B*). L—lumen; EP—epithelial cells; CT—connective tissue. (*From* Roberts *et al.* [4•]; with permission). **C**, Scanning electron micrograph of a group of isolated cholangiocytes after separation using immunomagnetic beads (M). Note the prominent microvilli (*arrowheads*) are limited to one side of the cells. (*From* Ishii *et al.* [12]; with permission). **D**, Phase contrast micrograph of a primary, confluent, monolayer culture of cholangiocytes 2 weeks after establishment demonstrating uniform epithelial morphology; original magnification x 500. (*From* Yang *et al.* [17••]; with permission).

proach involving immunoaffinity separation of cholangiocytes using a monoclonal antibody to a cholangiocyte surface component [12]. Using this technique, we consistently obtain 1 to 2×10^6 cholangiocytes from a normal rat liver that are pure 95% or more by specific markers and retain their morphologic polarity for a short term (Fig. 1*C*). A similar approach has also been used to separate cholangiocytes from human liver [13].

The development of long-term, primary cultures of cholangiocytes has provided another valuable tool with which to study cholangiocyte biology. Joplin *et al.* [13] reported culturing immunoaffinity-purified human cholangiocytes for up to 1 month using fibroblasts as a feeder layer; others have established primary monolayer cultures of cholangiocytes from humans [14] and rodents [15,16,17••] when plated on a suitable extracellular matrix substitute (*eg,* Matrigel; Collaborative Res., Lexington). Alternatively, Yang *et al.* [17••] reported the establishment of long-term, confluent, monolayer cultures of normal rat cholangiocytes using isolated segments of bile ducts as starting material that retain both morphologic polarity and cholangiocyte-specific phenotypes (Fig. 1*D*).

Several groups, including our own, have established primary cultures of human gallbladder epithelial cells [18,19•,20•]. Auth *et al.* [19•] recently reported that interferon-γ stimulates the expression of major histocompatibility complex (MHC) class II on human gall bladder epithelial cells in long-term primary culture [19•]. Similarly, we found that interferon-γ induces the expression of functional MHC class II protein on cultured rodent cholangiocytes, permitting cholangiocytes to behave as antigen-presenting cells [21•]. Both these *in vitro* models may represent important tools to investigate the interactions of biliary epithelia with the immune system.

Several carcinoma cell lines of human biliary epithelial origin have now been developed and characterized [22–25]. Many of these cell lines, in addition to being relatively easy to culture, retain specific cholangiocyte and epithelial phenotypes [23,24,26•]. These cell lines have already proven extremely useful for studying cholangiocyte biology, including ion secretion [26•] and cell secretory products (*eg,* membrane glycoproteins [22], growth factors [22], and tumor-associated proteins [23]).

Mechanisms of ductal bile secretion

Cholangiocytes play an important role in bile formation by modifying canalicular bile through the spontaneous and hormone-stimulated transport of both ions and water [27••]. Direct evidence for this concept comes from recent *in vivo* studies in rats with experimentally induced ductal hyperplasia showing that an increase in the number of cholangiocytes is associated with a massive increase in both spontaneous and secretin-stimulated bile flow [2,28]. Furthermore, the invariable increase in biliary HCO_3^- secretion, associated with secretin-stimulated choleresis [1,2,28], suggests that ductal HCO_3^- transport is closely linked to ductal water secretion.

Although the cellular mechanisms regulating ductal bile secretion are still unclear, several recent *in vitro* studies using the new experimental models described above have provided considerable mechanistic insight.

These findings include the following 1) the identification of the cystic fibrosis transmembrane conductance regulator (CFTR), a cyclic AMP–activated Cl^- channel, in cholangiocytes at the functional, gene, and protein level [29,30•]; 2) the immunohistochemical localization of CFTR to the apical region of human cholangiocytes [30•]; and 3) the functional identification of a Cl^-/HCO_3^- exchanger in rodent cholangiocytes [11•,31] and the demonstration that secretin stimulates the activity of this exchanger, probably via the activation of cyclic AMP-activated Cl^- channels [11•]. Additionally, other studies have shown the presence of secretin receptors on cholangiocyte plasma membranes [32] as well as demonstrating that secretin stimulates exocytosis in isolated cholangiocytes via a cyclic AMP-mediated mechanism [33].

Based on a growing body of evidence, it thus appears that secretin likely stimulates ductal HCO_3^- secretion by first binding to a receptor on the basolateral domain of cholangiocytes leading to increased activity of CFTR on the apical domain through the cyclic AMP, second messenger system. This sequence results in increased activity of an apical Cl^-/HCO_3^- exchanger in which lumenal Cl^- is exchanged for intracellular HCO_3^-, resulting in cholangiocyte HCO_3^- secretion (Fig. 2). This proposed mechanism for ductal HCO_3^- secretion is analogous to the apical mechanism regulating secretin-stimulated HCO_3^- secretion in intralobular pancreatic duct cells [34]. The role of exocytosis in ductal bile secretion remains largely speculative but may involve the hormone-regulated insertion of vesicles containing ion channels (*eg*, CFTR) into the apical plasma membrane or vacuolar H^+ pumps into the basolateral membrane of cholangiocytes [5•].

The mechanisms regulating ductal water secretion are even less well understood. Recently, Nielsen *et al.* [35•] using a polyclonal antibody and light microscopic immunocytochemistry, reported that aquaporin channel-forming integral membrane protein of 28 kD (CHIP), the prototypic water channel, is present at the apical and basolateral regions of human intrahepatic bile ducts. Further, we recently demonstrated that rodent cholangiocytes express aquaporin CHIP and transport water transcellularly via a channel-mediated mechanism [36]. These preliminary reports raise the possibility that aquaporin water channels are involved in the transcellular movement of water across cholangiocytes lining intrahepatic bile ducts; this water movement could theoretically occur at the apical domain in response to transient osmotic gradients created by secretin-induced ion secretion (Fig. 2).

Cholangiopathies

The cholangiopathies represent a group of diseases and syndromes of the biliary system at any site between the canals of Hering and the ampulla of Vater. These diseases may be classified in a variety of ways; in Table 1, we propose a classification based principally on known or postulated etiologies. Although a detailed description of these diseases is beyond the scope of this paper, a concise discussion of selected aspects relevant to cholangiocytes, with emphasis on the immune-mediated cholangiopathies, seems warranted given the recent progress in this area. For a complete and comprehensive discussion, readers should consult the excellent review article on this topic recently published [37••].

Pathogenesis of cholangiocyte injury

The major pathologic features of bile duct injury comprise cholangiocyte apoptosis, necrosis, and obliteration. In many cholangiopathies (*eg*, immune-mediated), cholangiocytes appear to undergo lysis or destruction by apoptosis (*ie*, programmed cell death) [38]. However, the precise mechanisms by which cholangiocyte apoptosis occurs are unclear and largely speculative. Cytokines released by peribiliary inflammatory cells have been suggested to contribute to this process either via a direct cytotoxic effect or via several possible indirect effects, including 1) increasing the expression of MHC class I and class II antigens on cholangiocytes, thus promoting targeting of cholangiocytes by the immune system, 2) decreasing the production of basement membrane matrix, and 3) stimulating the

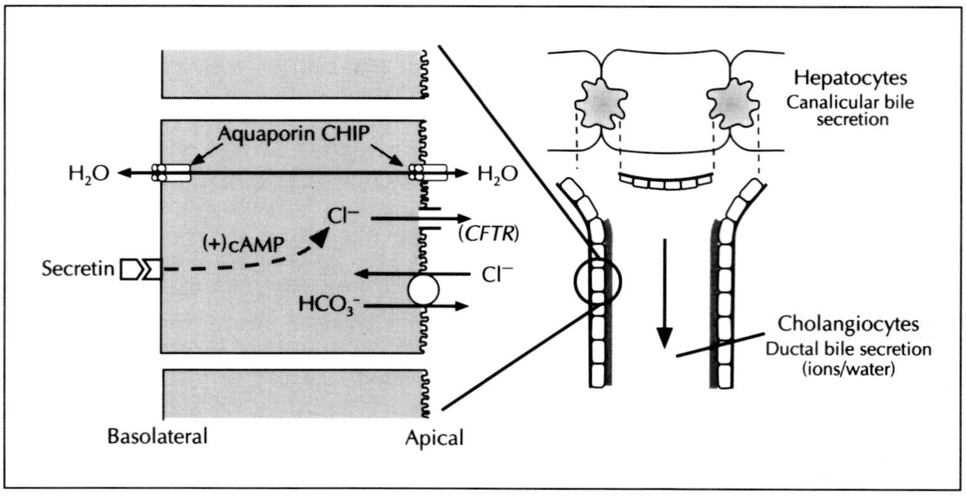

Fig. 2. Working model of the cellular mechanisms regulating ductal ion and water secretion. CHIP—channel-forming integral membrane protein of 28 kD. (*Adapted from* Cohn *et al.* [30•]; with permission.)

Table 1. Classification of the cholangiopathies*

Immune-mediated
Liver allograft rejection
Graft versus host disease
Primary biliary cirrhosis
Autoimmune cholangitis
Primary sclerosing cholangitis
Infectious
Viral, including HIV-associated cholangitis
Bacterial
Parasitic
Protozoan (HIV-associated)
Genetic and developmental
Cystic fibrosis
Allagille's syndrome
Ductal plate abnormalities (*eg*, Caroli's syndrome)
Tumors
Drug-induced
5-fluorouracil
Vascular
Idiopathic
Idiopathic adulthood ductopenia
Idiopathic childhood ductopenia
Biliary atresia
Sarcoidosis

*By convention, cholelithiasis and choledocholithiasis are excluded.

production of other pro-inflammatory mediators (such as eicosanoids) [37••]. The recent demonstration that pro-inflammatory cytokines increase the expression of MHC class I and class II molecules on human cholangiocytes *in vitro*, is consistent with the hypothesis that locally released cytokines play a pathogenetic role in the immune-mediated cholangiopathies [39•].

Damage to components of the hepatic artery, the exclusive blood supply of bile ducts [27••], can lead to fibroobliteration of bile ducts via ischemic injury and necrosis to cholangiocytes [37••]. Locally released cytokines may possibly contribute to this process by directly damaging endothelial cells lining the peribiliary plexi [37••]. Also, locally released endothelin-1, a potent vasoconstrictor, could potentiate this process given recent data showing that human gallbladder and hepatic cyst epithelial cells secrete this peptide [20•].

Little is known about the mechanisms responsible for progressive obliterative peribiliary fibrosis; cytokines may play an important pathogenetic role by stimulating fibroblast proliferation and collagen formation [37••]. Cholestasis (*ie*, the cessation or reduction of bile flow) usually accompanies bile duct injury and, hence, is an inherent feature of many of the cholangiopathies. However, the cellular mechanisms whereby cholangiocyte injury results in diminished ductal bile secretion are also unclear.

Also, cholangiocyte proliferation is commonly observed in human cholestatic liver diseases resulting from bile duct injury (*eg*, primary biliary cirrhosis) [27••,40,41] as well as in diseases associated with hepatic necrosis (*eg*, alcoholic liver disease or chronic hepatitis C) [42•,43•]. Although the ductal proliferation observed early in these diseases may be regular and limited to portal tracts (*ie*, type 1 or typical ductal proliferation) [41], prolonged cholestasis is often associated with "atypical" ductal hyperplasia [27••,40,41]. This latter process is characterized by irregular bile duct proliferation with formation of tortuous, poorly defined conduits that extend outside portal tract confines [40,41,44]. The epithelial cells lining these "atypical" bile ducts resemble normal cholangiocytes [44]. The cellular origin of this hyperplastic reaction is unknown; current evidence [27••,40,42•,44] favors either cholangiocyte metaplasia or retrodifferentiation of hepatocytes into cholangiocytes. Although the specific factors triggering cholangiocyte proliferation and differentiation are unknown, locally released inflammatory cytokines are potential candidates [37••].

Immune-mediated cholangiopathies

The immune-mediated cholangiopathies are conditions in which the cholangiocyte is thought to be the primary target of immune-mediated destruction by either alloimmune or autoimmune mechanisms. Liver allograft rejection after transplantation and the hepatic manifestations of chronic graft-versus-host disease after bone marrow transplantation exemplify putative alloimmune liver diseases, whereas primary biliary cirrhosis (PBC), autoimmune cholangitis, and primary sclerosing cholangitis (PSC), are putative autoimmune hepatobiliary diseases [37••]. Despite a surge of investigative activity into the autoimmune cholangiopathies, the pathogenesis of these diseases remains unclear, in part, because of the lack of experimental models. Attempts to produce an experimental model of immune-mediated cholangitis resembling PBC have been largely unsuccessful. Strategies reported include immunizing animals with a number of different "immunogens" including gallbladder mucous membranes, mitochondrial antigens, and peripheral blood lymphocytes from PBC patients [45•]. Similarly, a variety of approaches have been taken towards establishing an experimental model of PSC, again with limited success [46•]. Most of these have induced chronic hepatobiliary inflammation by initiating intestinal mucosal injury, either spontaneously (*ie*, cotton-topped tamarin model) or in response to toxins (*eg*, indomethacin, bacterial overgrowth) [46•]. Other approaches used include the repeated systemic administration of nonviable *Escherichia coli* or tumor necrosis factor [46•]. Recently, we reported a more direct approach to establishing an experimental model for immune-mediated cholangiopathies involving the active immunization of rats with purified rodent cholangiocytes [47•]. Immunized animals developed an unequivocal nonsuppurative cholangitis with portal tract infiltrates consisting principally of T lymphocytes. This model of immune cholangitis should prove useful in exploring the mechanisms by which the immune system targets and damages cholangiocytes.

Liver allograft rejection and graft-versus-host disease

Liver allograft rejection is characterized histologically by nonsuppurative destructive cholangitis (NSDC) and endotheliitis, and pathogenetically by immune-mediated injury to cholangiocytes and portal tract vasculature [37••,48,49••]. Cholangiocytes appear to be a major target for alloimmune-mediated destruction in rejection cholangitis based on 1) the demonstration that recipient T cells infiltrate the cholangiocytes lining interlobular bile ducts causing bile duct necrosis and destruction, 2) aberrant expression of HLA class II antigens by cholangiocytes, and 3) the progressive ductopenia characteristic of chronic allograft rejection [37••,48,49••,50]. A recent study demonstrating that destruction of portal microvasculature occurs early in rejection and precedes bile duct loss, suggests that ischemic injury to cholangiocytes may also play an important role in the pathogenesis of rejection-related ductopenia [51•].

Graft-versus-host disease after bone marrow transplantation frequently involves the liver and results in NSDC and loss of interlobular bile ducts [37••,52]. Several features of the hepatic manifestations of graft-versus-host disease are similar to PBC including the near-identical histology of NSDC lesions, the aberrant expression of HLA class II antigen on cholangiocytes, and the frequent development of autoantibodies including antimitochondrial antibodies, albeit in low titer [37••]. However, convincing evidence indicates that cholangiocyte injury in graft-versus-host disease is mediated by allogeneic T cells and not via autoimmune mechanisms [37••,52]. Although not proven, the cholangiocyte is the likely target cell for the alloimmune-mediated destruction. The recent development of mouse models of graft-versus-host disease with bile duct lesions induced by histocompatibility antigens may shed further insight into the pathogenetic processes involved [45•,53].

Primary biliary cirrhosis

Primary biliary cirrhosis is a chronic, idiopathic cholestatic liver disease characterized by the progressive inflammatory destruction of interlobular bile ducts [37••,54]. Although the pathogenesis of PBC is unclear, several lines of evidence suggest a central role for the autoimmune-mediated destruction of cholangiocytes, including 1) the frequent association of PBC with other autoimmune diseases, 2) the high frequency of serum autoantibodies, particularly antimitochondrial antibodies, 3) the increased frequency of the HLA-DRw8 haplotype, 4) the aberrant expression of HLA class II antigens by cholangiocytes in PBC, and 5) T-cell infiltration of interlobular bile duct epithelia causing destructive cholangitis [37••,54]. Also, splenic T lymphocytes taken from PBC patients at autopsy are cytotoxic against autologous bile duct cells, albeit at high effector-to-target ratios [55]. Recent data may shed new light on the pathogenesis of PBC. For example, the PBC-specific mitochondrial antigens (M2 antigens) have been identified; the E2 component of the pyruvate dehydrogenase complex (PDC-E2) is the major autoantigen [37••]. Nevertheless, the mechanism of autoantibody production and the pathogenetic importance of antimitochondrial antibodies in PBC remain unclear. Studies of the portal tract infiltrates in PBC have emphasized the role of cytotoxic T cells and B cells in the development of bile duct injury [56•,57]. Also, T cells from PBC livers that react against epitopes of M2 antigens have been cloned; this development may assist in defining the epitopes of PDC-E2 recognized by T-cell receptors [58•].

Immune-mediated bile duct destruction in PBC may involve T-cell recognition of the epitopes of microbial proteins, which resemble self-peptides presented by aberrantly expressed MHC class II on cholangiocytes [59]. This hypothesis, based on molecular mimicry between microbial proteins and self-peptides, is supported by two important factors: 1) the association between urinary tract infection with rough forms (mutants) of bacteria (*eg, E. coli*) and PBC-specific M2 antibody positivity [60], and 2) the homology between microbial proteins and self-peptide epitopes recognized by certain autoantibodies in PBC [61]. Recently, Van de Water [62•] demonstrated that one of eight mouse monoclonal antibodies and a human combinatorial antibody specific for PDC-E2 [63•] reacted strongly and specifically to the apical region of cholangiocytes in patients with PBC; seven other murine monoclonals gave typical mitochondrial staining. This suggests that a molecule cross-reactive with PDC-E2 is highly expressed in the lumenal region of cholangiocytes in PBC. Although these data also support the concept that molecular mimicry is important in PBC, the identity of this cross-reactive antigen and the mechanism by which it is presented by cholangiocytes and subsequently targeted by the immune system remains undefined.

Autoimmune cholangitis

Autoimmune cholangitis is a chronic cholestatic liver disease with features overlapping those of PBC and autoimmune chronic active hepatitis. The disease strongly resembles PBC, although serum antimitochrondrial antibodies are absent whereas high-titer serum antinuclear antibodies are present [37••,64•,65•]. The etiology and pathogenesis of autoimmune cholangitis are unknown, but autoimmune mechanisms are presumed. The classification of autoimmune cholangitis as a new disease entity, separate from antimitochrondral antibody-negative PBC, is controversial [37••], but is becoming increasingly accepted [64•,65•].

Primary sclerosing cholangitis

Primary sclerosing cholangitis, another chronic cholestatic liver disease, is characterized by fibrosing inflammation involving both intrahepatic and extrahepatic bile ducts with progression to biliary cirrhosis [37••,66]. A strong relationship between PSC and inflammatory bowel disease, particularly ulcerative colitis, is well established [37••,66]. The etiology of PSC is unknown, but autoimmunity has been implicated based on an association with other autoimmune diseases, the presence of circulating autoantibodies and the increased frequency of the HLA B8-DR3 haplotype [37••,66]. Also, a genetic predisposition is suggested by both family and haplotype studies. In a recent study of 83 patients with PSC, DR52a and Dw2 were the best candidate alleles for providing the known HLA association with PSC. Furthermore, possession of the HLA DR4 allele predisposed to rapid disease progression [67••].

An immune-mediated pathogenesis of PSC is suggested by numerous cellular and humoral immune abnormalities including decreased peripheral blood T lymphocytes [68], T-lymphocyte–predominant periportal infiltrates [68], increased circulating immune-complexes [69], and the presence of numerous circulating antibodies including antilactoferrin and antineutrophil antibodies [70,71•,72•]. Recent studies suggest that antineutrophil antibodies may have some diagnostic utility for PSC in adults [71•] and children [72•].

Current evidence suggests that cholangiocytes are target cells for immune-mediated destruction in PSC, although the data are perhaps less convincing than in PBC. Cholangiocytes have been shown to express an antigen that is recognized by an antibody that cross-reacts with a colonic epithelial cell protein from patients with ulcerative colitis [73]. Moreover, in a study of 16 patients with PSC, 10 had serum IgG autoantibodies against this cross-reactive peptide [74•]. Other evidence includes that peripheral blood lymphocytes from PSC patients are sensitized to unidentified biliary antigens and cholangiocytes aberrantly express MHC class II antigens at an early stage of the disease [37••]. Intercellular adhesion molecule (ICAM)-1, an important molecule for T-cell–mediated cell destruction, is expressed by cholangiocytes in end-stage PSC, suggesting that ICAM-1 is probably not involved in initiating this disease [75•]. As in PBC, bile duct destruction may be initiated by molecular mimicry against a bacterial, viral, or self-peptide crossreactive to an antigen expressed by cholangiocytes, although formal proof of this hypothesis is lacking.

Conclusions

Our understanding of the pathobiology of biliary epithelia has rapidly evolved because of the recent development of suitable experimental models. In particular, the ability to isolate and culture cholangiocytes has been instrumental in demonstrating that cholangiocytes 1) contribute to bile formation through hormone-induced water and electrolyte transport, and 2) represent the major cellular target of injury by the immune system in a variety of severe liver diseases. The anticipated refinement in current experimental models and a growing awareness of the importance of cholangiocytes should ensure that the pathobiology of biliary epithelia remains a focus of increasing attention.

References and recommended reading

Papers of particular interest, published within the annual period of review, have been highlighted as:

- • Of special interest
- •• Of outstanding interest

1. Tavoloni N: **The Intrahepatic Biliary Epithelium: An Area of Growing Interest in Hepatology.** *Semin Liver Dis* 1987, 7:280–292.
2. Alpini G, Lenzi R, Sarkozi L, Tavoloni N: **Biliary Physiology in Rats With Bile Ductular Cell Hyperplasia: Evidence for a Secretory Function of Proliferated Bile Ductules.** *J Clin Invest* 1988, **81**:569–578.
3. Ludwig J: **New Concepts in Biliary Cirrhosis.** *Semin Liver Dis* 1987, 7:293–301.
4. • Roberts SK, Kuntz SM, Gores GJ, LaRusso NF: **Regulation of Bicarbonate-Dependent Ductular Bile Secretion Assessed by Lumenal Micropuncture of Isolated Rodent Intrahepatic Bile Ducts.** *Proc Natl Acad Sci U S A* 1993, **90**:9080–9084.

Description of a novel *in vitro* experimental model that is an important tool for studying the physiology of intrahepatic bile ducts under normal and pathophysiologic conditions.

5. • Villanger O, Veel T, Raeder MG: **Secretin Causes H+ Secretion From Intrahepatic Bile Ductules by Vacuolar-Type H+-ATPase.** *Am J Physiol* 1993, **265**:G719–G724.

Study in microdissected pig bile ductules that implicates active basolateral H^+ transport in the regulation of ductal HCO_3^- secretion.

6. Benedetti A, Marucci L, Bassotti C, Mancini R, Contucci S, Jezequel AM, Orlandi F: **Tubulovesicular Transcytotic Pathway in Rat Biliary Epithelium: A Study in Perfused Rat Liver and in Isolated Intrahepatic Bile Duct.** *Hepatology* 1993, **18**:422–432.
7. Kumar U, Jordan T: **Isolation and Culture of Biliary Epithelial Cells From the Biliary Tract Fraction of Normal Rats.** *Liver* 1986, 6:369–378.
8. Gall JAM, Bhathal PS: **The Isolation of Intrahepatic Biliary Epithelial Cells From Normal Rat Livers.** *Cell Biol Int Rep* 1985, 9:315–322.
9. Yaswen P, Hayner NT, Fausto N: **Isolation of Oval Cells by Centrifugal Elutriation and Comparison With Other Cell Types Purified From Normal and Preneoplastic Livers.** *Cancer Res* 1984, 44:324–331.
10. Alpini G, Lenzi R, Zhai W-R, Liu MH, Slott PA, Paronetto F, Tavoloni N: **Isolation of a Nonparenchymal Liver Cell Fraction Enriched in Cells With Biliary Epithelial Phenotypes.** *Gastroenterology* 1989, 97:1248–1260.
11. • Alvaro D, Cho WK, Mennone A, Boyer JL: **Effect of Secretin on Intracellular pH Regulation in Isolated Rat Bile Duct Epithelial Cells.** *J Clin Invest* 1993, **92**:1314–1325.

A detailed study of rat cholangiocytes in short-term culture that provides potentially important mechanistic insight into the cellular mechanisms regulating agonist-induced ductal HCO_3^- secretion.

12. Ishii M, Vroman B, LaRusso NF: **Isolation and Morphologic Characterization of Bile Duct Epithelial Cells From Normal Rat Liver.** *Gastroenterology* 1989, 97:1236–1247.
13. Joplin R, Strain AJ, Neuberger JM: **Immuno-Isolation and Culture of Biliary Epithelial Cells From Normal Human Liver.** *In Vitro Cell Dev Biol* 1989, **25**:1189–1192.
14. Demetris AJ, Markus BH, Saidman S, Fung JJ, Makowka L, Graner S, Duquesnoy R, Starzl TE: **Isolation and Primary Cultures of Human Intrahepatic Bile Ductular Epithelium.** *In Vitro Cell Dev Biol* 1988, 24:464–470.
15. Mathis GA, Walls SA, Sirica AE: **Biochemical Characteristics of Hyperplastic Rat Bile Ductular Epithelial Cells Cultured "on Top" and "Inside" Different Extracellular Matrix Substitutes.** *Cancer Res* 1988, **48**:6145–6153.
16. Gall JAM, Bhathal PS: **Isolation and Culture of Intrahepatic Bile Ducts and Its Application in Assessing Putative Inducers of Biliary Epithelial Hyperplasia.** *Br J Exp Pathol* 1987, **68**:501–510.
17. •• Yang L, Faris RA, Hixson DC: **Long-Term Culture and Characteristics of Normal Rat Liver Bile Duct Epithelial Cells.** *Gastroenterology* 1993, 104:840–852.

Important paper that describes the methodology for establishing long-term primary cultures of normal rat cholangiocytes, as well as the morphologic, immunologic, and molecular characteristics of these cells.

18. Hoerl BJ, Vroman BT, Kasperbauer JL, LaRusso NF, Scott RE: **Biological Characteristics of Primary Cultures of Human Gallbladder Epithelial Cells.** *Lab Invest* 1992, **66**:243–250.
19. • Auth MKH, Keitzer RA, Scholz M, Blaheta RA, Hottenrott EC, Herrmann G, Encke A, Markus BH: **Establishment and Immunological Characterization of Cultured Human Gallbladder Epithelial Cells.** *Hepatology* 1993, **18**:546–555.

The inducible expression of HLA class II antigen and ICAM-1 on human gallbladder epithelial cells in long-term (> 6 weeks) culture suggests this experimental tool could be useful in studying the interaction of biliary epithelia with the immune system.

20. • Housset C, Carayon A, Housset B, Legendre C, Hannoun L, Poupon R: **Endothelin-1 Secretion by Human Gallbladder Epithelial Cells in Primary Culture.** *Lab Invest* 1993, 69:750–755.

Findings in this study raise the possibility that endothelin-1 may exert local biological and perhaps pathobiologic actions via a paracrine route.

21. • Phillips JO, Vroman B, Ueno Y, LaRusso NF: **Induction of Functional MHC Class II Protein Permits Rodent Cholangiocytes to Behave as Antigen Presenting Cells [Abstract].** *Gastroenterology* 1994, **106**:A961.

Although an abstract, the information contained within has important pathogenetic significance with respect to the immune-mediated cholangiopathies.

22. Yamaguchi N, Morioka H, Okhura H, Hirohashi S, Kawai K: **Establishment and Characterization of the Human Cholangiocarcinoma Cell Line HChol-Y1 in a Serum-Free, Chemically Defined Medium.** *J Natl Cancer Inst* 1985, **75**:29–35.

23. Sirisinha S, Tengchaisri T, Boonpucknavig S, Prempracha N, Ratanarapee S, Pausawasdi A: **Establishment and Characterization of a Cholangiocarcinoma Cell Line From a Thai Patient With Intrahepatic Bile Duct Cancer.** *Asia Pac J Allerg Immunol* 1991, 9:153–157.

24. Homma S, Nagamori S, Fujise K: **Human Bile Duct Carcinoma Cell Line Producing Abundant Mucin *In Vitro*.** *Gastroenterol Jpn* 1987, 22:74–79.

25. Knuth A, Gabbert H, Dippold W, Klein O, Sachsse W, Bitter-Suermann D, Prellwitz W, Meyer zum Buschenfelde KH: **Biliary Adenocarcinoma. Characterization of Three New Human Tumor Cell Lines.** *J Hepatol* 1985, 1:579–596.

26. • Basavappa S, Middleton J, Mangel AW, McGill JM, Cohn JA, Fitz JG: **Cl^- and K^+ Transport in Human Biliary Cell Lines.** *Gastroenterology* 1993, 104:1796–1805.

The demonstration that these cell lines retain certain biliary epithelial phenotypes as well as functional ion channels suggests that these experimental models may be used to study biliary fluid and ion transport.

27. •• Tarsetti F, Lenzen R, Salvi R, Schuler E, Dembitzer R, Tavoloni N: **Biology and Pathobiology of Intrahepatic Biliary Epithelium.** In *Hepatic Transport and Bile Secretion.* Edited by Tavoloni N, Berk PD. New York: Raven Press, Ltd.; 1993:619–635.

This comprehensive review includes 124 references. Special emphasis is given to the transport functions of cholangiocytes and the pathophysiology of bile duct injury.

28. Alpini G, Lenzi R, Zhai W, Slott PA, Liu MH, Sarkozi L, Tavoloni N: **Bile Secretory Function of Intrahepatic Biliary Epithelium in the Rat.** *Am J Physiol* 1989, **257**:G124–G133.

29. Fitz JG, Basavappa S, McGill J, Melhus O, Cohn JA: **Regulation of Membrane Chloride Currents in Rat Bile Duct Epithelial Cells.** *J Clin Invest* 1993, **91**:319–328.

30. • Cohn JA, Strong TV, Picciotto MR, Nairn AC, Collins FS, Fitz JG: **Localization of the Cystic Fibrosis Transmembrane Conductance Regulator in Human Bile Duct Epithelial Cells.** *Gastroenterology* 1993, **105**:1857–1864.

Elegant study that localizes CFTR in human liver to the lumenal membrane of cholangiocytes. Findings strongly suggest CFTR is intimately involved in ductal bile secretion.

31. Strazzabosco M, Mennone A, Boyer JL: **Intracellular pH Regulation in Isolated Rat Bile Duct Epithelial Cells.** *J Clin Invest* 1991, **87**:1503–1512.

32. Farouk M, Vigna SR, McVey DC, Meyers WC: **Localization and Characterization of Secretin Binding Sites Expressed by Rat Bile Duct Epithelium.** *Gastroenterology* 1992, **102**:963–968.

33. Kato A, Gores GJ, LaRusso NF: **Secretin Stimulates Exocytosis in Isolated Bile Duct Epithelial Cells by a Cyclic AMP-Mediated Mechanism.** *J Biol Chem* 1992, **267**:15523–15529.

34. Raeder MG: **The Origin of and Subcellular Mechanisms Causing Pancreatic Bicarbonate Secretion.** *Gastroenterology* 1992, **103**:1674–1684.

35. • Nielsen S, Smith BL, Christensen EI, Agre P: **Distribution of Aquaporin CHIP in Secretory and Resorptive Epithelia and Capillary Endothelia.** *Proc Natl Acad Sci U S A* 1993, **90**:7275–7279.

Although preliminary, the findings in this report have major implications with respect to water transport by cholangiocytes.

36. Roberts SK, Yano M, Pham L, Alpini G, Marks D, Phillips J, Ueno Y, Gores GJ, Agre P, LaRusso NF: **Intrahepatic Bile Duct Epithelial Cells Contain a Functional Water Channel, CHIP28 [Abstract].** *Hepatology* 1993, **18**:112A.

37. •• Woolf GM, Vierling JM: **Disappearing Intrahepatic Bile Ducts: The Syndromes and Their Mechanisms.** *Semin Liver Dis* 1993, **13**:261-275.

This detailed review summarizes current concepts regarding the pathogenesis of the human cholangiopathies. The references number 108.

38. Duval E, Wylie AH: **Death and the Cell.** *Immunol Today* 1986, 7:115–119.

39. • Ayres RCS, Neuberger JM, Shaw J, Joplin R, Adams DH: **Intercellular Adhesion Molecule-1 and MHC Antigens on Human Intrahepatic Bile Duct Cells: Effect of Pro-Inflammatory Cytokines.** *Gut* 1993, 34:1245–1249.

Indirect evidence suggesting that cytokines play a pathogenetic role in the immune-mediated cholangiopathies.

40. Desmet VJ: **Current Problems in the Diagnosis of Biliary Disease and Cholestasis.** *Semin Liver Dis* 1986, 6:233–245.

41. Nagore N, Howe S, Boxer L, Scheuer PJ: **Liver Cell Rosettes: Structural Differences in Cholestasis and Hepatitis.** *Liver* 1989, 9:43–51.

42. • Ray MB, Mendenhall CL, French SW, Gartside PS: **Bile Duct Changes in Alcoholic Liver Disease.** *Liver* 1993, **13**:36–45.

Further documentation by semiquantitative morphologic techniques of the extent of bile duct injury in this condition.

43. • Danque POV, Bach N, Schaffner F, Gerber M, Thung SN: **HLA-DR Expression in Bile Duct Damage in Hepatitis C.** *Mod Pathol* 1993, 6:327–332.

Absence of MHC class II antigen expression by cholangiocytes in hepatitis C–related bile-duct damage suggests an alternative mechanism of injury in this condition compared with the immune-mediated cholangiopathies.

44. Nakunuma Y, Ohta G: **Immunohistochemical Study on Bile Ductular Proliferation in Various Hepatobiliary Diseases.** *Liver* 1986, 6:205–211.

45. • Thiele DL, Williams FH: **Animal Models of Primary Biliary Cirrhosis.** In *Falk Symposium, 70th (1992: Basel Switzerland) Immunology and Liver.* Edited by Meyer zum Buschenfelde K-H, Hoofnagle JH, Manns M. Hingham, MA: Kluwer; 1993:410–422.

This review summarizes the published experimental models of PBC with emphasis on the authors' murine model of graft-versus-host disease.

46. • Sartor RB, Lichtman SN: **Animal Models of Sclerosing Cholangitis: Exploring Mechanisms of Hepatobiliary Inflammation Associated With Intestinal Injury.** In *Falk Symposium, 70th (1992: Basel, Switzerland) Immunology and Liver.* Edited by Meyer zum Buschenfelde K-H, Hoofnagle JH, Manns M. Hingham, MA: Kluwer; 1993:330–338.

This paper is a concise review summarizing the different experimental approaches used to establish an animal model of PSC.

47. • Ueno Y, Phillips JO, Ludwig J, LaRusso NF: **Nonsuppurative Cholangitis Induced in Rodents by Cholangiocyte Immunization: An Experimental Model for Immune Cholangiopathies [Abstract].** *Hepatology* 1993, **18**:170A.

The results of this abstract suggest a promising model of immune-mediated cholangitis. Full publication should follow.

48. Oguma S, Belle S, Starzl TE, Demetris AJ: **A Histometric Analysis of Chronically Rejected Human Liver Allografts: Insights Into the Mechanisms of Bile Duct Loss: Direct Immunologic and Ischemic Factors.** *Hepatology* 1989, 9:204–209.

49. •• Lowes JR, Hubscher SG, Neuberger JM: **Chronic Rejection of the Liver Allograft.** In *Gastroenterology Clinics of North America. Advances in Liver Transplantation.* Edited by Lake JR. Philadelphia: W.B. Saunders; 1993:401–420.

This review summarizes the classification, etiology, pathogenesis, clinical features, and management of chronic rejection of liver allograft and includes 82 references.

50. Weisner RH, Ludwig J, van Hoek B, Krom RAF: **Current Concepts in Cell-Mediated Hepatic Allograft Rejection Leading to Ductopenia and Liver Failure.** *Hepatology* 1991, 14:721–729.

51. • Matsumoto Y, McCaughan GW, Painter DM, Bishop GA: **Evidence That Portal Tract Microvascular Destruction Precedes Bile Duct Loss in Human Liver Allograft Rejection.** *Transplantation* 1993, **56**:69–75.

Study findings suggest that bile duct injury in rejection cholangitis may be related partly to cholangiocyte ischemia.

52. Shulman HM, McDonald GB: **Liver Disease After Marrow Transplantation.** In *The Pathology of Bone Marrow Transplantation.* Edited by Sale GE, Shulman HM. Chicago: Year Book Medical Publishers; 1984:104-135.

53. Saitoh T, Fujiwara M, Nomoto M: **Hepatic Lesions Induced by Graft-Versus-Host Reaction Across MHC Class II Antigens: An Implication for Animal Models of Primary Biliary Cirrhosis.** *Clin Immunol Immunopath*; 1988, **49**:166–172.

54. Kaplan MM: **Primary Biliary Cirrhosis.** *N Engl J Med* 1987, **316**:521–528.

55. Onishi S, Saibara T, Nakata S, Maeda T, Iwasaki S, Iwamura S, Miyazaki M, Yamamoto Y, Enzan H: **Cytotoxic Activity of Spleen-Derived Lymphocytes Against Autologous Biliary Epithelial Cells in Autopsy Patients With Primary Biliary Cirrhosis.** *Liver* 1993, **13**:188–192.

56. • Hashimoto E, Lindnor KD, Homburger HA, Dickson ER, Czaja AJ, Weisner RH, Ludwig J: **Immunohistochemical Characterization of Hepatic Lymphocytes in Primary Biliary Cirrhosis in Comparison With Primary Sclerosing Cholangitis and Autoimmune Chronic Active Hepatitis.** *Mayo Clin Proc* 1993, **68**:1049–1055.

These results substantiate previous findings of hepatic cellular infiltrates in PBC, although raising several questions about PBC's immunopathologic features.

57. Nakanuma Y: **Distribution of B Lymphocytes in Nonsuppurative Cholangitis in Primary Biliary Cirrhosis.** *Hepatology* 1993, **18**:570–575.

58. • Lohr H, Fleischer B, Gerken G, Yeaman SJ, Meyer zum Buschenfelde K-H, Manns M: **Autoreactive Liver-Infiltrating T Cells in Primary Biliary Cirrhosis Recognize Inner Mitochondrial Epitopes and the Pyruvate Dehydrogenase Complex.** *J Hepatol* 1993, **18**:322–327.

This study is an important step towards defining the epitopes of M2 antigens recognized by T-cell receptors. Further characterization of the autoreactive T-cell population described is now awaited.

59. Burroughs AK, Butler P, Sternberg MJE, Baum H: **Molecular Mimicry in Liver Disease.** *Nature* 1992, **358**:377–378.

60. Butler P, Valle F, Hamilton-Miller JMT, Brumfitt W, Baum H, Burroughs AK: **M2 Mitochondrial Antibodies and Urinary Rough Mutant Bacteria in Patients With Recurrent Bacteriuria.** *J Hepatol* 1993, **17**:408–414.

61. Nickowitz RE, Worman HJ: **Autoantibodies From Patients With Primary Biliary Cirrhosis Recognize a Restricted Region Within the Cytoplasmic Tail of Nuclear Pore Membrane Glycoprotein Gp210.** *J Exp Med* 1993, **178**:2237–2240.

62. •• Van de Water J, Turchany J, Leung PSC, Lake J, Munoz S, Surh CD, Coppel R, Ansari A, Nakanuma Y, Gershwin ME: **Molecular Mimicry in Primary Biliary Cirrhosis. Evidence for Biliary Epithelial Expression of a Molecule Cross-Reactive With Pyruvate Dehydrogenase Complex-E2.** *J Clin Invest* 1993, **91**:2653–2664.

This very elegant study provides evidence for molecular mimicry in PBC. Findings raise several important questions regarding the pathogenesis of this disease that are addressed in the discussion.

63. • Cha S, Leung PSC, Gershwin ME, Fletcher MP, Ansari AA, Coppel RL: **Combinatorial Autoantibodies to Dihydrolipoamide Acetyltransferase, the Major Autoantigen of Primary Biliary Cirrhosis.** *Proc Natl Acad Sci U S A* 1993, **90**:2527–2531.

This report details the isolation and characterization of human immunoglobulins specific to the human autoantigen, PDC-E2. Such reagents offer enormous potential to study antigen-antibody interaction in autoimmune disease.

64. • Taylor SL, Dean PJ, Riley CA: **Primary Autoimmune Cholangitis. An Alternative to Antimitochondrial Antibody-Negative Primary Biliary Cirrhosis.** *Am J Surg Pathol* 1994, **18**:91–99.

This paper reports on nine patients and reviews the literature.

65. • Ben-Ari Z, Dhillon AP, Sherlock S: **Autoimmune Cholangiopathy: Part of the Spectrum of Autoimmune Chronic Active Hepatitis.** *Hepatology* 1993, **18**:10–15.

Report of four patients, three of which responded to prednisolone.

66. LaRusso NF, Weisner RH, Ludwig J, MacCarty RL: **Primary Sclerosing Cholangitis.** *N Engl J Med* 1984, **310**:899–903.

67. •• Mehal WZ, Lo Y-MD, Wordsworth BP, Neuberger JM, Hubscher SC, Fleming KA, Chapman RW: **HLA DR4 Is a Marker for Rapid Disease Progression in Primary Sclerosing Cholangitis.** *Gastroenterology* 1994, **106**:160–167.

This paper details a haplotype study of 83 PSC patients from two populations that marks HLA DR52a and Dw2 as the primary HLA associations and HLA DR4 as a haplotype marker for rapid disease progression.

68. Snook JA, Chapman RW, Sachdev GK, Heryet A, Kelly PMA, Fleming KA, Jewell DP: **Peripheral Blood and Portal Tract Lymphocyte Populations in Primary Sclerosing Cholangitis.** *J Hepatol* 1989, 9:36-41.

69. Bodenheimer HCJ, LaRusso NF, Thayer WRJ, Charland C, Staples PT, Ludwig J: **Elevated Circulating Immune Complexes in Primary Sclerosing Cholangitis.** *Hepatology* 1983, 3:150–154.

70. Peen E, Almer S, Bodemar G, Ryden B-O, Sjolin C, Tejle K, Skogh T: **Anti-Lactoferrin Antibodies and Other Types of ANCA in Ulcerative Colitis, Primary Sclerosing Cholangitis, and Crohns Disease.** *Gut* 1993, 34:56–62.

71. • Hardarson S, LaBrecque DR, Mitros FA, Neil GA, Goeken JA: **Antineutrophil Cytoplasmic Antibody in Inflammatory Bowel and Hepatobiliary Diseases. High Prevalence in Ulcerative Colitis, Primary Sclerosing Cholangitis, and Autoimmune Hepatitis.** *Am J Clin Pathol* 1993, 99:277–281.

The presence of an autoantibody in 20 of 29 patients with PSC and in none of 33 patients with PBC, suggests this test might be useful in the differential diagnosis of these two conditions.

72. • Lo SK, Chapman RW, Cheeseman P, Charlton CPJ, Walker-Smith JA, Mieli-Vergani G, Fleming KA: **Antineutrophil Antibody: A Test for Autoimmune Primary Sclerosing Cholangitis in Childhood?** *Gut* 1993, 34:199–202.

In a blinded study of 72 children's sera, eight of 10 children with PSC were correctly identified by testing for a specific antineutrophil antibody.

73. Das KM, Vecchi M, Sakamaki S: **A Shared and Unique Epitope(s) on Human Colon, Skin, and Biliary Epithelium Detected by Monoclonal Antibody.** *Gastroenterology* 1990, **98**:464–469.

74. • Mandal A, Dasgupta A, Jeffers L, Squillante L, Hyder S, Reddy R, Schiff E, Das KM: **Autoantibodies in Sclerosing Cholangitis Aganist a Shared Peptide in Biliary and Colon Epithelium.** *Gastroenterology* 1994, **106**:185–192.

A circulating antibody was present in 10 of 16 patients with PSC and absent in patients with other cholestatic liver diseases.

75. • Broome U, Hultcrantz R, Scheynius A: **Lack of Concomitant Expression of ICAM-1 and HLA-DR on Bile Duct Cells From Patients With Primary Sclerosing Cholangitis and Primary Biliary Cirrhosis.** *Scand J Gastroenterol* 1993, **28**:126–130.

This paper demonstrates that ICAM-1 is not the adhesion molecule involved in the initiation of the putative cell-to-cell mediated destruction of bile ducts in these two cholangiopathies.

Nicholas F. LaRusso, MD, Center for Basic Research in Digestive Diseases, Mayo Medical School, Clinic and Foundation, 200 First Street, SW, Rochester, MN 55905, USA.

Biliary tract cancer

Olivier Farges, MD, and Henri Bismuth, MD, FACS

Paul Brousse Hospital, University Paris Sud, Villejuif, France

Biliary tract cancer is traditionally associated with a grim prognosis because of the difficulty in diagnosing at an early stage and the relative inefficiency of adjuvant treatments. However, a policy of extensive resection has been developed over the past few years, including resection of the extrahepatic bile duct, en bloc dissection of the regional lymph nodes and perineural tissue, and resection of the liver or pancreas when these are required to obtain tumor-free resection margins. The most significant recent advances are a better knowledge of the histologic spread of these tumors and the confirmation that improved survival and even a complete cure may be anticipated from radical surgery.

Current Opinion in Gastroenterology 1994, **10**:534–540

Epidemiology

There have been a number of ecologic and epidemiologic studies suggesting that gallstone was a risk factor for gallbladder cancer. A causative role for gallstones in the formation of carcinoma, however, has not been proven yet. The hypothetical link relates to repeated trauma and chronic inflammation of the mucosa. The recent study from Duarte *et al.* [1•], arising from Chile, a country where the prevalence of cholelithiasis is among the highest in the world, addresses this issue. The first relevant observation is the frequency (97%) of epithelial lesions found in the gallbladder of patients undergoing elective cholecystectomy for cholelithiasis, including antral metaplasia (95%), intestinal metaplasia (58%), hyperplasia (47%), dysplasia (16%), and *in situ* carcinoma (2.5%). The authors also found a significant association of intestinal metaplasia with hyperplasia and dysplasia, which is in agreement with the suggested sequence of intestinal metaplasia giving rise to dysplasia and subsequently carcinoma.

Gallstones have also been proposed to be a risk factor for cancer of the extrahepatic bile ducts, but again, direct evidence is lacking. An original approach has been used by Ekborn *et al.* [2•] to further support this hypothesis. Because gallstones are formed in the gallbladder, the authors analyzed whether the incidence of extrahepatic bile duct cancer was reduced in patients who had undergone a cholecystectomy. The standardized incidence ratio (SIR) of extrahepatic bile duct cancer (*ie*, ratio of observed to expected number of cancers) was 47 within a year of cholecystectomy (indicating that cholecystectomy serves as a screening process even when the cancer is missed at operation) but fell thereafter, being 0.8 from 5 to 10 years after cholecystectomy and 0.1 after 10 years. The SIR of primary liver cancer (used as a control for surveillance bias) was also increased during the 1st year after cholecystectomy (SIR = 6.9) but the number of cancers observed thereafter was similar to that expected (SIR = 0.8 to 1.5). This study demonstrates that cholecystectomy (and therefore removal of gallstones) is associated with a markedly reduced risk of extrahepatic bile duct cancer starting about 10 years after the operation. We believe this does not imply that patients with silent stones should undergo a cholecystectomy to lessen the risk of carcinoma, but that these patients should be regularly screened for the possible occurrence of this complication. Chijiiwa *et al.* [3] suggest that the same screening should be applied to patients with hepatolithiasis as these patients are also at risk to develop a cholangiocarcinoma (4% to 11%) even when calculi have been completely removed. What is remarkable in this situation is that the cancer may occur up to 14 years after desobstruction.

Besides gallstones, there has been increasing evidence, mainly from Japan, of a high association between an anomalous junction of the pancreatobiliary duct systems and cancer of the biliary tract through the reflux of pancreatic juice. Gallbladder carcinoma is a cancer with a previously reported incidence of 16% [4]; seven personal cases with 27 cases from the Japanese literature have been reviewed by Tanaka *et al.* [5]. One of the most interesting features of gallbladder cancer in this setting is the very low incidence of associated gallstones. The lack of gallstone-related symptoms probably accounts for the late discovery of these cancers and their grim prognosis (only two of 34 patients survived beyond 3 years). The authors therefore recommend a prophylactic cholecystectomy in patients with an anomalous junction without bile duct dilatation. We would in addition advocate a resection of the common bile duct and a biliojejunal anastomosis because these patients are also at risk of bile duct cancer [4].

Abbreviations

ERCP—endoscopic retrograde cholangiopancreatography; **PTC**—percutaneous transhepatic cholangiography; **SIR**—standardized incidence ratio.

 ISBN 1-85922-610-8 ISSN 0267–1379

Diagnosis of bile duct strictures

Several studies over the past years have stressed the difficulty in diagnosing biliary strictures. This may indeed be a real problem, as evidenced by a recent study showing that 11 of 82 patients who underwent resective surgery under the presumptive diagnosis of hilar cholangiocarcinoma in fact had benign fibrosing or localized sclerosing lesions [6]. The safety and efficacy of radiologic explorations, percutaneous sampling, and bile cytology have recently been reviewed in a leading article [7]. Bile cytology, fine-needle aspiration biopsy, cholangioscopy, and endosonography have in addition been the subjects of original articles over the past year.

Bile and brush cytology available at the time of endoscopic retrograde cholangiopancreatography (ERCP) or percutaneous transhepatic cholangiography (PTC) was evaluated by Kurzawinski *et al.* [8] in a series of 12 patients with benign strictures and 81 patients with malignant strictures. The sensitivity, specificity, and accuracy of bile cytology were 33%, 100%, and 40%, respectively, whereas after bile and brush cytology they were 69%, 100%, and 74%, respectively. The results of brushings were similar at ERCP and PTC and for the different cancer types (*ie*, ampulla, pancreas, and bile duct). Neither technique gave false-positive results, in contrast with previous studies, which is explained by the fact that bile was not sampled from the duodenum. The authors stress that a negative result warrants repeated sampling. One third of patients who had bile cytology alone and half the patients who had both bile and brush cytology had positive results after repeated sampling.

A more radical approach is the direct biopsy of the bile ducts under percutaneous cholangioscopy. Nimura [9•], who has performed this technique in 295 patients, recently showed the low morbidity and mortality rates of this technique (9% and 0%, respectively) as well as its sensitivity, 96% of the biopsies being positive in patients with bile duct carcinoma [9•].

The accuracy of fine-needle aspiration of pancreatic and biliary masses has also been recently reassessed based on an analysis of 82 patients, 61 of whom had a malignant lesion [10]. Sensitivity (90%), specificity (100%), accuracy (92%), positive predictive value (100%), and negative predictive value (74%) were similar to that reported in previous studies. Based on their experience and their analysis of the literature, the authors conclude that fine-needle aspiration biopsy is a safe technique (0.2% complication rate) that is particularly useful when it yields a positive response for malignancy [10]. On the contrary, a negative response for malignancy has a 16% to 26% chance of being incorrect, and should therefore not be used to supplant clinical judgment of malignancy in a potentially resectable lesion.

Tio *et al.* [11] have updated their experience with endosonography in the diagnosis and staging of Klatskin tumors. Accuracy of endosonography in diagnosing T2 and T3 common hepatic duct carcinoma was 70% and 91%, respectively, whereas it was 29% and 94% in the classification of N0 and N1 lymph nodes. The lower efficacy in the latter evaluation was mainly related to a high rate (32%) of false positivity.

Treatment of gallbladder carcinoma

Gallbladder carcinoma has traditionally been associated with a poor outcome. In a collected series published in 1978, the overall 5-year survival of nearly 6000 patients was 4.1% [12]. More recent studies, most from Japan, have shown that the efficacy of surgery in the treatment of gallbladder carcinoma is beginning to improve (Table 1), especially as a result of the use of more radical surgery including wedge resection of the gallbladder bed, resection of the suprahepatic segment of the extrahepatic bile duct, and en bloc dissection of the regional lymph nodes (including in the most recent series the interaortocaval nodes near the left renal vein) [13–15].

Ouchi *et al.* [16] compared a group of 25 patients operated on between 1979 and 1991 to a group of 26 patients treated at the same institution before 1979 (Table 1). Improvement in prognosis was related to the smaller size and the more limited invasion of the tumor, resulting in an increased incidence of curative re-

Table 1. Recent results with resection of gallbladder carcinoma

Study and year	Study period	Patients receiving operation, *n*	Curative resections, %	Survival, % 3-year	Survival, % 5 years
Ogura *et al.* [18], 1991	(1979–1988)	1686	58	43 (overall), 66 (radical)	30 (overall), 51 (radical)
Shirai *et al.* [14], 1992	(1981–1986)	40	80	—	65 (overall), 81 (curative)
Shirai *et al.* [19], 1992	(1981–1989)	98	—	—	40–100*
Ouchi *et al.* [16], 1993	(1979–1991)	25	76	72	61 (overall)

*5-year survival was 100% for patients with pT1 cancer (mucosa or muscular layer) and 40% for patients with pT2 cancer (perimuscular connective tissue without extension beyond serosa or into the liver) treated by cholecystectomy alone. Reoperation for radical surgery improved survival of pT2 patients to 90% at 5-year.

sections (76% vs 27%) through more aggressive surgery (bile duct resection: six of 25 vs four of 26; liver resection: 18 of 25 vs 13 of 26; and regional lymphadenectomy: 18 of 25 vs 13 of 26). Interestingly, the diagnostic accuracy of ultrasound, angiography, and computerized tomography scan between 1979 and 1991 were 36%, 33%, and 70% respectively, indicating that gallbladder cancers continue to be frequently misdiagnosed preoperatively.

Because removal of regional lymph node is an important component of radical resection, it is of interest to preoperatively assess lymphatic spread. This issue has been addressed by Ohtani *et al.* [17], who compared preoperative computerized tomography findings with pathologic findings in a series of 51 patients who underwent radical surgery for gallbladder carcinoma. Nodes most likely to be pathologically positive were those with an anteroposterior dimension of greater than 10 mm, a lobular shape, and a heterogeneous contrast enhancement. Overall, only 38% of the positive nodes had been visualized on computerized tomography scan, the least frequently recognized ones being the interaorto-caval (18%), cystic (20%), superior mesenteric (33%), and pericholedochal (36%). Two observations in this study deserve further attention. The first one is that the authors have documented pathologic spread into aortocaval nodes in five of 32 patients, into right celiac nodes in eight of 51 patients, along the common hepatic artery in 10 of 51 patients, and along the superior mesenteric artery in three of 51 patients. This suggests that lymphatic dissection should also include these regions. The second observation is that diagnostic sensitivity and positive predictive value of computerized tomography scan for posterosuperior pancreatoduodenal, retroportal, or right celiac nodes is among the highest. Preoperative computerized tomography scan may therefore aid in planning a pancreatoduodenectomy, if further trials prove that the additional risk associated with this procedure is worth being taken [14].

As for other cancers, over the past year there have been reports of tumor inoculation at the time of laparoscopic cholecystectomy [20,21,22•,23]. One of these studies [22•] reported on 10 patients in whom gallbladder cancer was discovered at laparoscopy yet who underwent a procedure that had the potential of spilling viable tumor cells. These patients underwent a reexploration 14 to 74 days (mean, 30 days) thereafter. Four patients were found to have gross intraperitoneal dissemination as a result of the initial operation or a tumor in a laparoscopic tract. We have had the same experience with patients in whom a gallbladder tumor was opened at the time of open-surgery cholecystectomy. These observations reinforce the idea that every effort should be made to prevent violation of gallbladder tumors and that patients with such tumors should undergo one-stage definitive therapy.

Previous experience with adjuvant chemotherapy has been disappointing and the occasionally reported improvement in survival probably relates to patient selection [24,25]. Intra-arterial chemotherapy with mitomycin initially seemed to yield encouraging results [26] but long-term outcome was not as expected, based on the analysis of 27 patients receiving 10 to 15 mg of mitomycin into the hepatic artery at 6-week intervals and an historical control group of 22 patients [27]. The cumulative 5-year survival for stage I to III tumors was not significantly different in the two groups and for more advanced tumors, no patient from either group survived more than 4 years. Of note, however, is that neither group underwent extensive resections, which might have precluded any beneficial effect from adjuvant therapy.

Treatment of bile duct cancer

Hilar cholangiocarcinomas are characterized by a usually slow growth rate and a low propensity for metastasis. However, they are located in close proximity to important vascular structures in the hilum of the liver and have a tendency to grow into the perineural tissue. Therefore, at the time these tumors are discovered, they may have already invaded the main hepatic artery or portal vein branches or spread for a considerable distance along the bile duct wall. Bismuth *et al.* [28] have shown that it is possible to improve survival, even achieve long-term, recurrence-free survival in patients who underwent a curative resection; this has been recently confirmed by several other groups (Table 2).

Surgical curability warrants that no microscopic residual tumor is present and therefore, knowledge of the histologic spread of the tumors is mandatory to help secure a clear upper margin. Recent studies have confirmed 1) the frequency (86%) of perineural infiltration [29•], possibly because of the ability of bile duct cells to secrete NCAM [30], 2) the distance (7.3 ± 3.5 mm in the hepatic direction; 3.4 ± 1.6 mm in the duodenal direction) that the tumor could spread along the bile duct wall [29•], and 3) the frequency (36% to 40%) with which the caudate lobe is involved [29•,31]. Interestingly, the only patients alive after 5 years in Ogura's series were those who had undergone a simultaneous caudate lobectomy [29•].

The clinicopathologic factors that significantly influence survival of patients with bile duct carcinoma have been studied by Bhuiya *et al.* [32•], who have one of the largest series of resected bile duct tumors in the world and have developed a policy of extensive resection. Based on an analysis of 70 patients whose bile duct carcinomas (52 upper, eight middle, and 10 lower) were resected between 1979 and 1990, they have by multivariate analysis shown that the two most prognostic variables were pancreatic invasion (46% vs 0%, 5-year survival) and perineural invasion (52% vs 19%, 5-year survival). Although this study may help identify patients who could best benefit from (yet undefined) adjuvant therapy, it is otherwise remarkable for 1) the high rate (73%) of curative resections and 2) the extent of resection performed (hepatectomy or pancreatoduodenectomy in 71% and 31% of the patients, respectively). Unfortunately, analysis was not stratified according to the location of the bile duct cancer.

This aggressive surgical approach to bile duct cancer is, however, associated with an increased mortality that

Table 2. Results of surgical treatment of Klatskin tumors

Study and year	Study period	Patients, *n*	Resectability, %	Curative resection, %	Survival, % 1-year	3-year	5-year
Nimura *et al.* [42], 1990	(1979–1989)	66	83	70	—	51*	38*
Reding *et al.* [43], 1991	(1955)	307	32 (10–51)	—	70†	30†	11†
Bismuth *et al.* [28], 1992	(1960–1990)	122	17	39	87	25	—
					100*	50*	—
Ogura *et al.* [29•], 1993	(1976–1991)	65	85	51	63	31	23
					83*	46*	29*
Tashiro *et al.* [31], 1993	(1975–1990)	46	74	53	61	46	24
					75*	59*	30*
Koyama *et al.* [38], 1993	NA	20	‡	—	80	33	26
					100*	67*	67*
Bhuiya *et al.*[32•], 1993	(1979–1990)	70	‡	—	—	—	25†
Gazzaniga *et al.* [44], 1993	(1970–1990)	100	43	58	70*	20*	20*
Nagorney *et al.* [45], 1993	(1976–1985)	79	§	15	51¶	—	13¶

*Survival is given for curative resections.
†Survival is given for palliative resection.
‡Study population comprises only patients undergoing resection. No information is available on the resectability rate.
§This study includes biliary carcinoma of all locations. Resectability rate is the group of patients with Klatskin tumors is not indicated.
¶Survival is given for the entire group whether resected or not.
NA—not available.

ranges in the most recent Japanese series between 4% and 33% [29•,33•], most of the deaths being related to hepatic failure. Nagino *et al.* [33•] have therefore, by discriminant analysis, computed a formula that predicts the risk of postoperative liver failure (score = - 0.768 + 0.014x [liver resection rate, %] + 1.093 [if a duodenopancreatectomy is performed] + 1.137 [if cholangitis is present] + 1.414 [if the oral glucose tolerance test pattern is linear] - 7.555x [indocyanine green disappearance test]; a score greater than 0 predicts the risk of postoperative liver failure with an 87% accuracy). It is noteworthy that serum total bilirubin level before drainage was not predictive of liver failure, probably because of the policy to systematically drain these patients preoperatively.

As stated by the authors [33•], prevention of posthepatectomy liver failure and extension of surgery are contradictory. Since 1991, this group has been developing a program of preoperative portal embolization to induce an atrophy of the embolized segments and therefore a compensatory hypertrophy of the liver segments anticipated to be spared by resection so as to prevent postoperative liver failure [34]. As well as Kinoshita *et al.* [35] and Makuuchi *et al.* [34], Nagino *et al.* [36•] have reported their experience with this procedure, using the percutaneous route and an ipsilateral approach (so as to prevent the hemorrhagic and carcinologic complications in the remaining liver) in 20 patients. There were no complications related to the procedure. In 16 patients with embolization of the right portal vein, the relative size of the left hepatic lobe, including the caudate lobe, increased after 2 weeks from a mean of 34% to 47% of the liver as assessed by computed tomography volumetry.

An alternative to liver resection associated with bile duct resection has been proposed in 1989 by Koyama *et al.* [37]. This includes targeting chemotherapy and intracavitary irradiation. Their experience now extends to 30 patients [38] and their 67% 5-year survival in the five patients receiving these treatments in addition to curative resection is impressive. The aggressive approach of Japanese surgeons is further supported by the report that long-term survival may be obtained after combined surgery and radiotherapy in patients with recurrent main hepatic duct cancer [39].

The lymphatic flow of distal bile duct cancer has also been recently reassessed by Kayahara *et al.* [40].

1) The frequency of nodal involvement in patients with distal bile duct cancer is 69%, a figure comparable to that of patients with pancreatic cancer (70.5%)

2) The degree of nodal involvement increases with increasing tumor infiltration into the pancreas; the pre- and perioperative assessment of pancreas invasion, however, underestimates histologic involvement

3) The most frequently involved lymph nodes are, by order of decreasing frequency the postero-superior pancreaticoduodenal lymph nodes (52%), the pericholedochal lymph nodes (28%), and lymph node around the superior mesenteric artery (22%); the practical implication of this is that nodal dissection around the superior mesenteric artery should also be performed in patients with distal bile duct cancer

Whether biliary bypass in patients with unresectable carcinoma should be performed surgically or nonoper-

Table 3. Results of pancreatoduodenectomy for the treatment of carcinoma of the ampulla of Vater published during 1989 to 1993

Study and year	Study period	Patients resected, *n*	Resectability, %	Operative mortality, %	Overall 5-year survival, %
Michelassi *et al.* [56], 1989	(1946–1987)	26	89	22	30
Shutze *et al.* [55], 1990	(1953–1988)	24	*	24	61
Martin *et al.* [54], 1990	(1979–1988)	24	NA	NA	43
Shyr *et al.* [51], 1993	(1965–1991)	102	*	17	26–54†
Willet *et al.* [46], 1993	(1981–1990)	41	*	5	55 (38–80)‡
Matory *et al.* [47], 1993	(1983–1990)	55	83	3	43
Klinkenbijl *et al.* [48], 1993	(1977–1988)	56	67	5	43

*Study refers only to patients who had undergone resection.
†5-year survival ranged from 26% for patients with aneuploid tumors to 54% for patients with diploid tumors.
‡5-year survival ranged from 38% for patients with high risk tumors to 80% for patients with low risk tumors.
NA—not available.

atively has been addressed over the past 8 years in four prospective controlled trials. The conclusion of these studies are similar, demonstrating that both techniques are equally effective in the short-term relief of jaundice. Of note, however, is that the mortality rates in the surgical arm were much greater than is usually reported. In addition, nonoperative palliation is frequently associated with late complications of recurrent jaundice and gastric outlet obstruction. Results of surgical palliation have recently been updated in a prospectively studied group of 118 patients undergoing a biliary bypass or a gastrojejunostomy [41•]. Although most of these patients had a tumor at the head of the pancreas, the results of this study are also relevant to biliary cancer. The in-hospital mortality rate was 2.5%, the mean postoperative stay was 14 days, and most of the postoperative complications were minor. Hospital readmission was required because of obstruction of the gastric outlet in five patients and because of recurrent jaundice or cholangitis in five patients. The 6-month and 1-year survival rates were 53% and 30%, respectively, with a mean survival of 7.7 months. Of relevant note is that 19% of the patients have survived at least 1 year.

Treatment of cancer of the ampulla of Vater

Cancer of the ampulla of Vater traditionally has a greater resectability rate and a better prognosis than other biliary cancers. Over the past 10 years, studies have suggested that the prognosis was significantly impaired by lymphatic invasion, regional nodal metastasis, higher tumor grade, invasion of the pancreas, and positive resection margin. Willet *et al.* [46] recently confirmed these findings, showing that patients with low-risk and high-risk tumors had a 80% and 38% 5-year survival, respectively, following pancreatoduodenectomy. Two other studies have however failed to demonstrate that positive lymph nodes, invaded surgical margins, tumor size, and extension into adjacent organs significantly influence survival [47,48].

In any case, these observations confirm that the best option for patients with cancer of the ampulla of Vater is resection, even it is only palliative [47,48], provided that it is associated with a low operative mortality (Table 3). The risk of mortality currently associated with pancreatoduodenectomy is approximately 5% or less. We believe this should remain the preferred technique of resection, local resection (the technique and results of which have recently been reviewed by Asbun *et al.* [49•]) should only be used as an alternative in elderly patients or in patients with benign or selected premalignant lesions, because of the greater risk of tumor recurrence [49•,50].

Preoperative radiotherapy may be beneficial in patients with cancer of the ampulla of Vater for several reasons: 1) bile duct (as well as pancreas) carcinoma is not (or is poorly) responsive to chemotherapy, 2) postoperative radiotherapy is associated with a trend toward better local control yet without improvement in survival, and 3) cancer of the ampulla of Vater initially has a locoregional spread, yet recurrence after pancreatoduodenectomy is mainly associated with distant metastasis, suggesting that tumor dissemination at the time of operative manipulation may occur that could be in some way prevented by preoperative radiotherapy [46].

Parameters that best define prognosis are those available on examination of the resected specimen. Shyr *et al.* [51] were able to demonstrate by multivariate analysis that DNA ploidy (which can be assessed by flow cytometry on fresh samples, *ie*, endoscopic biopsies performed before surgery) is an independent, and actually the best, predictor of survival of patients undergoing pancreatoduodenectomy for ampullary carcinoma.

Biliary drainage before surgery for biliary cancer

Whether jaundiced patients should undergo a biliary drainage before surgery for biliary cancer is still unresolved. Prospective controlled trials that have been conducted over the past 10 years [52•] have shown little or no advantages to this procedure, which has been consequently almost abandoned in Western countries. In Japan, however, it is still practiced. Indeed, percutaneous biliary drainage in Japan is associated with a very low rate of complications and the statement that the high incidence of biliary drainage–related complications would preclude its widespread use is probably outdated. In addition, the time interval between biliary drainage and surgery is longer in Japan than the usual 15- to 18-day duration used in Western countries. The shorter duration may be successful in relieving jaundice, but insufficent to allow full recovery of hepatocyte function. Obviously, the recovery of hepatocyte function is important in patients undergoing liver resection or major surgical procedures (such as an associated duodenopancreatectomy) but is of little relevance if a mere resection of the common bile duct is performed. It is therefore not surprising that little benefit of preoperative biliary drainage was reported from Western countries, when studies also included patients with benign lesions such as choledocolithiasis and few patients with curative resections. Finally, preoperative percutaneous drainage allows high-quality cholangiograms and an accurate assessment of the extent of cancer spread into each of the liver segments [9]. Two side effects of biliary drainage however, are, infrequently addressed: 1) it will result in the disappearance of the bile duct dilatation and therefore make the biliodigestive anastomosis more difficult, and 2) there is a risk of tumor seeding along the drain in 2% [9] to 6% [53] of the patients.

References and recommended reading

Papers of particular interest, published within the annual period of review, have been highlighted as:

- • Of special interest
- •• Of outstanding interest

1. • Duarte I, Llanos O, Domke H, Harz C, Valdivieso V: **Metaplasia and Precursor Lesions of Gallbladder Carcinoma.** *Cancer* 1993, **72**:1878–1884.

This paper provides an in-depth analysis of precursor lesions of gallbladder carcinoma from a country where the prevalence of biliary lithiasis is amongst the highest in the world.

2. • Ekborn A, Hsieh CC, Yuen J, Trichopoulos D, McLaughlin JK, Lan SJ, Adami HO: **Risk of Extrahepatic Bile Duct Cancer After Cholecystectomy.** *Lancet* 1993, **342**:1262–1265.

This was the first study to examine the incidence of extrahepatic bile duct cancer following cholecystectomy in a cohort of 62,734 patients who had undergone a cholecystectomy during 1965 to 1983 in the Uppsala region of Sweden.

3. Chijiiwa K, Ichimiya H, Kuroki S, Koga A, Nakayama F: **Late Development of Cholangiocarcinoma After the Treatment of Hepatolithiasis.** *Surg Gynecol Obstet* 1993, **177**:279–282.
4. Aoki H, Sugaya H, Shimazu M: **A Clinical Study on Cancer of the Bile Duct Associated With Anomalous Arrangements of the Pancreatobiliary Ductal System: Analysis of 569 Cases Collected in Japan.** *J Biliary Tract Pancreas* 1987, **8**:1539–1351.
5. Tanaka K, Nishimura A, Yamada K, Ishibe R, Ishizaki N, Yoshimine M, Hamada N, Taira A: **Cancer of the Gallbladder Associated With Anomalous Junction of the Pancreatobiliary Duct System Without Bile Duct Dilatation.** *Br J Surg* 1993, **80**:622–624.
6. Verbeek PCM, van Leeuwen DJ, de Wit LTh, Reeders JW, Smits NJ, Bosma A, Huibregtse K, van der Heyde MN: **Benign Fibrosing Disease at the Hepatic Confluence Mimicking Klatskin Tumors.** *Surgery* 1992, **112**:866–871.
7. Davidson BR: **Progress in Determining the Nature of Bile Duct Strictures.** *Gut* 1993, **34**:725–726.
8. Kurzawinski TR, Deery A, Dooley JS, Dick R, Hobbs KEF, Davidson BR: **A Prospective Study of Biliary Cytology in 100 Patients With Bile Duct Strictures.** *Hepatology* 1993, **18**:1399–1403.
9. • Nimura Y: **Staging of Biliary Carcinoma: Cholangiography and Cholangioscopy.** *Endoscopy* 1993, **25**:76–80.

This update on the staging of biliary carcinoma is from an author who has extensive experience with percutaneous cholangioscopy.

10. Earnhardt RC, McQuone SJ, Minasi JS, Feldman PS, Jones RS, Hanks JB: **Intraoperative Fine Needle Aspiration of Pancreatic and Extrahepatic Biliary Masses.** *Surg Gynecol Obstet* 1993, **177**:147–152.
11. Tio TL, Reeders WA, Sie LH, Wijers OB, Maas JJ, Colin EM, Tytgat GNJ: **Endosonography in the Clinical Staging of Klatskin Tumor.** *Endoscopy* 1993, **25**:81–85.
12. Piehler JM, Crichlow RW: **Primary Carcinoma of the Gallbladder.** *Surg Gynecol Obstet* 1978, **147**:929–942.
13. Shirai Y, Yoshida K, Tsukada K, Muto T, Watanabe H: **Early Carcinoma of the Gallbladder.** *Eur J Surg* 1992, **158**:545–548.
14. Shirai Y, Yoshida K, Tsukada K, Muto T, Watanabe H: **Radical Surgery for Gallbladder Carcinoma: Long Term Results.** *Ann Surg* 1992, **216**:565–568.
15. Shirai Y, Yoshida K, Tsukada K, Ohtani T, Muto T: **Identification of the Regional Lymphatic System of the Gallbladder by Vital Staining.** *Br J Surg* 1992, **79**:659–662.
16. Ouchi K, Suzuki M, Saijo S, Ito K, Matsno S: **Do Recent Advances in Diagnosis and Operative Management Improve the Outcome of Gallbladder Carcinoma?** *Surgery* 1993, **113**:324–329.
17. Ohtani T, Shirai Y, Tsukada K, Hatakeyama K, Muto T: **Carcinoma of the Gallbladder: CT Evaluation of Lymphatic Spread.** *Radiology* 1993, **189**:875–880.
18. Ogura Y, Mizumoto R, Isaji S, Kusuda T, Matsuda S, Tabata M: **Radical Operations for Carcinoma of the Gallbladder: Present Status in Japan.** *World J Surg* 1991, **15**:328–336.
19. Shirai Y, Yoshida K, Tsukada K, Muto T: **Inapparent Carcinoma of the Gallbladder: An Appraisal of a Radical Second Operation After Simple Cholecystectomy.** *Ann Surg* 1992, **215**:326–331.
20. Lucciarini P, Konigsrainer A, Eberl T, Margreiter R: **Tumour Inoculation During Laparoscopic Cholecystectomy.** *Lancet* 1993, **342**:59.
21. O'Rourke N, Price PM, Kelly S, Sikora K: **Tumour Inoculation During Laparoscopy.** *Lancet* 1993, **342**:368.
22. • Fong Y, Brennan MF, Turnbull A, Colt DG, Blumgart LH: **Gallbladder Cancer Discovered During Laparoscopic Surgery.** *Arch Surg* 1993, **128**:1054–1056.

This is an appraisal of the risks associated with laparoscopic management of gallbladder cancer.

23. Clair DG, Lautz DB, Brooks DC: **Rapid Development of Umbilical Metastases After Laparoscopic Cholecystectomy Fur Unsuspected Gallbladder Carcinoma.** *Surgery* 1993, **113**:355–358.
24. Falkson G, MacIntyre JM, Moertel CG: **Eastern Cooperative Oncology Group Experience With Chemotherapy for Inoperable Gallbladder and Bile Duct Cancer.** *Cancer* 1984, **54**:965–969.
25. Silk YN, Douglass HO Jr, Nava HR, Driscoll DL, Tartarian G. **Carcinoma of the Gallbladder: The Roswell Park Experience.** *Ann Surg* 1989, **210**:751–757.
26. Kairaluoma MI, Leinonen A, Niemelá R, Kivinieml H, Siniluoto T, Stahlberg M: **Superselective Intra-Arterial Chemotherapy With Mitomycin C in Liver and Gallbladder Cancer.** *Eur J Surg Oncol* 1988, **14**:45–50.
27. Mäkelä JT, Kairaluoma MI: **Superselective Intra-Arterial Chemotherapy With Mitomyin for Gallbladder Cancer.** *Br J Surg* 1993, **80**:912–915.
28. Bismuth H, Nakache R, Diamond T: **Management Strategies in Resection for Hilar Cholangiocarcinoma.** *Ann Surg* 1992, **215**:31–38.
29. • Ogura Y, Mizumoto R, Tabata M, Matsuda S, Kusuda T: **Surgical Treatment of Carcinoma of the Hepatic Duct Confluence: Analysis of 55 Resected Carcinomas.** *World J Surg* 1993, **17**:85–93.

This paper provides an in-depth analysis of the locoregional spread of Klatskin tumors.

30. Seki H, Tanaka JI, Sato Y, Kato Y, Umezawa A, Koyama K: **Neural Cell Adhesion Molecule (NCAM) and Perineural Invasion in Bile Duct Cancer.** *J Surg Oncol* 1993, **53**:78–83.
31. Tashiro S, Tsuji T, Kanemitsu K, Kamimoto Y, Hiraoka T, Miyauchi Y: **Prolongation of Survival for Carcinoma at the Hepatic Duct Confluence.** *Surgery* 1993, **113**:270–278.
32. • Bhuiya MMR, Nimura Y, Kamiya J, Kondo S, Nagino M, Hayakawa N: **Clinicopathologic Factors Influencing Survival of Patients With Bile Duct Carcinoma: Multivariate Statistical Analysis.** *World J Surg* 1993, **17**:653–657.

This multivariate analysis is from a group with the largest series of resected bile duct cancer ever studied.

33. • Nagino M, Nimura Y, Hayakawa N, Kamiya J, Kondo S, Sasaki R, Hamajima N: **Logistic Regression and Disciminant Analyses of Hepatic Failure**

After Liver Resection for Carcinoma of the Biliary Tract. *World J Surg* 1993, **17**:250–255.

This paper analyzes factors for postoperative hepatic failure in patients undergoing radical surgery for Klatskin Tumors.

34. Makuuchi M, Thai BL, Takayasu K, Takayama T, Kosuge T, Gunven P, Yamazaki S, Hasegawa H, Ozaki H: **Preoperative Portal Embolization to Increase the Safety of Major Hepatectomy for Hilar Bile Duct Carcinoma.** *Surgery* 1990, **107**:521–527.

35. Kinoshita H, Sakai K, Hirohashi K, Igawa S, Yamasaki O, Kubo S: **Preoperative Portal Vein Embolization for Hepatocellular Carcinoma.** *World J Surg* 1986, **10**:803.

36. • Nagino M, Nimura Y, Hayakawa N: **Percutaneous Transhepatic Portal Embolization Using Newly Devised Catheters: Preliminary Report.** *World J Surg* 1993, **17**:520–524.

This is one of the few studies to report the results of preoperative portal vein embolization of the liver segments to be resected, which allows a compensatory hypertrophy of the remaining segments in patients with carcinoma of the upper bile ducts.

37. Koyama K, Tanaka J, Kato S, Asanuma Y: **New Strategy for Treatment of Carcinoma of the Hilar Bile Duct.** *Surg Gynecol Obstet* 1989, **168**:523–530.

38. Koyama K, Tanaka J, Sato Y, Seki H, Kato Y, Umezawa A: **Experience in Twenty Patients With Carcinoma of Hilar Bile Duct Treated by Resection, Targeting Chemotherapy and Intracavitary Irradiation.** *Surg Gynecol Obstet* 1993, **176**:239–245.

39. Todoroki T, Fukuda Y, Kawamoto T, Saida Y, Ohara K, Iwasaki Y, Matsuzaki O: **Long-Term Survivors After Salvage Surgery Combined With Radiotherapy for Recurrence of Stage IV Main Hepatic Duct Cancer - Report of Two Cases.** *HepatoGastroenterology* 1993, **40**:285–293.

40. Kayahara M, Nagakawa T, Ueno K, Ohta T, Takeda T, Miyazaki I: **Lymphatic Flow in Carcinoma of the Distal Bile Duct Based on a Clinicopathologic Study.** *Cancer* 1993, **72**:2112–2117.

41. • Lillemoe KD, Sauter PK, Pitt HA, Yeo CJ, Cameron JL: **Current Status of Surgical Palliation of Periampullary Carcinoma.** *Surg Gynecol Obstet* 1993, **176**:1–10.

An update on the risk associated with surgical palliation of neoplasic strictures of the biliary tract.

42. Nimura Y, Hayakawa N, Kamiya J, Kondo S, Shionoya S: **Hepatic Segmentectomy With Caudate Lobe Resection for Bile Duct Carcinoma of the Hepatic Hilus.** *World J Surg* 1990, **14**:535.

43. Reding R, Buard JL, Lebeau G, Launois B: **Surgical Management of 552 Carcinomas of the Extrahepatic Bile Ducts (Gallbladder and Periampullary Tumors Excluded): Results of the French Surgical Association Survey.** *Ann Surg* 1991, **213**:236–241.

44. Gazzaniga GM, Filauro M, Bagarolo C, Ciferri E, Bondanza G: **Neoplasm of the Hepatic Hilum: The Role of Resection.** *Hepato Gastroenterol* 1993, **40**:244–248.

45. Nagorney DM, Donohue JH, Farnell MB, Schleck CD, Ilstrup DM: **Outcomes After Curative Resections of Cholangiocarcinoma.** *Arch Surg* 1993, **128**:871–879.

46. Willet CG, Warshaw AL, Convery K, Compton CC: **Patterns of Failure After Pancreaticoduodenectomy for Ampullary Carcinoma.** *Surg Gynecol Obstet* 1993, **176**:33–38.

47. Matory YL, Gaynor J, Brennan M: **Carcinoma of the Ampulla of Vater.** *Surg Gynecol Obstet* 1993, **177**:366–370.

48. Klinkenbijl JHG, Jeekel J, Schmitz PIM, Rombout PAR, Nix GAJJ, Bruining HA, van Blankenstein M: **Carcinoma of the Pancreas and Periampullary Region: Palliation Versus Cure.** *Br J Surg* 1993, **80**:1575–1578.

49. • Asbun HJ, Rossi RL, Munson JL: **Local Resection for Ampullary Tumors: Is There a Place for It?** *Arch Surg* 1993, **128**:515–520.

This paper relates the experience of the Lahey Clinic (including technique and results) with this uncommon surgical procedure.

50. Ricci JL: **Carcinoid of the Ampulla of Vater.** *Cancer* 1993, **71**:686–690.

51. Shyr YM, Su CH, Wu LH, Li AFY, Chiu JH, Lui WY: **DNA Ploidy as a Major Prognostic Factor in Resectable Ampulla of Vater Cancers.** *J Surg Oncol* 1993, **53**:220–225.

52. • Clements WDB, Diamond T, McCrory DC, Rowlands BJ: **Biliary Drainage in Obstructive Jaundice: Experimental and Clinical Aspects.** *Br J Surg* 1993, **80**:834–842.

A review of the physiopathologic consequences of jaundice and the benefits that may be anticipated from preoperative biliary drainage is provided.

53. Shorvon PJ, Leung JWC, Corcoran M, Mason RR, Cotton PB: **Cutaneous Seeding of Malignant Tumors After Insertion of Percutaneous Prosthesis for Obstructive Jaundice.** *Br J Surg* 1984, **71**:694–695.

54. Martin M, Rossi R, Dorucci V, Silverman ML, Braasch JW: **Clinical and Pathologic Correlations in Patients With Periampullary Tumors.** *Arch Surg* 1990, **125**:723–726.

55. Shutze W, Sack J, Aldrete JS: **Long-Term Follow-Up of 24 Patients Undergoing Radical Resection for Ampullary Carcinoma, 1953-1988.** *Ann Surg* 1990, **66**:1717–1720.

56. Michelassi F, Erroi F, Dawson PJ, Roncella M, Romagnoli J, Handcock M: **Experience With 647 Consecutive Tumors of the Duodenum, Ampulla, Head of the Pancreas, and Distal Common Bile Duct.** *Ann Surg* 1989, **210**:544–556.

Olivier Farges, MD, Centre Hépato-Biliaire, Hôpital Paul Brousse, 12, Avenue Paul Vaillant Couturier, B.P. 200, 94804 Villejuif Cedex, France.

Biliary imaging

Joseph T. Ferrucci, MD

Boston University Medical Center, Boston, Massachusetts, USA

Three new techniques highlight radiologic aspects of biliary tract disease. Percutaneous cholecystostomy using ultrasound guidance has proven a safe and effective technique for therapeutic drainage of acalculous cholecystitis. This technique is particularly appropriate for medically compromised patients who may be too ill to undergo formal surgical cholecystectomy. Chronic acalculous cholecystitis has also been the subject of successive investigation using cholecystokinin-stimulated cholescintigraphy. These patients, who are often considered to have "biliary dyskinesia," may be selected for cholecystectomy based on quantitative measures of gallbladder contractility. Magnetic resonance cholangiopancreatography affords a new method for noninvasive two-dimensional imaging of the biliary and pancreatic ducts that has significant advantages when compared with ultrasonography, computed tomography, and direct cholangiopancreatography by either endoscopic or retrograde routes.

Current Opinion in Gastroenterology 1994, **10**:541–545

Percutaneous cholecystostomy

During the past 10 years, percutaneous cholecystostomy has been increasingly used for both diagnosis and treatment of acute cholecystitis. The success rate has been high and the complication rate sufficiently low to be considered a suitable alternative to operative cholecystostomy or cholecystectomy, especially in high-risk patients. This is in contradistinction to a 25% mortality rate for cholecystectomy in patients with acute cholecystitis at high risk because of advanced age, sepsis, trauma, hyperalimentation, or other underlying disease.

Interventional radiologists perform percutaneous cholecystostomy under real-time ultrasound guidance for percutaneous single-step trochar or two-step Seldinger catheter drainage. The access approach is generally made transhepatically across intervening liver parenchyma through the nonperitonealized gallbladder fossa in order to contain bile leakage. Inspection of the bile drainage, real-time monitoring of the collapsing gallbladder after aspiration, and follow-up contrast cholecystocholangiography disclose the presence of infection, adequate gallbladder decompression, and the presence of calculi in the gallbladder of biliary ducts respectively (Fig. 1).

Vauthey *et al.* [1] refined the clinical indications in 21 elderly or critically ill patients undergoing percutaneous cholecystostomy for suspected acute cholecystitis. Ten (48%) were older than 65 years, nine (43%) were in intensive care units. Among the 21 patients, 18 had cholecystitis (eight calculous, and 10 acalculous). Sixteen of the 18 patients had immediate relief of symptoms and significant improvement of laboratory signs of cholecystitis. Among 10 patients with acalculous cholecystitis, only one underwent subsequent cholecystectomy. The other nine patients were alive and symptom-free with an intact gallbladder after a mean follow-up of 16 months. Of the eight patients with calculus cholecystitis, four underwent interval cholecystectomy, three died from underlying disease, and one patient had stones extracted percutaneously. The authors stress the versatility of percutaneous cholecystostomy in that it can be used either in the radiology department or in the intensive care unit. They emphasize that the natural history of patients with intercurrent illness and acalculous cholecystitis is such that those treated by percutaneous cholecystostomy do not require cholecystectomy or have further gallbladder symptoms. After a mean of 12 days, all patients in the acalculous group had a normal cholangiogram and the catheter was removed. Patients with calculous disease were treated selectively in relation to the course of their general medical condition. Half of the patients with calculous cholecystitis eventually underwent cholecystectomy because of persistent symptoms, recurrence or as definitive therapy. They conclude that the overall mortality rate of 5.5% compares favorably with the mortality rate of 20% to 30% for cholecystectomy in a similar group of critically ill patients.

Abbreviations

ERCP—endoscopic retrograde cholangiography; **MRCP**—magnetic resonance cholangiopancreatogram; **PTC**—percutaneous transhepatic cholangiography.

 ISBN 1-85922-610-8 ISSN 0267–1379

Creasy *et al.* [2] stressed the value of formal follow-up antegrade cholecystocholangiography to demonstrate gallstones or common duct stones after acute cholecystitis has been treated by percutaneous cholecystostomy. Obstructing cystic duct and common duct calculi were readily seen, including three patients in whom common duct calculi were visualized in nondilated ducts. Verbanck *et al.* [3] simplified the technique of percutaneous cholecystostomy to a single-stick needle aspiration, eliminating the requirement for longer term catheter drainage. In 18 high-risk patients with acute cholecystitis and severe intercurrent disease, simple gallbladder aspiration resulted in improvement in 17 of 18 cases, the only complication being local pain in two. Four of the 17 patients had an uncomplicated interval cholecystectomy; the remaining 13 who improved remained free from biliary symptoms during a mean follow-up of 14 months. Thus, single-stick percutaneous transhepatic gallbladder aspiration would seem a simpler and safer alternative to catheter drainage.

Lee *et al.* [4] applied percutaneous cholecystostomy for prophylactic biliary diversion and as a diagnostic test for acalculous cholecystitis in critically ill patients with sepsis of unknown cause. They performed a trial of percutaneous cholecystostomy in 24 patients in the intensive care unit having persistent, unexplained sepsis after complete clinical, laboratory, and radiologic search showed no alternative source of infection. They noted the unreliability of diagnostic tests in acute acalculous cholecystitis in this subset of patients, including poor sensitivity for clinical examination, ultrasonography, and biliary scintigraphy. Such patients are often obtunded and unresponsive; sonography often shows sludge and gallbladder distention and scintigraphy shows poor flow through the cystic duct due to bile stasis and sludge. Similarly, percutaneous aspiration with gram staining and culture of bile has also proven inadequate with a diagnostic sensitivity of less than 50%.

In this series [4] all patients were on ventilators, were receiving total parenteral nutrition, and were febrile. Fourteen patients showed dramatic improvements in clinical signs and symptoms, often within 24 hours. One patient died 3 weeks after percutaneous cholecystostomy of severe congestive cardiac failure and another underwent interval cholecystectomy. Therefore cholecystostomy was definitive therapy in 13 of 14 patients. No clinical response was observed in the other 10 patients. A respiratory source of infection was eventually found in three of the 10 nonresponders, but no definitive source was ever determined in the remaining seven. Five of these 10 patients eventually died of a combination of sepsis and multi-organ failure. The authors also confirmed a poor correlation between sonographic signs of sludge, wall thickening, pericholecystic fluid, and Murphy sign with the presence of a responsive or nonresponse. The authors conclude that in critically ill patients in an intensive care unit setting with persistent fever and a distended tense gallbladder on sonography, the threshold for percutaneous cholecystostomy should be exceptionally low. A positive response confirms the diagnosis, whereas a negative response eliminates the error of negative surgical exploration and also eliminates the gallbladder as a continuing concern.

Biliary dyskinesia syndrome

Despite the efficacy of cholecystectomy in relieving symptoms of patients with calculous gallbladder disease, surgeons have been reluctant to operate on patients with biliary-type pain in the absence of demonstrable gallstones. Patients suffering from this condition present as a diagnostic dilemma, usually in two types: typical biliary colic not associated with cholelithiasis or atypical right upper quadrant-epigastric pain accompanied by a host of negative investigations. Over the past several years there has been more acceptance of the entity of chronic acalculous cholecystitis as a cause of chronic abdominal pain, but there has been a distinct lack of ability, until recently, to accurately predict which patients are likely to benefit from cholecystectomy. However, the use of cholecystokinin-enhanced cholescintigraphy has now been clearly shown to accurately predict relief of symptoms with cholecystectomy.

In an informative review of cholecystokinin cholescintigraphy, Kloiber *et al.* [5] described the technical and clinical issues surrounding the documentation of gallbladder emptying. Inhibition of gallbladder motility and contractility is a well known precondition for development of gallbladder microcrystals and the actual gallstone nidus. Prior effects using cholecystokinin stimulation at oral cholecytography gave inconclusive results as to the ability to predict histologic abnormalities or relief of symptoms after cholecystectomy. However, these studies used an oral fatty meal resulting in poor control of gastric emptying and rather subjective radiologic estimates of cholecystographic ejection fraction.

Gallbladder emptying measured by scintigraphy with cholecystokinin stimulation is considerably more quantitative. Time activity curves can be constructed based on a region of interest over the gallbladder on digitized dynamic images. Background correction is done by subtracting radioactivity detected in a region of interest adjacent to the gallbladder region. Further refinement of the gallbladder contraction phase can be achieved by intravenous administration of cholecystokinin or its synthetic active octapeptide (sincalide; Kinevac, E.R. Squibb and Sons, Princeton, NJ). Intravenous physiologic infusion is preferred over dynamic bolus injection, as subjects rarely experience pain with the former.

Three recent studies illustrate a fairly consistent pattern of results. Zech *et al.* [6] reported on 59 patients who showed cholecystokinin-stimulated cholescintigraphy ejection fractions of less than 50% and underwent cholecystectomy with the following results: 54 (92%) had abnormal pathology and 56 (95%) had symptom relief (average follow-up, 1 year). Yap *et al.* [7] arbi-

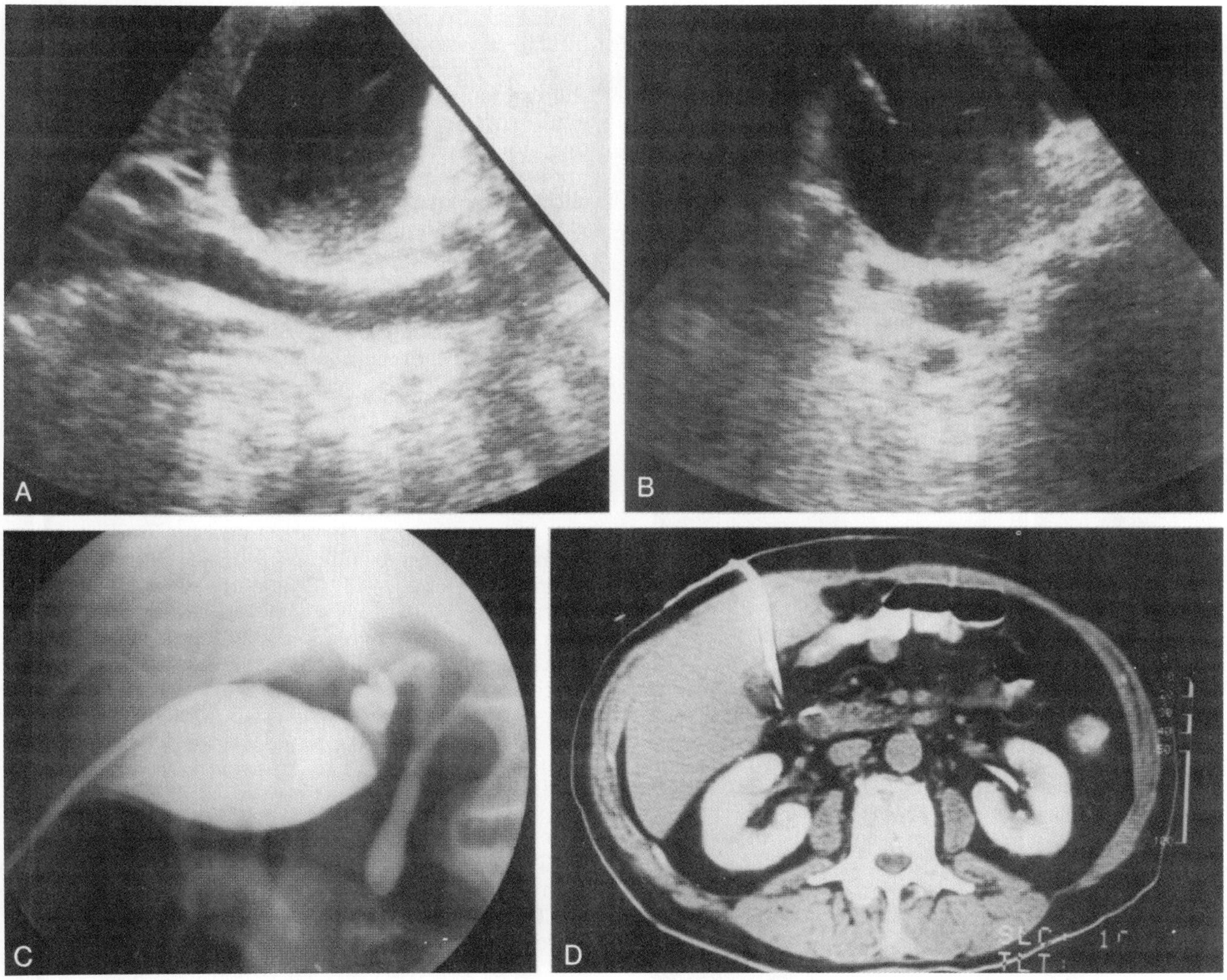

Fig. 1. Percutaneous cholecystostomy for therapeutic decompression in acute acalculous cholecystitis. **A,** Ultrasonogram showing a distended, sludge-filled gallbladder without stones. **B,** Needle aspiration/drainage under ultrasound guidance. Needle is seen entering percutaneously from 10 o'clock position. **C,** Catheter placed in the gallbladder fundus allows contrast medium to be injected for fluoroscopic filming. No stones are seen in the gallbladder or biliary ducts. **D,** Computed tomographic scan showing the catheter in place traversing the left lobe of the liver. The gallbladder is collapsed.

trarily defined the normal threshold as an ejection fraction of less than 40%. In 21 patients with an abnormally low ejection fraction randomly assigned to surgery, 11 were operated on, with 10 becoming asymptomatic and one having partial relief of symptoms. Of the 82 patients with normal ejection fractions in Yap's study group, 50 were asymptomatic on follow-up and 10 were symptomatic without specific treatment of biliary disease. Fourteen others had cholecystectomy and eight of these became symptomatic. In a third study, Reed *et al.* [8] used a lower ejection fraction of 35% as the discriminator. Of 30 patients undergoing cholecystectomy, 27 (90%) had pathologically abnormal gallbladders and 28 (94%) were relieved of symptoms over a follow-up period of 1 year.

It would appear therefore that in a patient with biliary-type symptoms and negative ultrasonography, cholecystokinin-enhanced cholescintigraphy with an abnormal ejection fraction should warrant cholecystectomy with a high expectation of symptomatic relief.

Magnetic resonance cholangiopancreatography

Three papers during the past year (two from Japan and one from the United Kingdom) [9–11] reported an exciting new method for obtaining three-dimensional magnetic resonance cholangiopancreatograms (MRCPs) that promises to have considerable impact on the diagnosis and management of biliary and pancreatic diseases. This is a bold statement, but the early results are striking.

Heretofore, magnetic resonance in the upper abdomen has been limited because of artifacts due to respiratory, peristaltic, and vascular motions. Most useful applications have been in the liver, where fairly reliable detection and characteristics of liver disease have been described. However, other methods such as ultrasound and computed tomography have been the stan-

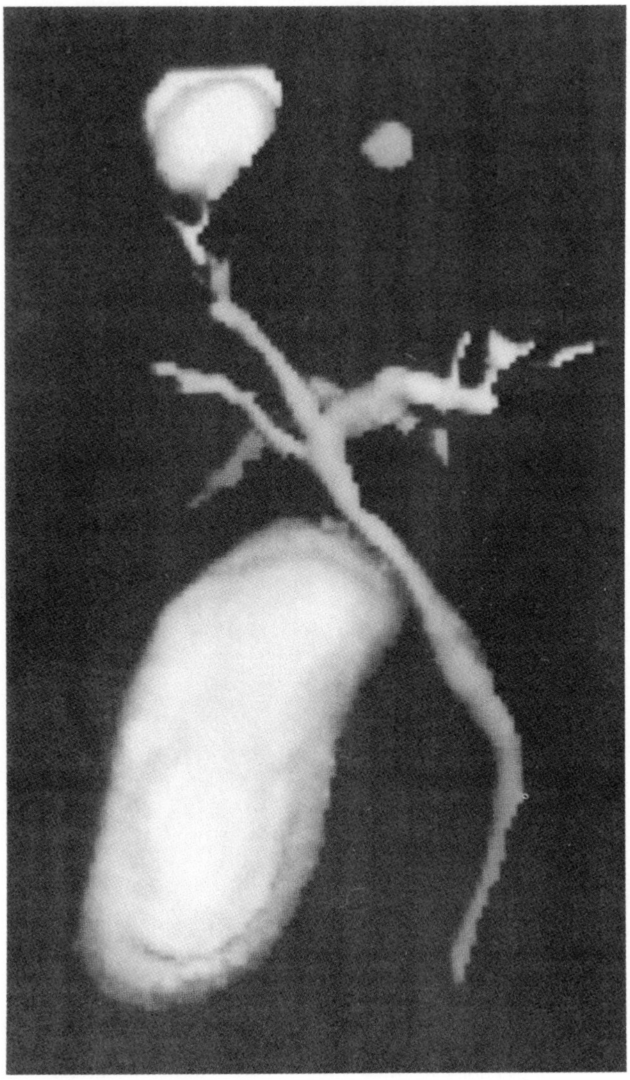

Fig. 2. Magnetic resonance cholangiogram. Normal caliber biliary ducts are evident as is the gallbladder. Two benign hepatic cysts are also displayed. No contrast medium was necessary for this study.

dard methods for evaluating the biliary tree and pancreas.

A recent study by Low *et al.* [12] from San Diego showed excellent detail of biliary duct disease when magnetic resonance images were obtained during a short breath-hold using gadolinium contrast enhancement. Dilated intrahepatic ducts were easily displayed as black tubular structures against a bright signal background of liver parenchyma and periductal extension of hilar cholangiocarcinomas was well seen. However, this study was merely an extension and refinement of heretofore standard liver magnetic resonance techniques.

In the first of the three papers on the new MRCP technique, Morimoto *et al.* [9] from Osaka were the first to show the potential of MRCP in 12 patients with malignant biliary obstruction using a three-dimension projection image. Their technique also used fast magnetic resonance breath-hold pulse sequences but used a projection image displaying the biliary duct as a frontal or coronal picture identical to a conventional direct cholangiogram obtained by percutaneous transhepatic cholangiography (PTC) or endoscopic retrograde cholangiopancreatography (ERCP). In addition, they employed postacquisition data processing by using a maximum intensity projection algorithm, which allowed the images to be viewed at a user selected angle. Individual image pixels were assigned a high signal to represent bile ducts and signal intensities were adjusted to give a volumetric appearance. In all 12 cases, dilatation and obstruction of the bile ducts were clearly demonstrated as bright signal structures analogous to conventional contrast cholangiography.

In a larger study of 40 patients, Hall-Craggs *et al.* [11] from Middlesex Hospital, London were able to acquire diagnostic cholangiograms in 39 of 40 cases. The static fluid in the biliary system appeared as a bright signal and allowed better demonstration of the peripheral biliary tree than that obtained by ERCP because of the limited direct filling owing to the risk of sepsis in those patients. MRCP demonstrated biliary ducts when ERCP was unsuccessful and, equally important, pancreatic duct, pancreatic pseudocysts, and common duct stones were well demonstrated. In two patients, magnetic resonance cholangiograms were manipulated at a three-dimensional work station, allowing the image to be rotated and pruned of peripheral branches so that the point of obstruction in the common duct could be more clearly demonstrated.

In a third study from Tokyo, Ishizaki *et al.* [12] found MRCP to precisely locate an obstructing biliary lesion with equal clarity as indirect cholangiography (PTC or ERCP). In addition, in one patient, common duct stones were shown by magnetic resonance that were overlooked by ERCP. On the other hand, MRCP could not differentiate carcinomas of the distal bile duct from the head of the pancreas.

Overall, the impact of MRCP could decrease the need for ultrasound, computed tomography, PTC, and ERCP as it provides a precise noninvasive three-dimensional coronal display of the biliary and pancreatic duct systems (Fig. 2). Disadvantages include less precise delineation of the length of the stricture because the distal duct systems are not as well dilated as with the direct injection. Similarly, image quality will be degraded by metallic surgical clips (cholecystectomy) or air in the biliary ducts (prior sphincterotomy). The method will be widely available because of the worldwide dissemination of magnetic resonance imaging equipment and further technical refinements are inevitable.

References and recommended reading

Papers of particular interest, published within the annual period of review, have been highlighted as:
- • Of special interest
- •• Of outstanding interest

1. • Vauthey JN, Lerut J, Martini M, Becker C, Gertsch P, Blumgart LH: **Indications and Limitations of Percutaneous Cholecystomy for Acute Cholecystitis.** *Surg Gynecol Obstet* 1993, 176:49–54.

This is an interesting study showing the applicability and safety of percutaneous cholecystostomy in elderly and critically ill patients.

2. Creasy TS, Gronvall S, Stage JG: **Assessment of the Biliary Tract by Antegrade Cholecystography After Percutaneous Cholecystostomy in Patients With Acute Cholecystitis.** *J Radiol* 1993, **66**:662–666.

3. Verbanck JJ, Demol JW, Ghillebert GL, Rutgeerts LJ, Surmont IP: **Ultrasound-Guided Puncture of the Gallbladder for Acute Cholecystitis.** *Lancet* 1993, **341**:1132–1133.

4. Lee MJ, Saini S, Brink JA, Hahn PF, Simeone JF, Morrison MC, Rattner D, Mueller PR: **Treatment of Critically Ill Patients With Sepsis of Unknown Cause: Value of Percutaneous Cholecystostomy.** *AJR Am J Roentgenol* 1991, **156**:1163–1166.

5. Kloiber R, Molnar CP, Shaffer EA: **Chronic Biliary-Type Pain in the Absence of Gallstones: The Value of Cholecystokinin Cholescintigraphy.** *AJR Am J Roentgenol* 1992, **159**:509–513.

6. Zech ER, Simmons LB, Kendrick RR, Soballe PW, Olcese JAM, Goff WB, Lawrence DP, Deweese RA: **Cholecystokinin Enhanced Hepatobiliary With Ejection Fraction Calculation As an Indicator of Disease of the Gallbladder.** *Surg Gynecol Obstet* 1991, **172**:21–24.

7. Yap L, Wycherley AG, Morphett AD, Toouli J: **Acalculous Biliary Pain: Cholecystectomy Alleviates Symptoms in Patients With Abnormal Cholescintigraphy.** *Gastroenterology* 1991, **101**:786–793.

8. • Reed DN, Fernandez M, Hicks PD: **Kinevac-Assisted Cholescintigraphy as an Accurate Predictor of Chronic Acalculous Gallbladder Disease and the Likelihood of Symptoms Relief With Cholecystectomy.** *Am Surg* 1993, **59**:273–277.

An ejection fraction of 35% or less is taken as a discriminator.

9. Morimoto K, Shimoi M, Shirakawa T, Aoki Y, Choi S, Miyata Y, Hara K: **Biliary Obstruction: Evaluation With Three-Dimensional MR Cholangiography.** *Radiology* 1992, **183**:578–580.

10. • Hall-Craggs MA, Allen CM, Owens CM, Theis BA, Donald JJ, Paley M, Wilkinson ID, Chong WK, Hatfield ARW, Lees WR, Russell CG: **MR Cholangiography: Clinical Evaluation in 40 Cases.** *Radiology* 1993, **189**:423–427.

This paper discusses a large series of 40 cases, including use of three-dimensional manipulation for multiplanar reformatting.

11. Ishizaki Y, Wakayama T, Okada Y, Kobayshi T: **Magnetic Resonance Cholangiography for Evaluation of Obstructive Jaundice.** *Am J Gastroenterol* 1993, **88**:2072–2077.

12. Low RN, Sigeti JS, Francis IR, Weinman D, Bower B, Shimakawa A, Foo FKF: **Evaluation of Malignant Biliary Obstruction: Efficacy of Fast Multiplanar Spoiled Gradient-Recalled MR Imaging vs. Spin-Echo MR Imaging, CT, and Cholangiography.** *AJR Am J Roentgenol* 1994, 162:315–323.

Joseph T. Ferrucci, MD, Professor and Chairman, Department of Radiology, Boston University Medical Center, 88 East Newton Street, Boston, MA 02118, USA.

Pathogenesis of cholesterol gallstones

Gwynneth D. Offner, PhD, and David P. Nunes, MD

Boston University School of Medicine and Boston City Hospital, Boston, Massachusetts, USA

Recent advances in the study of gallstone pathogenesis have focused on alterations in biliary lipids and proteins and on models of biliary hypomotility. The importance of both the concentration and composition of phospholipids in solubilizing cholesterol has been investigated. Several biliary proteins that promote cholesterol crystal nucleation and growth, including gallbladder mucin, immunoglobulins, aminopeptidase N, and α_1-acid glycoprotein have been further characterized. Animal models have provided increasing evidence for neuronal control of gallbladder motility. Studies in each of these areas have contributed to our still incomplete understanding of the mechanisms of cholesterol stone formation.

Current Opinion in Gastroenterology 1994, **10**:546–551

Gallstone disease is a multifactorial process caused by alterations in the lipid and protein composition of bile and defects in biliary motility (Table 1). In a recent review, Carey [1••] presents a concise summary of the pathogenic factors involved in both cholesterol and pigment stone formation. Changes in biliary lipids include increased cholesterol concentration with a relative reduction in the concentration of bile acids and phospholipids, resulting in cholesterol supersaturation, a prerequisite for cholesterol nucleation and stone growth. Numerous other changes are documented, including gallbladder mucin hypersecretion, alterations in the concentrations of both pro- and antinucleating proteins in bile, and reduced biliary motility. This review emphasizes recent papers that have advanced our knowledge in each of these areas with respect to the pathogenesis of cholesterol gallstone disease.

Biliary lipids and cholesterol gallstone disease

Cholesterol is carried in supersaturated bile in two principal forms: mixed micelles and cholesterol-enriched phospholipid vesicles. Although a third form of cholesterol carrier, lamellae, has been described by several laboratories, Cohen *et al.* [2•] have suggested that these structures may be an artifact of electron microscopy and are, in fact, multilamellar vesicles and mixed micelles. Cholesterol crystal nucleation, the initial phase of cholesterol gallstone formation, is thought to occur from the vesicular phase. The concentration of cholesterol in the vesicular phase increases with the concentration of bile.

Nakano and Chijiiwa [3•] have shown that hepatic bile taken from patients with cholesterol gallstones nucleates in half the time as hepatic bile taken from nongallstone patients. Concentration of bile in the gallbladder further reduced the crystal appearance time in cholesterol gallstone patients, whereas this effect was not seen in nongallstone patients. The shortened nucleation time of gallbladder bile was shown to be related to an increase in the proportion of cholesterol in the vesicular phase and is supported by the *in vitro* experiments of van Erpecum *et al.* [4•]. Together, these findings confirm the presence of a primary defect in hepatic bile that is further exacerbated by concentration in the gallbladder.

Phospholipids

There has been increased interest in the role of phospholipids in cholesterol crystal nucleation. Both the phospholipid concentration and the acyl group composition appear to be important modulators of cholesterol crystal appearance time *in vitro*. However, in human studies only minor differences in the acyl group composition of biliary phosphotidylcholine has been demonstrated. Approximately 95% of biliary phospholipid is phosphotidylcholine, 70% to 80% of the sn-1 group esterified with palmitic acid, and the majority of the sn-2 position esterified with linoleic, oleic, or arachidonic acid in that order.

Of particular importance is the report by Jungst *et al.* [5••], which demonstrates that the addition of phospholipid to rapidly nucleating bile results in an increase in the cholesterol crystal appearance time. This was associated with a transfer of cholesterol from the vesicular to the micellar phase. In contrast, addition of bile acids (such that the change in the cholesterol saturation index [CSI] was the same as that achieved through the addition of phospholipids) did not cause a similar effect. This strongly supports a pivotal role for phospholipids in stabilizing biliary cholesterol. The authors

Abbreviation

CSI—cholesterol saturation index.

 ISBN 1-85922-610-8 ISSN 0267–1379

Table 1. Proposed factors contributing to cholesterol gallstone disease

Hepatic factors
Genetic predisposition
Increased cholesterol secretion
High dietary cholesterol
Drugs
Reduced phospholipid secretion
Reduced bile salt secretion
Impaired gallbladder function
Reduced bile salt synthesis
Biliary factors
Bile salt composition
Small bowel disease
Phospholipid species and fatty acid composition
Gallbladder mucin hypersecretion
Phospholipases
Imbalance between pro- and antinucleating proteins
Biliary motility
Gallbladder hypomotility
Estrogen/progesterones
Reduced sensitivity to cholecystokinin
Neural mechanisms and brain peptides
Alterations in bile composition

suggest that increasing biliary phospholipid concentrations may be more effective than bile salts in gallstone prevention.

Previously, Halpern *et al.* [6] demonstrated that both the species of phospholipid and the fatty-acid composition at the sn-1 and sn-2 positions significantly affected whether cholesterol is carried in the vescular or micellar phase. Recently, Konikoff *et al.* [7•] showed that addition of lecithins containing short-chain and polyunsaturated fatty acids to a dilute, bile salt–rich, model bile resulted in the rapid formation of cholesterol filaments and monohydrate crystals. In contrast, "stiff" lecithins composed of saturated fatty acids significantly delayed the appearance of these early filamentous intermediates and crystals. The composition of the phospholipids absorbed to the surface of the cholesterol crystals was similar to that found in the vesicular phase of bile, lending support to the argument that cholesterol nucleation occurs from the vesicular phase. Their findings are supported by a second study demonstrating more rapid cholesterol crystal appearance in biles prepared with lecithins containing unsaturated fatty acid groups [8•].

If the composition of the acyl groups is important in determining the rate of cholesterol nucleation, then modulation of biliary phospholipid secretion could offer an important mechanism for the prevention of gallstone disease. Present data suggest that the hepatocyte selectively recruits 1-palmitoyl-2-linoleoyl-phosphatidylcholine to be secreted into bile and it is likely that this species is synthesized *de novo* in the hepatocyte. As bile acids are known to stimulate phosphatidylcholine synthesis, Shamburek and Schwartz [9•] studied the effects of bile acid administration on the secretion and composition of biliary phosphotidylcholines in rats. They found that there was a loss of selectivity in the secretion of phosphotidylcholine species as the rate of secretion increased, but this could not be related to bile acid hydrophobicity.

Bile salts

Bile salts are the major transporter of cholesterol in micelles but are also present as monomers in bile and in small quantities in vesicles. A study by Donovan *et al.* [10•] demonstrates that the distribution of bile salts between these three phases depends on the composition of the bile salts, the total lipid concentration of bile, and the bile salt–to-lecithin ratio. Hydrophilic bile salts are present in the intermicellar phase, whereas hydrophobic bile salts are preferentially distributed in mixed micelles. A report from Donovan and Jackson [11•] describes a simple ultrafiltration method for determining the intermicellar bile salt concentration. Use of these methods should help define the relationship between bile salt species, their effects on the partitioning of cholesterol between the micellar, vesicular, and nonmicellar/nonvesicular phases, and the resultant effect on cholesterol crystallization.

Animal models of gallstone disease

Animal models have been instrumental in defining many of the features of biliary physiology and biochemistry associated with gallstone formation. Cohen and Mosbach [12•] reviewed the history of the prairie dog and hamster models of cholesterol gallstone disease as well as their experience with these models. In hamsters, it has been noted that there are significant strain differences related to the propensity to form gallstones [12•,13•], which also depends on the type of triglyceride and concentration of cholesterol used to supplement the diet.

As in the hamster model, alterations in dietary fat may be an important modifier of cholesterol lithogenesis in the prairie dog. LaMorte *et al.* [14•] studied the effects of dietary fat on cholelithiasis in prairie dogs. They demonstrated that a high fat intake, in the form of corn oil, increased the incidence of gallstones. This was associated with higher plasma and biliary cholesterol concentrations, an increased ratio of biliary phospholipid to bile salts and an overall increase in the CSI of bile. Animals fed the high triglyceride diet were noted to have higher concentrations of linoleic acid, particularly at the sn-2 position, and a relatively lower concentration of palmitic acid. They propose that ω-6 polyunsaturated triglycerides augmented the formation of gallstones by increasing biliary cholesterol secretion.

Kim *et al.* [15•] studied the effects of cholestanol (5α-dihydrocholesterol) feeding on bile acid and cholesterol synthesis in mice and the development of gallstones using this model. During cholestanol feeding, 3-hydroxy-3-methylglutaryl coenzyme A reductase activity increased 51% (indicating increased *de novo* synthesis of cholesterol) while the activity of cholesterol 7α-hydroxylase, the rate-limiting enzyme for bile salt synthesis, fell. The combination of these effects promoted gallstone formation in this model.

Gallstones have been noted to occur with higher frequency in females, and at higher rates in multiparous women and women who take oral contraceptives. Previous studies have demonstrated that estrogens reduce bile salt secretion and in a recent paper, Gilloteaux *et al.* [16•] found that treatment of male hamsters with estrogen and medroxyprogesterone resulted in alterations to the gallbladder mucosa. Morphologic changes included increased mucus production, accumulation of apical granules, cytoplasmic vacuolation, and early gallstone formation. Furthermore, increases in serum lipids as well as an increase in liver and gallbladder weights were observed. Hence, estrogens, and progesterones may increase the propensity to form gallstones through several potentially important mechanisms.

Biliary proteins and cholesterol gallstone disease

Much recent work has focused on the biliary proteins that either promote or inhibit the nucleation of cholesterol crystals and it is widely assumed that one of the defects leading to the formation of gallstones is an imbalance in the concentrations of these pro- and antinucleating proteins. This field has seen rapid growth in the past several years and an overwhelming number of proteins that affect cholesterol crystal nucleation *in vitro* have been described (Table 2).

Gallbladder mucin

The large body of evidence for the involvement of gallbladder mucin in the pathogenesis of cholesterol gallstone formation has recently been summarized in an excellent review [17••]. Gallbladder mucin has been shown previously to promote cholesterol crystal nucleation, presumably through interactions of biliary lipids with hydrophobic binding sites on the mucin molecule. Recently, Afdhal *et al.* [18••] have shown that gallbladder mucin also affects the postnucleation phase of cholesterol crystal growth. Growth of seeded crystals in lithogenic model bile was accompanied by a decrease in both CSI and in crystal number. This suggests that mucin facilitates transfer of cholesterol to larger, more thermodynamically stable crystals. This paper is the first to directly demonstrate the effect of a protein on crystal size, rather than use turbidity measurements, which can not distinguish between increased crystal size or increased crystal number.

Although little is known about the primary structure of human gallbladder mucin, van Wijland *et al.* [19•] have demonstrated patient-to-patient variability in the carbohydrate moieties of gallbladder mucin. The same authors also analyzed mucin isolated from hepatic bile and found that the amino acid compositions of all samples were similar, as was the total carbohydrate content, but the glycan compositions were variable [20•]. Those mucin samples with lower *N*-acetyl-D-galactosamine content displayed increased potency in the nucleation time and vesicle fusion assays and the authors suggest that this effect could be due to either differential exposure of hydrophobic domains or alterations in mucin viscosity and gel-forming potential.

Mucin hypersecretion is an early and important event in the pathogenesis of cholesterol gallstone disease. The stimulus for mucin hypersecretion is poorly defined but is thought to be related to alterations in bile composition, which may in part be mediated through prostaglandins. Afdhal *et al.* [21•], using the prairie dog model, demonstrated that administration of prostaglandin E_1 alone caused a significant increase in mucin glycoprotein concentration but had no effect on the concentration of nonmucin glycoproteins. However, coadministration of prostaglandin E_1 and a cholesterol-supplemented diet significantly increased biliary total glycoprotein content, with an increase in both mucin and nonmucin proteins. The increase in nonmucin biliary glycoproteins is of particular interest, as there have been few studies demonstrating alterations in concentrations of these proteins in humans and the regulation of their synthesis or secretion into bile is poorly understood.

In a study from Sasaki *et al.* [22•], intraperitoneal administration of prostaglandin E_2 in guinea pigs resulted in a dose-dependent increase in both mucin glycoprotein and gallstone incidence. However, these animals developed primarily pigment stones, limiting the applicability to human cholesterol gallstone disease. Although the mechanism of this effect is not clear, the observed increase in both mucin and gallstone formation may be related to alterations in gallbladder motility induced by prostaglandin E_2.

Table 2. Major biliary proteins that promote cholesterol crystal nucleation and growth

Protein	Approximate M_r	Concentration in bile*	Assay	Study
Gallbladder mucin	2×10^6	0.5–4.0 mg/mL	Crystal growth	Afdhal *et al.* [18••]
IgM	80,000	100 µg/mL	NT	Upadhya *et al.* [23••]
IgG	53,000	200 µg/mL†	NT	Upadhya *et al.* [23••]
Aminopeptidase N	130,000	50 µg/mL	NT	Offner *et al.* [28•]
		40 µg/mL‡	NT	Nunez *et al.* [29•]
α-Acid glycoprotein	42,000	50 µg/mL	CCG	Abei *et al.* [26•]

*Concentrations shown were determined in gallbladder bile from cholesterol stone patients unless otherwise indicated.
†Concentration significantly higher than that found in control bile (≈20 µg/mL).
‡Concentration in hepatic bile.
NT—nucleation time or cholesterol crystal appearance time assay; CCG—cholesterol crystal growth assay measured turbidimetrically.

Nonmucin biliary concanavalin A–binding proteins

Many biliary proteins that bind the lectin concanavalin A have recently been reported to promote cholesterol crystal nucleation *in vitro*. The most thoroughly studied of these proteins are the biliary immunoglobulins. Upadhya *et al.* [23••] have extended their earlier studies by isolating each of these proteins and demonstrating that at physiologic concentrations, IgM was the most potent in nucleation time assays followed by IgG and IgA. They further showed that biliary IgG concentrations were significantly higher in cholesterol gallstone patients than in control subjects, whereas concentrations of IgM and IgA were similar. Highest IgG levels were found in patients with a CSI in the range of 1.2 to 1.4, leading the authors to suggest that changes in bile composition can cause increased IgG secretion, which may then promote nucleation and stone formation.

In another study, Lipsett *et al.* [24•] have isolated proteins from both cholesterol and pigment stones and identified two of these as immunoglobulin Fab fragments that promoted cholesterol crystal nucleation *in vitro*. Because commercially available Fab fragments had no effect, the authors suggest that an antigen-immunoglobulin complex may mediate cholesterol crystallization. However, Sanabria *et al.* [25•] found that fluorescein-conjugated albumin and IgG could diffuse into and out of nonfaceted cholesterol gallstones, suggesting that alterations in the protein composition of gallstones can occur during stone growth. These findings significantly alter the view that the proteins present in a mature gallstone necessarily play a significant pathogenic role in stone formation.

Another biliary protein that was further characterized recently is the 42-kD protein, identified by Abei *et al.* [26•] as α_1-acid glycoprotein. Three glycoforms of this acute-phase protein were isolated on concanavalin A sepharose and the authors found that only those forms that were bound or retained (containing biantennary glycans) promoted cholesterol crystal growth. The significance of this observation with respect to the interaction of α_1-acid glycoprotein with biliary lipids remains to be elucidated.

The protein that has received the most attention over the past year is the 130-kD protein identified as the canalicular enzyme aminopeptidase N [27]. In a study where all major concanavalin A–binding proteins were identified by amino-terminal sequence analysis, Offner *et al.* [28•] showed that aminopeptidase N from human gallbladder bile promoted cholesterol crystal nucleation at its physiologic concentration of approximately 50 μg/mL. Nunez *et al.* [29•] have also identified a 130-kD protein in human hepatic bile as aminopeptidase N. The protein was isolated from biliary vesicles and shown to promote cholesterol crystal nucleation *in vitro*. In a subsequent report [30•], these authors demonstrate that aminopeptidase N was associated with lamellar cholesterol carriers in supersaturated hepatic bile isolated from rats fed a diosgenin-simvastatin diet. It seems likely that aminopeptidase N is the 130-kD pronucleating protein first described by Groen *et al.* [31], although this has not been definitively established.

Abei *et al.* [32•] performed a comparative study that examined the effects of individual concanavalin A–binding proteins on crystal growth. They found that IgM was the most potent promoter followed by IgA, α_1-acid glycoprotein, and IgG. Surprisingly, aminopeptidase N was inactive in this study. Other experiments demonstrated that after removal of any of these proteins, the total concanavalin A–binding fraction still retained most of its promoting activity, suggesting that other unidentified proteins may be important in cholesterol crystallization.

Whereas the above studies have used crystal appearance time and crystal growth assays to investigate the pronucleating effects of biliary proteins, Luk *et al.* [33•] have used quantitative turbidimetric and fluorescence assays to examine the kinetics of phospholipase C–induced vesicle aggregation and fusion, a step which must occur prior to nucleation. Fusion was dependent on the formation of diacylglycerol, a product of lecithin hydrolysis by phospholipase C, which is known to destabilize lipid bilayers.

Mechanism of interaction of biliary proteins and cholesterol carriers

The mechanism whereby biliary proteins interact with biliary lipids is largely unknown, although it has been assumed that hydrophobic protein domains serve as binding sites. Evidence for this assumption has come from studies with gallbladder mucin [17••] and from the finding that certain biliary proteins, including aminopeptidase N, copurify with biliary vesicles [30•].

In a very interesting study, Ahmed *et al.* [34••] have proposed that the ability of a protein to promote nucleation is a function of its hydrophobicity, rather than a specific property of an individual protein. These authors empirically determined the hydrophobic indices of a number of proteins and tested them in cholesterol crystal nucleation assays. Surprisingly, they found that the most hydrophilic and most hydrophobic proteins were the most potent promoters and inhibitors of nucleation, respectively. Furthermore, they showed that the hydrophilic proteins were able to enhance the transfer of cholesterol from micellar to vesicular form and that hydrophobic proteins could reverse this process. These findings, although seemingly contrary to previous assumptions that hydrophobic domains on biliary proteins are responsible for lipid binding and nucleation, suggest that the overall hydrophobic/hydrophilic balance of biliary proteins influences cholesterol crystal nucleation by altering the cholesterol vesicular-to-micellar equilibrium.

Animal models of biliary motility

Alterations in gallbladder motility have been demonstrated to occur early in animal models of gallstone disease. The mechanism responsible for this change remains poorly understood, but it has been linked to changes in the CSI of bile. In a paper from Poston *et al.* [35], reduced gallbladder sensitivity to cholecystokinin and fewer cholecystokinin receptors were demonstrated in cholesterol-fed guinea pigs that developed stones compared with those that remained stone-free, suggesting that end-organ resistance to cholecystokinin is present in susceptible individuals. However, the observed differences were not statistically significant when either group was compared to the control group and further studies are needed before firm conclusions can be drawn.

In an interesting paper from Xu and Shaffer [36••], cisapride treatment of the Richardson ground squirrel fed a lithogenic diet resulted in normalization of biliary motility and biliary bile salt concentrations without increasing the size of the bile salt pool. The authors postulated that cisapride, by increasing gallbladder and intestinal motility, resulted in increased bile salt cycling, hence reducing the CSI towards normal. Cisapride probably enhances gallbladder motility by facilitating the response to cholinergic stimuli.

Recent data on biliary motility have suggested a more important role for neural pathways in the control of biliary motility than had previously been recognized. Cholinergic blockade increases the fasting volume of the gallbladder and reduces gallbladder emptying in response to both cholecystokinin and sham feeding. Cholecystokinin-induced gallbladder contraction is due to both a direct effect on the gallbladder and an effect mediated by cholinergic pathways. Gallbladder contraction has been shown to occur in association with phase II of the duodenal migrating motor complex and recently, neural projections between the duodenum and the gallbladder have been demonstrated.

A paper from Lenz *et al.* [37••] described the effects of 30 different neural peptides on cholecystokinin-induced gallbladder contraction. Three of these peptides, thyrotrophin-releasing hormone, vasoactive intestinal peptide, and calcitonin gene-related peptide, were all shown to modulate gallbladder contraction in response to both cholecystokinin and meals, predominantly through neural pathways as demonstrated by selective neural blockade. This study provides further evidence for the importance of central mechanisms in the control of biliary motility.

References and recommended reading

Papers of particular interest, published within the annual period of review, have been highlighted as:

- • Of special interest
- •• Of outstanding interest

1. •• Carey MC: **Pathogenesis of Gallstones.** *Am J Surg* 1993, **165**:410–419.

This is an integrated review of the pathogenesis of both cholesterol and pigment gallstones in which the author presents a unified theory assessing the relative importance of many of the proposed mechanisms involved in gallstone pathogenesis.

2. • Cohen DE, Kaler EW, Carey MC: **Cholesterol Carriers in Human Bile: Are "Lamellae" Involved?** *Hepatology* 1993, **18**:1522–1531.

This paper reviews experimental evidence for the existence of different cholesterol carriers in bile.

3. • Nakano K, Chijiiwa K: **Reduced Cholesterol Metastability of Hepatic Bile and its Further Decline in Gallbladder Bile in Patients With Cholesterol Gallstones.** *Gut* 1993, **34**:702–707.

Hepatic bile from cholesterol gallstone patients nucleates more rapidly than bile from nongallstone patients. The time to nucleation is further reduced following concentration of bile in the gallbladder.

4. • van Erpecum KJ, Stolk MJF, van den Broek AMWC, Renooij W, van den Heijning BJM, van Berge Henegouwen GP: **Bile Concentration Promotes Nucleation of Cholesterol Monohydrate Crystals by Increasing the Cholesterol Concentration in the Vesicles.** *Eur J Clin Invest* 1993, **23**:283–288.

Cholesterol crystal nucleation is enhanced by increasing the concentration of cholesterol in the vesicular phase without altering the cholesterol-to-phospholipid ratio.

5. •• Jungst D, Lang T, Huber P, Lange V, Paumgartner G: **Effect of Phospholipids and Bile Acids on Cholesterol Nucleation Time and Vesicular Micellar Cholesterol in Gallbladder Bile of Patients With Cholesterol Stones.** *J Lipid Res* 1993, **34**:1457–1464.

The effects of the addition of bile acids and phospholipids to rapidly nucleating human bile were studied. The addition of phospholipids significantly retarded the cholesterol crystal appearance time, whereas addition of bile acids had no effect.

6. Halpern Z, Moshkowitz M, Laufer H, Peled Y, Gilat T: **Effect of Phospholipids and Their Molecular Species on Cholesterol Solubility and the Nucleation in Human and Model Biles.** *Gut* 1993, **34**:110–115.

7. • Konikoff FM, Cohen DE, Carey MC: **Phospholipid Molecular Species Influence Crystal Habits and Transition Sequences of Metastable Intermediates During Cholesterol Crystallization from Bile Salt-Rich Model Bile.** *J Lipid Res* 1994, **35**:60–70.

The composition of phospholipid fatty acid side-chains significantly affects the cholesterol crystallization from model bile.

8. • Tao S, Tazuma S, Kajiyama G: **Fatty Acid Composition of Lecithin is a Key Factor in Bile Metastability in Supersaturated Model Bile Systems.** *Biochem Biophys Acta* 1993, **1167**:142–146.

Model biles prepared with lecithins rich in unsaturated fatty acids nucleate more rapidly than model biles prepared with lecithins containing saturated fatty acids.

9. • Shamburek RD, Schwartz CC: **Selective Composition of Biliary Phosphotidylcholines is Affected by Secretion Rate but not by Bile Acid Hydrophobicity.** *J Lipid Res* 1993, **34**:1833–1842.

Selectivity of phospholipid secretion is lost as phospholipid secretion increases within the physiologic range.

10. • Donovan JM, Jackson AA, Carey MC: **Molecular Species Composition of Inter-mixed Micellar/Vesicular Bile Salt Concentrations in Model Bile: Dependence Upon Hydrophilic-Hydrophobic Balance.** *J Lipid Res* 1993, **34**:1131–1141.

Hydrophobic bile salts are preferentially distributed in mixed micelles and vesicles whereas hydrophilic bile salts are present in the intermicellar phase.

11. • Donovan JM, Jackson AA: **Rapid Determination by Centrifugal Ultrafiltration of Inter-mixed Micellar/Vesicular (non-Lechithin Associated) Bile Salt Concentrations in Model Bile: Influence of Donnan Equilibrium Effects.** *J Lipid Res* 1993, **34**:1121–1129.

Validation of a centrifugal ultrafiltration technique for measuring the intermicellar concentration of bile salts.

12. • Cohen BI, Mosbach EH: **Cholesterol Cholelithiasis.** *Adv Vet Sci Comp Med* 1993, **37**:289–312.

A review of the hamster and prairie dog models of cholesterol gallstone disease with an emphasis on the authors' experience in the use of these models.

13. • Trautwein EA, Liang J, Hayes KC: **Cholesterol Gallstone Induction in Hamsters Reflects Strain Differences in Plasma Lipoproteins and Bile Acid Profiles.** *Lipids* 1993, **28**:305–312.

The authors studied the biliary lipid profiles and propensity to form gallstones in hamsters acquired from three sources. The major determinant of gallstone disease was found to be the source of hamster, though minor differences in biliary lipid composition and propensity to gallstone disease was demonstrated.

14. • LaMorte WW, O'Leary DP, Booker ML, Scott TE: **Increased Dietary Fat Content Accelerates Cholesterol Gallstone Formation in the Cholesterol-Fed Prairie Dog.** *Hepatology* 1993, **18**:1498–1503.

Supplementation of a cholesterol-enriched prairie dog diet with corn oil resulted in an increase in biliary cholesterol concentrations, a higher cholesterol saturation index, a higher proportion of biliary lecithins containing linoleic acid and increased incidence of gallstones. The authors conclude that gallstone formation is accelerated by feeding omega-6 polyunsaturated triglycerides.

15. • Kim K-S, Kano K, Hirabayashi N, Shefer S, Salen G, Seyama Y: **Gallstone Formation in Cholestanol-Fed Mice.** *J Biochem* 1993, **113**:420–424.

When fed to mice, cholestanol increased cholesterol synthesis and inhibited bile acid synthesis. Animals fed this diet had a higher incidence of gallstone formation and the alterations in cholesterol and bile salt metabolism were reversed when cholestanol feeding was discontinued.

16. • Gilloteaux J, Kosek E, Kelly TR: **Epithelial Surface Changes and Induction of Gallstones in the Male Syrian Hamster Gallbladder as a Result of a Two Month Sex Steroid Treatment.** *J Submicrosc Cytol Pathol* 1993, **25**:519–533.

Functional and morphologic changes of the gallbladder mucosa occur in male hamsters treated with medroxyprogesterone and estrogen. Changes included alterations in plasma lipids, increased mucin secretion, and early evidence of gallstone formation.

17. Klinkspoor JH, Tytgat GNJ, Groen AK: **Gallbladder Mucin and Cholesterol Gallstones.** *Eur J Gastroenterol Hepatol* 1993, **5**:226–234.
•• An excellent review of evidence for the role of gallbladder mucin in the pathogenesis of gallstones in experimental animals and humans as well as a discussion of gallbladder mucin secretion.

18. Afdhal NH, Niu N, Gantz D, Small DM, Smith BF: **Bovine Gallbladder Mucin Accelerates Cholesterol Monohydrate Crystal Growth in Model Bile.** *Gastroenterology* 1993, **104**:1515–1523.
•• Bovine gallbladder mucin was shown to promote cholesterol crystal growth, measured directly, in a lithogenic model bile seeded with cholesterol crystals. As the size of the crystals increased, the number of crystals decreased as did the CSI, suggesting a role for gallbladder mucin in the transfer of cholesterol.

19. van Wijland MJA, Klinkspoor JH, De Wit LT, Oude Elferink RPJ, Tytgat GNJ, Groen AK: **Heterogeneity of Human Gallbladder Mucin in Bile.** *Clin Sci* 1994, **86**:67–74.
• A report demonstrating that significant variability occurs in the carbohydrate moieties of gallbladder mucin isolated from different patients.

20. Klinkspoor JH, van Wijland MJA, Koelman CAM, van Dijk W, Tytgat GNJ, Groen AK: **Heterogeneity of Human Biliary Mucin: Functional Implications.** *Clin Sci* 1994, **86**:75–82.
• Heterogeneity in the carbohydrate moieties of mucin isolated from hepatic bile could be correlated with differences in the activity of mucin samples in cholesterol crystal nucleation assays and vesicle rupture assays.

21. Afdhal NH, Gong D, Niu Niu, Turner B, LaMont JT, Offner GD: **Cholesterol Cholelithiasis in the Prairie Dog: Role of Mucin and Non-Mucin Clycoproteins.** *Hepatology* 1993, **17**:693–700.
• The authors study the effects of exogenously administered prostaglandins on biliary mucin and nonmucin proteins using the prairie dog model. Prostaglandin E_1 increased the secretion of these proteins in association with cholesterol.

22. Sasaki H, Tazuma S, Kajiyama G: **Effects 16, 16-Dimethyl Prostaglandin E_2 on Biliary Mucous Glycoprotein and Gallstone Formation in Guinea Pigs.** *Scand J Gastroenterol* 1993, **28**:495–499.
• Biliary mucous glycoprotein and gallstone formation was increased in guinea pigs treated with prostaglandin E_2. However, pigment stones were the predominant gallstone type limiting the application of this model to human cholesterol gallstone disease.

23. Upadhya GA, Harvey PRC, Strasberg SM: **Effect of Human Biliary Immunoglobulins on the Nucleation of Cholesterol.** *J Biol Chem* 1993, **268**:5193–5200.
•• Comparison of the activity of isolated biliary immunoglobulins in cholesterol nucleation assays revealed that IgM was the most potent promoter followed by IgG and IgA. Higher concentrations of IgG, but not IgM or IgA, were detected in bile from cholesterol gallstone patients than in patients with pigment stones or in control subjects.

24. Lipsett PA, Hildreth J, Kaufman HS, Lillemoe KD, Pitt HA: **Human Gallstones Contain Pronucleating Nonmucin Glycoproteins that are Immunoglobulins.** *Ann Surg* 1994, **219**:25–33.
• Immunoglobulin Fab fragments were isolated from both cholesterol and pigment gallstones and found to accelerate cholesterol appearance time in nucleation assays.

25. Sanabria JR, Upadhya GA, Harvey PRC, Strasberg SM: **Diffusion of Substances into Human Cholesterol Gallstones.** *Gastroenterology* 1994, **106**:749–754.
• This report demonstrates that proteins can diffuse into and out of cholesterol gallstones, suggesting that the protein composition of stones can be altered during stone growth.

26. Abei M, Nuutinen H, Kawczak P, Schwarzendrube J, Pillay SP, Holzbach RT: **Identification of Human Biliary α1-Acid Glycoprotein as a Cholesterol Crystallization Promoter.** *Gastroenterology* 1994, **106**:231–238.
• This paper further characterizes the biliary 42-kD concanavalin A-binding protein. Three glycoforms of α_1-acid glycoprotein are described in which glycan composition could be correlated with the ability to promote crystal growth.

27. Offner GD, Gong D, Afdhal NH: **Aminopeptidase N is a 130 KD Pronucleating Glycoprotein in Human Hepatic and Gallbladder Bile [Abstract].** *Hepatology* 1991, **14**:92A.

28. Offner GD, Gong D, Afdhal NH: **Identification of a 130-Kilodalton Human Biliary concanavalin A Binding Protein as Aminopeptidase N.** *Gastroenterology* 1994, **106**:755–762.
• All major concanavalin A–binding biliary glycoproteins were identified by amino-terminal sequence analysis and the 130-kD protein identified as aminopeptidase N was isolated and found to promote cholesterol crystal nucleation at physiologic concentrations.

29. Nunez L, Amigo L, Rigotti A, Puglielli L, Mingrone G, Greco AV, Nervi F: **Cholesterol Crystallization-Promoting Activity of Aminopeptidase N Isolated from the Vesicular Carrier of Biliary Lipids.** *FEBS Lett* 1993, **329**:84–88.
• A 130-kD protein was isolated from hepatic biliary vesicles and identified as aminopeptidase N. This protein promoted nucleation of cholesterol crystals *in vitro*.

30. Rigotti A, Nunez L, Amigo L, Puglielli L, Garrido J, Santos M, Gonzalez S, Mingrone G, Greco A, Nervi F: **Biliary Lipid Secretion: Immunolocalization and Identification of a Protein Associated With Lamellar Cholesterol Carriers in Supersaturated Rat Bile.** *J Lipid Res* 1993, **34**:1883–1894.
• A model is described in which rats fed diosgenin/simvastatin develop supersaturated bile. Biliary lamellae isolated from these animals were found to contain the canalicular enzyme aminopeptidase N, suggesting a role for the canalicular membrane in biliary lipid secretion.

31. Groen AK, Noordam C, Drapers JAG, Egbers P, Jansen PLM, Tytgat GNJ: **Isolation of a Potent Cholesterol Nucleation-Promoting Activity from Human Gallbladder Bile: Role in the Pathogenesis of Gallstone Disease.** *Hepatology* 1990, **11**:525–533.

32. Abei M, Schwarzendrube J, Nuutinen H, Broughan TA, Kawczak P, Williams C, Holzbach RT: **Cholesterol Crystallization-Promoters in Human Bile: Comparative Potencies of Immunoglobulins, α1-Acid Glycoprotein, Phospholipase C and Aminopeptidase N.** *J Lipid Res* 1993, **34**:1141–1148.
• In this study, potential pronucleating proteins were isolated by immunoaffinity chromatography and IgM, IgA, and α_1-acid glycoprotein were found to be the most potent pronucleators. In addition, removal of these proteins from total concanavalin A-binding fraction showed only a partial loss of promoting activity, leading the authors to conclude that additional, yet uncharacterized, biliary proteins are important pronucleators.

33. Luk AS, Kaler EW, Lee SP: **Phospholipase C-Induced Aggregation and Fusion of Cholesterol-Lecithin Unilamellar Vesicles.** *Biochemistry* 1993, **32**:6965–6973.
• The effect of phospholipase C on vesicle aggregation and fusion was shown to be caused by diacylglycerol, a product of lecithin hydrolysis.

34. Ahmed HA, Petroni ML, Abu-Hamidiyyah M, Jazrawi RP, Northfield TC: **Hydrophobic/Hydrophilic Balance of Proteins: A Major Determinant of Cholesterol Crystal Formation in Model Bile.** *J Lipid Res* 1994, **35**:211–219.
•• The hydrophobic indices of a number of proteins were determined experimentally and found to be inversely related to the activity of these proteins in cholesterol crystal nucleation assays. In addition, the most hydrophilic proteins enhanced transfer of cholesterol from micellar to vesicular forms, whereas the most hydrophobic proteins reversed this process.

35. Poston GJ, Singh P, Dravian E, Yao CZ, Gomez G, Thompson JC: **Early Stages of Gallstone Formation in Guinea Pig are Associated With Decreased Biliary Sensitivity to Cholecystokinin.** *Dig Dis Sci* 1992, **37**:1236–1244.

36. Xu QW, Shaffer EA: **Cisapride Improves Gallbladder Contractility and Bile Lipid Composition in an Animal Model of Gallstone Disease.** *Gastroenterology* 1993, **105**:1184–1191.
•• Cisapride is shown to restore normal gallbladder contractility and to increase bile salt concentration in the bile of Richardson ground squirrels fed a lithogenic diet. The improvement in the CSI was probably secondary to increased cycling of bile through the enterohepatic circulation.

37. Lenz HJ, Zimmerman FG, Messmer B: **Regulation of Canine Motility by Brain Peptides.** *Gastroenterology* 1993, **104**:1678–1685.
•• Three brain peptides, thyrotrophin-releasing hormone, calcitonin gene-related peptide, and vasoactive intestinal peptide, alter gallbladder response to cholecystokinin and meal-stimulated gallbladder contraction. Use of neural blockade modulates their effects suggesting that these peptides mediate gallbladder contractility through neural pathways.

Gwynneth D. Offner, PhD, and David P. Nunes, MD, Section of Gastroenterology, Boston City Hospital, 818 Harrison Avenue, Boston, MA 02118, USA.

Gallstone epidemiology

Enrico Roda, MD, and Davide Festi, MD

University of Bologna, Bologna, and University Gabriele D'Annunzio, Chieti, Italy

In spite of many advances in the understanding of gallstone pathogenesis, knowledge of the natural history and risk factors for this very common disease is still incomplete. Furthermore, the availability of new surgical and nonsurgical therapeutic approaches makes it important to acquire this knowledge in order to identify the most appropriate treatment. In the past year, data on the natural history of gallstone disease were provided by epidemiologic studies on free-living populations; population or case-control studies evaluated some supposed risk factors of gallstone disease. Decision and quantitative analyses were performed to compare different therapeutic modalities.

Current Opinion in Gastroenterology 1994, **10:**552–557

The introduction of ultrasonography as a sensitive and accurate diagnostic tool for gallstone recognition began a new era in the study of gallstone epidemiology. In fact, previous approaches using clinically diagnosed cases or necroscopy data, although useful in performing historical comparisons of gallbladder disease rates and in identifying ethnic or racial differences, were unable to evaluate the true prevalence of the disease and suffered from potential referral bias and underestimation of clinically silent stones [1]. By using the ultrasound approach, cross-sectional and longitudinal studies were performed and initial data regarding prevalence, incidence, risk factors, and natural history of gallstone disease are now available. The results of population studies can be usefully employed in evaluating available therapeutic strategies and planning preventive programs. An agreed criteria [2,3••] to identify the best treatment of gallstone disease is particularly needed if we consider the different therapeutic options (surgical and nonsurgical) available today and the explosion in the use of laparoscopic cholecystectomy, the increased use of which seems to suggest a change in indications rather than resulting from risk-benefit ratio evaluation [4••]. This review focuses on recent acquisitions on gallstone epidemiology coming mainly from population studies; the use of these data in performing decision or quantitative analyses is also discussed.

Prevalence and incidence

The overall cost of epidemiologic studies is very high and a long time is required to obtain suitable results. For this reason the results available today are relatively few, as most of these are studies still ongoing. Necroscopy studies, such as the one recently reported by Mendez-Sanchez *et al.* [5], represent a different approach to gallstone epidemiology and their usefulness is in the evaluation of an historical trend in a specific area. However, some authors [6] claim the importance of necroscopy studies relates to the ability to identify diseases unsuspected or inactive during life.

In Italy, where the first epidemiologic studies were reported in the 1980s [7,8], a large multicenter study (MICOL [Multicenter Italian Study of Cholelithiasis]), is being performed [9]. This study involves 18 operative units covering almost all Italian regions and it has enrolled more than 33,000 subjects, from age 30 to 69 years. The cross-sectional phase is now over and the longitudinal one is ongoing. The available results confirm the earlier studies: the prevalence of gallstone disease was 13.8% (8.3% of gallstones; 5.5% of previous cholecystectomies for gallstone); the prevalence was higher in women (18.8%) than in men (9.5%) and increased linearly with age in both sexes. Parity, family history, obesity, and serum levels of triglycerides were significantly associated with gallstone disease, whereas the use of oral contraceptives and serum cholesterol levels appeared to be inversely related. The MICOL study confirmed that up to 80% of gallstones were asymptomatic. It was not possible to identify any predictive factors for symptom development.

Few data are available on the incidence of gallstones. In the Sirmione study [10•], the overall incidence of gallstone disease at 10 years was 4.6%; the incidence rate was higher in the first 5 years of observation (3.0%) than in the following 5 years. The incidence rate in the Sirmione study was similar to the one reported in Denmark by Jensen and Jorgensen [11] after a 5-year follow-up and somehow lower than the one calculated by using an epidemiologic method for converting prevalence rates into incidence rates [12]. An interesting result in the Sirmione study was that age, but not gender, was confirmed to be a true risk factor for gallstone development.

Risk factors

A main aim of epidemiologic studies of gallstones is to identify risk factors, because these could be used to design preventive programs. In the past year, some of

ISBN 1-85922-610-8 ISSN 0267–1379

the putative risk factors for gallstone disease have been evaluated by population or case-control studies.

Pregnancy

Epidemiologic and clinical evidence suggest that women are at higher risk for gallstones than men. Pregnancy and the use of female steroid hormones are also considered among the risk factors. Two studies have recently evaluated the relationship between pregnancy and gallstone formation. By studying women during the immediate postpartum period, Valdivieso *et al.* [13•] found a prevalence of gallstones (12.2%) higher than in nulliparous, age-matched volunteers (1.3%). In contrast to previous reports [8,14], a relationship between stone size (greater than 10 mm) and the appearance of biliary pain was documented. The frequency of biliary pain was high (31%); this was probably related to the earlier onset of gallstone disease and to the higher percentage of symptomatic gallstones in the Chilean population [15]. Patients with small stones were always asymptomatic and in 29% of them gallstones disappeared during the follow-up. The evaluation of bile lipid composition in patients with small stones documented an undersaturated bile with few cholesterol crystals during the follow-up period, whereas a bile supersaturated in cholesterol was present in controls. This observation suggests that gallbladder bile can improve rapidly after delivery even in patients with gallstones and this probably favors their dissolution.

That gallstones could represent a transient phenomenon during pregnancy is confirmed by the study of Maringhini *et al.* [16•], who prospectively followed women during pregnancy and after delivery to evaluate the frequency of biliary sludge and gallstone development. A total of 31% of subjects developed asymptomatic biliary sludge during pregnancy; in the majority of cases (61%), sludge disappeared during the follow-up period after delivery; 2% of subjects developed asymptomatic gallstones during pregnancy and in 28% of cases, mainly in those with small gallstones, these disappeared during the follow-up period. During pregnancy, biliary pain was present only in women with preexisting gallstones. An important result of this study is that patients with sludge at admission had a greater risk for developing new stones during pregnancy, probably indicating that biliary sludge may represent a pre-stone condition. Therefore, both studies [13,16•] provide evidence from large populations that pregnancy represents a risk factor for gallstone formation or for the development of symptoms when gallstones already exist. However they also indicate that the effect of pregnancy may be transient. This may explain the difference in results coming from studies on pregnancy and the risk of gallstone disease [1]; for this reason, Thijs *et al.* [17] stressed the need to consider the risk period when evaluating this possible relationship.

Nevertheless, pregnancy is an interesting model in which to study the pathophysiology of gallstone formation. A pathogenetic explanation has been proposed by Everson [18•]. Two hormone-induced mechanisms determine the presence of a supersaturated bile during pregnancy: the sluggish enterohepatic circulation of bile acids and the alteration of cholesterol balance. Impaired gallbladder emptying and increased intestinal transit time reduce the fractional turnover rate of the bile acid pool. Total bile acid pool size increases, but changes qualitatively (cholic acid pool increases and chenodeoxycholic and deoxycholic acid pools decrease), becoming more hydrophilic and hence having reduced capacity to solubilize cholesterol. Cholesterol synthesis increases, its conversion to bile acids decreases, and as a consequence, cholesterol secretion in bile increases. Further studies are needed to confirm this interesting hypothesis and to develop effective interventions in reducing the risk of gallstones in women.

Oral contraceptives

Studies of the relationship between oral contraceptive use and gallbladder disease have often yielded contradictory results [1]. Thijs *et al.* [19], evaluating the effect of oral contraceptives on the occurrence of gallstone disease in a case-control study, described the existence of a transient effect of oral contraceptives that did not extend beyond a 10-year use. To explain the observed differences in relation to age (a higher risk in younger than in older women) these authors postulated the existence of a subgroup of susceptible women in whom the occurrence of gallstone disease was accelerated by contraceptive use. They also came to a similar conclusion following a different methodological approach [20•]; all the controlled epidemiologic studies on oral contraceptives and the risk of gallbladder disease were reviewed by meta-analysis. Available data confirm a transient effect of oral contraceptive use on the rate of gallbladder disease, with a dose-effect relationship-noted with estrogen. Some results indicate that modern low-dose oral contraceptives have a smaller effect than older ones, even if the lack of a specified risk period makes this comparison difficult.

To investigate the relationship between the hormonal pattern and the presence of gallstone disease, Russo *et al.* [21] performed a case-control study using epidemiologic data and documented that in menopausal women with radiolucent and mixed stones, estradiol levels in the luteal phase were higher than in controls; men and postmenopausal women in the same conditions had lower luteinizing hormone levels than their respective controls. Although this observation indicates the existence of a relationship between endogenous sex hormones and gallstones, confirmation will require incidence studies on a larger population.

Two additional studies have tried to identify other factors accounting for differences in gallstone frequency between men and women. In an incidence study on newly formed gallstones, Rudnicki *et al.* [22] found that only women showed a positive correlation between gallstone development and serum levels of calcium, magnesium, bicarbonate, and parathyroid hormone. This result suggested a causal relationship between calcium homeostasis and gallstone disease: bound calcium and magnesium ions may increase the formation of gallstones in the form of bicarbonate-bound complexes. Unfortunately, no information was given on gallstone composition. Chijiwa *et al.* [23] studied cholesterol nucleation time but could not document any association with sex or age.

Obesity

Obesity is considered a confirmed risk factor for gallstone disease, particularly in women [24,25]. The lower prevalence of gallstone disease in men compared with women and a possible pathogenetic role of different regional fat distribution [26] could explain the difficulties in confirming the association of gallstone disease and obesity in men. An alternative hypothesis is that obesity does not represent the same risk in men as it does in women. During weight loss induced by surgery [27] or very low caloric diets [28•], the risk of gallstone formation further increases; in these settings, no differences were noted in relation to sex. Dieting does not seem to increase the risk of gallstone disease, at least acute gallstone disease [29].

Everhart [30•] reviewed the role of obesity and weight loss in gallstone formation. A total of 10% to 25% of obese subjects may develop gallstones within a few months after starting a very low caloric diet; about one third will develop biliary symptoms. In a small percentage of cases, gallstones spontaneously disappear during the follow-up period. High serum levels of triglycerides, a high initial body mass index, and a high absolute rate of weight loss represent the only identified risk factors for gallstone formation during weight loss. Prevention of gallstone formation during weight reduction has been achieved by oral administration of ursodeoxycholic acid and, to a lesser extent, aspirin [31]. No information is available on the effect of very low caloric diets on patients with preexisting gallstones. Obese patients during weight loss represent an interesting human model to study gallstone pathogenesis and prevention. However, further studies on larger populations are needed to identify the most suitable and safe diet in terms of nutrients, caloric contents, and eating habits. Furthermore, persons at particularly high risk of gallstone formation are appropriate for testing preventive measures.

Intestinal transit time and bowel habits

In a population survey, Heaton *et al.* [32•] evaluated the whole gut transit time in 15 of 48 women with gallstones and normal weight and observed that transit time was longer and the stool weight lower than in matched controls. This result confirmed the pathogenetic role of deoxycholic acid in gallstone formation, previously suggested by Marcus and Heaton [33]. The slower transit time caused an increased deoxycholic acid production and absorption and the increased biliary cholesterol secretion induced by this bile acid promoted gallstone formation. Moreover, this mechanism could also explain the higher prevalence of gallstones in females, because women had slower intestinal transit time and more constipation than men [34]. Although attractive, this hypothesis needs to be confirmed in men and in a larger study population.

Diabetes

Whether diabetes mellitus represents a risk factor for gallstone disease continues to be debated. Results from case-control and epidemiologic studies are conflicting and it is still unclear if the observed higher gallstone prevalence is related to diabetes itself or to the associated obesity. By evaluating clinical gallbladder disease in diabetic individuals identified during a population-based survey of diabetes and cardiovascular disease, Haffner *et al.* [35] documented that gallbladder disease was positively associated with the duration of diabetes. However, the prevalence of gallstones was not related to either plasma glucose levels or fasting insulin, suggesting a pathogenetic role of other factors linked to the diabetic or prediabetic state.

Socioeconomic status

The possible relationship between socioeconomic status and gallstone disease has been frequently evaluated [1] in order to identify potentially modifiable environmental factors. In a cohort study, Murray *et al.* [36] documented that cigarette smoking, parity, and lower social class represented risk factors for the development of symptomatic gallbladder disease. The use of oral contraception was associated with a small increase in risk that was limited to current users.

Gallbladder polyps

Gallbladder polyps represent a relatively frequent incidental finding during ultrasonography examination. The possible relationship between polyps and gallstones was recently evaluated by Shinchi *et al.* [37•], who studied the prevalence and risk factors of these lesions in a large population of males. Prevalence was 5.5% and no risk factors were identified, in particular those factors that are most frequently associated with gallstone disease. In very few cases both polyps and gallstones were present. These data confirm the results of a similar study made in Europe [38]. Moreover, polyps and gallstones seem to be different pathologic entities. However, because a higher incidence rate of gallstones was found in subjects with former polyps [11], further studies on a larger population, such as the MICOL study [9], are needed to confirm the role of polyps in gallstone formation.

Liver diseases

It is well known that liver diseases, particularly cirrhosis, are risk factors for gallstone formation, mainly pigmented stones. Conte *et al.* [39] prospectively evaluated 400 cirrhotic patients and demonstrated an overall gallstone incidence of 20% at 5 years and 38% at 8 years; symptoms were present in 10.2% at diagnosis and 16.1% during the follow-up. On multivariate analysis, high body mass index, female gender, and severe clinical deterioration were significantly related to a higher risk of developing gallstones.

Natural history

The knowledge of the natural history of gallstone disease represents a key factor in management decisions. Epidemiologic studies [7–9,10•] have clearly shown that asymptomatic gallstone patients represent the majority (up to 80%), and that the natural history of asymptomatic cases is generally benign [40]. In fact, a review of the available literature on the prognosis of asymptomatic and mild symptomatic gallstones [41••] indicates that serious symptoms and complications develop in about 1% to 2% of patients with asymptomatic gallstones annually, whereas these percentages are a little higher, about 1% to 3% per year, in patients with mild symptoms. No factors related to prognosis have been established. Complications such as acute cholecystitis, obstructive jaundice, pancreatitis, and cancer of the gallbladder are not frequent. The conclusions of the available studies confirm the advice of a working team [2] and of the American College of Physicians [42•], indicating that asymptomatic gallstones do not require treatment. This conclusion is further supported by a previous decision analysis [43] and by a recent review on the risks and benefits of gallstone therapy [44••].

The results of large longitudinal studies, such as the MICOL study [9], will probably provide answers to some unsolved questions regarding the natural history of asymptomatic gallstones, particularly as regards factors influencing prognosis.

Although the natural history of symptomatic gallstones is less benign (30% to 50% yearly rate of persisting pain), about 30% of patients who have had pain do not have further episodes of pain. It is generally agreed that symptomatic gallstones should be treated. However, quantitative analyses [45] have shown that the average amount of life expectancy gained by immediate surgical treatment in patients with symptomatic stones is only slightly higher than that achieved by expectant management, and may not be considered high enough to warrant therapy. The rates of biliary pain or of complications in symptomatic gallstones considered in these analyses came from a large multicenter study on gallstone dissolution [46]; they are higher and related to a shorter follow-up period than those observed in epidemiologic studies. Therefore, it is likely that quantitative analyses of epidemiologic data would indicate an even lower loss of life from conservative management.

Mortality

It is not the purpose of this article to review data concerning the relationship between gallstones and cancer; however a study recently published [47•] referring to an increased mortality from gallstones, should be discussed. Grimaldi *et al.* [47•] made a population-based prospective study among the Pima Indians, a population with a high prevalence of gallstones, to determine the association between gallstone disease and the overall rates and specific causes of death. The results indicated a higher death rate in patients with gallstone disease due to either malignancies (mostly of the digestive tract) or other nonneoplastic causes. In agreement with other reports [48], however, few subjects died directly from gallstone disease. These results, although not in agreement with a similar prospective population study from Rochester [49], suggest the need of a larger, more rigorous follow-up study of gallstones and mortality.

Prevention

The high frequency of gallstones, despite their low morbidity and nearly absent mortality makes gallstone disease a health problem whose prevention is desirable. The management of gallstone disease has a high cost and the advent of new treatments, such as laparoscopic cholecystectomy, does not seem to reduce this cost, at least over the short period. Hofmann [50••] has summarized the possibilities available to prevent this disease. Primary prevention is aimed at gallstone formation. An increased knowledge of prognostic factors in subjects belonging to high-risk groups (*eg*, obese patients during a weight reduction program or multiparous women at their last pregnancy) will probably allow identification of preventive treatments. In the general population, even in the absence of hard data, changes in lifestyle (a high-fiber, high-calcium, low saturated fatty-acid diet, regular consumption of three daily meals and a bedtime snack, along with a vigorous exercise program) should decrease cholesterol gallstone formation. No preventive measures have been identified for noncholesterol gallstones.

Secondary prevention aimed at the clinical manifestations of gallstones is mandatory. However, epidemiologic studies suggest that the natural history of symptomatic gallstones is probably more benign than previously thought. This allows physicians and patients to choose the best therapeutic approach in terms of medical indications and patient preference. Furthermore, the choice of treatments for gallstone disease depends not only on the presence of biliary symptoms but also on the functional characteristics of the gallbladder and the physicochemical properties of the stone. Information on the distribution of these characteristics in the general population can be employed in identifying the most appropriate treatment for individual patients as well as the most cost-effective one for the society.

Tertiary prevention against recurrence after successful gallstone dissolution or fragmentation must also be considered. Gallstone recurrence after these therapies is high (about 60% of patients) [51] and up to now no effective therapeutic regimen has been confirmed [51,52•], although some predictive factors, *eg*, the presence of multiple stones before therapy, have been identified [51]. Recent data [53] indicate that, although symptomatic gallstone patients successfully treated with oral bile acids are prone to gallstone recurrence, most of them do not develop biliary symptoms and, like asymptomatic gallstone patients, do not need further treatment.

Better knowledge of pathogenetic mechanisms, natural history, and risk factors of gallstone disease provided by large epidemiologic studies will probably answer many of the unsolved questions related to overall management of gallstone disease.

References and recommended reading

Papers of particular interest, published within the annual period of review, have been highlighted as:

- • Of special interest
- •• Of outstanding interest

1. Diehl AK: **Epidemiology and Natural History of Gallstone Disease.** *Gastroenterol Clin North Am* 1991, 20:1–19.

2. Paumgartner G, Carr-Locke DL, Roda E, Thistle JL: **Biliary Stones: Non-Surgical Therapeutic Approach.** *Gastroenterol Int* 1988, 1:17–25.

3. •• National Institute Health: **Consensus Development Conference Statement on Gallstones and Laparoscopy Cholecystectomy.** *Am J Surg* 1993, **165**:390–398.

This paper presents the results and the indications of a consensus panel for choosing the best surgical treatment for gallstone disease.

4. •• Legorreta AP, Silber JH, Costantino GN, Kobylinski RW, Zatz SL: **Increased Cholecystectomy Rate After the Introduction of Laparoscopic Cholecystectomy.** *JAMA* 1993, **270**:1429–1432.

This paper indicates that the use of laparoscopic cholecystectomy, a new technology touted as reducing health care costs, may result in an increased consumption of health care resources because of changes in the indications for gallbladder surgery.

5. Mendez-Sanchez N, Jessurun J, Ponciano-Rodriguez G, Alonso-De Ruitz P, Uribe M, Hernandez-Avila M: **Prevalence of Gallstone Disease in Mexico. A Necroscopy Study.** *Dig Dis Sci* 1993, **38**:680–683.

6. Simonovis NJ, Wells CK, Feinstein AR: **In-Vivo and Post-Mortem Gallstones: Support for Validity of the "Epidemiologic Necroscopy" Screening Technique.** *Am J Epidemiol* 1991, **133**:922–931.

7. Rome Group for Epidemiology and Prevention of Cholelithiasis (GREPCO): **Prevalence of Gallstone Disease in an Italian Adult Female Population.** *Am J Epidemiol* 1984, **119**:796–805.

8. Barbara L, Sama C, Morselli Labate AM, Taroni F, Rusticali AG, Festi D, Sapio C, Roda E, Banterle C, Puci A, Formentini F, Colasanti S, Nardin F: **A Population Study on the Prevalence of Gallstone Disease: The Sirmione Study.** *Hepatology* 1987, 7:913–917.

9. The MICOL Group: **Prevalence of Gallstone Disease in 18 Italian Population Samples: First Results From the MICOL Study.** In *Recent Advances in the Epidemiology and Prevention of Gallstone Disease.* Edited by Capocaccia L, Ricci G, Angelico F, Angelico M, Attili AF, Lalloni L. Dordrect: Kluwer Academic Publishers; 1991:37–44.

10. • Barbara L, Sama C, Morselli-Labate AM, Danesi GL, Festi D, Mastroianni A, Roda E, Venturoli N, Banterle C, Colasanti S, Formentini G, Nardin F, Nardin P, Pilia MC, Puci A: **10-Year Incidence of Gallstone Disease: The Sirmione Study.** *J Hepatol* 1993, **18(Suppl 1)**:S43.

This is the first report on gallstone incidence in a general population after 10 years of follow-up.

11. Jensen KH, Jorgensen T: **Incidence of Gallstones in a Danish Population.** *Gastroenterology* 1991, **100**:790–794.

12. Lowenfels AB, Velema JP: **Estimating Gallstone Incidence From Prevalence Data.** *Scand J Gastroenterol* 1992, **27**:984–986.

13. • Valdivieso V, Covarrubias C, Siegel F, Cruz F: **Pregnancy and Cholelithiasis: Pathogenesis and Natural Course of Gallstones Diagnosed in Early Puerperium.** *Hepatology* 1993, **17**:1–4.

This study indicates that pregnancy represents a risk factor for symptomatic gallstone development; however, gallstones often disappear after delivery.

14. Rome Group for the Epidemiology and Prevention of Cholelithiasis (GREPCO): **Radiologic Appearance of Gallstones and Its Relationship With Biliary Symptoms and Awareness of Having Gallstones: Observation During Epidemiological Studies.** *Dig Dis Sci* 1987, **32**:349–353.

15. Covarrubias C, Valdivieso V, Nervi F: **Epidemiology of Gallstone Disease in Chile.** In *Epidemiology and Prevention of Gallstone Disease.* Edited by Capocaccia L, Ricci G, Angelico F, Angelico M, Attili AF. Lancaster: MTP Press; 1984:26–30.

16. • Maringhini A, Ciambra M, Baccelliere P, Raimondo M, Orlando A, Tinè F, Grasso R, Randazzo MA, Barresi L, Gullo D, Mucicò M, Pagliaro L: **Biliary Sludge and Gallstones in Pregnancy: Incidence, Risk Factors, and Natural History.** *Ann Intern Med* 1993, **119**:116–120.

This study confirms that biliary sludge and gallstones are usually a transient phenomenon during pregnancy; patients with sludge may develop gallstones.

17. Thijs C, Knipschild P, Leffers P: **Pregnancy and Gallstone Disease: An Empiric Demonstration of the Importance of Specification of Risk Periods.** *Am J Epidemiol* 1991, **134**:186–19??

18. • Everson GT: **Pregnancy and Gallstones.** *Hepatology* 1993, **17**: 159–161.

A pathophysiologic explanation for pregnancy as a cholelithogenic state.

19. Thijs C, Leffers P, Knipshild P: **Oral Contraceptive Use and The Occurence of Gallstone Disease—A Case-Control Study.** *Prev Med* 1993, 22:122–131.

20. • Thijs C, Knipschild P: **Oral Contraceptives and the Risk of Gallbladder Disease: a Meta-Analysis.** *Am J Public Health* 1993, 8:1113–1120.

This study confirms the transient effect of oral contraceptive use on the rate of gallbladder disease, with a dose-effect relationship with estrogen.

21. Russo F, Cavallini A, Messa C, Mangini V, Guerra V, D'Amato G, Misciagna G, Di Leo A: **Endrogenous Sex Hormones and Cholesterol Gallstones: a Case-Control Study in an Echographic Survey of Gallstones.** *Am J Gastroenterol* 1993, **88**:712–717.

22. Rudnicki M, Jorgensen T, Jensen KH, Thode J: **Calcium, Magnesium, and Free Fatty Acids in the Formation of Gallstones: a Nested Case-Control Study.** *Am J Epidemiol* 1993, **137**:404–408.

23. Chijiwa K, Nakano K, Makino I, Noshiro H, Yamasaki T, Hirota I, Kiiyosawa R, Kurooki S, Ichimiya H: **Cholesterol Crystal Appearance Time of Gallbladder Bile in Middle-Aged Women.** *J Clin Gastroenterol* 1993, 16:195–198.

24. Stampfer MJ, Maclure KM, Colditz GA, Manson JE, Willett WC: **Risk of Symptomatic Gallstones in Women With Severe Obesity.** *Am J Clin Nutr* 1992, **55**:652–658.

25. Maglure KM, Hayes KC, Colditz GA, Stampfer MJ, Speizer FE, Willett WC: **Weight, Diet, and the Risk of Symptomatic Gallstones in Middle-Aged Women.** *N Engl J Med* 1989, **321**:563–568.

26. Heaton KW, Braddon FEM, Emmett PM, Mounford RA, Hughes AP, Bolton CH, Ghosh S: **Why Do Men Get Gallstones? Roles of Abdominal Fat and Hyperinsulinaemia.** *Eur J Gastroenterol Hepatol* 1991, 3:745–751.

27. Shiffman ML, Sugerman HJ, Kellum JM, Brewer WH, Moore EW: **Gallstone Formation After Rapid Weight Loss: A Prospective Study in Patients Undergoing Gastric Bypass Surgery For Treatment of Morbid Obesity.** *Am J Gastroenterol* 1991, **86**:1000–1005.

28. • **National Task Force on Prevention and Treatment of Obesity: Very Low-Calorie Diets.** *JAMA* 1993, **270**:967–974.

A comprehensive review on the safety and efficacy of very low caloric diets and a rational recommendation for their use.

29. Thijs C, Knipschild P, Leffers P: **Is Gallstone Disease Caused by Obesity or by Dieting?** *Am J Epidemiol* 1992, **135**:274–280.

30. • Everhart JE: **Contributions of Obesity and Weight Loss to Gallstone Disease.** *Ann Intern Med* 1993, **119**:1029–1035.

A review of the pathogenetic roles of obesity and weight loss in gallstone development.

31. Broomfield PH, Chopa R, Sheinbaum RC, Bonorris GG, Silverman A, Schoenfield LJ: **Effect of Ursodeoxycholic Acid and Aspirin on the Formation of Lithogenic Bile and Gallstones During Loss of Weight.** *N Engl J Med* 1988, **319**:1567–1572.

32. • Heaton KW, Emmett PM, Symes CL, Braddon FEM: **An Explanation for Gallstones in Normal-Weight Women: Slow Intestinal Transit.** *Lancet* 1993, **341**:8–10.

An interesting hypothesis to explain the higher gallstone prevalence in women.

33. Marcus SN, Heaton KW: **Deoxycholic Acid and the Pathogenesis of Gallstones.** *Gut* 1988, **29**:522–533.

34. Heaton KW, Radvan J, Cripps H, Mountford RA, Braddon FEM, Hughes AO: **Defecation Frequency and Timing, and Stool Form in the General Population - A Prospective Study.** *Gut* 1992, **33**:818–824.

35. Haffner SM, Diehl AK, Valdez R, Mitchell BD, Hazuda HP, Moraless P, Stern MP: **Clinical Gallbladder Disease in NIDDM Subjects. Relationship to Duration of Diabetes and Severity of Glycemia.** *Diabetes Care* 1993, **16**:1276–1284.

36. Murray FE, Logan RFA, Hannaford PC, Kay CR: **Cigarette Smoking and Parity As Risk Factors for the Development of Symptomatic Gallbladder Disease in Women: Results of the Royal College of General Practitioners' Oral Contraception Study.** *Gut* 1994, **35**:107–111.

37. • Shinchi K, Kono S, Honjo S, Imanishi K, Hirohata T: **Epidemiology of Gallbladder Polyps: An Ultrasonographic Study of Male Self-Defense Officials in Japan.** *Scand J Gastroenterol* 1994, **29**:7–10.

Polyp prevalence is similar in Japanese and Western populations, whereas gallstone prevalence is lower in Japan. Patients with polyps were not at increased risk of gallstones.

38. Jorgensen T, Jensen H: **Polyps in the Gallbladder. A Prevalence Study.** *Scand J Gastroenterol* 1990, **25**:281–286.

39. Conte D, Fraquelli M, Mandelli C, Braga M, Casarin P, Bodini P, Aimo GP, Borzio M, Barisani D: **Probability of Developing Gallstones and Related Risk Factors in 400 Cirrhotics.** *Eur J Gastroenterol Hepatol* 1994, 6:55–58.

40. Roda E, Taroni F, Festi D: **Gallstone Disease: A Clinical Lesson From Epidemiology.** *J Lithotripsy Stone Dis* 1990, 2:279–288.

41. Friedman GD: **Natural History of Asymptomatic and Symptomatic Gall-**
•• **stones.** *Am J Surg* 1993, **165**:399–404.
This paper provides a detailed review of available data on the prognosis of gallstone disease and a comparison of different treatment options.

42. American College of Physicians: **Guidelines for the Treatment of Gall-**
• **stones.** *Ann Intern Med* 1993, **119**:620–622.
This paper provides a good summary of decision making in treating gallstones.

43. Ransohoff DF, Gracie WA, Wolfenson LB, Neuhauser D: **Prophylactic Cholecystectomy or Expectant Management for Silent Gallstones. A Decision Analysis to Assess Survival.** *Ann Intern Med* 1983, **99**:199–204.

44. Ransohoff DF, Gracie WA: **Treatment of Gallstones.** *Ann Intern Med*
•• 1993, **119**:606–619.
This is a comprehensive review of the risks and benefits of treating asymptomatic and symptomatic gallstone patients.

45. Ransohoff DF, Gracie WA: **Management of Patients With Symptomatic Gallstones: A Quantitative Analysis.** *Am J Med* 1990, **88**:154–160.

46. Thistle JL, Cleary PA, Lachin JM, Tyor MP, Hersh T, The Steering Committee and the National Cooperative Gallstone Study Group: **The Natural History of Cholelithiasis: The National Cooperative Gallstone Study.** *Ann Intern Med* 1984, **101**:171–175.

47. Grimaldi CH, Nelson RG, Pettitt DJ, Sampliner RE, Bennett PH,
• Knowler WC: **Increased Mortality With Gallstone Disease: Results of a 20-Year Population Based Survey in Pima Indians.** *Ann Intern Med* 1993, **118**:185–190.
This study indicates an association between gallstone disease and an increased risk for malignancy and overall mortality in Pima Indians.

48. Cucchiaro G, Watters CR, Rossitch JC, Meyers WC: **Deaths From Gallstones. Incidence and Associated Clinical Factors.** *Ann Surg* 1989, **209**:149–151.

49. Maringhini A, Moreau JA, Melton LJ, Hench VS, Zinsmeister AR, DiMagno EP: **Gallstones, Gallbladder Cancer, and Other Gastrointestinal Malignancies. An Epidemiologic Study in Rochester, Minnesota.** *Ann Intern Med* 1987, **107**:30–35.

50. Hofmann AF: **Primary and Secondary Prevention of Gallstone Disease:**
•• **Implications for Patients Management and Research Priorities.** *Am J Surg* 1993, **165**:541–548.
This review reports on the current possibilities for gallstone prevention and the indications for future research.

51. Villanova N, Bazzoli F, Taroni F, Frabboni R, Mazzella G, Festi D, Barbara L, Roda E: **Gallstone Recurrence After Successful Oral Bile Acid Treatment. A 12-yr Follow Up Study and Evaluation of Long-Term Post-Dissolution Treatment.** *Gastroenterology* 1989, **97**:726–731.

52. Hood KA, Gleeson D, Ruppin DC, Dowling RH, and the British-
• Belgian Gall Stone Group: **Gallstone Recurrence and Its Prevention: The British/Belgian Gallstone Study Group's Post-Dissolution Trial.** *Gut* 1993, **34**:1277–1288.
This study documents that after medical dissolution, the risk of gallstone recurrence is not reduced by a high fiber, low refined-carbohydrate diet; recurrence may be lowered, but not abolished, by low-dose ursodeoxycholic acid.

53. Bazzoli F, Festi D, Zagari RM, Novelli V, Sangermano A, Fossi S, Morelli MC, Aldini R, Mazzella G, Roda E: **Gallstone Recurrence and History of Specific Biliary Symptoms During a Long-Term Post-Dissolution Follow-Up.** *Gastroenterology* 1992, **102**:302.

Enrico Roda, MD, Cattedra di Gastroenterologia, Policlinico S. Orsolo, Via Massarenti 9, 40100 Bologna, Italy.

Davide Festi, MD, Istituto di Fisiopatologia Medica, Ospedale SS Annunziata, via Valignani, 66100 Chieti, Italy.

Biliary motility

Marc F. Catalano, MD, and Walter J. Hogan, MD

Medical College of Wisconsin, Milwaukee, Wisconsin, USA

The control and operation of the gallbladder and sphincter of Oddi in modulating biliary pressure and bile flow continues to be elucidated and adapted to clinical situations. Prokinetic drugs may be useful in preventing stone formation in high-risk patients by promoting gallbladder emptying. Cholescintigraphy has been considered the most accurate test in evaluating acute cholecystitis. Now, cholecystokinin-assisted cholescintigraphy scans assess the gallbladder ejection fraction and detect chronic noncalculous gallbladder disease in the majority of these patients. Sphincter of Oddi manometric studies have helped in detecting sphincter of Oddi dysfunction and now better define patient groups and their outcomes to therapy. Finally, direct neural pathways have been demonstrated to connect the duodenum with the gallbladder and sphincter of Oddi, and the sphincter of Oddi with the gallbladder, confirming the existence of a highly integrated network that modulates biliary dynamics.

Current Opinion in Gastroenterology 1994, 10:558–566

Flow of bile into the duodenum involves a complex series of coordinated interrelationships between hepatocellular bile secretion and pressure differences generated between the gallbladder, cystic duct, and sphincter of Oddi. It is believed that functional disorders of bile flow may arise from a disturbance at any one of these locations.

During fasting, 75% of hepatic bile flow enters the gallbladder [1]. Periodic contraction of the gallbladder in conjunction with the migrating myoelectrical activity of the intestinal tract has been demonstrated [2]. Following a meal, a slow but sustained contraction of the gallbladder empties over 50% of its volume within 30 minutes. At the same time, resistance within the sphincter of Oddi decreases. Gallbladder filling takes place when a small negative pressure gradient occurring across the cystic duct coincides with simultaneous gallbladder relaxation and increased resistance to flow at the sphincter of Oddi.

The sphincter of Oddi demonstrates both tonic and rhythmic contractions that modulate the flow of bile into the duodenum in spurts rather than continuously. These myogenic contractions are modulated by neurohumoral stimuli. The rate of sphincter of Oddi phasic contractions changes synchronously with the gastrointestinal migrating motor complex and with meals.

The sphincter of Oddi can enhance common bile duct (CBD) outflow by a decrease in basal tone, an increase in rate of peristaltic contractions, or an increase in sphincter stroke volume. The sphincter may delay CBD outflow and promote gallbladder filling by an increase in basal tone, decrease in the proportion of antegrade peristalsis, or a decrease in sphincteric stroke volume.

Gallbladder contraction

Physiologic regulation of contraction

The principal stimulus for gallbladder contraction under normal conditions is ingestion of a meal. Fat-containing meals are the most powerful stimuli, although meals containing carbohydrate and protein produce some emptying. Following a liquid fat meal, minimum gallbladder volume is reached in 30 to 45 minutes and after a mixed solid-liquid meal, it may take up to 4 hours for the gallbladder to reach its minimum volume. Even during fasting, the gallbladder contracts periodically in rhythm with the gastrointestinal migratory motor complex, a phenomenon thought to be mediated by motilin [3•]. Long neural projections exist between the duodenum and gallbladder [4••]; these are most likely involved in the coordinated motility patterns of the gallbladder and intestine during fasting.

Under physiologic conditions, the most important controls of gallbladder emptying are cholinergic (vagal) nerves and cholecystokinin-mediated hormonal mechanism [5]. Cholinergic blockade achieved with atropine increases fasting gallbladder volume, suggesting a cholinergic role in maintaining fasting tone. Mourelle *et al.* [6] recently introduced the existence of a key L-arginine-nitric oxide pathway that regulated gallbladder contraction and reduces emptying following solid and liquid meals or in response to cholecystokinin. Atropine has been found to abolish gallbladder emptying in response to sham feeding, confirming that cephalic phase of gallbladder emptying depends on a cholinergic mechanism. Specific cholecystokinin antagonists similarly increase resting gallbladder volume and abolish postprandial contraction.

Abbreviations

CBD—common bile duct; **ERCP**—endoscopic retrograde cholangiopancreatography.

ISBN 1-85922-610-8 ISSN 0267–1379

Many peptides have been identified that in part, modulate gallbladder motility although with uncertain physiologic significance. Somatostatin in humans produces an increase in resting gallbladder volume and prevents contraction in response to sham feeding, test meals, cholinergic stimulation, and cholecystokinin infusion. Other peptides, including neurotensin, gastric-releasing peptide [7], substance P, and neuropeptide Y promote gallbladder contraction, whereas pancreatic polypeptide, peptide YY, calcitonin gene-related peptide [8], thyrotropin-releasing hormone [8], and vasoactive intestinal peptide promote gallbladder relaxation. Many of these peptides likely exert their effect indirectly by release of other peptides or via neurologic pathways.

Voltage-dependent calcium channel current, (L-type), is thought to be dominant in gallbladder smooth muscle cells in the guinea pig, but is unknown in humans [9]. Ishizuka *et al.* [10] recently suggested that both a reduced mobilization of intracellular calcium and a decreased muscle compliance are responsible, at least in part, for age-related reduced contraction of guinea pig gallbladder.

Radiologic evaluation

Knowledge of gallbladder emptying can be clinically important in the evaluation of patients with suspected gallstone disease, unexplained right upper quadrant abdominal pain, and biliary obstruction. Ultrasonography and roentgenography have been used to estimate gallbladder emptying and function. Radiographic methods estimate the rate of gallbladder emptying with serial planimetric measurements of radiopaque areas using formulas derived from theoretical geometric models but do not allow for the changing shape of the gallbladder as it contracts.

Cholescintigraphy has several advantages over these modalities. Gallbladder emptying following a test meal can be studied noninvasively, and quantitatively, with minimal radiation exposure. Two radionuclides commonly used are ^{99m}Tc diuisopropyliminodiacetic acid and ^{99m}Tc di-isopropylophenylocarbamoylmethiimino-diacetic acid (Hepatolite; DuPont Pharmaceutical, Billerica, MA). After intravenous administration of either of these agents count rates are determined continuously with a gamma counter for 45 to 60 minutes. Prompt and uniform uptake of radiotracer by the liver with excretion into the intrahepatic bile ducts, common bile duct, gallbladder, and finally the small intestine is seen in normal subjects.

Cholescintigraphy has been considered the most accurate test in the evaluation of acute cholecystitis, with a reported sensitivity and specificity as high as 95%. However, delayed images up to 4 hours postinjection of radiotracer may be required to achieve this level of accuracy. This delay in achieving the correct diagnosis is a disadvantage, and in some clinical settings it may not be feasible to acquire delayed images. Alternatively, use of morphine during hepatobiliary scintigraphy augments cholesctinigraphy scans in patients with suspected acute cholecystitis [11•]. The mechanism involves morphine contraction of the sphincter of Oddi, which increases intraductal pressure and diverts bile flow into the gallbladder if the cystic duct is patent. The use of morphine appears to help avoid delayed imaging without any loss of the accuracy of the test.

Another variation of the cholecystokinin-assisted cholescintigraphy scans in the assessment of the gallbladder ejection fraction. This test allows for diagnosing otherwise undetected chronic gallbladder disease in 90% of patients and allows selection of those patients likely to benefit from cholecystectomy with an equally high accuracy rate of 94% [12•].

Gallbladder dysmotility

Following drug therapy

Many drugs that affect gallbladder kinetics have been used therapeutically in different ways. Drugs that dilate the gallbladder and decrease intraluminal pressure may be used during biliary colic to decrease associated pain. Prokinetic drugs may be useful in preventing bile stagnation and stone formation. Treatment of acromegaly with somatostatin or its long-acting analogue, octreotide, has resulted in gallbladder dilation and impaired postprandial emptying [13]. This mechanism is believed to be a result of inhibition of gallbladder contraction mediated by a reduction of acetylcholine release, indicating an indirect effect on the gallbladder by the myenteric plexus [14]. Long-term treatment of acromegaly with octreotide has led to gallstone formation in up to 50% of cases [15].

Recently, Okano *et al.* [16] studied the effect of trimebutine maleate (2-dimethylamine-2-phenylbutyl-3, 4, 5-trimethozybenzoate hydrogen maleate) on gallbladder emptying. This drug has been used in the treatment of a variety of gastrointestinal dysmotility disorders, including irritable bowel syndrome, postoperative ilieus, and gastrectomy. These investigators found that trimebutine significantly inhibited fasting gallbladder emptying induced by neural reflex while it accelerated gallbladder emptying in the early phase of postprandial gallbladder contraction. No conclusions regarding possible therapeutic applications were mentioned.

A number of agents have been shown to have a prokinetic effect on the gallbladder including erythromycin [17••], cisapride [18], and cholestyramine [19]. The prevention of stone formation and sludge by promoting gallbladder emptying with oral prokinetic agents should be very useful in identifiable high-risk groups. These groups include obese patients on weight reduction diets, acromegalics taking octreotide, and patients receiving total parenteral nutrition, among others.

The most interesting prokinetic drug, erythromycin (a motilin receptor agonist) was studied by Catnach *et al.* [17••] and shown to have a pronounced effect on postprandial gallbladder emptying in patients with diabetic autonomic neuropathy, suggesting that the action of erythromycin on the gallbladder wall is predominately neurally mediated.

With pregnancy and steroid contraceptive use

Cholesterol cholelithiasis is more commonly seen in women than in men and is believed to be increased further in women during pregnancy, particularly in those who have had several pregnancies. This increased risk in women is poorly understood although estrogen and progesterone have been shown to increase biliary cholesterol saturation and impair the gallbladder response to exogenously administered cholecystokinin.

Gallbladder volume after an overnight fast is the net result of several variables, including the amount of bile secreted, its distribution between the gallbladder and intestinal tract, and the concentrating ability of the gallbladder. It has been speculated that increased gallbladder volume during fasting could be due to decreased water absorption by the gallbladder mucosa. The large amount of water that is normally absorbed from the gallbladder produces a 10-fold increase in the organic components of bile. Water absorption is dependent on the active absorption of sodium, which is mediated by the sodium pump (sodium-potassium ATPase) in the gallbladder epithelium. The activity of this pump is believed to be decreased by estrogen, which is present in large concentrations in the serum during late pregnancy.

Progesterone (a smooth muscle relaxant) also increases during pregnancy and has been shown to decrease gallbladder tone and increase receptive relaxation of the gallbladder resulting in dilatation of the gallbladder. It has also been shown that progesterone impairs the gallbladder response to exogenously administered cholecystokinin in animals.

Fasting gallbladder volumes have been determined and compared with postprandial volumes in women who were pregnant or using steroid contraceptives. After the first trimester, gallbladder fasting and residual volume after contraction are twice as great as controls and the rate of gallbladder emptying and the percentage of bile emptied are reduced. On the other hand, gallbladder emptying does not appear to be affected by contraceptive steroids.

Incomplete postprandial emptying of the gallbladder in the second or third trimester of pregnancy could contribute to cholesterol-gallstone formation. Because contraceptive steroids do not influence gallbladder function, one can only conclude that these drugs are not involved in emptying.

During fasting

Increased stone formation occurs in a number of patient groups with either temporary or permanent impairment of gallbladder motility. Patients receiving total parenteral nutrition do not empty their gallbladders regularly because of lack of cholecystokinin stimulation and therefore have a high incidence of biliary tract sludge and gallstones [20]. In persons receiving total parenteral nutrition, daily administration of intravenous cholecystokinin empties the gallbladder and prevents sludge formation [21]. Therefore, it is likely that correcting impaired emptying will prevent stone formation irrespective of the etiology of the motility defect.

Little and Avramovic [22] recently evaluated the rate of gallstone formation following major abdominal surgery. Seventy-three patients were studied with multiple abdominal ultrasound examinations. Twelve of 47 (28%) who underwent major abdominal surgery had gallstones within 14 to 36 months. Prolonged fasting after surgery was believed to be the predisposing factor for the formation of sludge and super-saturated bile.

In choledocholithiasis

For many years, investigators of the pathogenesis of gallstone disease have concentrated on the role of gallbladder motility as one potential cause. This has been facilitated by the availability of ultrasonographic and radionucleotide imaging [23]. Most studies have shown impaired gallbladder emptying in patients with known gallstones although other pathogenic factors have been implicated including cholesterol supersaturated bile, cholesterol crystal nucleating inhibitors and promoters, and secretion of mucin by the gallbladder mucosa.

The pathogenesis of gallbladder stasis has not been clearly delineated. It has been proposed that impaired cholecystokinin release, or inhibition of cholecystokinin stimulation during periods of prolonged fasting, total parenteral nutrition, or obstruction of extrahepatic bile ducts may cause gallbladder stasis. Other investigators have suggested that stasis may result from inflammation of the gallbladder wall prior to or following the formation of gallstones and in association with increased prostaglandin synthesis. Additional studies using gallbladder muscle strips exposed to bile with excess cholesterol showed impaired muscle contraction to cholecystokinin octapeptide, acetylcholine, and potassium even in the absence of gallstones compared with gallbladders with pigment stones. The mechanism of cholesterol-associated damage on the muscle cells, however, has not been investigated.

Behar *et al.* [24•], studying 19 human gallbladders with cholesterol stones and 11 with pigment stones, determined that muscle cells from gallbladders with cholesterol stones contract less than muscle cells from gallbladders with pigment stones. Furthermore, inositol triphosphate induced contractions of equal magnitude in cells from gallbladders with cholesterol and pigment stones, suggesting an impaired receptor activation of the mechanism for inositol triphosphate generation and release of stored calcium.

Schulz *et al.* [25] recently showed a significant contribution of the endogenous prostaglandin system to the cholecystokinin regulation of gallbladder motility. In large studies of gallstone patients, approximately 50% are shown to have impaired contractibility and many have abnormal emptying in response to both fatty meal and intravenous cholecystokinin. The impairment of gallbladder emptying is not the result of the physical presence of gallstones, as the defect does not correlate with the size or number of stones, and furthermore stone clearance with lithotripsy does not reverse the motility defect.

Berr *et al.* [26], in a study evaluating factors associated with early recurrence of cholesterol gallstones in a group of 20 patients successfully treated with bile acid litholytic therapy, found that gallbladders with recurrent stones emptied less completely in response to cholecystokinin compared with those without recurrent stones (Fig. 1). The median residual volume of these gallbladders after cholecystokinin infusion was more than twice as large in the recurrence group (7.5 mL) versus controls (3.2 mL) and the median fraction emptied tended to be less (64% vs 85%).

In diabetes

An increased incidence of gallbladder dysmotility has been described in patients with diabetes mellitus, including a higher incidence of gallstones [27], supersaturated bile, and a distended and poorly contracting gallbladder [28]. The mechanism of abnormal gallbladder emptying in diabetes is incompletely understood, although it is thought to represent a manifestation of denervation caused by visceral neuropathy referred to as *diabetic neurogenic gallbladder* [29]. However, other factors such as humoral mechanisms, *eg*, cholecystokinin blood levels, may be the cause of gallbladder dysmotility in diabetics [30,31]. Similarly, down-regulation of cholecystokinin receptors on gallbladder smooth muscle have been described in patients with poor gallbladder contraction [32]. In a study by Shaw *et al.* [33•], 50% of diabetics studied were found to have impaired gallbladder emptying following fat meal (Lipomal 1.5 mg/kg; Roberts Pharmaceutical Corp., Eatontown, NJ) that was not strictly corrected with diabetic neuropathy. Furthermore, it was not related to abnormal cholecystokinin release. One-year follow-up of those with impaired gallbladder contraction failed to demonstrate gallstone formation.

Gallbladder emptying and plasma hormone secretion cholecystokinin are significantly affected by blood glucose levels in response to sham and regular feeding [31]. In addition, these patients are shown to have decreased pancreatic polypeptide secretion compared with controls, suggesting depressed cholinergic tone during hyperglycemia [34]. The impaired gallbladder contraction during hyperglycemia in the gastrointestinal phase after regular feeding may result from impaired gastric emptying, impairing cholecystokinin secretion from the upper small intestine, or a diminished sensitivity of the gallbladder to cholecystokinin [35].

Wedmann *et al.* [36] evaluated gallbladder motility in diabetics with and without evidence of cardiovascular autonomic dysfunction and concluded that neuropathic dysfunction of the gallbladder is unlikely to play a major pathogenetic role in the development of gallstones in diabetic patients.

Sphincter of Oddi motility

Physiologic regulation

Sympathetic innervation of the sphincter of Oddi originates in the thoracic spinal segments 7 to 10 and the celiac ganglion, whereas parasympathetic fibers emerge from the vagus nerve. Adrenergic nerves may represent motor and inhibitory systems whereas parasympathetic cholinergic nerves may be responsible for motor sensory innervation of the sphincter of Oddi. Neural modulation of the sphincter of Oddi could represent the net effect of the excitatory and inhibitory neural input. These two sectors of the autonomic nervous system connect the central nervous system to a dense intrinsic neural network of myenteric neurons and ganglia cells located between the muscle layers of the sphincter of Oddi and the surface of the organ. Direct neural pathways have been shown to connect the duodenum with the gallbladder and the sphincter of Oddi, and the sphincter with the gallbladder. This implies that enteric nerve circuits participate in coordinating duodenal and biliary functions [4••].

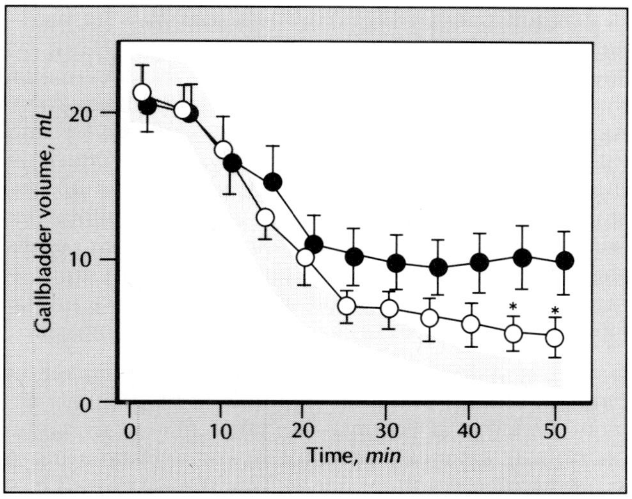

Fig. 1. Time course of gallbladder volume (mean ± SEM) during continuous infusion of cholecystokinin at a physiologic rate in 10 patients with recurrent gallstones (*solid circle*) and in 10 control patients (*open circle*) without recurrence of gallstones. Hatched area depicts the (mean ± 1 SEM) range of 15 previously studied healthy controls. *Asterisks* indicate data significantly different from control patients by Mann-Whitney test. (*Adapted from* Ohri *et al.* [75]; with permission.)

Many neurotransmitters have been identified in the extrahepatic biliary tree. Substance P–containing nerve terminals have been demonstrated in close proximity to cholinergic neurons and to the smooth muscle cells of the sphincter. Substance P may thus act on myocytes directly or indirectly through vagal cholinergic neurons sensitive to atropine blockade. Parodi *et al.* [37] were able to show the effect of substance P and calcium in significantly stimulating contractile frequency in the opossum sphincter of Oddi.

Numerous other peptides have been found recently to alter small bowel and biliary motor function. Of particular interest to biliary motility are cholecystokinin, bombesin-, gastrin-releasing peptide, neuropeptide Y, peptide YY, neurotensin, opioids, somatostatin, and vasoactive intestinal polypeptide [38].

Cholecystokinin has been the most extensively studied peptide; it is released after feeding and stimulates gallbladder contraction. Cholecystokinin, particularly its octapeptide, acts both directly on the sphincter of Oddi smooth muscle and indirectly via a neural mechanism. Both cholecystokinin forms relax the sphincter of Oddi by a tetrodotoxin-sensitive mechanism [39]. Cholecystokinin also has been shown to abolish phasic sphincter of Oddi contractions and decrease sphincter intraluminal pressure.

Neuropeptide Y has been identified in high concentrations in the biliary tree of pigs and dogs [40]. However, the physiologic action of this neuropeptide in biliary motility has not been characterized. Lillemoe *et al.* [41] found that neuropeptide Y stimulated sphincter of Oddi motility and increased gallbladder pressure in the prairie dog in a dose-related manner.

Neurotensin has been shown to contract the bile duct, ampulla, and gallbladder of the guinea pig in a dose-dependent manner [42]. The response may be mediated, in part, by a neural cholinergic mechanism, as suggested by a 70% to 85% reduction in the effect when the tissue was exposed to atropine and tetrodotoxin. Although neurotensin contracts the gallbladder and bile duct of the guinea pig, its physiologic effect on the biliary motility remains unclear. Gullo *et al.* [43] studied the effect of neurotensin on human gallbladder contraction by real-time ultrasonography. Their results showed a decrease in gallbladder contraction, suggesting the possibility of species-specific difference on the effect of neurotensin on gallbladder smooth muscle.

Glucagon has also been studied in the sphincter of Oddi and found to inhibit sphincter of Oddi motor activity. Ponce *et al.* [44] evaluated the effect of glucagon on human sphincter of Oddi motor activity using a manometric recording system. This study showed that glucagon significantly decreased the frequency of phasic sphincter of Oddi contractions. Basal sphincter of Oddi pressure, however, was not affected.

Nitric oxide has emerged as a key neurotransmitter throughout the gastrointestinal tract, including the biliary system. Nitric oxide might regulate sphincter of Oddi motility by activation of an enzymatic pathway present in sphincter of Oddi tissue homogenates [45]. Pauletzki *et al.* [46] recently suggested that baseline sphincter of Oddi motility is inhibited by a nitric oxide–sensitive pathway. Nitric oxide may play an important role in nonadrenergic, noncholinergic neurally mediated sphincter of Oddi relaxation [47].

Human and experimental studies on the sphincter of Oddi have established that the sphincter is not a simple, passive smooth muscle portion of the biliary system; rather, it plays an active role in modulating bile flow into the duodenum in both the fasted and postprandial states. Immunohistochemical studies have documented the presence of dense concentrations of neuropeptide-containing myenteric nerves in the sphincter of Oddi. Physiologic studies have confirmed that these peptides, in combination with the classic gastrointestinal hormones, exert significant effects on biliary motility.

Radiologic evaluation

Radiologic imaging has added substantially to our current knowledge of the sphincteric region and surrounding structures. Precise radiologic evaluation of the sphincter by ERCP requires a thorough knowledge of normal physiology and anatomy of the sphincter as well as an understanding of the morphologic and functional pathology encountered in this region. Computed tomography and ultrasound are also employed in the evaluation and follow-up of morphologic abnormalities of the sphincter region. Noninvasive functional evaluation of sphincter of Oddi, including fatty-meal sonography and quantitative hepatobiliary scintigraphy, are used at some institutions for screening patients with suspected sphincter of Oddi dysfunction or in follow-up of patients undergoing therapeutic sphincterotomy.

The primary goal of ERCP in patients with suspected sphincter Oddi dysfunction is to exclude structural CBD abnormalities such as choledocholithiasis, strictures, or tumors. Once these are excluded, attention is directed to the sphincteric segment. Findings suggestive of sphincter of Oddi disease include, dilation of the CBD (> 12 mm), delayed drainage of the CBD (> 45 minutes) dilated PD (> 6 to 7 mm) delayed drainage of the PD (≥9 minutes) or abnormalities in serum liver function tests.

There has been extensive controversy regarding the normal CBD diameter following cholecystectomy. Some have suggested slight dilatation of the CBD (>7 mm) is normal, as the duct assumes a reservoir function postcholecystectomy [48]. This has not been confirmed by other authors [49,50]. Fatty-meal sonography serves as a biliary stress test that theoretically distinguishes dilated nonobstructed from dilated obstructed symptoms. Fat (Lipomal 1.5 m/kg) in the duodenal lumen stimulates release of cholecystokinin by the intestinal mucosa. Cholecystokinin causes increased hepatic bile flow, contraction of the gallbladder (when present), and relaxation of the sphincter of Oddi. CBD measurements are made before the fatty meal and again 45 to 60 minutes following the meal [51]. A normal study is associated with no change or a decrease in the CBD diameter. A positive study is associated with an increase in the CBD diameter of 2 mm or more, following the fatty meal. Using these criteria, sensitivity of 74% and a specificity of 100% for partial CBD obstruction was reported by Darweesh *et al.* [51]. In patients in whom a positive fatty-meal sonography suggests partial CBD obstruction, ERCP with or without manometry should be considered.

Both quantitative and nonquantitative hepatobiliary scintigraphy have been used as the initial screen for partial CBD obstruction. Nonquantitative criteria for partial CBD obstruction is delayed liver-to-bowel transit time (>1 hour) or no significant decrease in biliary activity between 1 and 2 hours [52]. Quantitative hepatobiliary scintigraphy reports the time to peak hepatic activity and hepatic clearance (percent excreted at 45 to 60 minutes) as reliable indicators in sphincter of Oddi dysfunction. Darweesh *et al.* [53] reported 67% sensitivity and 85% specificity of quantitative hepatobiliary scintigraphy in patients with partial CBD obstruction. In their study, reduced hepatic isotope clearance

(<63%) at 45 minutes was the most sensitive indicator of a positive examination.

Manometric evaluation

Direct pressure recording of sphincter of Oddi motor activity during ERCP has become commonplace in many centers specializing in pancreaticobiliary disease. A European study, based on a retrospective review of patients with suspected pancreaticobiliary disorders, estimated that a single sphincter of Oddi manometric unit could service a population of 1.5 to 3 million people [54].

Benzodiazepine alone without opiates is the preferred form of premedication for sphincter of Oddi manometry. Recently midazolam, a newer, more rapidly eliminated benzodiazepine has been used in preference to diazepam for sphincter of Oddi manometry sedation. The influence of this drug on sphincter of Oddi motor function has been argued in two studies from the European continent. Rolney and Arleback [55] observed that midazolam lowered sphincter of Oddi tone if it were hypertensive, but did not effect sphincter of Oddi pressure if it was in the range of normal. On the other hand, Cuer *et al.* [56] found no evidence that midazolam had any effect on any elements of sphincter of Oddi motor activity in a group of 20 patients. While the debate continues, Allescher [57] contends diazepam is the sedative of choice for sphincter of Oddi manometry until midazolam has been more thoroughly evaluated. [57]

Elta and Barnett [58] reported on a prospective study evaluating the effects of meperidine on sphincter of Oddi motor function (1 ng/kg) that demonstrated no significant alteration of basal sphincter of Oddi pressure in a group of 18 patients. In an accompanying editorial, Sherman and Lehman [59] caution against routinely using meperidine analgesics while performing sphincter of Oddi manometry, until other centers validate these findings in larger groups of patients.

Finally, the reproducibility of sphincter of Oddi manometry in healthy subjects was once again demonstrated by Guelrud [60]. In his 1990 study, 10 healthy volunteers underwent sphincter of Oddi manometry on two separate occasions over a 1-week interval. At the first week, mean basal sphincter of Oddi pressure was 18.9±4.7 mm Hg (SD) whereas at the second study, mean basal sphincter of Oddi pressure was 17.6±5.0 mm Hg. Sphincter of Oddi manometry is a reproducible technique, at least in healthy subjects [61].

Sphincter of Oddi dysfunction

Sphincter of Oddi dysfunction can occur from two causes: a primary motor disturbance (dyskinesia) and a structural alteration (stenosis). The subsequent obstruction (albeit intermittent) to flow of bile could result in increased intraductal pressure, distention, and pain. It is often impossible to differentiate biliary dyskinesia papillary stenosis. Because of this difficulty, patients with suspected sphincter of Oddi dysfunction have been arbitrarily classified into three groups [62]. Characterized by biliary-type pain, abnormal liver function tests, and dilated or delayed CBD contrast drainage, type I patients are more likely to have sphincter of Oddi stenosis as a cause of their condition. Paradoxically, sphincter of Oddi manometric studies are reported to be normal in 15% [63], 35% [64], and 49% [65] of type I patients. These normal sphincter of Oddi pressure findings in type I patients, although disconcerting,

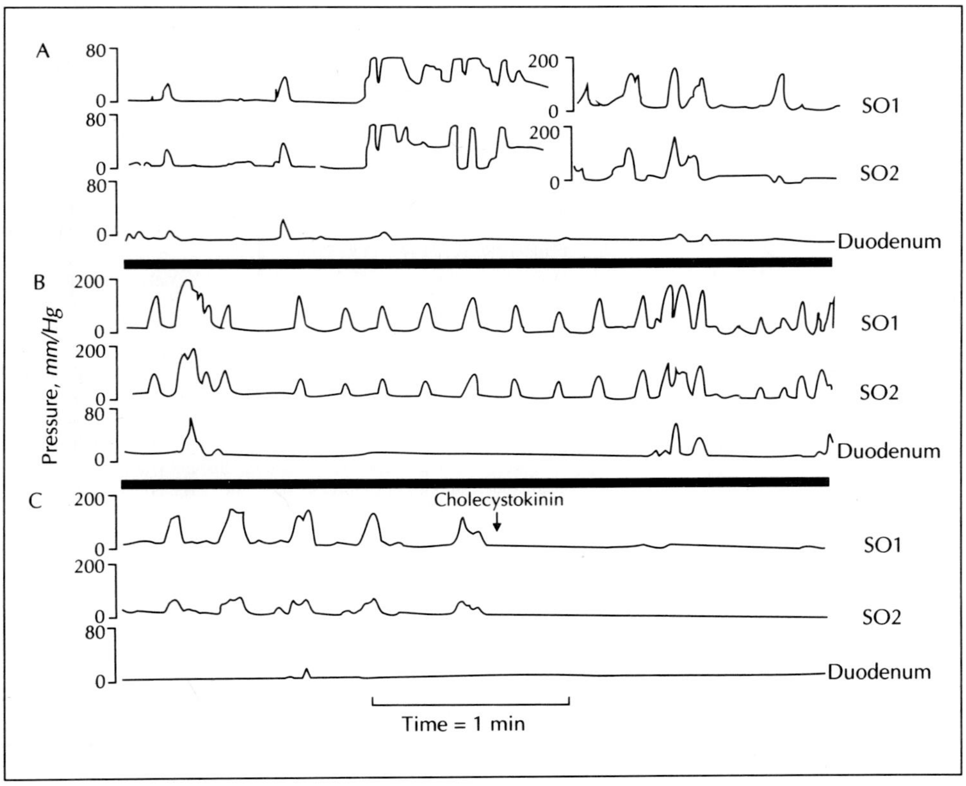

Fig. 2. Manometric tracings from the proximal (SO1) and distal (SO2) sphincter of Oddi and duodenum. **A**, The motility catheter is being pulled back from the duodenum with the proximal two sideholes entering the high-pressure zone of the sphincter. Note that the sensitivity scale for maximal pen deflection is changed from 0 to 80 to 0 to 200 mm Hg to capture the peaks of phasic sphincter of Oddi contractions. **B**, Duodenal contractions superimposed on the sphincter of Oddi. **C**, Response to an intravenous bolus of cholecystokinin. (*Adapted from* Richardson *et al.* [70•]; with permission.)

may be explained on the basis of sphincter of Oddi "noncompliance" rather than muscular spasm or true stricture [66]. Type II patients with suspected sphincter of Oddi dysfunction have biliary-type pain, but only one or two of the other objective criteria. A structural versus functional etiology for sphincter of Oddi dysfunction is difficult to separate in this patient group. Patients with elevated sphincter of Oddi pressure benefit from endoscopic sphincterotomy [67]. In one report, 85 type II patients with elevated basal sphincter of Oddi pressure (≥40 mm Hg) had an endoscopic sphincterotomy and were followed for a mean of 7±3 years. Subsequently, only four patients developed recurrent symptoms and postsphincterotomy restenosis (4.1% incidence) and this occurred within 4 months of the procedure. Repeat sphincterotomy effectively managed the situation and no further problems occurred during a mean follow-up of 25 months [68]. Sand *et al.* [69] reported the results of a treatment trial of nifedipine in a group of 13 type II patients in a double-blind, cross-over study. Ten of 12 patients had an abnormal quantitative cholecystogram but sphincter of Oddi pressures were not measured. Nifedipine (10 mg three times daily) significantly diminished the number of days of biliary pain and reduced the need for pain medication compared with placebo.

Sphincter of Oddi dysfunction may cause persistently elevated liver function tests and dilation of the distal common bile duct following orthotopic liver transplantation. Richards *et al.* [70] performed sphincter of Oddi motility studies through the T-tube tract in 10 patients at 3 months posttransplantation. Basal sphincter of Oddi pressure was normal in nine patients (16±5.8 mm Hg); phasic sphincter of Oddi characteristics were also normal (Fig. 2). One patient had abnormal pressures. All patients demonstrated a normal response to cholecystokinin-octapeptide with inhibition of phasic sphincter of Oddi contractile activity. In another group of five patients with liver transplantation and suspected sphincter of Oddi dysfunction, sphincter of Oddi manometry was also performed through a T-tube tract. Douzdjian *et al.* [71] detected two different manometric patters of sphincter of Oddi dysfunction. The first pattern, found in four patients, showed an elevated basal sphincter of Oddi pressure, infrequent phasic sphincter of Oddi activity, and an abnormal (paradoxic) response to cholecystokinin-OP. The second pattern, found in one patient, consisted of low basal sphincter of Oddi pressure and no phasic sphincter of Oddi activity.

The relationship of sphincter of Oddi dysfunction to an intact gallbladder was evaluated by Choudhry *et al.* [72]. A group of 35 patients with abnormal basal sphincter of Oddi pressure and intact gallbladder had an endoscopic sphincterotomy. However, only 15 of the 27 patients were improved at 1 month follow-up. Eleven of the unimproved patients, subsequently, underwent cholecystectomy and eight patients were improved. Prospective studies were urged to better define methods to discriminate sphincter of Oddi dysfunction from apparent gallbladder dysfunction in patients with chronic right upper quadrant pain. From the same center, Ruffolo *et al.* [73] evaluated the relationship of sphincter of Oddi dysfunction to the gallbladder ejection fraction in 81 type III patients with biliary pain. Abnormalities of sphincter of Oddi manometry or gallbladder ejection fraction were determined in 70% of these patients. However, sphincter of Oddi dysfunction was present in patients with similar frequency irrespective of the degree of gallbladder evacuation. Sphincter of Oddi and gallbladder dysfunction would appear to be independent factors.

Sphincter of Oddi motility was investigated in patients with bile duct stones by a percutaneous transhepatic route in 57 patients divided into three groups with common intrahepatic ductal stones, with intact gallbladders, or without intact gallbladders [74]. The investigators found no differences in basal sphincter of Oddi pressure, or phasic sphincter of Oddi contraction amplitude, frequency, or propagation duration among the three groups.

References and recommended reading

Papers of particular interest, published within the annual period of review, have been highlighted as:
- • Of special interest
- •• Of outstanding interest

1. Krishnamurthy GT, Bobba VA, Kingston E: **Radionuclide Ejection Fraction: A Technique for Quantitative Analysis of Motor Function of the Human Gallbladder.** *Gastroenterology* 1981, **80**:482–490.
2. Itoh Z, Takahashi I: **Periodic Contractions of the Canine Gallbladder During the Interdigestive State.** *Am J Physiol* 1981, **240**:6183–6189.
3. • Stolk MFJ, Van Expecum KJ, Smout AJPM, Akkermans LMA, Jansen JBMJ, Lamers CBHW, Peeters TL, Vanderge-Henegouwen GP: **Motor Cycles With Phase III Antrum Are Associated With High Motilin Levels and Prolonged Gallbladder Emptying.** *Am J Physiol* 1993, **264**:G596–G600.

This study discusses regulation of gallbladder motility during the interdigestive period-motor cycles. Phase III in antrum is associated with high motolin levels and prolonged gallbladder emptying.

4. •• Padbury RTA, Furness JB, Baker RA, Toouli J, Messenger JP: **Projections of Nerve Cells From the Duodenum to the Sphincter of Oddi and Gallbladder of the Australia Opossum.** *Gastroenterology* 1993, **104**:130–136.

Direct neural pathways have been shown to connect the duodenum with the gallbladder and the sphincter of Oddi, and the sphincter with the gallbladder, implying that the enteric nerve circuits participate in coordinating duodenal and biliary functions.

5. Tokunaga Y, Cox KL, Coleman R, Concepcion W, Nakazato P, Esquivel CO: **Characterization of Cholecystokinin Receptors on the Human Gallbladder.** *Surgery* 1993, **113**:155–162.
6. Mourelle M, Guarner F, Molero X, Moncada S, Malagelada JR: **Regulation of Gallbladder Motility of the Arginine-Nitric Oxide Pathway in Guinea Pigs.** *Gut* 1993, **34**:911–9115.
7. Beglinger C, Werth B, Hildebrande P, Luo H, Stalder GA: **Role of Gastric Releasing Peptide (GRP) in Contraction of the Human Gallbladder [Abstract].** *Gastroenterology* 1990, **98**:A244.
8. Lenz HJ, Zimmerman FG, Messmer B: **Regulation of Canine Gallbladder Motility by Brain Peptides.** *Gastroenterology* 1993, **104**:1678–1685.
9. Shimada T: **Voltage-Dependent Calcium Channel Current in Isolated Gallbladder Smooth Muscle Cells of Guinea Pigs.** *Am J Physiol* 1993, **264**:G1066–G1076.
10. Ishizuka J, Murakami M, Nichols GA, Cooper CW, Greeley GH, Thompson JC: **Age-Related Changes in Gallbladder Contractility and Cytoplasmic Ca+2 Concentration in the Guinea Pig.** *Am J Physiol* 1993, **264**:G624–G629.
11. • Kim CK, Juweid M, Woda A, Rothstein RD, Alavi A: **H Hepatobiliary Scintigraphy: Morphine-Augmented Versus Delayed Imaging in Patients With Suspected Acute Cholecystitis.** *J Nucl Med* 1993, **34**:506–509.

This study investigates the utility of morphine in augmenting the results of hepatobiliary scintigraphy in suspected cases of acute cholecystitis.

12. • Reed DN, Fernandez M, Hicks RD: **Kinevac-assisted Cholescintigraphy as an Accurate Predictor of Chronic Acalculus Gallbladder Disease and**

the Likelihood of Symptom Relief With Cholecystectomy. *Am Surg* 1993, **59**:273–277.

Cholecystokinin allows cholescintigraphy scans to detect unsuspected chronic gallbladder disease, allowing the appropriate selection of patients.

13. Stolk MFJ, Van Erpecum KJ, Koppeachaar HPF, de Braum WI, Jansen JBMJ, Lamers CBHW, Van Berge Henegouwen GP: **Postprandial Gallbladder Motility and Hormone Release During Intermittent Continuous Subcutaneous Actreotide Treatment in Acromegaly.** *Gut* 1993, **34**:808–813.

14. Nilsson BI, Svenberg T, Tollstrom T, Hellstrom PM, Samuelson K, Schnell PO: **Relationship Between Interdigestive Gallbladder Emptying, Plasma Motilin, and Migrating Motor Complex in Man.** *Acta Physiol Scand* 1990, **139**:55–61.

15. Plockinger U, Dienemann D, Quabbe HJ: **Gastrointestinal Side Effects of Octreotide During Long-Term Treatment of Acromegaly.** *J Clin Endocrinol Metab* 1990, **71**:1658–1662.

16. Okano H, Saeki S, Invi A, Kawai Y, Ohno S, Morimoto S, Ohmoto A: **Effect of Trimebutine Maleate on Emptying of Stomach and Gallbladder and Release of Gut Peptide Following a Solid Meal in Man.** *Dig Dis Sci* 1993, **38**:817–823.

17. •• Catnach SM, Ballinger AB, Stevens M, Faiclough PD, Trembath RC, Drury PL, Watkins PJ: **Erythromycin Induces Supranormal Gallbladder Contraction in Diabetic Anatomic Neuropathy.** *Gut* 1993, **34**:1123–1127.

This study clearly demonstrates the significant gallbladder promotility properties of erythromycin and its potential use in patients with autonomic neuropathy.

18. Marzio L, DiFelice F, Laico MG: **Gallbladder Hypokinesia and Normal Gastric Emptying of Liquids in Patients With Dyspeptic Symptoms: A Double Blind Placebo Controlled Trial With Cisapride [Abstract].** *Gastroenterology* 1990, **98**:A225.

19. Baldassarre G, Befiore A, Portincase P, Morelli N, Velardi A, Palmieri V: **Cholestyramine-Induced Prokinetic Effect on Human Gallbladder Motor Function: A Dose-Response Ultrasonographic Study [Abstract].** *Gastroenterology* 1990, **98**:A243.

20. Das JB, Cosentino CM, Levy MF, Ansari GG, Roffensperger JG: **Early Hepatobiliary Dysfunction During Total Parenteral Nutrition: An Experimental Study.** *J Pediatr Surg* 1993, **28**:14–18.

21. Sitzmann JV, Pitt HA, Steinborn PA, Pasha ZR, Sanders RC: **Cholecystokinin Prevents Parenteral Nutrition Induced Biliary Sludge in Humans.** *Surg Gynecol Obstet* 1990, **170**:25–31.

22. Little JM, Avramovic J: **Gallstone Formation After Major Abdominal Surgery.** *Lancet* 1991, **337**:1135–1137.

23. Bobba VR, Krishnamurthy GT, Kingston E, Turner FE, Brown PH, Langrell K: **Gallbladder Dynamics Induced by a Fatty Meal in Normal Subjects and Patients With Gallstones. Concise Communication.** *J Nucl Med* 1984, **25**:21–24.

24. • Behar J, Rhim BY, Thompson W, Biancani P: **Inositol Triphosphate Restores Human Gallbladder Motility Associated With Cholesterol Stones.** *Gastroenterology* 1993, **104**:563–568.

This study demonstrates that muscle cells from gallbladders with cholesterol stones contract less than cells from gallbladders with pigment stones.

25. Schulz M, Hanisch E, Guldutuna S: **In-Vitro-Kontraktilitatsverhalten Humaner Muskulatur Von Gallenblasen Nut und Ohne Steinnerkrankung-Relevanz Des Prostaglandin-Systems fur die CCK-Regulierte Motorik.** *Z Gastroenterol* 1993, **31**:376–387.

26. Berr F, Mayer M, Sackmann MF, Sauerbruch T, Holl J, Paumgartner G: **Pathogenic Factors in Early Recurrence of Cholesterol Gallstones.** *Gastroenterology* 1994, **196**:215–224.

27. Lieber MM: **The Incidence of Gallstone and Their Correlation With Other Diseases.** *Ann Surg* 1952, **135**:394–405.

28. Gitelson S, Oppenheim D, Schwartz A: **Size of the Gallbladder in Patients With Diabetes Mellitus.** *Diabetes* 1969, **18**:493–498.

29. Atkinson M, Hoskin DJ: **Gastrointestinal Complications of Diabetes Mellitus.** *Clin Gastroenterol* 1983, **12**:633–650.

30. Lilja P, Fagan CJ, Wiener I: **Infusion of Pure Cholecystokinin in Humans. Correlation Between Plasma Concentrations of Cholecystokinin and Gallbladder Size.** *Gastroenterology* 1982, **83**:256–261.

31. DeBoer SY, Masclee AM, Fan Lam W, Schipper J, Jansen JBMJ, Lamers CBHW: **Hyperglycemia Reduces Gallbladder Emptying and Plasma Hormone Secretion to Modified Sham Feeding and Regular Feeding.** *Hepatology* 1993, **17**:1022–1027.

32. Upp JR Jr, Nealon WH, Singh P, Fagan CJ, Jonas AS, Greeley GH Jr, Thompson JC: **Correlation of Cholecystokinin Receptors With Gallbladder Contractility in Patients with Gallstones.** *Ann Surg* 1987, **205**:641–648.

33. • Shaw SJ, Hajnal F, Lebovitz Y, Rolls P, Bauer M, Valenzuela J, Zeidler A: **Gallbladder Dysfunction in Diabetes Mellitus.** *Dig Dis Sci* 1993, **38**:490–496.

These investigators demonstrated that 50% of diabetics studied were found to have impaired gallbladder emptying following a fat meal, which was not strictly correlated with diabetic neuropathy.

34. DeBoer SY, Masclee AM, Jebbink MCW, Schipper J, Lemkes HHPJ, Jansen JBMJ, Lamers CBHW: **Effect of Acute Hyperglycemia on Gallbladder Contraction Induced by Cholecystokinin in Humans.** *Gut* 1993, **34**:1128–1132.

35. DeBoer SY, Masclee AM, Lamers CBHW: **Effect of Hyperglycemia on Gastrointestinal and Gallbladder Motility.** *Scand J Gastroenterol* 1992, **27**:13–18.

36. Wedmann B, Droge C, Armoiridis G, Schmidt-Heinevetter G, Wegener M, Ricken D: **Gallenblasenmotilit at bei Diabetikern Mit und Ohne Autonome Kardiale Neuropathie.** *Z Gastroenterol* 1992, **30**:519–524.

37. Parodi JE, Feldman MJ, Becker JM: **Substance P Stimulates the Opossum Sphincter of Oddi Through a Calcium Dependent Pathway.** *Surg Forum* 1990, **41**:157–159.

38. • Sand J, Tainio H, Nordback I: **Neuropeptides in Pig Sphincter of Oddi, Bile Duct, Gallbladder, and Duodenum.** *Dig Dis Sci* 1993, **38**:694–700.

This paper reviews the numerous peptides found to alter small bowel and biliary function.

39. Behar J, Biancani P: **Pharmacologic Characterization of Excitatory and Inhibitory Cholecystokinin Receptors of the Cat Gallbladder and Sphincter of Oddi.** *Gastroenterology* 1987, **92**:764–770.

40. Allen M, Gu J, Adrain JE: **Neuropeptide Y in the Guinea-Pig Biliary Tract.** *Experimental* 1984, **40**:765–767.

41. Lillemoe K, Webb TH, Pitt HA: **Neuropeptide Y. A Candidate Neurotransmitter for Biliary Motility.** *J Surg Res* 1988, **45**:254–260.

42. Yamasato T, Nakayama S: **Effects of Neurotensin on the Motility of the Isolated Gallbladder, Bile Duct and Ampulla in Guinea Pigs.** *Eur J Pharmacol* 1988, **148**:101–106.

43. Gullo L, Ancona D, Pezzilli R, Fusconi F, Bolondi L: **Study of the Effect of Neurotensin on Meal and Cerulein Induced Gallbladder Contraction.** *Digestion* 1992, **53**:67–72.

44. Ponce J, Garrigues V, Pertejo V: **Effect of Intravenous Glucagon and Glucagon-(1-21)-Peptide on Motor Activity of Sphincter of Oddi in Humans.** *Dig Dis Sci* 1989, **34**:61–64.

45. Mourelle M, Guarner F, Moncada S: **A Constitutive Nitric Oxide (NO) Synthase Present in Sphincter of Oddi Tissue Homogenates Modulates Its Motor Activity [Abstract].** *Gastroenterology* 1992, **102**:A324.

46. Pauletzki JG, Sharkey KA, Davison JS: **Nitric Oxide Synthase Products Mediate Neurally Induced Sphincter of Oddi Relaxation in the Guinea Pig [Abstract].** *Gastroenterology* 1992, **102**:A939.

47. Baker BRA, Saccone GTP, Toouli J: **Inhibition of Nitric Oxide Synthesis Attenuates Non-Adrenergic Non-Cholinergic Relaxation of the Australian Opossum Sphincter of Oddi [Abstract].** *Gastroenterology* 1992, **102**:A302.

48. Simeone JF, Butch RJ, Mueller PR: **The Bile Ducts After a Fatty Meal: Further Sonographic Observations.** *Radiology* 1985, **154**:763–768.

49. Mueller PR, Ferrucci JT Jr, Simone JF: **Postcholecystectomy Bile Duct Dilation: Myth or Reality?** *AJR Am J Roentgenol* 1981, **136**:355–359.

50. Wilson SA, Gosink BB, vanSonnenberg E: **Unchanged Size of a Dilated Common Bile Duct After a Fatty Meal: Results and Significance.** *Radiology* 1986, **160**:29–34.

51. Darweesh RMA, Dodds WJ, Hogan WJ: **Fatty-Meal Sonography for Evaluating Patients With Suspected Partial Common Duct Obstruction.** *AJR Am J Roentgenol* 1988, **151**:63–66.

52. Zeman RK, Burrell MI, Dobbins J: **Postcholecystectomy Syndrome: Evaluation Using Biliary Scintigraphy and Endoscopic Retrograde Cholangiopancreatography.** *Radiology* 1985, **156**:787–886.

53. Darweesh RMA, Dodds WJ, Hogan WJ: **Efficacy of Quantitative Hepatobiliary Scintigraphy and Fatty-Meal Sonography for Evaluating Patients With Suspected Partial Common Duct Obstruction.** *Gastroenterology* 1988, 94:779–786.

54. Ladas SD, Tassios PS, Katsogridakis J, Giorgiotis K, Tastemiroglou T, Raptis SA: **The Clinical Need for Sphincter of Oddi Manometry in Gastrointestinal Units.** *Endoscopy* 1993, **25**:387–391.

55. Rolney P, Arleback A: **Effect of Midazolam on Sphincter of Oddi Motility.** *Endoscopy* 1993, **25**:381–383.

56. Cuer JC, Dapoigny M, Bommelaer G: **The Effect of Midazolam Motility of the Sphincter of Oddi in Human Subjects.** *Endoscopy* 1993, **25**:384–386.

57. Allescher HD: **How to Sedate for Endoscopic Sphincter of Oddi Manometry.** *Endoscopy* 1993, **25**:399–400.

58. Elta GH, Barnett JL: **Meperidine Need Not be Prescribed During Sphincter of Oddi Manometry.** *Gastrointest Endosc* 1994, **40**:7–9.

59. Sherman S, Lehman G: **Opioids and the Sphincter of Oddi.** *Gastrointest Endosc* 1994, **40**:105–106.

60. Guelrud M: **Is Endoscopic Sphincter of Oddi Manometry a Reproducible Technique [Letter]?** *Dig Dis Sci* 1993, **38**:378.

61. Guelrud M, Mendoza S, Rossiter G, Villegas MI: **Sphincter of Oddi Manometry in Healthy Volunteers.** *Dig Dis Sci* 1990, **35**:38–46.

62. Hogan WJ, Geenen JE, Dodds WJ: **Dysmotility Disturbances of the Biliary Tract: Classification, Diagnosis and Treatment.** *Scand Liver Dis* 1987, 302–310.

63. Sherman S, Troiano FP, Hawes RH, O'Connor KW, Lehman GA: **Frequency of Abnormal Sphincter of Oddi Manometry Compared With the Clinical Suspicion of Sphincter of Oddi Dysfunction.** *Am J Gastroenterol* 1991, **86**:586–590.

64. Rolny P, Geenen JE, Hogan WJ, Venu RP: **Clinical Features, Manometric Findings and Therapy Results in Group I Patients With Sphincter of Oddi Dysfunction.** *Gastrointest Endosc* 1991, **37**:252.

65. Meshkinpour H, Mallot M: **Sphincter of Oddi Dysfunction and Unexplained Abdominal Pain; Clinical and Manometric Study.** *Dig Dis Sci* 1992, **37**:257–261.

66. Rolny P: **Normal Manometry Results in Group I Sphincter of Oddi Dyskinesia Patients [Reply].** *Gastroenterology* 1993, **104**:1243–1244.

67. Geenen JE, Hogan WJ, Dodds WJ, Toouli J, Venu RP: **The Efficacy of Endoscopic Sphincterotomy After Cholecystectomy in Patients With Sphincter of Oddi Dysfunction.** *N Engl J Med* 1989, **320**:82–87.

68. Manoukan AV, Schmalz MJ, Geenen JE, Hogan WJ, Venu RP, Johnson GK: **The Incidence of Post-Sphincterotomy Stenosis in Group II Patients With Sphincter of Oddi Dysfunction.** *Gastrointest Endosc* 1993, 39:496–498.

69. Sand J, Nordback I, Kaskinen M, Matikainen M, Lindhold TS: **Nifedipine for Suspected Type II Sphincter of Oddi Dyskinesia.** *Am J Gastroenterol* 1993, **88**:530–535.

70. • Richard RD, Yeaton P, Shaffer HA, Pambiancz DJ, Pruett TL, Stevenson WC, Mittal RK, McCallum RW: **Human Sphincter of Oddi Motility and Cholecystokinin Response Following Liver Transplantation.** *Dig Dis Sci* 1993, **38**:462–468.

A unique opportunity to study sphincter of Oddi function in a group of patients with transplanted livers was provided. Sphincteric motor function was generally normal in this group and sphincter of Oddi dysfunction is not a significant cause of biliary tract abnormalities in posthepatic transplantation.

71. Douzdjian V, Abecassis MM, Johlin FC: **Sphincter of Oddi Dysfunction Following Liver Transplantation. Screening by Bedside Manometry and Definitive Manometric Evaluation.** *Dig Dis Sci* 1994, **39**:253–256.

72. Choudhry J, Ruffolo T, Jamidar P, Hawes R, Lehman G: **Sphincter of Oddi Dysfunction in Patients with Intact Gallbladder: Therapeutic Response to Endoscopic Sphincterotomy.** *Gastrointest Endosc* 1993, 4:492–495.

73. Ruffolo TA, Sherman S, Lehman GA, Hawes RH: **Gallbladder Ejection Fraction and Its Relationship to Sphincter of Oddi Dysfunction.** *Dig Dis Sci* 1994, **39**:289–292.

74. Yuasa N, Nimura Y, Yasiu A, Akita Y, Odani K: **Sphincter of Oddi Motility in Patients With Bile Duct Stones: A Comparative Study Using Percutaneous Transhepatic Manometry.** *Dig Dis Sci* 1994, **39**:257–267.

75. Ohri SK, Somasundaram S, Koak Y, Macpherson A, Keogh BE, Taylor KM, Menzies IS, Bjarnason I: **The Effect of Intestinal Hypoperfusion on Intestinal Absorption and Permeability During Cardiopulmonary Bypass.** *Gastroenterology* 1994, **106**:318–323.

Marc F. Catalano, MD, and Walter J. Hogan, MD, Medical College of Wisconsin, 9200 West Wisconsin Avenue, Milwaukee, WI 53226, USA.

Biliary endoscopy

Jacques Devière, MD, and Michel Cremer, MD

Université Libre de Bruxelles, Hôpital Erasme, Brussels, Belgium

The diagnostic role of endoscopic retrograde cholangiopancreatography (ERCP) is improved by the use of brushing, according to samples analysis by flow cytometry, cell image analysis, or even molecular biology. Prevention of complications requires high expertise levels and ERCP should not be performed if it cannot be followed by the appropriate endoscopic therapy for logistic reasons. At present, it is clearly the first choice technique for treatment of gallstone pancreatitis, common bile duct (CBD) stones, treatment of benign biliary stricture, or palliation of biliopancreatic malignancies. The respective roles of classic and self-expanding metal stents are becoming more precise and new materials are still in development that might improve the long-term patency of the stents. Laparoscopic cholecystectomy is associated with an increase of postoperative CBD injuries and ERCP plays a major role in their management. The incidence of biliary injuries could be reduced by an optimization of surgical and endoscopic collaboration, limiting the necessity of perioperative approach to the CBD. Techniques like endoscopic ultrasonography or magnetic nuclear resonance could replace strictly diagnostic ERCP in selected situations.

Current Opinion in Gastroenterology 1994, **10**:567–572

Diagnostic role

Endoscopic retrograde cholangiopancreatography (ERCP) has outgrown its early limited diagnostic role to encompass an ever increasing number of diagnostic and therapeutic applications. Considerable efforts to enhance the sensitivity of biliary cytology in the diagnosis of bile duct strictures have been made.

A prospective study [1•] of biliary cytology in 100 patients with bile duct strictures has shown a greater sensitivity of combined bile and brushing samples (69%) compared with bile cytology alone (33%). However, 25% of patients in this series had no definitive diagnosis. Another study [2] reported a sensitivity of 56% for brush cytology with the Geenen brush system (Wilson Cook Medical, Winston-Salem, NC). Brushes introduced through double-lumen catheters are currently available. Brushing a stricture over a guide wire is possible, facilitating further dilatation and stenting (Microvasive, Watertown, MA). Salvage cytology, accomplished by rinsing the brush sheath with saline [3•], increases the cellular yield and thus sensitivity of the procedure. Endoscopic transpapillary biopsy has a reported sensitivity of 88% for cholangiocarcinoma and 71% for pancreatic cancer in a recent series [4]. However, in our experience, these forceps remain difficult to manipulate and should be used with caution, particularly in the pancreas.

In the era of molecular biology, the use of modern DNA analysis techniques to study biliary specimens is not surprising. Flow cytometry has been shown to improve the sensitivity of tumor detection but was associated with a greater false-positive rate than routine cytology [5•].

Differentiating malignant from inflammatory pancreatic strictures is an important clinical challenge, given the high risk of cancer in chronic pancreatitis. An elegant technique based on cell image analysis of brushing specimens has been described [6••], using a cell image processor that analysis morphometric, densitometric, and textural parameters on Feulgen-stained nuclei. A score is determined, based on the DNA histogram type, nuclear DNA content, and the percent proliferating cell population, allowing distinction of normal and inflammatory from malignant cytology specimens with 95% sensitivity and 100% specificity. Detection of cKi-*ras* gene mutations on codon 12 by the polymerase chain reaction in cytologic specimens from suspected pancreatic cancer has already acquired an important role in our diagnostic armamentarium. The technique has a sensitivity of 80% to 90% and 100% specificity [7,8].

Abbreviations

CBD—common bile duct; **ERCP**—endoscopic retrograde cholangiopancreatography; **SOD**—sphincter of Oddi dysfunction; **SOM**—sphincter of Oddi manometry.

 ISBN 1-85922-610-8 ISSN 0267–1379

Magnetic resonance cholangiography is a promising technique in the evaluation of obstructive jaundice. Adequate imaging is limited to patients with biliary dilatation and provides only a rough estimate of the level of obstruction [9,10•]. It could be of particular interest in cases of hilar malignant stricture.

Prevention of complications

Despite technical advances, the incidence of post-ERCP pancreatitis (1% to 2%) remains unchanged and the etiology is unclear. It might be a consequence of main pancreatic duct overinjection, but it can be observed after single common bile duct (CBD) opacification. Many drugs have been tested in the prevention of post-ERCP pancreatitis. Recently, the use of calcium-blocking drugs has been shown to prevent a model of post-ERCP pancreatitis in rats [11]. Indeed, verapamil (1 g/kg), administered before the induction of pancreatitis reduced elevation of serum amylase and improved histologic changes and survival.

In humans [12], the beneficial effects of calcium blockers using nifedipine at physiologic doses (20 mg, three times a day) on the incidence of post-ERCP pancreatitis were not confirmed. Prevention of pancreatitis has also been attempted by stenting the pancreatic duct after endoscopic sphincterotomy in high-risk patients (small CBD, precut sphincterotomy). Prophylactic stenting did not decrease the incidence of pancreatitis [13] and should not be recommended in clinical practice.

The safety of ERCP depends on the endoscopist's experience and knowledge of high-risk situations as well as the quality of the equipment. Prevention and treatment of complications were well described by Thornton and Axon [14•], emphasizing the risk of endoscopic sphincterotomy in nondilated ducts, the need for careful follow-up of patients with stents, the necessity of avoiding hypoxemia during ERCP, and the risk of precutting. The latter technique, in our opinion, is not an alternative to successful selective, deep CBD cannulation and should be necessary in less than 10% of cases.

Early detection of an infectious outbreak in ERCP centers is critical. Both detection and determination of the infectious source require an infection control unit, working independently to assess routinely the disinfection quality and the incidence of post-ERCP cholangitis or bacteremia. A recent study described a systematic approach to an outbreak of bacteremia and the use of DNA macrorestriction analysis to characterize the bacterial strains involved and determine the source of infection [15•]. In this case, it was due to an inefficient automated scope disinfector.

Duodenal perforation associated with endoscopic sphicterotomy occurs less frequently with increasing experience of the endoscopist. However, it must be recognized immediately because improvement of symptoms within 24 hours of medical treatment is correlated with recovery. Surgery should not be undertaken immediately, but only when symptoms do not improve after a brief period of nonoperative management [16]. This approach avoids unnecessary surgery in approximately two thirds of the patients who will respond to medical therapy.

Gallstone pancreatitis

The need for urgent therapeutic ERCP in patients with severe gallstone pancreatitis and its superiority to surgical exploration is well established. When the diagnosis of gallstone pancreatitis is made, sphincterotomy can be reasonably performed in all cases [17•]. In cases of mild pancreatitis, endoscopic sphicterotomy is indicated in the presence of CBD stones. The timing and definition of "urgent" ERCP are still unclear. Usually, ERCP performed within 48 hours of admission is considered urgent. Though not specifically proven to be beneficial, performance of ERCP within several hours after admission might improve its usefulness. This is suggested by an experimental study in the opossum [18••]: acute necrotizing pancreatitis was induced by obstructing the biliopancreatic system for 1 to 5 days. Duct decompression by removal of the balloon after 1 day prevented the increase in severity of all parameters of pancreatic injury compared with animals in which the balloon was left for 3 or 5 days. This study supports earlier studies of endoscopic decompression in clinical gallstone pancreatitis.

Common bile duct stone extraction

In experienced hands, endoscopic extraction of CBD stones has a success rate of 98% to 100% with less than 10% morbidity and a mortality around 0.5% [13,19•]. Published results from less experienced centers [20] are surprising, as complication and failure rates are comparable to those of early reports in the 1970s. This raises the problem of ERCP training and certification, as well as the criteria required for ERCP practice. It is certainly not reasonable to perform ERCP without having prior training in its therapeutic applications.

Recently, Binmoeller *et al.* [21••] reported their results in the management of 791 patients with CBD stones. Endoscopic sphicterotomy and endoscopic extraction were successful in 86% of patients without requiring lithotripsy techniques. In the remaining patients (n=108), the authors used mechanical lithotripsy if the stone was entrapped in the Dormia basket (n=33), peroral cholangioscopic electrohydraulic lithotripsy in other cases (n=6), and extracorporeal shock wave lithotripsy in intrahepatic stones (n=10). The overall success was 99% with 0.2% mortality. We use extracorporeal shock wave lithotripsy more frequently than electrohydraulic lithotripsy for CBD stones. Both techniques are efficient with a higher risk of CBD wall injury with electrohydraulic lithotripsy. The therapeutic approach should depend on the local facilities and expertise.

Binmoeller *et al.* [22•] also reported on 14 high-risk patients who underwent endoscopic treatment of Mirizzi syndrome by electrohydraulic lithotripsy under cholangioscopic guidance. Treatment was successful in all patients, requiring two ERCP sessions in only two patients with multiple stones. They observed only one complication (peritoneal leakage) resolved by endoscopic drainage and conservative management. This technique surely represents a good alternative to surgery. Endoscopic lithotripsy under visual control can also be performed with pulsed dye laser, with final CBD clearance in most cases and limited morbidity [23•]. Both electrohydraulic and laser lithotripsy could be used with a normal duodenoscope to clear impacted stones at the papilla. These techniques should be limited to failures of endoscopic extraction and mechanical lithotripsy, the latter remaining the first choice after initial failure of stone extraction [24•].

In small CBD stones, most complications are related to sphincterotomy. Therefore, May *et al.* [25•] have proposed stone extraction without sphincterotomy, after balloon sphincter dilatation. This approach could be useful in young patients with small single stones, but needs confirmation with analysis of the risk of pancreatitis after balloon dilatation. A prospective randomized study is ongoing.

A potential advantage of this approach, which leaves an intact papilla, is the prevention of bactobilia that may lead to CBD stone recurrence, as suggested by Cetta [26], who found a 9% recurrence of brown CBD stones within 4.3 years after sphincterotomy. However, this study did not provide evidence for the precise factors responsible for stone recurrence. In particular, the size of the CBD and the relative sphincterotomy size could be potentially important variables and require future study. In our experience, recurrent stones are often observed in older patients, with a large CBD and a relatively small sphincterotomy, suggesting that biliary stasis plays an important role. This observation would dictate performing large sphincterotomies depending on CBD and stone size.

Sphincter of Oddi dysfunction

Despite increasing use of sphincter of Oddi manometry (SOM) and the definition of criteria for normality, the selection of patients who could benefit from endoscopic treatment is difficult. SOM reliability is hampered by lack of true control groups, the intermittent nature of patients complaints, changes of sphincter of Oddi contractility induced by catheterization, and interobserver variability [27•].

The diagnosis of sphincter of Oddi dysfunction (SOD) should always be considered with caution, based on clinical and biochemical criteria and elevated sphincter of Oddi basal pressure. It probably involves multiple diseases for which the best treatment remains unknown. In a recent study, endoscopic sphincterotomy led to pain relief in 15 of 35 patients with SOD followed for 13 months [28]. Among nonresponders, 11 were cholecystectomized with subsequent improvement in eight. This study illustrates well the fact that, despite an apparent clear SOD definition on the basis of SOM findings, we are facing a poorly understood disease in which successive treatments are attempted without real knowledge of what we are treating.

Biliary stents

Benign strictures

Until recently, surgery was considered the mainstay treatment of benign postoperative biliary strictures. A retrospective analysis of 101 [29••] patients with benign strictures, treated either surgically or endoscopically, showed that stenting the bile duct is as efficient as surgery with less morbidity. Leaving a plastic stent in place for 1 year (with exchange every 3 months) yielded a definitive calibration of the stricture in 83% of the patients treated. Recurrent strictures occurred in 17% of patients in both groups. The authors [29••] rightly concluded that when cases of complete CBD transsection are excluded, endoscopic stenting is the initial treatment of choice in all patients with postoperative strictures. Self-expanding metallic stents have, in our opinion, no place in the management of these short and tight postsurgical strictures. In chronic pancreatitis, CBD strictures are virtually impossible to treat by prolonged stenting. In these cases, metallic stents could provide definitive biliary drainage [30].

Malignant strictures

Cholangitis is a major complication of prolonged stenting of CBD strictures. It is usually due to clogging of plastic stents but is also observed after tumor ingrowth or overgrowth in a metallic stent. A new self-expandable stent (Instent, Minneapolis, MN), consisting of a coil spring with closed loops made from a nickel titanium alloy, might prevent tumor ingrowth, offering longer patency [31•].

Our preliminary experience confirms the prolonged patency of these stents. The Instent is also theoretically removable but its retrieval is technically very difficult and must be done with caution to avoid endoscope damage. The high cost of metal stents still limits their use in many instances, especially in patients with poor prognosis. Hilar tumors and particularly slow growing cholangiocarcinomas, may benefit from drainage with metal stents (Wallstent, Schneider, Bulach, Switzerland). Treatment of hilar tumors requires placement of the two stents that can be done endoscopically by leaving a guide wire in both liver lobes and then successively pushing two stents over it, or by the stent through wire mesh technique [32].

A prospective study, involving a small number of patients, has compared the placement of two 14F plastic stents with two Wallstents in the palliation of hilar malignancies [33•]. The rate of technical success was higher and the incidence of further cholangitis lower with Wallstents. Wallstents are also associated with a reduction in days spent in the hospital for stent malfunction, decreasing in the global cost of patient care and therefore counterbalancing the initial high cost of the stent. The percutaneous approach to hilar malignancies has also become easier with metal stents, which are now preferred by radiologists [34].

It is clear that the establishment of a bacterial biofilm is a key event in biliary stent obstruction [35•]. Incorporation of antibiotics within stents has not been successful in preventing clogging, presumably because bacteria living in their biofilm are quite resistant to antibiotics. New polymers with ultrasmooth surface have been tested *in vitro* [36,37], showing promising results in preventing biofilm deposition and stent occlusion.

Complications of laparoscopic cholecystectomy

Literature abounds on laparoscopic cholecystectomy. Rarely has a technique been so widely accepted without prior clinical trials evaluating its specific complications. However, the technique seems responsible for an increased cholecystectomy rate because of changes in the indications for gallbladder surgery [38]. Early data suggested that the incidence of bile duct injury, which is one in 1000 after open cholecystectomy might be one in 100 after laparoscopic cholecystectomy.

The experience of endoscopists in managing postoperative bile duct injury has increased with the development of this technique. ERCP is the first choice treatment of most postoperative biliary leaks, CBD strictures, and stones, but it is limited in cases of complete CBD transection [39–41].

The latter complication is, in our opinion, the sole indication for reoperation. The treatment of CBD stones at the time of laparascopic cholecystectomy remains controversial. As far as ERCP is a proven technique in treatment of CBD stones, there is little reason to develop the laparoscopic transcystic approach to CBD stones, which is much more difficult and hazardous. Further studies should evaluate the criteria of patient selection for preoperative ERCP before laparoscopic cholecystectomy. Every surgical and endoscopic team should develop an algorithm to optimize the effectiveness of the combined approach and to minimize the necessity of intraoperative laparoscopic approach to the CBD [42].

Endoscopic ultrasonography

Staging of cholangiocarcinoma is difficult with all types of imaging techniques. Endoscopic ultrasonography findings were correlated with pathologic examination of resected specimens, showing an 86% accuracy in assessing depth of penetration [43]. The sensitivity for lymph node detection was above 90%, but specificity was lacking. The problem with cholangiocarcinoma is that such results can be expected when the tumor involves the CBD. In hilar tumors, endoscopic ultrasonography is much more difficult and results are often disappointing.

Endoscopic ultrasonography has also been compared with ultrasonography and computed tomography scan in the diagnosis of CBD stones [44••]. Diagnosis was confirmed by ERCP and endoscopic sphicterotomy or intraoperative findings. Sensitivity and specificity were, respectively, 25% and 100% for ultrasonography, 75% and 94% for computed tomography scan, and 97% and 100% for endoscopic ultrasonography. Endoscopic ultrasonography appears to be the best diagnostic tool for the diagnosis of choledocholithiasis compared with other noninvasive procedures (if endoscopic ultrasonography can be considered a noninvasive procedure).

Biliary tract disease after liver transplantation

The endoscopic approach to biliary complications after liver transplantation mainly concerns patients with choledococholedocostomies with either early anastomotic leak or late (most often after 1 month) anastomotic strictures [45]. Two papers [46•,47•] illustrate the unique role of ERCP in treating bile leaks after liver transplantation, providing a definitive treatment after one ERCP session (with endoscopic sphicterotomy, nasobiliary tube insertion, or stent placement) in 94% of patients [47•].

Strictures can also be treated with temporary plastic stents and, in our experience, calibration is often obtained in a shorter time than for postcholecystectomy CBD strictures. The need for reoperation is limited to these unusual cases of "tortuous" and redundant CBD.

Acknowledgments

The authors wish to thank C. Matthys and C. Azar, MD for typing and proofreading the manuscript.

References and recommended reading

Papers of particular interest, published within the annual period of review, have been highlighted as:
- • Of special interest
- •• Of outstanding interest

1. • Kurzawinski TR, Deery A, Dooley JS, Dick R, Hobbs KEF, Davidson BR: **A Prospective Study of Biliary Cytology in 100 Patients With Bile Duct Strictures.** *Hepatology* 1993, **18**:1399–1403.
This prospective study compares bile cytology alone with bile and brush cytology, demonstrating the higher sensitivity of the latter.

2. Ferrari AP Jr, Lichtenstein DR, Slivka A, Chang C, Carr-Locke DL: **Brush Cytology During ERCP for the Diagnosis of Biliary and Pancreatic Malignancies.** *Gastrointest Endosc* 1994, 40:140–145.

3. • Baron TH, Lee JG, Wax TD, Schmitt CM, Cotton PB, Leung JWC: **An In Vitro, Randomized, Prospective Study to Maximize Cellular Yield During Bile Duct Brush Cytology.** *Gastrointest Endosc* 1994, 40:146–149.
This paper describes the best techniques to maximize cellular yield during biliary brushing.

4. Kubota Y, Takaoka M, Tani K, Ogura M, Kin H, Fujimura K, Mizuno T, Inoue K: **Endoscopic Transpapillary Biopsy for Diagnosis of Patients With Pancreatobiliary Ductal Strictures.** *Am J Gastroenterol* 1993, **88**:1700–1704.

5. Ryan ME, Baldauf MC: **Comparison of Flow Cytometry for DNA**
• **Content and Brush Cytology for Detection of Malignancy in Pancreatobiliary Strictures.** *Gastrointest Endosc* 1994, **40**:133–139.
Flow cytometry for DNA content increases the diagnostic yield of brushings. In pancreatic cancer, increased survival is noted in case of diploid cell population compared with anenploid cell population.

6. Yeaton P, Kiss R, Devière J, Salmon I, Bourgeois N, Pasteels JL, Cre-
•• mer M: **Use of Cell Image Analysis in the Detection of Cancer From Specimens Obtained During Endoscopic Retrograde Cholangiopancreatography.** *Am J Clin Pathol* 1993, **100**:497–501.
A score system, based on nuclear parameters at cell image analysis, offers 95% sensitivity and 100% specificity in differentiating benign from malignant pancreatic lesions.

7. Barthelemy P, Bouisson M, Escourrou J, Vaysse N, Pradayral L: **Clinical Interest of Identification of Ki-ras Mutations in Pure Pancreatic Juice [Abstract].** *Gastroenterology* 1994, **106**:A886.

8. Van Laethem JL, Vertongen P, Devière J, Rickaert F, Cremer M, Robberecht P: **Detection of c Ki-ras Gene Codon 12 Mutations in Pancreatic Duct Brushing Samples in the Diagnostic Procedure of Pancreatic Tumors [Abstract].** *Gastroenterology* 1994, **106**:A447.

9. Ishizaki Y, Wakayama T, Okada Y, Kobayashi T: **Magnetic Resonance Cholangiography for Evaluation of Obstructive Jaundice.** *Am J Gastroenterol* 1993, **88**:2072–2077.

10. Hall-Craggs MA, Allen CM, Owens CM, Theis BA, Donald JJ, Paley M,
• Wilkinson ID, Chong WK, Hatfield ARW, Lees WR, Russell CG: **MR Cholangiography: Clinical Evaluation in 40 Cases.** *Radiology* 1993, **189**:423–427.
Magnetic resonance cholangiography appears useful for the assessment of complex strictures, in which conventional cholangiography carries a higher risk of sepsis.

11. Leahy AL, Darzi A, Pierce G, Qureshi A, Redmond P, Leader M, Bouchier-Hayes DJ, Broe P: **Verapamil Is Beneficial in a Model of Post-ERCP Pancreatitis.** *Eur J Gastroenterol Hepatol* 1993, **5**:467–469.

12. Sand J, Nordback I: **Prospective Randomized Trial of the Effect of Nifedipine on Pancreatic Irritation After Endoscopic Retrograde Cholangiopancreatography.** *Digestion* 1993, **54**:105–111.

13. Smithline A, Silverman W, Rogers D, Nisi R, Wiersema M, Jamidar, Hawes R, Lehman G: **Effect of Prophylactic Main Pancreatic Duct Stenting on the Incidences of Biliary Endoscopic Sphincterotomy-Induced Pancreatitis in High-Risk Patients.** *Gastrointest Endosc* 1993, 39:652–657.

14. Thornton J, Axon A: **Towards Safer Endoscopic Retrograde Cholan-**
• **giopancreatography.** *Gut* 1993, **34**:721–724.
A short leading article, pointing carefully the keys for quality ERCP.

15. Struelens MJ, Rost F, Deplano A, Maas A, Schwam V, Serruys E,
• Cremer M: **Pseudomonas Aeruginosa and Enterobacteriaceae Bacteremia After Biliary Endoscopy: An Outbreak Investigation Using DNA Macrorestriction Analysis.** *Am J Med* 1993, **95**:489–498.
An outbreak of septicemia after ERCP was characterized by DNA macrorestriction analysis and finally attributed to a defectuous automated desinfector.

16. Chung RS, Sivak MV, Roy Ferguson D: **Surgical Decisons in the Management of Duodenal Perforation Complicating Endoscopic Sphincterotomy.** *Am J Surg* 1993, **165**:700–703.

17. Neoptolemos JP: **Endoscopic Sphincterotomy in Acute Gallstone Pan-**
• **creatitis.** *Br J Surg* 1993, **80**:547–549.
A clear review of the place of ERCP and endoscopic sphincterotomy in acute gallstone pancreatitis.

18. Runzi M, Saluja A, Lerch MM, Dawra R, Nishino H, Steer ML: **Early**
•• **Ductal Decompression Prevents the Progression of Biliary Pancreatitis: An Experimental Study in the Opossum.** *Gastroenterology* 1993, **105**:157–164.
Suggesting that earlier is ductal decompression, better is the prognosis.

19. Assouline T, Liguory C, Ink O, Fritsch J, Choury AD, Lefebvre JF, Pel-
• letier G, Buffet C, Etienne JP: **Résultats Actuels de la Sphinctérotomie Endoscopique Pour Lithiase de la Voie Biliaire Principale.** *Gastroenterol Clin Biol* 1993, **17**:251–258.
Current results of endoscopic sphincterotomy and stone extraction in an experienced reference center.

20. Association Universitaire de Recherche en Chirurgie, Lenriot JP, Le Neel JC, Hay JM, Jaeck D, Millat B, Fagniez PL: **Cholangiopancréatographie Rétrograde Endoscopique et Sphinctérotomie Pour Lithiase Biliaire: Évaluation Prospective en Milieu Chirurgical.** *Gastroenterol Clin Biol* 1993, **17**:244–250.

21. Binmoeller KF, Bruckner M, Thonke F, Soehendra N: **Treatment of**
•• **Difficult Bile Duct Stones Using Mechanical, Electrohydraulic and Extracorporeal Shock Wave Lithotripsy.** *Endoscopy* 1993, **25**:201–206.
An excellent algorithm of "what we have to do" with CBD stones, highlighting the different techniques of lithotripsy.

22. Binmoeller KF, Thonke F, Soehendra N: **Endoscopic Treatment of**
• **Mirizzi's Syndrome.** *Gastrointest Endosc* 1993, 39:532–536.
This paper reports successful treatment of 14 Mirizzi's syndromes by endoscopic electrohydraulic lithotripsy under cholangioscopic guidance.

23. Neuhaus H, Hoffman W, Zillinger C, Classen M: **Laser Lithotripsy**
• **of Difficult Bile Duct Stones Under Direct Visual Control.** *Gut* 1993, 34:415–421.
Laser lithotripsy was performed using the mother-baby scope; this can be done through peroral cholangioscopy or percutaneous cholangioscopy.

24. Shaw MJ, Mackie RD, Moore JP, Dorsher PJ, Freeman ML, Meier
• PB, Potter T, Hutton SW, Vennes JA: **Results of a Multicenter Trial Using a Mechanical Lithotripter for the Treatment of Large Bile Duct Stones.** *Am J Gastroenterol* 1993, **88**:730–733.
A success rate of 92% was achieved by mechanical lithotripsy after failure of endoscopic extraction.

25. May GR, Cotton PB, Edmunds SEJ, Chong W: **Removal of Stones**
• **From the Bile Duct at ERCP Without Sphincterotomy.** *Gastrointest Endosc* 1993, 39:749–754.
Removal of small stones without sphincterotomy was successful in 24 patients, nine of them after sphincter dilatation.

26. Cetta F: **Do Surgical and Endoscopic Sphincterotomy Prevent or Facilitate Recurrent Common Duct Stone Formation.** *Arch Surg* 1993, **128**:329–336.

27. Blades EW, Sivak MV Jr: **Sphincter of Oddi Manometry: How Far Is**
• **the Leap of Faith?** *Gastrointest Endosc* 1993, 39:593–595.
This commentary on SOM facts and pitfalls was written by a skeptical enthusiast.

28. Choudhry U, Ruffolo T, Jamidar P, Hawes R, Lehman G: **Sphincter of Oddi Dysfunction in Patients With Intact Gallbladder: Therapeutic Response to Endoscopic Sphincterotomy.** *Gastrointest Endosc* 1993, 39:492–495.

29. Davids PHP, Tanka AKF, Rauws EAJ, Van Gulik TM, Van Leeuwen
•• DJ, De Wit LT, Verbeek PCM, Huibregtse K, Van Der Heyde MN, Tytgat GNJ: **Benign Biliary Strictures. Surgery or Endoscopy?** *Ann Surg* 1993, **217**:237–243.
Retrospective study of 101 patients with benign biliary strictures which strongly suggest that endoscopy is definitively the initial treatment of benign post operative strictures.

30. Devière J, Cremer M, Baize M, Love J, Sugai B, Vandermeeren A: **Management of Common Bile Duct Stricture Caused by Chronic Pancreatitis With Metal Mesh Self-Expandable Stents.** *Gut* 1994, **35**: 122-126.

31. Goldin E, Beyar M, Safra T, Globerman O, Verstandig A, Wengrower
• D, Fich A: **A New Self-Expandable and Removable Metal Stent for Biliary Obstruction. A Preliminary Report.** *Endoscopy* 1993, **25**:597–599.
A very interesting expandable stent. Its removal is however technically very difficult.

32. Neuhaus H, Gottlieb K, Classen M: **The "Stent Through Wire Mesh Technique" in Complicated Biliary Strictures.** *Gastrointest Endosc* 1993, 39:553–556.

33. Wagner HJ, Knyrim K, Vakil N, Klose KJ: **Plastic Endoprostheses**
• **Versus Metal Stents in the Palliative Treatment of Malignant Hilar Biliary Obstruction. A Prospective and Randomized Trial.** *Endoscopy* 1993, 25:213–218.
Prospective trial on a small number of patients with a trend to reduced morbidity, a significant reduction of costs with Wallstents.

34. Stoker J, Lameris JS, Van Blankenstein M: **Percutaneous Metallic Self-Expandable Endoprostheses in Malignant Hilar Biliary Obstruction.** *Gastrointest Endosc* 1993, 39:43–49.

35. Sung JY, Leung JWC, Shaffer EA, Lam K, Costerton JW: **Bacterial**
• **Biofilm, Brown Pigment Stone and Blockage of Biliary Stents.** *J Gastroenterol Hepatol* 1993, **8**:28–34.
A good review of pathogenesis of stent blockage.

36. McAllister EW, Carey LC, Brady PG, Heller R, Kovacs SG: **The Role of Polymeric Surface Smoothness of Biliary Stents in Bacterial Adherence, Biofilm Deposition, and Stent Occlusion.** *Gastrointest Endosc* 1993, 39:422–425.

37. Jansen B, Goodman LP, Ruiten D: **Bacterial Adherence to Hydrophilic Polymer-Coated Polyurethan Stents.** *Gastrointest Endosc* 1993, 39:670–673.

38. Legorreta AP, Silber JH, Costantino GN, Kobylinski RW, Zatz SL: **Increased Cholecystectomy Rate After the Introduction of Laparoscopic Cholecystectomy.** *JAMA* 1993, **270**:1429–1432.

39. Davids PHP, Ringers J, Rauws EAJ, De Wit LT, Huibregtse K, Van Der Heyde MN, Tytgat GNJ: **Bile Duct Injury After Laparoscopic Cholecystectomy: The Value of Endoscopic Retrograde Cholangiopancreatography.** *Gut* 1993, **34**:1250–1254.

40. Vitale GC, Stephens G, Wieman TJ, Larson GM: **Use of Endoscopic Retrograde Cholangiopancreatography in the Management of Biliary Complications After Laparoscopic Cholecystectomy**. *Surgery* 1993, **114**:806–814.

41. Manoukian AV, Schmalz MJ, Geenen JE, Hogan WJ, Venu RP, Johnson GK: **Endoscopic Treatment of Problems Encountered After Cholecystectomy**. *Gastrointest Endosc* 1993, **39**:9–14.

42. Cotton PB: **Endoscopic Retrograde Cholangiopancreatography and Laparoscopic Cholecystectomy**. *Am J Surg* 1993, **165**:474–478.

43. Tio TL, Reeders WA, Sie LH, Wijers OB, Maas JJ, Colin EM, Tytgat GNJ: **Endosonography in the Clinical Staging of Klatskin Tumor**. *Endoscopy* 1993, **25**:81–85.

44. •• Amouyal P, Amouyal G, Levy P, Tuzet S, Palazzo L, Vilgrain V, Gayet B, Belghiti J, Fekete F, Bernades P: **Diagnosis of Choledocholithiasis by Endoscopic Ultrasonography**. *Gastroenterology* 1994, **106**:1062–1067.

A prospective comparison of ultrasonography, computed tomography scan, and endoscopic ultrasonography, clearly demonstrating the superiority of the latter.

45. Donovan J: **Nonsurgical Management of Biliary Tract Disease After Liver Transplantation**. *Gastroenterol Clin North Am* 1993, **22**:317–336.

46. • Osorio RW, Freise CE, Stock PG, Lake JR, Laberge JM, Gordon RL, Ring EJ, Ascher NL, Roberts JP: **Nonoperative Management of Biliary Leaks After Orthotopic Liver Transplantation**. *Transplantation* 1993, **55**:1074–1077.

47. • Sherman S, Shaked A, Cryer HM, Goldstein LI, Busuttil RW: **Endoscopic Management of Biliary Fistulas Complicating Liver Transplantation and Other Hepatobiliary Operations**. *Ann Surg* 1993, **218**:167–175.

Two papers highlighting the unique role of endoscopy in treating bile leaks after transplantation.

Jacques Devière, MD, and Michel Cremer, MD, Department of Gastroenterology and Hepato-pancreatology, Université Libre de Bruxelles, Hôpital Erasme, Brussels, Belgium.

Stomach and duodenum

Editorial overview

Mitchell L. Schubert, MD

Medical College of Virginia and McGuire VAMC, Richmond, Virginia, USA

Current Opinion in Gastroenterology 1994, **10**:573–574

This section has been organized to highlight and provide expert review and commentary of the past year's major discoveries in the stomach and duodenum. An effort has been made to include both basic research and clinical papers because both approaches are necessary for a full understanding of the pathophysiology and treatment of gastroduodenal disorders. It is hoped that the reviews will provide much useful information for both investigators and practicing physicians, surgeons, and gastroenterologists.

In *Regulation of gastric secretion* (pp 575–588), I review recent advances in our understanding of the neural, paracrine, and hormonal pathways that regulate gastric exocrine (*ie*, acid and pepsinogen) and endocrine (*ie*, gastrin, histamine, somatostatin, and prostaglandin) secretion at the central, peripheral, and intracellular levels. The dorsomedial region of the nucleus tractus solitarius contains fenestrated capillaries with high permeability that may allow circulating peptides such as pancreatic polypeptide, peptide YY, and neuropeptide Y access to this region of the brain and neighboring dorsal motor nucleus where they may influence acid and pepsinogen secretion. The main stimulants of acid secretion are histamine (paracrine action), gastrin (hormonal action), and acetylcholine (neurocrine action); the main inhibitor is somatostatin (paracrine action). Techniques for purification and enrichment of fundic enterochromaffin-like cells have proven useful for identifying receptors regulating histamine secretion (*eg*, muscarine receptors, gastrin receptors, somatostatin receptors, and histamine H_2 autoreceptors). Molecular biological techniques have advanced our understanding of the post-translational processing of peptides (*eg*, gastrin and somatostatin) and the receptor subtypes to which they are coupled. Selective peptide antagonists (*eg*, the gastrin/cholecystokinin-B antagonist L365260) have proven useful tools with which to examine the pathways and receptors regulating secretion. With stimulation, parietal cells undergo a morphologic transformation in which resting intracellular tubulovesicles fuse with the canalicular membrane. At the same time, H^+K^+ATPase, the proton pump of the parietal cell, is translocated to the canalicular membrane and activated.

In *Gastroduodenal mucosal defense* (pp 589–594), John Wallace and Cameron Bell highlight the importance of impaired mucosal defense in the pathophysiology of peptic ulcer disease, particularly in regard to *Helicobacter pylori* and nonsteroidal anti-inflammatory drugs. Gastric mucus traps protons and scavenges toxic oxygen metabolites. Nitric oxide may enhance mucosal defense by stimulating mucus and bicarbonate secretion and increasing mucosal blood flow, especially at ulcer margins. Nonsteroidal anti-inflammatory drug–induced injury is mediated via leukocyte adherence to blood vessel walls through CD11/CD18 and intercellular adhesion molecule-1.

In *Medical management of peptic ulcer disease* (pp 595–599), David Ng and Roy Pounder review the efficacy and safety of histamine H_2 blockers and omeprazole for acute and maintenance therapy, and the conclusions of the National Institutes of Health Consensus Conference on the role of *H. pylori* in peptic ulcer disease. Although the conference recommended that ulcer patients with *H. pylori should* be treated with antimicrobial agents, my personal viewpoint is that such patient *may* be treated with antimicrobials. Until more effective and better tolerated antibiotic regimens are identified and validated, maintenance or even intermittent therapy with antisecretory drugs may be the most appropriate course in select patients.

In *Diagnosis and treatment with endoscopy* (pp 600–604), Eric Van Cutsem and Paul Rutgeerts review the positive yield of upper endoscopy in iron deficiency anemia, the beneficial role of therapeutic endoscopy (injection, heater probe, bicap, laser, and hemoclip) in bleeding ulcers, the efficacy of estrogen/progesterone for bleeding arteriovenous malformations, the safety and efficacy of percutaneous endoscopic gastrostomy for nutritional support, and the usefulness of endoscopic ultrasound to examine bleeding vessels and stage gastric cancer.

In *New trends in gastroduodenal surgery* (pp 605–609), Marek Rudnicki and Michael Gold report on the continued growth of laparoscopic surgery, the work-up and management of patients with Zollinger-Ellison Syndrome, and the utility of bariatric surgery. Early follow-up indicates that Nissen, Hill, and Toupet antireflux procedures can be performed laparoscopically with equivalent outcomes to open procedures. Laparoscopic parietal cell vagotomy, posterior truncal vagotomy with anterior seromyotomy, and truncal vagotomy combined with balloon pyloroplasty have been used successfully to decrease acid secretion. Even gastric resection and closure of perforation can be accomplished laparoscopically! Magnetic resonance imaging has proven especially useful for the detection of metastatic gastrinoma to the liver. Despite numerous procedures for weight reduction, none are optimal. Gastric bypass seems to provide greater weight loss and fewer complications than vertical gastroplasty.

In *Gastric cancer* (pp 610–617) Frank Sinicrope and Bernard Levin review the latest information regarding the epidemiology, pathogenesis, and treatment of gastric adenocarcinoma. Although the overall incidence of gastric cancer has declined in the United States, there has been a progressive increase in the incidence of adenocarcinoma of the proximal stomach and gastroesophageal junction. Risk factors implicated in the pathogenesis of gastric adenocarcinoma include a high salt diet, high intake of *N*-nitroso compounds, low intake of anti-oxidants such as ascorbic acid and carotenoids, and prior infection with *H. pylori.* The high prevalence of *H. pylori* infection in normal adults without gastric cancer underscores the fact that other factors besides *H. pylori* are necessary for the development of adenocarcinoma. Abnormalities in cellular adhesion molecules, such as E-cadherin or L-CAM, may portend tumor invasion and metastatic potential. Increased expression of CD44, a cell surface molecule involved in cell-to-cell interaction, appears to be associated with tumor progression, recurrence, and decreased survival. Despite new chemotherapeutic regimens including pre- and postoperative chemotherapy, *ie*, neoadjuvant therapy, the prognosis for gastric cancer remains poor with 5-year survival rates being less than 15%.

In *Gastroduodenal motility* (pp 618–622), Nicholas Talley discusses measurement and control of normal gastroduodenal motor function and treatment of gastric motility disorders, with an emphasis on functional dyspepsia. Functional dyspepsia afflicts more than 25% of the adult population. Its pathogenesis is unclear but may involve subtle abnormalities of gastric motor dysfunction or visceral hypersensitivity.

In closing, I would like to thank the Current Science staff, especially Kelly Streeter, for their invaluable assistance, the contributors for their excellent reviews, and Mary Beatty for her artwork.

Mitchell L. Schubert, MD, McGuire VAMC, Code 111N, Gastroenterology Division, 1201 Broad Rock Boulevard, Richmond, VA 23249, USA.

Regulation of gastric secretion

Mitchell L. Schubert, MD

Medical College of Virginia and McGuire VAMC, Richmond, Virginia, USA

This review of the past year's literature focuses on progress in the elucidation of the pathways and mechanisms controlling gastric exocrine (*ie*, acid and pepsin) and endocrine (*ie*, gastrin, histamine, and somatostatin) secretion at the central, peripheral, and intracellular levels by neural, hormonal, and paracrine agents. Molecular biological techniques continue to further our knowledge into the function of receptors regulating gastric secretion and the transduction pathways to which they are coupled. Techniques for purification and enrichment of fundic enterochromaffin-like cells have proven useful tools with which to examine the mechanisms regulating histamine secretion. Somatostatin, acting as a paracrine agent, is the main inhibitor of exocrine and endocrine secretion by the stomach and additional evidence is provided that the hypergastrinemia induced by *Helicobacter pylori* is mediated via a decrease in somatostatin secretion. The role of trefoil peptides and nitric oxide in the regulation of gastric secretion remains to be determined.

Current Opinion in Gastroenterology 1994, **10**:575–588

In vertebrates, parietal cells are the source of HCl. In some species, including humans, monkeys, rabbits, cats, guinea pigs, and oxen (but not rats, mice, or hogs) parietal cells also secrete intrinsic factor [1••]. Parietal cells develop in the neck region of the oxyntic gland and they migrate downward toward the base as they mature. The major stimulants of HCl secretion are gastrin, histamine, and acetylcholine. With stimulation, parietal cells undergo a morphologic transformation in which the resting intracellular tubulovesicular structures fuse with the canalicular membrane, greatly expanding its surface area and creating enormous villuslike infoldings. At the same time, H^+K^+-ATPase, the proton pump of the parietal cell, is translocated to the canalicular membrane and activated.

Parietal cells can be isolated and cultured to 100% purity [1••]. Such preparations have proven useful to examine receptors and the transduction pathways to which they are coupled. Other methods used to examine acid secretion, each with distinct advantages and disadvantages, include isolated apical membrane vesicles, isolated gastric glands, mucosal sheets in Using chamber, superfused mucosal segments, isolated whole stomach, and whole animal. Waisbren *et al.* [2•] describe a new technique in which single rabbit gastric glands can be perfused and both intracellular and intraluminal pH monitored. This technique should allow the environments at the apical and basolateral membranes of gastric glands to be separately controlled, and parietal and peptic cells to be monitored simultaneously in the same gland.

This review summarizes new knowledge published in the past year that contributes to our understanding of the 1) control of gastric acid secretion at the central, peripheral, and intracellular levels, 2) control of pepsinogen secretion, and 3) mechanisms whereby various neurotransmitters, paracrine agents, and hormones regulate acid secretion and are themselves regulated.

Central mechanisms

Stimulants

Pancreatic polypeptide, neuropeptide Y, and peptide YY

Pancreatic polypeptide, neuropeptide Y, and peptide YY form the pancreatic polypeptide family of structurally related brain-gut peptides. Although pancreatic polypeptide is present almost exclusively in endocrine cells of the pancreatic islets, high-affinity specific receptors for pancreatic polypeptide have been detected in the postrema, nucleus tractus solitarius (NTS), and dorsal motor nucleus (DMN) areas of the brain. These nuclei are directly involved in vagovagal regulation of gastrointestinal secretion. Vagal afferents from the gastrointestinal tract synapse on neurons within the NTS and area postrema. The NTS processes the sensory input and sends projections to the DMN. Vagal efferents from the DMN then project to enteric neurons within the gastrointestinal tract. The dorsomedial region of the NTS was recently shown to contain fenestrated capillaries with high permeability that may al-

Abbreviations

CGRP—calcitonin gene-related peptide; **DMN**—dorsal motor nucleus; **EGF**—epidermal growth factor; **GLP**—glucagon-like peptide; **GRP**—gastrin-releasing peptide; **MMC**—migrating motor complex; **NTS**—nucleus tractus solitarius; **PAM**—peptidyl-glycine α-amidating monooxygenase; **TGF**—transforming growth factor.

© 1994 Current Science ISBN 1-85922-611-6 ISSN 0267–1379

low circulating peptides such as pancreatic polypeptide access to the NTS and neighboring DMN. McTigue *et al.* [3•] microinjected picomolar amounts of pancreatic polypeptide into the dorsal vagal complex (*ie*, NTS and DMN) of anesthetized rats and observed an increase in gastric acid secretion. The response was blocked by bilateral cervical vagotomy or atropine, suggesting that intramedullary pancreatic polypeptide stimulates vagal cholinergic pathways.

Peptide YY is released from endocrine cells in the distal ileum and colon in response to luminal lipids and carbohydrates. Hernandez *et al.* [4] report that intravenous ^{125}I-labeled peptide YY also gains access to and binds to receptors in the dorsal vagal complex. Thus, peptide YY (and pancreatic polypeptide) may act centrally as endocrine neuromodulators in the dorsal vagal complex to regulate gastric acid secretion.

Neuropeptide Y is the most abundant peptidergic neurotransmitter in the brain and neuropeptide Y–containing fibers are directly connected to the dorsal vagal complex. Matsuda *et al.* [5] previously reported that intracerebroventricular injection of neuropeptide Y caused a concentration-dependent increase in acid secretion in rats that was abolished by vagotomy. Geoghegan *et al.* [6•] confirm and extend those findings by reporting that intracerebroventricular administration of neuropeptide Y increases basal as well as sham feeding– and meal-stimulated acid secretion in dogs. As above, the response was blocked by vagotomy, making neuropeptide Y a likely candidate to mediate the cephalic phase of gastric acid secretion. Neuropeptide Y–containing fibers may also be connected to the dorsal vagal complex indirectly via sensory neurons that have their cell bodies located in the nodose ganglion. These neurons have one process that terminates in the NTS and another that terminates in the innervated peripheral organ. Ghilardi *et al.* [7] report the presence of neuropeptide Y (Y1 and Y2) receptor binding sites on a discrete population of neurons in rat nodose ganglion. Possible sources of neuropeptide Y include the nodose ganglion cells themselves as well as sympathetic and parasympathetic neurons, for all three are capable of synthesizing and releasing neuropeptide Y.

The pancreatic polypeptide family of peptides is also present in spinal cord. Wager-Pagé *et al.* [8] report that intrathecal administration of pancreatic polypeptide and peptide YY increases whereas neuropeptide Y administration decreases gastric acid secretion. The inhibitory effect of neuropeptide Y was reversed by the α2 adrenergic receptor antagonist, yohimbine, implying that it was mediated via α2 adrenergic receptors.

Emotional stress

Psychologic factors have long been thought to play a role in the pathophysiology of peptic ulcer disease. Ten normal men and 10 men with inactive duodenal ulcer were randomly assigned to a dichotomous listening task (each ear received a different narrated passage from Defoe's *Robinson Crusoe* and subjects were asked to answer one or more specific questions based on the narration) or a control task (nondichotomous listening) and gastric acid secretion was determined [9]. Dichotomous listening attempts to mimic the experience of a busy person trying to perform several tasks at once. In the duodenal ulcer group, but not the normal group, emotional stress significantly increased basal acid output, by about 85%. These findings support a role for psychobiologic factors in the pathophysiology of duodenal ulcer disease.

Vagus

Welsh *et al.* [10], in an attempt to define the role of gastrin, histamine, and acetylcholine in vagally stimulated acid secretion, examined the acid response to electrical field stimulation in three, isolated, lumen-perfused stomach preparations (mouse, immature rat, and guinea pig). Field stimulation produced frequency-dependent stimulations of acid secretion in all three preparations that were abolished by the axonal blocker tetrodotoxin, indicating that they were neurally-mediated. In the mouse and guinea pig, the acid response was also abolished by atropine or famotidine, consistent with the notion that neurally released acetylcholine acted predominantly by releasing histamine. In the rat, however, individual antagonists only partly inhibited the response (the combination abolished the response), implying both direct cholinergic innervation of the parietal cell and noncholinergic release of histamine. Gastrin did not play a role, since the response was not inhibited by the gastrin antagonist, CI-988.

In concordance with the above observations, Watanabe *et al.* [11] also report that electrical vagal stimulation of the isolated mouse stomach induces an increase in acid secretion that can be abolished by tetrodotoxin, atropine, or cimetidine. As opposed to the previous study, however, 100 μmol/L of famotidine, a 10-fold greater dose than that required to abolish histamine-stimulated acid secretion in this preparation and five-fold greater than that used by Welsh *et al.* [10], inhibited vagally stimulated acid secretion by only 30%. The reason for the different responses to famotidine between the two studies is unclear.

Bäck *et al.* [12] reported that 10 days after vagotomy and pyloroplasty, the density of histamine cells in rat oxyntic mucosa was increased, the density of 5-hydroxytryptamine and somatostatin cells were unchanged, and the density of calcitonin gene-related peptide (CGRP) and bombesin/gastrin-releasing peptide (GRP) nerve fibers were decreased. The findings suggest that histamine cells and CGRP and bombesin/GRP nerve fibers are regulated by vagal activity. The increase in number and activity of histamine cells may be due to the decrease in acid secretion, hypergastrinemia, or loss of a normal vagal inhibitory influence on these cells.

Duodenal ulcer patients as a group have higher basal and maximal outputs of gastric acid and pepsin secretion than normal subjects. One hypothesis is that hypersecretion is due to vagal overactivity because basal secretion is largely eliminated by vagotomy. Hirschowitz and Groarke [13•] used modified sham feeding to study vagal activity in 144 patients with duodenal ulcer and 92 non-ulcer controls. Modified sham feeding raised basal acid output at least 15% and added amounts of acid equal to about 30% of peak acid output in all subjects. The speed and duration of responses were also similar in duodenal ulcer and control subjects. There was no significant change in serum gastrin. Although vagal stimulation by modified sham feeding produced quantitatively similar responses in non-ulcer women and men, as well as women with duodenal ulcer, men with duodenal ulcer did have evidence for vagal overactivity as manifest by elevated basal acid output and the ratios of basal acid output to peak acid output and sham acid output to maximal acid output as compared with all other groups. Thus, the hypersecretion described in duodenal ulcer patients appears to be derived largely from responses in men.

It should be noted that there is considerable variability in gastric secretory studies. Dalenbäck *et al.* [14••] continuously sampled gastric pH, PCO_2, and motility in eight healthy volunteers and demonstrated that late in migrating motor complex (MMC) phase II, acid output, bicarbonate output, and bile reflux increased significantly. Acid secretion reached a peak in association with MMC phase III (339 ±44 μmol/min) following which the gastric lumen was rapidly alkalinized because of both a decrease in acid and increase in bicarbonate secretion. The marked variability in acid secretion during the interdigestive motility cycle should be taken into account when performing gastric secretory studies (Fig. 1).

Inhibitors

Interleukin-1

In pylorus-ligated and in chronic gastric fistula rats, Saperas and Taché [15] reported that intracerebroventricular injection of interleukin-1β inhibits basal and pentagastrin-stimulated acid secretion. The effect can be abolished by intracerebroventricular injection of the interleukin-1 receptor antagonist, but not by peripheral administration of somatostatin monoclonal antibody, indicating that interleukin-1β interacts with specific interleukin receptors and acts independently of peripheral somatostatin. The interleukin-1 receptor antagonist, by itself, had no significant effect on acid secretion, indicating that central interleukin-1 does not exert a tonic influence on acid secretion. Saperas *et*

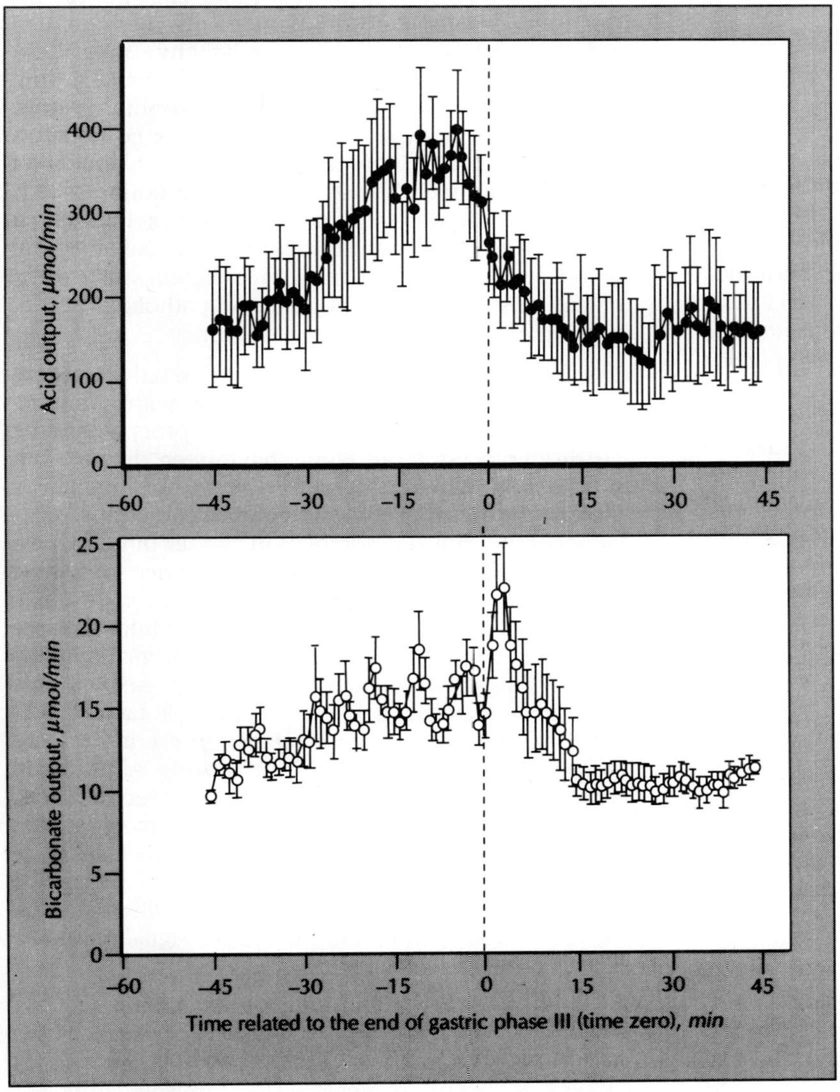

Fig. 1. Gastric acid output (*upper panel*) and bicarbonate output (*lower panel*) as related to the phase of the migrating motor complex (MMC). The end of motor phase-III activity (time zero) is indicated by a *vertical dotted line*. There is considerable variability in acid secretion with peak secretion occurring in association with phase III of the MMC. (*From* Dalenbäck *et al.* [14••]; with permission.)

al. [16] had previously reported that peripheral injection of indomethacin blocked the antisecretory effect of intracerebroventricular interleukin-1β, indicating that interleukin-1β exerts its effect via release of prostaglandins.

Neurotensin

Although the bulk of the body's content of neurotensin is present in the gastrointestinal tract, primarily in N cells of the ileum, this tridecapeptide was originally isolated from hypothalamus. Tsalis *et al.* [17] report that intracerebroventricular injection of neurotensin in dogs decreases gastric acid and increases gastrin secretion; there was no significant change in plasma neurotensin levels. The increase in gastrin may be due to the decrease in luminal acidity. Previous studies in rats suggest that the inhibitory effect of neurotensin may be mediated by dopaminergic neurons [18].

Dopamine

Dopamine receptors have been classified into at least five subtypes, designated D1-5. In the rat model, intraperitoneal injection of the D4 receptor antagonist clozapine inhibits basal acid secretion by 84% [19]. Because D4 receptors are present in high concentrations in mesolimbic brain regions, it is possible that dopamine acted via central mechanisms.

Neutral endopeptidase inhibitor-24.11

Neutral endopeptidase is a membrane-bound metalloprotease widely distributed throughout the body that is involved in the metabolism of various peptides. Quantitative immunoautoradiographic techniques indicate a moderate density of neutral endopeptidase-24.11 in the NTS and DMN [20]. Stephens *et al.* [21] reported that intracisternal injection of the neutral endopeptidase-24.11 inhibitor phosphoramidon produced a dose-dependent inhibition of gastric acid secretion in pylorus-ligated rats. The effect of the neutral endopeptidase inhibitor was not blocked by pretreatment with naloxone, a bombesin antagonist, or reserpine, indicating independence from mechanisms involving endogenous opiates, bombesin, or neurotensin. The endopeptidase inhibitor may have increased endogenous levels of tachykinins or interleukins, both of which have been shown to inhibit acid secretion after central injection [22]. Specific peptidase inhibitors as well as peptide receptor antagonists should prove useful tools with which to examine the central pathways regulating acid secretion.

Peripheral mechanisms

Stimulants

Gastrin

Gastrin is synthesized initially as a large precursor molecule, preprogastrin, which undergoes proteolytic cleavage by an endoprotease and a carboxypeptidase to a glycine-extended intermediate followed by amidation of the carboxyl terminal by peptidylglycine-α-amidating monooxygenase (PAM) to yield the biologically active peptide. PAM is a bifunctional protein that contains two separate enzyme activities, peptidylglycine-α-hydroxylating monooxygenase that catalyzes the conversion of glycine-extended peptides into peptidyl-α-hydroxyglycine intermediates and peptidyl-α-hydroxyglycine α-amidating lyase that cleaves the intermediate to form the peptide amide and glyoxylate. Using immunocytochemical and *in situ* hybridization techniques, Martínez *et al.* [23] showed that PAM is located in neurons of the myenteric and submucosal plexus and in mature gastrin cells. Amidated gastrin-17 is the major molecular form of gastrin in antral G cells.

Dickinson *et al.* [24•] mutated the wild-type Gly residue of progastrin to Ala or Ser and examined the expression of the three progastrin DNAs in *GH3* (rat pituitary tumor) and *MTC 6-23* (rat medullary thyroid carcinoma) endocrine cell lines. Replacement of the wild-type Gly with either amino acid abolished production of amidated gastrin, indicating that PAM has rigid substrate specificity for the glycine-extended precursor. In humans, gastrin-amide (active), gastrin-gly (inactive), and PAM may all coexist in plasma. Kapuscinski *et al.* [25] measured plasma concentrations of glycine extended and amidated gastrins and PAM in healthy subjects, patients with *MEN-1* with normal and high plasma gastrin, and patients with hypergastrinemic atrophic gastritis. The results demonstrated only very weak correlations between circulating PAM activity and gastrin amidation in plasma and were consistent with the notion that 1) gastrin amidation occurs mostly, if not exclusively, at the site of synthesis and storage and 2) circulating amidation activity does not contribute significantly to the amidation status of plasma gastrin in pathologic conditions characterized by hypergastrinemia.

Gastrin shares a common carboxy-terminal sequence, a domain critical for receptor binding, with cholecystokinin. Based on binding studies, receptors within the gastrin/cholecystokinin family have been divided into three major subtypes: cholecystokinin-A (alimentary), cholecystokinin-B (brain), and cholecystokinin-C (gastrin receptor). Small differences in agonist binding have created controversy regarding the existence of distinct cholecystokinin-B and gastrin receptor subtypes. The parietal cell gastrin and brain cholecystokinin-B receptors have recently been cloned and sequence analysis strongly suggests that both receptors are encoded by a single gene localized to chromosome 11 at bands p15.5 to p15.4 and that the two proteins represent the same receptor [26,27••,28,29••,30,31,32••]. Song *et al.* [32••], however, reported that the human cholecystokinin-B/gastrin receptor gene may be alternatively spliced to yield two different receptor isoforms that differ by five amino acids in the third intracellular loop. The isoforms may contribute to functional differences in gastrin- and cholecystokinin-mediated signal transduction or disease states.

A 78-kD protein (p78) from porcine gastric mucosal membranes that appears to be a component of the gastrin receptor has been purified and sequenced [33]. Cloning of the complementary DNAs revealed the presence of a protein related to the product of the *Escherichia coli fadB* gene, which possesses both enoyl-CoA hydratase and 3-hydroxyacyl-CoA dehydrogenase activity. The precise function of this protein remains to be determined.

Debate continues as to whether gastrin stimulates acid secretion directly or via release of histamine (Fig. 2). Thus far, the dog is the only species in which a direct action of gastrin on parietal cells has been firmly established. Cabero *et al.* [34] report that pentagastrin stimulates aminopyrine accumulation (a measure of acid secretion) in an enriched preparation of pig parietal cells (65% to 95%). The effect was not blocked by ranitidine, indicating a direct action of gastrin on the parietal cell. Gastrin, however, appeared to be dependent on endogenous cyclic AMP because the phosphodiesterase inhibitor isobutylmethylxanthine as well as dibutyryl-cyclic AMP augmented its effect and the protein kinase A inhibitor Rp-cyclic AMPs reduced its effect on aminopyrine accumulation.

In 14 volunteers, Zimmerhackl *et al.* [35] reported that famotidine (40 mg intravenous bolus) abolished basal and gastrin-17-stimulated acid secretion, suggesting that release of histamine mediates gastrin's effect. The response to gastrin was also partly blocked (72%) by atropine, implying perhaps that cholinergic tone is required for the full acid secretory response to histamine.

Gastrin secretion is stimulated by bombesin [36], cholinergic agonists, and adenosine A_2 agonists, and inhibited by somatostatin and adenosine A_1 agonists. Using canine antral gastrin cells in primary culture, Schepp *et al.* [37•] reported that prostaglandins exert both inhibitory and stimulatory influences on gastrin secretion. The synthetic prostaglandin analogue enprostil inhibited bombesin-, carbachol-, and forskolin (a receptor-independent activator of adenylate cyclase)-stimulated gastrin secretion via a pertussis toxin–sensitive mechanism. Prostaglandin E_2 also inhibited forskolin-stimulated gastrin secretion but had no significant effect on bombesin- or carbachol-stimulated secretion. However, in pertussis toxin–treated cultures, prostaglandin E_2 augmented bombesin-, carbachol-, and possibly forskolin-stimulated gastrin secretion. The exact mechanism responsible for the opposing actions of prostaglandins on gastrin release are unknown, but may involve selective activation of

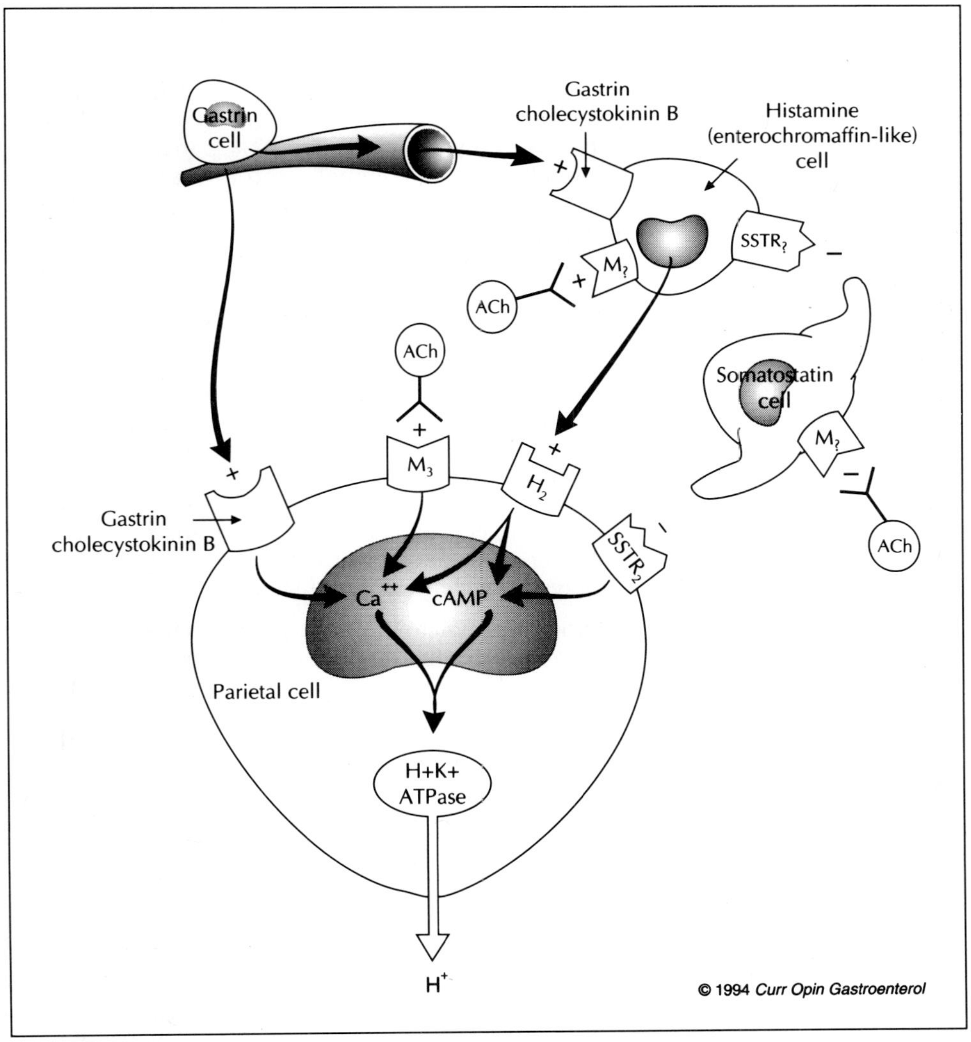

Fig. 2. Model for the neural and paracrine regulation of acid secretion in fundus of the stomach. The main inhibitor of acid secretion is somatostatin, which exerts a tonic restraint on acid secretion by the parietal cell and histamine secretion by the enterochromaffin-like cell. Cholinergic (ACh) neurons stimulate acid secretion directly via M_3 receptors on parietal cells as well as indirectly by stimulating histamine and inhibiting somatostatin secretion. In some species, gastrin acts predominantly by releasing histamine from mucosal stores. The parietal cell gastrin and acetylcholine receptors are coupled to increase in calcium, whereas the histamine (H_2) receptor is coupled both to increase in calcium and cyclic AMP. The somatostatin receptor on the parietal cell is likely of the SSTR2 subtype, which is coupled via a GTP-binding inhibitory protein (G_i) to a decrease in cyclic AMP. +, stimulatory signal; -, inhibitory signal; ?, receptor subtype not established.

specific subclasses of prostaglandin E receptors. At least three different subtypes of prostaglandin receptors have been defined pharmacologically and molecular biologically termed EP_1, EP_2, and EP_3 [38–40]. Activation of the EP_1 receptor is coupled to a rise in inositol triphosphate and intracellular calcium, activation of the EP_2 receptor to an increase in cyclic AMP, and activation of the EP_3 receptor to a decrease in cyclic AMP. The EP_2 messenger RNA is expressed in stomach [39].

Dockray *et al.* [41] reported that instillation of acid into the stomach of rats pretreated with omeprazole decreased plasma gastrin, confirming the notion that luminal acid inhibits gastrin secretion, an effect that may be mediated by release of somatostatin [42].

Renal insufficiency is associated with hypergastrinemia. Lichtenberger *et al.* [43•] demonstrated 30- to 40-fold elevations in gastric juice aliphatic amine concentrations in patients with acute renal failure. Because these amines have previously been shown to stimulate gastrin release from isolated gastrin cells and when orally fed to rats, it is possible that their accumulation may contribute to the hypergastrinemia associated with uremia.

Gastrin/cholecystokinin-B antagonists have proven to be useful tools with which to examine the role of gastrin in acid secretion. As opposed to the gastrin/cholecystokinin-B antagonist PD-136,450, which behaves as a partial secretory agonist *in vivo* [44], L365260 either inhibits or has no effect on basal acid secretion [45]. Varga *et al.* [45] report that the gastrin/cholecystokinin-B antagonist L365260 inhibits peptone-stimulated acid secretion in conscious rats by 50% [45], indicating a physiologic role for gastrin in meal-stimulated acid secretion. The findings support those previously reported by Lloyd *et al.* [46] using a gastrin monoclonal antibody. In humans, Murphy *et al.* [47] report that oral administration of L365260 has no effect on basal acid secretion, but inhibits pentagastrin-stimulated secretion in a dose-dependent manner. The gastrin/cholecystokinin-B receptor has been demonstrated to be present on both parietal and histamine-containing cells.

Histamine

Although histamine plays a key role in gastric acid secretion, the pathways regulating histamine release and the exact mechanism whereby histamine interacts with gastrin and acetylcholine to stimulate acid secretion remain controversial. Diaz *et al.* [48••] examined the cellular localization of H_2 receptors in rat stomach by *in situ* hybridization histochemistry using an antisense riboprobe for the rat H_2 receptor and autoradiographic distribution of the selective H_2 ligand, ^{125}I-aminopotentidine. In contrast to results discussed in last year's review [49], no labeling of the lamina propria was detected. Rather, consistent with current viewpoints, the H_2 receptor and its messenger RNA were detected in the isthmus of the glandular mucosa, in parietal cells.

It is likely that histamine, gastrin, and acetylcholine interact with specific receptors on the parietal cell and that a potentiating effect between secretagogues exist. In addition, gastrin and acetylcholine release histamine from mucosal stores (Fig. 2). The cellular source of histamine varies among species, with histamine stored mainly in enterochromaffin-like cells in rats and rabbits and in mastlike cells in dogs, pigs, and humans. In a preparation of isolated rabbit fundic mucosal cells enriched in mucous and endocrine cells but deficient in mast cells (*ie,* 12% histamine cells and 1% mast cells), Hollande *et al.* [50,51•] reported that gastrin and carbachol stimulate histidine decarboxylase activity (a measure of histamine synthesis) as well as histamine release. Carbachol was a less potent and slightly less efficient releaser of histamine than gastrin and its effect was blocked by pirenzepine (M_1 antagonist) but not by AFDX-116 (M_2 antagonist) or HHSiD (M_3 antagonist), suggesting that cholinergic stimulation involves an M_1 receptor. The stimulatory effect of gastrin was blocked by the gastrin antagonists L365260 and PD135666, implying that gastrin acts via a gastrin/cholecystokinin-B receptor. Activators of protein kinase C and the calcium ionophore A23187 stimulated histamine release, whereas activators of cyclic AMP (forskolin, IBMX, and dibutyryl-5′-cyclic AMP) were devoid of effect. Because this preparation contained various populations of cells, it is possible that concomitant release of somatostatin masked any direct effect of cyclic AMP activators on the histamine-containing cells. In support of this notion, Chuang *et al.* [52••] report, using an enriched and well-characterized cell culture of canine fundic mucosal cells (25% enterochromaffin-like cells, 0.6% mast cells, 3% somatostatin cells, 32% parietal cells, 11% chief cells, 27% mucous cells, and 1.4% serotonin cells), that addition of somatostatin antibody increased basal histamine release, suggesting that endogenous somatostatin exerts a paracrine inhibitory influence on histamine secretion.

Similar results were reported by Prinz *et al.* [53••] using a highly enriched (65-fold) suspension of enterochromaffin-like cells from rat fundic mucosa. Gastrin, carbachol, and active phorbol esters stimulated histamine release whereas somatostatin inhibited it. The cells were very sensitive to the stimulatory effect of gastrin, which was mediated via gastrin/cholecystokinin-B receptors. In contrast to results reported above with rabbit cells, forskolin and dibutyrl-5′-cyclic AMP stimulated histamine release.

Although acetylcholine and gastrin release histamine from enterochromaffin-like cells, a role for mast cells in the regulation of acid secretion should not be excluded. In the anesthetized rat [54] and pig [55], the mast cell stabilizer DS-4574 significantly inhibited (85%) carbachol- and pentagastrin-stimulated, but not histamine-stimulated acid secretion, suggesting a role also for mast cell–derived histamine.

Three subtypes of histamine receptors have been identified: H_1, H_2, and H_3. H_1 receptors are coupled to inositol phospholipid hydrolysis and release of intracellular calcium, H_2 receptors are coupled to stimulation of adenylate cyclase, and H_3 receptors are coupled to inhibition of a variety of neurotransmitters. In isolated enterochromaffin-like cells derived from rabbit [56•] and rat [53••] fundic mucosa, the H_3 agonist (r)-α-methylhistamine inhibited histamine synthesis and release whereas the H_3 antagonist thioperamide had the opposite effect, implying that histamine down-regulates its own synthesis and release via H_3 autoreceptors.

Acetylcholine

Studies using molecular cloning techniques have identified five subtypes of mammalian muscarinic receptor subtypes, designated m1 through m5. All possess seven putative, hydrophobic, transmembrane domains and belong to the G protein–coupled receptor family. The large cytoplasmic domain joining the fifth and sixth transmembrane segments plays a critical role in controlling the specificity of G protein signaling. The m1, m3, and m5 subtypes couple preferentially via a pertussis toxin–insensitive G protein to phosphoinositol hydrolysis, whereas m2 and m4 subtypes couple via a pertussis toxin-sensitive G protein, G_i, to inhibition of adenylate cyclase.

Acetylcholine stimulates acid secretion by binding to an m3 receptor on the parietal cell that is coupled to phospholipid hydrolysis with generation of 1,4,5-triphosphate and diacylglycerol (Fig. 2). The rise in 1,4,5-triphosphate leads to an increase in intracellular calcium, whereas the increase in diacylglycerol is associated with the translocation of protein kinase C from the cytosol to the membrane and its presumed activation.

By measuring the ability of substitution and deletion mutant derivatives of the m3 subtype to activate phospholipase C–dependent responses in RNA-injected Xenopus oocytes, Kunkel and Peralta [57] identified two clusters of charged residues near the fifth and sixth transmembrane segments that are required for normal signaling.

McKenna and Hanson [58] reported that a selective inhibitor of protein kinase C, Ro 31-8220, inhibits carbachol-stimulated aminopyrine accumulation in isolated rat parietal cells by 43% without any significant effect on the increase in intracellular calcium, implying that protein kinase C facilitates acid secretion.

Antidepressants may cause undesirable anticholinergic side-effects. Stanton *et al.* [59] expressed m1 to m5 muscarinic subtypes in Chinese hamster ovary cells and determined the affinity and selectivity of binding for 16 antidepressants and three H_1 antagonists. Many of the drugs were potent antagonists for one or more receptor subtypes; amitriptyline, nortriptyline, doxepin, and cyproheptadine were relatively potent (K_d 5 to 50 nmol/L) m3 receptor antagonists.

Ren and Harty [60•] reported that carbachol and the M1 antagonist pirenzepine inhibit and atropine enhances basal and stimulated acetylcholine release from rat antral mucosal/submucosal nerves. The findings suggest that acetylcholine release from antral mucosa is regulated by a negative autofeedback mechanism, probably involving M2 or M3 receptors, whereas M1 receptors facilitate release of neurotransmitter. Yokotani *et al.* [61] have further characterized the presence of an M3 autoreceptor in rat stomach that inhibits acetylcholine release. In the isolated vascularly perfused rat stomach, the following muscarinic antagonists, in order of decreasing potency, augmented electrical vagal-stimulated acetylcholine release: 4-DAMP (M3 antagonist), methoctramine (M2 antagonist), and pirenzepine (M1 antagonist). Because this preparation contains both myenteric and submucosal/mucosal neurons, one cannot say for certain that this receptor is the same one identified by Ren and Harty [60].

Electrical stimulation of periarterial gastric sympathetic nerves or infusion of clonidine inhibits vagal-stimulated acetylcholine release, implying that α2 adrenoreceptors mediate inhibition of acetylcholine release.

Meal

Anticipation of a meal activates central neurons whose input is relayed via the vagus nerve to postganglionic cholinergic and noncholinergic (bombesin/GRP and vasoactive intestinal peptide) neurons located within the submucosal plexus of the stomach. Upon ingestion of the meal, the same neurons are activated chemically by food components and mechanically by distension. These neurons regulate acid secretion directly by depositing various transmitters on parietal cells and indirectly by depositing transmitters on mucosal endocrine (*eg*, gastrin) or paracrine (*eg*, somatostatin and histamine) cells or other neurons (Fig. 2).

Antral distension may either decrease or increase gastrin secretion, depending on the grade of distension: low grades increase somatostatin and decrease gastrin secretion whereas high grades have the opposite effect, decreasing somatostatin and increasing gastrin secretion [62]. Hamlet *et al.* [63] report that 150-mL antral balloon distension inhibits pentagastrin-stimulated acid secretion by 30% in *Helicobacter pylori*–negative volunteers.

Dimaline *et al.* [64] report that fasting reduces and refeeding increases histidine decarboxylase, the enzyme responsible for converting histidine to histamine, messenger RNA in the gastric corpus of the rat. The increase in histidine decarboxylase could be blocked by gastrin antibody, indicating that its production is regulated by gastrin.

Pure ethanol in low concentrations (<5% vol/vol) is a mild stimulant of acid secretion, whereas at higher concentrations it has either no effect or a mildly inhibitory one [65•]. Ethanol has no significant effect on gastrin secretion in humans. Beer and wine, however, are strong stimulants of both gastrin and acid secretion, indicating that it is the nonethanolic components of these beverages that are responsible for stimulation of acid secretion.

Helicobacter pylori

In patients with duodenal ulcer disease, hypergastrinemia is largely related to gastric *H. pylori* infection [66]. The hypergastrinemia is due to a selective increase in gastrin-17, the predominant form of gastrin in the antrum [67]. A previous study by Moss *et al.* [68] suggested that the exaggerated meal-stimulated gastrin response to *H. pylori* was due to a decrease in antral somatostatin secretion. In support of this notion, Queiroz *et al.* [69] reported that antral somatostatin content was lower and gastrin content higher in 13 children positive for *H. pylori* infection, compared with seven children who tested negatively. With eradication, antral somatostatin content and D-cell density increased to within the normal range. Similar findings were reported in patients with duodenal ulcer, in that after *H. pylori* eradication, antral somatostatin concentration and D-cell density increased whereas antral and serum gastrin content decreased [70]. The findings suggest that the hypergastrinemia observed in *H. pylori*–positive patients may be due to a deficiency of antral somatostatin, which tonically inhibits the synthesis and release of gastrin.

Defects in histamine secretion may also be present in patients infected with *H. pylori* either as a direct result of the organism or secondary to changes in somatostatin or gastrin. Quieroz *et al.* [71] reported that the histamine content of the oxyntic mucosa of patients with duodenal ulcer increased after *H. pylori* eradication.

Inhibitors

Somatostatin

The biologic effects of somatostatin are mediated by a rapidly expanding family of receptors; at least five different subtypes of somatostatin receptors have now been cloned, termed SSTR1-5. The human SSTR1-4 receptors are somatostatin-14 selective whereas the rat SSTR2,3,5 and human SSTR5 receptors are somatostatin-28 selective [72–74]. Human SSTR3 has been mapped to chromosome 22 [73] whereas SSTR4-5 have been mapped to chromosome 20 [72,75]. The synthetic somatostatin analogue SMS201-995 binds human SSTR5 (and SSTR1) with low affinity and human SSTR4 with either high [76] or low affinity [74,77]. Bruno *et al.* [78] employed solution hybridization/nuclease protection analysis using subtype-specific complementary RNA probes to demonstrate that all subtypes except SSTR5 are expressed in rat stomach, in approximately equal proportions. Species differences may exist, for no hybridization signal for SSTR3 was detected in the human stomach [79]. Detailed *in situ* hybridization and immunohistochemistry studies will be necessary to determine the cellular localization of each receptor subtype. Patel *et al.* [80••] established stably transfected *CHO-K1* cells expressing human genes for SSTR1-5 and showed that all five human somatostatin subtypes are functionally coupled to inhibition of adenylate cyclase via pertussis toxin–sensitive G proteins. These findings have been confirmed by most [77,81–84], but not all, [76] investigators. Tomura *et al.* [82] reported that human SSTR2 not only inhibits adenylate cyclase via a pertussis toxin–sensitive mechanism but also stimulates phospholipase C and calcium mobilization in transfected COS-7 cells. Raynor *et al.* [76] reported that human SSTR1, SSTR2, and SSTR4 are not coupled to adenylate cyclase in transiently transfected *COS-1* and *CHO-K1* cells. Future studies should focus on the functional role of each subtype in the stomach.

Somatostatin is the main inhibitor of exocrine and endocrine secretion by the stomach and exerts a tonic restraint on acid secretion. This paracrine restraint is exerted on parietal cells, gastrin cells, and histamine cells (Fig. 2) [52••,85]. Campbell-Thompson and McGuigan [86] used antibodies to a synthetic peptide derived from the complementary messenger RNA sequence for somatostatin-14, to identify putative somatostatin-binding sites on plasma membranes of canine parietal cells.

Larsson and Houggaard [87••] used quantitative *in situ* hybridization combined with immunocytochemistry to demonstrate that gastrin cells in close contact with somatostatin cells express significantly lower levels of gastrin messenger RNA than other gastrin cells, thus providing the first direct microscopic evidence for paracrine inhibition of gastrin by somatostatin.

The two principal bioactive forms of somatostatin, somatostatin-14 and somatostatin-28, are derived from tissue-specific proteolytic processing of prosomatostatin. In the stomach, the predominant product is somatostatin-14, whereas in the intestine somatostatin-28 predominates. Prior studies in isolated mouse stomach have provided evidence for the existence of a feedback mechanism whereby an increase in luminal acid stimulates somatostatin secretion that, in turn, acts to attenuate acid secretion [88]. The findings have been confirmed by Greenberg *et al.* [89•] who reported that histamine- and gastrin-stimulated acid secretion is accompanied by the secretion of somatostatin-14 into the circulation of conscious dog. The somatostatin response was abolished by omeprazole or ranitidine, implying that luminal acidity contributes directly to stimulation of somatostatin-14. Ingestion of a meal caused approximately equivalent plasma elevations of somatostatin-14 and somatostatin-28. Release of somatostatin-28 could be abolished by pretreatment with the cholecystokinin-A antagonist MK-329, implying that secretion of somatostatin-28, unlike somatostatin-14, was dependent on release of cholecystokinin.

In humans [90], infusion of exogenous somatostatin-28 to mimic blood levels obtained after a meal has no significant effect on basal or pentagastrin-stimulated acid secretion, suggesting that postprandial plasma concentrations of somatostatin-28 are unlikely to regulate gastric acid secretion in man.

Calcitonin gene-related peptide

Calcitonin gene-related peptide (CGRP) is a 37 amino acid peptide product of alternative splicing of the human calcitonin/CGRP-1 pre-messenger RNA in nervous tissue [91]. In gastric mucosa, CGRP is localized to primary sensory neurons. Capsaicin, a sensory toxin capable of evoking neuropeptide release from peripheral sensory nerve endings, releases CGRP from rat antral mucosal/submucosal fragments [92••] and vascularly perfused whole stomach [93]. In antral segments, both exogenous CGRP and capsaicin stimulate somatostatin and inhibit gastrin and acetylcholine release; all responses are abolished by a CGRP antagonist, indicating that CGRP derived from sensory neurons may exert local effector actions to regulate antral neuroendocrine function.

Epidermal growth factor and transforming growth factor-α

Epidermal growth factor (EGF) and transforming growth factor (TGF)-α share 35% sequence identity and a nearly identical spectrum of biological activities. In all systems thus far studied, EGF and TGF-α appear to interact with the same membrane receptor. Orsini *et al.* [94], using the techniques of *in situ* hybridization and immunohistochemistry, have precisely localized the EGF/TGF-α receptor in human gastric mucosa to the basal cytoplasm and basolateral membranes of mucus neck cells, foveolar columnar cells, and surface epithelial cells as well as the basolateral membrane of parietal cells. Some faint staining was noted in the cytoplasm of some parietal cells. In accordance with these findings, EGF and TGF-α have been demonstrated to inhibit acid secretion in parietal cells isolated from various species [95] and in conscious rats and monkeys [96,97]. In isolated rat parietal cells, Ostrowski *et al.* [95] report that the ornithine decarboxylase inhibitor difluoromethylornithine blocks the inhibitory effect of EGF on acid production, suggesting that EGF acts through induction of ornithine decarboxylase activity and synthesis of polyamines.

Opioids

Opioids have been reported to have variable effects on gastric acid secretion, perhaps because of the existence of multiple opioid subtypes. Intorre *et al.* [98] report that the μ-agonist dermorphin stimulates acid secretion in dogs chronically fitted with both a gastric fistula and Heidenhain pouch, whereas the δ-agonist [D-Ala^2,D-Leu^5]enkephalin inhibits acid secretion, and the κ-agonist dynorphin-(1-13) has no significant effect. None of the agonists significantly modified the gastrin response induced by 2-deoxy-D-glucose, suggesting that the acid responses induced by the selective agonists occurred independently of gastrin release.

Leukotriene

Leukotrienes are arachidonic acid metabolites generated via the 5-lipoxygenase pathway. Leukotriene C_4 and leukotriene D_4 potentiate acid production by isolated rat parietal cells [99]. Huber *et al.* [100] report that leukotriene B_4 and leukotriene C_4 are both produced *in vitro* in the small cell fraction of isolated rat gastric mucosal cells. Although the exact cell type was not identified, it should be noted that this fraction is enriched in chromogranin A–positive neuroendocrine cells, including enterochromaffin-like cells.

Trefoil peptides

The trefoil peptides, so called because of the presence of one, or up to six, compact distinctive cysteine-rich domains arranged in a three-leafed structure, include pS2, spasmolytic polypeptide, and Xenopus laevis spasmolysin [101]. Although pS2 and spasmolytic polypeptide are expressed and secreted in normal rat and human antral and fundic mucosa [102,103], the specific functions of these trefoil peptides are unknown. It has been hypothesized that these peptides may serve as structural components of mucus or function in repair processes.

Nitric oxide

The formation of nitric oxide from L-arginine is catalyzed by the enzyme nitric oxide synthase, which has recently been shown to be present in the myenteric and submucosal plexi of rat gastric corpus [104•]. The nitric oxide donor, S-nitroso-*N*-acetyl-penicillamine, inhibits accumulation of the weak base aminopyrine, an index of acid secretory activity, in isolated rat parietal cells [105•]. In anesthetized rat, nitroprusside, another nitric oxide donor, inhibits histamine-stimulated acid secretion in a concentration-dependent manner [106]. The physiologic role of nitric oxide in regulation of acid secretion remains to be determined.

Enterogastrones

It has been postulated that a humoral factor is present in the small and large intestine, which, when released by food, is responsible for inhibition of acid secretion. Candidate enterogastrones include secretin, cholecystokinin, oxyntomodulin, glucagon-like peptide (GLP)-1, peptide YY, and neurotensin. Strong evidence, derived by the use of specific antiserum or selective antagonists, supports secretin and cholecystokinin as physiological enterogastrones [107,108]. Shiratori *et al.* [109] reported that triglyceride-induced inhibition of gastric acid secretion in rats was abolished by pancreatic juice diversion and restored by preincubation with lipase, suggesting that intestinal fat digestion is necessary for fat-induced inhibition of acid secretion.

Cholecystokinin is released from I-cells in the upper intestine in response to intraluminal nutrients [110]. Multiple pro-cholecystokinin posttranslational products have been identified including cholecystokinin-83, -58, -39, -33, -22, -8, and -5. There has been much debate concerning the exact molecular nature of cholecystokinin in plasma and species differences exist. Rehfeld [111] reported that postprandial plasma from rabbits contains mainly small molecular forms such as cholecystokinin-22 and cholecystokinin-8, whereas extracts of the duodenum in addition contain cholecystokinin-58, -39, and -33. Konturek *et al.* [112] reported that in humans, the cholecystokinin-A antagonist loxiglumide diminished the somatostatin response and increased further both the gastric acid and gastrin responses to a peptone meal, suggesting that cholecystokinin inhibits postprandial acid secretion, perhaps by releasing gastric somatostatin. Similar results were previously reported in dogs [113].

The gene encoding proglucagon is expressed in L-cells, located mainly in the distal small intestine and colon. Tissue-specific posttranslational processing yields glicentin, oxyntomodulin, and two GLPs, GLP-1 and GLP-2. GLP-1 immunoreactivity includes GLP-1-(1-37), GLP-1-(7-36)amide, GLP-1-(7-37), and GLP-1-(7-36)amide [114]. Bado *et al.* [115] reported that in cats the inhibition of gastric acid secretion induced by oxyntomodulin is accompanied by an increase in gastric somatostatin secretion, suggesting that this may account for the acid-inhibitory effect. On the other hand, in humans Wettergren *et al.* [116] report that the inhibition in postprandial and modified sham-feeding–stimulated acid secretion induced by GLP-1 was not accompanied by significant changes in plasma somatostatin.

Intracellular mechanisms

GTPases

GTPases, proteins that bind and hydrolyze GTP, can be classified into three major groups according to function and sequence homology: 1) eukaryotic initiation factors involved in protein synthesis, 2) α subunits of the heterotrimeric GTP-binding proteins, and 3) low molecular weight GTP-binding proteins, also known as Ras-like proteins, that are thought to act as specific regulators of membrane trafficking in exocytosis and endocytosis [117•]. A subset of low molecular weight GTP-binding proteins named Rab (for Ras-related rat brain) have been localized to particular compartments: Rab1B and Rab2 to an intermediate compartment between endoplasmic reticulum and golgi, Rab3a to synaptic vesicles, Rab4 to early endosomes, and Rab5 and Rab7 to early and late endosomes. Rab2, Rab11, and a new member of the Rab family named Rab 25 have been identified in rabbit parietal cells; Rab3a has been identified in rat chief cells. It is likely that these low molecular weight proteins are involved in the regulation of acid and pepsinogen secretion, perhaps by directing the processing of membranes into and out of the secretory canaliculus and the fusion of zymogen granules with the plasma membrane.

H^+K^+-ATPase

The canine gastric H^+K^+-ATPase has been cloned and shows 80% to 90% homology with the corresponding complementary DNAs previously identified in porcine and rodent stomach [118–121]. The enzyme, which is responsible for acid secretion by the parietal cell, consists of a large α subunit composed of about 1030 amino acids and a smaller β subunit consisting of about 290 amino acids. The α subunit functions in ATP hydrolysis and catalyzes the electroneutral exchange of intracellular H^+ for extracellular K^+. The precise function of the β subunit is not known, but it may function in membrane targeting of the enzyme, in modulating the conformation of the α subunit, in modulating the binding of K^+ to the enzyme [122], and as a target antigen in pernicious anemia [123]. *In situ* hybridization has localized both subunits to the parietal cell; older parietal cells at the base of the glands gave weaker hybridization signals than younger parietal cells closer to the surface [124]. In the resting state, H^+K^+-ATPase is immunolocalized to cytoplasmic tubulovesicles whereas in the stimulated state it is localized to the secretory canalicular membrane [125]. Electron microscopic autoradiography utilizing [^{3}H]omeprazole demonstrates that activation of the enzyme occurs only when it is present in the canalicular membrane, and not when present in the tubulovesicles [126]. Structurally related H^+K^+-ATPases have been identified in distal colon, renal collecting duct, uterus, and vascular smooth muscle [127].

Omeprazole inhibits acid secretion by blocking the α subunit, leading to an increase in α subunit messenger RNA. The effect of omeprazole on α subunit messenger RNA in rat appears to be mediated via histamine release induced by hypergastrinemia because the effect can be blocked by an H_2-receptor antagonist [128•]. Consistent with this notion, infusion of histamine increased α subunit messenger RNA by 144% [129]. In rabbits, omeprazole enhances degradation of H^+K^+-ATPase protein and degeneration of parietal cells [130,131]. To keep the parietal cell population in a steady state, their production is accelerated by an increase in preparietal cell production.

A cyclic AMP-dependent protein kinase product that enhances H^+K^+-ATPase activity, tentatively named "kayletin" because it allows K^+ influx into inside-out gastric microsomes, has been isolated from rabbit gastric microsomes [132]. It is possible that cyclic AMP-dependent protein kinase regulates the rate of H^+K^+-ATPase activity and thus the rate of acid secretion by inducing K^+ conductance through phosphorylation of this integral membrane-bound protein.

Chloride

The parietal cell apical secretory unit essential for acid secretion consists of H^+K^+-ATPase and parallel K^+ and Cl^- pathways. Acidification occurs as a result of primary active transport of H^+ through H^+K^+-ATPase, which exchanges cytosolic H^+ for luminal K^+. Concurrently, K^+ and Cl^- move from cell cytosol to lumen providing luminal K^+ to the H^+K^+-ATPase and Cl^- for HCl secretion. Cuppoletti *et al.* [133•] recently provided direct evidence for the existence of apical Cl^- channels in rabbit parietal cells. The channels were identified in gastric H^+K^+-ATPase–containing membrane vesicles reconstituted into lipid bilayers.

A Cl^-/HCO_3^- exchanger, also necessary for acid secretion, is present on the basolateral membrane of the parietal cell. This exchanger extrudes HCO_3^- to maintain intracellular pH and supplies Cl^- for secretion of HCl. 4,4′-Di-isothiocyanostilbene-2,2′-disulfonic acid (DIDS) competitively blocks the exchanger and as a result inhibits histamine-, bethanechol-, and gastrin-stimulated acid secretion in the mouse and rat [134]. Ammonia also inhibits this exchanger in frog oxyntopeptic cells [135].

Pepsinogen secretion

Cholecystokinin, gastrin, and muscarinic agonists stimulate pepsinogen secretion by mobilizing intracellular calcium whereas vasoactive intestinal peptide, secretin, and truncated GLP cause secretion by increasing intracellular cyclic AMP [136]. In rabbit gastric glands, cholecystokinin-8 and gastrin-17 interact with the same receptor, a cholecystokinin-A–type receptor [137]. The lower potency and efficacy of gastrin-17 was dependent both on the sulfation of a tyrosine residue and the position of the tyrosine residue relative to the

COOH-terminal phenylalanine amide. Using thapsigargin, a phorbol tumor promotor that causes influx of calcium and also depletes intracellular calcium by inhibiting calcium reuptake into intracellular stores, Kitsukawa *et al.* [138] reported that changes in intracellular calcium do indeed participate in the initial and sustained stimulation of pepsinogen secretion from guinea pig chief cells by cholecystokinin-8 and are responsible for cholecystokinin-8 potentiation of secretin-stimulated pepsinogen secretion.

In amphibians, acid and pepsinogen secretions are performed by one cell type, the oxyntopeptic cell, whereas in mammals, acid and pepsinogen secretions are performed by parietal and chief cells, respectively. In the amphibian oxyntopeptic cell, histamine, forskolin, and carbachol each stimulate acid and pepsinogen secretion; omeprazole abolishes acid but has little effect on pepsinogen secretion [139]. On the other hand, in the rat stomach, omeprazole strongly inhibits pepsinogen gene expression, synthesis, and secretion [140].

References and recommended reading

Papers of particular interest, published within the annual period of review, have been highlighted as:
- • Of special interest
- •• Of outstanding interest

1. Chew CS: **Parietal Cell Culture: New Models and Directions.** *Annu Rev Physiol* 1994, **56**:445–461.
••

A lucid review of the technique of isolated parietal cell culture from one of its pioneers.

2. Waisbren SJ, Geibel J, Boron WF, Modlin IM: **Luminal Perfusion of Isolated Gastric Glands.** *Am J Physiol* 1994, **266**:C1013–C1027.
•

A new technique is described for perfusing individual rabbit gastric glands. The technique allows simultaneous monitoring of intracellular and intraluminal pH and parietal and peptic cells.

3. McTigue DM, Edwards NK, Rogers RC: **Pancreatic Polypeptide in Dorsal Vagal Complex Stimulates Gastric Acid Secretion and Motility in Rats.** *Am J Physiol* 1993, **265**:G1169–G1176.
•

The dorsomedial region of the NTS contains fenestrated capillaries that may allow circulating gut peptides such as pancreatic polypeptide and peptide YY (and perhaps others) to gain access to the NTS and dorsal motor nucleus of the vagus. Thus, gut peptides in the systemic circulation may gain access to and regulate acid secretion via central mechanisms.

4. Hernandez EJ, Whitcomb DC, Vigna SR, Taylor IL: **Saturable Binding of Circulating Peptide YY in the Dorsal Vagal Complex of Rats.** *Am J Physiol* 1994, **266**:G511–G516.

5. Matsuda M, Aono A, Moriga M, Okuma M: **Centrally Administered NPY Stimulated Gastric Acid and Pepsin Secretion by a Vagally Mediated Mechanism.** *Regul Pept* 1991, **35**:31–41.

6. Geoghegan JG, Lawson DC, Cheng CA, Opara E, Taylor IL, Pappas TN: **Intracerebroventricular Neuropeptide Y Increases Gastric and Pancreatic Secretion in the Dog.** *Gastroenterology* 1993, **105**:1069–1077.
•

Central injection of neuropeptide Y increases basal as well as sham feeding– and meal-stimulated acid secretion in dogs. The response is blocked by vagotomy, making neuropeptide Y a likely candidate to mediate the cephalic phase of gastric acid secretion.

7. Ghilardi JR, Allen CJ, Vigna SR, Mcvey DC, Mantyh PW: **Cholecystokinin and Neuropeptide Y Receptors on Single Rabbit Vagal Afferent Ganglion Neurons: Site of Prejunctional Modulation of Visceral Sensory Neurons.** *Brain Res* 1994, **633**:33–40.

8. Wager-Pagé SA, Rosenbaum G, Veale WL, Davison JS: **Spinal and Peripheral Modulation of Gastric Acid Secretion and Arterial Pressure by Neuropeptide Y, Peptide YY, and Pancreatic Polypeptide in Rats.** *Peptides* 1993, **14**:1299–1308.

9. Bresnick WH, Rask-Madsen C, Hogan DL, Koss MA, Isenberg JI: **The Effect of Acute Emotional Stress on Gastric Acid Secretion in Normal Subjects and Duodenal Ulcer Patients.** *J Clin Gastroenterol* 1993, **17**:117–122.

10. Welsh NJ, Shankley NP, Black JW: **Comparative Analysis of the Vagal Stimulation of Gastric Acid Secretion in Rodent Isolated Stomach Preparations.** *Br J Pharmacol* 1994, **112**:93–96.

11. Watanabe K, Yano S, Yamamoto M, Kanaoka S: **Comparative Effects of Cimetidine and Famotidine on the Vagally Stimulated Acid Secretion in the Isolated Mouse Whole Stomach.** *Jpn J Pharmacol* 1993, **61**:229–236.

12. Bäck N, Ahonen M, Häppölä O, Kivilaakso E, Kiviluoto T: **Effect of Vagotomy on Expression of Neuropeptides and Histamine in Rat Oxyntic Mucosa.** *Dig Dis Sci* 1994, **39**:353–361.

13. Hirschowitz BI, Groarke J: **Vagal Effects on Acid and Pepsin Secretion and Serum Gastrin in Duodenal Ulcer and Controls.** *Dig Dis Sci* 1993, **38**:1874–1884.
•

Men with duodenal ulcer have evidence for vagal overactivity as manifested by elevated basal acid output, basal acid output to peak acid output, and sham acid output to maximal acid output.

14. Dalenbäck J, Mellander A, Olbe L, Sjövall H: **Motility-Related Cyclic Fluctuations of Interdigestive Gastric Acid and Bicarbonate Secretion in Man: A Source of Substantial Variability in Gastric Secretion Studies.** *Scand J Gastroenterol* 1993, **28**:943–948.
••

Acid secretion varies greatly during the interdigestive motility cycle. This should be taken into account when performing gastric secretory studies.

15. Saperas E, Taché Y: **Central Interleukin-1β-Induced Inhibition of Acid Secretion in Rats: Specificity of Action.** *Life Sci* 1993, **52**:785–792.

16. Saperas E, Yang H, Taché Y: **Interleukin-1 Acts at Hypothalamic Sites to Inhibit Gastric Acid Secretion in Rats.** *Am J Physiol* 1992, **263**:G414–G418.

17. Tsalis KG, Yovos JG, Botsios DS, Dadoukis D: **Intracerebroventricular Infusion of Neurotensin Suppresses Gastric Acid Secretion in Dogs.** *Eur J Surg Res* 1993, **25**:52–59.

18. Widerlov E, Breese GR: **Actions of Neurotensin on Dopaminergic and Serotonergic Pathways in Rat Brain.** *Ann N Y Acad Sci* 1982, **400**:428–430.

19. Glavin GB, Hall AM: **Clozapine, a Dopamine DA_4 Receptor Antagonist, Reduces Gastric Acid Secretion and Stress-Induced Gastric Mucosal Injury.** *Life Sci* 1994, **54**:PL261–PL264.

20. Pollard H, Bouthenet ML, Moreau J, Souil E, Verroust P, Ronco P, Schwartz JC: **Detailed Immunoautoradiographic Mapping of Enkephalinase (EC 3.4.24.11) in Rat Central Nervous System: Comparison With Enkephalins and Substance P.** *Neuroscience* 1989, **30**:339–376.

21. Stephens RL Jr, Lepard KJ, Mohammed JR, Ward PE: **Intracisternal Neutral Endopeptidase-24.11 Inhibitors Produce Inhibition in Gastric Acid Output: Independence From Opiate, Bombesin, or Neurotensin-Mediated Mechanisms.** *Regul Pept* 1993, **46**:549–555.

22. Improta G, Broccardo M: **Inhibitory Role on Gastric Secretion of a Central NK-3 Tachykinin Receptor Agonist, Senktide.** *Peptides* 1991, **12**:1433–1434.

23. Martínez A, Burrell MA, Kuijk M, Montuenga LM, Treston A, Cuttitta F, Polak JM: **Localization of Amidating Enzymes (PAM) in Rat Gastrointestinal Tract.** *J Histochem Cytochem* 1993, **41**:1617–1622.

24. Dickinson CJ, Daugherty D, Guo Y-J, Stadler B, Finniss S, Yamada T: **Substrate Specificity of the Gastrin-Amidating Enzyme.** *J Biol Chem* 1993, **268**:15929–15934.
•

As with many other peptide hormones, gastrin requires a carboxyl-terminal amide moiety for full biological activity. The posttranslational processing of the carboxyl terminus of gastrin begins with endoproteolytic cleavage of ^{94}Arg-^{95}Arg by a prohormone convertase. The carboxyl-terminal arginine residues are subsequently removed via the action of carboxypeptidase H, forming a glycine-extended intermediate that serves as the specific substrate for PAM to form the peptide amide.

25. Kapuscinski M, Green M, Sinha SN, Shepherd JJ, Shulkes A: **Peptide α-Amidation Activity in Human Plasma: Relationship to Gastrin Processing.** *Clin Endocrinol (Oxf)* 1993, **39**:51–58.

26. Kopin AS, Beinborn M, Lee Y-M, McBride EW, Quinn SM: **The CCK-B/Gastrin Receptor: Identification of Amino Acids That Determine Nonpeptide Antagonist Affinity.** *Ann N Y Acad Sci* 1994, **713**:67–78.

27. Lee YM, Beinborn M, McBride EW, Lu M, Kolakowski LF Jr, Kopin AS: **The Human Brain Cholecystokinin-B/Gastrin Receptor: Cloning and Characterization.** *J Biol Chem* 1993, **268**:8164–8169.
••

The parietal cell gastrin receptor and brain cholecystokinin-B receptor have been cloned and appear to be the same gene product.

28. Pisegna JR, De Weerth A, Huppi K, Wank SA: **Molecular Cloning of the Human Brain and Gastric Cholecystokinin Receptor: Structure, Functional Expression and Chromosomal Localization.** *Biochem Biophys Res Commun* 1992, **189**:296–303.

29. Miyake A, Mochizuki S, Kawashima H: **Characterization of Cloned Human Cholecystokinin-B Receptor as a Gastrin Receptor.** *Biochem Pharmacol* 1994, **47**:1339–1343.
••

Describes cloning of the human brain cholecystokinin-B receptor.

30. Ito M, Matsui T, Taniguchi T, Tsukamoto T, Murayama T, Arima N, Nakata H, Chiba T, Chihara K: **Functional Characterization of a Human Brain Cholecystokinin-B Receptor: A Trophic Effect of Cholecystokinin and Gastrin.** *J Biol Chem* 1993, **268**:18300–18305.

31. Zimonjic DB, Popescu NC, Matsui T, Ito M, Chihara K: **Localization of the Human Cholecystokinin-B/Gastrin Receptor Gene (CCKBR) to Chromosome 11p15.5-<p15.4 by Fluorescence In Situ Hybridization.** *Cytogenet Cell Genet* 1994, **65**:184–185.

32. •• Song I, Brown DR, Wiltshire RN, Gantz I, Trent JM, Yamada T: **The Human Gastrin/Cholecystokinin Type B Receptor Gene: Alternative Splice Donor Site in Exon 4 Generates Two Variant mRNAs.** *Proc Natl Acad Sci U S A* 1993, **90**:9085–9089.

The human cholecystokinin-B/gastrin receptor gene may be alternatively spliced to yield two different isoforms that differ by five amino acids in the third intracellular loop. The isoforms may contribute to functional differences in gastrin- and cholecystokinin-mediated signal transduction or disease states.

33. Baldwin GS, Chandler R, Grego B, Rubira MR, Seet KL, Weinstock J: **Isolation and Partial Amino Acid Sequence of a 78 kDa Porcine Gastrin-Binding Protein.** *Int J Biochem* 1994, **26**:529–538.

34. Cabero JL, Li Z-Q, Mårdh S: **Gastrin Action on Aminopyrine Accumulation in Isolated Pig Parietal Cells Requires cAMP.** *Biochim Biophys Acta Mol Cell Res* 1993, **1177**:245–252.

35. Zimmerhackl B, Wünsch E, Classen M, Schusdziarra V, Schepp W: **In Man Histamine and Muscarinergic Mechanisms Are Essential Mediators of Acid Secretion in Response to Synthetic Human Gastrin (1-17).** *Regul Pept* 1993, **46**:583–592.

36. Campbell BJ, Garner A, Dockray GJ, Hughes J, Dimaline R: **The Mechanism of Action of Gastrin Releasing Peptide (GRP) in Stimulating Avian Gastric Acid Secretion.** *Regul Pept* 1994, **49**:249–255.

37. • Schepp W, Chan CB, Giraud AS, Avedian D, Chen MCY, Chew P, Walsh JH, Soll AH: **Effects of Prostaglandins on Gastrin Release From Canine Antral Mucosal Cells in Primary Culture.** *Am J Physiol* 1994, **266**:G194–G200.

Enprostil inhibits gastrin release, whereas a stimulatory effect of prostaglandin E_2 can be unmasked in the presence of pertussis toxin. It is likely that these agents are acting on one or more different subtypes of prostaglandin receptors.

38. Bastien L, Sawyer N, Grygorczyk R, Metters KM, Adam M: **Cloning, Functional Expression, and Characterization of the Human Prostaglandin E_2 Receptor EP_2 Subtype.** *J Biol Chem* 1994, **269**:11873–11877.

39. Sando T, Usui T, Tanaka I, Mori K, Sasaki Y, Fukuda Y, Namba T, Sugimoto Y, Ichikawa A, Narumiya S, Nakao K: **Molecular Cloning and Expression of Rat Prostaglandin E Receptor EP_2 Subtype.** *Biochem Biophys Res Commun* 1994, **200**:1329–1333.

40. Sugimoto Y, Namba T, Honda A, Hayashi Y, Negishi M, Ichikawa A, Narumiya S: **Cloning and Expression of cDNA for Mouse Prostaglandin E Receptor EP3 Subtype.** *J Biol Chem* 1992, **267**:6463–6466.

41. Dockray GJ, Dimaline R, Forster ER, Evans D, Sandvik A, Varro A: **Gastrin Cell Responses to Acidification of the Achlorhydric Rat Stomach.** *Am J Physiol* 1993, **265**:G440–G444.

42. Schubert M: **Gastric Somatostatin: A Paracrine Regulator of Gastrin and Acid Secretion.** *Regul Pept Letter* 1991, 3:7–11.

43. • Lichtenberger LM, Gardner JW, Barreto JC, Dial EJ, Weinman EJ: **Accumulation of Aliphatic Amines in Gastric Juice of Acute Renal Failure Patients.** *Dig Dis Sci* 1993, **38**:1885–1888.

Aliphatic amines accumulate in the gastric juice of patients with acute renal failure and may contribute to the hypergastrinemia.

44. Schmassmann A, Garner A, Flogerzi B, Hasan MY, Sanner M, Varga L, Halter F: **Cholecystokinin Type B Receptor Antagonist PD-136,450 Is a Partial Secretory Agonist in the Stomach and a Full Agonist in the Pancreas of the Rat.** *Gut* 1994, **35**:270–274.

45. Varga G, Campbell DR, Bussjaeger LJ, Solomon TE: **Role of Gastrin and Cholecystokinin Receptors in Regulation of Peptone-Stimulated Gastric Acid Secretion in Conscious Rats.** *Eur J Pharmacol* 1993, **250**:37–42.

46. Lloyd KCK, Raybould HE, Taché Y, Walsh JH: **Role of Gastrin, Histamine, and Acetylcholine in the Gastric Phase of Acid Secretion in Anesthetized Rats.** *Am J Physiol* 1992, 262:G747–G755.

47. Murphy MG, Sytnik B, Kovacs TOG, Mertz H, Ewanik D, Shingo S, Lin JH, Gertz BJ, Walsh JH: **The Gastrin-Receptor Antagonist L-365,260 Inhibits Stimulated Acid Secretion in Humans.** *Clin Pharmacol Ther* 1993, **54**:533–539.

48. •• Diaz J, Vizuete M, Traiffort E, Arrang J, Ruat M, Schwartz J: **Localization of the Histamine H_2 Receptor and Gene Transcripts in Rat Stomach: Back to Parietal Cells.** *Biochem Biophys Res Commun* 1994, **198**:1195–1202.

In situ hybridization histochemistry and autoradiography were used to localize the H_2 receptor in rat stomach to the neck of the oxyntic glands, in parietal cells.

49. Mezey E, Palkovits M: **Localization of Targets for Anti-Ulcer Drugs in Cells of the Immune System.** *Science* 1992, **258**:1662–1665.

50. Hollande F, Gusdinar T, Bali J-P, Magous R: **Neurohormonal Regulation of Histamine Release From Isolated Rabbit Fundic Mucosal Cells.** *Agents Actions* 1993, **38**:149–157.

51. • Hollande F, Bali J-P, Magous R: **Neurohormonal Regulation of Histamine Synthesis in Isolated Rabbit Fundic Mucosal Cells.** *Am J Physiol* 1994, **266**:G395–G402.

A preparation of isolated rabbit fundic mucosal cells was used to show that gastrin (acting via gastrin/cholecystokinin-B receptor) and carbachol stimulate histidine decarboxylase activity and histamine release.

52. •• Chuang C-N, Tanner M, Lloyd KCK, Wong H, Soll AH: **Endogenous Somatostatin Inhibits Histamine Release From Canine Gastric Mucosal Cells in Primary Culture.** *Am J Physiol* 1993, **265**:G521–G525.

A well characterized cell culture of canine fundic mucosal cells enriched in enterochromaffin-like cells is described. Addition of somatostatin antibody increased basal histamine release, suggesting that endogenous somatostatin exerts a tonic inhibitory influence on histamine secretion.

53. •• Prinz C, Kajimura M, Scott DR, Mercier F, Helander HF, Sachs G: **Histamine Secretion From Rat Enterochromaffinlike Cells.** *Gastroenterology* 1993, **105**:449–461.

Gastrin, carbachol, and phorbol esters stimulated histamine release, whereas somatostatin inhibited histamine release, from a highly enriched (65-fold) suspension of enterochromaffin-like cells from rat fundic mucosa. H_3 autoreceptors that inhibit histamine release were identified.

54. Tabuchi Y, Furuhama K: **Inhibitory Effect of DS-4574, a Mast Cell Stabilizer With Peptidoleukotriene Receptor Antagonism, on Gastric Acid Secretion in Rats.** *Eur J Pharmacol* 1994, **255**:229–234.

55. Yamashika Y, Tabuchi Y, Kokue E: **Antisecretory Effect of DS-4574, a Mast Cell Stabilizer With Peptidoleukotriene Antagonism, on Gastric Acid Secretion in the Pig.** *Agents Actions* 1994, **41**:17–20.

56. • Hollande F, Bali J-P, Magous R: **Autoregulation of Histamine Synthesis Through H_3 Receptors in Isolated Fundic Mucosal Cells.** *Am J Physiol* 1993, **265**:G1039–G1044.

Identified H_3 autoreceptors that inhibit histamine release.

57. Kunkel MT, Peralta EG: **Charged Amino Acids Required for Signal Transduction by the m3 Muscarinic Acetylcholine Receptor.** *EMBO J* 1993, 12:3809-3815.

58. McKenna JP, Hanson PJ: **Inhibition by Ro 31-8220 of Acid Secretory Activity Induced by Carbachol Indicates a Stimulatory Role for Protein Kinase C in the Action of Muscarinic Agonists on Isolated Rat Parietal Cells.** *Biochem Pharmacol* 1993, **46**:583–588.

59. Stanton T, Bolden-Watson C, Cusack B, Richelson E: **Antagonism of the Five Cloned Human Muscarinic Cholinergic Receptors Expressed in CHO-K1 Cells by Antidepressants and Antihistaminics.** *Biochem Pharmacol* 1993, **45**:2352–2354.

60. • Ren J, Harty RF: **Presynaptic Muscarinic Receptors Modulate Acetylcholine Release From Rat Antral Mucosal/Submucosal Nerves.** *Dig Dis Sci* 1994, **39**:1099–1106.

Acetylcholine release from antral mucosa is regulated by a negative autofeedback mechanism, probably involving M2 or M3 receptors, whereas M1 receptors facilitate acetylcholine release.

61. Yokotani K, Okuma Y, Nakamura K, Osumi Y: **Release of Endogenous Acetylcholine From a Vascularly Perfused Rat Stomach In Vitro; Inhibition by M^3 Muscarinic Autoreceptors and *Alpha-2* Adrenoceptors.** *J Pharmacol Exp Ther* 1993, **266**:1190–1195.

62. Schubert ML, Makhlouf GM: **Gastrin Secretion Induced by Distention Is Regulated by Cholinergic and Vasoactive Intestinal Peptide Neurons in Rats.** *Gastroenterology* 1993, **104**:834–839.

63. Hamlet A, DalenbäckK J, Olbe L, Fändriks L: **Does Antral Distension Inhibit Gastric Acid Secretion or Stimulate Bicarbonate Secretion in 'Healthy' Subjects.** *Scand J Gastroenterol* 1993, **28**:999–1004.

64. Dimaline R, Sandvik AK, Evans D, Forster ER, Dockray GJ: **Food Stimulation of Histidine Decarboxylase Messenger RNA Abundance in Rat Gastric Fundus.** *J Physiol (Lond)* 1993, **465**:449–458.

65. • Chari S, Teyssen S, Singer MV: **Alcohol and Gastric Acid Secretion in Humans.** *Gut* 1993, 34:843–847.

Review of the effect of ethanol-containing beverages on gastrin and acid secretion.

66. Peterson WL, Barnett CC, Evans DJ, JR., Feldman M, Carmody T, Richardson C, Walsh J, Graham DY: **Acid Secretion and Serum Gastrin in Normal Subjects and Patients With Duodenal Ulcer: The Role of *Helicobacter pylori*.** *Am J Gastroenterol* 1993, **88**:2038–2043.

67. Mulholland G, Ardill JES, Fillmore D, Chittajallu RS, Fullarton GM, McColl KEL: ***Helicobacter pylori* Related Hypergastrinaemia Is the Result of a Selective Increase in Gastrin 17.** *Gut* 1993, 34:757–761.

68. Moss SF, Legon S, Bishop AE, Polak JM, Calam J: **Effect of *Helicobacter pylori* on Gastric Somatostatin in Duodenal Ulcer Disease.** *Lancet* 1992, 340:930–932.

69. Queiroz DMM, Moura SB, Mendes EN, Rocha GA, Barbosa AJA, De Carvalho AST: **Effect of *Helicobacter pylori* Eradication on G-cell and D-cell Density in Children.** *Lancet* 1994, 343:1191–1193.

70. Queiroz DMM, Mendes EN, Rocha GA, Moura SB, Resende LMH, Barbosa AJA, Coelho LGV, Passos MCE, Castro LP, Oliveira CA, Lima GF Jr: **Effect of *Helicobacter pylori* Eradication on Antral Gastrin- and Somatostatin-Immunoreactive Cell Density and Gastrin and Somatostatin Concentrations.** *Scand J Gastroenterol* 1993, 28:858–864.

71. Queiroz DMM, Mendes EN, Rocha GA, Moura SB, Resende LMH, Cunha-Melo JR, Coelho LGV, Passos MF, Oliveira CA, Lima GF, Castro LP: **Histamine Content of the Oxyntic Mucosa From Duodenal Ulcer Patients: Effect of *Helicobacter pylori* Eradication.** *Am J Gastroenterol* 1993, **88**:1228–1232.

72. Demchyshyn LL, Srikant CB, Sunahara RK, Kent G, Seeman P, Van Tol HHM, Panetta R, Patel YC, Niznik HB: **Cloning and Expression of a Human Somatostatin-14-Selective Receptor Variant (Somatostatin Receptor 4) Located on Chromosome 20.** *Mol Pharmacol* 1993, 43:894–901.

73. Corness JD, Demchyshyn LL, Seeman P, Van Tol HHM, Srikant CB, Kent G, Patel YC, Niznik HB: **A Human Somatostatin Receptor (SSTR3), Located on Chromosome 22, Displays Preferential Affinity for Somatostatin-14 Like Peptides.** *FEBS Lett* 1993, 321:279–284.

74. Yamada Y, Kagimoto S, Kubota A, Yasuda K, Masuda K, Someya Y, Ihara Y, Li Q, Imura H, Seino S, Seino Y: **Cloning, Functional Expression and Pharmacological Characterization of a Fourth (hSSTR4) and a Fifth (hSSTR5) Human Somatostatin Receptor Subtype.** *Biochem Biophys Res Commun* 1993, 195:844–852.

75. Yasuda K, Espinosa R, Davis E, Lebeau M, Bell G: **Human Somatostatin Receptor Genes: Localization of SSTR5 to Human Chromosome 20p11.2.** *Genomics* 1993, 17:785-786.

76. Raynor K, O'Carroll A-M, Kong H, Yasuda K, Mahan LC, Bell GI, Reisine T: **Characterization of Cloned Somatostatin Receptors SSTR4 and SSTR5.** *Mol Pharmacol* 1993, 44:385–392.

77. Rohrer L, Raulf F, Bruns C, Buettner R, Hofstaedter F, Schüle R: **Cloning and Characterization of a Fourth Human Somatostatin Receptor.** *Proc Natl Acad Sci U S A* 1993, 90:4196–4200.

78. Bruno JF, Xu Y, Song J, Berelowitz M: **Tissue Distribution of Somatostatin Receptor Subtype Messenger Ribonucleic Acid in the Rat.** *Endocrinology* 1993, 133:2561–2567.

79. Yamada Y, Reisine T, Law SF, Ihara Y, Kubota A, Kagimoto S, Seino M, Seino Y, Bell GI, Seino S: **Somatostatin Receptors, an Expanding Gene Family: Cloning and Functional Characterization of Human SSTR3, a Protein Coupled to Adenylyl Cyclase.** *Mol Endocrinol* 1992, 6:2136–2142.

80. Patel YC, Greenwood MT, Warszynska A, Panetta R, Srikant CB: **All •• Five Cloned Human Somatostatin Receptors (hSSTR1-5) Are Functionally Coupled to Adenylyl Cyclase.** *Biochem Biophys Res Commun* 1994, 198:605–612.

The human genes encoding SSTR1-5 were transfected into CHO-K1 cells and all five subtypes were shown to be coupled to inhibition of adenylate cyclase via a pertussis toxin–sensitive mechanism.

81. Hou C, Gilbert RL, Barber DL: **Subtype-Specific Signaling Mechanisms of Somatostatin Receptors SSTR1 and SSTR2.** *J Biol Chem* 1994, 269:10357–10362.

82. Tomura H, Okajima F, Akbar M, Majid M, Sho K, Kondo Y: **Transfected Human Somatostatin Receptor Type 2, SSTR2, Not Only Inhibits Adenylate Cyclase but Also Stimulates Phospholipase C and Ca^{2+} Mobilization.** *Biochem Biophys Res Commun* 1994, 200:986–992.

83. Xu Y, Song J, Bruno JF, Berelowitz M: **Molecular Cloning and Sequencing of a Human Somatostatin Receptor, hSSTR4.** *Biochem Biophys Res Commun* 1993, 193:648–652.

84. Bito H, Mori M, Sakanaka C, Takano T, Honda Z, Gotoh Y, Nishida E, Shimizu T: **Functional Coupling of SSTR4, a Major Hippocampal Somatostatin Receptor, to Adenylate Cyclase Inhibition, Arachidonate Release, and Activation of the Mitogen-Activated Protein Kinase Cascade.** *J Biol Chem* 1994, 269:12722–12730.

85. Kondo S, Shinomura Y, Kanayama S, Kawabata S, Miyazaki Y, Imamura I, Fukui H, Matsuzawa Y: **Somatostatin Inhibits Gastrin-Induced Histamine Secretion and Synthesis in the Rat.** *Regul Pept* 1993, 48:373–380.

86. Campbell-Thompson M, McGuigan JE: **Canine Parietal Cell Binding by Antibodies to the Complementary Peptide of Somatostatin.** *Am J Med Sci* 1993, 305:365–373.

87. Larsson L-I, Houggaard DM: **Evidence for Paracrine Somatostatinergic •• Regulation of Gastrin Gene Expression by Double-Staining Cytochemistry and Quantitation.** *J Histochem Cytochem* 1994, 42:37–40.

Quantitative *in situ* hybridization combined with immunocytochemistry was used to demonstrate that gastrin cells in close contact with somatostatin cells express significantly lower levels of gastrin messenger RNA than other gastrin cells, thus providing the first direct microscopic evidence for paracrine inhibition of gastrin by somatostatin.

88. Schubert ML, Edwards NF, Makhlouf GM: **Regulation of Gastric Somatostatin Secretion in the Mouse by Luminal Acid: A Local Feedback Mechanism.** *Gastroenterology* 1988, 94:317–322.

89. Greenberg GR, Fung L, Pokol-Daniel S: **Regulation of Somatostatin-14 • and -28 Secretion by Gastric Acid in Dogs: Differential Role of Cholecystokinin.** *Gastroenterology* 1993, 105:1387–1395.

Acid stimulates the secretion of somatostatin-14, whereas cholecystokinin stimulates the release of somatostatin-28.

90. Hildebrand P, Ensinck JW, Buettiker J, Drewe J, Burckhardt B, Gyr K, Beglinger C: **Circulating Somatostatin-28 Is Not a Physiologic Regulator of Gastric Acid Production in Man.** *Eur J Clin Invest* 1994, 24:50–56.

91. Van Oers CCM, Adema GJ, Zandberg H, Moen TC, Baas PD: **Two Different Sequence Elements Within Exon 4 Are Necessary for Calcitonin-Specific Splicing of the Human Calcitonin/Calcitonin Gene-Related Peptide I pre-mRNA.** *Mol Cell Biol* 1994, 14:951–960.

92. Ren J, Young RL, Lassiter DC, Harty RF: **Calcitonin Gene-Related Pep- •• tide Mediates Capsaicin-Induced Neuroendocrine Responses in Rat Antrum.** *Gastroenterology* 1993, 104:485–491.

The sensory toxin, capsaicin, releases CGRP from rat antral mucosal/submucosal fragments that in turn stimulates somatostatin and inhibits gastrin and acetylcholine release.

93. Gray JL, Bunnett NW, Orloff SL, Mulvihill SJ, Debas HT: **A Role for Calcitonin Gene-Related Peptide in Protection Against Gastric Ulceration.** *Ann Surg* 1994, 219:58–64.

94. Orsini B, Calabro A, Milani S, Grappone C, Herbst H, Surrenti C: **Localization of Epidermal Growth Factor/Transforming Growth Factor-α Receptor in the Human Gastric Mucosa: An Immunohistochemical and In Situ Hybridization Study.** *Virchows Arhc A Pathol Anat Histopathol* 1993, 423:57–63.

95. Ostrowski J, Wojciechowski K, Konturek SJ, Butruk E: **Inhibitory Effect of EGF on Secretory Response of Rat Parietal Cells Is Associated With an Induction of ODC.** *Am J Physiol* 1993, 264:C1428–C1433.

96. Rao RK, Chang H-H, Levenson S, Porreca F, Brannon PM, Davis TP, Koldovsky O: **Ontogenic Differences in the Inhibition of Gastric Acid Secretion by Epidermal Growth Factor.** *J Pharmacol Exp Ther* 1993, 266:647–654.

97. Guglietta A, Lesch CA, Romano M, McClure RW, Coffey RJ: **Effect of Transforming Growth Factor-α on Gastric Acid Secretion in Rats and Monkeys.** *Dig Dis Sci* 1994, 39:177–182.

98. Intorre L, Mengozzi G, Vanni E, Grassi F, Soldani G: **The Role of Peripheral Opioid Receptor Subtypes in the Modulation of Gastric Acid Secretion and Plasma Gastrin in Dogs.** *Eur J Pharmacol* 1993, 243:265–272.

99. Schepp W, Kath D, Tatge C, Zimmerhackl B, Schusdziarra V, Classen M: **Leukotrienes C^4 and D^4 Potentiate Acid Production by Isolated Rat Parietal Cells.** *Gastroenterology* 1989, 97:1420–1429.

100. Huber W, Trautmann M, Becker I, Schenck U, Peskar BM, Schepp W: **Leukotriene B^4 and C^4 Production in Isolated Rat Gastric Mucosal Cells.** *Am J Physiol* 1993, 265:G1021–G1028.

101. Poulsom R, Wright NA: **Trefoi—Peptides: A Newly Recognized Family of Epithelial Mucin-Associated Molecules.** *Am J Physiol* 1993, 265:G205–G213.

102. Jeffrey GP, Oates PS, Wang TC, Babyatsky MW, Brand SJ: **Spasmolytic Polypeptide: A Trefoil Peptide Secreted by Rat Gastric Mucous Cells.** *Gastroenterology* 1994, 106:336–345.

103. Hanby AM, Poulsom R, Singh S, Elia G, Jeffery RE, Wright NA: **Spasmolytic Polypeptide Is a Major Antral Peptide: Distribution of the Trefoil Peptides Human Spasmolytic Polypeptide and pS2 in the Stomach.** *Gastroenterology* 1993, 105:1110–1116.

104. Forster ER, Southam E: **The Intrinsic and Vagal Extrinsic Innervation • of the Rat Stomach Contains Nitric Oxide Synthase.** *Neuro report* 1993, 4:275–278.

The enzyme nitric oxide synthase, which catalyzes the formation of nitric oxide from L-arginine, is present in the myenteric and submucosal plexi of rat gastric corpus.

105. Brown JF, Hanson PJ, Whittle BJR: **The Nitric Oxide Donor, S- • Nitroso-N-Acetyl-Penicillamine, Inhibits Secretory Activity in Rat Isolated Parietal Cells.** *Biochem Biophys Res Commun* 1993, 195:1354–1359.

A nitric oxide donor inhibits acid production in isolated rat parietal cells.

106. Takeuchi K, Ohuchi T, Okabe S: **Endogenous Nitric Oxide in Gastric Alkaline Response in the Rat Stomach After Damage.** *Gastroenterology* 1994, **106**:367–374.

107. Lloyd KCK, Maxwell V, Kovacs TOG, Miller J, Walsh JH: **Cholecystokinin Receptor Antagonist MK-329 Blocks Intestinal Fat-Induced Inhibition of Meal-Stimulated Gastric Acid Secretion.** *Gastroenterology* 1992, **102**:131–138.

108. Rhee JC, Chang TM, Lee KY, Jo YH, Chey WY: **Mechanism of Oleic Acid-Induced Inhibition on Gastric Acid Secretion in Rats.** *Am J Physiol* 1991, **260**:G564–G570.

109. Shiratori K, Watanabe S-I, Takeuchi T: **Intestinal Fat Digestion Plays a Significant Role in Fat-Induced Suppression of Gastric Acid Secretion and Gastrin Release in the Rat.** *Dig Dis Sci* 1993, **38**:2267–2272.

110. Silvente-Poirot S, Dufresne M, Vaysse N, Fourmy D: **The Peripheral Cholecystokinin Receptors.** *Eur J Biochem* 1993, **215**:513–529.

111. Rehfeld JF: **The Molecular Nature of Cholecystokinin in Plasma.** *Scand J Gastroenterol* 1994, **29**:110–121.

112. Konturek JW, Gutwinska-Konturek M, Gabryelewicz A, Konturek SJ, Domschke W: **Cholecystokinin in the Control of Gastric Acid Secretion in Humans.** *J Clin Gastroenterol* 1993, **17(suppl 1)**:S40–S45.

113. Konturek SJ, Bilski J, Cieszkowski M: **Role of Cholecystokinin in the Intestinal Fat- and Acid-Induced Inhibition of Gastric Secretion.** *Regul Pept* 1992, **42**:97–109.

114. Campos RV, Lee YC, Drucker DJ: **Divergent Tissue-Specific and Developmental Expression of Receptors for Glucagon and Glucagon-Like Peptide-1 in the Mouse.** *Endocrinology* 1994, **134**:2156–2164.

115. Bado A, Cloarec D, Moizo L, Laigneau J-P, Bataille D, Lewin MJM: **Neurotensin and Oxyntomodulin-(30-37) Potentiate PYY Regulation of Gastric Acid and Somatostatin Secretions.** *Am J Physiol* 1993, **265**:G113–G117.

116. Wettergren A, Schjoldager B, Mortensen PE, Petersen H, Orskov C, Holst JJ: **Effect of GLP-1 on Gastric Motility and Gastric and Pancreatic Secretion in Man.** *Digestion* 1993, **54**:384–385.

117. • Wagner ACC, Williams JA: **Low Molecular Weight GTP-Binding Proteins: Molecular Switches Regulating Diverse Cellular Functions.** *Am J Physiol* 1994, **266**:G1–G14.

Excellent review of the role of low molecular weight GTP-binding proteins in gastroenterology.

118. Waldum HL, Brenna E, Kleveland PM, Sandvik AK, Syversen U: **Review Article: The Use of Gastric Acid-Inhibitory Drugs: Physiological and Pathophysiological Considerations.** *Aliment Pharmacol Ther* 1993, **7**:589–596.

119. Klaassen CHW, De Pont JJHHM: **Gastric H^+/K^+-ATPase.** *Cell Physiol Biochem* 1994, **4**:115–134.

120. Sachs G, Shin JM, Besancon M, Prinz C: **The Continuing Development of Gastric Acid Pump Inhibitors.** *Aliment Pharmacol Ther* 1993, **7(suppl 1)**:4–12.

121. Song I, Mortell MP, Gantz I, Brown DR, Yamada T: **Molecular Cloning and Structural Analysis of Canine Gastric H^+,K^+-ATPase.** *Biochem Biophys Res Commun* 1993, **196**:1240–1247.

122. Chow D-C, Forte JG: **Characterization of the β-Subunit of the H^+-K^+-ATPase Using an Inhibitory Monoclonal Antibody.** *Am J Physiol* 1993, **265**:C1562–C1570.

123. Song YH, Ma JY, Märdh S, Liu T, SjöstrandD SE, Rask L, Borch K, Huang GC, Barnett P, McGregor AM, Banga JP: **Localization of a Pernicous Anemia Autoantibody Epitope on the α-Subunit of Human H,K-Adenosine Triphosphatase.** *Scand J Gastroenterol* 1994, **29**:122–127.

124. Bamberg K, Nylander S, Helander KG, Lundberg LG, Sachs G, Helander HF: **In Situ Hybridization of mRNA for the Gastric H^+, K^+-ATPase in Rat Oxyntic Mucosa.** *Biochim Biophys Acta* 1994, **1190**:355–359.

125. Soroka CJ, Chew CS, Hanzel DK, Smolka A, Modlin IM, Goldenring JR: **Characterization of Membrane and Cytoskeletal Compartments in Cultured Parietal Cells: Immunofluorescence and Confocal Microscopic Examination.** *Eur J Cell Biol* 1993, **60**:76-87.

126. Scott DR, Helander HF, Hersey SJ, Sachs G: **The Site of Acid Secretion in the Mammalian Parietal Cell.** *Biochim Biophys Acta* 1993, **1146**:73–80.

127. Jaisser F, Coutry N, Farman N, Binder HJ, Rossier BC: **A Putative H^+-K^+-ATPase Is Selectively Expressed in Surface Epithelial Cells of Rat Distal Colon.** *Am J Physiol* 1993, **265**:C1080–C1089.

128. • Tari A, Yamamoto G, Sumii K, Sumii M, Takehara Y, Haruma K, Kajiyama G, Wu V, Sachs G, Walsh JH: **Role of Histamine[2] Receptor in Increased Expression of Rat Gastric H^+-K^+-ATPase α-Subunit Induced by Omeprazole.** *Am J Physiol* 1993, **265**:G752–G758.

Omeprazole inhibits acid secretion and thus stimulates gastrin secretion. Gastrin, in turn, stimulates histamine secretion which leads to an increase in expression of rat gastric H^+-K^+-ATPase α-subunit messenger RNA.

129. Tari A, Yamamoto G, Yonei Y, Sumii M, Sumii K, Haruma K, Kajiyama G, Wu V, Sachs G, Walsh JH: **Effect of Histamine on Rat Gastric H^+-K^+-ATPase α-Subunit Expression.** *Am J Physiol* 1994, **266**:G444–G450.

130. Crothers JM, Jr., Chow DC, Forte JG: **Omeprazole Decreases H^+-K^+-ATPase Protein and Increases Permeability of Oxyntic Secretory Membranes in Rabbits.** *Am J Physiol* 1993, **265**:G231–G241.

131. Karam SM, Forte JG: **Inhibiting Gastric H^+-K^+-ATPase Activity by Omeprazole Promotes Degeneration and Production of Parietal Cells.** *Am J Physiol* 1994, **266**:G745–G758.

132. Sack J: **Regulation of Gastric H^+-K^+-ATPase by cAMP-Dependent Protein Kinase.** *J Surg Res* 1993, **55**:223–227.

133. • Cuppoletti J, Baker AM, Malinowska DH: **Cl^- Channels of the Gastric Parietal Cell That Are Active at Low pH.** *Am J Physiol* 1993, **264**:C1609–C1618.

Direct evidence for the existence of apical Cl^- channels in rabbit parietal cells.

134. Horie S, Yano S, Watanabe K: **Inhibition of Gastric Acid Secretion *In Vivo* and *In Vitro* by an Inhibitor of Cl^--HCO_3^- Exchanger, 4,4′-Diisothiocyanostilbene-2,2′-Disulfonic Acid.** *J Pharmacol Exp Ther* 1993, **265**:1313–1318.

135. Yanaka A, Muto H, Ito S, Silen W: **Effects of Ammonium Ion and Ammonia on Function and Morphology of In Vitro Frog Gastric Mucosa.** *Am J Physiol* 1993, **265**:G277–G288.

136. Rai A, Singh G, Raffaniello R, Eng J, Raufman J-P: **Actions of *Helodermatidae* Venom Peptides and Mammalian Glucagon-Like Peptides on Gastric Chief Cells.** *Am J Physiol* 1993, **265**:G118–G125.

137. Tang LH, Miller MD, Goldenring JR, Modlin IM, Hersey SJ: **Partial Agonism by Gastrin for a Cholecystokinin Receptor Mediating Pepsinogen Secretion.** *Am J Physiol* 1993, **265**:G865–G872.

138. Kitsukawa Y, Felley C, Metz DC, Jensen RT: **Thapsigargin Defines Roles of Ca^{2+} in Initial, Sustained, and Potentiated Stimulation of Pepsinogen Secretion.** *Am J Physiol* 1994, **266**:G613–G623.

139. Ruiz MC, Acosta A, Abad MJ, Michelangeli F: **Nonparallel Secretion of Pepsinogen and Acid by Gastric Oxyntopeptic Cells of the Toad (Bufo marinus).** *Am J Physiol* 1993, **265**:G934–G941.

140. Kakei N, Ichinose M, Tsukada S, Tatematsu M, Tezuka N, Yahagi N, Matsushima M, Miki K, Kurokawa K, Takahashi K, Fukamachi H: **Omeprazole, a Proton Pump Inhibitor, Reduces the Secretion, Synthesis and Gene Expression of Pepsinogen in the Rat Stomach.** *Biochem Biophys Res Commun* 1993, **195**:997–1004.

Mitchell L. Schubert, MD, McGuire VAMC, Code 111N, Gastroenterology Division, 1201 Broad Rock Boulevard, Richmond, VA 23249, USA.

Gastroduodenal mucosal defense

John L. Wallace, PhD, and Cameron J. Bell, MB, BS, FRACP

University of Calgary, Alberta, Canada, and
Royal North Shore Hospital, St. Leonard's, New South Wales, Australia

The recognition that most peptic ulcer disease occurs as a consequence of either *Helicobacter pylori* infection or ingestion of nonsteroidal anti-inflammatory drugs has renewed interest in the hypothesis that ulcer disease occurs principally as a consequence of impaired mucosal defense. Studies published over the past year have advanced our understanding of the many complex interactions among the various components of mucosal defense, such as the microcirculatory response, mucus and bicarbonate secretion, and restitution. It is becoming increasingly clear that mediators such as nitric oxide, previously regarded solely as vasoactive substances, also affect the epithelium, parietal cells, and mast cells to produce effects that alter mucosal resistance to injury. Progress has also been made in understanding the influence of many mediators and growth factors on the ability of the mucosa to repair damage.

Current Opinion in Gastroenterology 1994, **10**:589–594

For much of this century, research on peptic ulcer disease has focused primarily on the concept that acid is responsible for initiating the tissue injury. However, in the past decade, it has become increasingly clear that acid hypersecretion alone seldom produces significant mucosal injury. There is now overwhelming evidence that infection with *Helicobacter pylori* and ingestion of nonsteroidal anti-inflammatory drugs (NSAIDs) are the most important causative factors in ulcer disease. Whereas these agents can affect gastric acid secretion and its delivery into the duodenum, it is likely that their effects on gastroduodenal mucosal defense are the most important in terms of producing mucosal injury. Thus, understanding the underlying mechanisms through which the mucosa resists and responds to injury has significant implications for the prevention and treatment of peptic ulcer disease. We have attempted to review some of the most important advances over the past year in our understanding of gastroduodenal mucosal defense.

Bicarbonate and mucus

The proposition that the mucus-bicarbonate layer is important in mucosal defense has received further support. In technically elegant studies wherein several parameters were simultaneously measured *in vivo*, Kaunitz *et al.* [1••] examined the resistance of rat gastric mucosa to physiologic concentrations of luminal acid. Consistent with previous studies of the effects of nicotine exposure on gastric mucus and susceptibility to injury, after acute nicotine infusion, the fall in intracellular pH following acid superfusion was blunted, mucus gel thickness was increased, and cell viability enhanced. Chronic nicotine exposure had opposite effects. Perhaps more importantly, the changes in concurrently measured parameters suggested that the mucus layer protected the gastric epithelium by impeding acid back-diffusion.

In addition to trapping protons, gastric mucus has previously been found to effectively scavenge toxic oxygen metabolites [2]. Hiraishi *et al.* [3•] expanded on this finding by demonstrating that mucus glycoprotein partially protected cultured rat gastric epithelial cells from oxygen radical–induced injury. A stimulant of mucus synthesis reduced xanthine oxidase–induced damage, whereas a mucolytic agent potentiated it, although the authors allow that properties of the two agents other than their effects on gastric mucus may have been operative. Their results suggest that gastric mucus plays a role in maintaining the integrity of the gastric mucosa against luminal oxidants.

The phenomenon whereby mild gastric injury causes an increased flux of bicarbonate into the gastric lumen has received further attention. Guttu *et al.* [4•] found that bicarbonate influx into the cat stomach increased immediately after injury with hyperosmolar saline, then returned to basal levels during epithelial restitution. With damage to the surface epithelium, bicarbonate probably entered passively from the mucosa. This study also suggested that bicarbonate leakage shortly after damage was dependent on gastric mucosal blood flow and availability of blood bicarbonate; omeprazole did not affect initial leakage but did impair recovery of luminal bicarbonate influx to predam-

Abbreviations

bFGF—basic fibroblast growth factor; **CGRP**—calcitonin gene-related peptide; **EGF**—epidermal growth factor; **ICAM-1**—intercellular adhesion molecule-1; **NSAID**—nonsteroidal anti-inflammatory drug.

 ISBN 1-85922-611-6 ISSN 0267–1379

age levels. The authors speculated that with less acid to neutralize after omeprazole, bicarbonate supplied by mucosal blood flow may have been free to contribute to luminal alkalinization. Thus, the mucosal hyperemia seen after gastric mucosal damage might be important in supplying bicarbonate to neutralize acid in the superficial mucosa as well as physically removing back-diffused protons. The role of this bicarbonate in tissue restitution is not clear, however, as restitution seemed to be more rapid in pentagastrin-stimulated animals.

In a related study, Takeuchi *et al.* [5•] provided evidence that endogenous NO (nitric oxide) was involved in regulating the alkaline response of the stomach to mild irritants. Mild injury of rat stomach increased luminal pH and decreased acid secretion. An inhibitor of NO biosynthesis attenuated the increase in luminal pH by diminishing the inhibitory effect of gastric irritation on acid secretion. The NO inhibitor did not affect the increased influx of bicarbonate into the gastric lumen. The authors speculated that irritation of the gastric mucosa might release NO, which in turn inhibits acid secretion, thus "enhancing" the gastric alkaline response, promoting an alkaline microenvironment, and favoring epithelial restitution. However, the contribution of NO to the mucus-bicarbonate barrier does not appear to be straightforward.

In uninjured rat gastroduodenal preparations, Takeuchi *et al.* [6••] reported that inhibition of NO biosynthesis increased bicarbonate secretion, suggesting that endogenous NO acts to suppress bicarbonate secretion. The effect of the NO inhibitor was dependent on vagal-cholinergic innervation and endogenous prostaglandins (but not on sensory afferent nerves). It was unclear, however, whether the effects on bicarbonate secretion were related to systemic effects of the NO synthesis inhibitor on blood pressure because another vasopressor, endothelin-1, also increased gastric bicarbonate secretion. Because NO has previously been shown to have a protective effect on the gastric mucosa and NO synthase inhibition has been shown to exacerbate injury due to other agents, Takeuchi *et al.* [6••] speculated that the role of endogenous NO in the gastroduodenal mucosa may be complex, with both protective [7] and deleterious effects. Finally, with regard to NO, Brown *et al.* [8] have expanded their previous demonstration that NO-releasing compounds increased mucus gel thickness in rat stomach. They have now shown that NO-releasing agents induce mucus secretion from isolated gastric mucosal cells, possibly via a direct effect of NO on the epithelial cells [9•].

Duodenal distension is recognized as influencing other aspects of gastroduodenal function but its effect on duodenal bicarbonate secretion has not been studied previously. Sababi and Nylander [10•] found that a small rise in intraluminal pressure (6 mm Hg) increased duodenal bicarbonate secretion by approximately 75% in perfused duodenal segments of anesthetized rats. The effect was dependent on nicotinic receptors and extrinsic nerves. Inhibitors of cyclooxygenase induced intermittent elevations of intraluminal pressure and similarly stimulated bicarbonate secretion (a finding at odds with studies in other species); their effect appeared to involve a similar though not identical, neural mechanism to that of distension. The authors hypothesized that luminal distension or duodenal contraction stimulates mechanoreceptors that enhance duodenal bicarbonate secretion via a neural mechanism.

Microcirculation

For many years, the importance of uninterrupted perfusion of the gastroduodenal mucosa has been recognized as a critical component of mucosal defense. In recent years, a great deal has been learned about the mediators and cells that regulate mucosal blood flow, particularly during periods of exposure of the mucosa to irritants or high concentrations of acid. In the past year, several studies have extended these findings. These studies can be subdivided into a number of categories: 1) studies demonstrating that cytoprotective agents mediate their effects at least in part through modulation of mucosal blood flow, 2) studies outlining the mechanisms regulating the hyperemic response to mucosal irritation or injury, and 3) studies focusing on the role of leukocytes and leukocyte-derived products in the production of mucosal injury. Each of these categories are reviewed below.

Mucosal protection and repair

The ability of epidermal growth factor (EGF) to reduce the severity of experimental ulcers in several models is well characterized, but the mechanism underlying this effect is not fully understood. Hui *et al.* [11•] provided evidence in support of a role for EGF in modulating gastric blood flow. They performed studies in both normal and sialoadenectomized rats under basal conditions and following topical absolute ethanol. Sialoadenectomy, which markedly reduces the delivery of endogenous EGF to the stomach, increased the severity of ethanol-induced damage but did not affect gastric blood flow. Exogenous EGF dose-dependently increased gastric blood flow and reduced the severity of ethanol-induced damage. As there was a good inverse relationship between these two effects, the authors suggested that the effects of EGF on gastric blood flow may contribute to its ability to reduce gastric damage. Although this point was not proven, the study of Howard *et al.* [12•] provides further evidence that elevation of gastric blood flow increases the resistance of the gastric mucosa to damage induced by ethanol. They demonstrated that administration of isoproterenol, at doses without systemic effects, could markedly reduce the severity of ethanol-induced gastric damage and could maintain gastric blood flow during the period of exposure to ethanol; prior treatment with propranolol prevented these effects.

NO is another vasodilator that has been implicated as an important mediator of gastric blood flow, but studies to date have focused entirely on the ability of this mediator to affect the susceptibility of the gastroduodenal mucosa to injury. Konturek *et al.* [13•] extended previous studies by assessing the role of NO in the healing of preexisting ulcers. They reported that in a gastric ulcer induced by acetic acid in the rat, healing was significantly delayed by inhibition of NO synthesis. Moreover, they showed that the NO synthase inhibitors reduced blood flow at the ulcer margin and the number of capillaries in the granulation tissue of the ulcer bed (indicative of angiogenesis). The effects of the NO synthase inhibitors could be partially reversed by administering L-arginine or a NO donor (*eg*, glyceryl trinitrate).

Hyperemic response to irritants

When an irritant is placed on the surface of the gastroduodenal mucosa, blood flow increases, presumably in an attempt to help dilute, buffer, or remove the irritant from the mucosal tissue. This response has been shown to be mediated largely by sensory afferent neurons within the mucosa, which release calcitonin gene-related peptide (CGRP) in the vicinity of submucosal arterioles, thereby causing vasodilation. This hypothesis is supported by the recent report from Peskar *et al.* [14•]

In addition to being a modulator of basal gastroduodenal blood flow, NO has been suggested to mediate the hyperemic response to irritants. This hypothesis was tested by Lugea *et al.* [15•] using a model of acid-induced adaptive cytoprotection in the rat duodenum. Exposure of the duodenum to a "mild" concentration of acid resulted in increased resistance to injury induced by subsequent exposure to a much higher concentration of acid. This was accompanied by increased duodenal mucosal blood flow. However, this increase in blood flow could be mimicked by a NO-releasing drug without reducing injury and acid-induced hyperemia could be attenuated by an inhibitor of NO synthesis without affecting the adaptive cytoprotection. Thus, Lugea *et al.* [15•] concluded that adaptive cytoprotection in this model was not due to increased blood flow and not mediated by NO.

Holzer *et al.* [16•] examined the role of NO in the hyperemia induced by exogenous CGRP. They reported that CGRP dose-dependently increased flow through the gastric artery. A NO synthase inhibitor significantly reduced both basal flow and CGRP-induced hyperemia. Some residual effect of CGRP was still observed following blockade of NO synthesis, suggesting both NO-dependent and -independent mechanisms for CGRP-induced dilation of extramucosal vessels.

Leukocytes and free radicals

Leukocytes, particularly neutrophils, have been implicated as playing an important role in both experimental ulcer and the ulcers associated with *H. pylori* infection. The role of neutrophils in the pathogenesis of gastric injury induced by nonsteroidal anti-inflammatory drugs was examined in the rat by Wallace *et al.* [17•] and Andrews *et al.* [18••], and in humans by Konturek *et al.* [19•]. By administering monoclonal antibodies directed against various adhesion molecules on the vascular endothelium and on leukocytes, Wallace *et al.* [17•] demonstrated that blockade of leukocyte adherence after indomethacin administration was accompanied by significant reductions in the severity of mucosal injury. These studies suggested that indomethacin-induced leukocyte adherence was mediated via CD11/CD18 and intercellular adhesion molecule-1 (ICAM-1). This conclusion was supported by the demonstration by Andrews *et al.* [18••] that following aspirin or indomethacin administration in the rat, there is a significant increase in the expression of ICAM-1 and CD11/CD18 within the gastric microcirculation. Studies similar to those of Wallace *et al.* [17•] were performed by Yoshida *et al.* [20•] using an *in vitro* system in which aspirin-induced neutrophil adherence to cultured endothelial cells was found to be mediated via CD11a/CD18 and ICAM-1. Konturek *et al.* [19•] attempted to examine the effects of aspirin administration on neutrophil adherence in humans. Aspirin was administered over 3 days to eight healthy male volunteers. Gastroscopy confirmed that the aspirin had produced gastric damage. When peripheral neutrophils and platelets were collected from the volunteers and assayed for adherence *in vitro*, it was found to be significantly increased over basal levels. Thus, these data support the animal studies suggesting augmented leukocyte adhesion following NSAID administration.

In the studies of Yoshida *et al.* [20•] discussed above, the adherence of neutrophils to the vascular endothelium was found to be in part mediated by leukotrienes, confirming earlier *in vivo* studies [21]. A role for leukotrienes in the pathogenesis of NSAID-induced gastric injury was further supported by the clinical study of Hudson *et al.* [22••]. They collected gastric biopsies from patients receiving long-term NSAID therapy. Biopsies from the patients taking NSAIDs made significantly more leukotriene B_4 than those from patients not taking NSAIDs who underwent endoscopy for dyspepsia (Fig. 1). There was a strong association between leukotriene B_4 synthesis and the presence of type C gastritis, which raises the possibility that the elevated leukotriene B_4 synthesis occurred purely as a consequence of the elevated numbers of inflammatory cells in the biopsy. However, Hudson *et al.* [22••] argued that there was a paucity of inflammatory cells in many biopsies from these patients, and that leukotriene B_4 synthesis was not elevated in patients with *H. pylori*–associated gastritis. They suggested that the elevated leukotriene B_4 synthesis in the NSAID users may have been a primary effect contributing to the gastropathy.

One of the mechanisms through which leukocytes can induce damage to the gastroduodenal mucosa is through the release of reactive oxygen metabolites, although it should be noted that other cells are also capable of producing these substances. Kozol *et al.* [23•] reported that incubation of rabbit gastric surface cells with nonstimulated neutrophils did not cause appreciable damage, but addition to this system of a bacterial formylated peptide, a neutrophil activator, resulted in widespread epithelial damage that was inhibited by superoxide dismutase and glutathione peroxidase, but not by protease inhibitors or dimethyl sulfoxide. Al-

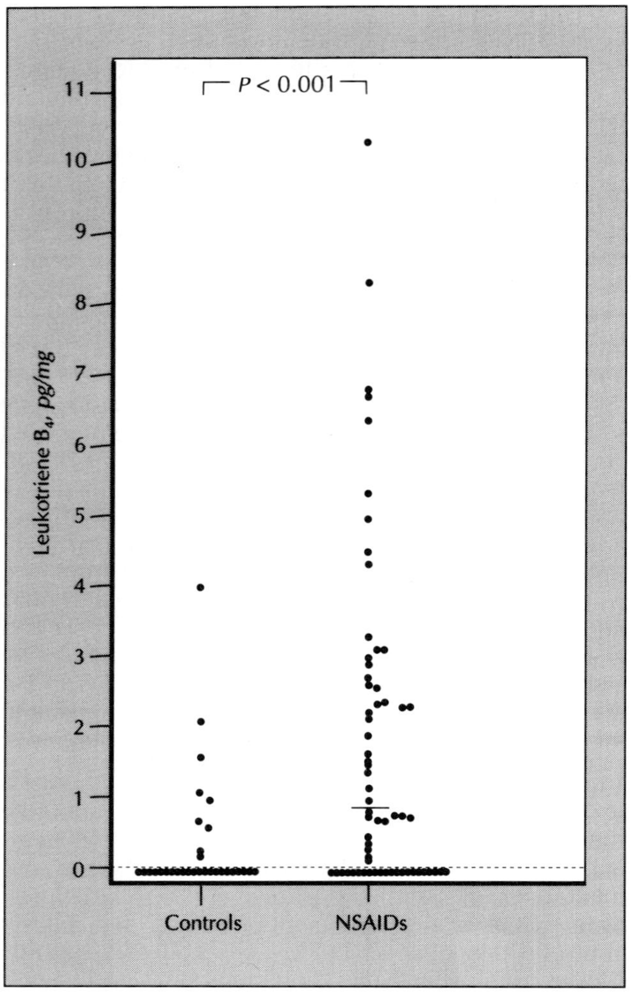

Fig. 1. Gastric mucosal synthesis of leukotriene B_4 in 65 patients with arthritis receiving long-term nonsteroidal anti-inflammatory drug (NSAID) treatment, compared with 23 control subjects. (*From* Hudson *et al.* [22••]; with permission.)

though these studies support a role for neutrophils in producing gastric epithelial injury, it should be noted that a very high ratio of neutrophils to gastric cells (20:1) was used, which seems unlikely to occur in an *in vivo* state.

Sensory afferents, mast cells, and neuropeptides

As discussed above, sensory afferent nerves in the gastroduodenal mucosa appear to mediate the hyperemic response to topical irritants through the release of CGRP [24]. This pathway was further examined by Peskar *et al.* [14•], who used a monoclonal antibody against CGRP in an attempt to immunoneutralize its actions. They observed that this antibody abolished the protective effects of capsaicin (which activates sensory afferent nerves) against ethanol-induced damage in the rat stomach.

In addition to causing vasodilation through the release of CGRP, capsaicin-induced activation of sensory afferent nerves has been shown to cause activation of mucosal mast cells, that contribute to vasodilation through the release of histamine [25]. In a very provocative paper, Gronbech and Lacy [26••] further examined the potential interactions among sensory afferent nerves, mast cells, and the mucosal microcirculation. They reported the intravascular administration of substance P attenuated the hyperemia caused by topical capsaicin administration. This effect of substance P was reversed by coadministration of a protease inhibitor or by ketotifen (a mast cell "stabilizer"), and these effects were correlated to preservation of stainable mast cells. These results suggest that substance P degranulates connective tissue mast cells, resulting in the release of proteases, which can attenuate the vasodilatory effects of capsaicin (by degrading CGRP).

Mast cell activation can also be modulated by NO, and this can have significant impact on gastrointestinal epithelial integrity. Kanwar *et al.* [27••] demonstrated that administration of a NO synthesis inhibitor resulted in mast cell activation within the gastrointestinal tract and in a significant increase in epithelial permeability. Stabilizers of mast cells as well as histamine H_1 and platelet-activating factor antagonists attenuated the effects of the NO synthase inhibitor (Fig. 2). These studies were supported by *in vitro* studies demonstrating that NO is released from mast cells, that this release can be markedly increased by interleukin-1, and that the NO can inhibit the release of platelet-activating factor [28••]

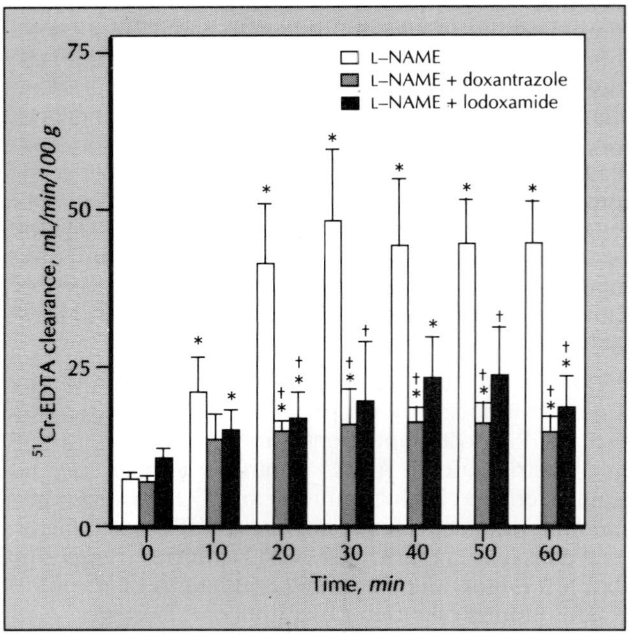

Fig. 2. Increase in intestinal epithelial permeability (measured by ^{51}Cr-EDTA flux from blood to lumen) following administration of a nitric oxide synthase inhibitor, N^{ω}-nitro-L-arginine methyl ester (L-NAME, given after the time zero measurement), and its attenuation by two mast cell stabilizers (doxantrazole and lodoxamide). *Asterisks* denote a significant increase above the basal level, whereas *daggers* denote a significant difference from the corresponding L-NAME group. (*From* Kanwar *et al.* [27••]; with permission.)

Restitution

As restitution is seen to be a critical component of the mucosal defensive response to superficial injury, there is a great deal of interest in substances that might accelerate this process. Paimela *et al.* [29•] examined the effects of basic fibroblast growth factor (bFGF) on restitution of bullfrog gastric mucosa mounted in Ussing chambers. They reported that luminally applied protamine or suramin, both of which are known to interfere with endogenous bFGF action, significantly inhibited electrophysiologic recovery following mucosal damage induced by hypertonic saline. Moreover, luminal sucralfate, which binds bFGF and prevents its degradation, allowed recovery of the epithelial damage to occur at a luminal of pH 3, at which repair usually does not occur. Luminal bFGF also permitted restitution to occur at pH 3.

Restitution *in vivo* is dependent to some extent on elevated mucosal blood flow. Because the hyperemic response in a healthy mucosa is mediated by sensory afferent nerves, Pabst *et al.* [30•] examined the importance of these nerves in the restitution process. They ablated sensory afferent nerves by treating rats with capsaicin, then administered ethanol orogastrically in order to produce mucosal injury. In rats in which sensory afferents were ablated with capsaicin, the damage caused by ethanol was significantly exacerbated relative to controls. However, rapid repair of the epithelial damage occurred normally, suggesting that blood flow to the damaged area must be mediated via mechanisms other than those mediated by sensory afferent nerves.

Trefoil peptides

A recently recognized family of molecules, the epithelial-derived trefoil peptides, have attracted a great deal of interest in the past few years. Poulsom and Wright [31•] have reviewed the subject and raised intriguing questions about the significance of these peptides in gastroduodenal ulceration. One trefoil peptide, spasmolytic polypeptide, inhibits gastric acid secretion, appears to be a growth factor, and is unusually resistant to enzymatic digestion. Spasmolytic polypeptide is produced by epithelial cells of the human gastric mucosa. Trefoil peptide expression is also associated with expression of mucin. Finally, in peptic ulceration and other chronic inflammatory or ulcerative gastrointestinal conditions, a so-called "ulcer-associated cell lineage" has recently been recognized. Cells in these structures express messenger RNA for different trefoil peptides, as well as the peptides themselves. Whether this family of molecules will emerge as a component of gastroduodenal mucosal defense remains to be determined.

Conclusions

As mentioned at the outset, the overwhelming evidence for an association between *H. pylori* infection and gastroduodenal ulcer formation has shifted much emphasis in research in this field from the regulation of acid secretion to better understanding the various components of mucosal defense. In the past year, several important advances have been made in this regard. In particular, the interactions among components of mucosal defense such as the microcirculation, sensory afferent nerves, mast cells, and the epithelium were the subject of a number of excellent studies. Significant progress has also been made in recognizing the contribution of various growth factors to the rapid repair of epithelial injury, as well as the contribution of vasoactive mediators such as NO in this process.

Acknowledgments

John L. Wallace, PhD, is a Medical Research Council of Canada Scientist and an Alberta Heritage Foundation for Medical Research Scientist.

References and recommended reading

Papers of particular interest, published within the annual period of review, have been highlighted as:

- • Of special interest
- •• Of outstanding interest

1. •• Kaunitz JD, Nishizaki Y, Kaneko K, Guth P: **Effect of Orogastric Nicotine on Rat Gastric Mucosal Gel Thickness, Surface Cell Viability and Intracellular pH.** *J Pharmacol Exp Ther* 1993, **265**:948–954.

These technically elegant experiments confirm previous studies of the effect of nicotine on gastric mucus secretion and susceptibility to injury. Perhaps more significantly, the simultaneous measurement of epithelial cell pH, gel thickness, and cell viability provide circumstantial support for the notion that the mucus-bicarbonate layer does serve to inhibit acid back-diffusion.

2. Grisham MB, Von Ritter C, Smith BF, Lamont JT, Granger DN: **Interaction Between Oxygen Radicals and Gastric Mucin.** *Am J Physiol* 1987, **253**:G93–G96.

3. • Hiraishi H, Terano A, Ota S, Mutoh H, Sugimoto T, Harada T, Razandi M, Ivey KJ: **Role for Mucous Glycoprotein in Protecting Cultured Rat Gastric Mucosal Cells Against Toxic Oxygen Metabolites.** *J Lab Clin Med* 1993, **121**:570–578.

These studies of cultured rat gastric cells show that the previously demonstrated ability of gastric mucus to scavenge oxyradicals translates into protection of gastric mucosal cells by mucous glycoprotein against toxic oxygen metabolites.

4. • Guttu K, Rosok B, Svanes K, Gronbech JE: **Release of Bicarbonate From Damaged and Restituted Gastric Mucosa in the Cat.** *Gastroenterology* 1993, **105**:74–83.

Complex studies of control, omeprazole-inhibited, and pentagastrin-stimulated cat stomach explore the relationship among time after injury, acid secretory status, and mucosal blood flow.

5. • Takeuchi K, Ohuchi T, Okabe S: **Endogenous Nitric Oxide in Gastric Alkaline Response in the Rat Stomach After Damage.** *Gastroenterology* 1994, **106**:367–374.

In this study using *ex vivo* rat stomach preparations, the authors demonstrate a role for NO in the gastric alkaline response following damage. Their data suggest that mucosal irritation releases NO which then serves to inhibit acid secretion, presumably contributing to repair of the damaged tissue.

6. •• Takeuchi K, Ohuchi T, Miyake H, Okabe S: **Stimulation by Nitric Oxide Synthase Inhibitors of Gastric and Duodenal HCO_3 Secretion in Rats.** *J Pharmacol Exp Ther* 1993, **266**:1512–1519.

The role of NO in regulating bicarbonate secretion in normal, rat stomach and duodenum was examined. Distinct from the situation after mild irritation or damage of the gastric mucosa, endogenous NO here seems to be involved in suppressing bicarbonate secretion.

7. MacNaughton WK, Cirino G, Wallace JL: **Endothelium-Derived Relaxing Factor (Nitric Oxide) Has Protective Actions in the Stomach.** *Life Sci* 1989, **45**:1869–1876.

8. Brown JF, Hanson PJ, Whittle BJR: **Nitric Oxide Donors Increase Mucus Gel Thickness in Rat Stomach.** *Eur J Pharmacol* 1992, **223**:103–104.

9. • Brown JF, Keates AC, Hanson PJ, Whittle BJR: **Nitric Oxide Generators and cGMP Stimulate Mucus Secretion by Rat Gastric Mucosal Cells.** *Am J Physiol* 1993, **265**:G418–G422.

In this study, the authors expand on their own previous work (Brown *et al.*, *Eur J Pharmacol* 1992, 223:103–104) and suggest an effector role for NO in mediating gastric mucus release.

10. Sababi M, Nylander O: **Elevation of Intraluminal Pressure and Cyclooxygenase Inhibitors Increases Duodenal Alkaline Secretion.** *Am J Physiol* 1994, **226**:G22–G30.
•
In perfused duodenal segments in anesthetized rats, the authors determine the effect of raising luminal pressure on duodenal bicarbonate secretion, simulating duodenal distension by food.

11. Hui WM, Chen BW, Kung AWC, Cho CH, Luk CT, Lam SK: **Effect of Epidermal Growth Factor on Gastric Blood Flow in Rats: Possible Role in Mucosal Protection.** *Gastroenterology* 1993, **104**:1605–1610.
•
This study demonstrates that protective actions of EGF in the rat stomach are accompanied by significant increases in gastric blood flow and suggests that there is a causal relationship between these two effects.

12. Howard TJ, Passaro E Jr, Guth PH: **Isoproterenol Prevents Ethanol-Induced Microvascular Stasis and Deep Histologic Injury in Rat Gastric Mucosa.** *Dig Dis Sci* 1993, **38**:1201–1209.
•
Isoproterenol administration significantly reduced gastric damage induced by ethanol, possibly by maintaining gastric microvascular perfusion during the period of exposure to the damaging agent.

13. Konturek SJ, Brzozowski T, Majka J, Pytko-Polonczyk J, Stachura J: **Inhibition of Nitric Oxide Synthase Delays Healing of Chronic Gastric Ulcers.** *Eur J Pharmacol* 1993, **239**:215–217.
•
Acetic acid–induced gastric ulcers healed significantly more slowly when an inhibitor of NO synthase was administered. This effect could be partially reversed by an NO-releasing drug or by administering the precursor of NO (L-arginine). Thus, NO may play a role in healing gastric ulcers.

14. Peskar BM, Wong HC, Walsh JH, Holzer P: **A Monoclonal Antibody to Calcitonin Gene-Related Peptide Abolishes Capsaicin-Induced Gastroprotection.** *Eur J Pharmacol* 1993, **250**:201–203.
•
Capsaicin-induced protection of the rat stomach against ethanol-induced injury could be attenuated by administration of an immunoneutralizing antibody directed against CGRP, reinforcing previous evidence that this peptide is an important mediator of gastric blood flow and mucosal defense.

15. Lugea A, Salas A, Guarner F, Malagelada J-R: **Adaptive Cytoprotection of the Rat Duodenum Is Not Dependent on Nitric Oxide-Induced Changes in Blood Flow.** *Am J Physiol* 1993, **264**:G994–G1000.
•
This study demonstrates that the adaptive response of the duodenum to acid, which results in increased resistance to injury, is not mediated by NO release or to increased mucosal blood flow.

16. Holzer P, Lippe IT, Jocic M, Wachter C, Erb R, Heinemann A: **Nitric Oxide-Dependent and -Independent Hyperaemia Due to Calcitonin Gene-Related Peptide in the Rat Stomach.** *Br J Pharmacol* 1993, **110**:404–410.
•
This study demonstrates that CGRP-induced vasodilation is only partly dependent upon NO release, since only a portion of the response was attenuated by an NO synthesis inhibitor.

17. Wallace JL, McKnight W, Miyasaka M, Tamatani T, Paulson J, Anderson DC, Granger DN, Kubes P: **Role of Endothelial Adhesion Molecules in NSAID-Induced Gastric Mucosal Injury.** *Am J Physiol* 1993, **265**:G993–G998.
•
This paper characterizes the endothelial adhesion molecules involved in NSAID-induced leukocyte adherence and gastric mucosal injury.

18. Andrews FJ, Malcontenti-Wilson C, O'Brien PE: **Protection Against Gastric Ischemia-Reperfusion Injury by Nitric Oxide Generators.** *Dig Dis Sci* 1994, **39**:366–373.
••
A rapid elevation in the expression of ICAM-1 and lymphocyte function-associated antigen-1 within the gastric microcirculation following administration of aspirin or indomethacin is demonstrated. The time frame within which these changes were observed was consistent with the leukocyte adherence observed following NSAID administration in previous studies.

19. Konturek JW, Dembinski A, Stoll R, Konturek M, Domschke W: **Gastric Mucosal Blood Flow and Neutrophil Activation in Aspirin-Induced Gastric Mucosal Damage in Man.** *Scand J Gastroenterol* 1993, **28**:767–771.
•
This provides supportive evidence for the hypothesis that NSAID administration results in increased adhesivity of leukocytes. Following a 3-day course of aspirin administration to healthy volunteers, neutrophil adherence to platelets was found to be significantly increased.

20. Yoshida N, Takemura T, Granger DN, Anderson DC, Wolf RE, McIntire LV, Kvietys PR: **Molecular Determinants of Aspirin-Induced Neutrophil Adherence to Endothelial Cells.** *Gastroenterology* 1993, **105**:715–724.
•
A characterization of the leukocyte and endothelial adhesion molecules that mediate aspirin-induced adherence of human neutrophils to cultured human umbilical vein endothelial cells is provided and a partial role for leukotrienes in this process is demonstrated.

21. Asako H, Kubes P, Wallace JL, Gaginella T, Wolf RE, Granger DN: **Indomethacin-Induced Leukocyte Adhesion in Mesenteric Venules: Role of Lipoxygenase Products.** *Am J Physiol* 1992, **262**:G903–G908.

22. Hudson N, Balsitis M, Everitt S, Hawkey CJ: **Enhanced Gastric Mucosal Leukotriene B_4 Synthesis in Patients Taking Non-Steroidal Anti-Inflammatory Drugs.** *Gut* 1993, **34**:742–747.
••
This carefully performed study evaluates the effects of long-term NSAID administration on gastric leukotriene synthesis. The authors provide strong evidence for elevated leukotriene B_4 synthesis being a primary effect of NSAID administration, rather than a secondary consequence of mucosal inflammation.

23. Kozol R, Kopatsis A, Fligiel SEG, Czanko R, Callewaert D: **Neutrophil-Mediated Injury to Gastric Mucosal Surface Cells.** *Dig Dis Sci* 1994, **39**:138–144.
•
This study demonstrates the ability of activated, but not resting, neutrophils to damage gastric epithelial cells.

24. Li DS, Raybould HE, Quintero E, Guth PH: **Role of Calcitonin Gene-Related Peptide in Gastric Hyperemic Response to Intragastric Capsaicin.** *Am J Physiol* 1991, **251**:G657–G661.

25. Wallace JL, McKnight GW, Befus AD: **Capsaicin-Induced Hyperemia in the Stomach: Possible Contribution of Mast Cells.** *Am J Physiol* 1992, **263**:G209–G214.

26. Gronbech JE, Lacy ER: **Substance P Attenuates Gastric Mucosal Hyperemia After Stimulation of Sensory Neurons in the Rat Stomach.** *Gastroenterology* 1994, **106**:440–449.
••
This elegant study focuses on the complex interactions among sensory nerves, mast cells, and the gastric microcirculation *in vivo*. The results suggest that substance P can attenuate the vasodilation induced by capsaicin by stimulating the release of proteases from mast cells, which can degrade CGRP.

27. Kanwar S, Wallace JL, Befus D, Kubes P: **Nitric Oxide Synthesis Inhibition Increases Epithelial Permeability Via Mast Cells.** *Am J Physiol* 1994, **266**:G222–G229.
••
This study demonstrates that inhibition of NO synthesis leads to activation of mast cells within the gastrointestinal tract, and that via the release of histamine and platelet-activating factor, this leads to a marked increase in epithelial permeability.

28. Hogaboam CM, Befus AD, Wallace JL: **Modulation of Rat Mast Cell Reactivity by IL-1β: Divergent Effects on Nitric Oxide and Platelet-Activating Factor Release.** *J Immunol* 1993, **151**:3767–3774.
••
Using an *in vitro* system in which release of NO and platelet-activating factor from isolated mast cells could be measured, this study showed that interleukin-1β could greatly augment NO release, leading to inhibition of platelet-activating factor release. Together with the findings of Kanwar *et al.* (*Am J Physiol* 1994, 266:G222–G229), this suggests that NO is an important physiologic regulator of mast cell reactivity in the gastrointestinal tract.

29. Paimela H, Goddard PJ, Carter K, Khakee R, McNeil PL, Ito S, Silen W: **Restitution of Frog Gastric Mucosa In Vitro: Effect of Basic Fibroblast Growth Factor.** *Gastroenterology* 1993, **104**:1337–1345.
•
This paper couples convincing electrophysiologic recordings that document recovery of epithelial integrity with some elegant morphology. The paper demonstrates that basic fibroblast growth factor is probably an important endogenous mediator of restitution of the gastric epithelium.

30. Pabst MA, Schoninkle E, Holzer P: **Ablatiln of Capsaicin Sensitive Afferent Nerves Impairs Defence But Not Rapid Repair of Rat Gastric Mucosa.** *Gut* 1993, **34**:897–903.
•
Whereas capsaicin-induced ablation of sensory afferent nerves greatly increases the susceptibility of the gastric mucosa to damage induced by ethanol, it does not interfere with the repair of this injury.

31. Poulsom R, Wright NA: **Trefoil Peptides: A Newly Recognized Family of Epithelial Mucin-Associated Molecules.** *Am J Physiol* 1993, **265**:G205–G213.
•
This comprehensive review article details current knowledge of this intriguing class of peptide molecules, raising as many questions as it answers.

John L. Wallace, PhD, Department of Pharmacology and Therapeutics, University of Calgary, Calgary, Alberta, T2N 4N1, Canada.

Medical management of peptic ulcer disease

David Ng, MB, MRCP(UK), and Roy Pounder, MA, MD, DSc(Med), FRCP

Royal Free Hospital School of Medicine, London, UK

Strong advice to stop smoking and careful prescription of nonsteroidal anti-inflammatory drugs remain basic steps in peptic ulcer management. Long-term, low-dose treatment with an H_2-blocker provides effective prophylaxis against recurrent ulceration, but most patients with peptic ulceration should now be offered treatment to eradicate infection with *Helicobacter pylori*. An H^+, K^+-APTase inhibitor is the treatment of choice for a patient with the Zollinger-Ellison syndrome. Treatment of peptic ulceration is usually safe, but there are concerns about increased hazards of enteric infection due to decreased gastric acid, and the accelerated development of gastric atrophy during long-term treatment with omeprazole. Finding an effective and convenient regimen for the eradication of *H. pylori* remains the major problem in the medical management of peptic ulceration.

Current Opinion in Gastroenterology 1994, **10**:595–599

There has been a worldwide decline in hospital admissions for peptic ulcer disease. In Australia, morbidity and mortality from peptic ulcer disease in those up to age 65 years fell between 1971 and 1987, with an especially large decrease in gastric and duodenal ulcer mortality in younger men. There was, however, an increase in duodenal ulcer mortality in elderly women [1]. A similar trend was seen in Scotland, with a 93% rise in duodenal ulcer perforation in women aged 65 years and older [2]. These data suggest that an environmental factor plays a role in elderly women to increase their risk of ulcer disease; nonsteroidal anti-inflammatory drugs (NSAIDs) are the main suspects. Smoking and stress are other possible environmental risk factors for peptic ulcer disease. Smoking increases the rate of ulcer recurrence and slows ulcer healing, possibly by an 80% decrease in acid-stimulated duodenal bicarbonate secretion [3•]. Stress increases gastric acid secretion in duodenal ulcer patients [4], but any link between stress and duodenal ulceration remains obscure [5]. Strong advice to stop smoking and careful prescription of NSAIDs remain basic steps in peptic ulcer management. NSAIDs should be used only in patients who do not respond to other analgesics, with the lowest possible dosage used and the least toxic NSAID selected [6••].

Treatment of peptic ulceration

Prior to the knowledge of the important role played by *Helicobacter pylori* and duodenal ulcer relapse, the only successful prophylaxis was by means of maintenance treatment with an H_2-antagonist [7]. Penston *et al.* [8] and Penston [9] in Scotland reported that long-term therapy with an H_2-antagonist for up to 9 years resulted in fewer hospital admissions, a decrease in the need for gastric surgery, and less ulcer bleeding. However, the natural course of duodenal ulceration remains unaltered by even prolonged treatment with an H_2-blocker. After an average of 7.5 years of continuous treatment with ranitidine, patients were randomly assigned to continue with either ranitidine or to receive placebo [10]. After 6 months of follow-up, 9% of the ranitidine group had developed symptom recurrence, compared with 48% in the placebo group [10].

A pharmaco-economic assessment of long-term management of peptic ulcer disease concluded that continuous treatment with an H_2-antagonist is a cost-effective management option [11]. A survey of 60,148 patients on the list of general practices identified 492 patients (0. 82%) were receiving long-term (>6 months) acid-suppressing treatment . Thirty-seven percent of the patients were being treated for duodenal ulceration and 24% for esophageal disease; however, 19% were being treated for undiagnosed abdominal pain. Seventy-four percent of patients found their treatment helpful, but 27% had a poor understanding of their diagnosis [12]. It is fortunate that H_2-antagonists have a good safety record [13].

There is some debate whether long-term treatment with an H_2-antagonist affects the natural history of duodenal ulceration. Penston [9] considers long-term continuous therapy almost mandatory, but Bardhan [14] argues that some patients are cured after a period of treatment with an H_2-antagonist. An important new study has demonstrated the effectiveness and safety of long-term maintenance therapy with an H_2-antago-

Abbreviation

NSAID—nonsteroidal anti-inflammatory drug.

© 1994 Current Science ISBN 1-85922-611-6 ISSN 0267–1379

nist for the prevention of recurrent hemorrhage in duodenal ulcer disease [15••]. Patients were randomly assigned to maintenance treatment with ranitidine (150 mg at night) or placebo, and were followed for up to 3 years. After a mean follow-up of 61 weeks, three of the 32 patients treated with ranitidine had recurrent hemorrhage, compared with 12 of the 33 given placebo, a significant difference (Fig. 1). Importantly, half of the episodes of recurrent bleeding were asymptomatic, demonstrating that patients cannot rely upon the return of ulcer symptoms to prevent them from suffering an unexpected hemorrhage. Eradication of *H. pylori* infection also decreases the risk of ulcer rehemorrhage [16•,17], although long-term H_2-blockade seems prudent for any vulnerable ulcer patient with a past history of hemorrhage.

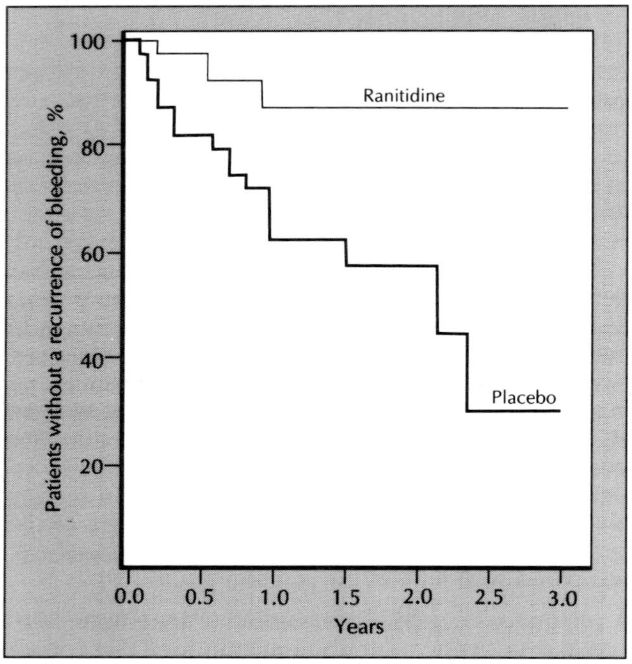

Fig. 1. Recurrence of duodenal ulcer hemorrhage in patients randomly assigned to maintenance daily treatment with ranitidine 150 mg or placebo. (*From* Jensen *et al.* [15••]; with permission.)

The development of H^+, K^+-ATPase (proton pump) inhibitors has introduced an entirely new range of treatment for patients with peptic ulceration [18]. Omeprazole was the first to be introduced into clinical practice, with the recent additions of lansoprazole [19•] and pantoprazole [20•]. The potential therapeutic advantage of proton pump inhibitors over an H_2-antagonist is their ability to cause a profound and unremitting decrease of intragastric acidity. As a result, when compared with H_2-antagonists, they tend to have a more rapid effect on symptoms, particularly in the daytime, and higher healing rates in the first weeks of treatment. New proton pump inhibitors are under development, including NC-1300-O-3 and TY-11345 [21–23].

Further changes can be expected in the management of peptic ulceration, although not all may necessarily be for the better. H_2-antagonists are now becoming available over-the-counter [24] and surgeons are exploring the opportunity for laparoscopic vagotomy [25].

Zollinger-Ellison syndrome

The management of a patient with a gastrinoma has been transformed in recent years by treatment with omeprazole, although emergency management may have to involve high doses of an intravenous histamine H_2-antagonist [26••]. A 9-year study described the efficacy of omeprazole in 116 patients [27]. Gastric acid secretion was controlled using 60 mg of omeprazole once daily in 46 (40%) of the patients, but 29 (25%) required twice daily dosing. Lansoprazole similarly controls gastric acid secretion, with a mean dose of 60 mg once or twice each day [28].

Acid inhibition safety

Four major safety issues have been debated recently concerning the pharmacologic control of gastric acid secretion. Firstly, it is now accepted that there is no clinically relevant interaction between H_2-antagonists and alcohol [29,30]. Secondly, treatment with H_2-antagonists may increase the risk of enteric infection, particularly in people over 65 years of age [31]. Thirdly, treatment with omeprazole often results in duodenal bacterial overgrowth involving both oral and fecal bacteria [32]. Finally, long-term treatment with omeprazole is associated with accelerated development of atrophic gastritis [33,34]. The rapid "aging" of the stomach during omeprazole treatment is most surprising—one might have expected gastrin-stimulated hyperplasia of the gastric mucosa. It has been argued this atrophy is not drug-related, but in one study of 443 patients, the prevalence of atrophic gastritis rose from 1.0% to 13.3% during approximately 1 year's treatment with omeprazole [33], an effect that could not be attributed to the passage of time between biopsies. Similarly, in another group of 74 patients (mean age 52.6 years), at the beginning of an average of 4 years' treatment with omeprazole, the prevalence of atrophic gastritis rose from 1.8% to 20.8% [34]. These authors claimed that it was "more disease- than drug-related" [34], which is most unlikely as disease was the indication for prescribing omeprazole, yet virtually no patients started treatment with gastric atrophy. Both of these studies demonstrated proliferation of enterochromaffin-like cells in patients treated with omeprazole, a change that was attributed to the loss of background mucosal cells during the development of atrophic gastritis.

Nonsteroidal anti-inflammatory drug–related disease

It is now accepted that NSAID treatment can result in diffuse damage to the gastrointestinal tract, not only in the gastroduodenum [6••] but also in the small and large intestine [35]. This damage can often be attenuated or reversed by misoprostol, a synthetic prostaglandin analogue [36]. The mechanism by which NSAIDs induce damage to the intestinal mucosa remains obscure. Recent studies have demonstrated the neutrophil adherence to the vascular endothelium may be a critical early event in the pathogenesis of this injury. A potential new strategy for the treatment of NSAID-related ulcers has been proposed; an antibody to CD-18 (a leukocyte adhesion molecule) completely prevented indomethacin-induced leukocyte adherence to gastric mucosal blood vessels, decreasing by 75% the severity of damage induced by indomethacin in the rat. Similarly, an antibody against intercellular adhesion molecule-1 decreased by 74% the severity of indomethacin-induced gastric injury, while also decreasing leukocyte adherence by 84%. Interactions at the leukocyte-endothelial interface may be critical in the pathogenesis of NSAID-induced mucosal injury, representing a new target for prevention of this form of injury [37].

Helicobacter pylori

Helicobacter pylori was the subject of an influential consensus conference at the National Institutes of Health in early 1994 [38]. This conference reached three important conclusions:

1. Ulcer patients with *H. pylori* infection require treatment with antimicrobial agents in addition to antisecretory drugs, whether on first presentation with illness or on recurrence

2. The value of treatment of patients with non-ulcer dyspepsia and *H. pylori* infection remains to be determined

3. The interesting relationship between *H. pylori* and gastric cancers requires further exploration

The one positive conclusion, recommending combination treatment for infected ulcer patients, tends to raise more questions than provide a clear answer for clinicians [39]. Although *H. pylori* is a bacterium that is highly sensitive to antibiotics in the laboratory, its eradication from the gastroduodenal mucosa has often proved difficult. The range and efficacy of various antibiotic combinations has been reviewed extensively [40,41], but at present there is no ideal therapeutic regimen. Omeprazole has been tested extensively with amoxycillin, and it can be generally concluded that large doses of both substances result in greater efficacy. However, the combination eradicates infection in only approximately two thirds of patients. Proton pump inhibitors alone have a modest bacteriostatic effect upon *H. pylori*, but they do not eradicate the infection [42]. The mechanism of its action when acting alone is unclear, but it may inhibit *H. pylori* urease activity, thereby affecting colonization [43]. Controlling intragastric acidity may also enhance the bioavailability of antibiotics [44]. Ranitidine added to metronidazole and amoxycillin produced one remarkable, placebo-controlled study where the combination not only resulted in an enhanced acute duodenal ulcer healing rate, but the eradication of the bacterium was also associated with prolonged duodenal ulcer remission (Fig. 2) [45•].

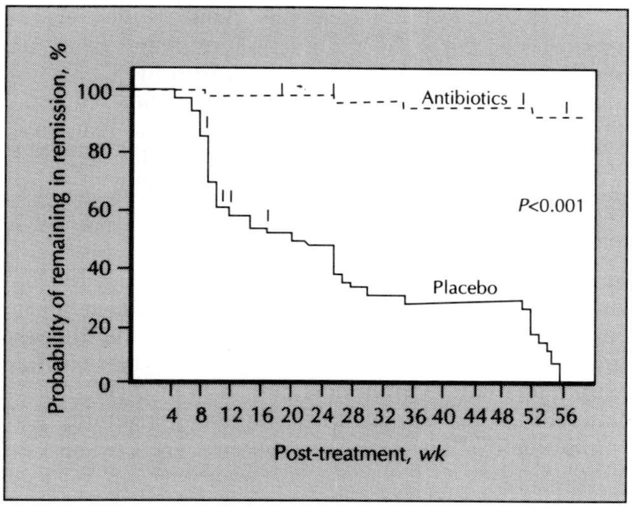

Fig. 2. Duodenal ulcer remission after healing with raniditine plus placebo, or ranitidine plus metronidazole and amoxycillin. The *tick marks* represent patients who, because of noncompliance, were considered to have withdrawn from the study. (From Hentschel *et al.* [45•]; with permission.)

At the moment, the most reliable regimen is triple therapy involving the use of a bismuth compound, together with metronidazole and oxytetracycline [40]. This is a difficult regimen that is unlikely to be promoted for three reasons: 1) neither bismuth subsalicylate nor tripotassium dicitrato bismuthate have completed modern, extensive animal and human toxicologic studies, 2) oxytetracycline must not be used by children or pregnant women, and 3) metronidazole often causes profound nausea in already dyspeptic subjects and primary resistance to this antibiotic results in almost inevitable failure of triple therapy to eradicate the bacterium [46]. Ranitidine bismuth citrate is a coprecipitate of ranitidine with bismuth citrate; it is a new chemical entity providing gastric acid antisecretory activity because of its ranitidine component together with bismuth activity against *H. pylori* [47]. Ranitidine bismuth citrate, when given orally after food, has an intrinsic activity against *H. pylori*, but it does not produce a reliable eradication of the bacterium when given as a single agent. When used with amoxycillin, oxytetracycline, or clarithromycin, however, it can produce a very high eradication rate [48].

Populations with a high prevalence of *H. pylori* infection also tend to have a high rate of gastric cancer [49••,50]. Both conditions occur more often in developing countries and in low socioeconomic groups. Familial clustering has been observed in both conditions and they are both associated with a marked chronic inflammatory response with chronic atrophic gastritis [51]. Although it is highly unlikely that *H. pylori* is the sole contributory factor to gastric carcinogenesis, it may produce an environment in which factors, such as a high-salt diet or frequent exposure to *N*-nitroso compounds, promote the occurrence of gastric cancer. In addition, the free-radical scavenger ascorbic acid is secreted less by a gastric mucosa that is infected with *H. pylori* [52]. Clearly, the potential association between

H. pylori and gastric cancer has major public health implications, particularly if a simple regimen could be developed for eradicating the bacterium from infected subjects. It appears that childhood is the most vulnerable time for the acquisition of infection, and that seroconversion is unusual in the adult population [53–55]. In the future, we may be offering eradication therapy for asymptomatic infected patients or immunization for uninfected children.

An association has been shown between colonization of the gastric mucosa by *H. pylori*, the acquisition of mucosa-associated lymphoid tissue, and the occurrence of primary B-cell gastric mucosa-associated lymphoid tissue lymphomas [56]. Anti-*H. pylori* treatment should now be given for patients presenting this lymphoma [57••].

References and recommended reading

Papers of particular interest, published within the annual period of review, have been highlighted as:

- • Of special interest
- •• Of outstanding interest

1. McIntosh JH, Byth K, Tsang N, Berman K, Holliday FM, Piper DW: **Trends in Peptic Ulcer Mortality in Sydney From 1971 to 1987.** *J Clin Gastroenterol* 1993, **16**:346–353.

2. Jibril JA, Redpath A, MacIntyre IM: **Changing Pattern of Admission and Operation for Duodenal Ulcers in Scotland.** *Br J Surg* 1994, **81**:87–89.

3. • Ainsworth MA, Hogan DL, Koss MA, Isenberg JI: **Cigarette Smoking Inhibits Acid-Stimulated Duodenal Mucosal Bicarbonate Secretion.** *Ann Intern Med* 1993, **119**:882–886.

This paper neatly demonstrates a significant ($P<0.\ 01$) decrease in acid-stimulated duodenal bicarbonate secretion by the duodenum with cigarette smoking.

4. Bresnick WH, Rask-Madsen C, Hogan DL, Koss MA, Isenberg JI: **The Effect of Acute Emotional Stress on Gastric Acid Secretion in Normal Subjects and Duodenal Ulcer Patients.** *J Clin Gastroenterol* 1993, **17**:117–122.

5. Piper DW, Tennant C: **Stress and Personality in Patients With Chronic Peptic Ulcer.** *J Clin Gastroenterol* 1993, **16**:211–214.

6. •• Langman MJS, Weil J, Wainwright P, Lawson DH, Rawlins MD, Logan RFA, Murphy M, Vessey MP, Colin-Jones DG: **Risks of Bleeding Peptic Ulcer Associated With Individual Non-Steroidal Anti-Inflammatory Drugs.** *Lancet* 1994, **343**:1075–1078.

This paper reports the rise of NSAID-related bleeding in 1144 patients of 60 years of age or older. There was an associated odds ratio of 4.5 for all NSAIDs, increasing with NSAID potency and dose.

7. Black J: **Reflections on the Analytical Pharmacology of Histamine H2-Receptor Antagonists.** *Gastroenterology* 1993, **105**:963–968.

8. Penston JG, Crombie IK, Waugh NR, Wormsley KG: **Trends in Morbidity and Mortality From Peptic Ulcer Disease: Tayside Versus Scotland.** *Aliment Pharmacol Ther* 1993, 7:429–442.

9. Penston JG: **A Decade of Experience With Long-Term Continuous Treatment of Peptic Ulcers With H2-Receptor Antagonists.** *Aliment Pharmacol Ther* 1993, 7 **(suppl 2)**:27–33.

10. Penston JG, Dixon JS, Boyd EJS, Wormsley KG: **A Placebo-Controlled Investigation of Duodenal Ulcer Recurrence After Withdrawal of Long-Term Treatment With Ranitidine.** *Aliment Pharmacol Ther* 1993, 7:259–265.

11. Ruszniewski P: **Pharmaco-Economic Considerations in the Long-Term Management of Peptic Ulcer Disease.** *Aliment Pharmacol Ther* 1993, 7(suppl 2):41–48.

12. Ryder SD, O'Reilly S, Miller R, Ross J, Acyna MR, Levi AJ: **Long Term Acid Suppressing Treatment in General Practice.** *BMJ* 1994, 308:827–830.

13. Sabesin SM: **Safety Issues Relating to Long-Term Treatment With Histamine H_2-Receptor Antagonists.** *Aliment Pharmacol Ther* 1993, 7(suppl 2):35–40.

14. Bardhan KD: **Can the H2 Receptor Antagonists Change the Natural History of Duodenal Ulcer Disease?** *Am J Gastroenterol* 1994, **89**:3–6.

15. •• Jensen DM, Ceng S, Kovacs TOG, Randall G, Jensen ME, Reedy T, Frankl H, Machicado G, Smith J, Silpa M, Van Deventer G: **A Controlled Study of Ranitidine for the Prevention of Recurrent Hemorrhage From Duodenal Ulcer.** *N Engl J Med* 1994, **330**:382–386.

The paper shows that after a mean follow-up of 61 weeks, three of 32 patients receiving maintenance ranitidine had recurrent bleeding. This was compared with 12 of 33 patients given placebo ($P<0.05$).

16. • Graham DY, Hepps KS, Ramirez FC, Lew GM, Saeed ZA: **Treatment of Helicobacter pylori Reduces the Rate of Rebleeding in Peptic Ulcer Disease.** *Scand J Gastroenterol* 1993, **28**:939–942.

Like the paper by Jensen *et al.* (*N Engl J Med* 1994, 330:382–386), this study shows that *H. pylori* eradication can effectively reduce the risk of recurrent peptic ulcer bleeding.

17. Labenz J, Borsch G: **Role of Hp Eradicaiton in the Prevention of Peptic Ulcer Bleeding Relapse.** *Digestion* 1994, **55**:19–23.

18. Sachs G, Shin JM, Besancon M, Prinz C: **The Continuing Development of Gastric Acid Pump Inhibitors.** *Aliment Pharmacol Ther* 1993, 7(suppl 1):4–12.

19. Arvanitakis C, Cassen M, Takemoto T: **Treatment of Acid Peptic Disease: Focus on Proton Pump Inhibitors.** *Aliment Pharmacol Ther* 1993, 7(suppl 1):2–75.

20. • Classen M, Della Fave G: **Management of Acid-Related Diseases: Focus on Pantoprazole.** *Aliment Pharmacol Ther* 1994, **8(suppl 1)**:1–70.

A good general overview of a new proton pump inhibitor.

21. Okabe S, Akimoto Y, Yamasaki S, Kuwahara K: **Effects of a New Benzimidazole Derivative, NC-1300-O-3, on Gastric Secretion and Gastroduodenal Lesions in Rats.** *Jpn J Pharmacol* 1991, **55**:477–491.

22. Igata H, Okabe S: **Effect of NC-1300-O-3 on Healing of Acetic Acid-Induced Gastric Ulcers in Rats.** *Jpn J Pharmacol* 1993, **62**:25–33.

23. Yamaguchi T, Aihara K, Yamada S, Narita S, Kogi K: **Biochemical and Pharmacological Properties of a Newly Synthesised Proton Pump (H+/K(+)-ATPase) Inhibitor, TY-11345 in Experimental Animals.** *Jpn J Pharmacol* 1993, 62:363–371.

24. Feldman M: **Pros and Cons of Over-the-Counter Availability if Histamine$_2$-Receptor Antagonists.** *Arch Intern Med* 1993, **153**:2415–2424.

25. Taylor TV, Bhandarkar DS: **Laparoscopic Vagotomy: An Operation for the 1990s?** *Ann R Coll Surg Engl* 1993, **75**:385–386.

26. •• Maton PN: **Review Article: The Management of Zollinger -Ellison Syndrome.** *Aliment Pharmacol Ther* 1993, 7:467–475.

Diagnostic awareness is emphasized in clinical presentation. The aims of treatment and safety of treatment are reviewed comprehensively and objectively.

27. Metz DC, Strader DB, Orbuch M, Koviach PD, Feigenbaum KM, Jensen RT: **Use of Omeprazole in Zollinger-Ellison Syndrome: A Prospective Nine-Year Study of Efficacy and Safety.** *Aliment Pharmacol Ther* 1993, 7:597–610.

28. Jensen RT, Metz DC, Koviack PD, Feigenbaum K: **Prospective Study of the Long-Term Efficacy and Safety of Lansoprazole in Patients With Zollinger-Ellison Syndrome.** *Aliment Pharmacol Ther* 1993, **7(suppl 1)**:41–50.

29. Fraser AG, Hudson M, Sawyer AM, Smith MSH, Sercombe J, Rosalki SB, Pounder RE: **Ranitidine Has No Effect Upon Post-Prandial Ethanol Absorption.** *Am J Gastroenterol* 1993, **88**:217–221.

30. Levitt MD: **Review Article: Lack of Clinical Significance of the Interaction Between H2-Receptor Antagonists and Ethanol.** *Aliment Pharmacol Ther* 1993, 7:131–138.

31. Neal KR, Brij SO, Slack CB, Hawkey CJ, Logan RFA: **Recent Treatment With H2-Antagonists and Antibiotics and Gastric Surgery As Risk Factors for Salmonella Infection.** *BMJ* 1994, **308**:176.

32. Fried M, Siegrist H, Frei R, Froehlich F, Duroux P, Thorens J, Blum A, Gonvers JJ, Gyr K: **Duodenal Bacterial Overgrowth During Treatment in Out-Patients With Omeprazole.** *Gut* 1994, **35**:23–26.

33. Solcia E, Fiocca R, Havu N, Dalvag A, Carlsson R: **Gastric Endocrine Cells and Gastritis in Patients Receiving Long-Term Omeprazole Treatment.** *Digestion* 1992, **51(suppl 1)**:82-92.

34. Lamberts R, Creutzfeldt W, Struber HG, Brunner G, Solcia E: **Long-Term Omeprazole Therapy in Peptic Ulcer Disease: Gastrin, Endocrine Cell Growth, and Gastritis.** *Gastroenterology* 1993, **104**:1356–1370.

35. Aabakken L: **Review Article: Non-Steroidal, Antiinflammatory Drugs: The Extending Scope of Gastrointestinal Side Effects.** *Aliment Pharmacol Ther* 1992, 6:143–162.

36. Fenn GC: **Controversies in NSAID-induced Gastro-Duodenal Damage: Do They Matter ?** *Aliment Pharmacol Ther* 1994, **103**:15–26.

37. Wallace JL, McKnight W, Miyasaka M, Tamatani T, Paulson J, Anderson DC, Granger DN, Kubes P: **Role of Endothelial Adhesion**

Molecules in NSAID-Induced Gastric Mucosal Injury. *Am J Physiol* 1993, **265**:G993–G998.

38. NIH Consensus Development Panel on Helicobacter pylori in peptic ulcer disease: **Helicobacter pylori in Peptic Ulcer Disease.** *JAMA* 1994, **272**:65–69.

39. Feldman M: **The Acid Test.** *JAMA* 1994, **272**:71–91.

40. Tytgat GNJ: **Review Article: Treatments That Impact Favourably Upon the Eradication of Helicobacter pylori and Ulcer Recurrence.** *Aliment Pharmacol Ther* 1994, **8**:359–369.

41. Penston JG: **Review Article: Helicobacter pylori Eradication: Understandable Caution but No Excuse for Inertia.** *Aliment Pharmacol Ther* 1994, **8**:370–391.

42. Kuipers EJ, Klinkenberg-Knol EC, Festen HPM, Lamers CBHW, Janse JBMJ, Snel P, Nelis F, Meuwissen GM: **Long Term Omeprazole Therapy Does Not Affect Hp Status in Most Patients.** *Scand J Gastroenterol* 1993, **28**:978–980.

43. Bugnoli M, Bayeli PF, Rappuoli R, Pannatii C, Figura N, Crabtree JE: **Inhibition of Helicobacter pylori Urease by Omeprazole.** *Eur J Gastroenterol Hepatol* 1993, **5**:683–685.

44. Westblom TU, Duriex DE: **Enhancement of Antibiotic Concentrations in Gastric Mucosa by H2-Receptor Antagonist.** *Dig Dis Sci* 1991, **36**:25–28

45. Hentschel E, Brandstatter G, Dragosics B, Hirschl AM, Nemec H,
• Schutze K, Taufer M, Wurzer H: **Effect of Ranitidine and Amoxycillin Plus Metronidazole on the Eradication of Helicobacter-pylori and the Recurrence of Duodenal Ulcer.** *N Engl J Med* 1993:**328**:308–312.

A well-designed trial of 104 patients receiving amoxicillin (750 mg three times a day) plus metronidazole (500 mg three times a day) for 12 days with ranitidine (300 mg at night) was compared with ranitidine and placebos alone. Eradication of *H. pylori* was achieved in 46 of 52 patients receiving antibiotics versus 1 of 52 of those given placebo. Ulcer healing was more rapid in the former group with lower relapse (1 of 46 vs 45 of 53).

46. Decross AJ, Marshall BJ, McCallum RW, Hoffman SR, Barrett LJ, Guerrant RL: **Metronidazole Susceptibility Testing for Helicobacter pylori: Comparison of Disk, Broth, and Agar Dilution Methods and Their Clinical Relevance.** *J Clin Microbiol* 1993, **31**:1971–1974.

47. Stables R, Campbell CJ, Clayton NM, Clitherow JW, Grinham CJ, McColm AA, McLaren A, Trevethick MA: **Gastric Anti-Secretory, Mucosal Protective, Anti-Pepsin and Anti-Helicobacter Properties of Ranitidine Bismuth Citrate.** *Aliment Phamacol Ther* 1993, 7:237–246.

48. Wyeth JW, Pounder RE, DeKoster E, Misiewicz JJ, O'Morain CA, Rauws EAJ, Duggan AE: **GR 122311X (Ranitidine Bismuth Citrate) in Antibiotics for the Eradication of H. pylori [Abstract].** *Gastroenterology* 1994, **106**:A212.

49. Eurogast Study Group: **An International Association Between Hp In-**
•• **fection and Gastric Cancer.** *Lancet* 1993, **341**:1359-1362.

A multicenter epidemiologic study revealed an approximate sixfold increase risk of gastric cancer in populations with 100% *H. pylori* infection compared with populations with no infection.

50. Nomura A, Stemmermann GN: **Helicobacter pylori and Gastric Cancer.** *J Gastroenterol Hepatol* 1993, **8**:294-303.

51. Sipponen P, Hyvarinen H: **Role of Helicobacter pylori in the Pathogenesis of Gastritis, Peptic Ulcer and Gastric Ulcer.** *Scand J Gastroenterol* 1993, **28(suppl 196)**:3–6.

52. Sobala GM, Schorah CJ, Shires S, Lynch DAF, Gallagher B, Dixon MF, Axon ATR: **Effect of Eradication of Helicobacter pylori on Gastric Juice Ascorbic Acid Concentrations.** *Gut* 1993, **34**:1038–1041.

53. Banatvala N, Mayo K, Jennings R, Deeks JJ, Feldman RA: **The Cohort Effect and Helicobacter pylori.** *J Infect Dis* 1993, **168**:219–221.

54. Blecker U, Hauser B, Anciers S, Peeters S, Suys B, Vandenplas Y: **The Prevalence of Helicobacter pylori-Positive Serology in Asymptomatic Children.** *J Pediatr Gastroenterol Nutr* 1993, **16**:226–256.

55. Kuipers EJ, Pena AS, van Kemp G, Uyterlinde AM, Pals G, Pels NFM, Kurz-Pohlmann E, Meuwissen SGM: **Seroconversion for Helicobacter pylori.** *Lancet* 1993, **342**:328–331.

56. Hussell T, Isaacson PG, Crabtree JE, Spenser J: **The Response of Cells From Low Grade B-Cell Gastric Lymphomas of Mucosa-Associated Lymphoid Tissue to Helicobacter pylori.** *Lancet* 1993, **342**:571–574.

57. Wotherspoon AC, Doglioni C, Diss TC, Pan L, Moschini A, de Boni M:
•• **Regression of Primary Low-Grade B-Cell Gastric Lymphoma of Mucosa-Associated Lymphoid Tissue After Eradication of Helicobacter pylori.** *Lancet* 1993, **342**:575–77.

A close correlation exists between B-cell gastric mucosa-associated lymphoid tissue lymphoma and *H. pylori*. This group demonstrates the regression of such tumors with *H. pylori* eradication.

David Ng, MB, MRCP(UK), and Roy Pounder, MA, MD, DSc(Med), FRCP, Royal Free Hospital School of Medicine, Rowland Hill Street, London, England, NW3 2PF, UK.

Diagnosis and treatment with endoscopy

Eric Van Cutsem, MD, PhD, and Paul Rutgeerts, MD, PhD

University Hospital Gasthuisberg, Leuven, Belgium

Upper gastrointestinal tract endoscopy plays a key role in the investigation of iron deficiency anemia and upper gastrointestinal hemorrhage. Therapeutic endoscopy improves the outcome in bleeding peptic ulcers, but better prognostic factors are needed for the selection of successful endoscopic hemostasis. A novel concept for predicting re-bleeding based on the appearance of the ulcer base has been proposed and transendoscopic Doppler has been used to examine vessels in ulcers. In variceal bleeding, transjugular intrahepatic portosystemic stent-shunt has been applied with increasing success, although the exact role of this technique has not been determined. Further evidence is given that estrogen-progesterone treatment is effective in the management of patients with severe, recurrent bleeding from gastrointestinal vascular malformations leading to high transfusion requirements. The role of endoscopic ultrasonography (mainly in the preoperative staging of gastric cancer) is further defined, suggesting that this technique, in certain situations, may be superior to radiologic staging methods.

Current Opinion in Gastroenterology 1994, **10**:600–604

Upper gastrointestinal bleeding

Role of upper tract endoscopy in anemia

Occult bleeding from the gastrointestinal tract is widely believed to be the most common cause of iron deficiency anemia in patients without an obvious source of blood loss. There are, however, no study-based guidelines for efficiently managing this disorder. Rockey and Cello [1•] prospectively studied 100 patients with iron-deficiency anemia, using upper gastrointestinal endoscopy and colonoscopy followed by small bowel enteroclysis, and found that endoscopy revealed at least one lesion potentially responsible for blood loss in 62 of 100 patients. Endoscopic examination of the upper gastrointestinal tract showed a bleeding source in 36 patients. Peptic ulceration was the most common cause (19 patients). The authors further conclude that detection of a likely source of blood loss during the initial examination may obviate further procedures, because they rarely found concomitant lesions in the upper and lower gastrointestinal tract [1•]. The data are in contrast with some of the guidelines proposed in a lucid review on iron deficiency anemia [2•]. Sayer and Long state that the lower gastrointestinal tract should be examined in all patients, regardless of upper gastrointestinal endoscopy findings, except in those patients found to have malignancy of the upper gastrointestinal tract [2•].

Ulcer bleeding

It is generally accepted that upper endoscopy provides an excellent diagnostic yield, identifying the source of bleeding in over 90% of cases, and that therapeutic endoscopy improves the outcome of certain bleeding ulcers, *ie*, ulcers with clinical evidence of major bleeding and endoscopic evidence of active bleeding or a nonbleeding, visible vessel. Several studies focus on the ability of endoscopy to predict outcome. Freeman *et al.* [3•] have advanced a novel concept for predicting re-bleeding on the basis of the appearance of the ulcer base at endoscopy. They developed a macroscopic classification of visible vessels: 1) clear, pale, or translucent vessels, 2) vessels with an attached clot, or 3) sentinel clots. Ten of 11 patients with vessels re-bled, whereas none of the seven sentinel clots re-bled [3•]. These findings are interesting, but further studies with a larger number of patients are certainly necessary, especially concerning interobserver agreement on the endoscopic interpretation and classification of these lesions [4].

Two quite similar, well-performed German studies [5•,6•] examined the assessment of bleeding risk in patients with bleeding ulcers as determined by the visual appearance of the ulcer base and by an endoscopic 20-MHz high-frequency Doppler probe. This pulsed Doppler can selectively examine vessels at different depths from the surface. These studies suggest that a pulsed Doppler probe may be more accurate than the endoscopic appearance in predicting the presence of a superficial vessel that is at increased risk of re-bleeding. The real issue, however, is whether using a Doppler probe to assess ulcer vessels and guide endoscopic hemostatic therapy will alter outcome. Therefore, a randomized controlled trial comparing therapy alternatives in two groups of bleeding patients, one guided by endoscopic appearance alone and one by endoscopic appearance and Doppler study, is needed. It seems reasonable that the Doppler may be more ac-

Abbreviations

PEG—percutaneous endoscopic gastrostomy; **TIPS**—transjugular intrahepatic portosystemic stent-shunt.

curate than the eye of the endoscopist, but more data are necessary [7].

In an excellent review on endoscopic hemostasis in nonvariceal bleeding, Gupta and Fleisher [8••] state that several equally efficacious modalities are presently available. Each endoscopist should choose one technique and use it constantly so as to develop ease and expertise. Although several studies compared different hemostatic treatment modalities for nonvariceal bleeding, only small differences, if any, were observed between treatment modalities. Rutgeerts *et al.* [9•] report that injection of absolute alcohol was more effective (but not significantly) than epinephrine-polidocanol in nonbleeding visible vessels. Lin *et al.* [10] concluded from a randomized study in patients with active ulcer bleeding that pure alcohol injection after an epinephrine injection can improve the hemostatic rate, compared with epinephrine alone. Chung *et al.* [11] found that epinephrine was as effective as a combination of epinephrine and 3% sodiumtetradecyl sulphate.

Another new addition to the armamentarium of the therapeutic endoscopist is the endoscopic metallic hemoclip, as described by Binmoeller *et al.* [12•]. Preliminary data in an uncontrolled study indicate that initial hemostasis was achieved in 78 patients with this hemoclip. Further studies are required to evaluate the efficacy and safety of hemoclips for controlling nonvariceal bleeding.

Three excellent reviews discuss the pathogenesis and treatment of gastrointestinal bleeding [8••,13•,14•].

Varices

Binmoeller *et al.* [15•] and Goff [16•] reviewed the treatment of bleeding esophageal varices. Endoscopic sclerotherapy is the procedure of choice for the management of bleeding esophageal varices. New therapeutic options such as endoscopic variceal ligation and transjugular intrahepatic portosystemic stent-shunt (TIPS) have entered the therapeutic arena. The first comparative studies have appeared and show promising results. Further studies are needed to distinguish subgroups of patients who are more likely to benefit from one of the techniques. TIPS may also be of value in the treatment of gastric varices, but further studies are needed to clarify its exact role.

Dieulafoy's lesions

The treatment of bleeding Dieulafoy's lesion remains controversial; many authors still favor surgical treatment. An uncontrolled study by Baettig *et al.* [17] suggests that endoscopic sclerotherapy with adrenaline and polidocanol is very effective in patients with active bleeding from Dieulafoy's lesions. Two articles [18,19] describe the use of transendoscopic Doppler ultrasound to identify arterial blood flow from these lesions and suggest that a high success rate can be obtained by Doppler-controlled endoscopic sclerotherapy.

Vascular malformations

Foutch [20••] reviews the clinical outlook, the difficulties in the diagnosis, and the treatment of angiodysplasia of the gastrointestinal tract. Endoscopic and hormonal treatment are discussed. Van Cutsem *et al.* [21••] report on the long-term outcome of a double-blind, randomized placebo-controlled, cross-over trial using 0.050 mg of ethinylestradiol and 1 mg of norethisterone in patients with severely bleeding lesions and high transfusion requirements. The study indicates that estrogen-progesterone treatment is effective in patients with severely bleeding vascular malformations and that the effect persists for a mean period of approximately 10 months. The mechanism of action, however, is not known. Stalder [22•] proposes a diagnostic and therapeutic algorithm for managing patients with bleeding arteriovenous malformations:

1. Search for vascular malformations by upper gastrointestinal endoscopy and colonoscopy and exclude other lesions responsible for bleeding
2. Attempt to treat all bleeding lesions endoscopically with laser, electrocoagulation, or injection sclerotherapy
3. If the bleeding cannot be identified, proceed to selective angiography or enteroscopy
4. If the bleeding lesion can be identified, but not treated, consider surgery. However, we have not had good experiences with the surgical treatment of vascular malformations, especially small bowel lesions, which are often spread throughout the bowel
5. If the above diagnostic and therapeutic means are not successful or if bleeding is recurrent, necessitating multiple transfusions, hormonal therapy should be attempted

Two uncontrolled trials, in a relatively small number of patients, suggest efficacy for the neodymium:yttrium-aluminum-garnet laser in treating bleeding watermelon stomach [23,24].

Portal hypertensive gastropathy and radiation-induced injury

Two studies from the Mayo Clinic report on relatively rare conditions associated with bleeding [25,26]. Gostout *et al.* [25] describe 12 patients with bleeding portal hypertensive gastropathy. The management of chronic and recurrent bleeding remains a problem. Further exploration of pharmacologic (*eg*, propranolol, nitrates), radiologic (TIPS), and surgical therapies (portosystemic shunt and transplantation) to control bleeding is needed. Zighelboim *et al.* [26] show that neodymium:yttrium-aluminum-garnet laser coagulation is an effective and safe treatment in bleeding radiation induced mucosal vascular lesions in the upper gastrointestinal tract and proximal colon in 15 patients.

Endoscopic feeding techniques

More than 10 years after its original description, percutaneous endoscopic gastrostomy (PEG) continues to be

Table 1. Accuracy of endoscopic ultrasonography in the preoperative determination of the T stage in 254 patients with gastric carcinoma*

Histopathologic T stage	Patients, *n*	EUS correct, *n(%)*	EUS overstaging, *n(%)*	EUS understaging, *n(%)*
pT1	27	22(81)	T2 5(19)	—
pT2	52	37(71)	T3 14(27)	T1 1(2)
pT3	151	132(87)	T4 8(5)	T2 11(7)
pT4	24	19(79)	—	T3 5(21)
All cases†	254	210(83)	27(11)	17(7)

**From* Dittler and Siewert [28••]; with permission.
†Accuracy 83%, overstaging 11%, understaging 7%, sensitivity 83%, specificity 94%.
EUS—endoscopic ultrasonography.

a subject of considerable interest. In a comprehensive review, Melliger and Ponsky [27••] discuss the technical aspects, safety, and complications of PEG. PEG is a safe and easy way of delivering nutritional support to patients who cannot swallow but have a normal gastrointestinal tract. Currently, much of the activity in the field of endoscopic feeding techniques has focused on jejunal access issues. Several abstracts describe percutaneous endoscopic jejunostomy techniques. Percutaneous endoscopic jejunostomy can be very useful in patients with gastroesophageal reflux or gastric evacuation problems, or in patients who have undergone a gastric resection, provided an easy and safe technique becomes available.

Endoscopic ultrasonography for gastric cancer

Two studies evaluated the accuracy of endoscopic ultrasonography for the preoperative staging of gastric cancer. Dittler and Siewert [28••] compared endoscopic ultrasonographic findings with postoperative histologic findings in 254 patients with gastric cancer who underwent surgery. They concluded that endoscopic ultrasonography was correct in determining the T and N stage in 83% and 66% of patients, respectively (Tables 1 and 2). Although endoscopic ultrasonography was accurate in determining the absence of lymph node metastases (accuracy in stage N0 = 93%), it was not reliable in determining N1 and N2 (64% and 52%, respectively). They suggested that the concomitant T stage may be an important criterion for assessing the nature of endosonographically visualized lymph nodes because 88% of all T3 and T4 tumors had lymph node metastases.

In a similar study, 147 patients who underwent surgery for gastric cancer, the accuracy of endoscopic ultrasonography was 78% in assessing tumor infiltration depth [29•]. The most frequent causes of misdiagnosis by endosonography were microscopic tumor invasion and peritumorous inflammatory changes. *In vitro* studies on lymph nodes removed from patients with esophageal and gastric cancer suggest that although the subjective assessment of internal echo patterns (homogeneity) and node margins by an experienced observer allow the accurate diagnosis of metastatic lymph nodes, there is a high proportion of false-positives (52%) and thus a relatively low specificity of the technique [30•].

Abe *et al.* [31] discussed various graphic classifications for the endoscopic ultrasonographic prediction of depth of transmural penetration of gastric cancer. In a comprehensive review of endoscopic ultrasonography, Rösch [32•] also discusses the value of endoscopic ultrasonography in the diagnosis of gastric lymphoma. It is suggested that endoscopic ultrasonography can be useful in monitoring the effect of chemotherapy in gastric lymphoma but not in gastric adenocarcinoma. In this article, the value of endoscopic ultrasonography in benign gastric disorders, such as portal hypertension and large gastric folds, is also discussed [32•].

Treatment of gastric cancer

A large Japanese study reports positive results from endoscopic laser treatment in early gastric cancer and

Table 2. Accuracy in the preoperative determination of the N stage in 254 patients with gastric carcinoma*

Histopathologic N stage	Patients, *n*	EUS correct, *n(%)*	EUS incorrect, *n(%)*
pN0	71	66(93)	N1 5(7) false-positive
pN1	51	33(65)	N0 18(35) false-negative
pN2	132	69(52)	N0 35(27) N1 28(21) false-negative
All cases†	254	168(66)	86(34)

**From* Dittler and Siewert [28••]; with permission.
†Accuracy for the N stage 66%, sensitivity 66%, specificity 93%.
EUS—endoscopic ultrasonography

from a combination of endoscopic mucosal resection and laser treatment [33]. Lambert [34•] reviews the indications and possibilities of endoscopic treatment of esophagogastric tumors.

Pathology

Ectors *et al.* [35•] report that more than half of patients with granulomatous gastritis have Crohn's disease, 25% have an isolated granulomatous gastritis, and 10% have a foreign body reaction.

Wolfsen *et al.* [36] examined 23 patients previously diagnosed as having Menetrier's disease and concluded that two distinct histologic entities with similar clinical manifestations may explain the variable finding of mucosal inflammation in Menetrier's disease. Patients with massive foveolar hyperplasia and minimal inflammation represent a form of hypertrophic gastropathy and should be designated as having Menetrier's disease, whereas patients with hypertrophic lymphocytic gastritis should be considered part of the spectrum of lymphocytic gastritis.

Two prospective, multicenter Italian studies [37•,38•] investigated the outcome in patients with moderate or severe gastric dysplasia and concluded that moderate gastric dysplasia shows a high risk of cancer development and requires a strict bioptic follow-up (*eg,* every 3 months). The finding of severe gastric dysplasia should warrant surgery because it is often associated with gastric cancer.

References and recommended reading

Papers of particular interest, published within the annual period of review, have been highlighted as:

- • Of special interest
- •• Of outstanding interest

1. Rockey DC, Cello JP: **Evaluation of the Gastrointestinal Tract in Patients**
• **With Iron-Deficiency Anemia.** *N Engl J Med* 1993, **329**:1691–1695.
Prospective study investigating the role and diagnostic value of gastrointestinal investigation in patients with iron-deficiency anemia. Detection of a likely source during upper endoscopy may obviate colonoscopy.

2. Sayer JM, Long RG: **A Perspective on Iron Deficiency Anaemia.** *Gut*
• 1993, **34**:1297–1299.
Review discussing the differential diagnosis of iron deficiency anemia. Colonoscopy should be performed in all patients, except those in whom upper endoscopy reveals malignancy.

3. Freeman ML, Cass OW, Peine CJ, Onstad GR: **The Non-bleeding Visible**
• **Vessel Versus the Sentinel Clot: Natural History and Risk of Rebleeding.** *Gastrointest Endosc* 1993, **39**:359–366.
Important study of natural history of stigmata of recent hemorrhage. The authors report that visible vessels have an extremely high likelihood of rebleeding, whereas sentinel clots did not.

4. Laine L: **Refining the Prognostic Value of Endoscopy in Patients Presenting With Bleeding Ulcers.** *Gastrointest Endosc* 1993, **39**:461–462.

5. Kohler LB, Riemann JF: **Endoscopic Injection Therapy of Forrest II and**
• **III Gastroduodenal Ulcers Guided by Endoscopic Doppler Ultrasound.** *Endoscopy* 1993, **25**:219–223.
Study showing that endoscopic Doppler appears to be a valuable diagnostic procedure in the assessment of bleeding ulcers.

6. Jaspersen D, Korner T, Schorr W, Wzatek J, Hammar C-H, Klingman
• R: **Diagnosis and Treatment Control of Gastroduodenal Ulcer Haemorrhage With an Endoscopic Doppler Device.** *Eur J Gastroenterol Hepatol* 1993, **5**:471–474.
Study stressing the value of endoscopic Doppler in the assessment of bleeding ulcers.

7. Silverstein F: **Ulcer Bleeding Stigmata: What is Better than the Endoscopist's Eye?** *Endoscopy* 1993, **25**:246–247.

8. Gupta PK, Fleischer D: **Endoscopic Hemostasis in Nonvariceal Bleed-**
•• **ing.** *Endoscopy* 1994, **26**:48–54.
Excellent review on endoscopic hemostasis in nonvariceal bleeding.

9. Rutgeerts P, Gevers AM, Hiele M, Broeckaert L, Vantrappen G: **Endo-**
• **scopic Injection Therapy to Prevent Rebleeding From Peptic Ulcers With a Protruding Vessel: A Controlled Comparative Trial.** *Gut* 1993, **34**:348–350.
Prospective randomized trial comparing the efficacy of alcohol with epinephrine polidocanol.

10. Lin HJ, Perng CL, Lee SD: **Is Sclerosant Injection Mandatory After an Epinephrine Injection for Arrest of Peptic Ulcer Haemorrhage? A Prospective, Randomised, Comparative Study.** *Gut* 1993, **34**:1182–1185.

11. Chung SS, Leung JW, Leong HT, Lo KK, Li AK: **Adding a Sclerosant to Endoscopic Epinephrine Injection in Actively Bleeding Ulcers: A Randomized Trial.** *Gastrointest Endosc* 1993, **39**:611–615.

12. Binmoeller KF, Thonke F, Soehendra N: **Endoscopic Hemoclip Treat-**
• **ment for Gastrointestinal Bleeding.** *Endoscopy* 1993, **25**:167–170.
This study evaluated the role of metallic clip for the treatment of nonvariceal gastrointestinal bleeding.

13. Laine L: **Rolling Review: Upper Gastrointestinal Bleeding.** *Aliment*
• *Pharmacol Ther* 1993, **7**:207–232.
Review of the different causes and treatment modalities of upper gastrointestinal bleeding.

14. Zuccaro G: **Bleeding Peptic Ulcer: Pathogenesis and Endoscopic Ther-**
• **apy.** *Gastroenterol Clin North Am* 1993, **22**:737–750.
This article reviewed the pathogenesis and endoscopic therapy of bleeding peptic ulcer.

15. Binmoeller KF, Vadeyar HJ, Soehendra N: **Treatment of Esophageal**
• **Varices.** *Endoscopy* 1994, **26**:42–47.
Excellent review on the treatment of esophageal varices.

16. Goff JS: **Gastroesophageal Varices: Pathogenesis and Therapy of Acute**
• **Bleeding.** *Gastroenterol Clin North Am* 1993 **22**:779–800.
The pathogenesis and therapy of acute variceal bleeding was reviewed.

17. Baettig B, Haecki W, Lammer F, Jost R: **Dieulafoy's Disease: Endoscopic Treatment and Follow-up.** *Gut* 1993, **34**:1418–1421.

18. Jaspersen D, Gaster CB, Koerner TH, Hammar CH: **Alimentary Tract and Pancreas. Doppler-Controlled Injection Treatment of Dieulafoy's Disease.** *J Gastroenterol Hepatol* 1993, **8**:267–269.

19. Jaspersen D: **Dieulafoy's Disease Controlled by Doppler Ultrasound Endoscopic Treatment.** *Gut* 1993, **34**:857–858.

20. Foutch PG: **Angiodysplasia of the Gastrointestinal Tract.** *Am J Gas-*
•• *troenterol* 1993, **88**:807–818.
Clinical review discussing the different aspects of angiodysplasia of the gastrointestinal tract.

21. Van Cutsem E, Rutgeerts P, Vantrappen G: **Long-term Effect of Hor-**
•• **monal Therapy for Bleeding Gastrointestinal Vascular Malformations.** *Eur J Gastroenterol Hepatol* 1993, **5**:439–443.
This double-blind randomized trial showed the effect of ethinylestradiol and progesterone in patients with high transfusion requirements due to bleeding gastrointestinal vascular malformations.

22. Stalder GA: **How to Treat Patients With Gastrointestinal Arterio-venous**
• **Malformations.** *Eur J Gastroenterol Hepatol* 1993, **5**:437–438.
This article proposes a concrete diagnostic and therapeutic work-up in patients with chronic bleeding vascular malformations.

23. Labenz J, Borsch G: **Bleeding Watermelon Stomach Treated by Nd-YAG Laser Photocoagulation.** *Endoscopy* 1993, **25**:240–242.

24. Potamiano S, Carter CR, Anderson JR: **Endoscopic Laser Treatment of Diffuse Gastric Antral Vascular Ectasia.** *Gut* 1994, **35**:461–463.

25. Gostout CJ, Viggiano TR, Balm RK: **Acute Gastrointestinal Bleeding From Portal Hypertensive Gastropathy: Prevalence and Clinical Features.** *Am J Gastroenterol* 1993, **88**:2030–2033.

26. Zighelboim J, Viggiano TR, Ahlquist DA, Gostout CJ, Wang KK, Larson MV: **Endoscopic Laser Coagulation of Radiation-Induced Mucosal Vascular Lesions in the Upper Gastrointestinal Tract and Proximal Colon.** *Am J Gastroenterol* 1993, **88**:1224–1227.

27. Mellinger JD, Ponsky JL: **Percutaneous Endoscopic Gastrostomy.** *En-*
•• *doscopy* 1994, **26**:55–59.
Article discussing the technical aspects and the complications of PEG.

28. Dittler HJ, Siewert JR: **Role of Endoscopic Ultrasonography in Gastric**
•• **Carcinoma.** *Endoscopy* 1993, **25**:162–166.
Extensive study in esophageal and gastric cancer staging, analyzing the T and N stages and the R classification. Surgical control with tumor removal is available in all cases.

29. • Grimm H, Binmoeller KF, Hamper K, Koch J, Henne-Bruns D, Soehendra N: **Endosonography for Preoperative Locoregional Staging of Esophageal and Gastric Cancer.** *Endoscopy* 1993, **25**:224–230.

A large experience of endoscopic ultrasound in the staging of esophageal and gastric cancer is reported.

30. • Heintz A, Mildenberger P, Georg M, Braunstein S, Junginger TH: **Endoscopic Ultrasonography in the Diagnosis of Regional Lymph Nodes in Esophageal and Gastric Cancer: Results of Studies In Vitro.** *Endoscopy* 1993, **25**:231–235.

In vitro study on the ultrasonographic appearance of malignant lymph nodes.

31. Abe S, Lightdale CJ, Brennan MJ: **The Japanese Experience With Endoscopic Ultrasonography in the Staging of Gastric Cancer.** *Gastrointest Endosc* 1993, **39**:586–591.

32. • Rösch T: **Endoscopic Ultrasonography.** *Endoscopy* 1994, **26**:148–168.

Comprehensive review on endoscopic ultrasonography.

33. Yasuda K, Mizuma Y, Nakajima M, Kawai K: **Endoscopic Laser Treatment for Early Gastric Cancer.** *Endoscopy* 1993, **25**:451–454.

34. • Lambert R: **Endoscopic Treatment of Esophago-Gastric Tumors.** *Endoscopy* 1994, **26**:28–35.

Review on the endoscopic treatment of esophagogastric tumors.

35. • Ectors NL, Dixon MF, Geboes KJ, Rutgeerts PJ, Desmet VJ, Vantrappen GR: **Granulomatous Gastritis: A Morphological and Diagnostic Approach.** *Histopathology* 1993, **23**:55–61.

This study examines the biopsies and the clinical and laboratory data in 71 patients with granulomatous gastritis. Crohn's disease was the most frequent etiology.

36. Wolfsen HC, Carpenter HA, Talley NJ: **Menetrier's Disease: A Form of Hypertrophic Gastropathy or Gastritis?** *Gastroenterology* 1993, **104**:1310–1319.

37. • Farinati F, Rugge M, Di Mario F, Valiante F, Baffa R: **Early and Advanced Gastric Cancer in the Follow-Up of Moderate and Severe Gastric Dysplasia Patients. A Prospective Study.** *Endoscopy* 1993, **25**:261–264.

Prospective multicenter study examining the significance of gastric epithelial dysplasia as precursor of gastric cancer.

38. • Fertitta AM, Comin U, Terruzzi V, Minoli G, Zambelli A, Cannatelli G, Bodini P, Bertoli G, Negri R, Brunati S, Fiocca R, Turpini F, Prada A, Ceretti E, Gullotta R, Cornaggia M: **Clinical Significance of Gastric Dysplasia: A Multicenter Follow-up Study.** *Endoscopy* 1993, **25**:265–268.

Prospective multicenter study examining the significance of moderate or severe gastric dysplasia.

Eric Van Cutsem, MD, PhD, and Paul Rutgeerts, MD, PhD, University Hospital Gasthuisberg, Herestraat 49, 3000 Leuven, Belgium

New trends in gastroduodenal surgery

Marek Rudnicki, MD, PhD, and Michael S. Gold, MD

The Mary Imogene Bassett Hospital, Cooperstown, New York, USA

Laparoscopic techniques continue to replace conventional open surgery in the treatment of many gastrointestinal disorders. Excellent results from the "minimal access" approach have been reported for gastroesophageal reflux and peptic ulcer disease. The incidence of gastric cancer continues to decline and lesions become more proximally located. However, aggressive surgical therapies have not resulted in increased cure rates. Treatment of pancreatic and extrapancreatic gastrinomas centers on surgical resection for potential malignancy. Gastric bypass seems to provide the best weight reduction in morbid obesity, with acceptably low side effects and complications.

Current Opinion in Gastroenterology 1994, **10**:605–609

Novel technologies, inventive techniques of visualization of gastrointestinal lesions, potency of pharmacologic agents, and advancements in perioperative care have given surgery a new perspective. Laparoscopic technology has already revolutionized operative treatment of gallstones. It may, in the near future, revolutionize gastroduodenal surgery.

Gastroesophageal reflux and hiatal hernia

Symptomatic gastroesophageal reflux continues to play an important role in surgical as well as gastroenterologic practice. Perioperative morbidity and long recovery after open Nissen fundoplication have caused most patients to choose long-term pharmacologic treatment. The development of laparoscopic techniques has allowed a reassessment of the surgical treatment of the incompetent lower esophageal sphincter. "Minimal access" technology uses well-established maneuvers to wrap the gastric fundus around the cardia. The first small series of laparoscopic Nissen fundoplications compare favorably with those of conventional fundoplications with respect to mortality, complications, and outcome, but with a more rapid recovery and less pain in the postoperative period [1,2••]. Early follow-up shows that Nissen, Hill, or Toupet (partial fundoplication) antireflux procedures can be performed successfully using a laparoscopic approach, with equivalent clinical outcome to open procedures [1,2••,3•,4•,5]. The cost of surgery is comparable with the expense of several years of treatment with gastric antisecretory drugs and repeated endoscopies. Laparoscopic surgery is now recommended in younger patients with documented symptomatic gastroesophageal reflux.

With further advancements in laparoscopic technology and surgical experience, this approach increases options available for repair of hiatal hernias. Excellent outcome without adverse sequela in early follow-up indicates that the laparoscopic approach will replace conventional open therapy in many patients [2••].

Peptic ulcer

With the availability of effective medication for control of gastric acidity, the need for elective surgical treatment of peptic ulcers has disappeared. In the past decade, there has been an 80% decrease in elective acid-reducing operations in the Western world. Eradication of *Helicobacter pylori* and potent antisecretory drugs successfully control and prevent the majority of peptic ulcers. The development of new laparoscopic techniques may shed a new light on the value of surgical treatment for peptic ulcer disease using procedures that carry low morbidity, short hospital stays, and rapid return to normal activities without the potential long-term consequences of medications [6••]. Cost analyses may prove that surgery is more cost-effective than long-term drug therapy to prevent symptomatic recurrence and acute complications [7]. Encouraging reports from a few centers seem to indicate that laparoscopic parietal cell vagotomy or posterior truncal vagotomy with anterior seromyotomy may be an alternative to medical treatment [8,9]. One should be cautious, however, not to repeat errors from the past by altering the indications for surgery simply because it can be performed laparoscopically. Balloon pyloroplasty can be successfully used with laparoscopic truncal vagotomy in the treatment of peptic ulcer in selected patients. With the development of new laparoscopic procedures, the approach to gastric surgery is changing. Reports are still very limited but it has been shown that laparoscopic gastric resection with Billroth II anastomosis can be performed safely [10•]. Laparoscopic resections result in decreased postoperative pain, quicker mobilization, fewer wound problems, better cosmesis, and quicker discharge.

Despite the reduced number of elective operations for peptic ulcer over the past several years, surgery remains the best treatment for gastric and duodenal perforations. Improved perioperative care allows a definitive approach, including gastric resection, in situations that previously would have been best treated with sim-

 ISBN 1-85922-611-6 ISSN 0267–1379

ple closure [11]. Successful closure of perforations with omental patch using a laparoscopic technique indicates that further development of this procedure should be anticipated [12]. However, in our zeal to embrace new technology, we must not be quick to abandon time-tested and proven procedures. Table 1 depicts several treatment modalities for peptic ulcer using laparoscopic techniques.

Table 1. Various laparoscopic approaches to peptic ulcer disease

Elective
- Laparoscopic truncal vagotomy + balloon pyloroplasty
- Transthoracic truncal vagotomy + balloon or open pyloroplasty
- Parietal cell vagotomy
- Posterior vagotomy + anterior parietal cell vagotomy
- Posterior vagotomy + anterior seromyotomy
- Billroth II gastrectomy with or without vagotomy

Urgent (for peptic ulcer perforation)
- Laparoscopic closure with sutures
- Laparoscopic omental patch
- Laparoscopic omental patch with truncal vagotomy (subsequent pyloroplasty)
- Laparoscopic closure with selective vagotomy

At the present time, a sensible "mini-invasive" laparoscopic approach has not been worked out for patients whose ulcers are actively bleeding. Endoscopic control of upper gastrointestinal bleeding has decreased the mortality and need for emergency operations (Table 2) [13•].

Table 2. Comparison of pretherapeutic endoscopy data on bleeding peptic ulcers*

Year	Patients, *n*	Age, *y*	Operation rate, *n/n*(%)	Mortality rate, *n/n*(%)
1982	908	64	245/980 (27)	54/245 (22)
1982	580	58	91/580 (15)	19/91 (21)
1993	1213	46	42/659 (6.4)	3/24 (7.1)

*From Williams *et al.* [13•]; with permission

Gastric cancer

As the biology and pattern of gastric cancer changes, it is hoped that new diagnostic and therapeutic strategies will influence long-term results. The incidence of gastric cancer continues to diminish in the United States [14••]. Previously, Asians were considered particularly prone to develop gastric cancer. Recently, the incidence of gastric carcinoma even in Japan has declined and shows a trend toward occurring later in life [15]. This decrease is mainly caused by the reduction of carcinoma of the well-differentiated type and is also highly correlated to the decline in carcinoma of the antrum, previously the most common type seen in Japan. A similar, significant shift of lesions to a proximal location was noted in a US study, which showed 31% of lesions in the upper third of the stomach, 14% in the middle third, and 26% in the distal third. This change in location suggests that as the incidence of the disease has decreased over time, the decline has been primarily in the cancers occurring in the distal part of the stomach, with a steady rise in the incidence of gastroesophageal carcinomas (Fig. 1) [16,17•].

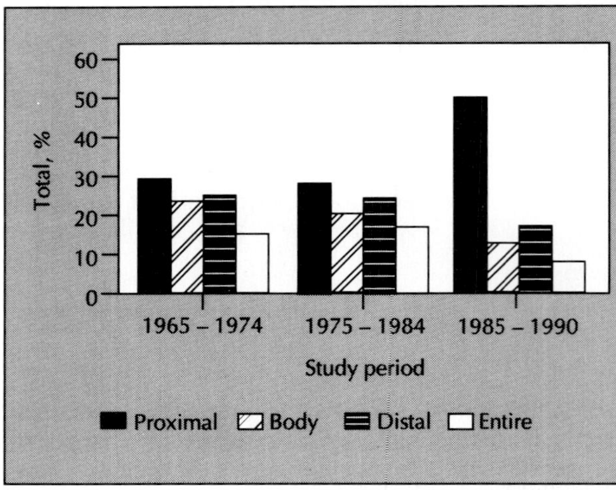

Fig. 1. Location of gastric cancers over the three study periods. *P*=0.0025. (*From* Salvon-Harmon *et al.* [17•]; with permission.)

A recent US review showed that 26% of 18,365 gastric cancer patients had a history of peptic ulcer [14••]. This high frequency of peptic ulcers emphasizes the need for aggressive diagnostic and therapeutic approaches to this entity and might indicate that gastric ulcers may be incorrectly diagnosed or perhaps undertreated. The following stages in the development of gastric cancer have been suggested: chronic gastritis, atrophy, intestinal metaplasia, and dysplasia [18]. It is suspected that prior infection with *H. pylori*, by causing chronic gastritis, may increase the susceptibility to develop gastric carcinoma. This view is supported by three arguments: 1) *H. pylori* infection causes chronic antral gastritis, 2) chronic antral gastritis may eventually lead to gastric atrophy and intestinal metaplasia, and 3) gastric atrophy and especially intestinal metaplasia are associated with an increased risk of cancer [19]. A sixfold increased risk of gastric cancer in populations with documented *H. pylori* infection compared with a population that had no infection was demonstrated in a European multicenter study [20••]. Interestingly, this infection is closely associated with differentiated gastric cancers, but not with undifferentiated types [21]. It is unlikely, however, that *H. pylori* is the sole contributing factor in the development of gastric cancer.

The effect of pregnancy and delivery on gastric cancer was examined in female patients 34 years of age or younger. Gastric cancer diagnosed within 2 years of pregnancy and delivery was more aggressive than that seen in young female patients with previous pregnancies or without children, or similar-aged male patients. The 5-year survival rate was also lower in this group (60%) versus control groups (83% to 85%). Eight patients became pregnant after gastrectomy for gastric cancer. Seven delivered healthy children without abnormalities, whereas one patient died during pregnancy. This study suggests that pregnancy or delivery in young women may accelerate the growth of gastric cancer [22].

Perineural invasion is an important route for local spread of gastric cancer. Immunohistochemical staining of laminin was used to visualize malignant cell infiltration into the perineurium or neural fasciculus in specimens of gastric cancers in which primary lesions extended to or through the muscularis propria. Five-year survival was 24% for patients in whom staining was positive for perineural invasion, whereas for patients with negative staining, 5-year survival rate was 71%. The presence of perineural invasion has a significant impact on prognosis of T2 tumors but not in those patients with T3 or T4 lesions [23•]. If further studies on different populations of patients confirm similar characteristics of perineural invasion, this method may be useful in determining the prognosis of advanced gastric cancer.

Adjuvant therapy after gastrectomy

The stage of disease and survival outcome after surgical resection for gastric cancer remains unchanged despite increased availability and sophistication of diagnostic techniques. Over the years there was hope that adjuvant therapy in addition to extensive surgical treatment would yield better long-term results. Meta-analysis of randomized trials published between 1980 and 1991 show that adjuvant chemotherapy regimens do not improve survival. Postoperative chemotherapy offered no additional survival benefit for patients with curatively resected gastric cancers [24••]. Intraperitoneal chemotherapy with cisplatin also proved ineffective in the treatment of advanced gastric cancer [25]. Preoperative and postoperative chemotherapy with etoposide, doxorubicin, and cisplatin demonstrated very limited effect on survival of patients with resectable gastric carcinoma, but was associated with substantial morbidity and mortality [26]. There is some hope that results of prospective studies of combined fluorouracil and leucovorin adjuvant therapy combined with upper abdominal irradiation can improve survival in patients who have undergone gastrectomy for gastric cancer [27••].

Zollinger-Ellison syndrome

Although it is almost 50 years since Zollinger and Ellison described the gastrinoma syndrome, little is known about the pathogenesis of these relatively well-differentiated endocrine tumors. Recently, it has been demonstrated that amplification of the *HER-2/neu* protooncogene occurs in gastrinoma tumors and gastrinoma cell lines. Because no alterations in *p53* or *ras* gene was shown, it may suggest that an amplified *HER2/neu* gene may be involved in the molecular tumorigenesis of these lesions [28••].

Functional pancreatic gastrinomas cause two problems: the control of the clinical manifestations related to overproduction of gastrin, and the malignant nature of tumors. The syndrome is characterized by intractable peptic ulcer, increased gastric acidity, and elevated serum gastrin. With the ability to control the effects of gastrin overproduction with potent antisecretory agents, malignant transformation remains the determinant of long-term survival after surgical excision.

The role of magnetic resonance imaging was compared with other imaging techniques in a prospective study of 43 patients with Zollinger-Ellison syndrome [29]. Results of preoperative tests were assessed at exploratory laparotomy or by liver biopsy. Magnetic resonance imaging had a sensitivity of 83% for 18 patients with metastatic gastrinoma to the liver, ultrasound 50%, computed tomography 56% (including contrast-enhanced dynamic computed tomography), and angiography 61%. For the localization of primary gastrinoma in 32 patients, magnetic resonance imaging had a sensitivity of 25%, ultrasound 19%, computed tomography 28%, and all three combined 38%, whereas angiography had 59%. Advances in magnetic resonance imaging have greatly improved its sensitivity for detection and assessment of the extent of metastatic gastrinoma to the liver [29].

Magnetic resonance imaging should be the primary study for detecting the presence of metastatic gastrinoma in the liver and their response to chemotherapy. Angiography remains the study of choice for detection, localization, and evaluation of resectability of primary gastrinomas. Abdominal ultrasound is not useful to visualize pancreatic or extrapancreatic endocrine tumors. Endoscopic ultrasound, however, seems to be promising in the localization of small submucosal neuroendocrine tumors of the gastrointestinal tract. This method makes it possible to observe the intramural structure of the stomach and duodenum in detail as cross-sectional images. The accuracy rate for lesions detectable by endoscopic ultrasonography reached 90%. Moreover, this method allowed direct detection of perigastroduodenal lymph node metastases [30]. Further use of this method raises the possibility of local endoscopic excision of small submucosal lesions with subsequent close follow-up. Extrapancreatic, mainly duodenal, lesions account for 23% of all gastrinomas [31••].

Flow cytometry has been used to determine whether DNA analysis may have a role in determining prognosis in gastrinoma. A strong correlation was found between extent of disease and both ploidy and S-phase percentage. High S-phase percentage was associated with widespread metastatic disease. Therefore it was suggested that multiple stem line aneuploid tumors with high S-phase percentages may have a poor prognosis whereas nontetraploid aneuploid tumors with low S-phase percentage may have a better outcome [32]. The same group suggested that fasting serum gastrin determinations and secretin-provocative testing at different postoperative times can be used to predict the probability of a patient remaining disease free at 3 years after surgery. The calcium-provocative test and imaging studies do not detect recurrences before changes in plasma gastrin levels are noted [33•].

Many patients with Zollinger-Ellison syndrome must undergo long-term gastric antisecretory treatment. Although omeprazole significantly inhibits gastric acid secretion, its prolonged use increases serum gastrin concentrations and fundic argyrophil cell densities in patients with gastrinoma. Exogenously induced hypochlorhydria may promote cell proliferation in the primary tumor, resulting in the growth of gastrinoma lesions [34•].

Obesity

Despite numerous procedures for weight reduction, none fulfill the criteria of low morbidity and ideal loss of weight. A preliminary report of a new method for surgical treatment of morbid obesity has recently been published from Duke University. Near-total intestinal bypass was performed in eight patients by anastomosing the proximal 25 to 30 cm of jejunum to transverse colon. A central venous catheter was placed for home infusion of fluids, minerals, vitamins, and protein to maintain adequate metabolism during the period of significant postoperative weight loss. After the desired body mass was achieved, the jejunocolostomy was taken down with construction of a vertical banded gastroplasty to assist in weight maintenance. The average weight loss was 1.5 kg/wk during the jejunocolostomy phase. Subsequent conversion to a vertical gastroplasty afforded maintenance of weight loss for up to 3.5 years [35]. Although the combination of two surgical procedures has some rationale, rates of complications for total treatment could be higher than for a single procedure. Combined treatment and prolonged use of supplementary infusions did not prevent increased liver steatosis as assessed by biopsy, although it did lessen the occurrence of abnormal liver function tests.

Age limits are being extended for many procedures, including bariatric surgery. Eighty-eight morbidly obese patients 55 years of age and older underwent Roux-en-Y gastric bypass or vertical gastroplasty [36]. Fifteen patients (17%) had a total of 30 early complications with no deaths within the first postoperative month. Sixteen patients (18%) developed late complications, which included staple-line disruption, incisional hernia, cholelithiasis, and peptic ulcer. Seven patients (8%) died from causes unrelated to surgery, although one suicide may have indicated the patient's dissatisfaction with the results of surgery. Surgical treatment resulted in an average of 57% excess body weight loss, reduction in medication required for obesity-related disorders, and a decreased body mass index to less than 30 kg/m^2 in 42% of patients [36]. These results are not different from those seen in younger patients. Although one should be very careful with recommendations for bariatric surgery for older patients, these data indicate that surgical therapy should not be withheld from appropriately selected patients in the older age groups. There seems to be general agreement that gastric bypass results in greater weight loss and less complications than after vertical gastroplasty [37••]. Gastric bypass is also the recommended reoperation after any failed weight reduction procedure [38•].

References and recommended reading

Papers of particular interest, published within the annual period of review, have been highlighted as:

- • Of special interest
- •• Of outstanding interest

1. Bittner HB, Meyers WC, Brazer SR, Pappas TN: **Laparoscopic Nissen Fundoplication: Operative Results and Short-Term Follow-Up.** *Am J Surg* 1994, **167**:193–198.

2. •• Cushieri A: **Laparoscopic Antireflux Surgery and Repair of Hiatal Hernia.** *World J Surg* 1993, **17**:40–45.

These are novel operations that use a modern laparoscopic approach for surgical treatment of gastroesophageal reflux and hiatal hernia.

3. • McKernan JB, Laws HL: **Laparoscopic Nissen Fundoplication for the Treatment of Gastroesophageal Reflux Disease.** *Am Surg* 1994, **60**:87–93.

Details technique of laparoscopic treatment for symptomatic gastroesophageal reflux disease refractory to conventional medical therapy.

4. • Aye RW, Hill LD, Kraemer SJM, Snopkowski P: **Early Results With the Laparoscopic Hill Repair.** *Am J Surg* 1994, **167**:542–546.

Follow-up of 40 patients after laparoscopic Hill repair for gastroesophageal reflux disease. It is concluded that Hill repair is safe, highly effective and has potential advantages over the laparoscopic Nissen procedure.

5. Swanstrom L, Wayne R: **Spectrum of Gastrointestinal Symptoms After Laparoscopic Fundoplication.** *Am J Surg* 1994, **167**:538–541.

6. •• Soper NJ, Brunt LM, Kerbl K: **Laparoscopic General Surgery.** *N Engl J Med* 1994, **330**:409–419.

A practical review of the present laparoscopic techniques used in gastrointestinal surgery.

7. Taylor TV, Bhandarkar DS: **Laparoscopic Vagotomy: An Operation for the 1990s?** *Ann R Coll Surg Engl* 1993, **75**:385–386.

8. Jensen PM, Wara P, Bardram L, Srage JG. **Laparoscopic Parietal Cell Vagotomy: Preliminary Results.** *Ugerskr Laeger* 1993, **155**:2603–2605.

9. Bailey RW, Zucker KA, Flowers JL: **Vagotomy.** In: *Laparoscopic Surgery.* Edited by Ballantyne GH, Leahy PF, Modlin IM. Philadelphia: WB Saunders Company; 1994: 405–419.

10. • Goh P, Kum CK: **Laparoscopic Billroth II Gastrectomy: A Review.** *Surg Oncol* 1993, **2(suppl 1)**:13–18.

Describes authors' initial experience with laparoscopic gastrectomy. Although this approach might be considered very controversial by many surgeons, mini-access techniques are gaining support.

11. Hamby LS, Zweng TN, Strodel WE: **Perforated Gastric and Duodenal Ulcer: An Analysis of Prognostic Factors.** *Am Surg* 1993, **59**:319–323.

12. Mouret P, Francois Y, Vignal J, Barth X, Lombard-Platet R: **Laparoscopic Treatment of Perforated Peptic Ulcer.** *Br J Surg* 1990, **70**:1006.

13. • Williams RA, Vartany A, Davis IP, Wilson SE: **Impact of Endoscopic Therapy on Outcome of Operation for Bleeding Peptic Ulcers.** *Am J Surg* 1993, **166**:712–715.

The study shows the benefit of endoscopic therapy for bleeding peptic ulcers. Since the introduction of therapeutic endoscopy, the mortality for emergent surgery for bleeding peptic ulcer disease has decreased.

14. •• Wanebo HJ, Kennedy BJ, Chmiel J, Steele G, Jr, Winchester D, Osteen R: **Cancer of the Stomach. A Patient Care Study By the American College of Surgeons.** *Ann Surg* 1993, **218**:583–592.

This is an excellent review of the status of gastric cancer and its treatment and survival trends in the United States.

15. Inoue M, Tajima K, Kitoh T, Sakamoto J, Yamamura Y, Sato T, Suzuki R, Koshikawa T, Nakamura S, Suchi T: **Changes in Histopathological Features of Gastric Carcinoma Over a 26-Year Period (1965-1990).** *J Surg Oncol* 1993, **53**:256–260.

16. Blot WJ, Devesa SS, Kneller RW, Fraumeni JF. **Rising Incidence of Adenocarcinoma of the Esophagus and Gastric Cardia.** *JAMA* 1991, **265**:1287–1289.

17. • Salvon-Harman JC, Cady B, Nikulasson S, Khettry U, Stone MD, Lavin P: **Shifting Proportions of Gastric Adenocarcinomas.** *Arch Surg* 1994, **129**:381–389.

A significant increase in the proportion of proximal gastric cancers was documented over 26 years of surgical treatment of 289 consecutive patients. Only slight improvement in survival rate is seen over this time.

18. Correa P: **Human Gastric Carcinogenesis: A Multistep and Multifactorial Process.** *Cancer Res* 1992, **52**:6735–6740.

19. Sipponen P, Hyvarinen H: **Role of Helicobacter pylori in the Pathogenesis of Gastritis, Peptic Ulcer and Gastric Cancer.** *Scand J Gastroenterol* 1993, **28(suppl)**:3–6.

20. •• The Eurogast Study Group: **An International Association Between *Helicobacter Pylori* Infection and Gastric Cancer.** *Lancet* 1993, **347**:1359–1362.

The multicenter epidemiologic study on the relation between prevalence of *H. pylori* and gastric cancer showed a sixfold increased risk of gastric cancer in patients with documented *H. pylori* infection.

21. Tatsuta M, Iishi H, Okuda S, Taniguchi H, Yokota Y: **The Association of *Helicobacter Pylori* With Differentiated-Type Early Gastric Cancer.** *Cancer* 1993, **72**:1841–1845.

22. Furukawa H, Iwanaga T, Hiratsuka M, Imaoka S, Oshikawa O, Kabuto T, Sasaki Y, Kameyama M, Ohigashi H, Nakamori S: **Gastric Cancer in Young Adults: Growth Accelerating Effect of Pregnancy and Delivery.** *J Surg Oncol* 1994, **55**: 3–6.

23. • Tanaka A, Watanabe T, Okuno K, Yasutomi M: **Perineural Invasion as a Predictor of Recurrence of Gastric Cancer.** *Cancer* 1994, **73**:550–555.

Gastric specimens were stained immunohistochemically for presence of laminin to evaluate perineural invasion of malignant cells. This method can be useful in determining the prognosis of gastric cancers without serosal invasion.

24. •• Hermans J, Bonekamp JJ, Boon MC, Bunt AMG, Ohyama S, Sasako M, Van De Welde CJH: **Adjuvant Therapy After Curative Resection for Gastric Cancer: Meta-Analysis of Randomized Trials.** *J Clin Oncol* 1993, **11**:1441–1447.

Meta-analysis of 2096 patients in 123 reports between 1980 and 1993 on adjuvant therapy for gastric cancer. Postoperative chemotherapy offers no additional survival benefit for patients with curatively resected gastric cancer.

25. Sautner T, Hofbauer F, Depisch D, Schiessel R, Jakesz R: **Adjuvant Intraperitoneal Cisplatin Chemotherapy Does Not Improve Long-Term Survival After Surgery for Advanced Gastric Cancer.** *J Clin Oncol* 1994, **12**:970–974.

26. Ajani JA, Mayer RJ, Ota DM, Steele GD, Evans D, Sugarbaker DJ, Dumas P, Gray C, Vena DA, *et al.*: **Preoperative and Postoperative Chemotherapy for Potentially Resectable Gastric Carcinoma.** *J Natl Cancer Inst* 1993, **85**:1839–1844.

27. •• Thompson GB, van Heerden JA, Sarr MG: **Adenocarcinoma of the Stomach: Are We Making Progress?** *Lancet* 1993, **342**:713–718.

An excellent, practical review of all aspects of gastric cancer including recent advances in the molecular basis of gastric cancer and its surgical management.

28. •• Evers BM, Rady PL, Sandoval K, Arany I, Tyring SK, Sanchez RL, Nealon WH, Townsend CM, Thompson JC: **Gastrinomas Demonstrate Amplification of the HER-2/*neu* Proto-oncogene.** *Ann Surg* 1994, **219**:596–604.

A new concept that alterations in protooncogenes may play a role in the pathogenesis of gastrinoma tumors. They can be identified by molecular biology techniques.

29. Pisegna JR, Doppman JL, Norton JA, Metz DC, Jensen RT: **Prospective Comparative Study of Ability of MR Imaging and Other Imaging Modalities to Localize Tumors in Patients With Zollinger-Ellison Syndrome.** *Dig Dis Sci* 1993, **38**:1318–1328.

30. Yoshikane H, Tsukamoto Y, Niwa Y, Goto H, Hase S, Mizutani K, Nakamura T: **Carcinoid Tumors of the Gastrointestinal Tract: Evaluation With Endoscopic Ultrasonography.** *Gastrointest Endosc* 1993, 39:375–383.

31. •• Farley DR, van Heerden JA, Grant CS, Thompson GB: **Extrapancreatic Gastrinomas: Surgical Experience.** *Arch Surg* 1994, **129**:506–512.

This report emphasizes extrapancreatic location of gastrinomas in 35 years experience in the Mayo Clinic. Patients with extrapancreatic gastrinomas have a favorable outcome.

32. Metz DC, Kuchnio M, Fraker DL, Venzon DJ, Jaffe G, Jensen RT, Stetler-Stevenson M: **Flow Cytometry and Zollinger-Ellison Syndrome: Relationship to Clinical Course.** *Gastroenterology* 1993, **105**:799–813.

33. • Fishbeyn VA, Norton JA, Benya RV, Pisegna JR, Venzon DJ, Metz DC, Jensen RT: **Assessment and Prediction of Long-Term Cure in Patients With the Zollinger-Ellison Syndrome: The Best Approach.** *Ann Intern Med* 1993, **119**:199–206.

The secretin provocative test and fasting serum gastrin levels are the best determinants of recurrent disease after gastrinoma resection.

34. • Cadiot G, Lehy T, Ruszniewski P, Bonfils S, Mignon M: **Gastric Endocrine Cell Evolution in Patients With Zollinger-Ellison Syndrome: Influence of Gastrinoma Growth and Long-Term Omeprazole Treatment.** *Dig Dis Sci* 1993, **38**:1307–1317.

Hypergastrinemia and increase in fundic argyrophil cell densities appears to be closely associated with gastrinoma growth in Zollinger-Ellison patients treated with omeprazole. It suggests that omeprazole-induced hypochlorhydia affects endocrine cell proliferation.

35. Grant JP: **Duke Procedure for Super Obesity: Preliminary Report With 3.5-Year Follow-up.** *Surgery* 1994, **115**:718–726.

36. Macgregor AMC, Rand CSW: **Gastric Surgery in Morbid Obesity: Outcome in Patients Aged 55 Years and Older.** *Arch Surg* 1993, **128**:1153–1157.

37. •• Sugerman HJ: **Surgery for Morbid Obesity.** *Surgery* 1993, **114**: 865–867.

A useful, critical review of recent advances in bariatric surgery with recommendations delineating the best surgical approach for treatment of excessive obesity.

38. • Behrns KE, Smith CD, Kelly KA, Sarr MG: **Reoperative Bariatric Surgery: Lessons Learned to Improve Patient Selection and Results.** *Ann Surg* 1993, **218**:646–653.

Some patients are not satisfied with their weight loss after bariatric surgeries, whereas others develop complications. This report retrospectively evaluates reoperative procedures for failed primary surgical treatment of morbid obesity. Gastric bypass provides more effective weight loss than vertical gastroplasty.

Marek Rudnicki, MD, PhD, Department of Surgery, The Mary Imogene Bassett Hospital, Cooperstown, NY 13326, USA.

Gastric cancer

Frank A. Sinicrope, MD, and Bernard Levin, MD

University of Texas M.D. Anderson Cancer Center, Houston, Texas, USA

Despite the decline in the incidence of gastric cancer in Western countries over the past four decades, adenocarcinoma of the proximal stomach and gastroesophageal junction are increasing steadily. Although little is known about the etiologic factors responsible for the increased incidence of these tumors, recent studies have identified molecular alterations in gastric cancers including mutations in oncogenes, tumor suppressor genes, and genes involved in cellular adhesion processes. Reduced expression and mutation of the cell adhesion molecule, E-cadherin, has been found in gastric cancers and may underlie their tendency toward invasion and metastasis. The carbohydrate-associated antigen sialosyl-Tn antigen has been shown to be of prognostic value in colon cancer and its role in the clinical behavior of gastric cancers is under evaluation. Interesting data on the use of chemopreventive agents have been obtained from a nutritional intervention trial in Linxian, China. Linxian has one of the highest rates of esophageal and gastric cardia cancer in the world and dietary deficiencies in vitamins and minerals are believed to contribute to cancer causation in this population. Regarding the treatment of local-regional gastric cancer, there is continued interest in combined pre- and postoperative chemotherapy in an effort to downstage disease prior to resection. However, more efficacious regimens are needed before the theoretical benefits of this approach can be fully realized. Chemotherapy for advanced disease remains experimental and current approaches aim to maximize existing regimens while the search for new agents continues.

Current Opinion in Gastroenterology 1994, **10**:610–617

Gastric carcinoma is the eighth leading cause of cancer death worldwide. In 1994 in the United States, 25,000 new cases will appear and 14,000 deaths secondary to this disease will occur [1]. Although the incidence of gastric cancer has declined in the United States over the past four decades, epidemiologic evidence indicates that adenocarcinoma of the proximal stomach and gastroesophageal junction have been increasing steadily since the mid-1970s [2,3]. Furthermore, the age-adjusted annual rate of increase among white men surpasses that of all other cancers [2]. A similar increase in the incidence of distal esophageal and gastric cardia cancer has been observed in Swedish and other European centers [3]. Proximal gastric cancers also appear to be clinically more aggressive than distal tumors [4]. Despite these observations, little is known about the etiologic factors responsible for the increased incidence of these tumors.

Chemoprevention of gastric cancer

Linxian County in rural north-central China has the one of the highest rates of esophageal and gastric cardia cancer in the world [5]. In this region, cancers of the esophagus are squamous cell in origin and gastric cardia tumors are adenocarcinomas. Case-control studies [6,7] from this region have failed to identify strong dietary or other environmental risk factors; however, intake of fresh fruits, leafy vegetables, and animal products are low in this population. Quantitation of blood micronutrients in Linxian residents has revealed low

Abbreviations

EAP—etoposide, doxorubicin, and cisplatin; **FAM**—fluorouracil, doxorubicin, and mytomycin C; **FAMe**—fluorouracil, doxorubicin, and methyl lomustine; **FAMTX**—high-dose fluorouracil, doxorubicin, and methotrexate; **FAP**—fluorouracil, doxorubicin, and cisplatin; **STn**—sialosyl-Tn antigen; **TNM**—tumor, node, metastasis; **UICC**—Union Internacional Contra la Cancrum.

 ISBN 1-85922-611-6 ISSN 0267–1379

levels of beta carotene, retinol, riboflavin, and vitamins C and E compared with Western subjects, although clinically manifest deficiencies of these micronutrients were uncommon [8••].

Dietary factors are believed to play a role in cancer causation and specifically, increased intake of fresh fruits and vegetables are associated with a reduced risk of esophageal, gastric, and other cancers [9]. Therefore, a large nutritional intervention trial was undertaken by the US National Cancer Institute [8••] to determine whether dietary supplementation of vitamins and minerals could reduce cancer incidence and mortality in Linxian, China. In this study, 29,584 subjects, 40 to 69 years of age, were randomly assigned to receive one of four nutrient combinations: 1) retinol and zinc, 2) riboflavin and niacin, 3) vitamin C and molybdenum, or 4) beta carotene, vitamin E, and selenium. An inverse relationship between blood levels of these nutrients and the risk of esophageal and gastric cancer had been observed in rural China [10–12]. During the 5.25-year follow-up period, there were 1300 cancer deaths, of which 681 were attributed to esophageal or gastric cancer. A significant reduction in total and cancer mortality, especially gastric cancer deaths (21% reduction), was observed among subjects receiving beta carotene, vitamin E, and selenium but not among those receiving other interventions. Furthermore, reductions in cancer incidence were noted to parallel reductions in cancer mortality. It is possible, however, that the study duration was not sufficient to detect a benefit from these other interventions.

Current evidence suggests that beta carotene is a cancer chemopreventive compound. In this regard, beta carotene has been shown to inhibit the development of carcinogen-induced carcinomas of the oral cavity and colon in experimental animals [13]. Furthermore, beta carotene and vitamin E have been shown to produce regression of oral leukoplakia, which is believed to be a precursor lesion of oral cancer [14–16]. Although retinoids have been shown convincingly to prevent development of second primary tumors in patients with squamous cell carcinoma of the head and neck [17], the Linxian trial failed to find a reduction in squamous cell esophageal cancer incidence or mortality in the retinol plus zinc group. The mechanisms by which these nutrients may reduce cancer incidence or mortality are largely unknown; however, data indicate that their antioxidant properties may be contributory [18]. In this regard, beta carotene can protect cells against DNA damage induced by reactive oxygen species. Furthermore, these nutrients may also inhibit formation of *N*-nitroso compounds that are carcinogenic in animals and may be of importance in the etiology of human esophageal and gastric cancers [19].

At the completion of the Linxian intervention trial, Wang *et al.* [20••] conducted an endoscopic survey in 391 subjects to determine if the nutritional interventions affected the prevalence of precancerous and cancerous lesions of the esophagus and stomach. Comparisons were made between asymptomatic subjects in the four intervention groups. Mucosal dysplasia or cancer was detected on endoscopic biopsy in 15% of subjects, nearly all of whom were asymptomatic. However, a statistically significant reduction in esophageal or gastric dysplasia or cancer was not observed for any of the interventions. The high prevalence of dysplasia and cancer found in this endoscopic study suggests the possibility that a significant percentage of patients in the Linxian intervention trial may have had precancerous or cancerous esophageal or gastric mucosal lesions at the beginning of the trial. Therefore, in some patients, the effect of nutrient supplementation on later stages of carcinogenesis or neoplastic progression may have been examined as opposed to their preventive effects on early carcinogenesis.

Li *et al.* [21••] examined the effects of nutrient supplementation on esophageal and gastric cancer mortality rates in patients with cytologically proven esophageal dysplasia. In this study, 3318 Linxian subjects were randomly assigned to receive daily supplementation with 14 vitamins and 12 minerals that were generally two to three times the US recommended daily allowances. Given the smaller number of subjects with dysplasia, it was not possible to study the micronutrients as was done in the large intervention trial by Blot *et al.* [8••]. Cancers were identified by balloon cytology and endoscopic examination in some subjects after 2.5 and 6 years. No significant effects on esophageal or gastric cardia cancer mortality or incidence rates were observed for subjects receiving supplements versus placebo. Therefore, although the results of the Linxian intervention trial are intriguing, studies with patients receiving baseline and follow-up endoscopic examinations, and the addition of biomarkers as intermediate endpoints, may aid in clarifying the potential benefits of these micronutrients. Furthermore, these results may not be directly applicable to the chemoprevention of esophageal and gastric cancers in the United States or other developed nations that have different epidemiologic risk profiles. Cancer chemoprevention is a rapidly growing field and we can look forward to future phase III studies in upper digestive tract malignancies.

Genotypic events

Current attention is focused on elucidating the molecular alterations in gastric cancer cells which influence tumor invasion and metastasis and therefore, determine clinical outcome. Recent evidence indicates that molecular alterations frequently found in colorectal carcinomas, such as mutations in the *APC, MCC,* and *DCC* genes, also occur in gastric cancers [22–25]. Interestingly, mutations in the *APC* gene have also been described in gastric adenomas [26]. Abnormalities in cellular adhesion processes are believed to underlie adhesion tumor invasion and metastatic potential and a class of cell adhesion molecules, known as cadherins, appear to figure prominently in this process [27]. Cadherins are calcium-dependent transmembrane glycoproteins that are localized to the lateral borders of epithelial cells and are involved in cell-to-cell adhesion [28]. Experiments in which the E-cadherin, also known as L-CAM, complementary DNA was introduced into cells by transfection resulted in suppression of invasive potential, whereas introduction of E-cadherin antisense oligonucleotides, which block messenger RNA translation, was shown to increase invasiveness [29].

Abnormalities in E-cadherin expression has been observed in several human cancers and are often associated with invasive and metastasizing tumors [30–33]. More recently, reduced E-cadherin expression has been detected in diffuse-type gastric carcinomas [34••,35] and gene mutations have been described in gastric cancer cells [36•]. In this regard, Oda *et al.* [36•], analyzed 10 loosely adherent human gastric adenocarcinoma cell lines for mutations in the *E-cadherin* gene. In MKN45 (poorly differentiated) and KATO III (invasive signet ring) cells, mutations in the *E-cadherin* messenger RNA sequence were detected that significantly reduced E-cadherin expression in the latter cell line. Moreover, in both cell lines, the wild-type allele was lost in addition to mutation. These abnormalities are similar to inactivation of the *p53* tumor suppressor gene whereby mutation and allelic loss are frequent events in human cancers [37].

In another study [34••], primary human gastric carcinomas were analyzed for E-cadherin using immunohistochemical methods and a specific monoclonal antibody. Compared with normal mucosa, 55 of 60 (92%) of primary tumors showed reduced E-cadherin immunostaining that was strongly correlated with decreased cellular differentiation and loss of glandular structures. However, E-cadherin immunostaining was not significantly related to tumor size, lymphatic vessel invasion, lymph node metastases, or patient survival by multivariate analysis. In contrast to intestinal-type cancers, diffuse tumors were uniformly negative for E-cadherin staining. The association between reduced E-cadherin expression and dedifferentiation [38] has led to speculation that abnormalities in E-cadherin may be involved in the development of diffuse-type tumors [39].

Tumor markers

Ongoing efforts are directed at identifying tumor markers that aid in diagnosis or predict clinical outcome in gastrointestinal cancers. One potential marker is sialosyl-Tn antigen (STn), which is a carbohydrate-associated antigen found on mucin-type glycoproteins. Expression of this antigen is absent in normal colonic mucosa but has been shown to be increased in colon carcinomas [40]. Moreover, STn expression has been shown to be an independent prognostic marker in colon carcinoma [41]. Recent studies have analyzed gastric tissues for STn expression to determine its clinical utility in this disease. STn expression was examined by immunohistochemical methods and a specific monoclonal antibody in 85 resected primary gastric cancers [42•]. Positive immunostaining was detected in 53 (62%) of carcinomas of different tumor stages and was significantly correlated with lymph vessel invasion, lymph node metastasis, and tumor stage. Five-year survival was significantly lower in STn-positive patients compared with STn-negative patients. A multivariate analysis revealed that tumor stage, depth of invasion, STn status, and lymph node metastasis were independent predictors of survival.

In another immunohistochemical study, 31 primary gastric carcinomas were examined [43•] and 21 (68%) stained positively for STn. No relationship between immunostaining and tumor stage or histologic grade were found. By univariate analysis, STn expression was found to be a significant adverse prognostic marker. However, the prognostic value of STn remains controversial and in this regard, David *et al.* [44] found no relationship between STn expression and clinicopathologic features of tumor aggressiveness or DNA ploidy in gastric cancers. Furthermore, the aforementioned studies included a relatively small number of patients with various tumor stages. Additionally, it can be argued that increased STn expression is an indicator of increased tumor burden and that extent of disease may not be fully detected by current staging methods. Whether or not STn expression influences biologic behavior or is simply a marker of tumor burden awaits further study. Therefore, these results must be interpreted with cautious skepticism until they are confirmed in a larger number of patient samples by multivariate analysis.

Recent studies have measured the STn antigen in the sera of patients with gastric cancer. A tumor marker that is frequently expressed and quantifiable in sera would aid in staging patients, in determining resectability, and in the early identification of recurrent disease. Takahashi *et al.* [45•] measured serum STn and carcinoembryonic antigen levels preoperatively in 349 Japanese gastric cancer patients and found elevated STn levels in 46 (13%) patients of which 22 (48%) had stage IV disease. Despite the advanced tumor stage of some patients, all underwent surgical resection. Patients testing positively for STn and carcinoembryonic antigen had more advanced disease at surgery and significantly shorter survival rates than those testing negative for both markers. In a previous publication, Takahashi *et al.* [46•] reported STn levels in this same patient cohort and large standard deviations were observed in the high STn group (> 45 U/mL). Furthermore, the aforementioned studies fail to answer the question of whether or not serum STn levels can predict clinical outcome independent of tumor stage, and therefore, further studies are needed to establish the clinical utility of this marker in gastric cancer.

CD44 is a cell surface molecule involved in cell-to-cell interaction that has recently been examined in gastric cancers [47]. Interest in the CD44 family of molecules developed as a result of a report demonstrating the presence of a CD44 isoform in metastatic but not in nonmetastatic cell lines [48]. Moreover, transfection of this CD44 isoform complementary DNA into rat sarcoma cells conferred metastatic potential [48]. In human diffuse large-cell lymphoma, increased CD44 expression was associated with a poor prognosis [49]. To determine if CD44 influences clinical outcome in a solid tumor, Mayer *et al.* [50••] examined benign and malignant gastric epithelia for CD44 expression using immunohistochemical methods and a specific monoclonal antibody. Normal gastric mucosa was negative for CD44; however, positive immunostaining was detected in basal epithelial cells in gastric glands in atrophic mucosa and intestinal metaplasia. Expression was observed in 30 of 61 (49%) primary gastric carcinomas and was positively correlated with histologic grade and distant metastasis (M-stage). In contrast to benign mucosa, CD44 immunoreactivity was not associated with inflammation, *ie*, leukocyte infiltration or HLA-DR expression. Among 31 patients resected for cure and followed for a mean of 17 months, CD44 expression was significantly associated with tumor recurrence and decreased survival. Despite the small number of patients, multivariate analysis revealed that CD44 expression was a significant independent prognostic marker. The mechanism by which CD44 might influence biological behavior of gastric cancer cells is unknown. CD44-positive stroma and polymorphonuclear leukocytes are frequently observed in the vicinity of gastric cancer cells and the latter are known sources of reactive oxygen species capable of inducing DNA damage [51]. Alternatively. the potential influence of CD44 in cell adhesion and cell-matrix interactions may underlie its association with tumor aggressiveness. In this regard, increased expressions of CD44 isoforms have been observed in human breast and colorectal carcinomas and have been shown to be associated with tumor progression [52,53]. The results of this study are very intriguing and further studies concerning the role of CD44 in the biology and clinical behavior of gastric cancers are anticipated.

Treatment

Surgery

The prognosis for gastric cancer remains extremely poor with 5-year survival rates ranging from 5% to 15% [1]. This is related to the fact that in Western countries, including the United States, the majority of patients are diagnosed with advanced disease. Factors known to influence clinical outcome in gastric cancer include location of the primary tumor, the presence or absence of lymph node involvement, and the depth of penetration of the gastric wall [54]. Curative resection remains the most effective treatment and includes removal of the primary tumor and regional lymph nodes with resection margins free of tumor. Unfortunately, only approximately 40% of patients are candidates for potentially curative surgery and despite this intervention, the majority of patients will develop locoregional disease and eventually die of metastatic disease [54,55]. For patients deemed resectable (*ie*, those with locoregional disease) who undergo curative resection, the median survival is 24 months with a projected 5-year survival of 20% [54,55].

Efforts to increase the cure rate in gastric cancer have focused on systematic lymph node dissection in an effort to completely excise the tumor. In a prospective, multicenter German study [56••], the prognostic significance of standard versus radical lymph node dissection was evaluated in 1654 patients undergoing resection. Standard lymph node dissection was defined as 26 or fewer nodes and radical as greater than 26 nodes, corresponding to the Japanese R_2 and R_1 procedures, respectively. Patients were staged according to the Union Internacional Contra la Cancrum (UICC) tumor, node, metastasis (TNM) classification (Table 1) [57] and mean follow-up was 48 months. Using the standard procedure, a median of 16 lymph nodes were removed in contrast to a median of 41 lymph nodes with the radical dissection. Of the 1654 resected patients, 1182 (71%) met criteria for an R_0 resection, *ie*, complete removal of macro- and microscopic tumor. By univariate and multivariate analyses, a significant improvement in survival rate was observed only for radically resected stages II and IIIa tumors compared with standard dissection. No significant differences in operative morbidity or mortality were found between patients undergoing standard versus radical procedures. This study was not randomized and approximately twice as many patients underwent radical dissection compared with the standard approach. It is possible that radical resection results in more accurate staging and may therefore have biased the results. Furthermore, several surgeons performed the resections given that the trial involved multiple centers. Despite these limitations, the results suggest that UICC stage II and IIIa patients may benefit from more extended lymph node dissection.

Table 1. Percent of patients diagnosed by stage and 5-year survival for gastric adenocarcinoma*

Stage UICC/TNM	5-year survival, %	Patients diagnosed, %
IA, T1, N0, M0	88	1–5
IB	80	1–5
T1, N1, M0		
T2, N0, M0		
II	55	10–15
T1, N2, M0		
T2, N1, M0		
T3, N0, M0		
IIIA	30	17–20
T2, N2, M0		
T3, N1, M0		
T4, N0, M0		
IIIB	9	17–20
T3, N2, M0		
T4, N1, M0		
IV, T4, N2, M+	—	72

*From Alexander *et al.* [73]; with permission.
TNM—tumor, node, metastasis; UICC—Union Internacional Contra la Cancrum.

The determination of nodal stage is currently based on the location of positive lymph nodes in both the TNM and Japanese classifications. Ichikura *et al.* [58•] compared the number of positive metastatic lymph nodes versus nodal stage in 772 Japanese patients who underwent potentially curative resection for gastric cancer. Patients were divided into three groups according to the depth of tumor invasion. By multivariate analysis in patients with four or more positive nodes, number of positive nodes was of greatest prognostic value followed by depth of invasion. Patients with one to three positive nodes had the same prognosis as patients without positive nodes. Although nodal stage and the number of positive nodes were closely related, nodal stage was not a significant prognostic indicator. The authors propose that current staging systems adopt the number of metastatic lymph node into their classification schemes and the aforementioned studies appear to provide support for this claim.

Neoadjuvant chemotherapy

Clinical staging of gastric cancer often results in understaging of patients who at exploration are found to have more extensive disease and are therefore at high risk for relapse. Recent efforts are focused on downstaging the disease using preoperative chemotherapy prior to potentially curative resection. Reducing tumor bulk preoperatively aims to make more patients resectable for cure and selects responders who are also more likely to benefit from postoperative systemic chemotherapy [59]. The use of pre- and postoperative chemotherapy is referred to as neoadjuvant therapy and aims to improve both resectability and overall survival (Table 2). Ajani *et al.* [60••] evaluated the combination of etoposide, doxorubicin, and cisplatin (EAP) as neoadjuvant therapy in 48 previously untreated patients with potentially resectable gastric cancer, 71% of whom had proximal gastric tumors. The selection of this regimen was based on promising results by Wilke *et al.* [61] whereby a 15% pathologic complete response rate was observed with EAP in unresectable patients. Patients received three courses of chemotherapy prior to resection and responders received two courses postoperatively. Dose reductions were required in 37 (77%) of patients, principally for myelosuppression. Nineteen patients (40%) required hospitalization for toxic effects: neutropenic fever in 15, grade 3 or 4 nausea and vomiting in 15, and grade 3 or 4 diarrhea in seven. Therapy was discontinued in one patient preoperatively and in six patients postresection. EAP in the doses and schedules employed was associated with substantial toxicity. Furthermore, a 31% response rate was observed with no pathologic complete responses and median survival was not superior to data for surgery alone. Therefore, more efficacious chemotherapy regimens are needed before the theoretical benefits of the neoadjuvant approach can be fully realized. Given that high-dose fluorouracil, doxorubicin, and methotrexate (FAMTX) has been shown to be at least as effective and significantly less toxic than EAP, it is undergoing phase II evaluation as neoadjuvant therapy at Memorial Sloan-Kettering Cancer Center.

Chemotherapy for advanced disease

Fluorouracil is the most commonly used drug in the treatment of gastric cancer with a response rate of 21% in collected studies [62]. Most studies employ intravenous bolus or short infusion therapy; however, recent trials have evaluated continuous infusion schedules. Although a randomized study of infusional therapy has yet to be performed, Moynihan *et al.* [63] observed a 31% response rate in a small number of patients. Given the modest response rates observed in single-agent chemotherapy studies, attention has focused on combination chemotherapy. Until recently, the most frequently employed drug combination has been fluorouracil, doxorubicin, and mitomycin C (FAM) and a response rate of 33% is derived from collected studies with an acceptable degree of toxicity [64].

Table 2. Theoretic advantages and disadvantages of neoadjuvant chemotherapy for locally advanced gastric carcinoma*

Advantages
Ability to assess individual patient responses by response of *in situ* primary
Opportunity to discontinue or change chemotherapy regimens in nonresponders
Decrease in primary tumor size, increase in resectability rate
Improvement in survival
Palliation of symptoms (dysphagia, obstruction, bleeding)
Disadvantages
Possibility of patient becoming incurable/unresectable by delaying operation
Unfavorable cell cycle kinetics in large primary tumors

*From Alexander *et al.* [73]; with permission.

The North Central Cancer Treatment Group (NCCTG) recently reported a study comparing fluorouracil, doxorubicin, and methyl lomustine (FAMe), fluorouracil, doxorubicin and cisplatin (FAP), and FAMe alternating with the antifolate compound triazinate compared with fluorouracil alone in 252 patients with locally unresectable or metastatic gastric cancer [65•]. The impetus for this study was previous data indicating that FAMe produced a survival advantage over fluorouracil plus doxorubicin [66] and a trend toward significant improvement over FAM [67]. These results previously led to the adoption of FAMe by the Gastrointestinal Tumor Study Group as standard therapy. A major objective of the NCCTG study [65•] was to attempt to modulate FAMe by the addition of triazinate, which in a phase II trial demonstrated a 15% objective response rate in previously treated patients [67]. The majority of patients in this study had nonmeasurable disease and survival was the primary endpoint. Three drug-related deaths occurred in the combination arms. None of the three regimens produced a survival advantage compared with fluorouracil alone and all three were more toxic.

Modifications of the FAM regimen have been developed including the substitution of high-dose methotrexate for mitomycin C (FAMTX). A randomized trial of FAMTX versus FAM found a superior response rate (41% vs 9%) and a survival advantage (42 vs 29 weeks) for FAMTX with an acceptable degree of toxicity [68]. This study established FAMTX as the control regimen to be employed in future randomized trials. Wilke *et al.* [69] developed the EAP regimen in the late 1980s and cumulative experience shows a response rate of approximately 50% [69,70]. In a randomized study comparing EAP and FAMTX, no difference in response was observed and the trial was terminated early due to a significant increase in toxicity and death with EAP [71].

Recent studies have replaced mitomycin C in the FAM regimen with cisplatin. A phase III randomized trial comparing fluorouracil and cisplatin, FAM, and fluorouracil alone was conducted in advanced disease [72•]. An acceptable degree of toxicity was observed for all three arms. Although the overall response rate was higher in the fluorouracil and cisplatin arm (51%) compared with the FAM (25%) and fluorouracil (26%) arms, the response duration was not significantly different. Moreover, no significant difference in overall survival (mean, 32 weeks) was seen among the three arms. The aforementioned studies emphasize the experimental status of therapy for advanced gastric cancer. Current approaches have attempted to maximize existing treatment modalities, however, the results thus far remain relatively poor. Until more efficacious therapies are identified, cost, toxicity and quality of life issues must be be seriously considered in the choice of treatment regimens outside of research protocols.

References and recommended reading

Papers of particular interest, published within the annual period of review, have been highlighted as:

- • Of special interest
- •• Of outstanding interest

1. Boring CC, Squires TS, Tong T, Montgomery S: **Cancer Statistics.** *CA Cancer J Clin* 1994, **44**:7–26.

2. Blot WJ, Devesa SS, Kneller RW, Fraumeni JF: **Rising Incidence of Adenocarcinoma of the Esophagus and Gastric Cardia.** *JAMA* 1991, **265**:1287–1289.

3. Hansson L-E, Sparen P, Nyren O: **Increasing Incidence of Carcinoma of the Gastric Cardia in Sweden From 1970 to 1985.** *Br J Surg* 1993, **80**:374–377.

4. Nakane Y, Okamura S, Boku T, Okusa T, Tanaka K, Hioki K: **Prognostic Differences of Adenocarcinoma Arising From the Cardi and the Upper Third of the Stomach.** *Am Surg* 1993, **59**:423–429.

5. Li JY: **Epidemiology of Esophageal Cancer in China.** *Monogr Natl Cancer Inst* 1982, **62**:113–120.

6. Li JY, Ershow AG, Chen ZJ, Wacholder S, Li GY, Guo W, Li B, Blot WJ: **A Case-Control Study of Cancer of the Esophagus and Gastric Cardia in Linxian.** *Int J Cancer* 1989, **43**:755–761.

7. Yu Y, Taylor PR, Li JY, Dawsey SM, Wang GQ, Guo WD, Wang W, Liu BQ, Blot WJ, Shen Q: **Retrospective Cohort Study of Risk Factors for Esophageal Cancer in Linxian, China.** *Cancer Causes Control* 1993, **3**:203–208.

8. •• Blot WJ, Li J-Y, Taylor PR, Guo W, Pawsey S, Wong G-Q, Yang CS, Zheng S-F, Gail M, Li G-Y, *et al.*: **Nutrition Intervention Trials in Linxian, China: Supplementation With Specific Vitamin/Mineral Combinations Cancer Incidence, and Disease-Specific Mortality in the General Population.** *J Natl Cancer Inst* 1993, **85**:1483–1491.

A randomized nutritional intervention trial was conducted among 29,584 residents of Linxian, China to determine the effect of vitamin and mineral supplements on esophageal and gastric cancer mortality in a high-risk population over a 5.25-year period. Significant reductions in cancer mortality and gastric cancer mortality were observed among those taking beta carotene, vitamin E, and selenium supplements.

9. Steinmetz KA, Potter JD: **Vegetables, Fruit and Cancer. I. Epidemiology.** *Cancer Causes Control* 1991, **2**:325–357.

10. Yu SY, Chu Y, Gang XL, *et al.*: **Regional Variation of Cancer Mortality and Its Relation to Selenium Levels in China.** *Biol Trace Elem Res* 1985, **7**:21–29.

11. Kneller RW, Guo WD, Hsing AW, Chen JS, Blot WJ, Li JY, Forman D, Faumeni JF: **Risk Factors for Stomach Cancer in Sixty-Five Chinese Counties.** *Cancer Epidemiol Biomarkers Prev* 1992, **1**:113–118.

12. Guo W, Li JY, Blot WJ, Hsing AW, Chen JS, Fraumeni JF: **Correlations of Dietary Intake and Blood Nutrient Levels With Esophageal Cancer Mortality in China.** *Nutr Cancer* 1990, **13**:121–127.

13. Birt DF: **Update on the Effects of Vitamins A, C, and E and Selenium on Carcinogenesis.** *Proc Soc Exp Biol Med* 1986, **183**:311–320.

14. Garewal HS, Meyskens FL Jr, Killen D, Reeves D, Kiersch TA, Elletson H, Strosberg A, King D, Steinbronn K: **Response of Oral Leukoplakia to Beta-Carotene.** *J Clin Oncol* 1990, **8**:1715–1720.

15. Stich FH, Rosin MP, Hornby AP: **Remission of Oral Leukoplakias and Micronuclei in Tobacco/Betel Quid Chewers Treated With Beta-Carotene and With Beta-Carotene Plus Vitamin A.** *Int J Cancer* 1988, 42:195–199.

16. Benner SE, Winn RJ, Lippman SM, Poland J, Hansen KS, Luna MA, Hong WK: **Regression of Oral Leukoplakia With α-Tocopherol: A Community Clinical Oncology Program Chemoprevention Study.** *J Natl Cancer Inst* 1993, **85**:44–47.

17. Hong WK, Lippman S, Itri LM, Karp DD, Lee JS, Byers RM, Schantz SP, Kramer AM, Lotan R, Peters LJ, *et al.*: **Prevention of Second Primary Tumors With Isoretinoin in Squamous-Cell Carcinoma of the Head and Neck.** *N Engl J Med* 1990, **323**:795–801.

18. National Research Council: *Diet and Health: Implications for Reducing Chronic Disease Risk.* Washington, DC: National Academy Press; 1989.

19. Mirvish SS: **The Etiology of Gastric Cancer: Intragastric Nitrosamide Formation and Other Theories.** *J Natl Cancer Inst* 1983, **71**:629–647.

20. •• Wang G-Q, Dawsey SM, Li J-Y, Taylor PR, Li B, Blot WJ, Weinstein WM, Liu F-S, Lewin KJ, Wang H: **Effects of Vitamin/Mineral Supplementation on the Prevalence of Histological Dysplasia and Early Cancer of the Esophagus and Stomach: Results From the General Population Trial in Linxian, China.** *Career Epidemiol Biomarkers Prev* 1994, 3:161-166.

At completion of Linxian nutritional intervention trial, a subset of subjects were examined endoscopically to determine the prevalence of precancerous or cancerous lesions of the esophagus or stomach relative to nutrient factor received. Cancer or dysplasia was diagnosed in 15% of subjects and differences between vitamin-mineral combinations were observed.

21. •• Li J-Y, Taylor PR, Li B, Dawsey S, Wang G-Q, Ershow AG, Guo W, Liu S-F, Yang CS, Shen Q, *et al.*: **Nutrition Intervention Trials in Linxian, China: Multiple Vitamin/Mineral Supplementation, Cancer Incidence, and Disease-Specific Mortality Among Adults With Esophageal Dysplasia.** *J Natl Cancer Inst* 1993, **85**:1492–1498.

A prospective nutritional intervention trial was performed in Linxian, China with subjects having esophageal dysplasia. Subjects were randomly assigned to receive daily supplements with 14 vitamins and 12 minerals or placebo and effects on cancer incidence and mortality were determined at a 6-year follow-up. No statistically significant reduction in cancer incidence or cancer mortality was observed.

22. Sano T, Tsujino T, Yoshida K, Nakayam H, Nakamura Y, Kajiyama G, Tahara E: **Frequent Loss of Heterozygosity on Chromosomes 1q, 5q and 17p in Human Gastric Carcinomas.** *Cancer Res* 1991, **51**:2926–2931.

23. Horii A, Nakatsuru S, Miyoshi Y, Ichii S, Nagase H, Kato Y, Yanagisawa A, Nakamura Y. **The APC Gene, Responsible for Familial Adenomatous Polyposis, Is Mutated in Human Gastric Cancer.** *Cancer Res* 1992, **52**:3231–3233.

24. Tahara E: **Growth Factors and Oncogenes in Human Gastrointestinal Carcinomas.** *J Cancer Res Clin Oncol* 1990, **116**:121–131.

25. McKie AB, Filipe MI, Lemoine NR: **Abnormalities Affecting the *APC* and *MCC* Tumour Suppressor Gene Loci on Chromosome 5q Occur Frequently in Gastric Cancer but not in Pancreatic Cancer.** *Int J Cancer* 1993, **55**:598–603.

26. Tamura G, Maesawa C, Suzuki Y, Tamada H, Satoh M, Ogasawara S, Kashiwaba M, Satodate R: **Mutations of the APC Gene Occur During Early Stages of Gastric Adenoma Development.** *Cancer Res* 1994, **54**:1149–1151.

27. Haynes BF, Liao H-X, Patton KL: **The Transmembrane Hyaluronate Receptor (CD44): Multiple Functions, Multiple Forms.** *Cancer Cells* 1991, 3:347–350.

28. Screaton GR, Bell MV, Jackson DG, Cornelis FB, Gerth U, Bell JI: **Genomic Structure of DNA Encoding the Lymphocyte Homing Receptor CD44 Reveals at Least 12 Alternatively Spliced Exons.** *Proc Natl Acad Sci U S A* 1992, **89**:12160–12164.

29. Vleminckx KL, Vakaet J, Mareel M, Fiers W, Roy FV: **Genetic Manipulation of E-Cadherin Expression by Epithelial Tumor Cells Reveals an Invasion Suppressor Role.** *Cell* 1991, **66**:107–119.

30. Eidelmann S, Damsky CH, Wheelock MJ, Damjanov J: **Expression of the Cell-Cell Adhesion Glycoprotein Cell-CAM 120/80 in Normal Human Tissues and Tumors.** *Am J Pathol* 1989, **135**:101–110.

31. Shimoyama Y, Kirohashi Sharano S, Noguchi M, Shimosata Y, Takeichi M, Abe O: **Cadherin Cell-Adhesion Molecules in Human Epithelial Tissues and Carcinomas.** *Cancer Res* 1989, 49:2128–2133.

32. Shimoyama Y, Hirohashi S: **Cadherin Intercellular Adhesion Molecule in Hepatocellular Carcinomas: Loss of E-Cadherin Expression in an Undifferentiated Carcinoma.** *Cancer Lett* 1991, **57**:131–135.

33. Schipper JH, Frixen UH, Behrens J, Unger A, Jahnke K, Birchmeier W: **E-Cadherin Expression in Squamous Cell Carcinomas of Head and Neck: Inverse Correlation With Tumor Dedifferentiation and Lymph Node Metastasis.** *Cancer Res* 1991, **51**:6328–6337.

34. •• Mayer B, Johnson JP, Leitl F, Jauch KW, Heiss MM, Schildberg W, Birchmeier W, Funke I: **E-Cadherin Expression in Primary and Metastatic Gastric Cancer: Down-Regulation Correlates With Cellular Dedifferentiation and Glandular Disintegration.** *Cancer Res* 1993, **53**:1690–1695.

Expression of the epithelial cell adhesion molecule, E-cadherin, was analyzed in gastric carcinomas using immunohistochemical methods. Reduced expression was found in 92% of primary tumors and was significantly associated with tumor recurrence and decreased survival.

35. Shimoyama Y, Hirohashi S: **Expression of E- and P-Cadherin in Gastric Carcinomas.** *Cancer Res* 1991, **51**:2185–2192.

36. • Oda T, Kanai Y, Oyama T, Yoshiura K, Shimoyama Y, Birchmeier W, Sugimura T, Hirohashi S: **E-Cadherin Gene Mutations in Human Gastric Carcinoma Cell Lines.** *Proc Natl Acad Sci U S A* 1994, 91:1858–1862.

Ten gastric carcinoma cell lines were analyzed for abnormalities in E-cadherin messenger RNA and protein expression. In two of these cell lines, mutations in the E-cadherin sequence were found with an associated loss of the E-cadherin wild-type allele, similar to inactivation of tumor suppressor genes.

37. Levine AJ, Perry ME, Chang A, Silver A, Dittmer D, Wu M, Welsh D: **The 1993 Walter Huber Lecture: The Role of the p53 Tumour-Suppressor Gene in Tumorigenesis.** *Br J Cancer* 1994, 69:409–416.

38. Shiozaki H, Tahata H, Oka H, Miyata M, Kobayashi K, Tamura S, Iihara K, Doki Y, Hirano S, Takeichi M, Mori T: **Expression of Immunoreactive E-Cadherin Adhesion Molecules in Human Cancers.** *Am J Pathol* 1991, **139**:17-23.

39. Tahara E: **Molecular Mechanism of Stomach Carcinogenesis.** *J Cancer Res Clin Oncol* 1993, **119**:265–272.

40. Itzkowitz SH, Yuan M, Montgomery CK, Kjeldsen T, Takahashi HK, Bigbee WL, Kim YS: **Expression of Tn, Sialosyl-Tn, and T Antigens in Human Colon Cancer.** *Cancer Res* 1989, 49:197–204.

41. Itzkowitz SH, Bloom EJ, Kokal WA, Modin G, Hakomori S, Kim YS: **Sialosyl-Tn: A Novel Mucin Antigen Associated With Prognosis in Colorectal Cancer Patients.** *Cancer* 1990, **66**:1960–1966.

42. • Ma XC, Terata N, Kodama M, Jancic S, Hosokawa Y, Hattori T: **Expression of Sialyl-Tn Antigen Is Correlated With Survival Time of Patients With Gastric Carcinomas.** *Eur J Cancer* 1993, **29A**:1820–1823.

Expression of STn was examined by immunohistochemical methods in 85 primary gastric carcinomas and positive staining was associated with clinicopathologic features of tumor aggressiveness.

43. • Werther JL, Rivera-MacMurray S, Bruckner H, Tatematsu M, Itzkowitz SH: **Mucin-Associated Sialosyl-Tn Antigen Expression in Gastric Cancer Correlates With an Adverse Outcome.** *Br J Cancer* 1994, 69:613–616.

Thirty-one gastric carcinomas were analyzed for expression of the carbohydrate-associated STn, using immunohistochemistry. Expression of STn was found in 68% of gastric cancers and was associated with a poor prognosis.

44. David L, Nesland JM, Clausen H, Carneiro F, Sobrinho-Simoes M: **Simple Mucin-Type Carbohydrate Antigens (Tn, Sialosyl-Tn, and T) in Gastric Mucosa, Carcinomas and Metastases.** *APMIS* 1992, **100**:162–172.

45. • Takahashi I, Maehara Y, Kusumoto T, Yoshida M, Kakeji Y, Kusumoto H, Furusawa M, Sugimachi K: **Predictive Value of Preoperative Serum Sialyl Tn Antigen Levels in Prognosis of Patients With Gastric Cancer.** *Cancer* 1993, 72:1836–1840.

The tumor marker potential of STn, a carbohydrate-associated antigen, was examined in 350 patients with gastric cancer. Patients were divided into two groups based on preoperative serum STn levels and correlation with clinicopathologic features was performed. High levels of STn were associated with an advanced tumor stage.

46. • Takahashi I, Maehara Y, Kusumoto T, Kohnoe S, Kakeji Y, Baba H, Sugimachi K: **Combined Evaluation of Preoperative Serum Sialyl-Tn Antigen and Carcinoembryonic Antigen Levels Is Prognostic for Gastric Cancer Patients.** *Br J Cancer* 1994, 69:163–166.

Serum STn antigen and carcinoembryonic antigen levels were determined in a previously reported (Takahashi *et al.*, *Cancer* 1993, 72:1836–1840) series of gastric cancer patients. Increased levels appear to reflect an increased tumor burden, however, whether or not STn has prognostic value independent of tumor stage awaits further study.

47. Haynes BF, Telen MJ, Hale LP, Denning SM. **CD44: A Molecule Involved in Leukocyte Adherence and T-Cell Activation.** *Immunol Today* 1989, **10**:423–428.

48. Günthert U, Hofmann M, Rudy W, Reber S, Zoller M, Haussmann I, Matzku S, Wenzel A, Ponta H, Herrlich P: **A New Variant of Glycoprotein CD44 Confers Metastatic Potential to Rat Carcinoma Cells.** *Cell* 1991, **65**:13–24.

49. Horst E, Meijer CJLM, Radaszkiewicz T, Ossekoppele GJ, van Krieken JHJM, Pals ST: **Adhesion Molecules in the Prognosis of Diffuse Large Cell Lymphoma: Expression of a Lymphocyte Homing Receptor (CD44), LFA-1 (CD11a/18) and ICAM-1 (CD54).** *Leukemia* 1990, 4:595–599.

50. •• Mayer B, Jauch KW, Günthert U, Figdor CG, Schildberg FW, Funke I, Johnson JP: **De-Novo Expression of CD44 and Survival in Gastric Cancer.** *Lancet* 1993, **342**:1019–1022.

Interesting report examining CD44 expression in primary gastric carcinomas using immunohistochemistry. By multivariate analysis, a significant association between increased CD44 immunostaining and reduced survival was observed.

51. Correa P: **Human Gastric Carcinogenesis: A Multistep and Multifactorial Process: First American Cancer Society Award Lecture on Cancer Epidemiology and Prevention.** *Cancer Res* 1992, **52**:6735–6740.

52. Matsumura Y, Tarin D: **Significance of CD44 Gene Products for Cancer Diagnosis and Disease Evaluation.** *Lancet* 1992, **340**:1053–1058.

53. Tababe KK, Ellis LM, Saya H: **Expression of CD44R1 Adhesion Molecule in Colon Carcinomas and Metastases.** *Lancet* 1993, **341**: 725–726.

54. Diehl JT, Hermann RE, Coopeerman AM, *et al.*: **Gastric Carcinona. A Ten-Year Review.** *Ann Surg* 1983, **198**:9–12.

55. Bizer LS: **Adenocarcinoma of the Stomach: Current Results of Treatment.** *Cancer* 1983, **51**:743–745.

56. •• Siewert JR, Böttcher K, Roder JD, Busch R, Hermanek P, Meyer HJ, and the German Gastric Carcinoma Study Group: **Prognostic Relevance of Systematic Lymph Node Dissection in Gastric Carcinoma.** *Br J Surg* 1993, **80**:1015–1018.

Prospective multicenter study evaluating standard versus radical lymph node dissection in patients with resectable gastric cancer. Radical dissection, defined as removal of 26 or more nodes, was shown by multivariate analysis to be an independent prognostic factor in UICC stage II and IIIA cancers. There was no significant difference in operative morbidity or mortality rates.

57. Hermanek P, Sobin LH, eds. *UICC TNM Classification of Malignant Tumours, edn 4.* Berlin: Springer; 1987:39–46.

58. • Ichikura T, Tomimatsu S, Okusa Y, Eefuji K, Tamakuma S: **Comparison of the Prognostic Significance Between the Number of Metastatic Lymph Nodes and Nodal Stage Based on Their Location in Patients With Gastric Cancer.** *J Clin Oncol* 1993, **11**:1894–1900.

Comparison of prognostic significance of nodal stage versus number of metastatic lymph nodes in 777 Japanese patients who underwent potentially curative resections. By multivariate analysis in patients with four or more positive nodes, the number of positive nodes was the most important prognostic marker followed by depth of invasion. Nodal stage was not significantly prognostic.

59. Kelsen D: **Neoadjuvant Therapy for Gastrointestinal Cancers.** *Oncology* 1993, 7:25–41.

60. •• Ajani JA, Mayer RJ, Ota DM, Steele GD, Evans D, Roh M, Sugarbaker DJ, Dumas P, Gray C, Vena DA, Stablein DM: **Preoperative and Postoperative Combination Chemotherapy for Potentially Resectable Gastric Carcinoma.** *J Natl Cancer Inst* 1993, **85**:1839–1844.

Evaluation of EAP as neoadjuvant therapy for local-regional gastric cancer. Curative resection was performed in 37 of 41 (77%); however, median survival was 15.5 months and no complete pathologic responses occurred. Regimen was associated with substantial toxicity.

61. Wilke H, Preusser P, Fink U, Gunzer U, Meyer J, Sewert JR, Achterrath W, Lenaz L, Kripp H: **Preoperative Chemotherapy in Locally Advanced and Nonresectable Gastric Cancer: A Phase II Study With Etoposide, Doxorubicin, and Cisplatin.** *J Clin Oncol* 1989, 7:1318–1326.

62. Comis R: **Integration of Chemotherapy Into Combined Modality Treatment of Solid Tumours.** *Cancer Treat Rev* 1974, **1**:22–33.

63. Moynihan T, Hansen R, Anderson T, Quebbeman E, Beatty P, Ausman R, Ritch P, Chitambar C, Vukelich M: **Continuous 5-Fluorouracil Infusion in Advanced Gastric Carcinoma.** *Am J Clin Oncol* 1988, 11:461–464.

64. Gohmann JJ, Macdonald JS: **Chemotherapy of Gastric Cancer.** *Cancer Invest* 1989, 7:39–52.

65. • Cullinan SA, Moertel CG, Wieand HS, O'Connell MJ, Poon MA, Krook JE, Mailliard JA, Tschetter LK for the North Central Cancer Treatment

Group: **Controlled Evaluation of Three Drug Combination Regimens Versus Fluorouracil Alone for the Therapy of Advanced Gastric Cancer.** *J Clin Oncol* 1994, **12**:412–416.

Randomized trial of FAMe, FAP, and FAMe alternating with triazinate compared with fluorouracil alone. No significant advantage of the other regimens over single-agent fluorouracil was observed.

66. Gastrointestinal Tumor Study Group: **Phase II-III Chemotherapy Studies in Advanced Gastric Cancer.** *Cancer Treat Rep* 1979, **63**:1871–1876.
67. Gastrointestinal Tumor Study Group: **Randomized Study of Combination Chemotherapy in Unresectable Gastric Cancer.** *Cancer* 1984, **53**:13–17.
68. Wils JA, Klein HO, Wagener DJ Bleiberg H, Reis H, Korsten F, Conroy T, Fickers M, Leyvraz S, Buyse M, *et al.* for the EORTC: **Sequential High-Dose Methotrexate and Fluorouracil Combined With Doxorubicin: A Step Ahead in the Treatment of Advanced Gastric Cancer. A Trial of the European Organization for Research and Treatment of Cancer Gastrointestinal Tract Cooperative Group.** *J Clin Oncol* 1991, **9**:827–831.
69. Wilke H, Preusser P, Fink U, Achterrath W, Meyer HJ, Stahl M, Lenaz L, Meyer J, Siewert JR, Geerlings H, *et al.*: **New Developments in the Treatment of Gastric Carcinoma.** *Semin Oncol* 1990, **17**:61–70.
70. Lerner A, Gonin R, Steele GD JR, Mayer RJ: **Etoposide, Doxorubicin, and Cisplatin Chemotherapy for Advanced Gastric Adenocarcinoma: Results of a Phase II Trial.** *J Clin Oncol* 1992, **10**:536–540.
71. Kelsen D, Atiq OT, Saltz L, Niedzwiecki D, Ginn D, Chapman D, Heelan R, Lightdale C, Vinciguerra V, Brennan M: **FAMTX Versus Etoposide, Doxorubicin, and Cisplatin: A Random Assignment Trial in Gastric Cancer.** *J Clin Oncol* 1992, **10**:541–548.
72. • Kim NK, Park YS, Heo DS, Suh C, Kim SY, Park KC, Kang YK, Shin DB, Kim HT, Kim HJ, *et al.*: **A Phase II Randomized Study of 5-Fluorouracil and Cisplatin Versus 5-Fluorouracil, Doxorubicin, and Mitomycin-C Versus 5-Fluorouracil Alone in the Treatment of Advanced Cancer.** *Cancer* 1993, **71**:3813–3818.

Randomized study demonstrating a higher response rate for fluorouracil and cisplatin versus FAM versus single-agent fluorouracil. However, no significant difference in survival was observed between the three study arms.

73. Alexander HR, Grem JL, Pass HI, Hamilton M, McAtee N, Fraker DL, Allegra CJ: **Neoadjuvant Chemotherapy for Locally Advanced Gastric Adenocarcinoma.** *Oncology (Huntingt)* 1993, **7**:37–42.

Frank A. Sinicrope, MD, Department of Gastrointestinal Medical Oncology and Digestive Diseases, The University of Texas M.D. Anderson Cancer Center, 1515 Holcombe Boulevard, Box 078, Houston, TX 77030, USA.

Gastroduodenal motility

Nicholas J. Talley, MD, PhD, FRACP

University of Sydney, Penrith, Australia

Gastroduodenal motility disturbances are considered to be of major importance in the pathogenesis of a number of diseases, including functional dyspepsia. The topics chosen for review this year highlight new advances in both physiology and pathophysiology. Human rather than animal studies were generally selected for review because of their direct relevance to human disease. Important contributions have included the development of new approaches for measuring gastric emptying and further insights into how gastric emptying occurs and is controlled. Useful studies of the epidemiology, classification, pathogenesis, and treatment of functional dyspepsia are also reviewed.

Current Opinion in Gastroenterology 1994, **10**:618–622

Measurement of motor function

Gastric emptying can be assessed by many different techniques. Although scintigraphy is now accepted as the reference method, it requires expensive equipment. Galil *et al.* [1•] reviewed their clinical experience with isotope emptying tests. They found that the results were often at variance with the clinical diagnosis but did not alter the treatment of patients with functional dyspepsia. Ghoos *et al.* [2••] described the development of a simple breath test to measure solid emptying using ^{14}C (radioactive)- or ^{13}C (nonradioactive)-labeled octanoic acid with egg yolk (in scrambled eggs). Upon reaching the duodenum, octanoic acid is oxidized, releasing labeled CO_2 that can be measured in the breath. This breath test could reliably measure solid emptying and accurately discriminate normal subjects from patients with delayed emptying.

Although occluding contractions (measured by manometry) and fundic tone (measured by the barostat) give indirect information, direct measures to quantify the propulsive force may be useful. Prather *et al.* [3•] applied a novel force transducer that measures only antegrade forces in healthy volunteers to quantitate propulsive forces after ingestion of a meal and in response to lipid and intravenous erythromycin. The results indicate that gastric axial forces provide an accurate assessment of overall gastric propulsion during solid emptying [3•].

Control of motor function

During the interdigestive state in the stomach, there is a cyclical pattern of motor activity referred to as the migrating motor complex (MMC). Currently there is an incomplete understanding of the mechanisms controlling phase III of the MMC (an activity front starting in the stomach characterized by a burst of high-amplitude, high-frequency rhythmic contractions that migrate down the small bowel). Motilin, a peptide hormone, is considered to play an important role in initiating the MMC, although this is still controversial. One study has reported that the selective serotonin type 3 receptor antagonist ondansetron suppressed the gastric component of phase III and abolished the normal rise in motilin preceding phase III in healthy volunteers [4•]. Furthermore, erythromycin, a motilin agonist, usually restored the gastric phase III. These results suggest that serotonin type 3 receptors are involved in the initiation of phase III activity through an effect on motilin.

Gastric emptying depends on the balance between propulsive forces and resistance to outflow. In an elegant ultrasonographic study, Brown *et al.* [5••] showed that the stomach slowly decants liquids while simultaneously allowing solids to fall to the pylorus (the most dependent part of the stomach); the pylorus did not allow large particles to pass until they were ground to a small size. The process of gastric accommodation allows the stomach to process meals of different sizes; tonic contraction of the fundus is considered to be a major factor in liquid emptying. Ropert *et al.* [6•] used the barostat to measure gastric fundic tone and simultaneously measured liquid emptying after three liquid meals; profound gastric relaxation was detected that increased with meal size but reversed with completion of emptying. Evidence has also been presented that voluntary suppression of defecation delays gastric emptying based on a study of 12 healthy male volunteers [7•], suggesting that a "cologastric brake" may exist. However, stress (which also may induce delayed gastric emptying) from attempts to voluntarily suppress defecation may have played a role.

Disturbed sensory perception in the stomach may be important in functional dyspepsia. Khan *et al.* [8•], in a study of male volunteers, carried out balloon dis-

Abbreviation

MMC—migrating motor complex.

 ISBN 1-85922-611-6 ISSN 0267–1379

tension at different rates to assess sensory perception mechanisms. They observed different results with ramp distension (inflating the balloon at constant rates from 20 to 200 mL/min) and rapid intermittent distensions (in which symptoms were induced at much reduced volumes). They concluded that the ramp distension response was consistent with the activation of stretch receptors situated parallel to muscle elements, whereas rapid intermittent distension may activate a separate group of rapidly adapting, possibly mucosal mechanoreceptors.

Edelbroek *et al.* [9•] investigated whether stimulation of duodenal mechanoreceptors alters distal gastroduodenal motor function in health. Balloon distension in the duodenum increased the number of isolated pyloric pressure waves during fasting but not postprandially, suggesting that stimulation of duodenal mechanoreceptors may partly control gastric emptying.

Nitric oxide

Nitric oxide is a gas that is poorly soluble in water and has a short half-life; it is generated from L-arginine by nitric oxide synthase. It is now known that nitric oxide is a key inhibitory neurotransmitter in the gut. Nitric oxide is considered important in mediating sphincter relaxation (*eg*, lower esophageal, pyloric, and internal anal sphincters), in accommodative and receptive relaxation (*eg*, the gastric fundus in response to a meal), and in regulation of phasic contractions in the antrum and small bowel, and the intestinal peristaltic reflex [10,11]. In animal studies, nitric oxide has been implicated in the regulation of gastroduodenal bicarbonate secretion [12] and the release of gastric mucus [13]. Another good review of this topic has appeared in the past year [14•].

Prokinetics

A number of designer drugs for motility disorders are now available [15•]. Cisapride is a serotonin type 4 receptor agonist that releases acetylcholine from postganglionic nerve endings in the myenteric plexus. However, it is poorly understood how cisapride promotes acceleration of gastric emptying in gastroparesis. An Australian group examined the effects of intravenous cisapride on the organization of antroduodenal contractions and pyloric motility in healthy control subjects and patients with gastroparesis [16•]. They found that cisapride stimulated antral pressure waves of 6 cm or greater in extent, which appeared to be important in promoting gastric emptying in gastroparesis; however, no placebo control was included.

The central role of *Helicobacter pylori* in peptic ulcer can no longer be denied. However, it has been suggested that prokinetics may be of value in ulcer treatment based on the hypothesis that dysmotility reduces acid clearance. Kerrigan *et al.* [17•] performed a careful double-blind study of 66 duodenal ulcer patients who were treated with cisapride or placebo; 34% of those taking cisapride relapsed versus 66% of the placebo group (a significant but not very striking difference). Testoni *et al.* [18] randomly allocated 60 patients with antral gastric ulcers to either cisapride, ranitidine, or both; healing rates at 8 weeks were similar in all groups (>88%) but no placebo arm was included, and the study was underpowered. Prokinetics are unlikely to play a role in ulcer therapy in the 1990s.

The value of cisapride in severe gastroparesis was investigated by Richards *et al.* [19•]. In a randomized, double-blind placebo-controlled trial of 43 patients, cisapride significantly increased solid-gastric emptying relative to baseline, but it did not improve symptom status relative to baseline or placebo. These findings suggest that patients with severe gastroparesis obtain little clinically relevant benefit from this compound.

Disturbances of electrical slow-wave rhythm have been linked to gastroparesis. This activity can be measured by the electrogastrogram. The effect of long-term prokinetic agent therapy on gastric dysrhythmias is not well established. One uncontrolled study evaluated cisapride (10 to 20 mg three times daily for 6 months) in patients with idiopathic (n=7) and diabetic (n=7) gastroparesis [20]. Baseline electrogastrograms were abnormal in 12 patients. After 6 months, two patients with bradygastria and two with tachygastria had reverted to normal three cycle per minute activity, and six other patients had some improvement. Although symptoms improved, there was no correlation between electrogastrogram results, gastric emptying values, and symptom scores.

Erythromycin, a motilin agonist, has prokinetic actions [21••]. Hill *et al.* [22] tested the effect of oral erythromycin in patients with a denervated stomach after esophagectomy. Erythromycin, but not cisapride, improved gastric emptying postoperatively compared with the preoperative values. In a controlled trial, Yeo *et al.* [23] report that intravenous erythromycin significantly accelerates gastric emptying after pancreaticoduodenectomy. However, long-term efficacy was not assessed in either study (tachyphylaxis has been observed to occur with erythromycin).

Functional dyspepsia

Epidemiology and classification

There has been a growing consensus that the term "chronic dyspepsia" should be restricted to mean recurrent or persistent pain or discomfort centered in the upper abdomen. Those with no obvious explanation for their symptoms are referred to as having functional or non-ulcer dyspepsia [24•].

New data on the epidemiology of functional upper gut symptoms has emerged. Drossman *et al.* [25••] evaluated 5430 US householders to assess symptoms, impact, and risk factors. They found that 26% had apparent functional gastroduodenal symptoms whereas 29% had "functional heartburn;" the prevalence was similar in men and women but higher in nonwhites. Only 23% of the householders had ever seen a doctor for functional gastroduodenal complaints, but nearly 9%

reported being too sick to go to work (compared with 4% without any functional gut complaints). However, this was not a random population–based survey (and therefore was potentially prone to bias) and some of the categories assessed may have overestimated functional disease (*eg*, "functional heartburn" is probably largely explained by gastroesophageal reflux disease). Population-based studies from Sweden and Denmark have also been published in the past year [26•,27]. A Scottish group reported on their extensive experience with dyspepsia in referred patients; they noted that clinicians were more confident in diagnosing structural disease but multiple diagnoses were common [28•].

The clinical value of classifying patients with dyspepsia into symptom subgroups (ulcer-like, dysmotility-like, and reflux-like) has continued to generate controversy. At the Mayo Clinic, 820 consecutive outpatients presenting for endoscopy were evaluated [29••]. Of the 162 patients with functional dyspepsia, 31% were classified into two or more subgroups, and 27% had nonspecific, unclassifiable complaints [29••]. Moreover, the subgroups could not usefully discriminate functional from structural disease. In 2253 dyspeptic patients, Mansi *et al.* [30] reported that patients with ulcer-like dyspepsia were more likely to have an abnormal endoscopy than patients with dysmotility-like dyspepsia, but the absolute differences were small. Overall, the data suggest that subclassifying dyspepsia by symptom type is not useful.

Pathogenesis

The pathogenesis of functional dyspepsia remains unclear. A lack of a link with smoking, alcohol, and nonsteroidal anti-inflammatory drugs has been confirmed in outpatients [31•] and in the general population [32•]. Gastric emptying of bland meals is abnormal in a subset, but this does not correlate with symptoms. Whether the use of more provocative test meals would identify a greater number of relevant abnormalities is unclear. Mangnall *et al.* [33•] evaluated the distribution of a radiolabeled liquid fatty meal; emptying was delayed and less of the meal was found in the proximal stomach in patients with functional dyspepsia compared with control subjects. Similar results were reported by Troncon *et al.* [34•] with a standard test meal. The relationship between intragastric distribution of a meal and symptom patterns in functional dyspepsia was also examined by Scott *et al.* [35•]. They found subtle abnormalities of gastric emptying in 48% of cases, but these did not correlate with symptoms. Therefore, intragastric distribution abnormalities are of questionable clinical significance.

Gastric-visceral hypersensitivity to balloon distension has been documented in up to 50% of patients with functional dyspepsia studied in specialized centers. Gut peptides, such as somatostatin, may modulate sensation. Kaneko *et al.* [36•] report that immunoreactive-somatostatin concentrations were significantly higher in the gastric mucosa of patients with ulcer-like dyspepsia than in other patients with functional dyspepsia or control subjects. Whether this finding could be explained by *H. pylori* status was not carefully addressed, and the pathogenic significance must await confirmatory studies.

Management

The treatment of functional dyspepsia remains unsatisfactory. In order to assess drug efficacy in dyspepsia, accurate measurement of outcome in clinical trials is of key importance, yet little attention has been paid to this issue. Dimenas *et al.* [37•] report on the development and validity of specific questionnaires to measure quality of life in dyspepsia. If confirmed, these findings represent a methodologic step forward for trials in this field.

Sucralfate was not superior to placebo in a well-performed double-blind trial [38•]. Fumagalli and Hammer [39] assessed the efficacy of cisapride versus metoclopramide in a randomized double-blind trial; at 4 weeks the overall response rate was similar (87% vs 77%), but 2 weeks after stopping treatment the response remained significantly better in the cisapride group (73% vs 47%). However, the lack of a placebo arm represents a major flaw and makes interpretation of the data very difficult.

Approximately 50% of patients with functional dyspepsia are infected with *H. pylori.* In a small, double-blind crossover trial of 48 patients, Frazzoni *et al.* [40] evaluated the efficacy of managing *H. pylori* with colloidal bismuth plus metronidazole versus placebo; in uninfected patients, cisapride versus placebo was assessed. No significant differences from placebo were detected, but the design of the study was flawed for several reasons, including inadequate accuracy. Finally, Hausken and Berstad [41•] studied 10 patients before and after administration of glyceryl trinitrate (which is known to generate nitric oxide). According to ultrasound results, the drug reduced the width of the antral area both during fasting and postprandially, but did not significantly reduce symptoms.

References and recommended reading

Papers of particular interest, published within the annual period of review, have been highlighted as:

- • Of special interest
- •• Of outstanding interest

1. • Galil MA, Critchley M, Mackie CR: **Isotope Gastric Emptying Tests in Clinical Practice: Expectation, Outcome, and Utility.** *Gut* 1993, **34**:916–919.

An audit of 472 gastric emptying tests carried out over 10 years.

2. •• Ghoos YF, Maes BD, Geypens BJ, Mys G, Hiele MI, Rutgeerts PJ, Vantrappen G: **Measurement of Gastric Emptying Rate of Solids by Means of a Carbon-Labeled Octanoic Acid Breath Test.** *Gastroenterology* 1993, **104**:1640–1647.

Describes a new, simple, and accurate noninvasive method for assessing solid gastric emptying; no radioactivity is required if ^{13}C is used. This method represents a diagnostic advance.

3. • Prather CM, Camilleri M, Thomforde GM, Forstrom LA, Zinsmeister AR: **Gastric Axial Forces in Experimentally Delayed and Accelerated Gastric Emptying.** *Am J Physiol* 1993, **264**:G928–G934.

Confirms that axial forces affect solid emptying.

4. • Wilmer A, Tack J, Coremmans G, Janssens J, Peeters T, Vantrappen G: **5-Hydroxytryptamine-3 Receptors Are Involved in the Initiation of Gastric Phase-3 Motor Activity in Humans.** *Gastroenterology* 1993, **105**:773–780.

A good physiologic study showing that serotonin type 3 receptors are involved in the initiation of gastric activity fronts in humans via the suppression of plasma motilin peaks.

5. •• Brown BP, Schulze-Delrieu K, Schrier JE, Abu-Yousef MM: **The Configuration of the Human Gastroduodenal Junction in the Separate Emptying of Liquids and Solids.** *Gastroenterology* 1993, **105**:433–440.

After a meal of chicken broth and beans in six healthy volunteers, the mechanisms by which the stomach "sieves" liquids from solids were evaluated by real-time ultrasound. This report is the first direct evidence of such processes in humans.

6. • Ropert A, Varannes SBD, Bizais Y, Roze C, Galmiche J-P: **Simultaneous Assessment of Liquid Emptying and Proximal Gastric Tone in Humans.** *Gastroenterology* 1993, **105**:667–674.

Suggests that gastric tone is not the major driving force in liquid emptying.

7. • Tjeerdsma HC, Smout AJPM, Akkermans LMA: **Voluntary Suppression of Defecation Delays Gastric Emptying.** *Dig Dis Sci* 1993, **38**:832–836.

Suggests that constipation may be a learned response in some patients, and that a cologastric brake may exist.

8. • Khan MI, Read NW, Grundy D: **Effect of Varying the Rate and Pattern of Gastric Distension on Its Sensory Perception and Motor Activity.** *Am J Physiol* 1993, **264**:G824–G827.

Suggests that two different populations of gastric mechanoreceptors exist, possibly in the mucosa and the muscle.

9. • Edelbroek M, Horowitz M, Dent J, Sun WM, Malbert C, Smout A, Akkermans L: **Effects of Duodenal Distension on Fasting and Postprandial Antropyloroduodenal Motility in Humans.** *Gastroenterology* 1994, **106**:583–592.

In 12 volunteers, duodenal balloon distension during fasting significantly increased the number of isolated pyloric pressure waves and basal pyloric pressure, with a greater response following more proximal distension; postprandially there was no significant increase of pyloric waves.

10. Bayguinov O, Sanders KM: **Role of Nitric Oxide As an Inhibitory Neurotransmitter in the Canine Pyloric Sphincter.** *Am J Physiol* 1993, **264**:G975–G983.

11. Barbier AJ, Lefebvre RA: **Involvement of the L-Argenine: Nitric Oxide Pathway in Nonadrenergic Noncholinergic Relaxation of the Cat Gastric Fundus.** *J Pharmacol Exp Ther* 1993, **266**:172–178.

12. Takeuchi K, Ohuchi T, Miyake H, Okabe S: **Stimulation by Nitric Oxide Synthase Inhibitors of Gastric and Duodenal HCO^{-}_{3}; Secretion in Rats.** *J Pharmacol Exp Ther* 1993, **266**:1512–1519.

13. Brown JF, Keates AC, Hanson PJ, Whittle BJR: **Nitric Oxide Generators and cGMP Stimulate Mucus Secretion by Rat Gastric Mucosal Cells.** *Am J Physiol* 1993, **265**:G418–G422.

14. • Brookes SJH: **Neuronal Nitric Oxide in the Gut.** *J Gastroenterol Hepatol* 1993, **8**:590–603.

A comprehensive and clear review.

15. • Gwee K-A, Read NW: **Disorders of Gastrointestinal Motility-Therapeutic Potentials and Limitations.** *Aliment Pharmacol Ther* 1994, **8**:105–118.

A good overview of the topic.

16. • Fraser RJ, Horowitz M, Maddox AF, Dent J: **Postprandial Antropyloroduodenal Motility and Gastric Emptying in Gastroparesis-Effects of Cisapride.** *Gut* 1994, **35**:172–178.

Suggests that in gastroparesis a disturbance of the relationship between antral, pyloric, and duodenal pressure waves is important.

17. • Kerrigan DD, Taylor ME, Read NW, Johnson AG: **Acid, Motility, and Ulcers: A Comparison of Cisapride With Placebo in the Prevention of Duodenal Ulcer Relapse.** *Gut* 1993, **34**:1042–1046.

A well-designed trial showing that a prokinetic drug produced a 35% reduction in duodenal ulcer relapse over 12 months.

18. Testoni PA, Bagnolo F, Buizza M, Masci E, Toti GL, Spinelli A, Manzi G: **Effectiveness of Cisapride in Gastric Ulcer: Results of a Double-Blind Randomized Trial Versus Ranitidine and Versus Cisapride Plus Ranitidine.** *J Clin Gastroenterol* 1993, **17**:5–9.

19. • Richards RD, Valenzuela GA, Davenport KG, Fisher KLK, McCallum RW: **Objective and Subjective Results of a Randomized, Double-Blind, Placebo-Controlled Trial Using Cisapride to Treat Gastroparesis.** *Dig Dis Sci* 1993, **38**:811–816.

Cisapride was not superior to placebo in symptom relief for patients with advanced gastroparesis.

20. Rothstein RD, Alavi A, Reynolds JC: **Electrogastrography in Patients With Gastroparesis and Effect of Long-Term Cisapride.** *Dig Dis Sci* 1993, **38**:1518–1524.

21. •• Peeters TL: **Erythromycin and Other Macrolides As Prokinetic Agents.** *Gastroenterology* 1993, **105**:1886–1899.

An excellent, comprehensive review.

22. Hill ADK, Walsh TN, Hamilton D, Freyne P, O'Hare N, Byrne PJ, Hennessy TPJ: **Erythromycin Improves Emptying of the Denervated Stomach After Oesophagectomy.** *Br J Surg* 1993, **80**:879–881.

23. Yeo CJ, Barry K, Sauter PK, Sostre S, Lillemoe KD, Pitt HA, Cameron JL: **Erythromycin Accelerates Gastric Emptying After Pancreatoduodenectomy: A Prospective, Randomized, Placebo-Controlled Trial.** *Ann Surg* 1993, **218**:229–238.

24. • Locke GR, Talley NJ: **Management of Non-Ulcer Dyspepsia.** *J Gastroenterol Hepatol* 1993, **8**:279–286.

A useful up-to-date review.

25. •• Drossman DA, Li Z, Andruzzi E, Temple RD, Talley NJ, Thompson WG, Whitehead WE, Janssens J, Funch-Jensen P, Corazziari E, Richter JE, Koch GG: U.S. **Householder Survey of Functional Gastrointestinal disorders: Prevalence, Sociodemography, and Health Impact.** *Dig Dis Sci* 1993, **38**:1569–1580.

Describes the prevalence and impact of functional gut symptoms as defined by the Rome criteria.

26. • Agreus L, Svardsudd K, Nyren O, Tibblin G: **The Epidemiology of Abdominal Symptoms: Prevalence and Demographic Characteristics in a Swedish Adult Population: A Report From the Abdominal Symptom Study.** *Scand J Gastroenterol* 1994, **29**:102–109.

Abdominal symptoms were reported by 54% of the population. These symptoms generally decreased with age and were more prevalent in women.

27. Kay L, Jorgensen T: **Epidemiology of Upper Dyspepsia in a Random Population: Prevalence, Incidence, Natural History, and Risk Factors.** *Scand J Gastroenterol* 1994, **29**:1–6.

28. • Crean GP, Holden RJ, Knill-Jones RP, Beattie AD, James WB, Marjoribanks FM, Spiegelhalter DJ: **A Database on Dyspepsia.** *Gut* 1994, **35**:191–202.

A detailed account of referred patients in Glasgow with dyspepsia (which was broadly defined).

29. •• Talley NJ, Weaver AL, Tesmer DL, Zinsmeister AR: **Lack of Discriminant Value of Dyspepsia Subgroups in Patients Referred for Upper Endoscopy.** *Gastroenterology* 1993, **105**:1378–1386.

In a consecutive sample of 820 outpatients, the proposed dyspepsia subgroups and other combinations of symptoms were not of clinical use in identifying functional dyspepsia or organic disease. The study suggests that the widely used dyspepsia subgroup classification should be discarded.

30. Mansi C, Savarino V, Mela GS, Picciotto A, Raffaella M, Celle G: **Are Clinical Patterns of Dyspepsia a Valid Guideline for Appropriate Use of Endoscopy? A Report on 2253 Dyspeptic Patients.** *Am J Gastroenterol* 1993, **88**:1011–1015.

31. • Talley NJ, Weaver AL, Zinsmeister AR: **Smoking, Alcohol, and Nonsteroidal Anti-Inflammatory Drugs in Outpatients With Functional Dyspepsia and Among Dyspepsia Subgroups.** *Am J Gastroenterol* 1994, **89**:524–528.

In a large outpatient study, smoking, alcohol, aspirin, nonaspirin nonsteroidal anti-inflammatory drugs, and acetaminophen were not associated with functional dyspepsia.

32. • Talley NJ, Zinsmeister AR, Schleck CD, Melton LJ III: **Smoking, Alcohol, and Analgesics in Dyspepsia and Among Dyspepsia Subgroups: Lack of an Association in a Community.** *Gut* 1994, **35**:619–624.

In a random population sample of uninvestigated dyspeptic patients and asymptomatic persons, smoking, alcohol, aspirin, and acetaminophen were not associated with dyspepsia when nongastrointestinal somatic complaints were taken into account.

33. • Mangnall YF, Houghton LA, Johnson AG, Read NW: **Abnormal Distribution of a Fatty Test Meal Within the Stomach of Patients With Non-Ulcer Dyspepsia.** *Eur J Gastroenterol Hepatol* 1994, **6**:323–327.

This paper shows that patients with functional dyspepsia during gastric emptying have abnormal distribution of a fatty-liquid meal.

34. • Troncon LEA, Bennett RJM, Ahluwalia NK, Thompson DG: **Abnormal Intragastric Distribution of Food During Gastric Emptying in Functional Dyspepsia Patients.** *Gut* 1994, **35**:327–332.

In 11 patients, three had delayed emptying, but there was significantly less of the meal distributed in the proximal half of the stomach.

35. • Scott AM, Kellow JE, Schuter B, Cowan H, Corbett AM, Riley JW, Lunzer MR, Eckstein RP, Hoschl R, Lam SK, Jones MP: **Intragastric Distribution and Gastric Emptying of Solids and Liquids in Functional Dyspepsia: Lack of Influence of Symptom Subgroups and *H. pylori*-Associated Gastritis.** *Dig Dis Sci* 1993, **38**:2247–2254.

In 75 patients, 48% had abnormal intragastric-scintigraphic patterns (fundal half-emptying time, antral maximal fraction); these patterns were more common in reflux-like dyspepsia.

36. • Kaneko H, Mitsuma T, Uchida K, Furusawa A, Morise K: **Immunoreactive-Somatostatin, Substance P, and Calcitonin Gene-Related Peptide Concentrations of the Human Gastric Mucosa in Patients With Nonulcer Dyspepsia and Peptic Ulcer Disease.** *Am J Gastroenterol* 1993, **88**:898–904.

Of 56 patients with functional dyspepsia, 34 had ulcer-like dyspepsia; immunoreactive-somatostatin concentrations in the gastric mucosa were higher in this subgroup.

37. Dimenas E, Glise H, Hallerback B, Hernqvist H, Svedlund J, Wiklund I:
• **Quality of Life in Patients With Upper Gastrointestinal Symptoms: An Improved Evaluation of Treatment Regimens?** *Scand J Gastroenterol* 1993, **28**:681–687.

The authors present data on the validity and responsiveness to change of quality of life instruments for dyspepsia. This study has important implications for future trials in the field.

38. Gudjonsson H, Oddsson E, Bjornsson S, Gunnlaugsson O, Theodors
• A, Jonasson TA, Bonnevie O, Thjodleifsson B: **Efficacy of Sucralfate in Treatment of Non-Ulcer Dyspepsia: A Double-Blind Placebo-Controlled Study.** *Scand J Gastroenterol* 1993, **28**:969–972.

Sixty-eight percent of patients on sucralfate had global improvement over 3 weeks compared with 69% of those on placebo.

39. Fumagalli I, Hammer B: **Cisapride Versus Metoclopramide in the Treatment of Functional Dyspepsia: A Double-Blind Comparative Trial.** *Scand J Gastroenterol* 1994, **29**:33–37.

40. Frazzoni M, Lonardo A, Grisendi A, Casa GD, Pulvirenti M, Ferrari AM, DiGregorio C, Melini L: **Are Routine Duodenal and Antral Biopsies Useful in the Management of "Functional" Dyspepsia? A Diagnostic and Therapeutic Study.** *J Clin Gastroenterol* 1993, **17**:101–108.

41. Hausken T, Berstad A: **Effect of Glyceryl Trinitrate on Antral Motility**
• **and Symptoms in Patients With Functional Dyspepsia.** *Scand J Gastroenterol* 1994, **29**:23–28.

Glyceryl trinitrate, which is known to generate nitric oxide, reduced abnormal antral filling ultrasonographically.

Nicholas J. Talley, MD, PhD, FRACP, Professor of Medicine, University of Sydney, Nepean Hospital, Penrith N.S.W. 2751, Australia.

Immunology

Editorial overview

W. Allan Walker, MD

Harvard Medical School, Boston, Massachusetts, USA

Current Opinion in Gastroenterology 1994, **10**:623–624

The field of mucosal immunology continues to grow at a logarithmic rate in large part because of the use of "new biology" approaches to more precisely define intestinal inflammation, immunophysiology, bacterial colonization, and the premalignant state. In this issue of *Current Opinion in Gastroenterology*, we cover four very important and evolving areas of immunology as they pertain to the gastrointestinal tract. Three reviews deal with the very important field of intestinal inflammation. These include an extensive review of the role of cytokines in experimental intestinal inflammation. An attempt is made to define the pattern of cytokine production in circumstances of acute, self-limited, and chronic inflammation and the role of specific subsets of mucosal T cells in regulatory cytokine release under conditions of inflammation. With the advent of more precise techniques for measuring cytokine production, *ie*, *in situ* hybridization, the role of the epithelium, endothelium, mesenchyme, and lymphoid elements can be more precisely determined *in vitro*. This improved approach to defining the pathogenesis of inflammation can help in the diagnosis and treatment of chronic inflammation, including inflammatory bowel disease.

In addition to a review of cytokines in inflammation, new and exciting animal models of intestinal inflammation are presented. Using techniques of genetic manipulation at the stem cell level, transgenic and "knockout" mice can be produced that either lack or overexpress certain inflammatory cytokines resulting in clinical manifestations of intestinal inflammation comparable to human inflammatory diseases. These *in vivo* models may help to further uncover a better understanding of complex mechanisms of acute and chronic inflammation and may help define the familial nature of inflammatory bowel disease and chronic infectious gastroenteritis. Finally, a detailed review of cytokine production by the gut of humans during inflammation helps to put the experimental cytokine studies and *in vivo* animal models of inflammation into perspective. The combination of *in vitro* cytokine studies, animal models, and human studies should provide a more complete approach to the treatment of inflammatory gastrointestinal disease states.

Additional information referring to the important area of mucosal immunophysiology is reviewed. This paper helps explain the role of myofibroblasts as an important effector cell in modulating the integrated actions of soluble mediators involved in gut absorption, secretion, motility, and blood flow. In addition, we have reviewed the defense factors in human milk as the basis for our understanding of intestinal host defense in infants and young children, as well as the development of the intestinal mucosal host defense system. Finally, we provide two reviews of bacteria and gut immunity and the role of malnutrition in altered bacterial/colonization and decreased intestinal host defenses. This important topic has expanded considerably in the past few years as approaches to microbial vaccines have become of more importance and the role of micronutrients dysfunctions in specific host defense deficiencies has been unraveled. The topics for this year's *Immunology* section were selected to highlight important new areas of rapidly evolving areas of mucosal immunology, of which an understanding is now essential to the subspecialty of gastroenterology.

Cytokine regulation of experimental intestinal inflammation

Hans Herfarth and R. Balfour Sartor (pp 625–632) provide an excellent and comprehensive review of the role of pro- and anti-inflammatory cytokines and specific subsets of mucosal T-helper cells (Th1 and Th2) in experimental intestinal inflammation. They emphasize that research in this field has provided a better understanding of the role of cytokines in the pathophysiology of intestinal inflammation. A delicate balance exists between protective and proinflammatory mediators that is necessary for an appropriate response to intestinal antigens, including bacterial antigens, for an effective healing mucosal injury and infection, rather than progressing to chronic inflammation. By understanding the role of subsets of T-helper cells, we can better understand immune regulation of chronic and acute self-limited inflammation and the genetic predisposition to one pattern or another. These studies have helped in the planning stage for development of *in vivo* animal models using transgenic or knockout mice.

New models of chronic intestinal inflammation

Atul Bhan, Emiko Mizoguchi, and Atsushi Mizoguchi (pp 633–638) reviewed another aspect of important breakthroughs in intestinal inflammation by summarizing the recent success in producing *in vivo* animal models using genetic manipulation of cytokine expression in transgenic and knockout mice models that spontaneously express chronic inflammation of the gastrointestinal tract. These models include mice mutant for interleukin-2, interleukin-10, and T-cell receptor genes. These models help define the role of these cytokines and the pathogenesis of chronic intestinal inflammation and may be important in defining the mucosal immune responses that must be controlled by new therapeutic

 ISBN 1-85922-611-6 ISSN 0267-1379

approaches to immunologically mediated inflammatory bowel disease.

Cytokine production in the human gastrointestinal tract during inflammation

Claudio Fiocchi, David Binion, and Jeffry Katz (pp 639–644) help to put the area of intestinal inflammation in perspective for the gastroenterologist by reviewing the recent literature that defines cytokine production and tissue levels in the intestine of humans with intestinal inflammatory states. They underscore the role of a recently described interleukin-1 receptor antagonist in down-regulating intestinal responses to inflammatory cytokines and emphasizing its importance in the prevention of chronic inflammation. The authors also stress the importance of measuring cytokines at the site of inflammation within the intestine, *ie*, intestinal secretions, *in situ* hybridization of intestinal biopsies, and colon versus small intestine, rather than in serum of stool collections. The latter approach may be misleading and unlikely to help define the precise mechanism of small intestinal versus colonic inflammatory states. They emphasize the importance of human data in devising new therapeutic approaches to the control of inflammation.

Intestinal subepithelial myofibroblasts as effector cells in mucosal immunophysiology

John Valentich and Don Powell (pp 645–651) further underscore our understanding of intestinal immunophysiology reviewing the role of myofibroblasts in this process. They stress the importance of defining the molecular basis of soluble mediator effects on intestinal epithelium in the normal process of absorption, secretion, and motility and the pathologic role of these mediator imbalances in intestinal inflammation and diarrhea. They define a family of phenotypically inter-related cells including pericryptal fibroblasts or subepithelial myofibroblasts as juxtaparenchmal cells and elaborate on their role in intestinal cellular proliferation, differentiation, inflammation, and modulation of immune responses. This comprehensive review of the relationship of various cell types in the intestine in injury and repair is important new information in the area of immunophysiology of the gut.

Defense factors in human milk

Agnes Wold and Lars Hanson (pp 652–658) draw on their extensive clinical experience in developing countries to underscore the importance of host defense factors in human milk for the passive and active protection of infants and young children against infectious and allergic intestinal disease states. They also make a case for these new data on passive protection of the intestine by human breast milk as an approach to understanding the development of intestinal host defenses and approaches to treatment of intestinal insults such as short bowel syndrome or chronic inflammation. Their review also helps to determine the role of cytokines in gut proliferation, differentiation, and normal physiologic function.

Bacteria and gut immunity

Shobha Char and Michael Farthing (pp 659–663) review the exciting new developments in our understanding of bacterial colonization and translocation, bacterial stimulus of mucosal immune responses, and the potential for development of new bacterial vaccines based on our understanding of the molecular interactions of bacterial with the gastrointestinal tract. They emphasize that "intestinal bacteria are considered to be vital for the maturation and maintenance of intestinal immunity in healthy individuals but may have harmful effects when the flora is modified by drugs such as the proton pump inhibitors that suppress gastric acid. Research continues to support the concept that a healthy flora can be maintained by certain bacterial species such as Lactobacilli, although their therapeutic role in disease states still has not been established." Finally, they review the new findings on bacterial stimulus to intestinal immune responses as the basis for developing an effective vaccine for therapeutic approach to epidemic bacterial gastrointestinal disease states (*eg*, *Shigella*, *Salmonella*, and *Helicobacter pylori* infection).

Malnutrition and gut immune function

Finally, Susanna Cunningham-Rundles (pp 664–670) provides a comprehensive review of recent studies that more precisely define the effect of malnutrition on gastrointestinal immune function. She emphasizes animal and human studies to define the intestinal immune dysfunctions with generalized and specific micronutrient deficiencies. These observations complement the previous review on bacterial interaction with the gut, an important component of the morbidity/mortality of malnutrition states. She concludes that "understanding the interaction between nutrients and the immune system in the gastrointestinal tract in the context of the highly differentiated nature of the gastrointestinal immune response, is vital for intervention and effective nutrient repletion."

W. Allan Walker, MD, Mucosal Immunology Laboratory, Massachusetts General Hospital-East, Building 149, 13th Street, Room 3004, Charlestown, MA 02129, USA.

Cytokine regulation of experimental intestinal inflammation

Hans H. Herfarth, MD, and R. Balfour Sartor, MD

University of North Carolina at Chapel Hill, Chapel Hill, North Carolina, USA

Cytokines are important mediators of intestinal inflammation and the local and systemic manifestations associated with gut injury. This review focuses on recent developments in cytokine regulation and activities in experimental intestinal inflammation with emphasis on the balance between pro- and anti-inflammatory cytokines. The influence of local expression of interleukin-1 and its physiological antagonist, the interleukin-1 receptor antagonist, as well as T-helper lymphocyte subsets in determining the chronicity of intestinal inflammation and infection is discussed along with genetic determinants of these balances. The effects of interleukin-1 on physiologic abnormalities associated with inflammation are summarized. The mechanisms by which cytokines regulate tissue injury and mediate genetic susceptibility in experimental intestinal inflammation provide new insights into the pathogenesis of inflammatory bowel disease.

Current Opinion in Gastroenterology 1994, **10**:625–632

Cytokines are soluble proteins produced by a variety of cells in response to injury, infection, or antigenic challenge. Through autocrine, paracrine, or endocrine functions, they mediate local and systemic manifestations of inflammation and help orchestrate numerous interactions between the immune system and physiologic processes. Recent advances have increased our knowledge of the regulation of cytokine production in intestinal inflammation, but we are only beginning to investigate the function of cytokines in pathophysiologic responses to gut injury. There is little doubt that cytokines play a key role in the pathogenesis of inflammatory bowel disease (IBD) [1••]. Animal models of intestinal inflammation provide a unique opportunity to study cytokine patterns of different stages of inflammation and to selectively block or amplify a particular cytokine to define its precise role in the inflammatory response.

Interleukin-1 family in animal models

Interleukin-1 has two structurally related isoforms, interleukin-1α and interleukin-1β. A key role of interleukin-1 in the pathogenesis of inflammation is based on increased concentrations at sites of injury, induction of many of the hallmarks of inflammation by exogenous administration, and diminished inflammation when its activity is blocked [2]. Interleukin-1 is produced by a variety of cell types that include monocytes, macrophages, platelets, fibroblasts, keratinocytes, endothelial cells, and smooth muscle cells. Interleukin-1 elicits systemic inflammatory reactions like fever, acute-phase protein synthesis, decreased plasma iron and zinc, and hypermetabolism; local release of interleukin-1 initiates inflammatory reactions including neutrophil tissue infiltration, edema, T- and B-cell activation, and induction of cytokine production.

The most recently described member of the interleukin-1 gene family is the interleukin-1 receptor antagonist, which binds to type I and II interleukin-1 receptors without agonist activity, thus blocking the biological activity of interleukin-1 [3]. This endogenous regulator of interleukin-1 bioactivity is produced by monocytes, macrophages, and epithelial cells in response to many of the same stimuli that induce interleukin-1 production (Fig. 1).

Tissue levels of interleukin-1 and interleukin-1 receptor antagonist

A number of studies have demonstrated a consistent increase in tissue levels of interleukin-1 messenger RNA and protein in experimental colitis; the measured tissue concentrations correlate with the degree of intestinal inflammation [1••]. Recently, two groups have shown a corresponding increase in interleukin-1 receptor antagonist during experimental colitis [4•,5•,6••]. Cominelli *et al.* [5•] and Ferretti *et al.* [6••] found interleukin-1 receptor antagonist in colonic tissues of healthy rabbits, whereas interleukin-1α was undetectable. A marked increase of interleukin-1α as well as interleukin-1 receptor antagonist was noted in inflamed tissues. Tissue interleukin-1 levels peaked at 48 hours after formalin-immune complex colitis, but interleukin-1 receptor antagonist remained elevated for 1 week [6••]. Interest-

Abbreviations

IBD—inflammatory bowel disease; **LPMC**—lamina propria mononuclear cells; **PAF**—platelet-activating factor; **Th1**—T-helper lymphocyte subset 1; **Th2**—T-helper lymphocyte subset 2.

 ISBN 1-85922-611-6 ISSN 0267–1379

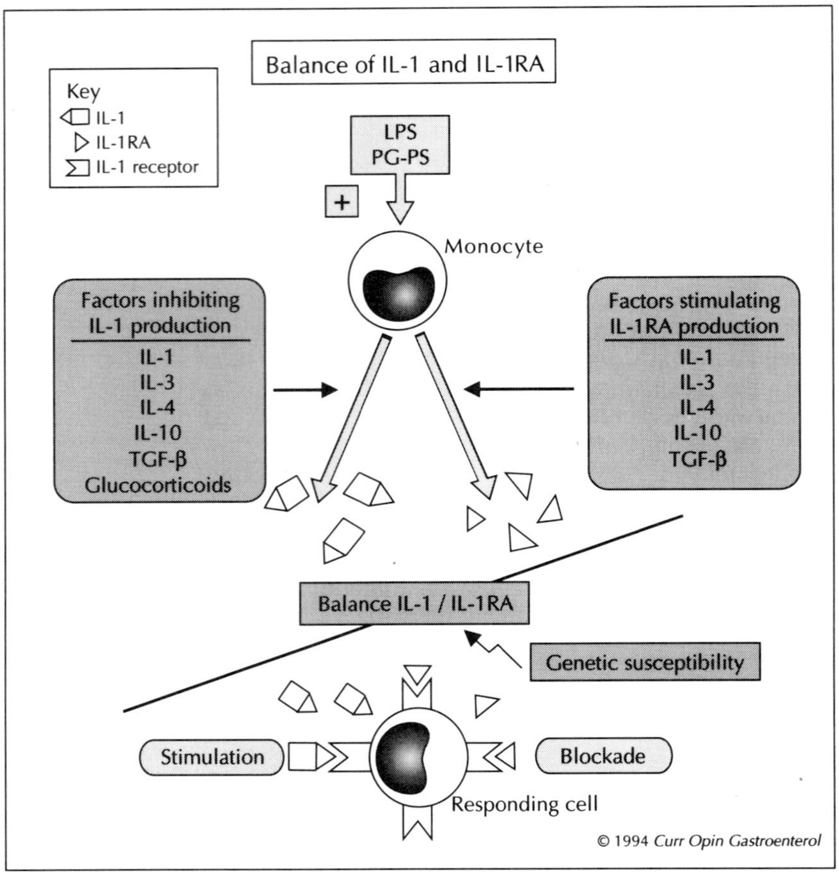

Fig. 1. Balance of interleukin-1 (IL-1) and its endogenous inhibitor interleukin-1 receptor antagonist (IL-1RA). IL-1 and IL-1RA are simultaneously secreted by monocytes stimulated with bacterial products. Several immunoregulatory factors differently influence the IL-1 and IL-1RA secretion. The relative balance of IL-1 and IL-1RA determines whether the IL-1 receptor is stimulated or blocked. A 50-fold molar excess of IL-1RA is required to completely block IL-1 bioactivity. LPS—lipopolysaccharide; PG-PS—peptidoglycan-polysaccharide; TGF—transforming growth factor.

ingly, treatment of the colitis with methylprednisolone significantly reduced interleukin-1α protein levels but had no effect on interleukin-1 receptor antagonist concentrations [5•], demonstrating differential regulation of interleukin-1 and interleukin-1 receptor antagonist by steroids. In contrast, interleukin-1 receptor antagonist messenger RNA tissue levels decreased significantly following corticosteroid therapy with no reduction of interleukin-1α messenger RNA expression. Similarly, McCall *et al.* [4•] demonstrated up-regulation of interleukin-1 receptor antagonist messenger RNA during acute and chronic phases of experimental granulomatous enterocolitis in rats; tissue concentrations of interleukin-1 receptor antagonist correlated with the degree of inflammation.

Balance of interleukin-1 and interleukin-1 receptor antagonist

Using the peptidoglycan-polysaccharide rat model, McCall *et al.* [4•] investigated the relative expression of interleukin-1 and interleukin-1 receptor antagonist in inflamed intestinal tissues to determine if dysregulation of the balance of these pro- and anti-inflammatory cytokines could determine the differential genetic susceptibility to chronic enterocolitis in inbred rat strains. In the peptidoglycan-polysaccharide model, chronic granulomatous intestinal inflammation is induced by subserosal (intramural) injection of bacterial cell wall fragments in susceptible rats [7,8]. In this model, only Lewis rats, which are susceptible to a number of chronic inflammatory conditions, develop chronic, spontaneously relapsing enterocolitis associated with arthritis, granulomatous hepatitis, and anemia; Buffalo and Fischer F344 rats, the latter major histocompatibility complex identical to Lewis rats, display only a transient intestinal inflammation with no systemic injury [4•]. Both interleukin-1 and interleukin-1 receptor antagonist messenger RNA tissue levels were increased during acute enterocolitis and correlated with inflammation in all rat strains. However, 4 weeks after peptidoglycan-polysaccharide injection only Lewis rats had sustained increases in interleukin-1 and interleukin-1 receptor antagonist messenger RNA expression, whereas tissue levels had returned to normal in the Buffalo and Fischer strains. The interleukin-1/interleukin-1 receptor antagonist ratio was increased during chronic inflammation in Lewis rats compared with the acute phase in low responding Fischer rats [4•].

Dysregulation of the balance of interleukin-1 and interleukin-1 receptor antagonist is demonstrated further by *in vitro* studies. Peptidoglycan-polysaccharide up-regulated both interleukin-1 and interleukin-1 receptor antagonist messenger RNA expression in peritoneal macrophages from Fischer and Lewis strains; after 8 hours there was still a high level of interleukin-1 messenger RNA in the Lewis peritoneal cells but a declining expression in macrophages from Fischer rats [4•]. Bristol *et al.* [9] showed that supernatants of peptidoglycan-polysaccharide–stimulated macrophages from susceptible Lewis rats contain relatively more interleukin-1β protein than supernatants of

Buffalo rat macrophages, whereas similar interleukin-1 receptor antagonist protein levels were reported.

These data suggest that the relative balance of interleukin-1 and interleukin-1 receptor antagonist, like the T-helper lymphocyte subset 1 (Th1) versus subset 2 (Th2) response, may play an important role in modulating the inflammatory response and that genetic factors can influence this balance. This hypothesis is supported by recent reports of different allelic representations of interleukin-1 receptor antagonist in patients with ulcerative colitis compared with controls [10] and increased tissue expression of interleukin-1 relative to interleukin-1 receptor antagonist in IBD patients compared with normal and inflammatory controls [11,12].

Effect of blocking interleukin-1

The key role of interleukin-1 in the pathogenesis of intestinal inflammation is demonstrated most convincingly by blockade of the inflammatory response by interleukin-1 receptor antagonist. Cominelli *et al.* [13,14] were the first to report that administration of interleukin-1 receptor antagonist inhibited intestinal injury in the rabbit formalin-immune complex colitis model. Similar results were achieved in the rat acetic acid–induced colitis model [15]. However, these animal models display an acute time course of inflammation rather than representing a chronic inflammatory event analogous to IBD. McCall *et al.* [4•] demonstrated that interleukin-1 receptor antagonist treatment attenuated both acute and chronic phases of peptidoglycan-polysaccharide–induced enterocolitis and its extraintestinal complications. These results not only implicate endogenous interleukin-1 as a key mediator of acute and chronic intestinal inflammation, but also provide evidence that exogenously administered interleukin-1 receptor antagonist may be an effective therapeutic agent in human IBD.

Effect of blocking endogenous interleukin-1 receptor antagonist

Blockade of endogenous interleukin-1 receptor antagonist by intravenous administration of neutralizing antibodies to interleukin-1 receptor antagonist increased mortality and prolonged intestinal inflammation in rabbits with formalin-immune complex–induced colitis [6••]. These results strongly support a protective role for endogenous interleukin-1 receptor antagonist in intestinal inflammation.

Physiologic responses to interleukin-1

Anorexia, weight loss, diarrhea, and abdominal cramps are cardinal clinical features of intestinal inflammation. Previous studies have reported weight loss and delayed gastric emptying after systemic administration of interleukin-1 or tumor necrosis factor [16,17]. Recent investigations in animal models of enterocolitis now demonstrate a role for endogenously produced interleukin-1 in the pathogenesis of weight loss and colonic motility changes associated with intestinal inflammation.

Interleukin-1β significantly suppresses the *in vitro* acetylcholine release and norepinephrine release [18•, 19] in jejunal longitudinal muscle-myenteric plexus preparations from normal rats, whereas in the same preparations interleukin-1β increased tissue levels of substance P [20]. These effects are indirect because protein synthesis was required, although interleukin-1 also had an acute direct effect on norepinephrine release. Collins *et al.* [21] have previously reported a marked suppression of acetylcholine release from myenteric nerves in the inflamed intestine of rats infected by *Trichinella spiralis* [21]. These results suggest that interleukin-1β is an important mediator of suppressed intrinsic nerve function and influences neuropeptide production in the inflamed intestine, which could explain the altered motility in patients with IBD [22].

Fargeas *et al.* [23] suggested a central nervous system action of interleukin-1 on intestinal motility, which was measured by electromyography in conscious rats. Intracerebroventricular interleukin-1β administration stimulated a migrating myoelectric complex pattern in the small intestine and cecocolonic spike bursts, which could be antagonized (only partly in the small intestine) by interleukin-1 receptor antagonist. The effects of interleukin-1 on colonic motility appeared to be secondary to induction of corticotropin-releasing hormone. Morteau *et al.* [24•] demonstrated a significant dysmotility of the proximal colon (non-inflamed portion) in rats after intrarectal administration of trinitrobenzene sulfonic acid. They proposed an involvement of interleukin-1 and platelet activating factor (PAF) in the disturbed colonic motility, because interleukin-1 receptor antagonist and PAF antagonists significantly improved the dysmotility.

A systemic regulatory role of interleukin-1 in the suppression of food intake in rats with experimental colitis was shown in several reports [25,26•]. Reduced food consumption was primarily due to a reduction in meal size rather than the number of meals, and was associated with delayed gastric emptying [26•]. The suppression in food intake was markedly attenuated by intracerebroventricular and, to a lesser extent, peripheral treatment with interleukin-1 receptor antagonist and cyclooxygenase inhibitors [25,27,28]. A corresponding inhibitory effect of interleukin-1 on gastric motility has been shown *in vitro* as well [29].

These data indicate that interleukin-1 acts not only by mediating and amplifying intestinal inflammatory events, but also is one important contributor to altered gastrointestinal motility and decreased food intake during inflammation. These effects appear to be centrally mediated as well as having a local effect and may be secondarily mediated by corticotropin-releasing hormone, PAF, and prostaglandins. It is clear that interleukin-1 now must be considered an important mediator in the brain-gut axis during intestinal inflammation.

Lymphokines in intestinal inflammation

Cytokines produced by activated T-helper lymphocytes are important regulators of the immune response.

Some cytokines amplify inflammation by activating lymphocytes, macrophages, epithelial cells, and endothelial cells; equally important, others suppress the immune response by inhibiting cellular proliferation and cytokine secretion [1••].

Interleukin-2 expression during experimental colitis

Interleukin-2, produced by activated T-helper lymphocytes, amplifies the immune response by inducing lymphocyte proliferation and activating several types of immunocytes.

Gurbindo *et al.* [30•] investigated the *in vitro* secretion of interleukin-2 by isolated colonic lamina propria mononuclear cells (LPMC) during the acute, chronic and resolution phases of colitis, induced by trinitrobenzene sulfonic acid and ethanol. Interleukin-2 activity was compared with macroscopic and microscopic evidence of colonic inflammation. Spontaneous interleukin-2 secretion was not increased by unstimulated cells in the acute or resolving phases. Significantly greater spontaneous interleukin-2 activity was observed in LPMC from the chronic phase compared with cells from control rats. The LPMC derived from animals with chronic or resolved colitis responded with enhanced interleukin-2 secretion to *in vitro* activation with concavalin A, in contrast to no increase over control values for LPMC isolated from the acute colitis group, suggesting an involvement of T lymphocytes in the chronic phase of colitis [30•]. These results are in accordance with those of Sartor *et al.* [31] who showed that T lymphocytes are involved in the chronic phase of peptidoglycan-polysaccharide–induced enterocolitis, but not in the acute phase [31]. However Matsumoto *et al.* [32] reported that cyclosporin A, which inhibits interleukin-2 and interferon-γ production by T-helper lymphocytes, prevented acute enteritis induced by indomethacin. These studies implicate T lymphocytes and their secreted cytokines in the pathogenesis of experimental intestinal inflammation, playing a greater role in the chronic phase than in the acute phase.

Concentrations of cytokines in homogenized tissues and supernatants of *in vitro*–stimulated cells must be evaluated in the context of relevant receptors and the activation state of secreting cells. Therefore the low interleukin-2 bioactivity observed by Gurbindo *et al.* [30•] in acute inflammation could be explained by maximal activation of the cells *in vitro* making them refractory to further activation *in vitro*, or high interleukin-2 receptor expression on LPMC that could bind interleukin-2 and remove it from the supernatant. Nevertheless, the results of measuring interleukin-2 in IBD are controversial, showing increased tissue messenger RNA and protein levels of interleukin-2 in

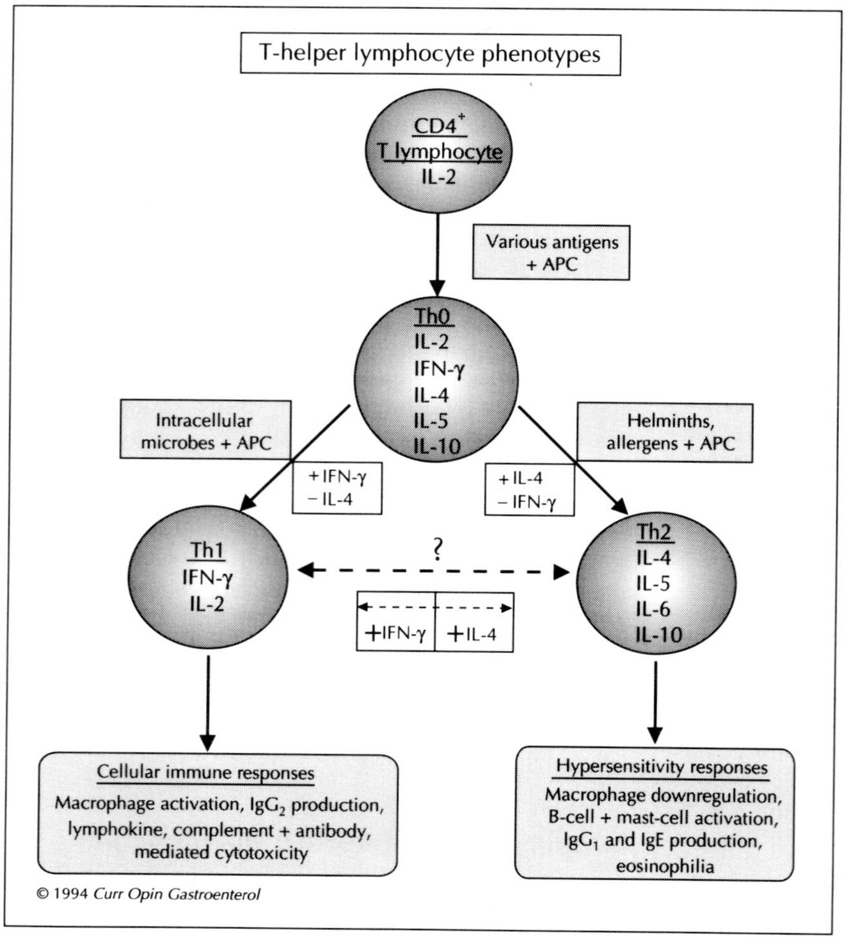

Fig. 2. T-helper cells (CD4+) cytokine secretion phenotypes, their regulation, and their interactions. Interferon-γ (IFN-γ) stimulates Th1 cells and inhibits Th2 cells, whereas interleukin (IL)-4 has reciprocal activities. APC—antigen-presenting cell.

Crohn's disease but not in ulcerative colitis [33,34], whereas *in vitro* production of interleukin-2 by isolated human LPMC in IBD is decreased [35,36].

Intestinal T-helper lymphocyte subset profiles

Two cytokine secretion patterns of $CD4^+$ lymphocytes have been described (Fig. 2): Th1 cells produce interleukin-2 and interferon-γ but not interleukin-4, interleukin-5, interleukin-6, or interleukin-10, whereas Th2 cells produce interleukin-4, interleukin-5, interleukin-6, and interleukin-10. Th1 cells mediate delayed-type hypersensitivity responses whereas Th2 cells regulate efficient B-lymphocyte immunoglobulin synthesis and allergic reactions. Both subsets of T cells produce interleukin-3 and granulocyte/monocyte colony stimulating factor. Th1 cells activate macrophages and promote production of opsonizing antibodies (IgG2a and IgG3), which are required to clear infection by intracellular organisms, whereas the cytokines excreted by Th2 cells down-regulate macrophages, promote isotype switching to cells producing IgE and IgG1, stimulate mast cells, and induce eosinophilia [37]. In addition to T-cell clones that fit into the Th1 or Th2 group, $CD4^+$ T-cell clones having the capacity to produce both sets of cytokines (Th0) have been reported [38].

The Th1 and Th2 pattern have not been extensively studied in experimental colitis models. Because of the high likelihood that regulation of these subsets will be important in chronic intestinal inflammation, we will briefly summarize the role of these T-cell subsets in determining host responses to experimental intestinal parasitic infections. The relevance of the Th1 and Th2 system to intestinal inflammation is that the balance of these cytokines may determine activity, chronicity, and host genetic susceptibility to inflammation. Moreover, the Th1 and Th2 profiles can be altered by early therapeutic interventions that dramatically change the course of inflammation.

Induction of Th1 versus Th2 response depends on the type of antigenic stimulation, duration of antigenic challenge, phase of inflammation, and host genetic background [39]. These responses have been most thoroughly evaluated in response to systemic infections, especially *Leishmania major*, and recently have been studied in intestinal parasitic infections.

A predominant Th2 pattern with elevated IgE levels and eosinophilia is seen during infection with intestinal helminths and is essential for immune-mediated worm expulsion. Svetic *et al.* [40] measured the Th1 and Th2 messenger RNA profiles in the spleen, mesenteric lymph nodes, and Peyer's patches of mice during various time points of intestinal infection with *Heligmosomoides polygyrus* [40]. *H. polygyrus* has a strictly enteric life cycle and invades the mucosa to molt several times before entering the upper small bowel lumen as a mature egg-laying worm. An early increase of interleukin-3, interleukin-5, and interleukin-9 12 hours after infection could be shown in cells from the Peyer's patches and mesenteric lymph nodes, followed by a marked increase of interleukin-4 after 4 days. Interleukin-2, interferon-γ, and interleukin-10 showed few changes during the time course of infection. This study suggests that a predominant Th2 pattern can be present shortly after infection and is not restricted to secondary infections or chronic inflammatory stimulation.

The protective role of Th2 cytokines in the *Nippostrongylus brasiliensis* model and the ability to alter lymphokine profiles by administration of cytokines early in the course of infection have been shown by Finkelmann *et al.* [41•]. Interleukin-12, which is known to stimulate endogenous interferon-γ production and to down-regulate the Th2 response by inhibiting interleukin-4 secretion [42,43], was administered to *N. brasiliensis*–inoculated mice. Interleukin-12 enhanced worm survival and egg production during the primary infection by down-regulating the Th2 response, thereby indicating a protective role for Th2 lymphokines in this infection [41•,44]. In the same model, treatment with interferon-α and interferon-γ increased the parasitic egg production and delayed the intestinal expulsion of adult worms, probably by suppressing an adequate Th2 response [45].

Genetic susceptibility to chronic intestinal parasitic infestation is determined by the type of lymphokine profile generated by infection. Else *et al.* [46••] reported that Balb/K mice were resistant to *Trichuris muris* infection, in that they cleared the whipworm infection by 35 days and demonstrated immunity to rechallenge. These mice generated a Th2 lymphokine profile to infection, in contrast to susceptible AKR mice, which mounted a Th1 response. Moreover, neutralization of interferon-γ or administration of interleukin-4 stimulated worm expulsion in the susceptible AKR strain and blockade of interleukin-4 resulted in persistent infection in Balb/K mice.

Similarly, Kopf *et al.* [47] showed that disruption of the murine interleukin-4 gene (interleukin-$4^{-/-}$ knockout mice) significantly reduces Th2 cytokine response to infection with *N. brasiliensis in vivo*, which was typically provoked by infection of control mice. Isolated $CD4^+$ cells from mesenteric lymph nodes of interleukin-$4^{-/-}$ mice after infection with *N. brasiliensis* produced significantly less interleukin-5 and interleukin-10 compared with cells from similarly infected interleukin-$4^{+/+}$ normal mice. Interferon-γ production was elevated in infected knockout mice compared with controls, suggesting a negative feedback role of interleukin-4 and interleukin-10 on Th1 cells [47]. Of note, Kühn *et al.* [48••] showed that the levels of interleukin-4 and interleukin-5 in interleukin-$10^{-/-}$ mice (interleukin-10 knockout mice) infected with *N. brasiliensis* were similar to control mice, suggesting that interleukin-10 is not necessary for the development of Th2 cells. This concept is supported by the observation that *in vitro* addition of anti–interleukin-10 antibody to *N. brasiliensis*–primed Th2 lymphocytes from normal mice could not switch the cytokine production from interleukin-4 (Th2) to interleukin-2 (Th1) [49].

The delicate balance of Th1 or Th2 responses is regulated not only by the type of antigen and the host genetic background but also by nutritional factors. Two studies show that vitamin A deficiency promotes a Th1 response and down-regulates the Th2 response [50,51].

These provocative studies clearly demonstrate the importance of genetic background in immune responses and the ability of therapeutic intervention with immunomodulatory cytokines and perhaps nutrition to shift the pattern of lymphokines. They also demonstrate the complexity of the immune response, where a Th1 cell–mediated response may be an appropriate reaction to certain infections (*eg*, intracellular bacteria or viruses), but a Th2 response is required for protection against other types of infections (*eg*, intestinal nematodes) [39]. In experimental visceral leishmaniasis a strong Th1 response leads to effective clearance of infection, whereas a Th2 profile results in uncontrolled disease [52]. The administration of interleukin-2 or interferon-γ has therapeutic effects in this model, whereas interleukin-4 has detrimental consequences [52,53].

In vivo deletion of cytokine genes

Overexpression or deletion of selected genes ("knockouts" generated by targeted deletion of genes in embryonic stem cells) in rodents creates animal models to study genetic diseases or the *in vivo* functions of the targeted gene. The results are sometimes unexpected, as demonstrated by the onset of spontaneous intestinal inflammation following targeted deletion of genes for the α or β T-cell receptor [54], interleukin-2 [55••] or interleukin-10 [48••].

These results have led to new insights into the pathogenesis of chronic intestinal inflammation and clearly illustrate an integral role for T-cell regulation of mucosal homeostasis [56•].

If mice deficient for interleukin-2 (interleukin-$2^{-/-}$) survive beyond 10 weeks of age, they develop an aggressive colitis. These mice suffer from progressive diarrhea, recurrent intestinal bleeding, and rectal prolapse, which leads to death within 10 to 25 weeks [55••]. Interleukin-10–deficient mice develop a panenterocolitis with the maximal involvement in the duodenum, proximal jejunum, and proximal colon [48••]. Interleukin-10 is a potent suppressor of effector functions of macrophages, T cells, and natural killer cells [57,58], prompting the authors to suggest that the intestinal inflammation is a result of defective down-regulation of the immune response to enteric antigens. Surprisingly, no intestinal inflammation was observed in interleukin-4 knockout mice [47], even though interleukin-4 displays equally potent down-regulatory functions and is more active than interleukin-10 in suppressing Th1 responses [59].

Results in these models suggest that the intestinal microbial flora play a critical role in the initiation and perpetuation of intestinal inflammation. Interleukin-2 and interleukin-10 knockout mice raised under pathogen-free conditions developed only minor inflammatory symptoms in the intestine. Interleukin-$2^{-/-}$ mice did not show any clinical signs of intestinal injury, but histologic and immunologic analyses of the colon revealed signs of mild colitis. Interleukin-$2^{-/-}$ mice reared under sterile conditions did not reveal any clinical or histologic signs of inflammation. Interleukin-$10^{-/-}$ mice raised in a pathogen-free environment displayed only right-sided colitis with no small intestine inflammation.

Development of spontaneous enterocolitis with deletion of certain Th1 or Th2 cytokines or functional T lymphocytes (T-cell receptor knockout mice) graphically demonstrates the complex regulatory functions of mucosal T cells. It appears that any derangement of immune homeostasis may be sufficient to induce inflammation when the mucosa is constantly exposed to the hostile microbial environment of the intestinal lumen.

Conclusions

The remarkable pace of research in this field has led to increased understanding of the role of the cytokine network in the pathophysiology of intestinal inflammation. Animal models provide an essential tool to study the *in vivo* interactions of cytokines with themselves, other inflammatory mediators, and the neuroendocrine system. *In vitro* experiments cannot approximate the complexity of the intact immune system and mechanistic human studies are difficult to conduct. Future investigations should focus on further clarifying the new leads discussed in this review.

First, a delicate balance between protective and proinflammatory mediators appears to be essential to maintain suppression of the immune response to ubiquitous luminal antigens, especially of bacterial origin, and to promote healing after mucosal injury or infection. Therefore, the cytokine patterns influencing chronic intestinal inflammation should be defined further, concentrating on the balance between suppressive and proinflammatory mediators. These investigations must be performed with the understanding that each inflammatory mediator has pleiotropic effects and that dysregulation of almost any component of the system can lead to intestinal injury. Conclusions can be drawn from modulating inflammation by cytokine blockade or changing the cytokine pattern (*ie*, from Th1 to Th2).

A second goal is to better understand the immunoregulatory mechanisms of genetic susceptibility to chronic intestinal inflammation. Dysregulation of the balance of interleukin-1 to interleukin-1 receptor antagonist in Lewis rats injected with bacterial cell wall polymers [4•] and Th1 to Th2 responses in inbred mice infected with nematodes [46••] are early examples of powerful insights that can be gained by examination of cytokine profiles in inbred rodent strains that display different susceptibilities to experimental colitis. The availability of genetically engineered rodents with specific deletion or overexpression of targeted immunoregulatory genes and the ability to backcross these gene alterations onto high and low responding inbred strains should dramatically accelerate our understanding of the immunogenetic basis of IBD.

Acknowledgments

This work was supported by the Deutsche Forschungsgemeinschaft (He 2379/1-1), the Crohn's and Colitis Foundation of America, and NIH grants DK 40249, DK 47700, DK 43735, and DK 34987.

References and recommended reading

Papers of particular interest, published within the annual period of review, have been highlighted as:

- • Of special interest
- •• Of outstanding interest

1. •• Sartor RB: **Cytokines in Intestinal Inflammation: Pathophysiological and Clinical Considerations.** *Gastroenterology* 1994, **106**:533–539.

This paper succinctly reviews the role of cytokines in the pathogenesis and clinical aspects of experimental and human intestinal inflammation.

2. Dinarello CA: **Interleukin-1 and Interleukin-1 Antagonism.** *Blood* 1991, **77**:1627–1652.

3. Arend WP: **Interleukin-Receptor Antagonist.** *Adv Immunol* 1993, **54**:167–227.

4. • McCall RD, Haskill S, Zimmermann EM, Lund PK, Thompson RC, Sartor RB: **Tissue Interleukin 1 and Interleukin-1 Receptor Antagonist Expression in Enterocolitis in Resistant and Susceptible Rats.** *Gastroenterology* 1994, **106**:960–972.

An analysis of the relative tissue expression of interleukin-1 and interleukin-1 receptor antagonist in acute and chronic phases of enterocolitis in high (Lewis) and low (Buffalo and Fischer) responding rat strains is provided.

5. • Cominelli F, Bortolami M, Pizarro TT, Monsacchi L, Ferreti M, Brewer MT, Eisenberg SP, Ng RK: **Rabbit Interleukin-1 Receptor Antagonist. Cloning, Expression, Functional Characterization, and Regulation During Intestinal Inflammation.** *J Biol Chem* 1994, **269**:6962–6971.

The measurement of interleukin-1 and interleukin-1 receptor antagonist tissue expression in inflamed and uninflamed colonic tissues of rabbits and analysis of the effects of glucocorticoid treatment on interleukin-1 and interleukin-1 receptor antagonist secretion during inflammation is discussed.

6. •• Ferretti M, Casini-Raggi V, Pizarro TT, Eisenberg SP, Nast CC, Cominelli F: **Neutralization of Endogenous IL-1 Receptor Antagonist Exacerbates and Prolongs Inflammation in Rabbit Immune Colitis.** *J Clin Invest* 1994, **94**:449–453.

This paper reports on the comparison of intestinal interleukin-1 and interleukin-1 receptor antagonist concentrations over 1 week in rabbit colitis and blockade of endogenous interleukin-1 receptor antagonist by neutralizing antibodies.

7. Yamada T, Sartor RB, Marshall S, Specian RD, Grisham MB: **Mucosal Injury and Inflammation in a Model of Chronic Granulomatous Colitis in Rats.** *Gastroenterology* 1993, **104**:759–771.

8. Sartor RB: **Animal Models of Intestinal Inflammation: Relevance to IBD.** In *Inflammatory Bowel Disease.* Edited by MacDermott RP, Stenson W. New York: Elsevier; 1991:337–354.

9. Bristol LA, Durum SK, Eisenberg SP: **Differential Regulation of Group A Streptococcal Peptidoglycan-Polysaccharide (PG-APS)-Stimulated Macrophage Production of IL-1 by Rat Strains Susceptible and Resistant to PG-APS-Induced Arthritis.** *Cell Immunol* 1993, **149**:130–143.

10. Mansfield JC, Holden H, Tarlow JK, Di Giovine FS, McDowell TL, Wilson AG, Holdsworth CD, Duff GW: **Novel Genetic Association Between Ulcerative Colitis and the Anti-Inflammatory Cytokine Interleukin-1 Receptor Antagonist.** *Gastroenterology* 1994, **106**:637–642.

11. Cominelli F, Kam L, Casini-Raggi V, Jin Y, Pizarro TT: **Specific Mucosal Imbalance of Interleukin-1 and Interleukin-1 Receptor Antagonist (IL-1RA) in IBD: A Potential Mechanism of Chronic Inflammation [Abstract].** *Gastroenterology* 1994, **106**:A667.

12. Isaacs KL, Sartor RB, Haskill S: **Cytokine Messenger RNA Profiles in Inflammatory Bowel Disease Mucosa Detected by Polymerase Chain Reaction Amplification.** *Gastroenterology* 1992, **103**:1587–1595.

13. Cominelli F, Nast CC, Clark BD, Schindler R, Llerena R, Eysselein VE, Thompson RC, Dinarello CA: **Interleukin-1 (IL-1) Gene Expression, Synthesis, and Effect on Specific IL-1 Receptor Blockade in Rabbit Immune Complex Colitis.** *J Clin Invest* 1990, **86**:972–980.

14. Cominelli F, Nast CC, Duchini A, Lee M: **Recombinant Interleukin-1 Receptor Antagonist Blocks the Proinflammatory Activity of Endogenous Interleukin-1 in Rabbit Immune Colitis.** *Gastroenterology* 1992, **103**:65–71.

15. Thomas TK, Will PC, Srivastava A, Wilson CL, Harbison M, Little J, Chesonis RS, Pignatello M, Schmolze D, Symington J, Kilian PL, Thompson RC: **Evaluation of an Interleukin-1 Receptor Antagonist in the Rat Acetic Acid-Induced Colitis Model.** *Agents Actions* 1991, **34**:187–190.

16. Otterness IG, Seymour PA, Golden HW, Reynolds JA, Dawny GO: **The Effects of Continuous Administration of Murine Interleukin-1α in the Rat.** *Physiol Behav* 1988, **43**:797–804.

17. Patton JS, Peters PM, McCabe J, Crase D, Hansen S, Chen AB, Ligitt D: **Development of Partial Tolerance to the Gastrointestinal Effects of High Doses of Recombinant Tumor Necrosis Factor-Alpha in Rodents.** *J Clin Invest* 1987, **80**:1587–1596.

18. • Main C, Blennerhassett P, Collins SM: **Human Recombinant Interleukin 1β Suppresses Acetylcholine Release From Ra1 Myenteric Plexus.** *Gastroenterology* 1993, **104**:1648–1654.

This paper provides a detailed study of the influence of interleukin-1 on acetylcholine release in muscle-myenteric plexus preparations *in vitro.*

19. Hurst S, Collins SM: **Interleukin-1β Modulation of Norepinephrine Release From Rat Myenteric Nerves.** *Am J Physiol* 1993, **264**:G30–G35.

20. Hurst SM, Stanisz AM, Sharkey KA, Collins SM: **Interleukin 1β-Induced Increase in Substance P in Rat Myenteric Plexus.** *Gastroenterology* 1993, **105**:1754–1760.

21. Collins SM, Blennerhassett PA, Blennerhassett MG, Vermillion DL: **Impaired Acetylcholine Release From the Myenteric Plexus of Trichinella Infected Rats.** *Am J Physiol* 1989, **257**:G898–G903.

22. Snape WJ, Matarazzo SA, Cohen S: **Abnormal Gastrocolonic Response in Patients With Ulcerative Colitis.** *Gut* 1980, **21**:392–396.

23. Fargeas M-J, Fioramonti J, Bueno L: **Central Action of Interleukin 1β on Intestinal Motility in Rats: Mediation by Two Mechanism.** *Gastroenterology* 1993, **104**:377–383.

24. • Morteau O, More J, Pons L, Bueno L: **Platelet-Activating Factor and Interleukin 1 Are Involved in Colonic Dysmotility in Experimental Colitis in Rats.** *Gastroenterology* 1993, **104**:47–56.

This is an interesting report about the colonic motility changes in the TNBS model, which could be attenuated by interleukin-1 receptor antagonist or PAF antagonist. This suggests an involvement of interleukin-1 and PAF in colonic dysmotility during experimental inflammation.

25. McHugh KJ, Weingarten HP, Keenan C, Wallace JL, Collins SM: **On the Suppression of Food Intake in Experimental Models of Colitis in the Rat.** *Am J Physiol* 1993, **264**:R871–R876.

26. • McHugh K, Castonguay TW, Collins SM, Weingarten HP: **Characterization of Suppression of Food Intake Following Acute Colon Inflammation in the Rat.** *Am J Physiol* 1993, **265**:R1001–R1005.

A meticulous analysis of changes in the food consumption of rats after induction of experimental colitis is provided.

27. McHugh JK, Weingarten HP, Thompson RC, Collins SM: **Interleukin-1β Mediates the Anorexia and Weight Loss in Experimental Colitis in Rats [Abstract].** *Gastroenterology* 1992, **102**:A663.

28. McHugh KJ, Weingarten HP, Collins SM: **Anorexia in Experimental Colitis Is Mediated by Interleukin-1 at Both a Peripheral and Central Level [Abstract].** *Gastroenterology* 1993, **104**:A1051.

29. Montuschi P, Preziosi P, Navarra P: **Interleukin-1αand Tumor Necrosis Factor Inhibit Rat Gastric Fundus Motility In Vitro.** *Eur J Pharmacol* 1993, **233**:303–304.

30. • Gurbindo C, Russo P, Sabbah S, Lohoues MJ, Seidman E: **Interleukin-2 Activity of Colonic Lamina Propria Mononuclear Cells in a Rat Model of Experimental Colitis.** *Gastroenterology* 1993, **104**:964–972.

This was the first report of changes of interleukin-2 secretion of lamina propria mononuclear cells in the acute, chronic and resolving phase of experimental colitis.

31. Sartor RB, Bender DE, Allen JB, Zimmerman EM, Holt LC: **Chronic Experimental Enterocolitis and Extraintestinal Inflammation Are T Lymphocyte Dependent [Abstract].** *Gastroenterology* 1993, **104**:775A.

32. Matsumoto T, Lida M, Nakamura S, Hizawa K, Kuroki F, Fujishima M: **Preventive Effect of Immunosuppressive Agents Against Indomethacin-Induced Small Intestinal Ulcers in the Rat.** *Dig Dis Sci* 1994, **39**:787–795.

33. Breese E, Braegger CP, Corrigan CJ, Walker SJA, MacDonald TT: **Interleukin-2 and Interferon-Gamma-Secreting T Cells in Normal and Diseased Human Intestinal Mucosa.** *Immunology* 1993, **78**:127–131.

34. Mullin GE, Lazenby AJ, Harris MI, Bayless TM, James SP: **Increased Interleukin-2 mRNA in the Intestinal Mucosal Lesions of Crohn's Disease But Not Ulcerative Colitis.** *Gastroenterology* 1992, **103**:1620–1627.

35. Matsuura T, Fiocchi C: **Cytokine Production in the Gastrointestinal Tract During Inflammation.** In *Immunophysiology of the Gut.* Edited by Walker AW, Harmatz PR, Wershil BK. San Diego: Harcourt Brace & Co., 1993:145–163.

36. Matsuura T, West GA, Youngman KR, Klein JS, Fiocchi C: **Immune Activation Genes in Inflammatory Bowel Disease.** *Gastroenterology* 1993, **104**:448–458.

37. Mosmann TR, Coffman RL: **TH1 and TH2 Cells: Different Patterns of Lymphokine Secretion Lead to Different Functional Properties.** *Annu Rev Immunol* 1989, 7:145–173.

38. Street NE, Mosmann TR: **Functional Diversity of T-Lymphocytes Due to Secretion of Different Cytokine Patterns.** *FASEB J* 1991, **5**:171–177.

39. Romagnani S: **Induction of Th1 and Th2 Responses: A Key Role for the Natural Immune Response?** *Immunol Today* 1992, **13**:379–381.

40. Svetic A, Madden KB, Zhou XD, Lu P, Katona IM, Finkelman FD, Urban JF, Gause WC: **A Primary Intestinal Helminthic Infection Rapidly Induces a Gut-Associated Elevation of Th2-Associated Cytokines and IL-3.** *J Immunol* 1993, **150**:3434–3441.

41. Finkelmann FD, Madden KB, Cheever AW, Katona IM, Morris SC,
• Gately MK, Hubbard BR, Gause WC, Urban JF: **Effects of Interleukin 12 on Immune Responses and Host Protection in Mice Infected With Intestinal Nematode Parasites.** *J Exp Med* 1994, **179**:1563–1572.

Interleukin-12 administration promotes a Th1 response in experimental infection with *N. brasiliensis* thereby preventing a protective Th2 response. This study points out the possibilities of immunomodulatory therapy.

42. Morris SZ, Madden KB, Adamovicz JJ, Gause WC, Hubbard BR, Gately MK, Finkelman FD: **Effects of IL-12 on In Vivo Cytokine Gene Expression and Ig-Isotype Selection.** *J Immunol* 1994, **152**:1047–1056.

43. McKnight AJ, Zimmer GJ, Fogelman I, Wolf SF, Abbas AK: **Effects of IL-12 on Helper T Cell-Dependent Immune Responses In Vivo.** *J Immunol* 1994, **152**:2172–2179.

44. Urban JF, Katona IM, Paul WE, Finkelman FD: **Interleukin 4 Is Important in Protective Immunity to a Gastrointestinal Nematode Infection in Mice.** *Proc Natl Acad Sci U S A* 1991, **88**:5513–5517.

45. Urban JF, Madden KB, Cheever A, Trotta PP, Katona IM, Finkelman FD: **IFN Inhibits Inflammatory Responses and Protective Immunity in Mice Infected With the Nematode Parasite *Nippostrongylus brasiliensis*.** *J Immunol* 1993, **151**:7086–7094.

46. Else KJ, Finkelman FD, Maliszewski CR, Grencis RK: **Cytokine-Medi-**
•• **ated Regulation of Chronic Intestinal Helminth Infection.** *J Exp Med* 1994, **179**:347–351.

This study demonstrates the correlation between the genetic susceptibility and the pattern of cytokine response to infection. Balb/K mice generated a protective Th2 response to Trichuris muris infection, whereas AKR mice, which maintain a chronic infection, respond with a Th1 secretion pattern. Blocking interleukin-4 in Balb/k mice led to persistent infection and depletion of interferon-γ in susceptible AKR mice allowed worm expulsion.

47. Kopf M, Le Gros G, Bachmann M, Lamers MC, Bluethmann H, Köhler G: **Disruption of the Murine IL-4 Gene Blocks Th2 Cytokine Responses.** *Nature* 1993, **362**:245–247.

48. Kühn R, Löhler J, Rennick D, Rajewsky K, Müller W: **Interleukin-10-**
•• **Deficient Mice Develop Chronic Enterocolitis.** *Cell* 1993, **75**:263–274.

Spontaneous enterocolitis develops in interleukin-10 knockout mice, suggesting an immunoregulatory role for interleukin-10 in the intestine. Important animal model for further research in the pathophysiology of intestinal inflammation.

49. Saito S, Dorf M, Watanabe N, Tadakuma T: **Preferential Induction of IL-4 Is Determined by the Type and Duration of Antigenic Stimulation.** *Cell Immunol* 1994, **153**:1–8.

50. Cantorna MT, Nashold FE, Hayes CE: **In Vitamin A Deficiency Multiple Mechanisms Establish a Regulatory T-Helper Cell Imbalance With Excess Th1 and Insufficient Th2 Function.** *J Immunol* 1994, **152**:1515–1522.

51. Wiedermann U, Hanson LA, Kahu H, Dahlgren UI: **Aberrant T-Cell Function *In Vitro* and Impaired T-Cell Dependent Antibody Response *In Vivo* in Vitamin A-Deficient Rats.** *Immunology* 1993, **80**:581–586.

52. Sher A, Gazzinelli RT, Oswald IP, Clerici M, Kullberg M, Pearce EJ, Berzofsky JA, Mosmann TR, James SL, Morse HC, Shearer GM: **Role of T-Cell Derived Cytokines in the Downregulation of Immune Responses in Parasitic and Retroviral Infection.** *Immunol Rev* 1992, **127**:183–204.

53. Murray HW, Miralles GD, Stoeckle MY, McDermott DF: **Role and Effect of IL-2 in Experimental Visceral Leishmaniasis.** *J Immunol* 1993, **151**:929–938.

54. Mombaerts P, Mizoguchi E, Grusby MJ, Glimcher MH, Bhan AK, Tonegawa S: **Spontaneous Development of Inflammatory Bowel Disease in T Cell Receptor Mutant Mice.** *Cell* 1993, **75**:275–282.

55. Sadlack B, Merz H, Schorle H, Schimpl A, Feller AC, Horak I: **Ulcerative**
•• **Colitis-Like Disease in Mice With a Disrupted Interleukin-2 Gene.** *Cell* 1993, **75**:253–261.

Interleukin-2 knockout mice develop colonic ulcerations and bloody diarrhea, resembling ulcerative colitis. Like the interleukin-10 knockout mice, these mice are important animal models for future research in the pathophysiology of intestinal inflammation.

56. Strober W, Ehrhardt RO: **Chronic Intestinal Inflammation: An Unex-**
• **pected Outcome in Cytokine or T Cell Receptor Mutant Mice.** *Cell* 1993, **75**:203–205.

This editorial discusses the results and the implications of the experimental gene targeted disruption of the interleukin-2, interleukin-10, and T-cell receptor gene in mice for inflammatory bowel disease.

57. Moore KW, O'Garra A, de Waal Malefyt R, Vieira P, Mosmann TR: **Interleukin-10.** *Annu Rev Immunol* 1993, **11**:165–190.

58. Bogdan C, Nathan C: **Modulation of Macrophage Function by Transforming Growth Factor β, Interleukin-4, and Interleukin-10.** *Ann N Y Acad Sci* 1993, **685**:713–739.

59. Romagnani S: **Regulatory Role of IL4 and Other Cytokines in the Function and Development of Human T-Cell Clones.** *Res Immunol* 1993, **144**:625–628.

R. Balfour Sartor, MD, Division of Digestive Diseases and Nutrition, School of Medicine, CB#7080, Room 326 Burnett-Womack Building, University of North Carolina at Chapel Hill, Chapel Hill, NC 27599-7080, USA.

New models of chronic intestinal inflammation

Atul K. Bhan, MD, Emiko Mizoguchi, MD, and Atsushi Mizoguchi, MD

Massachusetts General Hospital and Harvard Medical School, Boston, Massachusetts, USA

Gene-targeting technology in embryonic stem cells has allowed creation of animals transgenic or mutant for a number of molecules. The presence of spontaneous chronic intestinal inflammation in mice mutant for interleukin-2, interleukin-10, and T-cell receptor genes has provided new models of chronic intestinal inflammation. By crossing mice mutant for different genes with each other, it is possible to generate mice deficient for a group of specific cytokines, adhesion molecules, or lymphocyte subsets. These models will not only help clarify the role of factors considered important in the pathogenesis of chronic intestinal inflammation, but they also permit precise dissection of mucosal immune responses and may help develop new therapeutic approaches to human inflammatory bowel disease.

Current Opinion in Gastroenterology 1994, **10**:633–638

Finding the cause of chronic intestinal inflammation in human inflammatory bowel disease (IBD), *ie*, Crohn's disease and ulcerative colitis, has been the major quest of investigators in gastrointestinal research. It is clear that the pathogenesis of these disorders is complex and may involve a number of factors including genetics, alteration of intestinal epithelial cells and mucin glycoprotein, mucosal immune mechanisms, and responses to bacterial and nonbacterial antigens in the lumen [1]. Alteration of mucosal immunity has remained a possible pathogenetic mechanism of these disorders [2,3,4•].

Because most of the human studies are carried out at a time when the disease is well established, it is difficult to separate secondary changes from primary events. Therefore, the availability of suitable experimental models would permit the study of events at different stages of disease. A number of experimental models have been developed over the years [1,5,6,7•]. These include injection of immune complexes, sensitization of animals to bacterial and synthetic antigens, and production of inflammation with chemical irritants. Most of these models primarily represent acute mucosal injury and inflammation and do not resemble chronic inflammation of human IBD [8••]. The recognition of spontaneous colitis, resembling ulcerative colitis, in cotton-top tamarins (*Saguinus oedipus*) received considerable attention as a suitable model of IBD [1]. A heritable form of colitis in mice has been reported [9]. The recent introduction of gene-targeting technology has helped create genetically altered animals (primarily mice and rats) with either an extra copy of a specific gene (transgenic) or disruption ("knockout") of a specific gene [10–13,14••,15••]. These animals provide powerful models with which to study functions of the molecules encoded by the altered genes. Interestingly, some of these animals develop chronic intestinal inflammation that resembles human IBD. These potential models of human IBD are discussed (Table 1).

HLA-B27–associated chronic intestinal inflammation

The association of HLA-B27, a serologically defined allele of human HLA-B locus, with ankylosis spondylitis was tested by creating transgenic rats expressing human HLA-B27 and β_2 microglobulin [11]. Rats from one transgenic line spontaneously develop inflammatory lesions in many organs resembling the HLA-B27–associated human disorders [11]. The inflammation is most prevalent in the gastrointestinal tract and is associated with diarrhea. The chronic inflammation is present in the stomach and small and large intestine; the colon is most consistently affected. The colonic lesions are characterized by epithelial hyperplasia and increased depth of crypts, depletion of mucus-secreting cells, mononuclear cell infiltration of the lamina propria, and formation of crypt abscesses. The susceptibility to develop inflammatory lesions in the transgenic rat appears to correlate with the level of HLA-B27 expression [10]; HLA-B27 expression is mostly restricted to lymphoid cells with minimal expression on gut epithelial cells.

In a recent study, the transfer of bone marrow cells from disease-prone transgenic rats to irradiated disease-resistant transgenic and nontransgenic rats led to development of multisystem inflammatory disease. The inflammatory lesions were most prominent in the

Abbreviations

IBD—inflammatory bowel disease; **MHC**—major histocompatibility complex; **TCR**—T-cell receptor; **TNF**—tumor necrosis factor.

 ISBN 1-85922-611-6 ISSN 0267-1379

Table 1. Models of chronic intestinal inflammation in transgenic and mutant ("knockout") animals

Model	Peripheral lymphoid tissue	Site of chronic inflammatory lesions	Other observations
HLA-B27, β_2m transgenic rats	T and B cells present Expression of HLA-B27 by bone marrow–derived cells	Gastrointestinal tract, peripheral and vertebral joints, skin, nails, male genital tract, heart Colon most consistently involved	Disease can be transferred with bone marrow cells
IL-2–mutant mice	T and B cells present	Colon, rectum	Disease not present in germ-free mice
IL-10–mutant mice	T and B cells present	Small intestine, colon	Inflammation restricted to proximal colon in specific pathogen-free conditions
TCR-mutant mice			
TCR-α	No TCR-$\alpha\beta^+$ T cells*; TCR-$\gamma\delta^+$ T cells and B cells present	Colon, rectum	Severe disease
TCR-β	No TCR-$\alpha\beta^+$ T cells; TCR-$\gamma\delta^+$ T cells and B cells present	Colon, rectum	Mild-to-moderate disease
TCR-δ	No TCR-$\gamma\delta^+$ T cells; TCR-$\alpha\beta^+$ T cells and B cells present	None	—
TCR-β×TCR-δ	No TCR-$\alpha\beta^+$ or TCR-$\gamma\delta^+$ T cells†; B cells present	Colon, rectum	Mild disease
Class II MHC–mutant mice	Absence of CD4+, TCR-$\alpha\beta^+$ T cells†; TCR-$\gamma\delta^+$ T cells and B cells present	Colon, rectum	Disease also present in TCR-α- or TCR-β- × class II MHC–mutant mice

*A minor population of CD4+, dull TCR-β^+ T cells present.
†A small population of CD4+ TCR-$\alpha\beta^+$ T cells present.
IL—interleukin; MHC—major histocompatibility complex; TCR—T-cell receptor.

colon, and reportedly did not resemble graft-versus-host disease [16••]. Interestingly, remission of the inflammatory lesions in transgenic rats could be induced by radiation followed by engraftment of nontransgenic bone marrow. The studies so far indicate that high expression of HLA-B27 on bone marrow–derived cells, in particular macrophages and antigen-presenting cells, is essential for the disease transfer [16••].

Interleukin-2–mutant mice

Interleukin-2, a product of activated T cells, is a key lymphokine that has been shown to regulate the activity of a number of cells including T cells, B cells, macrophages, natural killer cells, and lymphokine-activated killer cells. In particular, it is involved in T-cell proliferation and activation of cytotoxic responses. Mice deficient in interleukin-2 were developed by creating a targeted mutation in the interleukin-2 gene by homologous recombination in pluripotent mouse embryonic stem cells [13,17••]. These mice have normal thymus development and composition of peripheral T cells at 4 weeks of age. However, T-cell responses to mitogens are reduced. A marked increase of IgG1 and IgE levels in the serum suggests an abnormality of B-cell differentiation, perhaps through Th2-dependent pathway. These mice, after the age of 3 to 4 weeks become sick (*eg*, splenomegaly, lymphadenopathy, severe anemia) and about 50% die between 4 and 9 weeks after birth [17••]. The remaining mice of either sex present with chronic diarrhea, intermittent intestinal bleeding, and frequent rectal prolapse by 6 and 15 weeks of age. The most striking findings are present in the colon, which is rigid with thickened walls and shows mucosal ulceration. Microscopically, the crypt architecture is altered with the presence of epithelial regeneration and dysplasia, crypt branching, and crypt abscesses. The lamina propria contains an infiltrate of lymphocytes and plasma cells admixed with some neutrophils.

Immunohistochemical studies so far have revealed a predominance of T cells in the infiltrate and an increased number of intraepithelial CD8$^+$ T cells [17••]. There appears to be a marked decrease in double-negative CD4$^-$, CD8$^-$ intraepithelial lymphocyte population. The mucosal T cells express activation markers (CD44, CD69) and increase in the proportion of proliferating cells as compared with controls. IgA- and IgG1-secreting cells (B cells) are markedly increased in the colon with substantial increase in serum IgA levels. Preliminary studies also reveal the presence of circulating antibodies reactive with colonic epithelium [17••]. Overall, the colonic abnormalities in interleukin-2–mutant mice resemble human ulcerative colitis.

Interleukin-10–mutant mice

The cytokine interleukin-10 is produced by a variety of cells including T cells (Th2 subset), B cells, macrophages, thymocytes, and keratinocytes. It has multiple activities and participates in the growth, differentiation, and function of several cell types including T cells, B cells, and macrophages [14••,18•]. One of the important roles of interleukin-10 may be regulating immune response; interleukin-10 produced by Th2 cells suppresses development of Th1 type response (delayed-type hypersensitivity reactions) [14••,18•]. Interleukin-10–deficient mice were generated by gene targeting technology in murine embryonic stem cells [14••]. Development of T and B cells in these mice appears to be normal.

Most interleukin-10–mutant mice raised under conventional conditions have growth retardation and anemia by 4 to 8 weeks prior to their death. The animals show histologic findings of enterocolitis with involvement of enteric intestine. The inflammatory changes are more severe in the duodenum, proximal jejunum, and proximal colon [14••]. The mucosal abnormalities include branched and fused villi, enlarged and branched crypts, and formation of inflammatory polyps. The mucosa shows extensive infiltration by lymphocytes, plasma cells, macrophages, neutrophils, and occasionally multinucleated giant cells. Numerous IgA^+ plasma cells are present. Overall, the enterocolitis observed in interleukin-10–mutant mice does not resemble any specific human disease [14••].

T-cell receptor–mutant mice

The T-cell receptor (TCR) on the majority of T cells for antigens associated with major histocompatibility complex (MHC) molecules is a heterodimer of two polypeptide chains, α and β. A small number of T cells express TCR composed of γ and δ chains. Several strains of TCR-mutant mice have been generated by targeting various TCR genes in embryonic stem cells [15••,19,20•,21••]. Mice mutant for TCR-β are deficient in TCR-$\alpha\beta^+$ T cells, but contain TCR-$\gamma\delta$ T cells in the peripheral lymphoid tissue. Mice mutant for TCR-α are deficient in TCR-$\alpha\beta^+$ T cells, but contain TCR-$\gamma\delta$ and a small population of $CD4^+$ cells that stain faintly for CD3-ε and TCR-β. TCR-δ–mutant mice are deficient in TCR-$\gamma\delta$ T cells, but contain TCR-$\alpha\beta$ T cells. By crossing TCR-β–mutant mice and TCR-δ–mutant mice, mice deficient in both TCR-$\alpha\beta^+$ and TCR-$\gamma\delta$ T cells have been developed. All the TCR-mutant mice contain B lymphocytes in the peripheral lymphoid tissue.

Spontaneous chronic inflammatory disease of the colon develops with age (4 to 6 months) in TCR-α, TCR-β and TCR-$\beta \times$TCR-δ double-mutant mice but not in TCR-δ-mutant mice [15••]. The disease is characterized by marked thickening of rectum and colon with shortening of the large bowel in the most severe cases. The disease is more severe in the rectum than the proximal part of colon and the small intestine is not involved. The crypts in the diseased colon show hyperplasia and elongation with presence of branching and cystic dilatation in most severe cases. Goblet cells are depleted and crypt abscesses can be identified. The lamina propria contains an infiltrate of lymphocytes and plasma cells admixed with neutrophils; TCR-$\gamma\delta^+$ T cells and IgA^+ plasma cells are predominant in the infiltrate. Although there is no obvious mucosal ulceration or blood in the stools, the colonic disease is more reminiscent of ulcerative disease rather Crohn's disease. Features characteristic of Crohn's disease such as granulomas and transmural fissures are absent.

The presence of the colonic disease in TCR-mutant mice correlates with the absence of TCR-$\alpha\beta^+$ T cells. TCR-$\gamma\delta$ T cells most likely do not play an essential role in the initiation of the disease as indicated by the presence of disease in TCR-$\beta \times$TCR-δ double-mutant mice. Because the disease is mild in these double-mutant mice and there are many TCR-δ^+ cells in colonic lesions of TCR-α–mutant mice, TCR-$\gamma\delta^+$ cells may play a secondary role in the pathogenesis of this disease. Because all the TCR mice with colonic disease contain B cells [21••] and RAG-1–mutant mice [12] (lacking both T and B cells) do not develop the disease, B cells may play a role, perhaps by generation of autoantibodies, in the pathogenesis of chronic IBD.

Class II major histocompatibility complex–mutant mice

Expression of class II MHC molecules by intestinal epithelium in inflammatory conditions has generated a lot of interest [22]. It is not clear whether this merely represents a byproduct of inflammation (induction of class II molecules by cytokines produced during inflammation) or if it plays an important role in the pathogenesis of IBD. The colonic epithelium in the inflamed colonic tissue in the models discussed above (interleukin-2–mutant, interleukin-10–mutant, and TCR-mutant) express class II MHC molecules, [14••,15••,17••] in contrast to normal controls where normal colonic epithelium is negative for class II molecules. The importance of class II molecules in the development of intestinal inflammation was tested by cross breeding TCR-α or TCR-β mice with mice mutant for class II MHC [15••]. TCR-α or TCR-$\beta \times$class II MHC-mutant mice, which do not express class II molecules, developed chronic inflammation in the colon. Interestingly, class II MHC-mutant mice also develop marked colitis similar to that present in TCR-mutant mice [15••]. These experiments indicate that class II MHC expression is not critical in the pathogenesis of chronic intestinal inflammation.

Causes of chronic intestinal inflammation

Role of microorganisms

Because all of the mutant mice including interleukin-10–mutant, interleukin-2–mutant, and TCR-mutant mice have a deficiency in their immune system, one obvious cause of chronic inflammation is likely to be the presence of pathogenic microorganisms in the colony. However, in none of these mutant mice has a specific pathogen been isolated so far. A possible role of nonpathogenic microorganisms in enteric flora is suggested by studies in mice kept in a defined microbial environment. An attenuated form of intestinal inflammation restricted to proximal colon was present in interleukin-10–mutant mice in a specific pathogen-free environment, and interleukin-2–mutant mice did not develop the colonic inflammatory disease when kept in a germ-free or specific pathogen-free facility. Although IBD in TCR-mutant mice was observed in mice kept in specific pathogen-free conditions, the effect of a germ-free environment on the development of the disease has not yet been determined.

It is quite likely that the normal mucosal immune responses to enteric microorganisms and luminal antigens are altered in these models. This altered immune response possibly leads either to induction of mucosal injury due to imbalance of cytokines present at the mucosal sites or to the generation of autoimmune response.

Cytokine dysregulation and imbalance

The intestinal mucosa contains a variety of inflammatory cells that are capable of secreting a spectrum of cytokines. Intestinal epithelial cells are also capable of producing cytokines and expressing cytokine receptors [23•,24•]. These cytokines can be divided broadly into immunoregulatory (*eg*, interleukin-2, interleukin-4, interleukin-5, interleukin-10, interferon-γ, and transforming growth factor-β) and proinflammatory (*eg*, interleukin-1,interleukin-6, tumor necrosis factor [TNF]-α) cytokines; these functional differences are not absolute and the actions of different cytokines is often influenced by other cytokines. The controlled immune response normally present in the mucosa could be easily disturbed by alteration in the regulation or balance of cytokines, subsequently leading to chronic inflammation [8••,25•]. The presence of chronic inflammation in interleukin-2– and interleukin-10–mutant mice supports this possibility. In TCR-mutant mice, the absence of TCR-αβ T cells is also likely to lead to absence or decreased production of cytokines made primarily by this major subset of T cells. The abnormal cytokine milieu could either lead to enhanced production of certain cytokines or allow the effect of certain cytokines to go unchecked. Generation of autoimmune mechanisms may result from alteration of immunoregulatory cytokines, whereas tissue damage may result from increased production of proinflammatory cytokines. Abnormality of interleukin-2 production by the mucosal lymphocytes in IBD has been reported [3,4•]. Increased production of interleukin-6 [26•,27•] and TNF-α [27•] has been detected in colonic tissues of patients with IBD. Interleukin-1α has been implicated in the pathogenesis of enteropathy of graft-versus-host disease in mice [28•]. The study of cytokines in chronic inflammation is complicated by the fact that changes in receptors of these cytokines may also contribute to pathogenesis of the disease process [29]. Interleukin-1 receptor antagonist has been shown to reduce inflammation in experimental models of intestinal inflammation [30,31].

Autoimmune mechanism

A possible autoimmune mechanism in the pathogenesis of IBD, particularly in ulcerative colitis, has been suspected for a long time. Circulating antibodies to colonic epithelial cells and heat shock proteins have been demonstrated in ulcerative colitis, but convincing evidence in support of their pathogenic role has not been forthcoming [32,33,34]. The distinctive antineutrophilic cytoplasmic antibody present in ulcerative colitis patients represents an autoantibody of diagnostic value but of no pathogenic significance [35]. Circulating antibodies and IgG eluted from diseased colonic tissue reactive with a 40-kD protein belonging to tropomyosin family and present on colonic epithelial cells have been demonstrated in ulcerative colitis, but not in Crohn's disease [32,36•]. It is possible that antibodies generated under abnormal immunoregulation to bacterial or luminal antigen may crossreact with antigens normally located in colonic tissue or in other cells. Antibodies reactive with colonic epithelial cells have been identified in interleukin-2–mutant mice and more than 80% of TCR-α–mutant mice have been reported to develop antinuclear antibodies [37•]. It is possible that autoantibodies are important in the pathogenesis of chronic inflammatory lesion in these mutant mice. By crossing these mutant mice with mice deficient in B cells [38,39], the role of antibodies in these inflammatory lesions can be tested. Autoantibodies may cause mucosal injury at the mucosal site by activating complement system or by mechanisms involving antibody-dependent, cell-mediated cytotoxicity. Injury once initiated may involve other factors such as bacterial invasion and increased permeability of luminal antigens. Inflammatory cells including T cells, macrophages, natural killer cells, granulocytes, and mast cells may participate in the development of chronic inflammation.

Changes in other mutant mice

Because gene targeting technology in embryonic stem cells provides a powerful tool to study the function of molecules, it is not surprising that an increasing number of mice mutant for different types of molecules are becoming available. Mice mutant for interleukin-4 [40], interferon-γ [41], interferon-γ receptor [42], intercellular adhesion molecule 1 [43], and transforming growth factor-β_1 genes [44] have been created. Mice mutant for transforming growth factor-β_1 develop mixed inflammatory cell infiltrates in numerous organs including the heart, stomach, liver, lung, salivary gland, conjunctiva, and pancreas [44]. Inflammatory ocular lesion (blepharitis) with histologic features of allergic reaction have been observed in interleukin-4 transgenic mice, which overexpress interleukin-4 in T cells [45]. Chronic intestinal inflammation in these mutant mice has not been reported.

Conclusions

Because inflammatory lesions in TCR-mutant mice, interleukin-2–mutant mice, and interleukin-10–mutant mice are restricted to intestine, it is clear that T-cell and cytokine abnormalities can manifest as chronic intestinal inflammation without involvement of other organs [46••]. The absence of the inflammatory disease in germ-free interleukin-2–mutant mice suggests an important role of microorganisms in the initiation of intestinal inflammation, possibly through autoimmune mechanisms. Even though the pathogenesis of chronic intestinal inflammation in mice and humans may not turn out to be the same, these models will not only provide clues to the pathogenesis of human IBD, but also allow the role of factors such as genetics, abnormalities of epithelial cells and mucin, dietary factors, bacterial antigens and inflammatory mediators considered to be important in the pathogenesis of IBD to be elucidated. These mice will also serve to test therapeutic strategies for amelioration of chronic intestinal inflammation [46••].

Acknowledgments

Supported by grants from the National Institutes Health and Crohn's and Colitis Foundation of America.

References and recommended reading

Papers of particular interest, published within the annual period of review, have been highlighted as:

- • Of special interest
- •• Of outstanding interest

1. Podolsky DK: **Inflammatory Bowel Disease.** *N Engl J Med* 1991, **325**:928–937.

2. MacDermott RP, Stenson WF: **Alterations of the Immune System in Ulcerative Colitis and Crohn's Disease.** *Adv Immunol* 1988, 42:285–328.

3. Kusugami K, Matsuura T, West GA, Youngman KR, Rachmilewitz D, Fiocchi C: **Loss of Interleukin-2-Producing Intestinal CD4+ T Cells in Inflammatory Bowel Disease.** *Gastroenterology* 1991, **101**:1594–1605.

4. • Matsuura T, West GA, Youngman KR, Klein JS, Fiocchi C: **Immune Activation Genes in Inflammatory Bowel Disease.** *Gastroenterology* 1993, 104:448–456.

The expression of interleukin-2, interleukin-2 receptor α, and interleukin-2 receptor β messenger RNA was significantly higher in intestinal lamina propria cells isolated from tissue specimens of Crohn's disease and ulcerative colitis patients and health controls than from circulating peripheral blood cells. Lamina propria cells from IBD specimens produced similar higher interleukin-2 receptor α and interleukin-2 receptor β messenger RNA than the controls, but expressed significantly lower interleukin-2 messenger RNA. Thus the defect of interleukin-2 activity in IBD is probably related to decreased interleukin-2 transcription.

5. Okayasu I, Hatakeyama S, Yamada M, Ohkusa T, Inagaki Y, Nakaya R: **A Novel Method in the Induction of Reliable Experimental Acute and Chronic Ulcerative Colitis in Mice.** *Gastroenterology* 1990, 98:694–702.

6. Sartor RB: **Animal Models of Intestinal Inflammation.** In *Inflammatory Bowel Disease.* Edited by McDermott RP, Stenson WF. New York: Elsevier; 1992: 337–353

7. • Gurbindo C, Russo P, Sabbah S, Lohoues M-J, Seidman E: **Interleukin-2 Activity of Colonic Lamina Propria Mononuclear Cells in a Rat Model of Experimental Colitis.** *Gastroenterology* 1993, **104**:964–972.

Intracolonic administration of trinitrobenzene sulfonic acid was used to develop acute and chronic inflammation in the colon of rats. *In vitro* production of interleukin-2 by isolated lamina propria mononuclear cells was significantly increased in chronic but not acute or resolved colitis groups. Interleukin-2 activity after conconvalin A activation of lamina propria cells was highest in the groups with resolved or chronic colitis. The study indicates that interleukin-2 production of lamina propria cells varies according to the severity and duration of colitis.

8. •• Shanahan F: **Pathogenesis of Ulerative Colitis.** *Lancet* 1993, **342**:407–411.

An excellent review of pathogenesis of ulcerative colitis.

9. Birkenmeier EH, Sundenberg JP, Elson CO: **A Heritable Form of Colitis in Mice.** *Gastroenterology* 1992, 102:A596.

10. Taurog JD, Maika SD, Simmons WA, Breban M, Hammer RE: **Susceptibility to Inflammatory Disease in HLA-B27 Transgenic Rat Lines Correlates With the Level of B27 Expression.** *J Immunol* 1993, **150**:4168–4178.

11. Hammer R, Maika SD, Richardson JA, Tang J-P, Taurog JD: **Spontaneous Inflammatory Disease in Transgenic Rats Expressing HLA-B27 and Human β_2m: An Animal Model of HLA-B27-associated Human Disorders.** *Cell* 1990, **63**:1099–1112.

12. Mombaerts P, Iacomini J, Johnson RS, Herrup K, Tonegawa S, Papaioannou VE: **RAG-1-Deficient Mice Have No Mature B and T Lymphocytes.** *Cell* 1992, **68**:869–877.

13. Schorle H, Holtschke T, Hunig T, Schimpe A, Horak I: **Development and Function of T Cells in Mice Rendered Interleukin-2 Deficient by Gene Targeting.** *Nature* 1991, **352**:621–624.

14. •• Kühn R, Löhler J, Rennick D, Rajewsky R, Müller W: **Interleukin-10 Deficient Mice Develop Chronic Enterocolitis.** *Cell* 1993, **75**:263–274.

A study of the effects of interleukin-10 deficiency in mice mutant for interleukin-10 genes. Although the lymphocyte development and antibody responses are normal, most animals are growth retarded and anemic and develop chronic enterocolitis.

15. •• Mombaerts P, Mizoguchi E, Grusby MJ, Glimcher LH, Bhan AK, Tonegawa S: **Spontaneous Development of Inflammatory Bowel Disease in T Cell Receptor Mutant Mice.** *Cell* 1993, **75**:275–282.

The study describes spontaneous development of chronic colonic inflammation resembling human ulcerative colitis in mice mutant for TCR receptors. Chronic colitis was present in mice mutant for TCR-α, TCR-β, TCR-$\beta \times \delta$ or class II MHC but not in mice mutant for TCR-δ or RAG-1. This paper discusses the role of mucosal immune system in the pathogenesis of chronic intestinal inflammation in these mice.

16. •• Breban M, Hammer RE, Richardson JA, Taurog JD: **Transfer of the Inflammatory Disease of HLA-B27 Transgenic Rats by Bone Marrow Engraftment.** *J Exp Med* 1993, **178**:1607–1616.

Rats transgenic for human HLA-B27 and β_2 microglobulin develop inflammatory lesions in many organs including the intestine. The study describes the transfer of this inflammatory disease from disease-prone transgenic rats to irradiated disease-resistant transgenic rats or nontransgenic rats by bone marrow cells expressing HLA-B27.

17. •• Sadlack B, Merz H, Schorle H, Schimpl A, Feller AC, Horak I: **Ulcerative Colitis-Like Disease in Mice With a Disrupted Interleukin-2 Gene.** *Cell* 1993, **75**:253–261.

Description of ulcerative colitis–like disease in mice mutant for interleukin-2 genes. The data provides evidence for a primary role of immune system in the pathogenesis of chronic colonic inflammation.

18. • Moore KW, O'Garra A, de Waal Malefyt R, Vera P, Mosmann TR: **Interleukin 10.** *Ann Rev Immunol* 1993, **11**:165–190.

An excellent review of interleukin-10.

19. Mombaerts P, Clarke AR, Rudnicki MA, Iacomini J, Itohara S, Lafaille JJ, Wang L, Ichikawa Y, Jaenisch R, Hooper ML, Tonegawa S: **Mutations in T-cell Antigen Receptor Genes α and β Block Thymocyte Development at Different Stages.** *Nature* 1992, **360**:225–231.

20. • Itohara S, Mombaerts P, LaFaille J, Iacomini J, Nelson A, Clarke AR, Hooper ML, Farr A, Tonegawa S: **T Cell Receptor δ Gene Mutant Mice: Independent Generation of $\alpha\beta$ T Cells and Programmed Rearrangements of $\gamma\delta$ TCR Genes.** *Cell* 1993, 72:337–348.

Analysis of mice mutant for TCR-δ genes and generation of TCR-$\alpha\beta$ T cells without expression of TCR-$\gamma\delta$ genes.

21. •• Mombaerts P, Mizoguchi E, Ljunggren HG, Iacomini J, Ishikawa H, Wang L, Grusby MJ, Glimcher LH, Winn HJ, Bhan AK, Tonegawa S: **Peripheral Lymphoid Development and Function in TCR Mutant Mice.** *Int Immunol* 1994, 6:1061–1070.

Analysis of the peripheral lymphoid tissue development in mice mutant for TCR genes and RAG-1 genes. The study includes immunohistologic and flow cytometric characteristics of lymphoid cells and functional studies of T cells, B cells, and natural killer cells.

22. Mayer L, Eisenhardt D, Salomon P, Bauer W, Plous R, Piccinini L: **Expression of Class II Molecules on Intestinal Epithelial Cells in Humans: Differences Between Normal and Inflammatory Bowel Disease.** *Gastroenterology* 1991, **100**:3–12.

23. • Ciacci C, Mahida YR, Dignass A, Koizumi M, Podolsky DK: **Functional Interleukin-2 Receptors on Intestinal Epithelial Cells.** *J Clin Invest* 1993, 92:527–632.

The presence of interleukin-2 receptors on intestinal epithelial cells was detected by binding of ^{125}I-interleukin-2 to IE6 cell line established from normal rat crypt epithelium and to rat primary intestinal epithlial cells. In addition, messenger RNA for the interleukin-2 receptor β chain was demonstrated by Northern blot analysis of messenger RNA from primary rat intestinal epithelial cells. The interleukin-2 receptors appeared to be functional.

24. • Jones SC, Trejdosiewicz LK, Banks RE, Howdle PD, Axon ATR, Dixon MF, Whicher JT: **Expression of Interleukin-6 by Intestinal Enterocytes.** *J Clin Pathol* 1993, 46:1097–1110.

Demonstration of interleukin-6 by immunofluorescence on intestinal epithelial cells in small and large intestines of patients with IBD and celiac disease and in histologically normal mucosa.

25. • Lichtman SN, Sartor RB: **Examining the Role of Inflammatory Cytokines in Chronic Inflammatory Bowel Disease.** *J Pediatr Gastroenterol Nutr* 1993, 16:239–240.

An editorial review of the role of inflammatory cytokines in chronic IBD.

26. • Hyams JS, Fitzgerald JE, Treem WR, Wyzga N, Kreutzer DL: **Relationship of Functional and Antigenic Interleukin 6 to Disease Activity in Inflammatory Bowel Disease.** *Gastroenterology* 1993, **104**:1285–1292.

Compared with controls, raised serum interleukin-6 levels were found in patients with IBD; the levels were higher in Crohn's disease than in ulcerative colitis. Increase in disease activity in Crohn's disease was related to raised interleukin-6 levels rather than functional activity as judged by enzyme-linked immunsorbent assay.

27. • Jones SC, Haidar A, Hagan P, Crabtree JE, Banks RE, Axon ATR, Dixon MF, Whicher JT: **Cytokine Production in the Mucosa of Patients With Inflammatory Bowel Disease.** *Eur J Gastroenterol Hepatol* 1993, **5**:607–612.

Mucosal biopsies from patients with IBD and controls were cultured for 24h and the interleukin-6 and TNF-α in the culture medium was determined by enzyme-linked immunsorbent assay. *In vitro* production of interleukin-6 and TNF-α was found to be greater in patients with active ulcerative colitis than in patients with inactive ulcerative colitis or Crohn's disease or in healthy controls.

28. • Mowat A MCI, Hutton AK, Garside P, Steel M: **A Role for Interleukin-1α in Immunologically Mediated Intestinal Pathology.** *Immunology* 1993, **80**:110–115.

Discusses the role of interleukin-1α in immunologicallly mediated intestinal inflammation. The intestinal lesions of mice with graft-versus-host reaction showed increased production of interleukin-1α and treatment of these mice with anti-interleukin-1α antibodies abolished the crypt hyperplasia in jejunem.

29. Cominelli F, Fiocchi C, Eisenerg SP, Bortolami M: **Imbalance of IL-1 and IL-1 Receptor Antagonist in the Intestinal Mucosa of Crohn's Disease and Ulcerative Colitis Patients: A Novel Pathogenetic Mechanism.** *Gastroenterology* 1992, **102**:A609.

30. Cominielli F, Nast C, Clark BD, Schindler R, Lierena R, Eysselein VE, Thompson RC, Dinarello CA: **Interleukin 1 (IL-1) Gene Expression, Synthesis and Effect of Specific IL-l Receptor Blockage in Rabbit Immune Complex Colitis.** *J Clin Invest* 1990, **86**:972–980.

31. McCarthy PL, Ahyankar S, Neben S, Newman G, Sieff C, Thompson RC, Burakoff SJ, Ferrara JL: **Inhibition of Interleukin-1 by Interleukin-1 Receptor Antagonist Prevents Graft-vs-Host Disease.** *Blood* 1991, **78**:1915–1918.

32. Takahashi F, Shah HS, Wise LS, Das KM: **Circulating Antibodies Against Human Colonic Extract Enriched With a 40 kDa Protein in Patients With Ulcerative Colitis.** *Gut* 1990, **31**:1016-1020.

33. Elsaghier A, Prantera C, Bothamley G, Wilkins E, Jindal S, Ivanyi J: **Disease Association of Antibodies to Human and Mycobacterial hsp 70 and hsp 60 Stress Proteins.** *Clin Exp Immunol* 1992, **89**:305–309.

34. Stevens TR, Winrow VR, Blake DR, Rampton DS: **Circulating Antibodies to Heat-Shock Protein 60 in Crohn's Disease and Ulcerative Colitis.** *Clin Exp Immunol* 1992, **90**:271–274.

35. Shanahan F, Duerr RH, Rotter JI, Yang H, Sutherland LR, McElree C, Landers CJ, Targan SR: **Neutrophil Autoantibodies in Ulcerative Colitis: Familial Aggregation and Genetic Heterogeneity.** *Gastroenterology* 1992, **103**:456–461.

36. • Das KM, Dasgupta A, Mandal A, Geng X: **Autoimmunity to Cytoskeletal Protein Tropomyosin.** *J Immunol* 1993, **150**:2487–2493.

A 40-kD protein, P40, was purified from human colonic tissue. Two peptides were sequenced after proteolytic digestion of P40 and the protein was demonstrated to belong to the tropomyosin family. Sera from 95 % of patients with ulcerative colitis was found reactive with tropomyosin, suggesting that a cytoskeletal microfilament protein belonging to tropomyosin family may act as autoantigen in patients with ulcerative colitis.

37. • Wen LI, Roberts SJ, Viney JL, Wong FS, Mallick C, Findly RC, Peng Q, Craft JE, Owen MT, Hayday AC: **Immunoglobulin Synthesis and Generalized Autoimmunity in Mice Congenitally Deficient in αβ(+) T Cells.** *Nature* 1994, **369**:654–658.

Demonstration of high serum concentration of IgE and IgG1 in TCR-α–mutant mice as compared with control mice. In addition, sera from more than 80% of TCR-α–mutant mice were positive for antinuclear antibody (IgG) by immunofluorescence. A possible role of TCR-γδ cells providing "help" to B cells in the production of autoantibodies is discussed.

38. Kitamura D, Roes J, Kuhn R, Rajewsky R: **A B Cell-Deficient Mouse by Targeting Disruption of the Membrane Exon of the Immunoglobulin μ Chain Gene.** *Nature* 1991, **350**:423-426.

39. Chen J, Trounstine M, Alt FW, Young F, Kurahara C, Loring JF, Huszar D: **Immunoglobulin Gene Rearrangement in B Cell Deficient Mice Generated by Targeted Deletion by the JH Locus.** *Int Immunol* 1993, **5**:647–656.

40. Kühn R, Rajewsky K, Müller W: **Generation and Analysis of Interleukin-4 Deficient Mice.** *Science* 1991, **254**:707–710.

41. Dalton DK, Pitts-Meek S, Keshav S, Figari IS, Bradley A, Steward TA: **Multiple Defects of Immune Cell Function in Mice With Disrupted Interferon-γ Genes.** *Science* 1993, **269**:1739–1752.

42. Huang S, Hendriks W, Althage A, Hemmi S, Bluethmann H, Kamijo R, Vilcek J, Zinkernagel RM, Aguet M: **Immune Response in Mice That Lack the Interferon-γ Receptor.** *Science* 1993, **259**:1742–1745.

43. Sligh JE Jr, Ballantyne CM, Rich SS, Hawkins HK, Smith CW, Bradley A, Beaudet AL: **Inflammatory and Immune Responses Are Impaired in Mice Deficient in Intercellular Adhesion Molecule 1.** *Proc Natl Acad Sci U S A* 1993, **90**:8529–8533.

44. Shull MM, Ormsby I, Kier AB, Pawlowski S, Diebold RJ, Yin M, Allen R, Sidman C, Proetzel G, Calvin D, Annunziata N, Doetschman T: **Targeted Disruption of the Mouse Transforming Growth Factor-β1 Gene Results in Multifocal Inflammatory Disease.** *Nature* 1992, **359**:693–699.

45. Tepper RI, Levinson DA, Stanger BZ, Campos-Torres J, Abbas AK, Leder P: **IL-4 Induces Allergic-Like Inflammatory Disease and Alters T Cell Development in Transgenic Mice.** *Cell* 1990, **62**:457–467.

46. •• Strober W, Ehrhardt RO: **Chronic Intestinal Inflammation: An Unexpected Outcome in Cytokine or T Cell Receptor Mutant Mice.** *Cell* 1993, **75**:203–205.

A brief review of pathogenesis of human IBD and an excellent discussion of chronic intestinal inflammation present in TCR-mutant and cytokine-mutant mice.

Atul K. Bhan, MD, Emiko Mizoguchi, MD, Atsushi Mizoguchi, MD, Immunopathology Unit, Department of Pathology, Cox-5, Massachusetts General Hospital, Boston, MA 02114, USA.

Cytokine production in the human gastrointestinal tract during inflammation

Claudio Fiocchi, MD, David G. Binion, MD, and Jeffry A. Katz, MD

Case Western Reserve University, Cleveland, Ohio, USA

Cytokines are immunoregulatory and proinflammatory products secreted by a variety of cells, particularly those of the immune system. Cytokines play a pivotal role in the intestinal immune system in health and disease. During intestinal inflammation, the concentration, source, and function of these molecules are altered. No abnormality is specific for any particular type of bowel inflammation, because similar changes occur in diseases of different etiology and pathogenesis. Thus, simple measurement of any cytokine in the gut, or more so in the circulation, is of limited value when trying to understand diseases where multiple cells and complex functional interactions occur. In spite of this, the study of cytokines has contributed the most towards expanding our knowledge of gut inflammation. Not only will further investigation of these mediators ultimately uncover the intimate mechanisms of normal and pathologic mucosal immunity, but understanding their modulation will be the key to truly effective anti-inflammatory therapies.

Current Opinion in Gastroenterology 1994, **2**:639–644

Cytokines and mucosal immunity

Inflammation is the most common response of the organs of the body to incoming insults. The gastrointestinal tract is particularly susceptible to inflammation because of its enormous surface area in contact with the external environment, and its exposure to a variety of dietary and bacterial antigens. Owing to their presence, the gut mucosa is in a permanent state of "physiologic intestinal inflammation," represented by the abundant mononuclear cells (T cells, B cells, plasma cells, macrophages, and so forth) infiltrating the epithelium and the immediate subepithelial space (lamina propria). When the tightly regulated number of immune cells becomes excessive, pathologic inflammation ensues with consequences that vary depending on the cause and the mechanisms involved. Intestinal inflammation is a complex phenomenon in which different cell types are implicated, including epithelial, mesenchymal (fibroblasts, muscle cells), endothelial, nervous, and immune cells [1•]. Most secrete soluble factors, but this is most typical when immune cells are activated, producing a variety of substances collectively named cytokines. These molecules are key regulators of mucosal immunity, and play a fundamental role in all types of acute and chronic inflammation. Other noncytokine products are also involved, such as prostaglandins, leukotrienes, platelet-activating factor, and several growth factors. A list of mediators relevant to intestinal inflammation is presented in Tables 1, 2, and 3. Because of the required focus on the current literature, only some of them will be discussed here, but comprehensive reviews are available [2•].

Because of their transient and self-limited nature, relatively little is known about production of cytokines in acute intestinal inflammatory responses. Thus, most of the information contained in this review is based on data derived from chronic conditions where intestinal tissues or cells can be readily obtained for study, such as inflammatory bowel disease (IBD). Cytokines have become the central focus of attention in human intestinal inflammation because of their relevance to pathogenesis and potential therapeutic implications. Nevertheless, human studies have limitations and knowledge of gut cytokines must be complemented with insights gained from animal models of intestinal inflammation [3]. These are discussed in detail in other papers in this issue.

Interleukin-1β

Interleukin-1β is the most potent pro-inflammatory cytokine and its marked elevation in both Crohn's disease and ulcerative colitis intestine is well documented [2•]. Some of the most recent reports have investigated its specific localization and disease association. Unlike other cytokines that are produced by various cells within the gut mucosa, interleukin-1β bioactiv-

Abbreviations
IBD—inflammatory bowel disease; **TNF**—tumor necrosis factor.

© 1994 Current Science ISBN 1-85922-611-6 ISSN 0267–1379

ity, immunoreactivity, and messenger RNA are largely confined to lamina propria mononuclear cells and are not expressed by epithelial cells [4]. This cytokine is one of the main products of activated macrophages in both normal and inflamed tissue, but its enhanced production is not restricted to IBD. In active pouchitis, interleukin-1β is significantly higher than in normal pouches or normal ileal mucosa, its levels correlating with the degree of tissue infiltration by epithelioid and tingible body macrophages [5].

Perhaps of greater importance than interleukin-1β itself is interleukin-1 receptor antagonist, a natural antagonist that binds to the same target cell receptors as interleukin-1β without triggering an inflammatory cascade. The final outcome of interleukin-1β's biological effect may actually depend on the relative proportions of these two cytokines, the so-called interleukin-1 receptor antagonist/interleukin-1 balance. An excess of interleukin-1 or a relative lack of interleukin-1 receptor antagonist may cause an imbalance predisposing to mucosal inflammation. The existence of gene polymorphism, *ie*, the preferential use of specific alleles for the interleukin-1β and the interleukin-1 receptor antagonist gene, may also be a determining factor of how much inflammation is generated or how efficiently the host can defend against it, a concept probably applicable to most cytokines. A recent study shows that allele 2 of interleukin-1 receptor antagonist is over-represented in ulcerative colitis patients, perhaps leading to an increased risk for more severe or extensive colitis [6••].

Interleukin-2

Interleukin-2, exclusively produced by T lymphocytes, is the prototypical immunoregulatory cytokine and several studies have investigated its level in IBD. The results have been rather contradictory, with enhanced, normal, or decreased mucosal levels being reported by different laboratories. These discrepancies are the likely result of the widely disparate methodologies employed. In spite of this controversy, a more uniform picture is emerging regarding dissimilarities in the production of and response to interleukin-2 between the two forms of IBD. Confirming previous observations [7], levels of interleukin-2 bioactivity or messenger RNA are significantly greater in Crohn's disease than in ulcerative colitis [8,9]. This is important, because it demonstrates how each form of intestinal inflammation is associated with a differential induction or response to the same cytokine, pointing to distinct immunopathogenic mechanisms. In addition, a prominent role of interleukin-2 in Crohn's disease is reinforced by the symptomatic exacerbations seen in patients receiving high-dose interleukin-2 for treatment of malignancies [10•].

Table 1. Target cells and functional properties of mediators relevant to intestinal inflammation*

	IFN-α	IFN-β	IFN-γ	TNF-α	LT	IL-1α	IL-1β	IL-1ra
Macrophages	yes	yes	yes	yes	—	—	—	yes/no
Granulocytes	—	yes	yes	yes	yes	yes	yes	—
Eosinophils	no	—	—	yes	—	yes	yes	—
Natural killer	yes	yes	yes/no	no	—	yes	yes	—
LAK activity	yes	yes	yes	yes/no	—	—	—	—
B cell								
Activation	—	—	yes	yes	—	yes	yes	—
Proliferation	yes	yes	yes	yes/no	yes	yes	yes	yes/no
Differentiation	yes	—	yes	yes/no	yes	yes	yes	—
Ig isotype switching	—	—	IgG2a	—	—	—	—	—
T cell								
Activation	—	—	—	—	—	yes	yes	—
Proliferation	yes	—	no	yes	—	yes	yes	yes/no
Differentiation	—	—	—	—	—	—	—	—
Endothelium	—	—	yes	yes	yes	yes	yes	yes/no
Extracellular matrix	—	—	yes	yes	yes	yes	yes	yes/no
Cytotoxicity	yes	yes	yes	yes	yes	yes	yes	—
MHC class I/II	I/II	I/II	I/II	I	I	no	no	—
Chemotaxis	yes	—	yes	yes	—	yes	yes	—
Adhesion molecules	—	—	yes	yes	—	yes	yes	—
ROM/NO production	—	—	yes	yes	yes	yes	yes	yes/no
Pyrogenesis	yes	yes	yes	yes	—	yes	yes	yes
Acute-phase reaction	—	—	yes	yes	—	yes	yes	yes
Angiogenesis	—	—	—	yes	yes	—	—	—

**Adapted from* Burke *et al.* [37]; with permission.
IFN—interferon; Ig—immunoglobulin; IL—interleukin; IL-1ra—interleukin-1 receptor antagonist; LAK—lymphokine-activated killer; LT—lymphotoxin; MHC—major histocompatibility complex; NO—nitric oxide; ROM—reactive oxygen metabolite; TNF—tumor necrosis factor.

Table 2. Target cells and functional properties of mediators relevant to intestinal inflammation*

	IL-2	IL-3	IL-4	IL-5	IL-6	IL-7	IL-8†	IL-9
Macrophages	yes	—	yes	—	—	yes	yes	—
Granulocytes	—	—	—	yes/no	—	—	yes	—
Eosinophils	no	yes	yes	yes	—	—	—	—
Natural killer	yes	yes	yes	—	yes	yes	—	—
LAK activity	yes	yes	yes/no	—	no	yes	—	—
B cell								
Activation	—	—	yes	yes	—	—	—	—
Proliferation	yes	yes	yes	yes/no	—	yes	—	—
Differentiation	yes	yes	yes	yes/no	yes	yes	—	—
Ig isotype switching	—	—	IgE, IgG1	IgA	—	—	—	—
T cell								
Activation	yes	—	yes	—	yes	yes	—	—
Proliferation	yes	—	yes	—	yes	yes	—	yes
Differentiation	yes	—	yes	—	yes	yes	—	—
Endothelium	—	—	yes	—	—	—	yes	—
Extracellular matrix	—	—	yes	—	—	—	yes	—
Cytotoxicity	—	—	yes	—	yes	—	—	—
MHC class I/II	—	II	II	I	—	—	—	—
Chemotaxis	yes	yes	yes	yes	—	—	yes	—
Adhesion molecules	yes	yes	yes	yes	yes	yes	yes	—
ROM/NO production	yes	yes	yes	—	yes	—	yes	—
Pyrogenesis	yes	—	—	—	—	—	yes	—
Acute-phase reaction	—	—	—	—	yes	—	yes	—
Angiogenesis	—	—	—	—	—	—	yes	—

**Adapted from* Burke *et al.* [37]; with permission.
†IL-8—and related chemokines
Ig—immunoglobulin; IL—interleukin; LAK—lymphokine-activated killer; MHC—major histocompatibility complex; NO—nitric oxide; ROM—reactive oxygen metabolite.

Interleukin-6

Interleukin-6 is a cytokine with a wide spectrum of biological functions, some of which are shared with those of other pro-inflammatory cytokines, such as interleukin-1β and tumor necrosis factor (TNF)-α. Previously, two separate studies have described elevated serum interleukin-6 levels in Crohn's disease but not ulcerative colitis patients [11,12]. This observation has been recently confirmed by another group of investigators, who stressed the importance of studying both bioactive (functional) and immunoreactive (antigenic) interleukin-6 in the context of clinical parameters [13]. In colonic Crohn's disease, functional and antigenic serum interleukin-6 levels were greater than in disease limited to the small bowel, whereas increased disease severity was reflected by bioactive but not immunoreactive cytokine in both Crohn's disease and ulcerative colitis. Enhanced intestinal synthesis of interleukin-6 correlating with disease severity was also found in the rectosigmoid of ulcerative colitis patients submitted to a unique perfusion technique [14], as well as in supernatants of isolated lamina propria mononuclear cells and organ cultures [15,16].

In addition to levels, the localization of individual cytokines in the gut is also important. In a study utilizing an immunofluorescence technique, interleukin-6 distribution was investigated in the small and large bowel of patients with IBD and celiac disease and in control subjects [17]. Surprisingly, interleukin-6 was found predominantly in enterocytes and colonocytes, but not in lamina propria mononuclear cells, without marked differences between inflamed and noninflamed mucosa. Increased interleukin-6 production is not limited to classical IBD, as a significantly enhanced concentration of this product can also be found in cultures of antral biopsies of patients with *Helicobacter pylori*–associated gastritis [18]. These studies underscore the importance of defining in detail, not only the patients, but also the methods, tissues, and cell types when evaluating cytokines in gut inflammation.

Interleukin-8

Interleukin-8 is a member of the chemokine family, a group of cytokines whose main function consists of attracting leukocytes, making these molecules directly relevant to gut inflammation. Interleukin-8 is perhaps the most potent inducer of polymorphonuclear neutrophil chemotaxis, with some activity for T cells, and its role in IBD is justifiably the focus of intense investigation. After initial reports of enhanced synthesis of interleukin-8 in the mucosa of ulcerative colitis patients [19,20], elevated levels of this cytokines were also found in Crohn's disease [21]. However, in spite of similarly elevated amounts of this chemokine

Table 3. Target cells and functional properties of mediators relevant to intestinal inflammation*

	IL-10	IL-11	IL-12	CSF	TGF-α	TGF-β	PDGF
Macrophages	yes	—	—	yes	—	—	—
Granulocytes	—	—	—	yes	—	—	—
Eosinophils	—	—	—	yes	—	—	—
Natural killer	—	—	yes	—	—	yes	yes
LAK activity	yes	—	yes	—	—	no	—
B cell							
Activation	—	—	—	—	—	—	—
Proliferation	—	—	—	—	—	yes	—
Differentiation	yes	—	—	—	—	yes	—
Ig isotype switching	yes	—	IgE	—	—	IgA	—
T cell							
Activation	—	—	—	—	—	yes	—
Proliferation	yes	—	yes	yes	—	yes	—
Differentiation	—	—	—	—	—	yes	—
Endothelium	—	—	—	—	—	yes	—
Extracellular matrix	—	—	—	—	yes	yes	yes
Cytotoxicity	—	—	—	—	—	yes/no	—
MHC class I/II	II	—	—	—	—	II	—
Chemotaxis	yes	—	—	yes/no	—	yes/no	yes
Adhesion molecules	—	—	—	yes	—	yes	—
ROM/NO production	yes	—	—	yes	—	yes	—
Pyrogenesis	—	—	—	—	—	—	—
Acute-phase reaction	—	yes	—	—	—	—	—
Angiogenesis	—	—	—	yes	yes	yes	—

**Adapted from* Burke *et al.* [37]; with permission.
CSF—colony-stimulating factor (include granulocyte-, macrophage- and granulocyte-macrophage-CSF); Ig—immunoglobulin; IL—interleukin; LAK—lymphokine-activated killer; MHC—major histocompatibility complex; NO—nitric oxide; PDGF—platelet-derived growth factor; ROM—reactive oxygen metabolite; TGF—transforming growth factor.

in the inflamed mucosa, an accompanying increase of tissue myeloperoxidase (a major enzymatic product of neutrophils) was found only in ulcerative colitis but not Crohn's disease, again suggesting distinct cellular events in the two forms of IBD. Fluids from colorectal perfusions of patients with ulcerative colitis also contain high concentration of interleukin-8 and myeloperoxidase [22]. These remarkable changes at the level of the diseased organ are not necessarily translated to the peripheral circulation, where serum levels are seldom detectable and bear a marginal correlation with parameters of clinical activity [23]. This stresses the importance of assessing the difficult to obtain but more dependable tissue levels rather than the easily accessible but unreliable peripheral blood levels, when trying to understand intestinal inflammation.

As already reported for interleukin-6, there is some evidence that intestinal interleukin-8 may be produced by epithelial cells, potentially converting them from passive to active participants of gut inflammation. In fact, immunoreactive interleukin-8 and its messenger RNA can be easily detected in several colon cancer epithelial cell lines *in vitro* [24•,25]. Whether or not interleukin-8 is actually produced by enterocytes or colonocytes *in vivo* under physiologic or pathologic conditions is still unresolved.

Tumor necrosis factor-α

Among all cytokines evaluated in the gut, TNF-α is by far the most controversial. This preferential product of macrophages is also a multipotent mediator sharing many biological activities with interleukin-1β and interleukin-6, and the bowel is particularly susceptible to its inflammatory and tissue damaging capacity, making it very significant to gut inflammation.

A rise in serum TNF-α concentration was initially reported in children with active ulcerative or Crohn's colitis [26], but this was not confirmed in a comparable pediatric population, where no correlation was found with disease activity or growth parameters [27]. Contradictory results on TNF-α tissue concentrations have also been reported. Two studies using immunohistochemical staining of endoscopically derived or resected samples showed a significant increase of TNF-α–positive mucosal mononuclear cells in children with IBD [28,29], whereas another study found cellular localization by *in situ* hybridization in Paneth cells but not lamina propria cells in infants with acute necrotizing enterocolitis [30]. Polymerase chain reaction amplification failed to detect TNF-α messenger RNA in most adult IBD samples in an additional study [31]. In any case, a rise in tissue or even stool TNF-α during gut inflammation is nonspecific, because this occurs in Crohn's disease, ulcerative colitis, various forms of virus- or bacteria-induced diarrhea, and in chronic gastritis [18,32,33]. Despite these contradictory results, secretion of TNF-α can be specifically induced *in vitro* from mononuclear cells of infants allergic to cow's milk when challenged by this antigen [34••]. Furthermore, culture supernatants from the stimulated cells could trigger electrogenic chloride secretion in an experimental epithelial barrier system, suggesting that an antigenic stimulation *in vivo* may lead to a TNF-α–mediated increase in intestinal permeability or perhaps mucosal inflammation.

Conclusions

It is obvious that knowledge of cytokines in intestinal inflammation must be extended far beyond what has been presented here. Because of their large number and multiple overlapping functions, studying cytokines even in simple experimental systems is a complex task, which is made more difficult in the setting of human patients with diseases having different etiologies and mechanisms. Several well-characterized cytokines likely to have important roles in various steps of gut inflammation, such as interleukin-4, -5, -10, -12, and -13 have been described only in abstract form, and have yet to receive the full attention they deserve. For instance, accumulation of interleukin-5 messenger RNA has been described in the gut mucosa of patients with celiac disease but this allergy-related cytokine has not been explored in any other type of bowel inflammation [35]. Newer cytokines (interleukin-14, interleukin-15) are constantly being added to a long list of immunoregulatory and proinflammatory factors, widening the gap between simple awareness of their existence and concrete acquisition of data about their function in the gut. Methodologic problems in assessing mucosal cytokines plague the field, including subjective criteria for patient selection, assessment of disease severity, measurement of serum versus culture supernatant versus whole tissue concentrations, and utilization of complementary but not comparable methods relying on immunostaining, bioactivity, immunoreactivity, or RNA isolation.

Given these considerable limitations, it is remarkable that no other area of investigation has contributed so much to expanding our knowledge of gut inflammation as the study of cytokines has. Their contribution is not limited to basic cellular and molecular mechanisms, but extends into clinical assessment and differential diagnosis, as well as into the therapeutic arena [2•]. In regard to the latter, it is almost certain that the most dramatic advances in new treatment modalities of gut inflammation will come from understanding how cytokines work in the gut and how their secretion and activity can be modulated or neutralized by new drugs or natural immunomodulators [36].

References and recommended reading

Papers of particular interest, published within the annual period of review, have been highlighted as:

- • Of special interest
- •• Of outstanding interest

1. • Castro GA, Arntzen CJ. **Immunophysiology of the Gut: A Research Frontier for Integrative Studies of the Common Mucosal Immune System.** *Am J Physiol* 1993, **265**:G599–G610.

An excellent review article focused on the close and crucial inter-relationships among the various cellular components of the bowel, and the importance of integrating mucosal immune and nonimmune systems for local homeostasis.

2. • Fiocchi C. **Cytokines.** In *Inflammatory Bowel Disease. From Bench to Bedside.* Edited by Targan SR, Shanahan F. Baltimore: Williams & Wilkins; 1994:106–122.

A comprehensive review of cytokines in human IBD, discussing the physiologic role of individual mediators, abnormalities in Crohn's disease and ulcerative colitis, and implications in pathogenic, clinical, and therapeutic aspects of these entities.

3. Fiocchi C: **Cytokines and Animal Models: A Combined Path to Inflammatory Bowel Disease Pathogenesis.** *Gastroenterology* 1993,**104**:1202–1219.
4. Youngman KR, Simon PL, West GA, Cominelli F, Rachmilewitz D, Klein JS, Fiocchi C: **Localization of Intestinal Interleukin 1 Activity, Protein and Gene Expression to Lamina Propria Cells.** *Gastroenterology* 1993, **104**:749–758.
5. Gionchetti P, Campieri M, Belluzzi A, Paganelli GM, Bertinelli E, Ferretti M, Lauri A, Biasco G, Poggioli G, Miglioli M, Barbara L: **Macrophage Subpopulations and Interleukin-1b Tissue Levels in Pelvic Ileal Pouches.** *Eur J Gastroenterol Hepatol* 1994, **6**:217–222.
6. •• Mansfield JC, Holden H, Tarlow JK, DiGiovane FS, McDowell TL, Wilson AG, Holdsworth CD, Duff GW: **Novel Genetic Association Between Ulcerative Colitis and the Anti-inflammatory Cytokine Interleukin-1 Receptor Antagonist.** *Gastroenterology* 1994,**106**:637–642.

The first report on cytokine gene polymorphism in IBD. Particularly relevant are the potential implications of differential cytokine gene expression for the variable clinical manifestations of gut inflammation.

7. Kusugami K, Youngman KR, West GA, Fiocchi C: **Intestinal Immune Reactivity to Interleukin 2 Differs Among Crohn's Disease, Ulcerative Colitis and Control.** *Gastroenterology* 1989, **97**:1–9.
8. Mullin GE, Lazenby AJ, Harris ML, Bayless TM, James SP: **Increased Interleukin-2 Messenger RNA in the Intestinal Mucosal Lesions of Crohn's Disease but Not Ulcerative Colitis.** *Gastroenterology* 1992, **102**:1620–1627.
9. Gurbindo C, Sabbah S, Menezes J, Justinich C, Marchand R, Seidman EG: **Interleukin-2 Production in Pediatric Inflammatory Bowel Disease: Evidence for Dissimilar Mononuclear Cell Function in Crohn's Disease and Ulcerative Colitis.** *J Pediatr Gastroenterol Nutr* 1993, **17**:247–254.
10. • Sparano JA, Brandt LJ, Dutcher JP, DuBois JS, Atkins MB: **Symptomatic Exacerbation of Crohn Disease After Treatment With High-Dose Interleukin-2.** *Ann Intern Med* 1993, **118**:617–618.

A brief but intriguing case report on the *in vivo* administration of interleukin-2 to patients with Crohn's disease, its clinical effects, and its implications for disease pathogenesis.

11. Mahida YR, Kurlak L, Gallagher A, Hawkey CJ: **High Circulating Levels of Interleukin 6 in Active Crohn's Disease but Not Ulcerative Colitis.** *Gut* 1991, **32**:1531–1534.
12. Gross V, Andus T, Caesar I, Roth M, Scholmerich J: **Evidence for Continuous Stimulation of Interleukin-6 Production in Crohn's Disease.** *Gastroenterology* 1992, **102**:514–519.
13. Hymas JS, Fitzgerald JE, Treem WR, Wyzga N, Kreutzer DL: **Relationship of Functional and Antigenic Interleukin 6 to Disease Activity in Inflammatory Bowel Disease.** *Gastroenterology* 1993, **104**:1285–1292.
14. Raab Y, Hallgren R, Gerdin B: **Enhanced Intestinal Synthesis of Interleukin-6 Is Related to Disease Severity and Activity in Ulcerative Colitis.** *Digestion* 1994, **55**:44–49.
15. Reinecker H-C, Steffen M, Witthoeft T, Pflueger I, Schreiber S, MacDermott RP, Raedler A: **Enhanced Secretion of Tumour Necrosis Factor-alpha, IL-6, and IL-1β by Isolated Lamina Propria Mononuclear Cells From Patients With Ulcerative Colitis and Crohn's Disease.** *Clin Exp Immunol* 1993, **94**:174–181.
16. Jones SC, Haidar A, Hagan P, Crabtree J, Banks RE, Axon ATR, Dixon MF, Whicker JT: **Cytokine Production in the Mucosa of Patients**

With Inflammatory Bowel Disease. *Eur J Gastroenterol Hepatol* 1993, 5:607–612.

17. Jones SC, Trejdosiewicsz LK, Banks RE, Howdle PD, Axon ATR, Dixon MF, Whicher JT: **Expression of Interleukin-6 by Intestinal Enterocytes.** *J Clin Pathol* 1993, 46:1097–1110.

18. Crabtree JE, Shallcross TM, Heatley RV, Wyatt JI: **Mucosal Tumour Necrosis Factor α and Interleukin-6 in Patients With Helicobacter Pylori Associated Gastritis.** *Gut* 1991, 32:1473–1477.

19. Mahida YR, Ceska M, Effenberger F, Kurlak L, Lindley I, Hawkey CJ: **Enhanced Synthesis of Neutrophil-Activating Peptide-I/Interleukin-8 in Active Ulcerative Colitis.** *Clin Sci (Colch)* 1992, 82:273–275.

20. Izzo RS, Witkon K, Chen AI, Hadjiyane C, Weinstein MI, Pellecchia C: **Interleukin-8 and Neutrophil Markers in Colonic Mucosa From Patients With Ulcerative Colitis.** *Am J Gastroenterol* 1992, 87:1447–1452.

21. Izzo RS, Witkon K, Chen AI, Hadjiyane C, Weinstein MI, Pellecchia C: **Neutrophil-Activating Peptide (Interleukin-8) in Colonic Mucosa From Patients With Crohn's Disease.** *Scand J Gastroenterol* 1993, 28:296–300.

22. Raab Y, Gerdin B, Ahlstedt S, Hallgren R: **Neutrophil Mucosa Involvement Is Accompanied by Enhanced Local Production of Interleukin-8 in Ulcerative Colitis.** *Gut* 1993, 34:1203–1206.

23. Jones SC, Evans SW, Lobo AJ, Ceska M, Axon ATR, Whicher JT: **Serum Interleukin-8 in Inflammatory Bowel Disease.** *J Gastroenterol Hepatol* 1993, 8:508–512.

24. • Eckmann L, Jung HC, Schurer-Maly C, Panja A, Morzycka-Wroblewska E, Kagnoff MF: **Differential Cytokine Expression by Human Intestinal Epithelial Cell Lines: Regulated Expression of Interleukin 8.** *Gastroenterology* 1994, 105:1689–1697.

A detailed study showing that intestinal epithelial cells can produce a variety of cytokines that until recently were considered the exclusive product of immune cells.

25. Schuerer-Maly C-C, Eckmann L, Kagnoff MF, Falco MT, Maly F-E: **Colonic Epithelial Cell Lines as a Source of Interleukin-8: Stimulation by Inflammatory Cytokines and Bacterial Lipopolysaccharide.** *Immunology* 1994, 81:85–91.

26. Murch SH, Lamkin VA, Savage MO, Walker-Smith JA, MacDonald TT: **Serum Concentrations of Tumour Necrosis Factor α in Childhood Chronic Inflammatory Bowel Disease.** *Gut* 1991, 32:913–917.

27. Hymas JS, Treem WR, Eddy E, Wyzga N, Moore RE: **Tumor Necrosis Factor-α Is Not Elevated in Children With Inflammatory Bowel Disease.** *J Pediatr Gastroenterol Nutr* 1991, 12:233–236.

28. Olson AD, Ayass M, Chensue S: **Tumor Necrosis Factor and IL-β Expression in Pediatric Patients With Inflammatory Bowel Disease.** *J Pediatr Gastroenterol Nutr* 1993, 16:241–246.

29. Murch SH, Braegger CP, Walker-Smith JA, MacDonald TT: **Location of Tumor Necrosis Factor α by Immunohistochemistry in Chronic Inflammatory Bowel Disease.** *Gut* 1993, 34:1705–1709.

30. Tan X, Hsueh W, Gonzales-Crussi F: **Cellular Localization of Tumor Necrosis Factor (TNF)-α Transcripts in Normal Bowel and in Necrotizing Enterocolitis.** *Am J. Pathol* 1993, 142:1858–1865.

31. Isaacs KL, Sartor RB, Haskill S: **Cytokine Messenger RNA Profiles in Inflammatory Bowel Disease Mucosa Detected by Polymerase Chain Reaction Amplification.** *Gastroenterology* 1992, 103:1587–1595.

32. Nicholls S, Stephens S, Braegger CP, Walker-Smith JA, MacDonald TT: **Cytokines in Stools of Children With Inflammatory Bowel Disease or Infective Diarrhea.** *J Clin Pathol* 1993, 46:757–760.

33. Breese EJ, Michie CA, Nicholls SW, Murch SH, Williams CB, Domizio P, Walker-Smith JA, MacDonald TT: **Tumor Necrosis Factor-α Producing Cells in the Intestinal Mucosa of Children With Inflammatory Bowel Disease.** *Gastroenterology* 1994, 106:1455–1466.

34. •• Heyman M, Darmon N, Dupont C, Dugas B, Hirribaren A, Blaton M-A, Desjeux J-F: **Mononuclear Cells From Infants Allergic to Cow's Milk Secrete Tumor Necrosis Factor α, Altering Intestinal Function.** *Gastroenterology* 1994, 106:1514–1523.

A very well done study demonstrating that production of pro-inflammatory cytokines can occur when immune cells are exposed to an antigen to which the cells are specifically sensitized. The secretory products of activated immune cells can alter epithelial barrier function, implicating them in diarrhea, altered mucosal permeability, and intestinal inflammation. This work is important because it demonstrates possible consequences of stimulation of mucosal immunity on key intestinal functions.

35. Desreumaux P, Janin A, Colombel JF, Prin L, Plumas J, Emilie D, Torpier G, Capron A, Capron M: **Interleukin 5 Messenger RNA Expression by Eosinophils in the Intestinal Mucosa of Patients With Coeliac Disease.** *J Exp Med* 1992, 175:293–296.

36. Wallace JL: **Inflammatory Mediators in Inflammatory Bowel Disease: Clues for Designer Therapy.** *Can J Gastroenterol* 1993, 7:121–126.

37. Burke F, Naylor MS, Davies B, Balkwill F: **The Cytokine Wall Chart.** *Immunol Today* 1993, 14:165–170.

Claudio Fiocchi, MD, Case Western Reserve University. School of Medicine (BRB), Gastroenterology Division, 10900 Euclid Avenue, Cleveland, OH 44106-4952, USA.

Intestinal subepithelial myofibroblasts and mucosal immunophysiology

John D. Valentich, PhD, and Don W. Powell, MD

University of Texas Medical Branch, Galveston, Texas, USA

A major challenge in gastrointestinal immunophysiology is to define the mucosal cells and soluble mediators whose integrated actions modulate gut absorption, secretion, motility, and blood flow. This knowledge has immense significance not only for attaining an in-depth understanding of normal physiology, but also for evolving insight into the molecular etiology and pathogenesis of gastrointestinal inflammatory disease. This article summarizes current knowledge of specialized mucosal cells commonly referred to as pericryptal fibroblasts or subepithelial myofibroblasts. Subepithelial myofibroblasts are members of a family of phenotypically interrelated cells that we collectively call juxtaparenchymal cells. Recognized morphologically for more than 25 years, the role of juxtaparenchymal cells in mucosal function remains an enigma. Given their strategic location at the interface between the epithelium and lamina propria, juxtaparenchymal cells may modulate information transfer between these tissue compartments and play a pivotal role in mucosal immunophysiology.

Current Opinion in Gastroenterology 1994, **10**:645–651

Mucosal paracrine cell interactions

Paracrine mediators, together with endocrine, immune, and neural inputs, are major regulators of mucosal physiology in both normal and pathologic states [1,2•,3•]. Fundamental processes such as cell proliferation and apoptosis, terminal differentiation, inflammation, and repair and modulation of the immune response are initiated, maintained, and terminated by local interactions between soluble mediators and target cells. In mucosal tissues such as the intestine, a myriad of subepithelial cell types, permanently or transiently resident in the lamina propria, engage in complex bidirectional signaling networks, both with one another and with overlying epithelial cells. These cells include neutrophils, eosinophils, macrophages, mast cells, several subsets of lymphocytes, endothelial cells, smooth muscle cells, fibroblasts, and neurons. The role of these cells in mucosal physiology and inflammation has been the subject of recent meetings and reviews [1,2•,3•,4]. This article focuses on the subepithelial juxtaparenchymal cells, whose participation in mucosal immunophysiology has received limited attention.

Myofibroblasts as juxtaparenchymal cells

In nonpathologic conditions, myofibroblast-like cells intercalate between parenchymal cells and the stromal cells comprising an organ's supporting structural matrix. The most intensively studied examples include glomerular mesangial cells, capillary pericytes, hepatic Ito cells, and pulmonary interstitial fibroblasts [5-7]. Because of their strategic location between parenchymal cells and adjacent neural, immune, and endocrine tissues, myofibroblasts may play a crucial role in modulating information flow between these compartments (Fig. 1).

Myofibroblasts are members of a family of phenotypically polymorphic cells displaying structural, biosynthetic, antigenic, and functional characteristics of both connective tissue fibroblasts and smooth muscle cells [8,9]. Both of the latter cell types, in addition to macrophages, are postulated progenitors of myofibroblasts [8,10]. Myofibroblasts probably represent only one point in a continuum of possible phenotypes that these cells may assume in different physiologic or pathophysiologic states. Tissue injury, inflammation, and neoplasia are frequently associated with myofibroblast activation [8]. Cytokines and growth factors, extracellular matrix components, adhesion molecules, lipid mediators, neurotransmitters, and physical stretch may promote phenotypic transitions. Therefore, we refer to all members of this family of cells collectively as *juxtaparenchymal cells*, irrespective of their prevailing phenotypic state and in recognition of their physical proximity and known or putative functional interactions with organ parenchymal cells.

Juxtaparenchymal cells in inflammation and fibrosis

Data from studies employing cultured Ito cells, mesangial cells, and lung interstitial fibroblasts provide in-

Abbreviations

ANP—atrial natriuretic peptide; **ICC**—interstitial cells of Cajal.

 ISBN 1-85922-611-6 ISSN 0267–1379

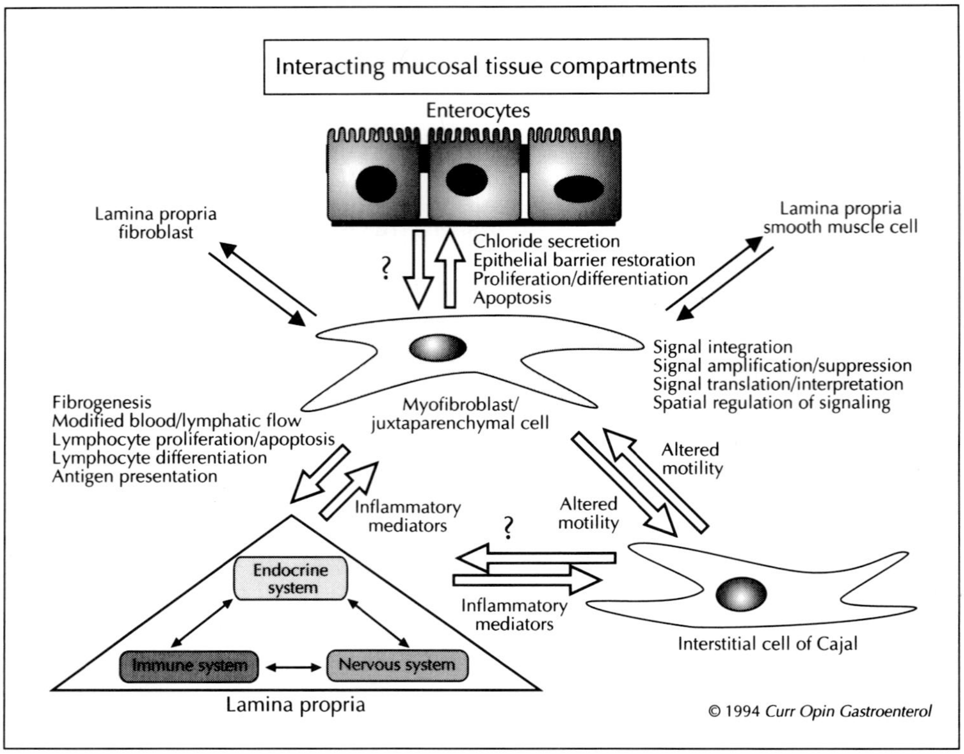

Fig. 1. Hypothetical pathways for signaling between intestinal juxtaparenchymal cells and enterocytes, interstitial cells of Cajal and lamina propria cells (*open arrows*). Pathways of possible phenotypic transition between lamina propria fibroblasts, smooth muscle cells, and juxtaparenchymal cells (*solid arrows*). Juxtaparenchymal cells may exhibit multiple phenotypes depending on local paracrine or juxtacrine inputs from cells and extracellular matrix molecules.

sight into the molecular mechanisms through which juxtaparenchymal cells may affect intestinal mucosal immunophysiology. The former cells are components of autocrine, paracrine, and juxtacrine signaling networks that exert profound effects on tissue physiology and pathophysiology [5,6,11]. Cytokines, growth factors, peptide hormones, extracellular matrix molecules, lipid mediators, oxygen radicals, and nitric oxide are important effector molecules in these networks. Because activation of juxtaparenchymal cells *in vivo* is correlated with leukocyte infiltration and the initiation and progression of hepatic, glomerular, and pulmonary fibrosis, it is possible that intestinal juxtaparenchymal cells display similar effector functions.

Small intestinal and colonic juxtaparenchymal cells

Juxtaparenchymal cell proliferation, differentiation, migration, and death

A sheath of juxtaparenchymal cells, some of which express phenotypic features of myofibroblasts, underlies the crypt, villus, and surface epithelium in the small intestine and colon [12,13]. Early ultrastructural descriptions of these cells referred to them as the "pericryptal fibroblastic sheath" or the "subepithelial reticulohistiocytic complex" [14,15]. Juxtaparenchymal cells in these intestinal microdomains differ in shape, cytoplasmic organelle content, and contractile protein expression. A three-dimensional network of myofibroblast-like cells extends laterally from the pericryptal region into the lamina propria [12,13]. The functional or lineage relationships between pericryptal and lamina propria myofibroblasts and mucosal smooth muscle cells are unresolved.

In the crypt region, juxtaparenchymal cells overlap with one another and exhibit a flattened "fried egg" shape [14]. Coincident with migration to the surface or villus tip, the cells elaborate long attenuated processes and assume a highly stellate morphology [14,16]. Ultrastructural analysis with ^{3}H-thymidine kinetic autoradiography experiments demonstrates a pattern of proliferation, migrating, and cytodifferentiation in juxtaparenchymal cells, paralleling that found in the overlying epithelium [14,17–19]. The complement of cytoplasmic organelles in colonic and jejunal juxtaparenchymal cells range from that of undifferentiated cells at the base of crypts to biosynthetically active cells at the mouth of the crypt and under the surface epithelium. These data led to the concept of an integrated epithelial-mesenchymal unit exhibiting coordinated cell proliferation and differentiation from the base to the surface of rabbit colonic crypts [17]. These findings were not confirmed in rat and mouse colon and mouse small intestine, where a more complex relationship between juxtaparenchymal cells and epithelial cells may exist [19,20]. The latter data indicate that juxtaparenchymal cell and epithelial proliferation kinetics are independent, and respond differently to starvation/feeding and circadian rhythms [21]. However, ongoing epithelial-mesenchymal interactions in adult intestinal mucosa are likely.

Intercellular contacts

Gap junctions and macular adherens junctions are found between the cytoplasmic processes of intestinal juxtaparenchymal cells [12,13,16]. Hemidesmosome-like attachment bodies are also observed on the contra-epithelial side of subepithelial myofibroblasts [13]. Colonic juxtaparenchymal cells form synaptic-like contacts with nerve terminals containing clear (cholinergic) and dense core (adrenergic/peptidergic) vesicles and exhibit gap-junction contacts with lamina propria smooth muscle cells [12,16,22]. Formation of synaptic contacts between juxtaparenchymal cells and neurons is consistent with the observation that receptors for the muscarinic agonist carbachol are coupled to prostaglandin E_2 production in 18Co cells, a human colonic subepithelial myofibroblasts-like cell line [23•,24]. Interestingly, embryonic, postnatal, and adult duodenal juxtaparenchymal cells exhibit close (< 10.0 nm) contacts with processes that extend from overlying epithelial cells and transverse the basal lamina [25]. In addition, penetration of the epithelial basal lamina by juxtaparenchymal cell processes has been described [15]. This diversity of intercellular contacts confers on juxtaparenchymal cells the potential for mediating electrical, paracrine, and juxtacrine signaling between epithelial and lamina propria cells. Coordinated electrical or metabolic activity of cells comprising the juxtaparenchymal cell sheath may occur through their extensive coupling via gap junctions. Finally, adherens junctions and hemidesmosomes could allow transmission throughout the villus of contractile force generated by subepithelial myofibroblasts.

Extracellular matrix proteins and receptors

Colonic juxtaparenchymal cells contain immunoreactive type IV collagen and are sometimes surrounded by a discontinuous basal lamina [12,22]. *In situ* hybridization shows that α_1(I), α_2(I), α_1(III), α_1(IV), and α_2(V) procollagen genes are expressed in colonic juxtaparenchymal cells [26]. The extracellular matrix glycoprotein tenascin is associated with juxtaparenchymal cells in adult intestine and its developmental apppearance is correlated with mucosal smooth muscle and subepithelial myofibroblast differentiation [27]. Tenascin exhibits both morphoregulatory and immunoregulatory functions. Together with other molecules such as hepatocyte growth factor/scatter factor, epimorphin, Neu differentiation factor, and fibroblast activation protien, it may be a member of an evolving family of mesenchymally derived paracrine mediators involved in epithelial-mesenchymal interactions in both developing and adult tissues.

Human small intestine and colonic juxtaparenchymal cells, together with muscularis mucosa and villus core smooth muscle cells, express integrin VLA (very late activation)-1,-3, and -5 α-chains. However, VLA-2 and -4 α-chain expression is restricted to juxtaparenchymal cells and villus core smooth muscle cells [28]. This study also noted continuity between VLA-positive cells in the muscularis mucosa and the pericryptal juxtaparenchymal cell sheath.

Cytoskeletal elements and contractile proteins

Colonic juxtaparenchymal cells contain bundles of microfilaments and intermediate filaments as well as individual thick filaments [12,13]. Filaments are especially prominent in cell processes. Focal densities found in microfilament bundles may represent the dense bodies associated with myofiloments in smooth muscle cells. An immunocytochemical study of contractile proteins by Joyce *et al.* [13] distinguished three classes of colonic juxtaparenchymal cells: pericryptal juxtaparenchymal cells containing high levels of smooth muscle tropomyosin and smooth muscle myosin, villus juxtaparenchymal cells containing intermediate levels of these proteins, and lamina propria juxtaparenchymal cells with low levels of both proteins. Also found in pericryptal juxtaparenchymal cells are α-smooth muscle actin, the actin-binding protein filamin, and the intermediate filament protein desmin [22,29]. α-Smooth muscle actin is expressed by myofibroblasts in numerous tissues [8]. Connective tissue fibroblasts contain none of the above smooth muscle contractile proteins.

Plasma membrane receptors for peptides, amines, and nucleotides

Following intravascular injection of rats with ^{125}I-endothelin-1 or ^{125}I-atrial natriuretic peptide (ANP), autoradiography of histologic sections of small intestine demonstrates peptide binding to villus juxtaparenchymal cells [30,31]. Similarly, autoradiography of sections of human colon incubated with ^{125}I-endothelin-1 shows preferential concentration of silver grains in the lamina propria immediately beneath colonocytes [32]. Endothelin-1–stimulated contraction of myofibroblasts in granulation tissue [33], hepatic Ito cells [34], and glomerular mesangial cells *in vitro* [35] suggests a possible physiologic function for juxtaparenchymal cell endothelin receptors. Colocalization of endothelin and ANP receptors raises the possibility that these peptides have antagonistic effects on juxtaparenchymal cell functions as in smooth muscle and mesangial cells. ANP increases cyclic GMP formation in 18Co cells [23•] and cytochemical studies demonstrate cyclic GMP–dependent protein kinase immunoreactivity in pericryptal and subepithelial juxtaparenchymal cells [13]. These data suggest a role for cyclic GMP–mediated signaling in intestinal juxtaparenchymal cell activation.

In primary cultures of rat intestinal juxtaparenchymal cells and in 18Co cells, endothelin-1 rapidly (< 15 minutes) induces flattening and cytoskeletal reorganization in cells previously induced by cyclic AMP to assume a stellate morphology [23•,36••]. These *in vitro* cell shape changes may reflect the *in situ* transition of intestinal juxtaparenchymal cells from a flattened polygonal shape in the pericryptal region to a stellate morphology in villus and surface regions [14]. Fibroblasts in ocular and synovial tissue, which may participate in immune functions at these locations, also assume a stellate or dendritic morphology following stimulation by prostaglandin E_2 or elevation of intracellular cyclic AMP levels [37,38•].

Furuya *et al.* [39•] have recently demonstrated that endothelins, substance P, angiotensin II, ATP, bradykinin, and 5-hydroxytryptamine increase cytosolic calcium levels in cultured rat lamina propria fibroblasts. The latter two agonists also stimulate prostaglandin E_2

formation in a porcine jejunal myofibroblast-like cell line [40].

Relationships between intestinal juxtaparenchymal cells, macrophages, and interstitial cells of Cajal

Organized layers of interstitial cells of Cajal (ICC) are associated with neuronal plexes at the interface between the longitudinal and circular muscle layers and at the submucosal surface of the circular muscle layer of the intestine [41]. Like mucosal juxtaparenchymal cells, ICC are highly pleiomorphic cells. They exhibit an extensively ramified stellate morphology and, via gap junctions between adjacent cells, form an integrated syncytial network. ICC also develop gap junctions with smooth muscle cells and display synaptic contacts with neuronal varicosities in the submucosal and myenteric plexus [41,42]. ICC exhibit oscillations in membrane potential and intracellular calcium levels and may play a role in generating intestinal electrical rhythmicity [43]. They may also serve as mechanosensitive stretch receptors responding to distension of the bowel wall [41,42] or participate in inhibitory nonadrenergic, noncholinergic neurotransmission [42].

Morphologic and immunocytochemical studies demonstrate that ICC exhibit numerous similarities to intestinal juxtaparenchymal cells (Table 1). Such commonalties suggest that these cells also have analogous functions. This raises the intriguing possibility that together they form a bidirectional link mediating the flow and integration of information between the mucosal, submucosal, and muscular layers of the intestine. Interestingly, in his original studies, Cajal also described cells exhibiting the staining properties of ICC in the lamina propria.

Participation of juxtaparenchymal cells in intestinal immunophysiology

The descriptive ultrastructural and histochemical data summarized previously allow limited inferences about the participation of juxtaparenchymal cells in mucosal inflammation. The recent characterization of 18Co cells, a human colonic cell line exhibiting an array of phenotypic characteristics of subepithelial myofibroblasts, provides a powerful investigative tool for defining the physiologic functions of intestinal juxtaparenchymal cells at the cellular and molecular levels [23•,24].

Following mucosal injury in the ileum, alterations in the organization of subepithelial myofibroblast cytoplasmic actin filaments accompanied by ATP-dependent villus shortening suggest that subepithelial myofibroblasts mediate villus contraction [44]. Villus contraction may be important in rapidly reducing the area of mucosa denuded of epithelium and restoring epithelial barrier faction. In addition to wound repair, myofibroblast-mediated villus motility may also influence normal mucosal blood and lymph flow and solute transport [45].

Although juxtaparenchymal cells have not been specifically investigated, gut mesenchymal cells enhance intestinal epithelial proliferation and differentiation *in vitro* and may contribute to wound reepithelialization *in vivo* [46]. Intestinal lamina propria cells as well as α–smooth muscle actin–positive myofibroblast-like cells at the periphery of granulomas in a rat model of colitis express insulin-like growth factor 1 [47–49]. These data suggest that juxtaparenchymal cells may be a source of mitogens for both epithelial and lamina propria cells [50].

Table 1. Relationships between intestinal subepithelial myofibroblasts and interstitial cells of Cajal

Similar morphology [14,16,41]*
Stellate shape
Discontinuous basal lamina
Numerous surface caveolae
Cytoplasmic dense bodies
Sub plasma membrane dense bands
Commone cytoskeletal elements and contractile proteins [12,13,22,29,41,73••]
Smooth muscle α-actin expressed
Abundant thin filaments, particularly in cell processes
Abundant intermediate filaments
Intercellular junctions and contacts [12,13,41]
Gap junctions formed with one another and with smooth muscle cells
Synaptic-like contacts with neuronal varicosities
Contain guanylate cyclase and cyclic GMP–dependent protein kinase [13,74]
Similar intercellular topographical relationships [12–14,41]
SEMF: epithelium ←→ SEMF ←→ lamina propria cells + neurons
ICC: smooth muscle ←→ ICC ←→ neurons + lamina propria cells?
Possible origin from smooth muscle cells or fibroblasts [8,41]
Physical or lineage relationship to macrophage-like cells [10,14,15,41]
Endothelin, substance P and ATP receptors expressed [30,32,39••,43]†
Oscillations in cytosolic calcium concentration dependent on influx of extracellular calcium [39••,43]
Adjacent to endothelin-producing parenchymal cells [32,57]
SEMF: epithelium
ICC: submucosal and myenteric neurons

*Numbers in brackets represent reference numbers of relevant studies.
†The conclusion that ICC contain endothelin receptors is inferential and based on the observation that ^{125}I-endothelin binds to myenteric plexes but not to myenteric neurons.
ICC—interstitial cells of Cajal; SEMF—subepithelial myofibroblast.

Fibrosis is a common sequelae of mucosal inflammation and intestinal juxtaparenchymal cells may participate in this process. Expression of the procollagen genes α_1(I), α_2(I), α_1(III), α_1(IV), and α_2(V) is enhanced in juxtaparenchymal cells in ulcerative colitis, whereas in Crohn's disease only α_1(I) and α_1(III) message levels are elevated [26]. Ultrastructural studies suggest that juxtaparenchymal cells are responsible for inordinate subepithelial collagen deposition in mucosal inflammatory diseases such as collagenous colitis [51], ulcerative colitis [52], and bronchial asthma [53•].

Intestinal inflammation is frequently associated with debilitating diarrhea resulting from excessive and uncontrolled epithelial salt and water secretion. Several studies demonstrate juxtaparenchymal cell modulation of epithelial chloride secretion. Coculture or acute juxtaposition of P2JF porcine jejunal myofibroblast-like cells with T84 colonocytes up-regulates the responsiveness of the latter to mast cell–derived and neutrophil-derived chloride secretagogues [40]. Acutely juxtaposed 18Co cells sensitize T84 cells to calcium-dependent secretagogues by a prostaglandin E_2–mediated mechanism [24].

The proinflammatory cytokines interleukin-1 and tumor necrosis factor-α activate expression of both the COX-1 and COX-2 isoforms of the cyclooxygenase gene in 18Co cells [23•]. In addition, interleukin-1 stimulates interleukin-6 and prostaglandin-E_2 production in these cells. Interleukin-1, interferon-γ, and lipopolysaccharide also enhance cytokine, procollagen, and adhesion molecule gene expression in cultured human intestinal fibroblasts [54••,55•]. These data indicate that intestinal juxtaparenchymal cells are capable of both producing and responding to cytokines that have pivotal roles in modulating local inflammatory responses.

Intestinal epithelial and enterochromaffin cells may be sources of endothelin and ANP, respectively [56,57]. Endothelin-1, -2, and -3 are present in colonic mucosal extracts [58]. In addition, monocytes, macrophages, neutrophils, and endothelial cells express endothelin immunoreactivity or messenger RNA and secrete endothelin in response to cytokines or lipopolysaccharide [59–62]. In inflammatory bowel disease, the percentage of lamina propria and submucosal cells expressing immunoreactive endothelin is increased [63]. The presence of receptors for ANP and endothelin on juxtaparenchymal cell plasma membranes suggests the existence of a paracrine signaling mechanism that may play a role in ANP- and endothelin-activated epithelial chloride secretion in the normal or inflamed intestine. Both peptides stimulate intestinal salt secretion by an ill-defined mechanism that does not involved direct action on epithelial cells.

Several studies demonstrate interactions between juxtaparenchymal cells and lamina propria lymphocytes. Primary cultures of lamina propria fibroblasts enhance the survival and proliferation of co-cultured autologous lamina propria TCR$\alpha\beta^+$ lymphocytes [55•]. In colonic hyperplastic polyps, juxtaparenchymal cells express the class II major histocompatibility complex molecule HLA-DR on their surfaces [64]. Subepithelial stellate-shaped cells expressing class II molecules and phenotypic markers of macrophages or dendritic cells are found in normal human and mouse intestine [65–67]. Uncharacterized human intestinal fibroblasts *in vitro* display cell surface HLA-DR molecules whose expression is enhanced in ulcerative colitis or following interferon-γ stimulation [68•]. Juxtaparenchymal cells in the lung interstitium and the glomerular mesangium also express class II molecules [11,69]. Interestingly, the original ultrastructural descriptions of the subepithelial region of intestinal mucosa noted the presence of macrophage-like cells in this tissue compartment [14,15]. It is possible that a lineage relationship between myofibroblasts and macrophages exits [10]. In hyperplastic polyps, HLA-DR$^+$ juxtaparenchymal cells are in close contact with CD4$^+$ lymphocytes [64]. CD4 antigen is also expressed in mesangial cells and lung interstitial fibroblasts [70,71]. These data suggest that intestinal juxtaparenchymal cells participate in mucosal antigen presentation and may play a role in T-cell memory by promoting the survival of sensitized lamina propria or intraepithelial lymphocytes.

Juxtaparenchymal cells and ICC may comprise a communication pathway crucial for coordinating ion transport and motility in the intestine. Interconnections between ICC in the longitudinal and circular muscle layers support their involvement in nonneuronal vertical communication across the intestinal wall, perhaps operating in parallel with nerve fibers projecting from myenteric ganglia to submucoal ganglia and into the mucosa [41]. Intestinal anaphylaxis is accompanied by modified excitability and synaptic transmission in myenteric neurons and altered patterns of smooth muscle motility [3•,72]. The impact of intestinal inflammation on ICC function has not been investigated.

Conclusions

There are compelling reasons to suspect that intestinal juxtaparenchymal cells have significant roles in intestinal mucosal immunophysiology. Through direct cell-cell contact or via soluble mediators, juxtaparenchymal cells can interact with adjacent epithelial and lamina propria cells. Because of their localization at the epithelial–lamina propria interface, juxtaparenchymal cells may mediate signal transmission between these compartments. Dysfunction of signal transmission may be a crucial determinant in the pathogenesis of intestinal inflammatory disease. To critically test this hypothesis, the biological functions of intestinal juxtaparenchymal cells at the cellular and molecular levels must be elucidated.

Acknowledgments

Supported by grant DK-15350 from the National Institute of Diabetes, Digestive, and Kidney Diseases.

References and recommended reading

Papers of particular interest, published within the annual period of review, have been highlighted as:
- • Of special interest
- •• Of outstanding interest

1. Powell DW: **Immunophysiology of Intestinal Electrolyte Transport**. In *Absorptive and Secretory Processes of the Intestine. Handbook of Physiology, The Gastrointestinal System IV*. Edited by Frizzell RA, Field M. Bethesda: American Physiological Society; 1991:591–641.

2. • Cooke HJ: **Neuroimmune Signalling in Requisition of Intestinal Ion Transport**. *Am J Physiol* 1994, **266**:G167–G178.

This is an authoritative synthesis of the interactions between neurons, enterocytes, and immune mediators that collectively modulate intestinal ion transport.

3. • Castro GA, Powell DW: **The Physiology of the Mucosal Immune System and Immune-Mediated Responses in the Gastrointestinal Tract**. In *Physiology of the Gastrointestinal Tract*. Edited by Johnson LR. New York: Raven Press; 1994.

This provides a comprehensive review of intestinal immunophysiology from the perspective of organs and organisms.

4. Stead RH, Perdue MH, Cooke H, Powell DW, Barrett KE: **Neuro-Immuno-Physiology of the Gastrointestinal Mucosa**. *Implications for*

Inflammatory Diseases. New York: New York Academy of Sciences; 1992.

5. Sedor JR, Konieczkowski M, Huang S, Gronich JH, Nakazato Y, Gordon G, King CH: **Cytokines, Mesangial Cell Activation and Glomerular Injury.** *Kidney Int* 1993, **39**(suppl):S65–S70.

6. Friedman SL: **The Cellular Basis of Hepatic Fibrosis.** *N Engl J Med* 1993, **328**:1828–1835.

7. Leslie KO, Mitchell J, Low R: **Lung myofibroblasts.** *Cell Motil Cytoskeleton* 1992, **22**:92–98.

8. Skalli O, Gabbiani G: **The Biology of the Myofibroblast: Relationship to Wound Contraction and Fibrocontractive Diseases.** In *The Molecular and Cellular Biology of Wound Repair*, Edited by Clark RAF, Henson PM. New York: Plenum Press; 1988:373–402.

9. Komuro T: **Re-evaluation of Fibroblasts and Fibroblast-Like Cells.** *Anat Embryol (Berl)* 1990, **182**:103–112.

10. Bhawan J, Majno G: **The Myofibroblast: Possible Derivation From Macrophages in Xanthogranuloma.** *Am J Dermatopathol* 1989, **11**:255–258.

11. Froneck MJ, Derdak S, Felch ME, Silvera MR, Watts HB, Phipps RP: **Cellular and Molecular Characterization of Thy-1+ and Thy-1- Murine Lung Fibroblasts.** In *Pulmonary Fibroblast Heterogeneity*. Edited by Phipps RP. Boca Raton: CRC Press; 1992:135–198.

12. Guldner F-H, Wolff JR, Keyserlingk DG: **Fibroblasts as a Part of the Contractile System in Duodenal Villi of Rat.** *Z Zellforsch* 1972, **135**:349–360.

13. Joyce NC, Haire MF, Palade GE: **Morphologic and Biochemical Evidence for a Contractile Cell Network Within the Rat Intestinal Mucosa.** *Gastroenterology* 1987, **92**:68–81.

14. Kaye GI, Lane N, Pascal RR: **Colonic Pericryptal Fibroblast Sheath: Replication, Migration, and Cytodifferentiation of a Mesenchymal Cell System in Adult Tissue. II. Fine Structural Aspects of Normal Rabbit and Huamn Colon.** *Gastroenterology* 1968, **54**:852–865.

15. Donnellan WL: **The Structure of the Colonic Mucosa: The Epithelium and Subepithelial Reticulohistiocytic Complex.** *Gastroenterology* 1965, **49**:496–514.

16. Desaki J, Fujiwara T, Komuro T: **A Cellular Reticulum of Fibroblast-Like Cells in the Rat Intestine: Scanning and Transmission Electron Microscopy.** *Arch Histol Jap* 1984, **47**:179–186.

17. Pascal RR, Kaye GI, Lane N: **Colonic Pericryptal Fibroblast Sheath: Replication, Migration, and Cytodifferentiation of a Mesenchymal Cell System in Adult Tissue. I. Autoradiographic Studies of Normal Rabbit Colon.** *Gastroenterology* 1968, **54**:835–851.

18. Marsh MN, Trier JS: **Morphology and Cell Proliferation of Subepithelial Fibroblasts in Adult Mouse Jejunum. I. Structural Features.** *Gastroenterology* 1974, **67**:622–635.

19. Marsh MN, Trier JS: **Morphology and Cell Proliferation of Subepithelial Fibroblasts in Adult Mouse Jejunum. II. Radioautographic Studies.** *Gastroenterology* 1974, **67**:634–645.

20. Neal JV, Potten CS: **Description and Basic Cell Kinetics of the Murine Pericryptal Fibroblast Sheath.** *Gut* 1981, **22**:19–24.

21. Neal JV, Potten CS: **Circadian Rhythms in the Epithelial Cells and the Pericryptal Fibroblast Sheath.** *Gut* 1981, **22**:19–24.

22. Richman PI, Tilly R, Jass JR, Bodmer WF: **Colonic Pericrypt Sheath Cells: Characterisation of Cell Type With New Monoclonal Antibody.** *J Clin Pathol* 1987, **40**:593–600.

23. • Valentich JD, Saada JI, Powell DW: **Interleukin-1α (IL-1) Stimulates Prostaglandin H Synthase (PGHS) Gene Expression in a Human Colonic Myofibroblast-Like Cell Line [Abstract].** *Gastroenterology* 1994, **106**:A787.

Describes the initial characterization of 18Co cells, an established human colonic cell line that displays numerous phenotypic properties of subepithelial myofibroblasts including stellate morphology, expression of the smooth muscle isoform of α-actin and functional receptors for endothelin-1 and -3, ANP, and carbachol. This cell line will be an important tool for defining the cellular and molecular biology of intestinal juxtaparenchymal cells.

24. Valentich JD, Powell DW: **Interleukin-1α(IL-1) Treatment of a Myofibroblast-Like Cell Line (18Co) Enhances Sensitization of Juxtaposed T84 Cells to Secretagogues [Abstract].** *Gastroenterology* 1994, **106**:A278.

25. Komuro T, Hashimoto Y: **Three-Dimensional Structure of the Rat Intestinal Wall (Mucosa and Submucosa).** *Arch Histol Cytol* 1990, **53**:1–21.

26. Matthes H, Herbst H, Schuppan D, Stallmach A, Milani S, Stein H, Riecken E-O: **Cellular Localization of Procollagen Gene Transcripts in Inflammatory Bowel Diseases.** *Gastroenterology* 1992, **102**:431–442.

27. Beaulieu J-F, Jutras S, Durand J, Vachon PH, Perreault N: **Relationship Between Tenacin and α-Smooth Muscle Actin Expression in the Developing Human Small Intestinal Mucosa.** *Anat Embryol* 1993, **188**:149–158.

28. Choy M-Y, Richman PI, Horton MA, MacDonald TT: **Expression of the VLA Family of Integrins in Human Intestine.** *J Pathol* 1990, **160**:35–40.

29. Sappino A-P, Dietrich P-Y, Skalli O, Widgren S, Gabbiani G: **Colonic Pericryptal Fibroblasts: Differentiation Pattern in Embryogenesis and Phenotypic Modulation in Epithelial Proliferative Lesions.** *Virchows Arch A Pathol Anat Histopathol* 1989, **415**:551–557.

30. Furuya S, Naruse S, Nakayama T, Nokihara K: **^{125}I-Endothelin Binds to Fibroblasts Beneath the Epithelium of Rat Small Intestine.** *J Electron Microsc (Tokyo)* 1990, **39**:264–268.

31. Bianchi C, Thibault G, De Lean A, Genest J, Cantin M: **Atrial Natriuretic Factor Binding Sites in the Jejunum.** *Am J Physiol* 1989, **256**:G436–G441.

32. Inagaki H, Bishop AE, Escrig C, Wharton J, Allen-Mershi TG, Polak JM: **Localization of Endothelinlike Immunoreactivity and Endothelin Binding Sites in Human Colon.** *Gastroenterology* 1991, **101**:47–54.

33. Appleton I, Tomlinson A, Chander CL, Willoughby DA: **Effect of Endothelin-1 on Croton Oil-Induced Granulation Tissue in the Rat: A Pharmacologic and Immunohistochemical Study.** *Lab Invest* 1992, **67**:703–710.

34. Zhang JX, Pegoli W Jr., Clemens MG: **Endothelin-1 Induces Direct Constriction of Hepatic Sinusoids.** *Am J Physiol* 1994, **266**:G624–G632.

35. Simonson MS, Dunn MJ: **Endothelin-1 Stimulates Contraction of Rat Glomerular Mesangial Cells and Potentiates β-Adrenergic-Mediated Cyclic Adenosine Monophosphate Accumulation.** *J Clin Invest* 1990, **85**:790–797.

36. •• Furuya S, Furuya K: **Characteristics of Cultured Subepithelial Fibroblasts of Rat Duodenal Villi.** *Anat Embryol (Berl)* 1993, **187**:529–538.

This paper demonstrates cyclic AMP induction and endothelin reversal of stellate morphology in primary cultures of duodenal lamina propria fibroblasts. Other markers were not investigated to verify the assumed subepithelial origin of the cultured cells.

37. Goto M, Sasano M, Yamanaka H, Miyasaka N, Kamatani N, Inoue K, Nishioka K, Miyamoto T: **Spontaneous Production of an Interluekin 1-Like Factor by Cloned Rheumatoid Synovial Cells in Long-Term Culture.** *J Clin Invest* 1987, **80**:786–796.

38. • Smith TJ, Wang H-S, Hoog MG, Henrikson RC, Keese CR, Giaever I: **Prostaglandin E_2 Elicits a Morphological Change in Cultured Orbital Fibroblasts From Patients With Graves Ophthalmopathy.** *Proc Natl Acad Sci U S A* 1994, **91**:5094–5098.

This shows that orbital, but not dermal, fibroblasts assume a highly stellate shape when stimulated with prostaglandin E_2 or cyclic AMP. This morphologic response appears to be identical to that observed in intestinal subepithelial myofibroblasts and in synovial cells. Although its significance is unknown, stellate transformation may denote functional similarities between these cells, all of which are proposed to play a role in the immunophysiology of the tissues in which they are located.

39. •• Furuya K, Furuya S, Yamagishi S: **Intracellular Calcium Responses and Shape Conversions INduced by Endothelin in Cultured Subepithelial Fibroblasts of Rat Duodenal Villi.** *Pflugers Arch* 1994, **428**:97–104.

This reports that intestinal fibroblasts express receptors for endothelins, substance-P, angiotensin-II, bradykinin, and ATP coupled to the elevation of intracellular calcium. These data give functional significance to the autoradiographic localization of endothelin and ANP receptors on subepithelial myofibroblasts *in situ* and suggest that subepithelial myofibroblasts may be the direct targets of mediators that modulate intestinal ion transport.

40. Berschneider HM, Powell DW: **Fibroblasts Modulate Intestinal Secretory Responses to Inflammatory Mediators.** *J Clin Invest* 1992, **89**:484–489.

41. Thuneberg L: **Interstitial Cells of Cajal.** In *Handbook of Physiology, The Gastrointestinal System, Motility and Circulation, Section 6, Volume I, Part 1*. Edited by Wood JD. Baltimore: Waverly Press; 1989:349–386.

42. Daniel EE, Berezin I: **Interstitial Cells of Cajal: Are They Major Players in Control of Gastrointestinal Motility?** *J Gastrointest Mot* 1992, **4**:1–24.

43. Publicover NG, Horowitz NN, Sanders KM: **Calcium Oscillations in Freshly Dispersed and Cultured Interstitial Cells From Canine Colon.** *Am J Physiol* 1992, **262**:C589–C597.

44. Moore R, Carlson S, Madara JL: **Villus Contraction Aids Repair of Intestinal Epithelium After Injury.** *Am J Physiol Gastrointest Liver Physiol* 1989, **257**:G274–G283.

45. Womack WA, Kvietys PR, Granger DN: **Villous Motility.** In *Handbook of Physiology, The Gastrointestinal System, Motility and Circulation, Section 6, Volume I, Part 2*. Edited by Wood JD. Baltimore: Waverly Press; 1989:975–986.

46. Evans GS, Flint N, Potten CS: **Primary Cultures for Studies of Cell Regulation and Physiology in Intestinal Epithelium.** *Annu Rev Physiol* 1994, **56**:399–417.

47. Han VKM, D'Ercole AJ, Lund PK: **Cellular Localization of Somatomedin (Insulin-Like Growth Factor) Messenger RNA in the Human Fetus.** *Science (Washington DC)* 1987, **236**:193–197.

48. Zimmermann EM, Sartor RB, McCall RD, Pardo M, Bender D, Lund PK: **Insulinlike Growth Factor 1 and Interleukin 1β Messenger RNA in a Rat Model of Granulomatous Entercolitis and Hepatitis.** *Gastroenterology* 1993, **105**:399–409.

49. Zimmermann EM, McNaughton K, Sartor RB, Lund PK: **IGF-1 Is Overexpressed in Cells With Smooth Muscle Phenotype in Peptidoglycan-Polysaccharide Induced Chronic Enterocolitis in the Rat.** *Gastroenterology* 1993, **104**:A808.

50. Ryan J, Costigan DC: **Determination of the Histological Distribution of Insulin Like Growth Factor 1 Receptors in the Rat Gut.** *Gut* 1993, **34**:1693–1697.

51. Hwang WS, Kelly JK, Shaffer EA, Hershfield NB: **Collagenous Colitis: A Disease of Pericryptal Fibroblast Sheath?** *J Pathol* 1986, **149**:33–40.

52. Balazs M, Egerszegi P, Vadasz G, Kovacs A: **Collagenous Colitis: An Electron Microscopic Study Including Comparison With the Chronic Fibrotic Stage of Ulcerative Colitis.** *Histopathology* 1988, **13**:319–328.

53. • Holgate ST, Djukanovic R, Howarth PH, Montefort S, Roche W: **The T Cell and the Airway's Fibrotic Response in Asthma.** *Chest* 1993, **103**:125S–128S.

This summarizes studies from the authors' laboratory suggesting that subepithelial myofibroblasts in the distal airway are targets of proinflammatory cytokines and are responsible for mucosal fibrosis in asthma.

54. •• Pang G, Couch L, Batey R, Clancy R, Cripps A: **GM-CSF, IL-1α, IL-1β, IL-6, IL-8, IL-10, ICAM-1 and VCAM-1 Gene Expression and Cytokine Production in Human Duodenal Fibroblasts Stimulated With Lipopolysaccharide, IL-1α and TNFα.** *Clin Exp Immunol* 1994, 96:437–443.

Currently, this is the most comprehensive study of the cytokine repertoire of intestinal fibroblasts. Additional phenotypic characterization of the fibroblast cultures used in this study is required to associate cytokine production with specific lamina propria mesenchymal cell types.

55. • Ina K, Binion D, West GA, Fiocchi C: **Human Intestinal Fibroblasts Prevent Mucosal T-Cell Apoptosis [Abstract].** *Gastroenterology* 1994, **106**:A704.

A preliminary study suggesting that intestinal fibroblasts promote lymphocyte survival. If confirmed and extended, these data will have significant implications for the evolution of memory T cells in chronic inflammation.

56. Gerbes AL, Nathrath W, Cantin M, Denecke H: **Presence of Atrial Natriuretic Factor Prohormone in Enterochromaffin Cells of the Human Large Intestine.** *Gastroenterology* 1991, **101**:424–429.

57. Reddix RA, Cooke HJ: **Endothelin-1 Immunohistochemical Distribution and Receptors Mediating Secretion in Guinea Pig Distal Colon [Abstract].** *Gastroenterology* 1994, **106**:A1046.

58. Takahashi K, Jones PM, Kanse SM, Lam H-C, Spokes RA, Ghatei MA, Bloom SR: **Endothelin in the Gastrointestinal Tract: Presence of Endothelinlike Immunoreactivity, Endothelin-1 Messenger RNA, Endothelin Receptors, and Pharmacological Effect.** *Gastroenterology* 1990, 99:1660–1667.

59. Sessa WC, Kaw S, Hecker M, Vane JR: **The Biosynthesis of Endothelin-1 by Human Polymorphonuclear Leukocytes.** *Biochem Biophys Res Commun* 1991, **174**:613.

60. Ehrenreich H, Anderson RW, Fox CH, Rieckmann P, Hoffman GS, Travis WD, Coligan JE, Kehrl JH, Fauci AS: **Endothelins, Peptides With Potent Vasoactive Properties Are Produced by Human Macrophages.** *J Exp Med* 1990, **172**:1741–1748.

61. Yoshizumi M, Kurhara H, Morita T, Yamashita T, Oh-Hashi Y, Sugiyama T, Takaku F, Yanagisawa M, Masaki T, Yazaki Y: **Interleukin-1 Increases the Production of Endothelin-1 by Cultured Endothelial Cells.** *Biochem Biophys Res Commun* 1990, **166**:324–329.

62. Salh B, Zhou A, Freeman H, Kwan WC: **Characterization of Endothelin (ET) Release by Normal and Crohns' Disease (CD) Monocytes [Abstract].** *Gastroenterology* 1994, **106**:A765.

63. Murch SH, Braegger CP, Sessa WC, MacDonald TT: **High Endothelin-1 Immunoreactivity in Crohn's Disease and Ulcerative Colitis.** *Lancet* 1992, **339**:381–385.

64. Bedossa P, Poynard T, Bacci J, Naveau S, Lemaigre G, Chaput JC, Martin E: **Expression of Histocompatibility Antigens and Characterization of the Lymphocyte Infiltrate in Hyperplastic Polyps of the Large Bowel.** *Hum Pathol* 1990, **21**:319–324.

65. Selby WS, Poulter LW, Hobbs S, Jewell DP, Janossy G: **Heterogeneity of HLA-DR-Positive Histiocytes in Human Intestinal Lamina Propria: A Combined Histochemical and Immunohistochemical Analysis.** *J Clin Pathol* 1983, **36**:379–384.

66. Mayrhofer G, Pugh CW, Barclay AN: **The Distribution, Ontogeny and Origin in the Rat of Ia-Positive Cells With Dendritic Morphology and of Ia Antigen in Epithelia, With Special Reference to the Intestine.** *Eur J Immunol* 1983, **13**:112–122.

67. Matsumoto S, Setoyama H, Umesaki Y: **Differential Induction of Major Histocompatibility Complex Molecules on Mouse Intestine by Bacterial Colonization.** *Gastroenterology* 1992, **103**:1777–1782.

68. • Ina K, Klein JS, Strong SA, West GA, Fiocchi C: **Human Intestinal Fibroblasts Express Adhesion Molecules for and Modulate the Function of Mucosal T Cells [Abstract].** *Gastroenterology* 1994, **106**:A704.

A preliminary study showing that intestinal fibroblasts express adhesion molecules involved in inflammatory reactions and differentially modulate the proliferation of T cells derived from normal, Crohn's disease, and ulcerative colitis lamina propria.

69. Radeke HH, Emmendorffer A, Uciechowski P, Von Der Ohe J, Schwinzer B, Resch K: **Activation of Autoreactive T-Lymphocytes by Cultured Syngeneic Glomerular Mesangial Cells.** *Kidney Int* 1994, **45**:763–774.

70. Karlsson-Parra A, Dimeny E, Fellstrom B, Klareskog L: **HIV Receptors (CD4 Antigen) in Normal Human Glomerular Cells.** *N Engl J Med* 1989, **320**:741.

71. Derdak S, Dixon P, Watts H, Penney D, Phipps R: **CD4 Expression in Lung Fibroblasts.** *Lancet* 1991, **337**:374.

72. Palmer JM: **Immunomodulation of Electrical and Synaptic Behavior of Myenteric Neurons of Guinea Pig Small Intestine During Infection With *Trichinella spiralis*.** In *Effects of Immune Cells and Inflammation on Smooth Muscle and Enteric Nerves.* Edited by Snape WJ Jr, Collins SM. Boca Raton: CRC Press; 1991:181–195.

73. •• Torihashi S, Kobayashi S, Gerthoffer WT, Sanders KM: **Interstitial Cells in Deep Muscular Plexus of Canine Small Intestine May Be Specialized Smooth Muscle Cells.** *Am J Physiol* 1993, **265**:G638–G645.

This immunocytochemical study demonstrates that interstitial cells of Cajal contain smooth muscle actin as well as myosin thick filaments. The data suggest that interstitial cells of Cajal may share functional or lineage relationships with subepithelial myofibroblasts.

74. Shuttleworth CW, Xue C, Ward SM, De Vente J, Sanders KM: **Immunohistochemical Localization of 3', 5'-Cyclic Quanosine Monophosphate in the Canine Proximal Colon: Responses to Nitric Oxide and Electrical Stimulation of Enteric Inhibitory Neurons.** *Neuroscience* 1993, **56**:513–522.

John D. Valentich, PhD, and Don W. Powell, MD, Department of Internal Medicine, University of Texas Medical Branch, 301 University Boulevard, Galveston, TX 77555-0567, USA.

The authors welcome discussion of the issues raised in this publication via e-mail at valentich@beach.utmb.edu.

Defense factors in human milk

Agnes E. Wold, MD, PhD, and Lars Å. Hanson, MD, PhD

University of Göteborg, Göteborg, Sweden

The newborn infant is more susceptible to infections than older children or adults. This is because all three lines of defense against microbial invasion, *ie*, barrier functions, innate immunity, and specific immunity, are to a greater or lesser extent immature at birth. Nature's response to the immaturity of the infant's immune system is to provide ready-made defense factors from the mother. This is achieved first by the transplacental passage of IgG antibodies, and later via the breast milk. Breastfeeding has been shown to decrease morbidity in gastroenteritis, septicemia, otitis media, urinary tract infection, and necrotizing enterocolitis. Breast milk contains a wide variety of defense factors, *ie*, immunoglobulins, leukocytes, hormones, cytokines, and complex oligosaccharides in free form or bound to macromolecules. These factors are reviewed and their potential protective effects in the abovementioned clinical states are discussed.

Current Opinion in Gastroenterology 1994, **10:**652–658

The newborn infant is more susceptible to infections than older children or adults because all three lines of defense against microbial invasion (barrier functions, innate immunity, and specific immunity) are to a greater or lesser extent immature at birth. The *physical barriers* are more permeable than those of adults. Both the skin and mucosal membranes are thin, and they are not yet covered by a normal protective flora. The *innate immune system* is also not fully developed at birth. Complement components are often low in newborn infants, especially premature infants. Phagocyte levels in the blood are as high as in adults, but the total pool of granulocytes that can be mobilized on infection is small. The *specific immune system* is fairly well-developed at birth, with the exception of the antibody response of the IgG2 and IgG4 subclasses. However, although the newborn infant has the capacity to react with specific immunity to almost all antigens, a primary immune response has to take place for each new antigen that is encountered. This takes a longer time to develop, is lower in magnitude, and has a different isotype pattern than a secondary response. Consequently, the newborn infant is at risk of developing overwhelming infection before the specific immune response is fully activated.

Nature's response to the immaturity of the infant's immune system is to provide ready-made defense factors from the mother. This is achieved first by the transplacental passage of IgG antibodies, and later via the breast milk. The milk is probably designed to be sufficient as the sole food source until 6 to 8 months of age, when teeth have developed and the infant becomes interested in picking up pieces of food with the use of the pinch grip. Exclusive breastfeeding for this period of time is, however, rare in many cultures. In some developing countries, cultural traditions prescribe a number of additional feeds, often heavily contaminated, to the newborn infant [1•].

Because the immunoglobulins in human breast milk are not taken up into the blood, breastfeeding was not believed to contribute to defense against infection in infants. The reduced infection rate seen among breastfed infants in developing countries was ascribed solely to feeding of contaminated fluids to the non-breastfed babies. In 1979, however, a study performed in a rural community in the state of New York showed a striking increase of the relative risk of severe morbidity in bottlefed infants: 16 at 0 to 2 months of age, four at 0 to 4 months, and two at 0 to 12 months [2].

Today, breastfeeding has been proven to reduce the morbidity in diarrheal disease, sepsis, pneumonia, otitis media, urinary tract infection, and necrotizing enterocolitis (Table 1). As evident from Table 1, similar degrees of protection are achieved in developing and highly developed countries. The influence of breastfeeding on infant mortality has not been studied in the industrialized countries after World War II [3], but it is highly significant in less developed countries. Thus, in southern Brazil, the relative risk of dying during the 1st year of life because of diarrheal infection was 4.2 in infants receiving formula in addition to breast milk and 14.2 in infants receiving only bottle feed [4]. There is no *a priori* reason why a decreased mortality among breastfed babies could not occur also in developed countries, especially among high-risk infants where infection is a major cause of mortality.

Abbreviations

TGF—transforming growth factor; **TNF**—tumor necrosis factor.

 ISBN 1-85922-611-6 ISSN 0267–1379

Table 1. Diseases in which breastfeeding has been proven to exert protection

Disease and country	Risk ratio	Study
Gastroenteritis		
Developing countries	2–10	Reviewed in Jason *et al.* [67]
Industrialized countries	2–8	Reviewed in Kovar *et al.* [3]
Sepsis		
Pakistan	18	Ashraf *et al.* [59]
Sweden	ND	Winberg and Wessner [68]
Pneumonia (deaths)		
Brazil	4	Victora *et al.* [4]
Otitis media		
Finland	>3*	Saarinen [69]
United States	2	Duncan *et al.* [70]
Urinary tract infection		
Italy	3–5†	Piscane *et al.* [65]
Sweden	ND	Mårild *et al.* [66]
Necrotizing enterocolitis		
Great Britain	20‡	Lucas and Cole [71]

*Relative risk three times greater for falling ill before 1 year of age, comparing children breastfed 6 months or more versus bottlefed infants. Before 6 months of age 0% of the fully breastfed infants fell ill, versus 10% in the bottlefed group.
†Relative risk five times greater if considering feeding mode at referral, three times greater if considering ever breastfed versus never breastfed.
‡In infants born after at least 30 weeks' gestation.
ND—not determined.

The following review will outline some of the defense factors present in human breast milk, and discuss some potential mechanisms for their protective effects.

Immunoglobulins

Human breast milk contains enormous amounts of secretory IgA, 5 to 10 g/L in the early colostrum and 0.3 to 1 g/L in the mature milk. Thus, the fully breastfed baby is supplied with 0.5 to 1 g/d or 0.2 to 0.3 g/kg of secretory IgA. This is five times more IgA per body weight than an adult person synthesizes, and thus a much higher concentration is encountered on the mucosal surfaces of breastfed infants as compared with adults. The supplementation with IgA is probably most important in the premature infant who has received insufficient amounts of IgG via transplacental passage. IgM and IgG antibodies are found in much lower quantities, approximately 0.06 and 0.1 g/L in colostrum and 0.06 and 0.01 g/L in mature milk. Although insignificant compared with other species such as the pig and the rat, there is probably a low degree of absorption of milk immunoglobulin during the earliest days of life [5].

Secretory IgA is formed by the combination of dimeric IgA with secretory component exposed on the basolateral aspect of the mammary gland epithelial cells [6]. The whole complex is internalized, and released to the milk as secretory IgA. The secretory component–mediated transport system exceeds that of the IgA production, especially during the first period of lactation. The milk therefore contains free secretory component, in addition to secretory IgA.

The antibodies in human milk are directed against a wide variety of bacterial and viral antigens, and also against food proteins in the mother's diet. These antibodies are produced by plasma cells in the mammary gland, most of which derive from the Peyer's patches of the small intestine. Antigen is sampled from the intestinal lumen by specialized cells called M cells and presented to B and T cells in the patches. Those B and T cells that have specificity for the antigen in question proliferate, mature, and leave the patches for other mucosal sites, including the lactating mammary gland [6]. It seems as if not only blasts homing to mucosal surfaces are attracted by the mammary gland during lactation, but also blasts participating in systemic immune responses [7]. Therefore, the milk will contain a very broad range of antibodies, reflecting ongoing mucosal as well as systemic responses. There is evidence from cell transfer studies in rats that not only IgA- but also IgG- and IgM-producing blasts home to the mammary gland [8]. Thus, the IgG antibodies in milk are probably also locally produced in the mammary gland, which explains the difference in IgG subclass distribution between milk and serum. The IgG2 and IgG4 subclasses, which are characteristically present during mucosal immune responses, are selectively enriched in the milk compared with serum [9].

In addition to classic antibody activity, milk immunoglobulins may interact with microorganisms by other mechanisms. The N-linked oligosaccharide chains of secretory IgA function as receptors for type 1–fimbriated *E. coli*, thereby reducing their attachment to colonic epithelial cells [10]. The two subclasses of IgA found in humans, IgA1 and IgA2, occur in approximately equal proportions in breast milk. IgA1 possesses O-linked oligosaccharide chains, in addition to the N-linked chains found in all immunoglobulin classes. *Pseudomonas aeruginosa* and bacteria making up dental plaques are examples of bacteria that recognize the O-linked oligosaccharides of the structure Galβ1-3GalNAc, found in IgA1 [11]. The N-linked chains also differ slightly between the subclasses, with more completely glycosylated chains on IgA1 [12]. The oligosaccharide chains of secretory component are extremely complex [13] and inhibit the adherence of *Helicobacter pylori* to gastric epithelium [14].

Not only antibodies are transferred to the infant via the breast milk, but also antigens from the mother's diet [15]. Antigens and antibodies delivered via the milk have been shown in various experimental animal models to either prime the offspring or render it tolerant [15], but the significance in humans is unknown.

Cells

Colostrum contains approximately 5 $\times 10^6$ leukocytes/mL, which decreases to 10^5/mL in mature milk. With the increase in milk volume, the infant is supplied by an almost constant amount of cells throughout the lactation period. The dominant cell types are polymorphonuclear neutrophils and macrophages, which together make up 90% of the milk cells. Lymphocytes account for the remaining 10%, of which T cells ac-

higher counts of staphylococci (*Staphylococcus aureus* and *Staphylococcus epidermidis*) in breastfed infants [49–51], and the 100-fold higher counts of enterococci in bottlefed infants [49,51,52]. Higher counts of *E. coli* in bottlefed compared with breastfed babies are found in some studies [53], but not in others [54]. In general, these differences are less than one log in magnitude, and *E. coli* is a major colonizer during the first period of life in both groups (Table 2). Breastfed infants, however, carry a less variable *E. coli* flora than the bottlefed ones, with fewer serotypes being represented in a fecal sample [55]. Breastfeeding also reduces the colonization with other members of the *Enterobacteriaceae* family than *E. coli, eg, Klebsiella* and *Enterobacter* [56,57]. Because *Klebsiella* is the dominant cause of gram-negative septicemia in community-acquired as well as hospital-acquired sepsis in Pakistan [58], the reduced frequency of sepsis recorded in this country among breastfed infants [59] could, in part, be mediated by this effect.

Some studies have found higher frequencies of colonization with bifidobacteriae in breastfed than bottlefed infants, but when bottlefed infants are colonized with bifidobacteria, they have the same counts as breastfed ones [52]. However, with marginally higher counts of bifidobacteria and marginally lower counts of other species, a higher percentage of the breastfed infants may have bifidobacteria as their "dominant species" [63]. It is a common misunderstanding that high counts of bifidobacteria would result in low counts of *E. coli*, but no such association exists [52,54]. In some recent studies performed in Western countries, a very low degree of colonization with bifidobacteria was found [49,50]. This may relate to excessive hygienic measures during delivery in Western countries, which prevent transfer of anaerobic microflora from mother to infant. In fact, only a minority of infants born in Western hospitals acquire their *E. coli* from the mother [61].

It should be noted that although small differences are seen between breastfed and bottlefed infants with regard to groups of bacteria that colonize their intestine, the outcome of the colonization may differ profoundly. For example, fully breastfed infants may be colonized with several diarrheal pathogens and still remain healthy [62]. This may depend on the different agents in breast milk that protect against intestinal secretion and inflammation.

Effect on receptor expression

The effect of supplying receptor analogues for adhering bacteria, sometimes in very large amounts, on the microbial flora is not self-evident. It could reduce the advantage of bacterial adherence. Alternatively, however, the binding to soluble receptors could be beneficial for bacteria by some unknown mechanism. In fact, we have found up-regulation of type 1–fimbriation in *E. coli* colonizing breastfed compared with bottlefed infants [63]. In contrast, there was a lower incidence of *E. coli* displaying mannose-resistant hemagglutination and adherence to intestinal epithelial cells among the breastfed infants (Slaviková *et al.*, Unpublished data). Similarly, a lower frequency of colonization with *E. coli* strains expressing a mannose-resistant hemagglutination of human and bovine erythrocytes [64] and P-fimbriated is seen in breastfed infants [56]. A reduction of P-fimbriated clones of *E. coli* in the intestinal flora may be responsible for the protection of breastfeeding against urinary tract infection. This interpretation is favored by the fact that the protection by breastfeeding lasted for a period of time after termination of breastfeeding [65,66].

Table 3. Mechanisms and factors believed to be responsible for the protective effect of breastfeeding in different clinical entities

Clinical entity	Mechanism	Factor responsible
Gastroenteritis	Toxin neutralization	Antibodies, oligosaccharides
	Antiadherence	Oligosaccharides
	Antisecretion	Antisecretory factor
Sepsis	Modulation of intestinal microflora	?
	Antiadherence	Oligosaccharides
	Anti-inflammation	?
Necrotizing enterocolitis	Modulation of intestinal microflora	?
	Antiadherence	Oligosaccharides
	Anti-inflammation	?
Urinary tract infection	Modulation of intestinal microflora	?
Otitis media	Antiadherence	Oligosaccharides

Conclusions

Breastfeeding has a well-documented protective effect against a number of diseases in the infant. Some tentative mechanisms for the protection are summarized in Table 3. Thus, mechanisms that may be involved in the protection against diarrhea include antitoxin antibodies, oligosaccharide structures that prevent adherence by toxins or whole microorganisms, or antisecretory factors or other hormones. Future research will delineate which role is played by which components in milk for the protection afforded by breastfeeding.

References and recommended reading

Papers of particular interest, published within the annual period of review, have been highlighted as:

- • Of special interest
- •• Of outstanding interest

1. • Ashraf RN, Jalil F, Khan SR, Zaman S, Karlberg J, Lindblad BS, Hanson LÅ: **Early Child Health in Lahore, Pakistan: V. Feeding Patterns.** *Acta Paediatr Suppl* 1993, **390**:47–61.

Feeding practices of children from four different socioeconomic groups in Pakistan were studied during the 1st year of life. The results showed that although breastfeeding is highly prevalent, exclusive breastfeeding is very rare in this culture. Moreover, before breastfeeding is initiated, most children receive other feeds, often contaminated.

2. Cunningham AS: **Morbidity in Breast-Fed and Artificially Fed Infants. II.** *J Pediatr* 1979, **95**:685–689.

3. Kovar MG, Sedula MK, Marks JS, Frase DW: **Review of the Epidemiologic Evidence for and Association Between Infant Feeding and Infant Health.** *Pediatrics* 1984, 74:615–638.

4. Victora CG, Smith PG, Vaughan JP, Nobre LC, Lombardi C, Teixeira AMB, Fuchs SMC, Moreira LB, Gigante LP, Barros FC: **Evidence for Protection by Breast-Feeding Against Infant Deaths From Infectious Diseases in Brazil.** *Lancet* 1987, ii:319–321.

5. Ogra SS, Weintraub D, Ogra PL: **Immunologic Aspects of Human Colostrum and Milk. III. Fate and Absorption of Cellular and Soluble Components in the Gastrointestinal Tract of the Newborn.** *J Immunol* 1977, **119**:245–248.

6. Hanson LÅ, Brandtzaeg P: **The Mucosal Defense System.** In *Immunological Disorders in Infants and Children,* 3rd edn. Edited by Stiehm ER, Philadelphia: Saunders; 1989:116–155.

7. Parmely MJ, Manning LS: **Cellular Determinants of Mammary Cell-Mediated Immunity in the Rat: Kinetics of Lymphocyte Subset Accumulation in the Rat Mammary Gland During Pregnancy and Lactation.** *Ann N Y Acad Sci* 1983, **409**:517–533.

8. Dahlgren UI, Wold AE, Hanson LÅ, Midtvedt T: **The Secretory Antibody Response in Milk and Bile Against Fimbriae and LPS in Rats Monocolonized or Immunized in the Peyer's Patches With *Escherichia coli*.** *Immunology* 1990, **71**:295–330.

9. Kim K, Keller MA, Heiner DC: **Immunoglobulin Subclasses in Human Colostrum, Milk and Saliva.** *Acta Paediatr* 1992, **81**:113–118.

10. Wold AE, Mestecky J, Tomana M, Kobata A, Ohbayashi H, Endo T, Svanborg Edén C: **Secretory Immunoglobulin A Carries Oligosaccharide Receptors for *Escherichia coli* Type 1 Fimbrial Lectin.** *Infect Immun* 1990, **58**:3073–3077.

11. Borén T, Landys D, Strömberg N: **Secretory Immunoglobulin A Heavy Chains Present Galβ/GalNAcβ-Saccharide Receptors for *Actinomyces naeslundi*.** 1994, in press.

12. Wold AE, Motas C, Svanborg C, Mestecky J: **Lectin Receptors on IgA Isotypes.** *Scand J Immunol* 1994, **39**:195–201.

13. Mizoguchi A, Mizouchi T, Kobata A: **Structure of the Carbohydrate Moieties of Secretory Component Purified From Human Milk.** *J Biol Chem* 1982, **257**:9612–9621.

14. Borén T, Falk P, Roth KA, Larsson G, Normark S: **Attachment of *Helicobacter pylori* to Gastric Epithelium Mediated by Blood Group Antigens.** *Science* 1994, **262**:1892–1895.

15. Hanson LÅ, Telemo E, Wiedermann U, Dahlman A, Saalman R, Ahlstedt S, Friman V, Holmgren J, Czerkinsky C, Dahlgren U: **Sensitization and Development of Tolerance Via the Gut.** *Pediatr Allergy Immunol* 1993, 4:16–20.

16. Jain N, Mathur NB, Sharma VK, Dwarkadas AM: **Cellular Composition Including Lymphocyte Subsets in Preterm and Full Term Human Colostrum and Milk.** *Acta Paediatr Scand* 1991, **80**:395–399.

17. Wirt DP, Adkins LT, Palkowetz KH, Schmalstiegh FC, Goldman AS: **Activated and Memory T Lymphocytes in Human Milk.** *Cytometry* 1992, **13**:282–290.

18. Gibson CE, Eglinton BA, Penttila IA, Cummins AG: **Phenotype and Activation of Milk-Derived and Peripheral Blood Lymphocytes From Normal and Coeliac Subjects.** *Immunol Cell Biol* 1991, 69:387–393.

19. Bertotto A, Gerli R, Castellucci G, Crupi S, Scalise F, Spinozzi F, Fabietti G, Forenza N, Vaccaro R: **Mycobacteria-Reactive Gamma/Delta T Cells Are Present in Human Colostrum From Tuberculin-Positive, But Not From Tuberculin-Negative Nursing Mothers.** *Am J Reprod Immunol* 1993, **29**:131–134.

20. Skansen-Saphir U, Lindfors A, Andersson U: **Cytokine Production in**
• **Mononuclear Cells of Human Milk Studied at the Single-Cell Level.** *Pediatr Res* 1993, **34**:213–216.

This paper provides methodologically elegant demonstration of cytokine production by milk macrophages. Spontaneous cytokine production was occasionally seen, most frequently observed for interleukin-8, but also sometimes for interleukin-1, TNF-α, and interleukin-6. Stimulation of milk mononuclear cells with lipopolysaccharide-induced an extensive production of interleukin-1α, interleukin-1β, interleukin-1 receptor antagonist, interleukin-6, interleukin-8, and TNF-α, and less often interleukin-10 and granulocyte-macrophage colony-stimulating factor. The lymphocytes did not spontaneously produce cytokines, but could be induced to synthesize interleukin-2, interleukin-3, interleukin-4, interleukin-10, interferon-γ, and TNF-α.

21. Keeney SE, Schmalstieg FC, Palkowetz KH, Rudloff HE, Le BM, Goldman AS: **Activated Neutrophils and Neutrophil Activators in Human Milk: Increased Expression of CD11b and Decreased Expression of L-Selectin.** *J Leukoc Biol* 1993, **54**:97–104.

22. Lucas A, Mitchell MD: **Prostaglandins in Human Milk.** *Arch Dis Child* 1980, **55**:950–952.

23. Shimizu T, Niklasson A, Strandvik B: **Leukotriene B4 and C4 Generation by Human Colostral Macrophages In Vitro.** *Biol Neonate* 1993, **63**:65–69.

24. Robinson G, Volovitz B, Passwell JH: **Identification of a Secretory IgA Receptor on Breast-Milk Macrophages: Evidence for Specific Activation Via These Receptors.** *Pediatr Res* 1991, **29**:429–434.

25. Clemente J, Leyva-Cobián F, Hernández M, García-Alonso A: **Intracellular Immunoglobulins in Human Milk Macrophages: Ultrastructural Localization and Factors Affecting the Kinetics of Immunoglobulin Release.** *Int Arch Allergy Immunol* 1986, **80**:291–299.

26. Jain L, Vidyasagar D, Xantou M, Ghai V, Shimada S, Blend M: **In Vivo Distribution of Human Milk Leukocytes After Ingestion by Newborn Baboons.** *Arch Dis Child* 1989, 64:930–933.

27. Schlesinger JJ, Covelli HD: **Evidence for Transmission of Lymphocyte Response to Tuberculin by Breast-Feeding.** *Lancet* 1977, 2:529–532.

28. Deroche A, Nepomnaschy I, Torello S, Goldman A, Piazzon I: **Regulation of Parental Alloreactivity by Reciprocal F1 Hybrids. The Role of Lactation.** *J Reprod Immunol* 1993, **23**:235–245.

29. Campbell Jr DA, Lorber MI, Sweeton JC, Turcotte JG, Niederhuber JE, Beer AE: **Breast Feeding and Maternal-Donor Renal Allografts.** *Transplantation* 1984, **37**:340–344.

47. Buescher ES, McIlheran SM, Frenck RW: **Further Characterization of Human Colostral Antioxidants.** *Pediatr Res* 1989, **25**:266–270.

30. Söder O: **Isolation of Interleukin-1 From Human Milk.** *Int Arch Allergy Immunol* 1987, **83**:19–23.

31. Rudloff HE, Schmalstieg FC, Mushtaha AA, Palkowetz KH, Liu SK, Goldman AS: **Tumor Necrosis Factor-Alpha in Human Milk.** *Pediatr Res* 1992, **31**:29–33.

32. Bocci V, Von Bremen K, Corradeschi F, Franchi F, Luzzi E, Paulesu L: **Presence of Interferon-Gamma and Interleukin-6 in Colostrum of Normal Women.** *Lymphokine Cytokine Res* 1993, **12**:21–24.

33. Saito S, Yoshida M, Ichijo M, Ishizaka S, Tsujii T: **Transforming Growth Factor-Beta (TGF-β) in Human Milk.** *Clin Exp Immunol* 1993, 94:220–224.

34. Ramsay AJ, Husband AJ, Ramshaw IA, Bao S, Matthaei KI, Koehler G, Kopf M: **The Role of Interleukin-6 in Mucosal IgA Antibody Responses In Vivo.** *Science* 1994, **264**:561–563.

35. Kunz C, Rudloff S: **Biological Functions of Oligosaccharides in Human**
•• **Milk.** *Acta Paediatr* 1993, **82**:902–912.

A characterization is given of the free complex oligosaccharides that are found in large quantities (4 to 6 g/L) in human milk, but are virtually lacking in cow's milk–based formula. The possible biologic effects of these oligosaccharides are discussed.

36. Holmgren J, Svennerholm AM, Lindblad M: **Receptor-like Glycocompounds in Human Milk That Inhibit Classical and El Tor Vibrio Cholerae Cell Adherence (Hemagglutination).** *Infect Immun* 1983, 39:147–154.

37. Andersson B, Porras O, Hanson LÅ, Lagergård T, Svanborg Edén C: **Inhibition of Attachment of *Streptococcus pneumoniae* and *Haemophilus influenzae* by Human Milk and Receptor Oligosaccharides.** *J Infect Dis* 1986, **153**:232–237.

38. Schroten H, Plogmann R, Hanish FG, Hacker J, Nobis-Bosch R, Wahn V: **Inhibition of Adhesion of S-Fimbriated *E. coli* to Buccal Epithelial Cells by Human Skim Milk Is Predominantly Mediated by Mucins and Depends on the Period of Lactation.** *Acta Paediatr* 1993, **82**:6–11.

39. Koldovsky O, Thornburg W: **Hormones in Milk.** *J Pediatr Gastroenterol Nutr* 1987, 6:172–176.

40. Uany R, Stringel G, Thomas R, Quan R: **Effect of Dietary Nucleotides on Growth and Maturation of the Developing Gut in the Rat.** *J Pediatr Gastroenterol* 1990, **10**:597–603.

41. Carver JD, Pimentel B, Cox WI, Barness LA: **Dietary Nucleotide Effects Upon Immune Function in Infants.** *Pediatrics* 1991, **88**:359–363.

42. Lönnroth I, Lange S, Skadhauge E: **The Antisecretory Factors: Inducible Proteins Which Modulate Secretion in the Small Intestine.** *Comput Biochem Physiol* 1988, **90A**:611–617.

43. Lönnroth I, Martinsson K, Lange S: **Evidence of Protection Against Diar-**
• **rhoea in Suckling Piglets by a Hormone-Like Protein in the Sow's Milk.** *J Vet Med Sci* 1988, **35**:628–635.

An interesting new principle for protection against diarrhea is suggested: the presence of a hormone-like activity in milk that will block secretion in the offspring via an action directly on intestinal secretion.

44. Brock JH, Pickering MG, McDowell MC, Deacon AG: **Role of Antibody and Enterorbactin in Controlling the Growth of *Escherichia coli* in Human Milk and Acquisition of Lactoferrin and Transferrin-Bound Iron by *Escherichia coli*.** *Infect Immun* 1983, 40:453–459.

45. Blau H, Passwell JH, Levanon M, Davidson J, Kohen F, Ramot B: **Studies on Human Milk Macrophages: Effect of Activation on Phagocyto-**

sis and Secretion of Prostaglandin E_2 and Lysozyme. *Pediatr Res* 1983, 17:241–245.

46. Murphey DK, Buescher ES: **Human Colostrum Has Anti-Inflammatory Activity in a Rat Subcutaneous Air Pouch Model of Inflammation.** *Pediatr Res* 1993, 34:208–212.

48. Bjorge L, Skeie Jensen T, Vedeler CA, Ulvestad E, Kristofferson EK, Matre R: **Soluble CD59 in Pregnancy and Infancy.** *Immunol Lett* 1993, 36:233–234.

49. Simhon A, Douglas JR, Drasar BS, Soothill JF: **Effect of Feeding on Infants' Faecal Flora.** *Arch Dis Child* 1982, **57**:54–58.

50. Lundequist B, Nord CE, Winberg J: **The Composition of the Faecal Microflora in Breastfed and Bottle Fed Infants From Birth to Eight Weeks.** *Acta Paediatr Scand* 1985, 74:45–51.

51. Balmer SE, Wharton BA: **Diet and Faecal Flora in the Newborn: Breast Milk and Infant Formula.** *Arch Dis Child* 1989, 64:1672–1677.

52. Stark PL, Lee A: **The Microbial Ecology of the Large Bowel of Breast-Fed and Formula-Fed Infants During the First Year of Life.** *J Med Microbiol* 1982, **15**:189–203.

53. Balmer SE, Hanvey LS, Wharton BA: **Diet and Faecal Flora in the Newborn: Nucleotides.** *Arch Dis Child* 1992, 70:F137–F140.

54. Hewitt JH, Rigby J: **Effect of Various Milk Feeds on Numbers of *Escherichia coli* and *Bifidobacterium* in the Stools of New-Born Infants.** *J Hyg Camb* 1976, 77:129–139.

55. Ørskov F, Biering Sørensen K: ***Escherichia coli* Serogroups in Breast-fed and Bottle-Fed Infants.** *Acta Path Microbiol Scand Sect B* 1975, **83**:25–30.

56. Tullus K: **Fecal Colonization With P-Fimbriated *E. coli* Between 0 and 18 Months of Age.** *Epidemiol Infect* 1988, **100**:185–191.

57. Adlerberth I, Carlsson B, de Man P, Jalil F, Khan SR, Larsson P, Mellander L, Svanborg C, Wold AE, Hanson LÅ: **Intestinal Colonization With *Enterobacteriaceae* in Pakistani and Swedish Hospital-Delivered Infants.** *Acta Paediatr Scand* 1991, 80:602–610.

58. Bhutta ZA, Naqvi SH, Muzaffar T, Farooqui BJ: **Neonatal Sepsis in Pakistan.** *Acta Pediatr Scand* 1991, **80**:596–601.

59. Ashraf RN, Jalil F, Zaman S, Karlberg J, Khan SR, Lindblad BS, Hanson LÅ: **Breast Feeding and Protection Against Neonatal Sepsis in a High Risk Population.** *Arch Dis Child* 1991, 66:488–490.

60. Roberts AK, Chierici R, Sawatzki G, Hill MJ, Volpato S, Vigi V: **Supplementation of an Adapted Formula With Bovine Lactoferrin: 1. Effect on the Infant Faecal Flora.** *Acta Paediatr* 1992, **81**:119–124.

61. Gothefors L, Carlsson B, Ahlstedt S, Hanson LÅ, Winberg J: **Influence of Maternal Gut Flora and Colostral and Cord Serum Antibodies on Presence of *Escherichia coli* in Faeces of the Newborn Infant.** *Acta Paediatr Scand* 1976, 65:225–232.

62. Mata LJ, Urrutia JJ: **Intestinal Colonization of Breast-Fed Children in a Rural Area of Low Socioeconomic Level.** *Ann N Y Acad Sci* 1971, 176:93.

63. Lodinová-Zádníková R, Slavíková M, Tlaskalová-Hogenová H, Adlerberth I, Hanson LÅ, Wold A, Carlsson B, Svanborg C, Mellander L: **The Antibody Response in Breast-Fed and Non-Breast-Fed Infants After Artificial Colonization of the Intestine with *Escherichia coli* 083.** *Pediatr Res* 1991, **29**:396–399.

64. Giugliano LG, Meyer CJ, Arantes LC, Ribeiro ST, Giugliano R: **Mannose-Resistant Hemagglutination (MRHA) and Haemolysin Production of Strains of *Escherichia coli* Isolated From Children With Diarrheoa: Effect of Breastfeeding.** *J Trop Pediatr* 1993, 39:183–187.

65. Piscane A, Graziano L, Mazzarella G, Scarpellino B, Zona G: **Breast-Feeding and Urinary Tract Infection.** *J Pediatr* 1992, 120:87–89.

66. Mårild S, Jodal U, Hanson LÅ: **Breast-Feeding and Urinary-Tract Infection.** *Lancet* 1990, 336:942.

67. Jason JM, Nieburg P, Marks JS: **Mortality and Infectious Disease Associated With Infant-Feeding Practices in Developing Countries.** *Pediatrics* 1984, 74:702–727.

68. Winberg J, Wessner G: **Does Breast Milk Protect Against Septicemia in the Newborn?** *Lancet* 1971, i:1091–1094.

69. Saarinen UM: **Prolonged Breast Feeding as Prophylaxis for Recurrent Otitis Media.** *Acta Paediatr Scand* 1982, **71**:567–571.

70. Duncan B, Ey J, Holberg CJ, Wright AL, Martinez FD, Taussig LM: **Exclusive Breast-Feeding for at Least 4 Months Protects Against Otitis Media.** *Pediatrics* 1993, **91**:867–872.

71. Lucas A, Cole TJ: **Breast Milk and Neonatal Necrotising Enterocolitis.** *Lancet* 1990, 336:1519–1523.

Agnes E. Wold, MD, and Lars Å. Hanson, MD, Department of Clinical Immunology, Guldhedsgatan 10, S-413 46 Göteborg, Sweden.

Bacteria and gut immunity

Shobha Char, PhD, and Michael J.G. Farthing, MD, FRCP

The Medical College of St. Bartholomew's Hospital, London, UK

The interaction between the intestinal microflora and the host mucosal immune system is complex. Intestinal bacteria are considered vital for the maturation and maintenance of intestinal immunity in healthy individuals but may have harmful effects when the flora is modified by drugs such as the proton pump inhibitors, which suppress gastric acid. Research continues to support the concept that a healthy flora can be maintained by certain bacterial species such as *Lactobacillus,* although their therapeutic role in disease states has not yet been established. Translocation of bacteria across the gut wall occurs in certain disease states in which epithelial integrity is disrupted, particularly during intravenous nutrition and small bowel transplantation. Impairment of mucosal immunity has recently been documented in HIV infection and AIDS, including a deficit in antigen presentation. Modulation of gut immune responses is the cornerstone of vaccine development for intestinal infections. New antigen delivery systems are being developed that may assist in promoting protective immune responses rather than the development of oral tolerance.

Current Opinion in Gastroenterology 1994, **10**:659–663

Intestinal microflora

The human gastrointestinal tract contains 10^{14} bacterial cells (an equivalent of 1 kg). There is a marked variation in the number and pattern of bacterial flora at different levels of the tract. The number of ingested bacteria is reduced dramatically by gastric acid. A low concentration of organisms is maintained in the small bowel by intestinal motility that ensures that nonadherent organisms are constantly cleared from the small intestine. Despite this clearing, the concentration of bacteria increases from the jejunum through the ileum, with a marked increase in the colon. The bacterial content of duodenal fluid following acid inhibition by the proton pump inhibitor omeprazole was examined in a controlled prospective study [1•]. Duodenal bacterial overgrowth of both oral- and fecal-type bacteria occurred frequently in ambulatory patients treated with omeprazole. Further studies are needed to determine the clinical significance during long-term treatment with omeprazole. Shindo *et al.* [2•] found evidence of overgrowth of bacteria capable of deconjugating bile salts in the jejunum of seven of 27 patients with liver cirrhosis who had a positive bile acid breath test. Bacterial overgrowth in these patients was attributed to the shift to alkaline pH in the gastric juice.

The dominant populations of bacteria in the intestine are members of the genera *Bacteroides, Eubacterium, Bifidobacterium, Clostridium, Lactobacillus,* and *Fusobacterium. Escherichia coli* and aerotolerant streptococci constitute the accompanying flora. Various microorganisms are eliminated from the intestine by a "barrier effect" exerted by the normal microflora. The normal microflora thus supports the immune system by providing colonization resistance against pathogenic exogenous microorganisms. *Lactobacillus* sp has been shown to inhibit the growth of potentially pathogenic organisms such as *Staphylococcus, Pseudomonas, Salmonella,* and *Helicobacter pylori in vitro.* It has been suggested that *Lactobacillus* might contribute to the maintenance of colonization resistance through the production of lactic and acetic acids, hydrogen peroxide, and antimicrobial substances. It is thus considered important to maintain the levels of *Lactobacillus* in the intestinal flora because several other studies also indicate a protective effect against potential pathogens [3••].

Bacterial translocation

In normal situations, the only bacteria that readily translocate from the intestinal lumen to mesenteric lymph nodes (MLNs) and other viscera are facultative intracellular pathogens such as *Salmonella* spp and *Listeria* spp. It is well known that this tendency is increased in patients with impaired T-cell function, such

Abbreviations

GVHD—graft-versus-host disease; **MLN**—mesenteric lymph node; **TNF**—tumor necrosis factor.

 ISBN 1-85922-611-6 ISSN 0267–1379

as those with AIDS or lymphomas, or organ transplant recipients. Lim *et al.* [4•] studied the effect of HIV infection on intestinal lamina propria macrophage subsets in 41 patients at various stages of HIV infection. The results show that there was no difference in overall density of macrophages, but there was a significant decrease in dendritic cells in all clinical stages of HIV. Thus, the antigen-presenting arm of mucosal immune defenses may be seriously compromised in HIV infection, and this loss represents a further insult to mucosal immunity already impaired as a result of loss of $CD4^+$ T lymphocytes. These factors may contribute to the development of opportunistic infection in the gut.

In the context of mechanisms involved in immune response, bacterial translocation through specialized absorptive cells, called M cells, appears to be a part of the antigen-sampling process resulting in the development of gut-associated lymphoid tissue [5]. The term *bacterial translocation* has been used to describe the passage of bacteria from the gut lumen through the mucosa to the MLNs and other organs. The main factors promoting bacterial translocation include virulence and pathogenicity of the bacterial strain, increased numbers of the bacterial strain in the gut because of disturbances in the indigenous intestinal microflora, permeability of the intestinal mucosa, and a lowered immune status of the host.

Translocation has not been shown directly in healthy individuals. However, translocation enables contact of bacteria or bacterial fragments with the immune system and consequently leads to the production of systemic antibacterial antibodies. Indeed such antibodies have been detected in healthy individuals directed against their own anaerobic fecal bacteria [6] and a facultatively anaerobic *E. coli* strain that colonized the gastrointestinal tract after oral ingestion [7]. Apperloo-Renkema *et al.* [8••] demonstrate a decrease in the colonization resistance of intestinal microflora in patients with the autoimmune disease systemic lupus erythematosus. A lower colonization resistance theoretically increases the risk of translocation of more bacterial species, which may trigger the polyclonal and antigen-specific B-cell activation that leads to the production of multiple autoantibodies in systemic lupus erythematosus.

Bacterial translocation has been identified as a possible mechanism for the development of sepsis in various experimental conditions and in surgery, obstructive jaundice, acute pancreatitis, and burn patients. Runkel *et al.* [9•] examined the hypothesis that prolonged intestinal transit time may disrupt the luminal microflora of the gut and thereby promote bacterial translocation in an animal model. Following administration of morphine, which is known to inhibit bowel transit, samples were obtained from the MLNs, blood, spleen, liver, duodenum, jejunum, ileum, and cecum for standard bacteriology. The bacterial counts increased significantly in each intestinal segment following morphine treatment. Bacteria translocated to the MLNs in five, and to distant sites in four of eight morphine-tested animals. The authors concluded that the morphine-induced prolongation in bowel transit promotes bacterial translocation secondary to an overgrowth of enteric bacteria in the intestinal lumen. Thus, bacterial overpopulation of the bowel is an important promoter of translocation. Further studies are needed to determine whether therapeutic stimulation of motility might be a possible means of managing sepsis and whether the use of drugs that slow bowel motility are clinically important in the pathogenesis of sepsis. Price *et al.* [10••] assessed the effects of rejection, graft-versus-host disease (GVHD) and immunosuppression after heterotopic small bowel transplantation in rats. Isografts, allografts with and without immunosuppression, and the semiallogenic parent to the F1 hybrid GVHD model were studied. Intestinal microflora in graft and host loops and bacterial translocation to host organs and the graft MLNs were determined. Bacterial translocation was not detected in isografted animals, but was observed in all other animal groups. These data show that bacterial translocation from the intestine occurs in the presence of acute rejection and GVHD and that immunosuppression to prevent rejection does not prevent translocation.

Bacterial lipopolysaccharide has been speculated to facilitate bacterial translocation by a mechanism involving physical disruption of the gut mucosal barrier. Wells *et al.* [11••] used polarized, cultured intestinal epithelial cells (Caco2 cells) to study the effect of lipopolysaccharide on enterocyte structure, viability, and susceptibility to bacterial invasion and found no discernible effect. Thus, lipopolysaccharide-induced bacterial translocation might not involve loss of epithelial viability or facilitated entry of bacteria into intestinal epithelial cells.

Nord [12] has reviewed the ecologic effects of penicillins, cephalosporins, macrolides, tetracyclines, nitroimidazoles, and quinolines on the human intestinal microflora. The disturbances in normal intestinal microflora can cause bacterial overgrowth and emergence of resistant microorganisms, which may lead to serious infections and also encourage transfer of resistance factors among bacteria.

Intestinal immune system

The intestine is the largest immune organ in the body. It has been estimated that gut-associated lymphoid tissue contains 40% of the immune effector cells in the body, possibly representing up to 25% of the intestinal mucosal mass. Intestinal immune cells are found in one of three compartments: as aggregates in follicles and Peyer's patches, distributed within the mucosa as diffuse elements of the lymphoid network, and in the epithelium [13]. Various interleukins and other cytokines that contribute to interactions among cellular components of the immune system are produced by cells within the lamina propria. Conversely, cellular constituents of the lamina propria mucosae have been found to respond to various cytokines. Pang *et al.*

[14•] reported the presence of interleukin-2–activated large granular lymphocytes in the lamina propria of human duodenal mucosa that secrete an array of cytokines and may thus regulate cells of myeloid and monocytic lineages. The intestinal epithelium is where the host encounters a myriad of different environmental antigens and pathogens. A number of recent reports demonstrate that intestinal epithelial cells are a potentially important source of a number of cytokines that may modulate the immune response at the intestinal mucosa. Intestinal epithelial cell populations have been found to express or respond to interleukin-1, interleukin-2 [15•], interleukin-6 [16•], tumor necrosis factor (TNF), interferon-γ, and transforming growth factor-β[15•]. Nicholls *et al.* [17•] have shown that there is a constant low-grade production of TNF-α in the intestines of healthy people and attribute this production to the possible leaking of antigenic products of the normal flora across normal epithelium, leading to continual stimulation of the intestinal immune system. Using immunohistochemistry, they have documented cells containing TNF-α the subepithelial lamina propria mucosae of colonic biopsy specimens from children with no detectable gut disease [18•].

The use of cytokines in nonspecific therapy of bacterial infections has been reviewed by Vogels and van der Meer [19]. Administration of TNF-α or interleukin-1 and interleukin-6 to mice before infection with *Salmonella typhimurium* and *Listeria monocytogenes,* respectively, protected them from an otherwise lethal infection. Interferon-γ inhibits the replication of *L. monocytogenes* in hepatocytes [20•]. Baqar *et al.* [21•] have shown that orally administered cytokines interleukin-2, interleukin-5, or interleukin-6 offered protection in mice challenged with *Campylobacter jejuni*. Although the mechanism involved in developing such immunity is not yet known, the oral administration of cytokines could minimize many of the problems associated with the systemic administration of these molecules.

Mucosal vaccines

Secretory IgA represents the primary immune barrier against pathogens. Gut-associated lymphoid tissue secretes 40 mg/kg body weight of IgA daily, compared with 30 mg/kg of IgG produced by the total immune system. Intestinal B cell activation, although quite variable after oral cholera vaccination, is in the rank order IgA, IgG, and IgM. Nilssen *et al.* [22•] report that in IgA-deficient individuals, IgG antibodies are elicited as compensation for the impaired IgA response following oral cholera vaccination. Although the vaccine might be of importance for enhancing mucosal immunity in IgA-deficient individuals, the authors caution that in patients with chronic gut disease it could enhance IgG-mediated immunopathology in the absence of anti-inflammatory IgA antibodies.

Many groups are currently working on the development of enteric vaccines for the prevention of both intestinal and systemic infections. McGhee *et al.* [23•] have reviewed areas that are currently receiving extensive research attention and will be of major importance for development of mucosal and systemic immunity following oral vaccination. The use of delivery systems such as biodegradable microspheres incorporating an array of antigens is reviewed by Elridge *et al.* [24•]. Orr *et al.* [25•] evaluated an acellular approach to induce type-specific anti-*Shigella* immunity using the proteosome delivery system. Proteosomes are preparations of neissarial outer membrane protein vesicles that have previously been shown to enhance the parenteral immunogenicity of peptides. Their new candidate vaccine for shigellosis was composed of *Shigella* lipopolysaccharide complexed with proteosome. Their data demonstrate that proteosomes can be used as an effective mucosal vaccine delivery system and that orally or intranasally administered acellular vaccines can protect against *Shigella* infections. Hornquist and Lycke [26•] demonstrate that cholera toxin given orally as an adjuvant with antigen-promoted antigen priming of both the helper T-cell subsets Th1 and Th2 of $CD4^+$ T precursor cells. Further information will no doubt be forthcoming in the next few years regarding optimal mucosal vaccine delivery systems and protocols for mucosal immunization.

References and recommended reading

Papers of particular interest, published within the annual period of review, have been highlighted as:
• Of special interest
•• Of outstanding interest

1. • Fried M, Siegrist H, Frei R, Froehlich F, Duroux P, Thorens J, Blum A, Bille G, Gonvers JJ, Gyr K: **Duodenal Bacterial Overgrowth During Treatment With Omeprazole.** *Gut* 1994, 35:23–26.

The extent of bacterial overgrowth during the profound inhibition of acid secretion that occurs with omeprazole treatment is unknown. This controlled prospective study examined the bacterial content of duodenal aspirates of patients treated with omeprazole. The results indicate that duodenal bacterial overgrowth of both fecal and oral type bacteria occurs often in ambulatory patients treated with omeprazole.

2. • Shindo K, Machida M, Miyakawa K, Fukumura M: **A Syndrome of Cirrhosis, Achlorhydria, Small Intestinal Bacterial Overgrowth, and Fat Malabsorption.** *Am J Gastroenterol* 1993, **88**:2084–2091.

Twenty-seven patients with liver cirrhosis, tested by a breath analysis technique using glycine-1-^{14}C–labeled glycocholate, showed a marked increase of $^{14}CO_2$-specific activity. Bacterial overgrowth was found in the jejunal fluid of these patients. The majority of the bacterial species that were identified deconjugated bile acids. There was a good correlation between $^{14}CO_2$ activity and gastric pH. The authors conclude that some patients with liver cirrhosis have bacterial overgrowth in the proximal small intestine, which is probably associated with the shift to alkaline pH in gastric juice.

3. •• Lidbeck A, Nord CE: **Lactobacilli and the Normal Human Anaerobic Microflora.** *Clin Infect Dis* 1993, **16**:S181–S187.

The normal human microflora is a complex and usually stable ecosystem. Administration of antimicrobial agents may disrupt the normal microflora, leading to a decrease in colonization resistance. Lactobacilli are part of the normal gram-positive anaerobic microflora. Several studies have indicated the protective effect of lactobacilli against potential pathogens in the gastrointestinal tract. Thus, it is considered important to maintain or increase their levels in the intestinal microflora.

4. • Lim SG, Condez A, Poulter LW: **Mucosal Macrophage Subsets of the Gut in HIV: Decrease in Antigen-Presenting Phenotype.** *Clin Exp Immunol* 1993, 92:442–447.

The aim of this study was to investigate alterations in macrophage subpopulations in patients at different stages of HIV disease and their relevance to the associated decrease in mucosal immunity. The result suggests that the antigen-presenting arm of mucosal immune defenses may be seriously compromised in HIV infection.

5. Wells CL, Maddaus MA, Simmons RL: **Proposed Mechanisms for the Translocation of Intestinal Bacteria.** *Rev Infect Dis* 1988, **10**:958–978.

6. Apperloo-Renkema HZ, Wilkinson MFH, van der Waaij D: **Circulating Antibodies Against Faecal Bacteria Assessed by Immunomorphometry: Combining Quantitative Immunofluorescence and Image Analysis.** *Epidemiol Infect* 1992, **109**:497–506.

7. Apperloo-Renkema HZ, van der Waaij D: **Study of Colonization Resistance for *Enterobacteriaceae* in Man by Experimental Contamination and Biotyping as Well as the Possible Role of Antibodies in the Clearance of These Bacteria From the Intestines.** *Epidemiol Infect* 1991, **107**:619–626.

8. Apperloo-Renkema HZ, Bootsma H, Mulder BI, Kallenberg CG,
•• van der Waaij D: **Host–Microflora Interaction in Systemic Lupus Erythematosus (systemic lupus erythematosus): Colonization Resistance of the Indigenous Bacteria of the Intestinal Tract.** *Epidemiol Infect* 1994, **112**:367–373.

There is increasing evidence that in autoimmune disease–prone animals, the composition of the indigenous intestinal microflora might play an important role in the expression of autoimmune disorders. In this study, colonization resistance (the defense capacity of the indigenous microflora against colonization of the intestines by foreign bacteria) was measured in healthy individuals and patients with the autoimmune disease systemic lupus erythematosus by a comprehensive biotyping technique. colonization resistance tended to be lower in patients with active systemic lupus erythematosus than in healthy individuals. The authors suggest that this difference could indicate that, in systemic lupus erythematosus, more and different bacteria translocate across the gut wall, some of which could serve as polyclonal B-cell activators or as antigens cross reacting with DNA.

9. Runkel NSF, Moody FG, Smith GS, Rodriguez LF, Chen Y,
• Larocco MT, Miller TA: **Alterations in Rat Intestinal Transit by Morphine Promote Bacterial Translocation.** *Dig Dis Sci* 1993, **38**:1530–1536.

This study examined the role of altered bowel transit in influencing intestinal bacteriostasis and bacterial translocation using morphine as a pharmacologic inhibitor of transit and concluded that the morphine-induced prolongation in bowel transit promotes bacterial translocation secondary to an overgrowth of enteric bacteria in the intestinal lumen.

10. Price BA, Cumberland NS, Ingham Clark CL, Pockley AG, Lear
•• PA, Wood RFM: **The Effect of Rejection and Graft-Versus-Host Disease on Small Intestinal Microflora and Bacterial Translocation After Rat Small Bowel Transplantation.** *Transplantation* 1993, **56**:1072–1076.

The effects of rejection, GVHD, and immunosuppression on intestinal microflora and bacterial translocation after heterotropic rat small bowel transplantation were assessed in this study. The results demonstrate that rejection and GVHD are associated with shifts in intestinal microflora toward potentially pathogenic organisms and that bacterial translocation into recipient tissues poses a major threat for the development of sepsis.

11. Wells CL, Jechorek RP, Olmsted SB, Erlandsen SL: **Effect of**
•• **LPS on Epithelial Integrity and Bacterial Uptake in the Polarized Human Enterocyte-Like Cell Line Caco2.** *Circ Shock* 1993, **40**:276–288.

Bacterial lipopolysaccharide has been speculated to facilitate bacterial translocation by a mechanism involving physical disruption of the gut mucosal barrier. Using a polarized, cultured intestinal epithelial cell line (Caco2), this study demonstrated that lipopolysaccharide-induced bacterial translocation might not involve loss of epithelial viability or facilitated entry of bacteria into intestinal epithelial cells.

12. Nord C: **The Effect of Antimicrobial Agents on the Ecology of the Human Intestinal Microflora.** *Vet Microbiol* 1993, **35**:193–197.

13. Kagnoff MF: **Immunology of the Intestinal Tract.** *Gastroenterology* 1993, **105**:1275–1280.

14. Pang G, Buret A, Batey RT, Chen QY, Couch L, Cripps A, Clancy
• R: **Morphological, Phenotypic and Functional Characteristics of a Pure Population of CD56+ CD16–CD3– Large Granular Lymphocytes Generated From Human Duodenal Mucosa.** *Immunology* 1993, 79:498–505.

This study has shown for the first time that CD56+ CD16–CD3–large granular lymphocytes can be generated from histologically normal duodenal mucosa by culturing the biopsy-obtained tissue in the presence of recombinant interleukin-2. These cells may be related to classic NK cells and may produce an array of cytokines and direct cytotoxicity against tumor cells. The results provide evidence for an important role of gut mucosal large granular lymphocytes in the induction and regulation of inflammation and immunity in the gut.

15. Ciacci C, Mahida YR, Koizumi M, Podolsky DK: **Functional**
• **Interleukin-2 Receptors on Intestinal Epithelial Cells.** *J Clin Invest* 1993, **92**:527–532.

This paper reports the presence of intermediate- and low-affinity functional receptors for the cytokine interleukin-2 in the IEC-6 cell line established from normal crypt epithelium. The relevance of observations in the IEC-6 cell line to intestinal mucosa *in vivo* was supported by the demonstration of a gradient of expression of the interleukin-2 receptor in primary rat intestinal epithelial cells. These results suggest that the range of cellular targets of interleukin-2 is broader than appreciated, and interleukin-2 may serve to integrate epithelial and lymphocyte responses in the intestinal mucosa.

16. McGee DW, Beagley KW, Aicher WK, McGhee JR: **Transforming**
• **Growth Factor-β and IL-1β Act in Synergy to Enhance IL-6 Secretion by the Intestinal Epithelial Cell Line, IEC-6.** *J Immunol* 1993, **151**:970–978.

The regulation of interleukin-6 secretion by intestinal epithelial cells was studied using the IEC-6 cell line as a model. Interleukin-1 was found to be a potent inducer of interleukin-6 secretion by the IEC-6 cell line. Transforming growth factor-β and interleukin-1β act in synergy to enhance interleukin-6 secretion by the IEC-6 cell line. These results suggest that the intestinal epithelial cell may be an important interleukin-6 producing cell in mucosal immune responses.

17. Nicholls S, Stephens S, Braegger CP, Walker-Smith J, Macdonald
• TT: **Cytokines in Stools of Children with Inflammatory Bowel Disease or Infective Diarrhoea.** *J Clin Pathol* 1993, **46**:757–760.

The concentrations of interleukin-6 and TNF-α were measured in feces from 14 healthy children, 32 children with inflammatory bowel disease, and 23 children with acute diarrhea. TNF-α was detected in the stools of all healthy children. Raised values of TNF-α were indicative of mucosal inflammation, but were not specific. Stool interleukin-6 was of little use in assessing mucosal inflammation because immunoreactivity is rapidly lost in stool samples.

18. Murch SH, Braegger CP, Walker-Smith JA, MacDonald TT: **Loca-**
• **tion of TNF-α Immunohistochemistry in Chronic Inflammatory Bowel Disease.** *Gut* 1993, **34**:1705–1709.

The location and tissue density of cells immunoreactive for TNF-α in intestinal specimens from 24 patients with chronic inflammatory bowel disease was studied. There was increased density of TNF-α immunoreactive cells in the lamina propria mucosae of both ulcerative colitis and Crohn's disease specimens that might contribute to the pathogenesis of these diseases.

19. Vogels MTE, van der Meer JWM: **Use of Immune Modulators in Nonspecific Therapy of Bacterial Infections.** *Antimicrob Agents Chemother* 1992, **36**:1–5.

20. Gregory SH, Wing EJ: **IFN-γ Inhibits the Replication of**
• ***Listeria monocytogenes* in Hepatocytes.** *J Immunol* 1993, **151**:1401–1409.

Hepatocytes constitute the principal site of listerial replication in the livers of nonimmune mice whereas in immune mice the bacteria are rapidly eliminated. This paper reports that interferon gamma produced during primary infections exerts a significant inhibitory effect on the replication of *Listeria* within the parenchymal cells of the liver. *In vitro* experiments indicate that interferon gamma–stimulated hepatocytes possess the elevated capacity to kill intracellular *Listeria* organisms.

21. Baqar S, Pacheco ND, Rollwagen FM: **Modulation of Mucosal**
• **Immunity Against *Campylobacter jejuni* by Orally Administered Cytokines.** *Antimicrob Agents Chemother* 1993, **37**:2688–2692.

This is the first report of a study in which animals were given oral cytokines and challenged with an enteric pathogen. Using a murine model of infection, the authors found enhanced clearance of bacteria and increased *C. jejuni*–specific serum and secretory immunoglobulin levels after oral cytokine feeding. The data presented suggest that interleukin-2, interleukin-5, and interleukin-6 may each have different roles or functions in the induction and subsequent regulation of protective immune responses.

22. Nilssen DE, Friman V, Theman K, Bjorkander J, Kilander A,
• Holmgren J, Hanson LA, Brandtzaeg P: **B-Cell Activation in Duodenal Mucosa After Oral Cholera Vaccination in IgA Deficient**

Subjects With or Without IgG Subclass Deficiency. *Scand J Immunol* 1993, **38**:201–208.
Alterations in duodenal immunoglobulin-producing cells induced by two cholera vaccines were studied in mucosal tissue sections from adults with selective IgA deficiency. The results showed that oral cholera vaccination preferentially activates intestinal IgG-producing cells in these subjects and that IgG rather than IgM antibodies are elicited as compensation for a lacking IgA response.

23. McGhee JR, Fujihashi K, Xu-Amano J, Jackson RJ, Elson CO,
• Beagley KW, Kiyono H: **New Perspectives in Mucosal Immunity With Emphasis on Vaccine Development.** *Semin Hematol* 1993, **30**:3–15.
The focus in this review is on five areas that are currently receiving extensive research attention and will be of major importance for development of mucosal and systemic immunity to oral vaccines. These five areas include the following: helper T cell subsets (Th) and cytokines for mucosal IgA responses, Th1- and Th2-type subsets in regulation of mucosal IgA responses, antigen uptake and presentation in the mucosal immune system, the importance of memory in mucosal immunity to vaccines, and the determination of whether oral immunization alone induces immunity in all mucosal effector tissues.

24. Elridge JH, Staas JK, Chen D, Marx PA, Tice TR, Gilley RM:
• **New Advances in Vaccine Delivery Systems.** *Semin Hematol* 1993, **30**:16–24.
This review focuses on the use of microspheres composed of the biodegradable and biocompatible copolymer poly DL-lactide-co-glycolide as a promising approach to the delivery of vaccines, combining adjuvant activity with controlled release and effective presentation to mucosally associated lymphoid tissues.

25. Orr N, Robin G, Cohen D, Arnon R, Lowell GH: **Immunogenic-**
• **ity and Efficacy of Oral or Intranasal *Shigella flexneri* 2a and *Shigella sonnei* Proteosome-Lipopolysaccharide Vaccines in Animal Models.** *Infect Immun* 1993, **61**:2390–2395.
A new acellular candidate vaccine for shigellosis composed of purified *Shigella flexneri* 2a and *Shigella sonnei* lipopolysaccharide hydrophobically complexed with group C type 2b *Neisseria meningitidis* outer membrane protein proteosomes has been tested. Immunization of mice either orally or intranasally with this complex induced specific homologous anti-lipopolysaccharide antibodies in both intestinal and respiratory secretions as well as in sera. These data demonstrate that proteosomes can be used as an effective mucosal vaccine delivery system.

26. Hornquist E, Lycke N: **Cholera Toxin Adjuvant Greatly Promotes**
• **Antigen Priming of T Cells.** *Eur J Immunol* 1993, **23**:2136–2143.
This study was undertaken to investigate if cholera toxin administered together with keyhole limpet hemocyanin would act to promote or inhibit priming of keyhole limpet hemocyanin–specific T cells and whether the adjuvant effect of cholera toxin is strictly an effect on intestinal antigen processing or is a generalized phenomenon. The results clearly show that cholera toxin adjuvant strongly promotes antigen-specific priming of $CD4^+$ T lymphocytes. The adjuvant effect of cholera toxin was not restricted to mucosal immune responses but was also evident following a single parenteral immunization with keyhole limpet hemocyanin and cholera toxin.

Shobha Char, PhD, and Michael J.G. Farthing, MD, FRCP, The Medical College of St. Bartholomew's Hospital, Digestive Diseases Research Centre, Charterhouse Square, London EC1M 6BQ, UK.

Malnutrition and gut immune function

Susanna Cunningham-Rundles, PhD

New York Hospital, Cornell University Medical Center, New York, New York, USA

Malnutrition produces atrophy of lymphoid organs and impaired function leading to susceptibility to environmental pathogens, viral reactivation, and development of opportunistic infections. Key aspects of nutrient modulation of immune response are related to micronutrient interactions that are often deficient in generalized infections, in chronic illness, during parenteral nutrition, and in the very young or elderly. Malnutrition is closely associated with mucosal atrophy and poor intestinal absorption. Although immune response to gastrointestinal microflora is usually considered in defensive terms, it now seems likely that an important consequence of this interaction is the production of growth factors, cytokines, and regulatory molecules that selectively control regional immune function. Malnutrition may directly affect cytokine production and cytokines produced in response to infection, interleukin-1, interleukin-6, and tumor necrosis factor can be a direct cause of malnutrition and wasting. Malnutrition is an important factor in many infections, including AIDS, because cytokine network interactions critical to host defense may be altered by nutrient status. In addition, current studies suggest that cytokine patterns thought to mediate host defense in peripheral blood are characteristic of an inflammatory response in the gastrointestinal tract and therefore may precipitate altered nutrient metabolism, potentially leading to malnutrition and impaired host defense.

Current Opinion in Gastroenterology 1994, **10**:664–670

Malnutrition is a major cause of secondary (acquired) immunodeficiency and ranked first in the world before the appearance of HIV [1]. Severe protein-calorie malnutrition (PCM), marasmus and marasmic kwashiorkor, involves vitamin and mineral deprivation and produces wasting and stunting, whereas protein insufficiency kwashiorkor, with or without infection, causes edema associated with hepatomegaly from fatty infiltration of the liver. Primary malnutrition is associated with atrophy of lymphoid organs and function, leading to susceptibility to pathogens, reactivation of viral infections, and development of opportunistic infections [2,3•,4••]. Mild malnutrition also may be directly associated with increased susceptibility to infectious disease [5]. The recent report of vitamin A deficiency in maternal to fetal transmission of HIV [6••] is a dramatic instance of nutrient deficiency as a risk factor in immune response and disease pathogenesis.

Although the potential relationship between nutrients and immune response was envisioned 20 years ago [7], the technical tools to explore this interaction have become available only comparatively recently, especially for human studies. Newer approaches are likely to allow this field to progress from characterization of phenomena to investigation of mechanism [8•,9,10•] and will potentially provide a basis for rational intervention.

Malnutrition is closely associated with mucosal atrophy and poor intestinal absorption. Although immune response to gastrointestinal microflora is usually considered in defensive terms, it now seems likely that an important consequence of this interaction is the production of growth factors and regulatory molecules. Recent studies suggest that human T cells, like those of the mouse, may be functionally divided according to patterns of cytokine production that mediate host defense [11] and may vary significantly in different compartments of the immune system. Malnutrition may directly affect cytokine production and cytokines produced in response to infection [12•] can be a direct cause of malnutrition and wasting.

Immune response

The specificity of nutrient interaction in immune response is highly affected by nutrient level and length of exposure to a particular level. Undernutrition, especially PCM, has long been associated with increased susceptibility to infections and with greater morbidity from infections [13••,14]. Recent studies in the rat have shown that dietary protein has a direct effect on mucosal IgA, secretory component, number of IgA containing cells, and level of IgG. This effect was not related to caloric restriction because protein deprivation alone affected gut immune expression in a dose-dependent fashion and could be reversed by refeeding [15]. Refeeding experiments in a different, murine

Abbreviations

PCM—protein-calorie malnutrition; **Th1**—helper T-cell subset 1; **Th2**—helper T-cell subset 2; **TNF**—tumor necrosis factor.

 ISBN 1-85922-611-6 ISSN 0267–1379

model after a protein-free diet have indicated that nucleotides also contribute to restoration of mucosal T-lymphocyte function [16].

In environments where exposure to potential pathogens is less prevalent, there has been concern that protein insufficiency could lead to poorer response to immunization, but data remain unclear on this point. In general, low protein has a more profoundly depressing effect on thymus-dependent, cell-mediated immunity than on humoral immunity [17]. Recent studies of influenza immunization of elderly persons similarly suggest that low protein status did not prevent development of a protective antibody response, although reduced IgM response did correlate with lower protein [18].

Human states of undernutrition may be complicated by other lifestyle factors, such as smoking or alcohol use, that also may affect immune response. For example, increased bacterial infections in alcoholics has been linked to poor nutrition. Recent studies in a murine model have shown that ethanol consumption produces an increase in $CD8^+$ T cells in the lamina propria independent of nutritional status [19].

Current studies suggest that some of the negative effects of PCM are related to attendant trace element deficiency [9]. Micronutrient deficiencies of vitamins and trace elements associated with impaired immune response have been found in chronically ill patients, hospitalized or institutionalized persons, and in the very young or elderly [2,20•,21,23•]. Persons receiving parenteral nutrition are particularly vulnerable to immune impairment from micronutrient insufficiency, such as selenium deficiency [24]. The potential value of micronutrient repletion is indicated by the recent report from China on the impact of vitamin A supplementation on childhood diarrhea, and respiratory infections [13••]. In a study in Linxian, China, the benefit of vitamin and mineral supplementation, especially the combination of beta-carotene, vitamin E, and selenium, was observed [25••]. This latter study suggests that the high risk of cancer of the esophagus and colon in this region may have been related to suboptimal dietary intake.

There are few single-nutrient deficiency syndromes in humans other than Menkes syndrome, which involves altered copper metabolism, and acrodermatitis enteropathica, a genetically based syndrome of zinc deficiency that blocks immune development, allowing intractable and even fatal infections. Zinc is essential for the development of normal immune function because it is required for the biological activity of thymic hormone necessary for T-cell maturation [26•]. Secondary zinc deficiency can sometimes mimic primary deficiency as observed in association with prematurity, intravenous hyperalimentation, and artificial feeding [27,28]. Secondary zinc deficiency may be a significant complication of gastrointestinal disturbances including regional enteritis, celiac disease, and diarrhea, as well as the more widely recognized conditions of IgA deficiency, fetal alcohol syndrome, and hyperzincuria in sickle cell disease. However, the use of zinc supplementation in inflammatory bowel disease, where zinc deficiency has been reported, remains controversial [29••]. Current consensus is that micronutrients are also vital for protection against free radicals generated during normal metabolism and in association with immune response [30•,31•]. The relationship of micronutrients to antioxidant defense is shown in Table 1.

Table 1. Tumor necrosis factor and malnutrition

Mechanisms
Direct effect
Hypothalmus
Increased catabolism, energy expenditure
Lipid, protein depletion
Hypertriglyceridemia
Acute-phase protein biosynthesis
Magnitude increased by
Interleukin-1
Interferon-γ
Endotoxin

Although iron deficiency is the most common nutrient deficiency in the world including the United States, excess iron repletion may enhance bacterial growth. Although iron is required for the development of the immune system, iron overload can inhibit some immune effector functions. In β-thalassemia, iron uptake in the gastrointestinal tract is significantly enhanced, even in heavily transfused patients with associated iron overload, presumably as an inappropriate adaptive response to the chronic anemia that would have occurred in the absence of transfusion. Strategies to remove iron through use of chelating agents, however, may affect zinc levels and may thus down-regulate immune response [32•].

Malnutrition other than undernutrition may have equal or greater impact on the immune response. The negative effect of overnutrition, especially fats and lipids, has come to be appreciated. Calorie restriction, alone, has been shown to have overall value in reducing risk of neoplasia in certain tumor susceptible animal models [33•] and reduction of calories derived from fat has shown efficacy in certain genetically susceptible disease models [34]. These studies may have a significant bearing on approaches to enteral and parenteral nutrition in some cases where the use of certain lipid formulations has been found to have a negative effect on immune response [35••].

Regional host defense in the gastrointestinal tract

The influence of malnutrition on gut immune response has become increasingly apparent from studies on regional immunity in host defense [8•,20•,36••,37,38•]. Infection involving the gut directly can trigger an inflammatory immune response, affect nutrient absorption, and lead to malabsorption and malnutrition [39,40]. These relationships are interdependent and reciprocal. Impaired mucosal immune response directly affects the integrity of the gastrointestinal mucosal barrier, which may lead to bacterial translocation and to increased dietary protein absorption. Current understanding of the significance of excess absorption of dietary proteins from the gastrointestinal tract has come from studies in primary humoral immune deficiency, especially selective IgA deficiency, where it leads to chronic immune challenge with profound consequences for host defense [41••]. Local mucosal IgA subclass deficiency may also be caused by certain bacteria that produce IgA proteases. Subclass deficiency that fails to block invasion can then cause increased susceptibility to infection [42] and affect nutrient uptake at the macromolecular level.

The antigenic potential of dietary substances has been studied mainly in defined clinical settings such as IgA deficiency where uptake is massively increased and gluten sensitive enteropathy where normal oral stimulation of the mucosal immune system fails to lead to tolerance. Suppression of the IgG response with maintenance of the IgA response is fundamental to mucosal immunity. Current thinking suggests that the development of nonresponsiveness is actually an active process [43••] and may be elicited repeatedly by dietary substances during a lifetime. Recent data suggest that malnutrition and wasting, induced experimentally by bacterial infection, can impair the oral tolerance response [44], implying that tolerance could be impaired by malnutrition.

Prolonged contact with dietary protein may affect gut permeability as shown recently in a suckling rat model where supplementation of maternal milk with cow milk was used to induce intestinal permeability to intact proteins. Addition of lactobacilli elicited an immune response and thereby reestablishment of the mucosal barrier [45•]. There is current interest in the development of a fermented oatmeal soup containing human *lactobacillus* suitable for human use in both enteral and parenteral nutrition [46••] with the goal of restoring normal human flora and reestablishing the mucosal barrier.

Dietary nutrients may also directly act on intestinal permeability through effects on gastrointestinal microflora [47•] where immune protection may be insufficient to withstand challenge. In the critically ill, malnourished patient, bacterial translocation may be triggered by low levels of endotoxin. Recent studies in the rat [48•] suggest that enteral diet with bulk-forming and nonfermentable dietary fiber may decrease the translocation process which then reduces challenge to the immune system.

Diet has also been shown to affect gut immune response in experimental systems by affecting microflora and gastric secretions specifically through increased immune driven hypersensitivity [10•] and inflammatory response. In humans, one episode of infection may predispose one to a second because of effects mediated both by impaired immunity and nutritional status. In a thoughtful recent study, Baqui *et al.* [49••] have investigated the link between diarrhea and malnutrition in Bangladesh children. Both malnutrition and cellular immune deficiency, defined by immune response to a skin test panel, were independent risk factors such that anergic children, either well or poorly nourished, had a significantly higher incidence of diarrhea. Other studies [8•] suggest that immune damage caused by unknown antigens (perhaps mediated by cytokines?) may be responsible for the observed lack of consistent relationship between mucosal damage and clinical severity or risk of repeated attack. Interestingly in this study, nutritional rehabilitation was effective in improving intestinal crypt cell proliferative activity [8•].

Nutrition is especially important to host defense in the neonate where the immune system is both undeveloped and engaged in primary exposure to a wide range of potential pathogens. Antigen-specific secretory IgA, antibodies in milk can be protective against gastrointestinal symptoms such as diarrhea related to giardia infection [50•], although infection is not prevented. Because infants depend upon IgA antibodies from maternal milk, there has been interest in how maternal nutrient support might affect level and avidity of specific milk antibodies. Recent studies suggest that although moderate malnutrition does not impair the level of milk antibodies and supplementation does not enhance the level, supplementation may prevent decline in total milk secretory IgA and affect antibody avidity [51•]. Nutrients that specifically enhance mucosal IgA response have not been identified, and although recent studies suggest that glutamine addition to parenteral solution may enhance the ability of intestinal tissue to produce an antigen-specific secretory IgA response [52], this remains controversial [53].

Enteric infections can lead directly to malnutrition through mucosal dysfunction, impaired digestion, and absorption. Further, as described in the following section, cytokines triggered by immune activation may directly produce malnutrition.

Cytokine-mediated malnutrition

Cytokines produced in association with infection, inflammatory response, stress including starvation, and cancer, are essential mediators of host defense, but can also mediate the syndrome of septic shock and cause loss of lean tissue and body fat. Interleukin-1, interleukin-6, and tumor necrosis factor (TNF)-α, have been implicated in this process [54••]. Experimental infusion of TNF-α, also known as cachectin, into human volunteers, has been shown to induce all of these effects as a single agent. Mechanisms of TNF related malnutrition are shown in Table 2.

In contrast to systemic immunity, the primary activity of mucosal immune response is to protect the mucosa by blocking microbial, toxin, and antigen entry through secretion and transport of IgA to the lumen of the gut, a process mediated by a special type of memory T cells with reduced proliferative capacity capable of providing B-cell help. Both lamina propria T lymphocytes and intraepithelial T lymphocytes develop in relative independence of the thymus, and function differently from peripheral blood T cells in using the CD2 signal transduction pathway rather than the T-cell receptor/CD3 pathway.

Table 2. Antioxidant host defense

Role of micronutrients
- Antioxidant vitamins E, C, and beta carotene (provitamin A) have vital antioxidant effects within cell membranes
- Reduction of oxygen species within cells is caused by the activity of enzymes with associated trace elements
  - Superoxide dismutases
    - Copper
    - Zinc
    - Manganese
  - Glutathione peroxidase, a selenoenzyme
  - Iron-containing catalase

Recent studies suggest that normal mucosa may down-regulate mucosal T-cell reactivities [55••]. Triggering of these cells, however, can produce an inflammatory response. The diarrhea, body wasting, and villus atrophy and crypt hyperplasia accompanying experimentally induced graft-versus-host reaction are known to be T-cell–dependent and it seems that analogous immune processes are involved in inflammatory enteropathies. Further, normal intestinal growth at weaning may be mediated through T-cell activation by food substances and microbial flora [56•]. These studies suggest that macromolecular transport and solvent drag effects probably allow frequent stimulation and activation of the gut immune system in the absence of an infecting agent or obvious barrier damage and that the inflammatory response may be down-regulated rather than dormant or inactivated. New studies show that genes for inflammatory cytokines, including TNF-α, exist in lymphoid cells of the human gastrointestinal tract [57] and that recombinant interleukin-1 can induce intraepithelial lymphocyte proliferation [58••].

Systemic cellular immune function appears to be regulated through functionally distinct helper T-cell cytokine patterns, such that when helper T-cell subset 1 (Th1) cytokines interleukin-2 and interferon-γare produced, cellular immune host defense is favored and when helper T-cell subset 2 (Th2) cytokines (Th2) interleukin-4, interleukin-5, interleukin-6, and interleukin-10 are produced, B-cell response is induced. Recent studies indicate that elicitation of cytokine patterns is signal-specific and furthermore, may be regionally compartmentalized [11,59,60]. Studies have shown that Th2 cytokines interleukin-5 and interleukin-6 are selectively induced and signal Peyer's patch B cells to produce secretory IgA following oral immunization [61••]. Absence of interleukin-10 in gene-targeted mice, a cytokine that down-regulates Th1 cytokines has been found cause severe inflammation and growth retardation [62••]. This effect was lessened under germ-free conditions.

Tumor necrosis factor is another Th1 cytokine that exists in both membrane-bound and secreted forms regulated by at least two receptors, which can also exist in soluble form and regulate expression. Probert *et al.* [63••] have shown recently that a lethal wasting syndrome can be demonstrated in mice expressing T-cell–targeted human TNF transgenes. The magnitude of the effect was directly related to level of constitutive expression of TNF and the wasting effect was neutralized by monoclonal antibodies directed against human TNF. Recent data suggests that increased levels of TNF are produced in inflammatory bowel disease and in infective diarrhea, but that low levels are also produced by the intestines of healthy people [64•]. These data suggest that the inflammatory response in the gastrointestinal tract does involve TNF production and is normally down-regulated.

Malnutrition is an important manifestation of HIV infection and in fact there are many parallels between immune changes in AIDS and PCM as outlined in Table 3. The connection between PCM and HIV enteropathy, which can produce an intractable wasting syndrome, is likely to be the deregulation of cytokine production in association with opportunistic infection. It has been suggested that a Th1 to Th2 switch in cytokine pattern in the peripheral blood compartment precedes loss of $CD4^+$ T cells [65] and favors progression. Recent studies, however, also suggest that much of the HIV viral burden is located in regional lymph nodes rather than in peripheral blood [66]. Studies of mucosal $CD4^+$ T-cell level in HIV have suggested early, quantitative loss of these cells [67], whereas other studies have shown that mucosal antibody response to cholera vaccine in HIV-positive persons, even those with low $CD4^+$ T-cell levels, is conserved in the context of hyporesponsiveness at the peripheral level [68•]. Although Th1 response is normally down-regulated in the gastrointestinal tract, the possibility that HIV replication may be favored in $CD4^+$ T cells producing Th2 cytokines [69] could lead to a gradual Th2 to Th1 switch through cellular attrition, thus initiating an inflammatory process and increased TNF production in the gastrointestinal tract.

Table 3. Protein calorie malnutrition and AIDS

Comparable immune changes
- Decreased total T lymphocytes
- Decreased helper T lymphocytes
- Hypergammaglobulinemia
- Thymic atrophy
- Skin test anergy
- Poor response to immunization
- Depressed T lymphocyte and T-dependent B-lymphocyte activity
- Decreased natural killer cell activity

These interactions may have an important bearing on the phenomenon of growth retardation and the HIV-related wasting syndrome in general [70••] and in pediatric HIV disease, which in contrast to adults appears early in the course of congenital HIV infection. About one third of otherwise asymptomatic children with a relatively intact peripheral blood $CD4^+$ T-cell compartment fail to thrive or show velocity of growth below the fifth percentile [71]. In addition to the fact that growing children may have increased caloric needs in the context of chronic infection compared with adults, it is likely that immaturity of the immune system in the infected neonate may increase vulnerability to cytokine deregulation [72]. TNF up-regulation has been observed in HIV infection, in general, and has prognostic significance in children [73,74]. Inflammatory reactions in the mucosa and increased TNF production in association with regional HIV infection may compromise gastrointestinal absorption. Thus, understanding the interaction between nutrients and the immune system in the gastrointestinal tract in the context of the highly differentiated nature of the gastrointestinal immune response is vital for intervention and effective nutrient repletion.

Acknowledgments

Work described by the author was supported by National Institutes of Health NCI 29502, Pediatric AIDS Foundation Grant #500384-14-PG, National Institutes of Health RO1 AI35517, the Helena Rubenstein Foundation, the Aaron Diamond Foundation, and the Children's Blood Foundation.

References and recommended reading

Papers of particular interest, published within the annual period of review, have been highlighted as:

- • Of special interest
- •• Of outstanding interest

1. Cunningham-Rundles S: **Effect of Nutritional Status on Immunological Function.** *Am J Clin Nutr* 1981, **35**:1202–1210.

2. Chandra RK: **Nutrition and the Immune System.** *Proc Nutr Soc* 1993, **52**:77–84.

3. • Ozkan H, Olgun N, Sasmaz E, Abacioglu H, Okuyan M, Cevik N: **Nutrition, Immunity and Infections: T Lymphocyte Subpopulations in Protein-Energy Malnutrition.** *J Trop Pediatr* 1993, **39**:257–260.

Data show that PCM produced elevated immunoglobulin levels and reduced $CD3^+$ T-cell levels compared with controls, indicating an effect on both cell-mediated and humoral immunity.

4. •• Keusch GT: **Malnutrition and the Thymus Gland.** In *Nutrient Modulation of Immune Response.* Edited by Cunningham-Rundles S. New York: Marcel Dekker; 1993:283–299.

This article provides an excellent overview of thymic changes in human malnutrition at the level of thymic microenvironment. Data on the effect of thymic factor replacement and the level of thymic factor responsive cells in peripheral blood of malnourished subjects are of particular interest.

5. Bloem MW, Wedel M, Egger RJ, Speek AJ, Schrojver J, Saowakontha S, Schreurs WH: **Mild Vitamin A Deficiency and Risk of Respiratory Tract Diseases and Diarrhea in Preschool and School Children in Northeastern Thailand.** *Am J Epidemol* 1992, **131**:332–339.

6. •• Semba RD, Miotti PG, Chiphangwi JD, Saah AJ, Canner JK, Dallabetta GA, Hoover DR: **Maternal Vitamin A Deficiency and Mother to Child Transmission of HIV-1.** *Lancet* 1994, **343**:1593–1596.

This large scale investigation of maternal to fetal transmission of HIV showed that as maternal vitamin A concentrations fell, rate of infant infection increased from 7% at the minimum to 32% at the maximum. Although there was some nonuniformity in data obtained, the data are provocative and likely to engender additional studies.

7. Smythe PM, Schonland M, Brereton-Stiles GG, Coovadia HM, Grace HJ, Loening WEK, Mafoyne A, Parent MA, Vos GH: **Thymolymphatic Deficiency and Depression of Cell-Mediated Immunity in Protein-Calorie Malnutrition.** *Lancet* 1971, ii:939–943.

8. • Sullivan PB, Marhs MN: **Small Intestinal Mucosal Histology in the Syndrome of Persistent Diarrhoea and Malnutrition: A Review.** *Acta Paediatr Suppl* 1994, **381**:72–77.

This review presents evidence, partly based on computer-assisted modeling of morphologic data that different sources of injury to the intestinal mucosa (nutritional, infectious, and allergic), act through a common mechanism of cell-mediated immune damage.

9. Good RA, Lorenz E: **Nutrition and Cellular Immunity.** *Int J Immunopharmacol* 1992, **14**:361–366.

10. • Ferguson A: **Immunological Functions of the Gut in Relation to Nutritional State and Mode of Delivery of Nutrients.** *Gut* 1994, **35**(suppl 1):S10–S12.

This article provides a fresh and interesting perspective.

11. Yamamura MK, Uyemura RJ, Deans K, Weinberg TH, Rea B, Bloom B, Modlin RL: **Defining Protective Responses to Pathogens: Cytokine Profiles in Leprosy Lesions.** *Science* 1991, **254**:277–279.

12. • Beisel WR: **Impact of Infectious Disease on the Interaction Between Nutrition and Immunity.** In *Nutrient Modulation of Immune Response.* Edited by Cunningham-Rundles S. New York: Marcel Dekker; 1993:475–480.

The role of acute generalized infection and the nutritional cost of the acute-phase response are discussed in terms of the pathogenesis of altered body composition, malnutrition, and host defense.

13. •• Lie C, Ying C, Wang EL, Brun T, Geissler C: **Impact of Large-Dose Vitamin A Supplementation on Childhood Diarrhoea, Respiratory Disease and Growth.** *Eur J Clin Nutr* 1993, **47**:88–96.

Vitamin E and Vitamin A supplementation in children under 3 years of age in China was associated with decreased incidence and severity of diarrhea and respiratory disease and increased levels of serum retinol and IgA, suggesting a positive effect on the mucosal immune system.

14. Vijayakumar M, Bhaskaram P, Hemalatha P: **Malnutrition and Childhood Tuberculosis.** *J Trop Pediatr* 1990, **36**:294–298.

15. Sullivan DA, Vaerman JP, Soo C: **Influence of Severe Protein Malnutrition of Rat Lacrimal, Salivary and Gastrointestinal Immune Expression During Development, Adulthood and Ageing.** *Immunology* 1993, **78**:308–317.

16. Pizzini RP, Kumar S, Kulkarni AD, Rudolph FB, Van Buren CT: **Dietary Nucleotides Reverse Malnutrition and Starvation-Induced Immunosuppression.** *Arch Surg* 1990, **125**:86–89.

17. Woodward BD, Woods JW, Crouch DA: **Direct Evidence That Primary Acquired Cell-Mediated Immunity Is Less Resistant Than Is Primary Thymus-Dependent Humoral Immunity to the Depressive Influence of Wasting Protein-Energy Malnutrition in Weanling Mice.** *Am J Clin Nutr* 1992, **55**:1180–1185.

18. Pozzetto B, Odelin MF, Bienvenu J, Defayolle M, Aymard M: **Is There a Relationship Between Malnutrition, Inflammation, and Post-Vaccinal Antibody Response to Influenza Viruses in the Elderly?** *J Med Virol* 1993, **41**:39–43.

19. Lopez MC, Watzl B, Hebert AR, Murphy L, Huang DS, Watson RR: **Ethanol-Induced Changes in the Intestinal Mucosa-Associated Immune System of Young and Mature Mice.** *Alcohol* 1993, **10**:555–557.

20. • Prindull G, Ahmad M: **The Ontogeny of the Gut Mucosal Immune System and the Susceptibility to Infections in Infants of Developing Countries.** *Eur J Pediatr* 1993, **152**:786–792.

A detailed and informative review of the development of mucosal immunity and how this could be affected by malnutrition.

21. Shronts EP: **Basic Concepts of Immunology and Its Application to Clinical Nutrition.** *Nutr Clin Practice* 1993, **8**:177–183.

22. Rognum TO, Thrane PS, Stoltenberg L, Vege A, Brandtzaeg P: **Development of Intestinal Mucosal Immunity in Fetal Life and the First Postnatal Months.** *Pediatr Res* 1992, **32**:145–149.

23. • Chandra RK: **Influence of Nutrition on Immunocompetence in the Elderly.** In *Nutrient Modulation of Immune Response.* Edited by Cunningham-Rundles S. New York: Marcel Dekker; 1993:455–468.

Evaluation of nutrient deficiencies in the elderly is demonstrated in association with reduced immune response. In addition the article describes the benefit of controlled supplementation on immune response.

24. Peretz A, Neve J, Duchateau J, Siderova V, Huygen K, Famaey JP, Carpentier YA: **Effects of Selenium Supplementation on Immune Parameters in Gut Failure Patients on Home Parenteral Nutrition.** *Nutrition* 1991, **7**:215–221.

25. •• Blot WJ, Li JY, Taylor PR, Guo W, Dawsey S, Wang GQ, Yang CS, Zheng SF, Gail M, Li GY, Yu Y, Liu B, Tangrea J, Sun Y, Liu F, Fraumeni JF Jr, Zhang YH, Li B: **Nutrition Intervention Trials in Linxian, China: Supplementation With Specific Vitamin/Mineral Combinations, Cancer Incidence, and Disease Specific Mortality in the General Population.** *J Natl Cancer Inst* 1993, **85**:1483–1491.

This nutrient intervention study demonstrated on overall survival benefit from beta-carotene, vitamin E, and selenium supplementation after 5 years. The effect appeared to be mainly due to lower mortality from stomach cancer. The setting of this study, in an area with increased stomach cancer incidence and persistently lower micronutrient intake is likely to have been critical to the overall benefit observed.

26. • Dardenne M, Bach JF: **Rationale for the Mechanism of Zinc Interaction in the Immune System.** In *Nutrient Modulation of Immune Response.* Edited by Cunningham-Rundles S. New York: Marcel Dekker;1993: 501–510.

Commentary provides a model for the effect of zinc on the immune system, covering clinical deficiency syndromes and the biochemical interaction of zinc with thymulin, the thymic hormone.

27. Buehning LJ, Goltz RW: **Acquired Zinc Deficiency in a Premature Breast-Fed Infant.** *J Am Acad Dermatol* 1993, **28**:499–501.

28. Kanekura T, Tashiro M: **Zinc Deficiency: Report of Three Cases.** *Cutis* 1991, **48**:161–164.

29. •• Van de Wal Y, Van Der Sluys Veer A, Verspaget HW, Mulder TPJ, Griffioen G, Van Tol EAF, Pena AS, Lamers CBHW: **Effect of Zinc Therapy on Natural Killer Cell Activity in Inflammatory Bowel Disease.** *Aliment Pharmacol Ther* 1993, 7:281–286.

This study appeared to show that prolonged zinc administration did not affect disease activity in inflammatory bowel disease. Zinc levels were low at the beginning and increased during the study; however a depressing effect on natural killer cell activity was noted. Given the small sample size and some uncertainties about data interpretation, additional studies will be needed to clarify interpretation.

30. • Johnston CS, Meyer CG, Srlakshmi JC: **Vitamin C Elevates Red Blood Cell Glutathione in Healthy Adults.** *Am J Clin Nutr* 1993, **58**:103–105.

Healthy adults who had undergone a period of reduced, self-selected vitamin C intake were given either placebo or two doses (500 and 2000 mg) of vitamin C. The results showed that red cell glutathione levels were increased with either dose compared with placebo.

31. • Bendich A: **Issues in Retinoid and Carotenoid Research.** In *Nutrient Modulation of Immune Response.* Edited by Cunningham-Rundles S. New York: Marcel Dekker; 1993:469–473.

The article presents current controversies in approaching studies of antioxidant vitamins. Questions of how to distinguish between immune enhancement and antioxidant effects and these relationships in conditions where there may be increased free-radical burden are discussed.

32. • Cunningham-Rundles S, Giardina PJ, Hilgartner MW: **Effect of Therapeutic Chelation on Immune Response in Transfusion Dependent Thalassemia.** In *Nutrient Modulation of the Immune Response.* Edited by Cunningham-Rundles S. New York: Marcel Dekker; 1993:411–421.

Studies in patients with beta thalassemia undergoing continual therapeutic chelation for iron overload are presented, showing that zinc levels are also reduced and cause reduction in natural killer cells with long-term implications for immune response.

33. • Lorenz E, Good RA: **Nutritional Indications for Cancer Prevention-Calorie Restriction.** In *Nutrient Modulation of the Immune Response.* Edited by Cunningham-Rundles S. New York: Marcel Dekker; 1993:481–490.

The beneficial effects of caloric restiction on life span and mammary tumor incidence in murine models is presented. A mechanism of action associated with reduction in prolactin levels is discussed.

34. Morrow WJ, Homsy J, Levy JA, Swanson C: **The Influence of Nutrition on Experimental Autoimmune Disease.** In *Nutrient Modulation of the Immune Response.* Edited by Cunningham-Rundles S. New York: Marcel Dekker; 1993:153–167.

35. •• Gillou PJ, Monson JR, Sedman PC, Brennan TG: **Modification of Lymphocyte Function by Fatty Acids: Biological and Clinical Implications.** In *Nutrient Modulation of the Immune Response.* Edited by Cunningham-Rundles, S. New York: Marcel Dekker; 1993:369–391.

Data are presented showing the results of a continuing series of investigations into the effects of lipid emulsions in total parenteral nutrient support of tumor-bearing patients. These studies first appeared to indicate a beneficial effect on interleukin-2 production and $CD3^+$ T cells. Subsequent studies showed that longer treatment was associated with reduced interluekin-2 production and diminished cytotoxicity toward tumor targets. Studies are discussed in the context of total parenteral nutrition support of patients with gastrointestinal malignancy.

36. •• Flo J, Massouh EJ, Roux ME: **Long Term Effects of Malnutrition During Lactation on GALT.** *Reg Immunol* 1993, **5**:100–105.

This study demonstrated that malnutrition during lactation in the rat caused a transient decrease in intestinal lymphocytes, specifically secretory α+ B cells and also IgA level. In addition there were long-term effects on response to immunization that may have been linked to decreases in T cells.

37. Castro GA, Arntzen CJ: **Immunophysiology of the Gut: A Research Frontier for Integrative Studies of the Common Mucosal Immune System.** *Am J Physiol* 1993, **265**:G599–G610.

38. • Kagnoff MF: **Immunology of the Intestinal Tract [Review].** *Gastroenterology* 1993, **105**:1275–1280.

This article is an interesting and well written overview with a historical perspective.

39. Mata L: **Diarrheal Disease As a Cause of Malnutrition.** *Am J Trop Med Hyg* 1992, **47**:16–27.

40. Gendrel D, Richard-Lenoble D, Kombila M, Gahouma D, Barbet JP, Walter P: **Decreased Intraepithelial Lymphocytes in the Intestinal Mucosa in Children With Malnutrition and Parasitic Infections.** *Ann Pediatr* 1992, 39:95–98.

41. •• Cunningham-Rundles C: **Macromolecular Antigen Absorption From the Gastrointestinal Tract in Humoral Immunodeficiency.** In *Nutrient Modulation of the Immune Response.* Edited by Cunningham-Rundles S. New York: Marcel Dekker; 1993:339–358.

Studies on the effect of physiologic levels of milk ingestion in IgA deficiency provide a novel approach to questions on the immunologic consequences of excess dietary protein absorption. The data demonstrate the existence of a regulatory circuit involving antigen antibody complex formation and the generation of anti-idiotypes that control this response.

42. Brandtzaeg P: **Humoral Immune Response Patterns of Human Mucosae: Induction and Relation to Bacterial Respiratory Tract Infection.** *J Infect Dis* 1992, **165(suppl 1)**:S167–S176.

43. •• Strober W: **Dietary Antigens and Regulation of the Mucosal Immune Response.** In *Nutrient Modulation of the Immune Response.* Edited by Cunningham-Rundles S. New York: Marcel Dekker; 1993:533–540.

This commentary addresses the immune basis of oral tolerance and how this may be linked to protection against auto immune responsiveness. The importance of T-cell suppression in mucosal immunity is discussed in the context of how a break in this activity is central to gluten sensitive enteropathy.

44. Garcia-Tomayo F, Fierro L, Rivera R: **Oral Tolerance Impairment in Mice With Staphylococci-Induced Wasting Syndrome.** *Arch Med Res* 1992, 23:33–37.

45. • Fleming AL, Field EH, Tolaymat N, Cowdery JS: **Age Influences Recovery of Systemic and Mucosal Immune Responses Following Acute Depletion of CD4 T Cells.** *Clin Immunol Immunopathol* 1993, 69:285–291.

In this suckling rat model, maternal milk supplemented with cow milk caused increased intestinal permeability to intact proteins. This was reversed by addition of lactobacilli, leading to reestablishment of the mucosal barrier. The protective nature of immune response was indicated by increase in cells secreting antibodies to β-lactoglobulin.

46. •• Johansson ML, Molin G, Jeppsson B, Nobaek S, Ahrne S, Bengmark S: **Administration of Different Lactobacillus Strains in Fermented Oatmeal Soup: In Vivo Colonization of Human Intestinal Mucosa and Effect on the Indigenous Flora.** *Appl Environ Microbiol* 1993, **59**:15–20.

Colonization of the gastrointestinal tract was achieved in healthy volunteers, suggesting that this approach may be used to reestablish normal flora in sepsis, which might affect immune nutrient interactions.

47. • Isolauri E, Majamaa H, Arvola T, Rantala I, Virtanen E, Arvilomm H: **Lactobacillus Casei Strain GG Reverses Increased Intestinal Permeability Induced by Cow Milk in Suckling Rats.** *Gastroenterology* 1993, **105**:1643–1650.

This study of cow milk ingestion by suckling rats showed that gastrointestinal permeability to intact proteins caused by prolonged challenge colloid be reversed by *Lactobacillus casei* γ-globulin. The data suggest the importance of immune response in establishing and maintaining the mucosal barrier.

48. • Deitch EA: **Bacterial Translocation: The Influence of Dietary Variables.** *Gut* 1994, **35 (suppl 1)**:S23–S27.

Transmucosal passage of bacteria was found to be enhanced by preexisting malnutrition and in response to subethal endotoxin challenge. Enteral feeding with bulk forming, nonfermentable fiber was beneficial.

49. •• Baqui AH, Black RE, Sack RB, Chowdhury HR, Yunus M, Siddique AK: **Malnutrition, Cell Mediated Immune Deficiency, and Diarrhea: A Community-Based Longitudinal Study in Rural Bangladeshi Children.** *Am J Epidemiol* 1993, **137**:335–365.

This study reports a link between diarrhea and malnutrition on Bangladeshi children. Both malnutrition and cellular immune deficiency were found to be risk factors. Anergic children, both well nourished and undernourished, had a significantly higher incidence of diarrhea even when data were controlled for recent history of diarrhea, age, and socioeconomic factor.

50. • Walterspeil JN, Morrow AL, Guerrero ML, Ruiz-Palacios GM, Pickerling LK: **Secretory Anti-Giardia Lambia Antibodies in Human Milk: Protective Effect Against Diarrhea.** *Pediatrics* 1994, 93:28–31.

The study supports the significance of dietary milk in preventing diarrhea although not infection in the neonate. The amount of anti-*Giardia* secretory IgA in mothers' milk was directly associated with protection against symptoms of infection in the infants.

51. • Herias MV, Cruz JR, Gonzalez-Cossio T, Nave F, Carlsson B, Hanson LA: **The Effect of Caloric Supplementation on Selected Milk Protective Factors in Undernourished Guatemalan Mothers.** *Pediatr Res* 1993, 34:217–221.

Caloric supplementation of undernourished mothers was evaluated in terms of milk anti bodies against tetanus toxoid and *E. coli* antigens. Supplementation was found to increase mainly total secretory IgA compared with non-supplemented mothers, suggesting that milk antibody levels are conserved in moderate malnutrition.

52. **Glutamine in Parenteral Solutions Enhances Intestinal Mucosal Immune Function in Rats.** *Nutr Rev* 1993, **51**:152–155.

53. Spaeth G, Gottwald T, Haas W, Holmer M: **Glutamine Peptide Does Not Improve Gut Barrier Function and Mucosal Immunity in Total Parenteral Nutrition.** *J Parenter Enteral Nutr* 1993, **17**:317–323.

54. •• Moldawer LL, Lowry SF: **Interactions Between Cytokine Production and Inflammation: Implications for Therapies Aimed at Modulating the**

Host Defense to Infection. In *Nutrient Modulation of Immune Response.* Edited by Cunningham-Rundles S. New York: Marcel Dekker; 1993:511–522.

This current commentary discusses the autocrine, paracrine, and endocrine activities of cytokines at the tissue level. There is an informative presentation of how cytokines involved in response to infection produce pathologic effects as well as those beneficial to host defense.

55. •• Qiao L, Schurmann G, Autschbach F, Wallich R, Meuer SC: **Human Intestinal Mucosa Alters T-Cell Reactivities.** *Gastroenterology* 1993, **105**:814–819.

This interesting article presents data on the difference between peripheral blood T-cell and mucosal T-cell activation pathways and some preliminary findings suggesting that specific nonprotein mucosal substances regulate this pathway.

56. • Marsh MN, Cummins AG: **The Interactive Role of Mucosal T Lymphocytes in Intestinal Growth, Development and Enteropathy.** *J Gastroenterol Hepatol* 1993, **8**:270–278.

This article provides an interesting commentary on how mucosal T cells interact at the level of intestinal structure and function and how this may affect growth.

57. Pang G, Buret A, Batey RT, Chen QY, Couch L, Cripps A, Clancy R: **Morphological, Phenotypic and Functional Characteristics of a Pure Population of CD56+ CD16- CD3- Large Granular Lymphocytes Generated From Human Duodenal Mucosa.** *Immunology* 1993, **79**:498–505.

58. •• Mowat AM, Hutton AK, Garside P, Steel M: **A Role for Interleukin-1 alpha in Immunologically Mediated Intestinal Pathology.** *Immunology* 1993, **80**:110–115.

In this animal model, interleukin-1 was found to play a direct role in intestinal enteropathy in the mouse and should be considered a key effector molecule.

59. Barnes PF, Shuzhuang L, Abrams JS, Wang E, Yamamura M, Modlin RL: **Cytokine Production at the Site of Disease in Human Tuberculosis.** *Infect Immun* 1993, **61**:197–203.

60. Barnes PF, Abrams JS, Lu S, Sieling PA, Rea TH, Modlin RL: **Patterns of Cytokine Production by Mycobacterium-Reactive Human T-Cell Clones.** *Infect Immun* 1993, **61**:197–203.

61. •• Xu-Amano J, Kiyono H, Jackson RJ, Staats HF, Fujihashi K, Burrows PD, Elson CO, Pilliai S, McGhee JR: **Helper T-Cell Subsets for Immunoglobulin A Responses: Oral Immunization With Tetanus Toxoid and Cholera Toxin As Adjuvant Selectively Induces Th2 Cells in Mucosa Associated Tissues.** *J Exp Med* 1993, **178**:1309–1321.

Mucosal immune response characterized by helper T-cell subset 2 cytokines was induced using oral immunization with a T-dependent protein antigen and a mucosal adjuvant indicating the selectivity of this interaction.

62. •• Kuhn R, Lohler J, Rennick D, Klaus R, Muller W: **Interleukin-10-Deficient Mice Develop Chronic Enterocolitis.** *Cell* 1993, **75**:263–274.

Studies show that interleukin-10 is a key regulatory cytokine in the interstinal tract and suggests that growth retardation is produced if cytokine production favoring an inflammatory response is not downregulated.

63. •• Probert L, Keiffer J, Corbella P, Cazlaris H, Patsavoudi E, Stephens S, Kaslaris E, Kioussis D, Kollias G: **Wasting, Ischemia, and Lymphoid Abnormalities in Mice Expressing T-Cell-Targeted Human Tumor Necrosis Factor Transgenes.** *J Immunol* 1993, **151**:1894–1906.

Studies using a transgenic murine system showed that TNF expression that was constitutively up-regulated under the influence of the T-cell specific, locus control region of the human CD2 gene, produced a lethal wasting syndrome. All pathologic changes were neutralized by monoclonal antibody directed against human TNF.

64. • Nicholls S, Stephens S, Braegger CP, Walker-Smith JA, MacDonald TT: **Cytokines in Stools of Children With Inflammatory Bowel Disease or Infective Diarrhoea.** *J Clin Pathol* 1993, **46**:757–760.

Datza are presented showing that there is a constant production of TNF in the intestine that is increased in inflammation.

65. Clerici M, Shearer: **A$T_H1 \rightarrow T_H2$ Switch Is a Critical Step in the Etiology of HIV Infection.** *Immunol Today* 1993, **14**:107–110.

66. Panteleo G, Graziosi C, Demarest JF, Butini L, Montroni M, Fox CH, Orenstein JM, Kotler DP, Fauci AS: **HIV Infection Is Active and Progressive in Lymphoid Tissue During the Clinically Latent Stage of Disease.** *Nature* 1993, **362**:355–362.

67. Lim SG, Condez A, Lee CA, Johnson MA, Elia C, Poulter LW: **Loss of Mucosal CD4 Lymphocytes Is an Early Feature of HIV Infection.** *Clin Exp Immunol* 1993, **92**:448–454.

68. • Erikkson K, Kilander A, Hagberg L, Norkrans G, Holmgren J, Czerkinsky C: **Intestinal Antibody Responses to Oral Vaccination in HIV-Infected Individuals.** *AIDS* 1993, **7**:1087–1091.

Data indicate that peripheral blood T-cell responsiveness and mucosal immune responsiveness are independently affected by HIV infection and that mucosal response is relatively conserved.

69. Maggi E, Mazzetti M, Ravina A, Annunziato F, DeCarli M, Peirre Piccinni M, Manetti R, Carbonari M, Pesce AM, DelPrete G, Romagnani S: **Ability of HIV to Promote a T_H1 to T_H0 Shift and to Replicate Preferentially in T_H2 and T_H0 Cells.** *Science* 1994, **265**:244–248.

70. •• Nahlen BL, Chu SY, Nwanyanwu OC, Berkelman RL, Martinez SA, Rullan J: **HIV Wasting Syndrome in the United States.** *AIDS* 1993, **7**:183–188.

This report on the current status of the HIV wasting syndrome in US patients provides data on incidence and risk factors.

71. Cunningham-Rundles S, Noroski L, Cervia JS: **Malnutrition As a Cofactor in HIV Disease.** *J Infect Dis* 1994, in press.

72. Cunningham-Rundles S, Chen C(X), Bussel JB, Blankenship C, Veber MB, Sanders- Laufer D, Hinds T, Cervia JS, Edelson P: **Human Immune Development: Implications for Congenital HIV Infection.** *Ann NY Acad Sci* 1993, **693**:20–34.

73. Scott Algara D, Wuiller T, Marasescu M, deSaint Martin J, Dighiero G: **Serum Levels of IL-2, IL-1α, TNA-α and Soluble Receptor of IL-2 in HIV-1 Infected Patients.** *AIDS Res Human Retroviruses* 1991, 7:381.

74. Mintz M, Rapport R, Oleske JM, Connor EM, Koenigsberger MR, Denny T, Epstein LG: **Elevated Serum Levels of Tumor Necrosis Factor Are Associated With Progressive Encephalopathy in Children With Acquired Immunodeficiency Syndrome.** *Am J Dis Child* 1989, **143**:771.

Susanna Cunningham-Rundles, PhD, The New York Hospital/Cornell University Medical Center, 1300 York Avenue, New York, NY 10021, USA.

Index to authors

Volume 10 1994

© 1994 Current Science ISBN 1-85922-611-6 ISSN 0267–1379

Cumulative index to subjects

Volume 10 1994

© 1994 Current Science ISBN 1-85922-611-6 ISSN 0267–1379